VOLUME ONE HUNDRED AND NINE

ADVANCES IN PARASITOLOGY

Toxocara and Toxocariasis

VOLUME ONE HUNDRED AND NINE

ADVANCES IN PARASITOLOGY

Toxocara and Toxocariasis

Edited by

DWIGHT D. BOWMAN

*Department of Microbiology and Immunology,
College of Veterinary Medicine, Cornell University,
Ithaca, NY, United States*

ELSEVIER

ACADEMIC PRESS
An imprint of Elsevier

Academic Press is an imprint of Elsevier
125 London Wall, London EC2Y 5AS, United Kingdom
The Boulevard, Langford Lane, Kidlington, Oxford OX5 1GB, United Kingdom
50 Hampshire Street, 5th Floor, Cambridge, MA 02139, United States
525 B Street, Suite 1650, San Diego, CA 92101, United States

First edition 2020

ISBN: 978-0-12-820958-5
ISSN: 0065-308X

For information on all Academic Press publications
visit our website at https://www.elsevier.com/books-and-journals

Publisher: Zoe Kruze
Acquisitions Editor: Ashlie M. Jackman
Editorial Project Manager: Ana Claudia Garcia
Production Project Manager: Abdulla Sait
Cover Designer: Matthew Limbert

Typeset by SPi Global, India

Contents

PART IV
Dogs (and cats) disease, diagnosis, prevalence of infection, and treatment

Contributors

Ahmed Awad Adeel
Independent Consultant, Lawrenceville, GA, United States

Lyudmila V. Akhmadishina
Martsinovsky Institute of Medical Parasitology, Tropical and Vector-Borne Diseases, Sechenov University, Moscow, Russia

Norsyahida Arifin
Institute for Research in Molecular Medicine, Universiti Sains Malaysia, Gelugor, Pulau Pinang, Malaysia

H. Auer
Medical Parasitology, Institute of Specific Prophylaxis and Tropical Medicine, Center of Pathophysiology, Infectiology and Immunology, Medical University Vienna, Vienna, Austria

Herbert Auer
Department of Medical Parasitology, Center of Pathophysiology, Infectiology and Immunology, Institute of Specific Prophylaxis and Tropical Medicine, Medical University Vienna, Vienna, Austria

Hamed Behniafar
Department of Parasitology and Mycology, School of Medicine, Shahid Beheshti University of Medical Sciences, Tehran, Iran

Dwight D. Bowman
Department of Microbiology and Immunology, College of Veterinary Medicine, Cornell University, Ithaca, NY, United States

Richard S. Bradbury
School of Health and Life Sciences, Federation University Australia, Berwick, VIC, Australia

Ellen P. Carlin
EcoHealth Alliance, New York, NY, United States

Bill C.H. Chang
Department of Veterinary Biosciences, Melbourne Veterinary School, Faculty of Veterinary and Agricultural Sciences, The University of Melbourne, Parkville, VIC, Australia

Jenny Jovana Chaparro-Gutiérrez
CIBAV Research Group, Medicine Veterinary School, Agrarian Sciences Faculty, University of Antioquia, Medellín, Colombia

Nozyechi Ngulube Chidumayo
Clinical Studies Department, School of Veterinary Medicine, University of Zambia, Lusaka, Zambia

Chia-Mei Chou
Department of Molecular Parasitology and Tropical Diseases, School of Medicine, College of Medicine, Taipei Medical University, Taipei, Taiwan

Carlos Roberto Silveira Correa
Departamento de Saúde Coletiva, Faculdade de Ciências Médicas, São Paulo, Brazil

Carmen Cretu
Department of Parasitology, Carol Davila University of Medicine and Pharmacy, Colentina Clinical Hospital, Bucharest, Romania

Filipe Dantas-Torres
Department of Immunology, Aggeu Magalhães Institute, Oswaldo Cruz Foundation (Fiocruz), Recife, Pernambuco, Brazil

Christoph F. Dietrich
Department of Internal Medicine (DAIM), Kliniken Hirslanden Beau Site, Salem und Permanence, Bern, Switzerland

Yi Dong
Department of Ultrasound, Zhongshan Hospital, Fudan University, Shanghai, China

Maryam Ebrahimi
Department of Parasitology and Mycology, School of Medicine, Shahid Beheshti University of Medical Sciences, Tehran, Iran

David A. Elsemore
IDEXX Laboratories, Inc., Westbrook, ME, United States

Yadolah Fakhri
Department of Environmental Health Engineering, Student Research Committee, School of Public Health, Shahid Beheshti University of Medical Sciences, Tehran, Iran

Chia-Kwung Fan
Department of Molecular Parasitology and Tropical Diseases, School of Medicine; Research Center of International Tropical Medicine; Tropical Medicine Division, International PhD Program in Medicine, College of Medicine, Taipei Medical University, Taipei, Taiwan

Paula Mayara Matos Fialho
Institute of Medical Sociology, Centre for Health and Society, Medical Faculty, University of Duesseldorf, Duesseldorf, Germany

Magdalena Figlerowicz
Department of Infectious Diseases and Child Neurology, Karol Marcinkowski University of Medical Sciences, Poznań, Poland

Shawn D. Gale
Department of Psychology; The Neuroscience Centre, Brigham Young University, Provo, UT, United States

Robin B. Gasser
Department of Veterinary Biosciences, Melbourne Veterinary School, Faculty of Veterinary and Agricultural Sciences, The University of Melbourne, Parkville, VIC, Australia

V. Gnani Charitha
Department of Veterinary Parasitology, College of Veterinary Science, Sri Venkateswara Veterinary University, Tirupati, Andhra Pradesh, India

Jeffrey K. Griffiths
Department of Public Health and Community Medicine, Tufts University, Massachusetts

Martin Peter Grobusch
Department of Infectious Diseases, Centre of Tropical Medicine and Travel Medicine, Amsterdam University Medical Centers, location AMC, University of Amsterdam, Amsterdam, The Netherlands

Dawson W. Hedges
Department of Psychology; The Neuroscience Centre, Brigham Young University, Provo, UT, United States

Charlotte V. Hobbs
Children's of Mississippi, University of Mississippi Medical Center, Jackson, MS, United States

Andreas Hofmann
Department of Veterinary Biosciences, Melbourne Veterinary School, Faculty of Veterinary and Agricultural Sciences, The University of Melbourne, Parkville, VIC, Australia

Peter J. Hotez
Texas Children's Hospital Center for Vaccine Development, Departments of Pediatrics and Molecular Virology & Microbiology, National School of Tropical Medicine, Baylor College of Medicine; Department of Biology, Baylor University, Waco; Hagler Institute for Advanced Studies at Texas A&M University, College Station; James A Baker III Institute of Public Policy, Rice University, Houston; Scowcroft Institute of International Affairs, Bush School of Government and Public Service, Texas A&M University, College Station, TX, United States

David J. Jenkins
School of Animal and Veterinary Sciences, Charles Sturt University, Wagga Wagga, NSW, Australia

Emily J. Jenkins
Zoonotic Parasite Research Unit, Department of Veterinary Microbiology, Western College of Veterinary Medicine, University of Saskatchewan, Saskatoon, SK, Canada

Jennifer K. Ketzis
Department of Biomedical Sciences, Ross University School of Veterinary Medicine, Basseterre, St. Kitts and Nevis, West Indies

Ling Kong
Department of Pathogen Biology, Guangdong Provincial Key Laboratory of Tropical Disease Research, School of Public Health, Southern Medical University, Guangzhou, China

Karen K. Kyuregyan
Russian Medical Academy of Continuous Professional Education; Mechnikov Research Institute for Vaccines and Sera, Moscow, Russia

Manigandan Lejeune
Department of Population Medicine and Diagnostic Sciences, Animal Health Diagnostic Center, College of Veterinary Medicine, Cornell University, Ithaca, NY, United States

Susana Zevallos Lescano
Universidade de São Paulo, Instituto de Medicina Tropical de São Paulo—FMUSP, Laboratório de Imunopatologia da Esquistossomose, São Paulo, Brazil

Guo-Hua Liu
Hunan Provincial Key Laboratory of Protein Engineering in Animal Vaccines, College of Veterinary Medicine, Hunan Agricultural University, Changsha, China

Sara López-Osorio
CIBAV Research Group, Medicine Veterinary School, Agrarian Sciences Faculty, University of Antioquia, Medellín, Colombia

Felix Lötsch
Division of Infectious Diseases and Tropical Medicine, Department of Medicine, Medical University of Vienna, Vienna, Austria

Araceli Lucio-Forster
Department of Microbiology and Immunology, Cornell University College of Veterinary Medicine, Ithaca, NY, United States

Alexander N. Lukashev
Martsinovsky Institute of Medical Parasitology, Tropical and Vector-Borne Diseases, Sechenov University, Moscow, Russia

Maria A. Lukasheva
Martsinovsky Institute of Medical Parasitology, Tropical and Vector-Borne Diseases, Sechenov University, Moscow, Russia

Guangxu Ma
Department of Veterinary Biosciences, Melbourne Veterinary School, Faculty of Veterinary and Agricultural Sciences, The University of Melbourne, Parkville, VIC, Australia

Calum N.L. Macpherson
School of Graduate Studies, School of Veterinary Medicine, St. George's University, WINDREF, Grenada, West Indies

Anna Mania
Department of Infectious Diseases and Child Neurology, Karol Marcinkowski University of Medical Sciences, Poznań, Poland

Mario Noé Martínez-Gordillo
Laboratorio de Parasitología Experimental del Instituto Nacional de Pediatría, Mexico City, Mexico

C. Mathivathani
Department of Veterinary Parasitology, Rajiv Gandhi Institute of Veterinary education and Research, Pondicherry University, Puducherry, India

Katarzyna Mazur-Melewska
Department of Infectious Diseases and Child Neurology, Karol Marcinkowski University of Medical Sciences, Poznań, Poland

Mikhail I. Mikhailov
Russian Medical Academy of Continuous Professional Education; Mechnikov Research Institute for Vaccines and Sera, Moscow, Russia

Andrew D. Miller
Department of Biomedical Sciences, Section of Anatomic Pathology, Cornell University, Ithaca, NY, United States

Hamed Mirjalali
Foodborne and Waterborne Diseases Research Center, Research Institute for Gastroenterology and Liver Diseases, Shahid Beheshti University of Medical Sciences, Tehran, Iran

Lapo Mughini-Gras
Division of Veterinary Public Health, Faculty of Veterinary Medicine, Institute for Risk Assessment Sciences, Utrecht University, Utrecht; National Institute for Public Health and the Environment, Centre for Infectious Disease Control (CIb), Bilthoven, The Netherlands

Alessandra Nicoletti
Department G.F. Ingrassia, Section of Neurosciences, University of Catania, Catania, Italy

Rolf Nijsse
Department of Infectious Diseases and Immunology, Faculty of Veterinary Medicine, Utrecht University, Utrecht, The Netherlands

Rahmah Noordin
Institute for Research in Molecular Medicine, Universiti Sains Malaysia, Gelugor, Pulau Pinang, Malaysia

Paul Overgaauw
Division of Veterinary Public Health, Faculty of Veterinary Medicine, Institute for Risk Assessment Sciences, Utrecht University, Utrecht, The Netherlands

Indu S. Panicker
School of Health and Life Sciences, Federation University Australia, Berwick, VIC, Australia

Felipe Penagos-Tabares
CIBAV Research Group, Medicine Veterinary School, Agrarian Sciences Faculty, University of Antioquia, Medellín, Colombia

Hong-Juan Peng
Department of Pathogen Biology, Guangdong Provincial Key Laboratory of Tropical Disease Research, School of Public Health, Southern Medical University, Guangzhou, China

Harm Ploeger
Department of Infectious Diseases and Immunology, Faculty of Veterinary Medicine, Utrecht University, Utrecht, The Netherlands

Martha Ponce-Macotela
Laboratorio de Parasitología Experimental del Instituto Nacional de Pediatría, Mexico City, Mexico

Marie-Kristin Raulf
Institute for Parasitology, Centre for Infection Medicine; Immunology Unit & Research Center for Emerging Infections and Zoonoses, University of Veterinary Medicine Hannover, Hanover, Germany

V.C. Rayulu
Department of Veterinary Parasitology, College of Veterinary Science, Sri Venkateswara Veterinary University, Tirupati, Andhra Pradesh, India

Seyed Mohammad Riahi
Department of Epidemiology and Biostatistics, Faculty of Health, Cardiovascular Diseases Research Center, Birjand University of Medical Sciences, Birjand, Iran

Ali Rostami
Infectious Diseases and Tropical Medicine Research Center, Health Research Institute, Babol University of Medical Sciences, Babol, Iran

Maria N. Ruzina
Martsinovsky Institute of Medical Parasitology, Tropical and Vector-Borne Diseases, Sechenov University, Moscow, Russia

Mahdi Sepidarkish
Department of Epidemiology and Biostatistics, School of Medicine, Babol University of Medical Sciences, Babol, Iran

Wojciech Sluzewski
Department of Infectious Diseases and Child Neurology, Karol Marcinkowski University of Medical Sciences, Poznań, Poland

Adel Spotin
Immunology Research Center, Tabriz University of Medical Sciences, Tabriz, Iran

Andrea Springer
Institute for Parasitology, Centre for Infection Medicine, University of Veterinary Medicine Hannover, Hanover, Germany

Christina Strube
Institute for Parasitology, Centre for Infection Medicine, University of Veterinary Medicine Hannover, Hanover, Germany

Ali Taghipour
Department of Parasitology, Faculty of Medical Sciences, Tarbiat Modares University, Tehran, Iran

Siti Naqiuyah Tan Farrizam
Institute for Research in Molecular Medicine, Universiti Sains Malaysia, Gelugor, Pulau Pinang, Malaysia

Aysegul Taylan-Ozkan
Department of Medical Microbiology, Hitit University School of Medicine, Corum, Turkey; Department of Medical Microbiology and Clinical Microbiology, Near East University School of Medicine, Nicosia, Cyprus

Donna L. Tyungu
University of Oklahoma Health Sciences Center, Oklahoma City, OK, United States

Patrick Waindok
Institute for Parasitology, Centre for Infection Medicine, University of Veterinary Medicine Hannover, Hanover, Germany

J. Walochnik
Medical Parasitology, Institute of Specific Prophylaxis and Tropical Medicine, Center of Pathophysiology, Infectiology and Immunology, Medical University Vienna, Vienna, Austria

Tao Wang
Department of Veterinary Biosciences, Melbourne Veterinary School, Faculty of Veterinary and Agricultural Sciences, The University of Melbourne, Parkville, VIC, Australia

Timothy Wu
Department of Biomedical Sciences, Section of Anatomic Pathology, College of Veterinary Medicine, Cornell University, Ithaca, NY, United States

Muhammad Hafiznur Yunus
Institute for Research in Molecular Medicine, Universiti Sains Malaysia, Gelugor, Pulau Pinang, Malaysia

Wen-Bin Zheng
State Key Laboratory of Veterinary Etiological Biology, Key Laboratory of Veterinary Parasitology of Gansu Province, Lanzhou Veterinary Research Institute, Chinese Academy of Agricultural Sciences, Lanzhou; Hunan Provincial Key Laboratory of Protein Engineering in Animal Vaccines, College of Veterinary Medicine, Hunan Agricultural University, Changsha, China

Xing-Quan Zhu
State Key Laboratory of Veterinary Etiological Biology, Key Laboratory of Veterinary Parasitology of Gansu Province, Lanzhou Veterinary Research Institute, Chinese Academy of Agricultural Sciences, Lanzhou; Jiangsu Co-innovation Center for the Prevention and Control of Important Animal Infectious Diseases and Zoonoses, Yangzhou University College of Veterinary Medicine, Yangzhou; Hunan Provincial Key Laboratory of Protein Engineering in Animal Vaccines, College of Veterinary Medicine, Hunan Agricultural University, Changsha, PR, China

Yang Zou
State Key Laboratory of Veterinary Etiological Biology, Key Laboratory of Veterinary Parasitology of Gansu Province, Lanzhou Veterinary Research Institute, Chinese Academy of Agricultural Sciences, Lanzhou, China

Preface

Toxocariasis is a scourge. In the United States, it has been estimated that approximately 70 persons per year are blinded by this disease (Lum et al., 2011), but the true burden of disease is not known. Toxocariasis is caused by human infection with the larval roundworms of the genus Toxocara, principally *T. canis* and also *T. cati* from domestic dogs and cats, although other species of Toxocara may also cause human disease. Larval parasites may persist for years, causing damage as they wander through the human host. Toxocariasis causes significant neurological and generalized disease due to the intense immune response sometimes engendered by these lost larval forms. In many locations, it is a significant zoonosis that leads to asthma, other diseases linked to hypereosinophilia, and neuropsychiatric illness. Children are at elevated risk of infection because of their close contacts with pets, and because of their occasional ingestion of soil with Toxocara eggs. Chapters in this tome provide superb reviews of the pathology, +diagnostic testing for, and clinical illness produced by Toxocara in human and animal hosts.

The reports herein provide an unprecedented view of the global scope of this disease. It is estimated that ~1.4 billion persons globally are infected with, or exposed, to Toxocara species. Toxocariasis is a genuine neglected tropical disease as the true global disease extent and burden of disease are unknown. Serological data is used to impute the burden of disease, and in many locations, seroprevalence is increasing. Chapters in this volume discuss the seroprevalence and incidence of human and animal disease in a diverse set of locations: Africa, Australia, Brazil, Canada, China, Europe, India, Mexico, Turkey, Russia, South America, and the United States. Remarkable differences in seroprevalence are reported, representing the interplay of the environment, and human and animal behaviour. In addition, laboratory techniques and animal models for studying the life cycle, molecular biology, and diagnosis of this parasite are provided. This volume represents a landmark in the assembly of such information.

Children are not the only group of concern. People who work with soil, such as farmers, are at risk. In some locations, increasing age, animal and soil contact, and low socioeconomic status predict seropositivity. However, many groups of people have contact with soil. For example, domestic pets are a source of comfort and joy, and increasingly prevalent in middle income countries. Parks, playgrounds, and recreational spaces are often contaminated. Soil (and water) are often contaminated by *Toxocara* eggs which are capable of surviving in the environment for years. As the world becomes wealthier, more urban, and warmer, the potential for exposure may paradoxically be increasing for many persons.

At the end of the day, toxocariasis is largely preventable by treating domestic pets to rid them of these roundworms. Once cured of the infection then ongoing contamination of soil with *Toxocara* eggs ceases, although they may survive for years. Increasing awareness of this disease, and increasing routine deworming of cats and dogs, could substantially reduce the global burden of disease. Adoption of a 'One Health' approach, that recognizes both human and animal infections and the opportunities for prevention, could fuel a global decrease in this neglected tropical disease. I for one, as a clinician, hope never to see another child or adult with blindness or neurological disease caused by this disease. Treatment of ocular disease fails to prevent blindness in the majority of people. All too frequently, people with neurological disease due to toxocariasis suffer from delayed diagnosis, sometimes for years. The contributors to this volume are to be saluted for this remarkable compendium.

Reference

Lum, F.C., Hoskins, H.D., Moorthy, R.S., Read, R.W., Starr, M.C., et al., 2011. Ocular toxocariasis—United States, 2009–2010. Morb. Mortal. Wkly Rep. 60 (22), 734–736.

Jeffrey K. Griffiths
Department of Public Health and Community Medicine
Tufts University, Massachusetts

PART I

The organism and the recognition of the disease

CHAPTER ONE

Toxocara: Protecting pets and improving the lives of people

Ellen P. Carlin[a,*,†], **Donna L. Tyungu**[b,†]
[a]EcoHealth Alliance, New York, NY, United States
[b]University of Oklahoma Health Sciences Center, Oklahoma City, OK, United States
[*]Corresponding author: e-mail address: carlin@ecohealthalliance.org

Contents

Abstract

Toxocara sp. are zoonotic parasitic roundworms that cause infection and morbidity in both developed and developing countries. In humans, infection is thought to be most common in children, particularly those living in poverty, and usually results from consumption of soil contaminated with parasite eggs deposited by dog or cat faeces. Infection in humans results in different clinical manifestations, some more overt like visceral or ocular larva migrans and others more cryptic like neurocognitive delay. Despite its pervasiveness, toxocariasis has become a neglected infection. We review the dynamics of the human-animal interface in the context of this parasite, discuss the challenges in controlling transmission to humans, and cite key areas of research that could enable improved interventions. With political will and proper resource allocation, we propose that effective interventions are possible in the near term.

1. Introduction

Toxocariasis is a significant zoonotic parasitic infection in the United States and globally. This roundworm's many hosts include animals both domestic and wild, with dogs and cats being the primary source of infection

† Each author contributed equally to this manuscript.

Advances in Parasitology, Volume 109
ISSN 0065-308X
https://doi.org/10.1016/bs.apar.2020.01.001

for humans. The domestic dog (*Canis familiaris*) is a definitive host for *Toxocara canis* and the domestic cat (*Felis catus*) for *T. cati*. Humans are paratenic hosts—that is, they are not required for the parasite to complete its life cycle, but the larvae can migrate through human tissue, causing significant damage in the process. The U.S. Centers for Disease Control and Prevention (CDC) lists larval toxocariasis as one of the Neglected Parasitic Infections (NPI) of the United States, along with Chagas disease, cysticercosis, toxoplasmosis, and trichomoniasis (Parise et al., 2014). Soil-transmitted helminthiases, which include *Toxocara*, are listed by the World Health Organization (WHO) among the 17 diseases that affect more than 1 billion people worldwide (WHO, 2012), and were the subject of a 2001 resolution by the World Health Assembly endorsing steps to reduce its morbidity and mortality (WHA, 2001).

Researchers, clinicians, and public health officials have thus worked for decades to understand infection prevalence in these host populations and the dynamics of how the parasites transmit infection within and between species. Yet work done to date to aggressively and systematically control or eliminate toxocariasis from developed and developing countries is variable at best across countries and, in general, insufficient to meet the need. As described in this issue, adult worms in animals generally cause minor to moderate gastrointestinal upset, but migrating larvae in a human host can cause significant damage to multiple systems including visceral, ocular, and neurological, resulting in significant mortality that can lead to permanent end-organ damage. Eliminating remaining questions about transmission risk and developing and implementing protocols for breaking the transmission cycle is both requisite and feasible.

2. The dynamics of zoonotic transmission and infection

The most common form of transmission of *Toxocara* eggs to animals and people is via ingestion of egg-contaminated soil (Lee et al., 2010). *Toxocara* sp. eggs are resistant to extreme environmental weather changes and, within a few weeks of infected dogs and cats contaminating soil with egg-laden faeces, the deposited eggs embryonate and become infectious L3 larvae. Dogs and cats may ingest these infective eggs from which the larvae hatch then moult into adult worms in the animals' gastrointestinal tract, and the cycle repeats. Dogs and cats may also become infected through the ingestion of paratenic hosts (Holland, 2017; Strube et al., 2013), animals that ingest their meals on or in the soil, and can simultaneously ingest the offending eggs and pass them on; examples include rodents, rabbits, chickens, other birds, and even snails (Campos-da-Silva et al., 2015; Cardillo et al., 2016).

Human infections are generally caused by inadvertent ingestion of contaminated soil (Congdon and Lloyd, 2011; Walsh and Haseeb, 2014). Thus, it is not necessarily pet ownership which poses a risk but rather the overall environmental burden of eggs to which one is exposed, although pet ownership is a risk factor (Berrett et al., 2017). Human infection can also occur via ingestion of paratenic hosts (Holland, 2017; Strube et al., 2013). Ingestion of contaminated meat or vegetables poses another transmission route; raw or undercooked meat contaminated with encysted larvae (e.g. escargot, chicken) or raw uncleaned vegetables can put consumers at increased risk (Campos-da-Silva et al., 2015; Cardillo et al., 2016; Merigueti et al., 2018; Sharghi et al., 2001; Taira et al., 2012; Zibaei et al., 2017). Finally, the coats of dogs and cats may sometimes be contaminated with the infective eggs of these parasites and may serve as another potential transmission risk to pet owners and others who interact with them (Aydenizoz-Ozkayhan et al., 2008; Bakhshani et al., 2019; Keegan and Holland, 2010; Roddie et al., 2008).

Human infection events occur most frequently in children, minority, and immigrant populations, and in those residing in impoverished areas including rural farming communities, or poor urban neighbourhoods (Congdon and Lloyd, 2011; Walsh and Haseeb, 2014). The risk of transmission in humans is greater in younger age groups due to geophagia or pica, a normal stage of human development. Immigrants and those living in poor or rural areas at higher risk due to increased parasite burden in those communities. An analysis of immigrants to Spain showed that immigrants from poorer tropical and subtropical Latin American countries had increased rates of *Toxocara* seropositivity, some countries as high as 34% (Turrientes et al., 2011). In the United States, evaluation of 2011 to 2014 NHANES data showed that immigrants had higher seroprevalence as compared to nonimmigrants (12.4% vs. 3.7%) (Berrett et al., 2017).

While the most common clinical manifestation in dogs and cats is gastrointestinal upset, human symptoms can be severe. The clinical manifestations of toxocariasis were historically categorized into two syndromes: visceral larva migrans (VLM) and ocular larva migrans (OLM). Other recognized clinical syndromes are neurotoxocariasis and covert toxocariasis. Neurotoxocariasis refers to parasitic migration with resultant damage to brain tissue. An additional syndrome with more subtle symptomatology is recognized as 'covert toxocariasis' and the majority of individuals infected are thought to have this form, but due to lack of symptoms may go undiagnosed (Holland, 2017). A small percentage of people, mainly children, develop the severe symptomatic form of disease and may suffer significant and permanent ocular or neurological damage. Ocular pathology is associated with inflammation due to larval migration and can result in decreased visual acuity, uveitis, macular edema, granulomas and even unilateral blindness (Despreaux et al., 2016; Liu et al., 2016). The migratory nature of the parasite also results in the potential for epidermal damage and, more seriously, visceral damage including in the liver and spleen. Less frequent and covert clinical manifestations of toxocariasis include myositis, internal abscesses, and cardiac damage (Bolivar-Mejia et al., 2013; Walsh et al., 1988). Other conditions that need further study in controlled settings include resultant neurocognitive delay or regression as a result of infection, as well as the association of toxocariasis with psychiatric diagnoses (Alvarado-Esquivel et al., 2014; Cong et al., 2014; Fan et al., 2015; Kaplan et al., 2008). *Toxocara* has been described as an enigmatic parasite, and more research is needed to truly understand all the ways in which the human body is affected (Holland, 2017).

3. Interfacing with animals: Prevalence, pets, and the human-animal bond

Serological studies in people can reveal evidence of past exposure and are thus a common way to assess the overall burden of exposure. Seroprevalence rates vary markedly from country to country, with higher income nations often reporting much lower rates than less industrialized nations (McGuinness and Leder, 2014). In an extreme case, the seroprevalence of the population of the island of La Réunion (Magnaval et al., 1994) was 92.8% positive. In the United States, national surveys produced seroprevalence range estimates of: 4.6–7.3% of children aged one to 11 years were positive in a 1971–1973 CDC survey (Herrmann et al., 1985); 13.9% of individuals at least 6 years of age in the CDC's 1998–1994 survey (Won et al., 2008); and 5.1% of individuals aged 6 years and older were seropositive in a 2011–2014 study (Berrett et al., 2017). Prevalence rates were dependent on the population studied, particularly with respect to sociodemographic factors, with some subpopulations reaching well into the double-digits. Different studies also use different serologic testing techniques to identify rates. Seropositivity has been found to increase with age, to be more common in males, to be inversely related to socioeconomic status and level of education attained, and to be associated with dog ownership (Berrett et al., 2017; Won et al., 2008). *Toxocara* seroprevalence in people remains high with age, suggesting life-long infections or regular reinfection. Increased seroprevalence rates are associated with familial poverty (Berrett et al., 2017; Inagaki et al., 2019; Lee et al., 2014; Walsh, 2011). The presence of specific antibodies to these infections indicates that very large numbers of people are infected, and the majority of these infections likely occur from the accidental ingestion of infective eggs from soil. (See chapter "Global and regional seroprevalence estimates for human toxocariasis—A call for action" by Ma and Gasser and other chapters in this issue for detailed explorations of human seroprevalence.)

The prevalence of toxocariasis (and not just antibody evidence of infection) in companion animals has been more directly studied owing to the commonality of routine and research-based faecal examination of dogs and cats. In the United States, a survey of shelter animals reported a 15.2% prevalence of ascarids (*T. canis* or *Toxascaris leonina*) in the nationwide shelter dog population (Blagburn et al., 1996), compared to a range of 1.6–2.8% in the owned pet population (Little et al., 2009). (See detailed discussion in later chapters in this issue on canine and feline prevalence.) Veterinary intervention to prevent and treat toxocariasis in canine and feline patients is a mainstay of clinical veterinary practice. These interventions, which generally include faecal flotation (in-house or sent to a diagnostic laboratory) and preventive or therapeutic administration of a de-worming pharmaceutical are as much about the health of the animal patients as they are about safeguarding public health.

Given the sharing of eggs between companion animals and people, in the developed world the question of breaking the transmission cycle becomes one of intervening somewhere along the transmission spectrum between pets and their guardians. In the United States, pet ownership increased 6.1% from 2014 to 2016, amounting to 84.6 million households, with millennials representing the largest pet-owning demographic according to a biennial survey (JAVMAnews, 2017). One source finds nearly 57% of all U.S. homes owning a pet in 2018 (Burns, 2018). Sixty-two percent of respondents to a U.S. Harris poll cite pet ownership; 71% of these individuals owned dogs and 49% owned cats (HarrisPoll, 2015). Ninety-five percent of those surveyed consider their pets to be members of their family; 71% frequently or occasionally allow their pets to sleep in their beds. Other surveys reveal that more than half of all people surveyed across 22 countries report owning at least one pet, with 33% owning a dog and 23% a cat (GFK, 2016).

Pet ownership is distributed relatively evenly across income brackets in the United States, implying that of the many people who own pets, a proportion of them likely cannot afford access to basic veterinary care, which often includes routine faecal diagnostics and deworming. According to the Humane Society of the United States, the percentage of pets in underserved communities who have never been seen by a veterinarian is 77% (Humanesociety.org, 2019). This deficit in care poses the potential for serious problems. It increases the risk of infection of family members, especially children. Higher transmission rates can, in turn, perpetuate the cycle of poverty due to the potential stunting effects on cognitive development in infected children (Hotez, 2014; Walsh and Haseeb, 2012). Knowledge of toxocariasis by pet owners is insufficient, with many not understanding the risk of infection or the potential for zoonotic transmission, resulting in decreased deworming efforts (Michalczyk et al., 2019).

The presence of street animals or strays may also correlate to increased infection risk through environmental contamination. In the developing world, stray, street, or otherwise peridomestic dogs may be more common than owned animals; the numbers of such dogs are not known but undoubtedly number in at least the hundreds of millions (Otranto et al., 2017).

4. Veterinary intervention and its public health implications

Toxocariasis is not a reportable disease in companion animals or humans in the United States, and in general global data are available on an ad hoc basis based on serological estimates. The monitoring system presently in place in the United States for examining the prevalence of these infections in dogs and cats relies on voluntary sharing of data or information by veterinarians and/or diagnostic laboratories. The Companion Animal Parasite Council monitors incidence in the United States and Canada of roundworm (*T. canis, T. cati*, or *T. leonina*) infection as diagnosed by positive centrifugal flotation tests by two major diagnostic laboratories, using the data to create risk maps (Companion Animal Parasite Council, 2019) (Fig. 1).

The volume of samples submitted from U.S. laboratories for these tests can reach over 7 million individual tests annually for dogs and more than 1 million for cats, resulting in the most comprehensive platform for incidence and estimation of prevalence in these populations, and providing a basis from which to measure the impact of interventions.

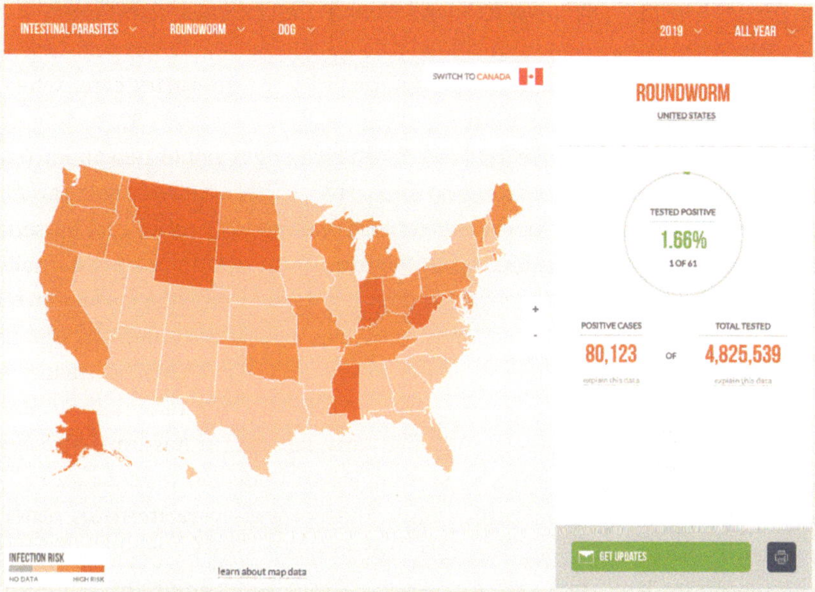

Fig. 1 Roundworm prevalence map from the Companion Animal Parasite Council. The interactive website allows users to toggle parasite type, host species, state, and county to view prevalence estimates. *Retrieved from capcvet.org/maps/#2019/all/roundworm/dog/united-states/11August2019.*

Despite the clinical and scientific community's substantial knowledge about the biology, epidemiology, and means of treatment of these parasites, they have been difficult to eradicate in companion animal populations. Reasons for this are likely multifactorial. Earlier misconceptions about the lifecycle of the parasites in companion animals implied that adult dogs were less susceptible to infection than juveniles (Lee et al., 2010), which may have impacted screening or deworming decisions for adults. In one survey-based study in Western Canada, although small animal veterinarian perception of zoonotic concern ranked as 'medium-significant' for *T. canis* and *T. cati* and was the highest for these compared to seven other parasites included in the survey, that concern dropped for adult animals compared to juveniles; 65% of veterinarians reported recommending at least annual prophylactic deworming for adult dogs and cats, leaving more than 1/3 of veterinarians not recommending routine deworming for adults (Stull et al., 2007). Practical challenges in eradication also stem from the existence of stray and street populations, and lack of access to care among pet owners who cannot afford it or chose not to take advantage of it. On the positive side, the veterinary medical community does have excellent means for removing *Toxocara* from dogs and cats through wide availability of effective and inexpensive dewormers, creating ample opportunity for intervention and control, if not complete eradication.

Despite this, larval toxocariasis has faced challenges gaining acceptance as a disease worthy of greater attention and control. The reality of toxocariasis as an NPI in the United States and other developed countries is, from one perspective, enigmatic. Its biology and transmission dynamics are well studied. The worm was first described in dogs by Werner in 1782 and in cats by Shrank in 1788; and the first case report of suspected human toxocariasis was published in 1947 (Perlingiero and Gyorgy, 1947). The zoonotic transmission routes and effective interventions in animals that can break the transmission cycle are well understood. The very fact that it has been publicly labelled by the WHO and CDC as a neglected infection should rationally spur spending to counteract this reality, but competing interests for other, higher-profile diseases—malaria, HIV, tuberculosis—may cannibalize available resources. It is not a lower exposure rate that diminishes its perceived importance—indeed, based on seroprevalence estimates, hundreds of millions of people worldwide are or have been infected including many in industrialized countries, thus rivalling malaria cases in absolute numbers. It is rather the lower biologic profile of the parasite, which often manifests covertly or asymptomatically, and its lower political profile, which subjugates it to other more deadly infections, that may be resulting in the relative inattention paid to it.

Parise et al. (2014) describe three factors that the U.S. CDC's NPIs have in common (and which also apply globally): the surprisingly large numbers of persons infected or at risk; a lack of clinician awareness and poor availability of optimal diagnostic tests; and the dearth of interventions that can prevent or cure illness. The last of these at least as it relates to prevention is not strictly applicable to toxocariasis—we actually do know how to intervene to prevent the transmission of this parasite. Of the five infections on the CDC NPI list, *Toxocara* is the single parasite among them for which excellent methods for monitoring infection levels and routine methods of treating source animals are available. The veterinary community has reliable means—including highly effective and inexpensive anthelmintics—for removing *Toxocara* from dogs and cats. Diminution of the incidence and ultimately prevalence of the disease in people will require an accepted mandate for the rigorous and 100% routine removal of this parasite from dogs and cats. Although there has been no such mandate to date and thus no elimination of the parasite from dogs and cats, the targeting of control to these hosts would be likely to impact the human infection rate, as has occurred during the success of targeted canine treatment in the reduction or eradication of cystic hydatid disease (Craig and Larrieu, 2006; Irabedra et al., 2016).

5. Research and intervention steps toward control and eradication

Toxocariasis in people has been overlooked as a disease worth studying and eradicating, a state that both results from and is perpetuated by a lack of funding. This is as true in the United States as elsewhere. More work on diagnostics would advance the human medical community's efforts toward identifying infected individuals, leading to more work on the clinical implications of toxocariasis, and would ultimately enable better evaluation and treatment of infected patients, preventing the devastating end-organ damage and clinical manifestations discussed above. This work would define a picture of risk that should be deemed unacceptable and worthy of intervention.

Resolving the paucity of data and knowledge in some areas could advance progress. These areas notably include: (1) quantifying the relative contribution by different host species and the environmental distribution of eggs in different geographic locations (Macpherson, 2013; Morgan et al., 2013); (2) human subjects research particularly exploring the parasite's effect on neurocognitive deficits as well as other long-term effects of infection; and (3) improved diagnostic techniques to identify acutely infected individuals and to enable quality research studies involving human subjects in the future. Diagnosis is presently made by reliance on recognition of a constellation of symptoms and nonspecific lab studies, namely, leukocytosis, eosinophilia (not consistently present in all forms of the disease), and hypergammaglobulinemia (IgE). Detection of these signs and symptoms may lead to additional testing via enzyme-linked immunosorbent assay (TES-ELISA) for antibodies, a test that does not differentiate between species causing infection or current versus past infection. Additionally, the test was developed using excretory and secretory antigens of larval *T. canis*, leaving questions regarding *T. cati* cross-reactivity and inability to delineate etiologic species after a positive test (Fillaux and Magnaval, 2013; Meghji and Maizels, 1986; Poulsen et al., 2015). Physicians are also largely unaware of the effects of *Toxocara* infection, resulting in the majority of diagnoses being made after end-organ damage (e.g. unilateral blindness) has already occurred. Improved diagnostics including new biomarkers may help establish evidence of infection earlier and improve recognition of this disease. Through the continuation of research efforts that are currently underway, such as national geo-prevalence studies to elucidate community transmission risk, animal model research to help better understand the clinical effects of infection, and through new efforts to address gaps in epidemiological, diagnostics, and human subjects research, we can achieve an improved understanding of the parasite's effect on the human body and develop improved treatment strategies.

Fundamentally, the ultimate solutions to toxocariasis will lie in preventive efforts. Decades of study of transmission routes of the parasite into animal and human populations have elucidated the dynamics of the infection process; the answers to how to prevent infection are thus already available, if not the funding to implement intervention studies. The straightforward mode of *Toxocara* infection—human ingestion of contaminated animal faeces—is such that a reduction in human burden would be directly related to the reduction of the presence of the parasite in companion animals. This relatively simple epidemiological reality, therefore, presents an opportunity to intervene in a direct way.

The control and virtual eradication of human toxocariasis is an achievable outcome. Despite the knowledge gaps described, interventions are possible today with political will and resource allocation. Much is understood about key factors in transmission and key populations at risk, such that concerted efforts to break transmission through aggressive animal deworming, animal monitoring, and geosurveillance coupled with human serosurveys that could be designed and piloted in the near term would likely facilitate substantial progress.

The human-animal bond has been postulated to result in health benefits for both animal and owner. Improved cognitive development in children (Endenburg and Van Lith, 2011), increased time outdoors and walking for older adults (Curl et al., 2017), and companionship for veterans suffering from post-traumatic stress (Lafollette et al., 2019) may all result from pet ownership. Given the benefits of the human-animal bond; the reality of sustained and even increasing pet ownership in the developed world; and the ubiquity of peridomestic dog populations in developing countries, solutions that acknowledge the importance of human-animal interactions while operating to break transmission cycles between humans and animals will be most effective. The monitoring system already in place for pets on a national level in the United States could enable a relatively easy means to monitor the success of intervention in the animal population. Further, the renewed national and global emphasis on One Health approaches offers a timely opportunity to mitigate the zoonotic spread of this parasite. Sustained collaborative efforts among the medical, veterinary, and public health communities to undertake applied toxocariasis research efforts will reduce infection rates in people and animals and diminish the burden of this neglected disease.

References

Alvarado-Esquivel, C., Hernandez-Tinoco, J., Sanchez-Anguiano, L.F., Cisneros-Martinez, J.A., 2014. Low seroprevalence of Toxocara infection in schizophrenic inpatients in Durango, Mexico: a case control study. Int. J. Biomed. Sci. 10, 269–271.

Aydenizoz-Ozkayhan, M., Yagci, B.B., Erat, S., 2008. The investigation of Toxocara canis eggs in coats of different dog breeds as a potential transmission route in human toxocariasis. Vet. Parasitol. 152, 94–100.

Bakhshani, A., Maleki, M., Haghparast, A., Parande Shirvan, S., Borji, H., 2019. A survey on Toxocara cati eggs on the hair of stray cats: a potential risk factor for human toxocariasis in Northeastern Iran. Comp. Immunol. Microbiol. Infect. Dis. 64, 10–13.

Berrett, A.N., Erickson, L.D., Gale, S.D., Stone, A., Brown, B.L., Hedges, D.W., 2017. Toxocara seroprevalence and associated risk factors in the United States. Am. J. Trop. Med. Hyg. 97, 1846–1850.

Blagburn, B.L., Lindsay, D.S., Vaughn, J.K., Rippey, N.S., Wright, J.C., Lynn, R.C., Kelch, W.J., Ritchie, G.C., Hepler, D.I., 1996. Prevalence of canine parasites based on fecal flotation. Comp. Cont. Ed. Pract. Vet. 18, 483–509.

Bolivar-Mejia, A., Rodriguez-Morales, A.J., Paniz-Mondolfi, A.E., Delgado, O., 2013. Cardiovascular manifestations of human toxocariasis. Arch. Cardiol. Mex. 83, 120–129.

Burns, K., 2018. Pet ownership stable, veterinary care variable, AVMA sourcebook details pet ownership numbers and how veterinary care varies by pet species and other factors. JAVMAnews.

Campos-da-Silva, D.R., Da Paz, J.S., Fortunato, V.R., Beltrame, M.A., Valli, L.C., Pereira, F.E., 2015. Natural infection of free-range chickens with the ascarid nematode Toxocara sp. Parasitol. Res. 114, 4289–4293.

Cardillo, N., Prous, C.G., Krivokapich, S., Pittaro, M., Ercole, M., Perez, M., Pasqualetti, M., Farina, F., Rosa, A., Gatti, G., Ribicich, M., 2016. First report of *Toxocara Cati* in the domestic land snail *Rumina Decollata*. Rev. Argent. Microbiol. 48, 206–209.

Companion Animal Parasite Council, 2019. Parasite Prevalence Maps [Online]. Available: https://capcvet.org/maps/#2019/all/roundworm/dog/united-states/. Accessed Aug 11 2019.

Cong, W., Zhang, X.X., Zhou, N., Yu, C.Z., Chen, J., Wang, X.Y., LI, B., Qian, A.D., Zhu, X.Q., 2014. Toxocara seroprevalence among clinically healthy individuals, pregnant women and psychiatric patients and associated risk factors in Shandong Province, Eastern China. PLoS Negl. Trop. Dis. 8, e3082.

Congdon, P., Lloyd, P., 2011. Toxocara infection in the United States: the relevance of poverty, geography and demography as risk factors, and implications for estimating county prevalence. Int. J. Public Health 56, 15–24.

Craig, P.S., Larrieu, E., 2006. Control of cystic echinococcosis/hydatidosis: 1863-2002. Adv. Parasitol. 61, 443–508.

Curl, A.L., Bibbo, J., Johnson, R.A., 2017. Dog walking, the human-animal bond and older adults' physical health. Gerontologist 57, 930–939.

Despreaux, R., Fardeau, C., Touhami, S., Brasnu, E., Champion, E., Paris, L., Touitou, V., Bodaghi, B., Lehoang, P., 2016. Ocular Toxocariasis: clinical features and long-term visual outcomes in adult patients. Am. J. Ophthalmol. 166, 162–168.

Endenburg, N., Van Lith, H.A., 2011. The influence of animals on the development of children. Vet. J. 190, 208–214.

Fan, C.K., Holland, C.V., Loxton, K., Barghouth, U., 2015. Cerebral Toxocariasis: silent progression to neurodegenerative disorders? Clin. Microbiol. Rev. 28, 663–686.

Fillaux, J., Magnaval, J.F., 2013. Laboratory diagnosis of human toxocariasis. Vet. Parasitol. 193, 327–336.

GFK, May 2016. Pet ownership: global GFK survey. Available at: https://www.gfk.com/fileadmin/user_upload/website_content/Global_Study/Documents/Global-GfK-survey_Pet-Ownership_2016.pdf.

Harrispoll, T., 2015. More Than Ever, Pets are Members of the Family [Online]. Available: https://theharrispoll.com/whether-furry-feathered-or-flippers-a-flapping-americans-continue-to-display-close-relationships-with-their-pets-2015-is-expected-to-continue-the-pet-industrys-more-than-two-decades-strong/ Accessed Aug 8 2019.

Herrmann, N., Glickman, L.T., Schantz, P.M., Weston, M.G., Domanski, L.M., 1985. Seroprevalence of zoonotic toxocariasis in the United States: 1971-1973. Am. J. Epidemiol. 122, 890–896.

Holland, C.V., 2017. Knowledge gaps in the epidemiology of Toxocara: the enigma remains. Parasitology 144, 81–94.

Hotez, P.J., 2014. Neglected infections of poverty in the United States and their effects on the Brain neglected infections of poverty viewpoint. JAMA Psychiat. 71, 1099–1100.

Humanesociety.Org, 2019. Pets by the numbers U.S. pet ownership, community cat and shelter population estimates [Online]. Available: https://www.humanesociety.org/resources/pets-numbers, Accessed Aug 10 2019.

Inagaki, K., Kirmse, B., Bradbury, R.S., Moorthy, R.S., Arguello, I., McGuffey, C.D., Tieu, B., Hobbs, C.V., 2019. Case report: ocular Toxocariasis: a report of three cases from the Mississippi Delta. Am. J. Trop. Med. Hyg. 100, 1223–1226.

Irabedra, P., Ferreira, C., Sayes, J., Elola, S., Rodrlguez, M., Morel, N., Segura, S., Santos, E.D., Guisantes, J.A., 2016. Control programme for cystic echinococcosis in Uruguay. Mem. Inst. Oswaldo Cruz 111, 372–377.

JAVMANEWS, 2017. Millennials now primary pet-owning demographic [Online]. J. Am. Vet. Med. Assoc. Am. Vet. Med. Assoc. Available: https://www.avma.org/News/JAVMANews/Pages/170515g.aspx. Accessed Aug 9 2019.

Kaplan, M., Kalkan, A., Kuk, S., Demirdag, K., Ozden, M., Kilic, S.S., 2008. Toxocara seroprevalence in schizophrenic patients in Turkey. Yonsei Med. J. 49, 224–229.

Keegan, J.D., Holland, C.V., 2010. Contamination of the hair of owned dogs with the eggs of Toxocara spp. Vet. Parasitol. 173, 161–164.

Lafollette, M.R., Rodriguez, K.E., Ogata, N., O'haire, M.E., 2019. Military veterans and their PTSD service dogs: associations between training methods, PTSD severity, dog behavior, and the human-animal bond. Front. Vet. Sci. 6, 23.

Lee, A.C., Schantz, P.M., Kazacos, K.R., Montgomery, S.P., Bowman, D.D., 2010. Epidemiologic and zoonotic aspects of ascarid infections in dogs and cats. Trends Parasitol. 26, 155–161.

Lee, R.M., Moore, L.B., Bottazzi, M.E., Hotez, P.J., 2014. Toxocariasis in North America: a systematic review. PLoS Negl. Trop. Dis. 8, e3116.

Little, S.E., Johnson, E.M., Lewis, D., Jaklitsch, R.P., Payton, M.E., Blagburn, B.L., Bowman, D.D., Moroff, S., Tams, T., Rich, L., Aucoin, D., 2009. Prevalence of intestinal parasites in pet dogs in the United States. Vet. Parasitol. 166, 144–152.

Liu, Y., Zhang, Q., Li, J., Ji, X., Xu, Y., Zhao, P., 2016. Clinical characteristics of pediatric patients with ocular Toxocariasis in China. Ophthalmologica 235, 97–105.

Macpherson, C.N., 2013. The epidemiology and public health importance of toxocariasis: a zoonosis of global importance. Int. J. Parasitol. 43, 999–1008.
Magnaval, J.F., Michault, A., Calon, N., Charlet, J.P., 1994. Epidemiology of human toxocariasis in La Réunion. Trans. R. Soc. Trop. Med. Hyg. 88, 531–533.
McGuinness, S.L., Leder, K., 2014. Global burden of Toxocariasis: a common neglected infection of poverty. Curr. Trop. Med. Rep. 1, 52–61.
Meghji, M., Maizels, R.M., 1986. Biochemical properties of larval excretory-secretory glycoproteins of the parasitic nematode Toxocara canis. Mol. Biochem. Parasitol. 18, 155–170.
Merigueti, Y., Da Silva Raposo, R., Zampieri, B.P., De Lima Cerazo, L.M., Pereira, L., Santarem, V.A., 2018. Dispersion and infectivity of Toxocara canis eggs after passage through chicken intestine. Parasitol. Res. 117, 3481–3486.
Michalczyk, M., Sokol, R., Galecki, R., 2019. Internal parasites infecting dogs in rural areas. Ann. Parasitol. 65, 151–158.
Morgan, E.R., Azam, D., Pegler, K., 2013. Quantifying sources of environmental contamination with Toxocara spp. eggs. Vet. Parasitol. 193, 390–397.
Otranto, D., Dantas-Torres, F., Mihalca, A.D., Traub, R.J., Lappin, M., Baneth, G., 2017. Zoonotic parasites of sheltered and stray dogs in the era of the global economic and political crisis. Trends Parasitol. 33, 813–825.
Parise, M.E., Hotez, P.J., Slutsker, L., 2014. Neglected parasitic infections in the United States: needs and opportunities. Am. J. Trop. Med. Hyg. 90, 783–785.
Perlingiero, J.G., Gyorgy, P., 1947. Chronic eosinophilia; report of a case with necrosis of the liver, pulmonary infiltrations, anemia and ascaris infestation. Am. J. Dis. Child. 73, 34–43.
Poulsen, C.S., Skov, S., Yoshida, A., Skallerup, P., Maruyama, H., Thamsborg, S.M., Nejsum, P., 2015. Differential serodiagnostics of Toxocara canis and Toxocara cati—is it possible? Parasite Immunol. 37, 204–207.
Roddie, G., Stafford, P., Holland, C., Wolfe, A., 2008. Contamination of dog hair with eggs of Toxocara canis. Vet. Parasitol. 152, 85–93.
Sharghi, N., Schantz, P.M., Caramico, L., Ballas, K., Teague, B.A., Hotez, P.J., 2001. Environmental exposure to Toxocara as a possible risk factor for asthma: a clinic-based case-control study. Clin. Infect. Dis. 32, E111–E116.
Strube, C., Heuer, L., Janecek, E., 2013. Toxocara spp. infections in paratenic hosts. Vet. Parasitol. 193, 375–389.
Stull, J.W., Carr, A.P., Chomel, B.B., Berghaus, R.D., Hird, D.W., 2007. Small animal deworming protocols, client education, and veterinarian perception of zoonotic parasites in western Canada. Can. Vet. J. 48, 269–276.
Taira, K., Saitoh, Y., Okada, N., Sugiyama, H., Kapel, C.M., 2012. Tolerance to low temperatures of Toxocara cati larvae in chicken muscle tissue. Vet. Parasitol. 189, 383–386.
Turrientes, M.C., Perez De Ayala, A., Norman, F., Navarro, M., Perez-Molina, J.A., Rodriquez-Ferrer, M., Garate, T., Lopez-Velez, R., 2011. Visceral larva migrans in immigrants from Latin America. Emerg. Infect. Dis. 17, 1263–1265.
Walsh, M.G., 2011. Toxocara infection and diminished lung function in a nationally representative sample from the United States population. Int. J. Parasitol. 41, 243–247.
Walsh, M.G., Haseeb, M.A., 2012. Reduced cognitive function in children with toxocariasis in a nationally representative sample of the United States. Int. J. Parasitol. 42, 1159–1163.
Walsh, M.G., Haseeb, M.A., 2014. Small-area estimation of the probability of toxocariasis in New York City based on sociodemographic neighborhood composition. PLoS One 9, e99303.
Walsh, S.S., Robson, W.J., Hart, C.A., 1988. Acute transient myositis due to Toxocara. Arch. Dis. Child. 63, 1087–1088.
WHA, 2001. WHA54.19 Schistosomiasis and soil-transmitted helminth infections, 54th World Health Assembly, Agenda item 13.3, May 22.

WHO, 2012. World Health Organization. Accelerating Work to Overcome the Global Impact of Neglected Tropical Diseases: A Roadmap for Implementation. Executive Summary. World Health Organization, Geneva, Switzerland.
Won, K.Y., Kruszon-Moran, D., Schantz, P.M., Jones, J.L., 2008. National seroprevalence and risk factors for zoonotic Toxocara spp. infection. Am. J. Trop. Med. Hyg. 79, 552–557.
Zibaei, M., Sadjjadi, S.M., Maraghi, S., 2017. The occurrence of Toxocara species in naturally infected broiler chickens revealed by molecular approaches. J. Helminthol. 91, 633–636.

CHAPTER TWO

History of *Toxocara* and the associated *larva migrans*

Dwight D. Bowman*
Department of Microbiology and Immunology, College of Veterinary Medicine, Cornell University, Ithaca, NY, United States
*Corresponding author: e-mail address: ddb3@cornell.edu

Contents

Abstract

This review covers the systematics and nomenclature of the Ascaridoid genus toxocara, and more specifically the species *Toxocara canis* and *Toxocara cati*. Also discussed is the discovery of the persistence of these larvae in the tissues of paratenic hosts, and the role that other species of this genus might or could play in other such hosts; including those where the life cycle has been described, i.e., *Toxocara vitulorum*, *Toxocara pteropodis*, Toxocara mackerrasae, and *Toxocara tanuki*. Also examined is the work that led to the realization that the larval stage leaving the egg actually being a third rather than a second stage larva. Also discussed on the work showing that the larvae can persist in paratenic host with remarkable longevity without undergoing any morphological change for years and that these larvae can be transmitted from one paratenic host to another by ingestion. People are usually infected by the ingestion of eggs containing third-stage larvae, but infections also occur on occasions from the ingestion of uncooked paratenic hosts.

1. Systematics and nomenclature

Werner (1782) described *Lumbricus canis* of the dog, the worm that is now known as *Toxocara canis*. Getting from the initial binomen of *Lumbricus*

Advances in Parasitology, Volume 109
ISSN 0065-308X
https://doi.org/10.1016/bs.apar.2020.01.037

canis to that of *Toxocara canis* was a long and twisted tale that has been described in detail in two papers by JFA Sprent (1956, 1958). Things were long confused as to whether *Toxocara canis* was the same as *Toxocara cati*, and whether *Toxascaris* was the same as *Toxocara*. Arguments raged as to the proper name for the species and the genus, but things seemed to finally settle down sometime in the 1930s when it was decided through papers published by Stiles and Hassall (1905), Johnston (1916), and as discussed by Warren (1970b), the name was introduced and has since remained as *Toxocara canis*. Sprent (1958) listed the synonyms for *T. canis* as *Belascaris triquetra* (Schrank, of Rudolphi) Leiper, 1907; *Belascaris marginata* (Rudolphi) Railliet and Henry, 1911; *Belascaris masculior* Railliet and Henry, 1911; *Toxocara vulpis* (Froelich) Yorke and Maplestone, 1926; and *Toxocara masculior* Railliet and Henry, 1911; Yorke and Maplestone, 2918.

Sprent (1958) also reported that the hosts other than *Canis lupus familiaris* that served as final host for *Toxocara canis* included the dingo, jackal, wolves, the spotted hyaena, the Fennec fox, the African wild dog (*Lycaon pictus*), the raccoon dog (*Nyctereutes procyonoides*), and numerous species of foxes of the genus *Vulpes*. Since the appearance of Sprent's publication, *T. canis* has also been reported from coyotes, *Canis latrans* (Redman et al., 2016). Based on scat samples with *Toxocara* eggs, it has also been reported in a number of South American canids, i.e., the bush dog, *Speothos venaticus*, in Argentina (Vizcaychipi et al., 2016); the maned wolf, *Chrysocyon brachyurus*, and crab eating fox, *Cerdocyon thous*, in Minas Gerais, Brazil (Santo et al., 2012); and Darwin's fox, *Pseudalopex fulvipes*, in Chile (Jiménez et al., 2012).

At the same time, membership in the genus *Toxocara* has continued to grow by either the relocating of existing species originally described as being within other genera or by descriptions of new *Toxocara* species. Warren (1970a,b) in his careful examination of the makeup of the genus *Toxocara*, redefined the genus such that it contained what were considered 11 valid *Toxocara* species. Warren also carefully outlined various features of taxonomic importance for species differentiation within the genus, such as, differences in lip morphology, the shape of lateral alae, spicules, egg size, and size of the surface pits found on the eggs of different species. Warren could find no significant reason to separate the species from ruminants within the genus *Neoascaris*, which like *Toxocara* had an obvious ventriculus at the base of the oesophagus, based solely on their having ruminant hosts, and therefore, Warren subjugated these species within the genus *Toxocara*. Also, he classified four species that had been described as being within *Toxocara* as being *species inquirendae*. These four species were *Toxocara cynonycteridis* of bats, *Toxocara elephantis* of Asian elephants that had been housed in European zoos, *Toxocara manzadiensis* from a young bovine, and *Toxocara pearsei* that was described from a snapping shrimp, *Synalpheus brooksi*, by Chitwood (1935).

After the subjugation of *Neoascaris* and the removal of the four *species inquirendae*, Warren recognized 11 species within the genus *Toxocara* with (1) *Toxocara canis* (Werner, 1782) Stiles, 1905, being the type genus and species. The other 10 species he recognized were (2) *Toxocara alienata* (Rudolphi, 1819) Warren, 1970 from the ring-tailed coati, *Nasua nasua rufa,* crab eating racoon *Procyon cancrivorus*, and peccary *Tayassus torquatus* of South America; (3) *Toxocara apodemi* (Olsen, 1957) Warren, 1970 from the Korean field mouse, *Apodemus peninsulae*; (4) *Toxocara cati* (Schrank, 1788) of felids worldwide; Brumpt, 1927; (5) *Toxocara mackerrasae* (Sprent, 1957), Warren, 1970 of the bush rat, *Rattus fuscipes,* and the water rat, *Hydromys chrysogaster,* of Australia; (6) *Toxocara paradoxura* Kou, 1958 from a palm civet, *Paradxurus minor exitis* (=*Paradoxurus hermaphorditus*) in China; (7) *Toxocara pteropodis* Baylis, 1936 from a suckling fruit bat *Pteropus geddiei* in the French Republic of Vanuatu; (8) *Toxocara suricattae* (Ortlepp, 1940), Warren, 1970 from meerkats, *Suricata suricatta*, in South Africa; (9) *Toxocara tanuki* Yamaguti, 1941 from the Japanese raccoon dog, *Nyctereutes procyonoides viverrinus*; (10) *Toxocara vincenti* Puylaert, 1967 from the African civet, *Civettictis civetta* and a Tanzanian genet *Genetta stuhlmanni*; and (11) *Toxocara vitulorum* (Goeze, 1782) Warren, 1970 of bovines.

An additional 8 species that have been added to the list of 11 species cited in the 1970 publication by Warren include: (12) *Toxocara vajrasthirae* described from the mustelid hog-badger, *Arctonyx collaris*, of Thailand (Sprent, 1972); two additional species described in a single publication (Warren, 1972): (13) *Toxocara genettae* from the common genet, *Genetta felina*, of South Africa, which has since also been found in Europe (Alvarez et al., 1990; Casanova et al., 2000), and (14) *Toxocara sprenti* from the small Indian civet *Viverricula indica* (Warren, 1972). In 1974 the species, (15) *Toxocara warreni* was named for worms collected from a water chevrotain or fanged deer, *Hyemoschus aquaticus*, in Gabon (Durette-Desset and Chabaud, 1974). Maung (1975) erected the new species (16) *Toxocara hippopotami* for a species that had been originally described by Canavan (1931) from a hippopotamus in the Philadelphia Zoological Garden as *Ascaris hippopotami* basing the new description also on specimens that had been collected from a *Hippopotamus amphibius* from Lake Edward in Uganda. In 1981, a species, (17) *Toxocara indica*, was described for worms collected from a greater bandicoot rat,

Bandicota indica, in Nagpur, India (Naidu, 1981). Macchioni (1999) described a species, (18) *Toxocara lyncis,* from 4 of 9 *Lynx caracal* in Somalia; this species resembled *T. cati,* which has been reported previously from *L. caracal,* but it had narrower cervical alae. Gibbons et al. (2001) described a new species in cats in Malaysia that had initially thought to be *T. canis* using the name (19) *Toxocara malaysiensis*: this species has since been found also in cats in China (Li et al., 2006) and in Vietnam (Le et al., 2016).

The genus and species of the cat *Toxocara* that commonly occurs in the domestic cat and that is now known as *Toxocara cati* had a taxonomic history that was as convoluted and twisted as that of *Toxocara canis*. *Toxascaris leonina* (von Linstow, 1902) Leiper, 1907 the other common ascaridoid of the cat and also dogs, was recognized as being in a genus that was different than the genus *Toxocara*; this was due to its lack of an oesophageal ventriculus and narrow cervical alae. The systematics and taxonomy of both these genera and the synonymies are described in careful detail in two publications by Sprent (1956, 1959) on their biology and development. The *Toxocara* of the domestic cat had been given the name *Ascaris cati* by Schrank in 1788, and in the end, it came to rest with the possession of the binomen *Toxocara cati* (Schrank, 1788) Brumpt, 1927. For those interested in the nomenclatural details of the names of the species of large roundworms of dogs and cats, the three papers by Sprent and a fourth paper by Sprent and Barrett (1964) discussing both genera are a good place to start.

2. Discovery of the persistence of Ascaridoidean Nematodes in host tissues

In 1949 at an annual meeting of the American Society of Parasitologist, Tiner (1949) presented a paper discussing an experimental infections of rodents with ascaridoid eggs that caused a deadly disease in wild rodents (It was later shown that Tiner was working with eggs of species shown to be in the genus *Baylisascaris* that migrate to the rodents brains growing larger as they migrate.). At the same time this was occurring, Sprent was performing similar work using a series of different ascaridoids nematodes. These two authors both published papers on the topic of migrating ascaridoid larvae in 1952 and 1953 (Sprent, 1952, 1953 and Tiner, 1952). In the midst of these publications, was the first case report on visceral larva migrans by Beaver et al. (1952), where *Toxocara canis* larvae were recovered from three children presenting with an eosinophilia associated disease syndrome in New Orleans, Louisiana. Thus, the puzzle was coming together as the various disjointed pieces were being individually assembled.

Prior to this case report by Beaver and coworkers and the contemporary research by Sprent and Tiner, the life cycle of the ascaridoids of terrestrial mammals, other than that of the monoxenous life cycles of the medically and veterinary important species of *Ascaris lumbricoides* of people, *Ascaris suum* of pigs, and *Parascaris equorum* of the horse. These species were monoxenous, and in various studies, when eggs containing larvae of these three species were fed to rodents or lagomorphs, there were no lasting stages of these parasites in the tissues of the infected animals. The major impetus for the additional work on these parasites was that fact that these other worms of dogs and other animals could serve as sources for disease in animals other than their final hosts. This was not a totally novel concept. In fact, in 1921, Fülleborn (1921) had suggested that these types of infection might occur due to these other ascaridoids. In his studies of "ascarid infection by eating encapsulated larvae", he noted that many ascarid larvae, such as the herring worm (Anisakis), pass as encysted larvae through different hosts to get to the final host. Fülleborn also described nodules with *Toxocara* larvae in the tissues of dogs, rabbits, and guinea pigs, and showed that he could infect puppies in utero if he infected the pregnant mother with larvae recovered from guinea pig lungs. This ultimately led Fülleborn to provide foreshadowing of the discovery of the existence of visceral larva migrans: Based on the common "frequency of *Belascaris* (= *Toxocara*) eggs, animals—and certainly humans too—often have the opportunity to ... form such *Belascaris* nodules like guinea pigs and mice. On the potential pathological meaning of *Belascaris* (= *Toxocara*) nodules in liver, kidney, brain, lung etc. possibly in humans, I will not enter here. [translated from the German]".

Thus, with the discovery of the human syndrome and the realization that many species of ascaridoid nematodes have larvae in hosts other than the final host, work progressed rapidly on detailing nuances of the life cycles of these parasites. Relative to *Toxocara*, two pairs of papers works were very important. The pair of papers by Sprent (1952, 1953) on the distribution and longevity of the larvae of the canine *Toxocara* and other Ascaridoidea in the bodies of experimentally infected mice, and the pair by Nichols (1956a,b) describing the diagnostic morphology of *Toxocara canis* and *Toxocara cati* in experimentally infected mice and compared it with that of the morphology of larvae from mice infected with *Ascaris lumbricoides*, *Necator americanum*, *Strongyloides stercoralis*, and *Ancylostoma caninum*.

In the work by Sprent (1952, 1953), mice were fed infective eggs of different Ascaridoid species, i.e., *Ascaris lumbricoides* from humans, *Ascaris suum* from pigs, *Parascaris equorum* from horses, *Toxocara canis* from the dog and fox (*Vulpes vulpes*), *Toxascaris leonina* from a lynx (*Lynx canadensis*) and a wolf (*Canis lupus lycaon*), *Ascaris* (now *Baylisascaris*) *columnaris* from the skunk (*Mephitis mephitis*), an *Ascaris* species from the fisher (*Martin pennanti*) (now = *Baylisascaris devosi* Sprent, 1968), and *Toxascaris* (now *Baylisascaris*) *transfuga* from a black bear (*Euarctos americanus*). In this work, the larvae of *A. lumbricoides*, *A. suum*, and *P. equorum* made a liver-lung migration and then were no longer found in the mice after 2 weeks. All other species had larvae that entered the tissues of the carcass and remained for months (Noted here is the fact that this did also occur with *Toxascaris leonina*; the persistence of the larvae of this fairly common nematode in the larvae of paratenic hosts is often not considered as a potential agent of visceral larva migrans.). The work of Nichols, also showed similar to postinfection persistence of the larval parasites, results relative to larval persistence were similar to that shown by Sprent, i.e., the larvae of *T. canis* and *T. cati* persisted in the tissues, while the larvae of *A. lumbricoides*, *S. stercoralis*, and *N. americanus* were not found in mice after several weeks. Nichols also found that the larvae of the canine hookworm, *A. caninum*, did persist for extended periods in the tissues of infected mice. He also showed that in histological sections that the larvae of *T. canis* could be differentiated from the larvae of *A. caninum*; also, the larvae of *T. cati* were shown in histologic sections to be thinner than were the larvae of *T. canis* (in the sections, the maximum diameter for *T. canis* was 14–20 μm and *T. cati* it was 12–16 μm). A good number of years later an examination of the biology of *Toxocara vitulorum* relative to zoonotic importance was performed. Warren (1971) examined the persistence of larvae in experimentally infected mice. In this case, the larvae migrated through the liver and lungs, but only a few entered the carcass and only a very small percentage of the infective dose was found in the carcass tissues 1–3 months after infection.

3. Modes of infection and larval development of *Toxocara* species in their typical final hosts

The life cycles of only a few of the *Toxocara* species occurring in different final hosts have been examined, i.e., *Toxocara canis*, *Toxocara cati*, *Toxocara vitulorum*, *Toxocara pteropodis*, *Toxocara mackerrasae,* and *T. tanuki* of the raccoon dog. A brief summary of the generalities of the described life cycles is presented in the following; the biology of the remaining 13 species has not yet been reported.

Toxocara canis: The larval development of *Toxocara canis* is dogs was reviewed most recently by Schnieder et al. (2011), and the following is a summary of the account of these authors. Upon the ingestion of eggs, third-stage larvae hatched from the eggs within 2–4 h after infection, and then after penetrating the intestinal wall, they enter lymph vessels, make their way to the mesenteric lymph nodes, and enter the venous capillaries and via the portal circulation are carried to the liver where they arrive about 24 h after infection. They then move via the *vena cava* to the lungs via the pulmonary artery with most being in the lungs between 72 and 96 h post infection. Those that remain in the liver are found within small granulomas. The larvae that reach the lungs follow two different routes depending on the immune status and age of the infected dogs. In naïve and young dogs, the larvae typically enter alveoli and via bronchioles are carried to the pharynx where they are swallowed and then grow to adult worms in the small intestine—following much the same developmental pattern as that of *Ascaris suum* and *Ascaris lumbricoides*. In dogs that are older and/or previously infected, many of the *T. canis* larvae will re-enter the circulatory system and be carried to somatic tissues where they persist. The immune response seems directed mainly against third-stage larvae (more below about which larval stage is the infective stage that leaves the egg) by showing that if these larvae were introduced into the intestine of a previously infected dogs the larvae tended not to develop, while some 50% of fourth-stage larvae introduced directly into the small intestine developed to adulthood. The dose of eggs that a dog ingests also impacts the ability of worms to develop to the adult stage. When only 100 or less eggs are ingested by a dog, even adult dogs, there is a very high probability that patent infections will develop than when dogs are given larger doses. It appears, that as in *Ascaris* where the moult to the fourth-stage occurs when larvae leave the lungs and the return to the intestine, this event occurs at the same point in *T. canis* larvae that go onto develop into adult worms within the dog. Adults females typically produce eggs approximately 4–5 weeks after infection, and the adults live on average somewhere around 4 months.

The infection of dogs with larvae from paratenic hosts were summarized from experiments numerous experimental studies, and overall it was shown that after passing through a mouse, the larvae tend not to undergo a somatic tissue migration with development occurring mainly within the intestinal tract. The first such report was that of Fülleborn as was noted above where dogs were infected using larvae from the tissues of guinea pigs. Sprent (1958) found that he could infect dogs by feeding them infected mice, and that in these cases, the larvae did not undergo somatic migrations after infection. Warren (1969) found that with mice that had been infected with 25,000 eggs 4 days prior to feeding their larval containing murine tissues to dogs that the larvae underwent a tracheal migration following their ingestion then developed to the adult stage in the small intestine. Similar result were reported by Herschel (1981) who inoculated 11 dogs with 100 larvae that had been in mice for 28 days and produced patent infections in 6 of the dogs with worm burdens of 15 adults or less; somatic migration did appear to occur in a female dog upon necropsy that was given 150,000 larvae that had migrated through four layers of filter paper. Pahari and Sasmal (1990a,b) fed 60-day-old *T. canis* larvae from infected quail to 3 dogs (400 each) and had 2 unfed controls. Forty days later the dogs were necropsied, and the 3 dogs fed larvae shed young maturing worms in their faeces on day 33 after infection, eggs in their faeces 38 days after infection, and at necropsy 74, 85, and 102 adult worms were found in each of the intestines of the 3 infected dogs.

In dogs, it was long suspected and has been corroborated that infection occurs prenatally. Also, it has been shown that the infection occurs primarily by transplacental or intrauterine infection of the puppies, rather than by transmammary or lactational transmission. It has been shown that larvae can live for a year in dogs and that larvae can be passed from mother to puppies in three successive litters. Lactogenic transmission can occur, but it is not a major means of transmission from mother to puppies when compared to the transplacental infection of puppies. The comparison of infections in groups of dogs that had or had not acquired patent prenatal infections has shown that those infected prenatally are not protected against developing patent *T. canis* infections later in life if they are infected with small numbers of infective eggs (Fahrion et al., 2008).

Toxocara cati: The first work on the life cycle of *T. cati* in the final host was that of Sprent (1956) who examined infections in the feline host and in mice. After infection with eggs, the larvae migrated to the liver and lungs and then returned to the intestine via the trachea. After the tenth day, the larvae were in the stomach wall and could also be recovered from muscle tissues. When cats were fed infected mice, they seemed to develop almost exclusively within the digestive tract. In egg-infected cats, fourth-stage larvae first appeared after 19 days in the intestinal wall and intestinal contents; in mouse infected cats, fourth-stage larvae appeared in these same sites in 20 days. The moult to the adult stage occurred in the intestinal lumen when the larvae were 4.3–6.5 mm long. Eggs were first observed beginning 56 days after the infection. Sprent fed infective eggs to a pregnant queen during the last 4 weeks of gestation and did not recover larvae from the kittens examined after birth. Swerczek et al. (1971) examined 78 kittens at birth from 20 naturally infected queens and 14 kittens from 7 queens that were experimentally infected with 300–2000 eggs per day from day 2 to 56 prepartum, and no larvae were found in the organs of the kittens when they were examined. When 12 kittens were examined 2–3 weeks after natural delivery from 5 queens that had been orally fed 2000 *T. cati* eggs for 1–10 day prepartum a total of almost 8000 larvae were recovered mainly from the gastrointestinal tract; while no larvae were found in 5 kittens (1 from each litter) that was not allowed to nurse. These authors also found larvae in the mammary glands and went on to show that 19 kittens derived by caesarean section from 6 queens that were raised colostrum-free to maturity remained free of *T. cati*. Coati et al. (2004) reexamined vertical transmission of *T. cati* to kittens in three experiments: Experiment 1 contained four naturally infected queens that maintained their patent infections for the 38 weeks of the study period wherein they were each mated twice to produce two consecutive litters. Half the kittens from each queen were examined directly after caesarean delivery, while the others were reared by their mothers. In the litters produced by the second mating, all the kittens remained with their mothers. The kittens were found not to be infected, and no larvae were found in the mammary glands of the queens. Experiment 2 contained four parasite-naïve queens that were experimentally infected with eggs during late pregnancy (2000 eggs daily beginning 10 days prior to expected date of delivery). All the queens developed patent infections 6–7 weeks after the first egg inoculation, and of the 952 larvae recovered, 98% were found in the gastrointestinal tract. Experiment 3 contained two of the queens from Experiment 2 that had been dewormed with pyrantel and no eggs were shed prior to delivery of the kittens. These cats were mated, allowed to give birth, and suckle their young. All members of 1 L of kittens developed patent infections beginning 44 days after delivery, and the other litter remained free of infection. Both queens became patent on day 56 post-partum. Thus, the work was stated to show that infection of nursing kittens is most likely to occur only if the mothers are infected during lactation with chronic infections being atypical sources of post-natal lactogenic transmission.

Toxocara vitulorum: This is a parasite of *Bos taurus* cattle and the buffalo, *Bubalus bubalis*. There have been reports from sheep and goats, but particularly with goats, it is considered that some of the eggs in the faeces may be due to coprophagia. An in-depth review of all aspects of this parasite including the taxonomy, distribution, life cycle, and more was presented by Roberts as a Review in the Commonwealth Agriculture Bureau Abstracts (1993). For a long time, this species that parasitizes the cow and the buffalo was considered to be the same as or equivalent to *Ascaris suum* but things changed with a publication by Neumann (1883). However, it remained in its own genus, *Neoascaris*. As work on the life cycle continued, many initially thought it was transmitted directly in the same manner as *A. suum* and *A. lumbricoides*, but no evidence could be produced. Others thought it might be transferred transplacentally as Fülleborn had shown for the dog, ascarid *T. canis*. After the discovery by Olsen and Lyons (1962) of the transmission of nematode larvae through the milk of the mother, this seemed to the many veterinarians who dealt with this infection and saw only infections in young animals as an excellent possibility. Ultimately, through work by several authors and groups (Mia et al., 1975; Roberts, 1990; Skryabin and Schulz, 1937; Warren, 1971), it has become clear that this is mainly a disease of calves that become infected through larvae in their mother's milk; and hence its disappearance on large dairy farms where calves are bottle raised. When a cow ingests the infective eggs, the larvae migrate to the liver where most remain, but a percentage go onto the lungs, and a few go to the muscle, brain, kidney, and peripheral lymph nodes. Over the next 3–7 weeks the larvae in the liver increase in size by about 10%, but not until the cow becomes pregnant, do they grow significantly and migrate. They become about 500–600 μm long and then make their way to the mammary gland where they grow to a length of 1.05–1.50 mm. These larvae ad are passed in the milk. Very few larvae are passed in the colostrum, and the passage in the milk stops after about the first 8 days of lactation. All development takes places in the intestinal tract of the calves. It seems almost impossible to induce patent infections in adult cattle, but there is some suspicion that it might be possible to infect naïve calves if they are infected the first day of life.

Toxocara pteropodis: This parasite was thought at one time to be the potential cause of a hepatic syndrome outbreak in people that was described as "Palm Island mystery disease" (Prociv, 1983). Eggs of this parasite were found on mangos that the patients in the outbreak had been eating, and this led to *T. pteropodis* being considered as a potential cause of this disease (Moorhouse, 1982) and work being performed on this parasite's life cycle. Other causes were also considered, e.g., algal intoxication due to an algal bloom in a nearby lake that was treated with copper sulphate 5 days before cases occurred, and people who drank the water had signs of the disease.

After the work described below, it was stated that *T. pteropodis* was an unlikely cause of the disease, and that the real cause may have been multifactorial and that this might have been one of the factors in the outbreak (Prociv et al., 1986).

In the research performed, the parasite was found to infect all four species of Australia's flying fox species, genus *Pteropus*, i.e., *Pteropus poliocephalus*, *Pteropus alecto*, *Pteropus. conspicillatus*, and *Pteropus scapulatus*. Studies were published dealing with the infection of different hosts, including *P. poliocephalus* (Prociv, 1983); mice, rats, guinea pigs, and long-tailed macaques (Prociv, 1983, 1986; Prociv and Brindley, 1986a,b; Prociv and Mak, 1987). In the bats, adult worms were found only in parturient females, while in other bats larvae were found only in the livers. Following parturition, larvae were found in the mammary glands for up to 2 weeks post-partum. Developing larvae were found only in the intestines of young bats beginning at 2 days of age without any signs of lung migration. The young bats passed eggs in their faeces at 2 months of age, and when about 5-months old, the adult worms were passed in the faeces. The authors also report, without describing the studies, that rabbits, pigs, chickens, and ducklings were refractory to infection. Adult rats were refractory to infection, but suckling rats could be infected at lower levels than mice. When mice were infected orally with eggs, the larvae went to the liver and grew from 430 to 600 μm; the same result occurred when eggs were inoculated subcutaneously or intraperitoneally (Prociv, 1985a,b). Comparing *T. pteropodis* migration to different *Toxocara* spp. in guinea pigs, it was found that when guinea pigs were fed *T. pteropodis* eggs, the larvae entered the liver, but disappeared within 25 days. In the case of *Toxocara canis*, the larvae entered the liver, then the lungs, and finally entered the muscles and appeared to increase in number in the brains over a period of 7 months. In the case of *T. cati*, the larvae tended to stay within the somatic musculature. In bat studies with *T. pteropodis*, when they were infected orally or subcutaneously the larvae were mainly in the liver, while bats infected with *T. canis* had larvae that appeared in the musculature and then appeared in the brain. In the long-tailed macaque, *Macaca fascicularis*, that were given 200,000 *T. pteropodis* eggs once, 5000 followed by 15,000 eggs, or 10 daily doses of 2000 eggs, an eosinophilia developed and almost all larvae were found in the liver, but in most cases the larvae died within granulomas (Prociv and Mak, 1987).

Toxocara mackerrasae: Warren (1970a,b) examined the life cycle of *T. mackerrasae* in mice and laboratory rats, and the natural rat host, *Rattus fuscipes*, and found that there was no somatic migration. There was very little success in obtaining adult worms in any of the hosts, but Warren pointed out that even in the wild, of 585 rats examined, only 105 (18%) were found to be infected with 1–6 (mean 2.8%) adult *T. mackerrasae* in each. Of the 291 *T. mackerrasae* collected, the adults were only found in larger rats, i.e., rats greater than 14.0 cm in length. Also, of these 291 helminth specimens, only 16 were gravid females, and they were found only in 9 of the rats.

Toxocara tanuki: The biology of this species with adults in raccoon dogs, *Nyctereutes procyonoides*, has been examined relative to its behaviour in mice. Kondo et al. (1975) reported in an abstract that in egg-infected mice the larvae behaved quite differently than those of *T. canis* and *T. cati*. The larvae migrated to the liver and then remained in the liver, only rarely migrating to other viscera. This was also reported by Okamoto (1986) when mice examined for on days 1, 2, 3, 5, 7, 14, 21, 28, 35 and 49 after being given 300, 3000, or 30,000 *T. tanuki* infective eggs, almost all recovered larvae were from the liver, and only rarely were larvae found in lungs, brain, or carcass. It was also found that more larvae were recovered from the livers of athymic nude mice than from heterozygotic littermates.

4. Number of moults by the larva within the eggshell

It was only recently accepted by most that there are two moults within the eggshell as part of the the life history of the Ascaridoid nematodes (see Schnieder et al., 2011). Ransom and Foster (1920) in their description of work on the life cycle of *Ascaris lumbricoides* and *A. suum*, stated that there was a single moult in the egg that the a second moult apparently occurred before the larva reached the stage where it migrates from the lungs to the intestine of the host. Work by others over the years supported this claim relative to other genera in other hosts, e.g., Ortlepp (1922) on the life cycles of the Ascaridoidea of snakes, *Ophidascaris* and *Polydelphis*; Goodey and Cameron (1923) on the biology of *Ascaris* (now *Baylisascaris*) *columnaris* of skunks; Roberts (1934) and Alicata (1935) again with *A. suum* and *A. lumbricoides*; Wright (1935) for *Toxascaris leonina*, and Markowski (1937) with *Contracaecum* (now *Hysterothylacium*) *aduncum*, and Huizinga (1969) with *Contracaecum multipapillatum*. There were a few dissenters claiming two moults within the egg: Skryabin and Schulz (1937, cited by Roberts, 1993) with *Toxocara vitulorum* of the cow; Thomas (1937) with *Contracaecum spiculigerum* having adults in piscivorus birds; and Dubinin (1948; cited in

1968 translation of Mozgovoi, 1953) with *Ascaris tarbagan* (now *Baylisascaris laevis*) of the marmot. However, the dogma remained that there was only a single moult of the larva in the egg, although the second moult that supposedly occurred in the host was almost never described and often when it was, what was described was not an actual moult but variations in morphology or size.

In 1966, Thust (1966) published images on the electron microscopy of *Ascaris suum* in the egg and line drawing showing two moults occurring within the eggshell. However, folks were either unaware of the publication (not published in a typical parasitology source journal) or doubtful of the results, and also, the early work by Beaver, Sprent, Warren, and Nichols had seemingly supported the "one molt in the egg" dogma. Then, in 1971, Araujo (1971) published work on the life cycle of the ascaridoids of snakes (*Polydelphis*, *Hexametra*, and *Ophidascaris*) and stated that there were two moults in the egg and that the first was very thin and usually not present in larvae that had already moulted to the third stage after weeks of culture and that the first sheath was easily destroyed when the larvae were pressed from the eggshells for examination. Araujo (1972a) next published descriptions of two moults in the eggs *A. lumbricoides*, *A. suum*, and *T. canis*, and also in *Polydelphis* (now *Travassosascaris*) *quadrangularis* (Araujo, 1972b). Maung (1978) verified the work of Araujo with *A. lumbricoides* and *A. suum*. Smith et al. (1983) using the very distinctive head and tail of the larva that leaves the egg, found no moults by *Lagochilascaris sprenti* in mice unless they occurred relative to the odd larva that decided to mature within the murine muscle tissues to the adult stage, Finally, the very well-done and excellently illustrated publication on moulting by the larva within the eggshell by Bruňaska et al. (1995) was published, and although it took time to catch on, it ultimately convinced most that there are two moults in the eggs of the terrestrial Ascaridoidea and many of the aquatic forms as well.

The "one-moult" dogma had been intensely defended, and a lot of folks spent a good deal of time explaining why they could not find moulting forms or ignored the question. Schacher (1957) illustrated (figs 5–7) a larva of *T. canis* pressed from the eggshell with two cuticles 2 and reported that "Since this feature was only occasionally evident, it apparently does not indicate 2 separate molts within the egg, but rather a splitting or swelling of the cuticle". People had claimed that the thin outer cuticle sometimes seen on the larva in an eggshell was the remnants of the vitelline membrane; however, Foor (1967) clearly showed (figs 13–17) that the vitelline layer was basically on the outside of the eggshell and under the external albuminous layer produced by the uterus of the female, and not at all associated with the external surface of the developing larva. Nichols (1956a,b) in his work with the larvae of *T. canis*, *T. cati*, and *A. lumbricoides* never found a moulting larval stage with two cuticles. The fact that there is not a moult from a second stage to a third stage within the different hosts actually fits well with these life cycles that are dependent on the utilization of paratenic hosts and long-term survival and passage by ingestion of tissues of *Toxocara canis* and *Toxocara cati* larvae without their undergoing any further development. It should be noted, that in the case of *Baylisascaris*, *Toxascaris*, *Lagochilascaris*, *Ophidascaris*, *Hexametra*, and other Ascaridoidea, the larvae in the paratenic hosts can grow, even to lengths of several inches in the case of those with adults in snakes and birds, but these larvae grow but do not moult within their paratenic hosts.

5. Paratenesis

A "paratenic host" was defined by Baer in his text *Ecology of Animal Parasites* in 1951 as "An optional intermediate host is one which the larvae usually enters passively, along with ingested food. The larvae are able to survive for considerable time without the new environment affecting in any way their ontogeny. Such larvae will invariably remain at the same stage of development as when first swallowed by this host". "...the designation paratenic host is proposed since being derived from the Greek παρατείνω—"to prolong, to draw out, i.e., to complicate the life cycle, ... The basis for this concept is one of ontogeny, as no larval form undergoes any development in a paratenic host". [This last statement carefully allows for the fact that the larvae can grow, as long as, they do not develop. The plerocercoid of *Dibothriocephalus* can grow massively, but it does not develop to another stage. Thus, whether or not a moult (or in other phyla, an ontogenetic change) occurs in the host is important relative to whether or not the term paratenesis applies to larval toxocariasis.]

This concept of paratenesis has led to a series of studies where the larvae of *T. canis* and *T. cati*, have been recovered from one murine host or another host species and used to orally infect mice or rats to show that the larvae are acting as they would in a paratenic host, i.e., having the potential to pass from one host to the next, persisting without undergoing any development. Larvae have been passed form mouse, chicken, quail, piglets, and macaques to mice in different studies.

Studies in support of the concept of paratenesis have dealt with the passage of larvae of *T. canis* from host to host without any development occurring unless the host is a canid. Smith and Beaver (1953) report that Nichols in his thesis successfully showed that larvae in murine tissue could migrate into and persist in the tissues of mice fed larvae from infected mice. Ishii (1959) examined mouse to mouse transmission by successfully passing larvae by oral infection from mice infected with *T. canis* to secondarily infected mice, and larvae could then be passed to a third set of mice. Beaver (1962) reported on a long-term study of *T. canis* larvae in two experimentally infected rhesus macaques (*Macaca mulatta*) and stated: "At 7 years, biopsies from both monkeys still contained larvae in relatively large numbers, and when fed to a mouse the larvae migrated to the tissues in the normal manner". Pahari and Sasmal (1990a,b) described the infection of Japanese quail (*Coturnix japonica*) with 5000 eggs of *T. canis*, and then 60 days after infection, 50 larvae obtained from the birds at necropsy were given to mice that were examined 6 and 12 days later. On both days, slightly more than 50% of the larvae were recovered from liver, lungs, viscera, brain, and muscles of the mice. Sasmal et al. (2008) infected piglets with *T. canis* eggs, and then 15 days later fed 5 g of liver to each of 5 mice; the larval burdens in the mice upon examination 10 days after feeding revealed mean numbers of larvae per gram of the infected 5 mice to be 20 (liver), 17 (lungs), 3 (heart), 12 (brain), and 30 (carcass).

Others looked to see if this event occurred with *T. cati*. Dubey (1968) fed larvae from the carcasses of *T. cati* egg-infected mice to a rat and 2 mice. In the rat given 4500 larvae from mice, he recovered 1384 larvae 40 h post-feeding (906 larvae in the gut wall and 352 in the muscle); from the 2 mice each given 2000 larvae, he recovered a total of 1462 larvae post-feeding with 1455 of the larvae being recovered from the muscle tissue of the carcass.

Okoshi and Usui (1968) experimentally successfully orally transferred the larvae or *T. canis* recovered from the carcass and brain of mice and livers of chickens to mice. In the case of *T. cati*, larvae also could be transferred from infected mice to mice and infected chickens to mice. The oral transfer of larvae of *Toxascaris leonina* from the carcass of one mouse to a second and third mouse did occur, but only if the larvae were in the first mouse 20 days or less, these larvae. *T. leonina* larvae do grow in the tissues of mice, and by 32 days, the larvae will have grown to lengths of about 0.7 mm long (Bowman, 1987). Okosh and Usui also transferred *T. canis* larvae from infected earthworms to mice and then to chickens. In the case of *T. cati*, they transferred larvae from earthworms to mice, but they recovered no larvae from chickens receiving larvae from mice. Henson (1975) showed that the African night crawler, *Eudrilus eugeniae* could be infected and maintain larval *T. canis* for at least 30 days. There has been a case visceral larva migrans in an adolescent who developed the syndrome after having eaten an earthworm on a dare (Cianferoni et al., 2006). Hoffmeister et al. (2007) describe a case of cerebral toxocariasis after the ingestions of raw duck liver, and they also present information on earlier described cases that appear to be from the ingestion of raw liver from chickens, cattle, and sheep. Cases from raw liver ingestion have continued to appear amongst those choosing to eat raw liver (Choi et al., 2012; Hiramatsu et al., 2017; Yoshikawa et al., 2008).

6. Larval longevity

Considerable attention has been paid to the length of time that the larvae survive in paratenic hosts. When one examines human serology, the antigen levels to the larval excretory-secretory proteins seem to persist for extended periods, perhaps the life of the human host (Won et al., 2008). It remains at this time impossible to tell whether this is due to persistent larvae being present in the human hosts or to reinfections resulting in elevated antibody levels. A number of studies have examined the longevity of larvae in different paratenic hosts held for extended periods after infection. These studies of extended periods have been performed in birds, rodents, and primates.

The larvae seem to remain viable in their paratenic hosts for years. In birds, Galvin (1964) reported that in chickens and pigeons at about 5 months post infection that he could recover 30% of the infective dose from the liver of chickens and about 18% of the dose from pigeons. In rodents, Sprent (1953) reported on the distribution and longevity of larvae of *T. canis* and *T. cati* in mice were given 2500 infective eggs. *T cati* was only examined at a maximum of 2 months postinfection, and there was a total of 730 larvae found in the carcass (110 in the head, 380 in the anterior portion, and 240 in the posterior portion), no larvae were found at 1 or 2 months in the brain. In the case of *T. canis*, similar numbers of larvae were recovered in all mice examined monthly, and at 6 months postinfection there was a total of 300 larvae recovered from the carcass (140 head, 100 anterior portion, and 90 posterior portion) with an additional 170 being found in the brain. Bardón et al. (1994), showed that in mice given 1000 infective eggs, a mean of 78.6% larvae were recovered from tissues 1-month post infection and that 29% larvae were recovered 1-year post infection. As already stated above, *T. canis* and *T. cati* larvae in infected guineas pigs were shown to still be present in muscle 7 months after infection (Prociv and Mak, 1987).

In primates the larvae also seem to persist for long periods. Glickman and Summers (1983) inoculated 20 male cynomolgus macaques (*Macaca fascicularis*) with 45,000 eggs. In the examination of six animals at necropsy, at 220 days postinfection, larvae, apparently viable, were found in histologic sections of liver tissue. For the brain, it was estimated based on the examination of pressed tissues between slides that it contained somewhere between 0.9 and 8.2 larvae per gram of tissue. Again, in 1966, Beaver described the long-term follow-up on two experimentally infected macaques that were followed for 10 years. Beaver describes finding larvae in these monkeys, and suggests that larvae can survive for 9 or 10 years: "The monkeys referred to were a male and a female, inoculated with massive doses of infective *T. canis* larvae in 1954 and 1955. Biopsies of the liver were taken at 6-month, and later at yearly, intervals. Active, apparently infective larvae were found in all biopsies through 1964, but when the animals were sacrificed in 1965 no larvae were found, in the liver or elsewhere".

7. Concluding remarks

Toxocara canis and *Toxocara cati* are, in much of the world, the most common intestinal parasites of dogs and cats. Human serology and larval persistence within paratenic hosts would suggest that larval toxocariasis is possibly the most common helminth parasite living in people on the planet. Fortunately, in most people, the larvae do not cause clinical signs except when present in massive numbers or when they invade areas such as the retina where a single larva can cause significant disease. The means of controlling human infections is through the reduction of infections in our favourite animal companions, dogs and cats; in order to reduce the presence of eggs in the environment. Alternate approaches would be vaccines to render the infection of pets and people unlikely or the routine drug treatment of people with compounds active against the larvae, but these two strategies seem unlikely to receive marked attention for an infection without more routine serious outcomes in typical human paratenic hosts who often suffer from no significant demonstrable outcomes of the infection.

References

Alicata, J.E., 1935. Early Developmental Stages of Nematodes Occurring in Swine. United States Department of Agriculture, p. 91, Technical Bulletin 489.

Alvarez, F., Iglesias, R., Bos, J., Tojo, J., Sanmartin, M.L., 1990. New findings on the helminth fauna of the common European genet (*Genetta genetta* L.): first record of *Toxocara genettae* Warren, 1972 (Ascarididae) in Europe. Ann. Parasitol. Hum. Comp. 65, 244–248.

Araujo, P., 1971. Considérations sur la deuxième mue des larves d'Ascarides parasites de serpents. Ann. Parasitol. Hum. Comp. 46, 605–612.

Araujo, P., 1972a. Observações pertinents às primeras ecdises de larvas de *Ascaris lumbricoides*, *A. suum* e *Toxocara canis*. Rev. Inst. Med. trop. S. Paulo 14, 83–90.

Araujo, P., 1972b. Observations sur le cycle biologique de l'Ascaride Polydelphis quandrangularis (Schneider 1866) parasite du serpent crotale. Ann. Parasitol. Hum. Comp. 47, 91–120.

Baer, J.G., 1951. Ecology of Animal Parasites. University of Illinois Press, Urbana, IL, USA, p. 12.

Bardón, R., Cuéller, C., Guillén, J.L., 1994. Larval distribution of *Toxocara canis* in BALBc/mice at nine weeks and one year post-inoculation. J. Helminthol. 68, 359–360.

Beaver, P.C., 1962. Toxocarosis (visceral larva migrans) in relation to tropical eosinophilia. Bull. Soc. Pathol. Exot. 55, 555–576.

Beaver, P.C., Snyder, C.H., Carrera, G.M., Dent, J.H., Lafferty, J.W., 1952. Chronic eosinophilia due to visceral larva migrans. Report of three cases. Pediatrics 9, 7–19.

Bowman, D.D., 1987. Diagnostic morphology of four larval ascaridoid nematodes that may cause visceral larva migrans: *Toxascaris leonina*, *Baylisascaris procyonis*, *Lagochilascaris sprenti*, and *Hexametra leidyi*. J. Parasitol. 73, 1198–1213.

Bruňaska, M., Dubinský, P., Reiterová, K., 1995. *Toxocara canis*—ultrastructural aspects of larval moulting in the maturing eggs. Int. J. Parasitol. 25 (6), 683–690.

Canavan, W.P.N., 1931. Nematode parasites of vertebrates in the Philadelphia Zoological Garden and vicinity. II. Parasitology 23, 196–229.

Casanova, J.C., Feliu, C., Miquel, J., Torres, J., Spakulova, M., 2000. Faunistic and ecological trends on the helminthic community of *Genetta genetta* Linnaeus, 1758 (Carnivora: Viverridae) in the Iberian Peninsula. Helminthologia 37, 223–228.

Chitwood, B.J., 1935. Nematodes parasitic in, and associated with, Crustacea, and descriptions of some new species and a new variety. Proc. Helminthol. Soc. Wash. 2, 93–96.

Choi, D., Lim, J.H., Choi, D.C., Lee, K.S., Paik, S.W., Kim, S.H., Choi, Y.H., Huh, S., 2012. Transmission of Toxocara canis via ingestion of raw cow liver: a cross-sectional study in healthy adults. Korean J. Parasitol. 50, 23–27.

Cianferoni, A., Schneider, L., Schantz, P.M., Brown, D., Fox, L.M., 2006. Visceral larva migrans associated with earthworm ingestion: clinical evolution in an adolescent patient. Pediatrics 117, 336–339.

Coati, N., Schnieder, T., Epe, C., 2004. Vertical transmission of *Toxocara cati Schrank* 1788 (Anisakidae) in the cat. Parasitol. Res. 92, 142–146.

Dubey, J.P., 1968. Migration of *Toxocara cati* larvae in mice. Tropic. Geogr. Med. 20, 172–176.

Dubinin, V.B., 1948. Ascaridata of Animals and Man and the Diseases Caused by them. Part 1. Izdatel'stvo Akademii Nauk SSSR, Moskva. English translation appeared 1968, US Dept Commerce, cited in Mozgovoi, A.A. (1953).

Durette-Desset, M.-C., Chabaud, A.G., 1974. Trois nouveaux Nématodes parasites du Chevrotain aquatique: *Hyemoschus aquaticus* au Gabon (collection G. Dubost). Bull. Mus. Natl. Hist. Nat. 135, 75–87.

Fahrion, A.S., Staebler, S., Deplazes, P., 2008. Patent *Toxocara canis* infections in previously exposed and in helminth-free dogs after infection with low numbers of embryonated eggs. Vet. Parasitol. 152, 108–115.

Foor, W.E., 1967. Ultrastructural aspects of oocyte development and shell formation in *Ascaris lumbricoides*. J. Parasitol. 53, 1245–1261.

Fülleborn, F., 1921. Askarisinfektion durch Verzehren eingekapselter Larven und über gelungene intrauterine Askarisinfektion. Arch. f. Schiffs u. Tropenhyg. 25, 367–375, (In German).

Galvin, T.J., 1964. Experimental *Toxocara canis* infections in chickens and pigeons. J. Parasitol. 50, 124–127.

Gibbons, L.M., Jacobs, D.E., Sani, R.A., 2001. Toxocara malaysiensis n. sp. (Nematoda: Ascaridoidea) from the domestic cat (*Felis catus* Linnaeus, 1758). J. Parasitol. 87, 660–665.
Glickman, L.T., Summers, B.A., 1983. Experimental Toxocara canis infection in cynomolgus macaques (*Macaca fascicularis*). Am. J. Vet. Res. 44, 2347–2354.
Goodey, T., Cameron, T.W.M., 1923. Observations on the morphology and life history of *Ascaris columnaris* Leidy, a nematode parasite of the skunk. J. Helminthol. 1, 1–8.
Henson, R.N., 1975. Experimental infection of the African night crawler *Eudrilus eugenieae* (Kinberg) with the common dog ascarid *Toxocara canis* (Werner). Tex. J. Sci. 26, 598–599.
Herschel, A.-M., 1981. Zum Verhalten der Larven von Toxocara canis Werner 1782 (Anisakidae) aus paratenischen Wirten im Hund (Beagle). Inaugural-Dissertation Doctor Medicine Veterinariae, Tierärztlichen Hochschule Hannover, Deutschland, p. 65.
Hiramatsu, Y., Yoshimura, M., Saigo, R., Arata, H., Okamoto, Y., Matsuura, E., Maruyama, H., Takashima, H., 2017. *Toxocara canis* myelitis involving the lumbosacral region: a case report. J. Spinal Cord Med. 40, 241–245.
Hoffmeister, B., Glaeser, S., Flick, H., Pornschlegel, S., Suttorp, N., Bergmann, F., 2007. Cerebral toxocariasis after consumption of raw duck liver. Am. J. Trop. Med. Hyg. 76, 600–602.
Huizinga, H.W., 1969. The life cycle of *Contracaecum multipapillatum* (von Drasche, 1882) Lucker, 1941 (Nematoda Heterocheilidae). J. Parasitol. 53, 368–375.
Ishii, T., 1959. Studies on larva migrans (2) Comparative studies on migratory behaviour and larval morphology of *Toxocara canis* and *Ascaris suilla*, concerning with their re-infectivity. Jpn. J. Parasitol. 8, 558–566, Japanese, English summary.
Jiménez, J.E., Briceñoc, C., Alcaíno, H., Vásqueze, P., Funk, S., González-Acuña, D., 2012. Coprologic survey of endoparasites form Darwin's fox (*Pseudalopex fulvipes*) in Chiloé, Chile. Arch. Med. Vet. 44, 93–97.
Johnston, T.H., 1916. A census of the endoparasites recorded as occurring in Queensland, arranged under their hosts. Proc. R. Soc. Queensland 28, 31–79.
Kondo, K., Kurimoto, H., Shimada, Y., Oda, K., 1975. Experimental studies on genus *Toxocara* and it related nematodes. 2. The migration and parasitic behavior of *Toxocara tanuki* larvae in mice. Jpn. J. Parasitol. 24 (Suppl. 2), 45, (Abstract from Annual Meeting) [In Japanese].
Le, T.H., Anh, N.T., Nguyen, K.T., Nguyen, T.T., Thuy do, T.T., Gasser, R.B., 2016. *Toxocara malaysiensis* infection in domestic cats in Vietnam—an emerging zoonotic issue? Infect. Genet. Evol. 37, 94–98.
Li, M.-W., Zhu, X.-Q., Gasser, R.B., Liu, R.-Q., Sani, R.A., Lun, Z-R., Jacobs, D.E., 2006. The occurrence of *Toxocara malaysiensis* in cats in China, confirmed by sequence-based analyses of ribosomal DNA. Parasitol. Res. 99, 554–557.
Macchioni, G., 1999. A new species, *Toxocara lyncis*, in the caracal (*Lynx caracal*). Parassitologia 41, 529–532.
Markowski, S., 1937. Ueber die Entwicklungsgeschichte und Biologie des Nematoden *Contracaecum aduncum* (Rudolphi 1802). Bull. Internat. Acad. Polon. Sc. et Lett., Cracovie, Cl. Sc. Math. et Nat., ser. B: Sc. Nat. (II) 2 (5–7), 227–247.
Maung, M., 1975. An ascaridoid nematode from a hippopotamus. Int. J. Parasitol. 5, 431–439.
Maung, M., 1978. The occurrence of the second moult of *Ascaris lumbricoides* and *Ascaris suum*. Int. J. Parasitol. 8, 371–378.
Mia, S., Dewan, M.L., Uddin, M., Chowdury, U.A., 1975. The route of infection of buffalo calves by *Toxocara* (*Neoascaris*) *vitulorum*. Trop. Anim. Health Prod. 7, 153–156.
Moorhouse, D.E., 1982. Toxocariasis a possible cause of the Palm Island mystery disease. Med. J. Aust. 1, 172–173.
Mozgovoi, A.A., 1953. Ascaridata of animals and man and the diseases caused by them. Part 1. In: Skrjbin, K.I. (Ed.), Vol. 2 Essentials of Nematodology. Translated from Russian, Israel Program for Scientific Translations Ltd, Jerusalem, Israel, pp. 111–116, 1968.

Naidu, T.S.V., 1981. Two new ascarid nematodes from vertebrate hosts from India. Folia Parasitol. 28, 327–334.
Neumann, M.G., 1883. Sur l'Ascaride des bêtes bovines. Rev. Vet. (Toulouse) Aout, 1–20.
Nichols, R.L., 1956a. The etiology of Visceral larva migrans. I. Diagnostic morphology of infective second-stage *Toxocara* larvae. J. Parasitol. 42, 349–362.
Nichols, R.L., 1956b. The etiology of visceral Larva migrans: II. Comparative larval morphology of *Ascaris lumbricoides*, *Necator americanus*, *Strongyloides stercoralis* and *Ancylostoma caninum*. J. Parasitol. 42, 363–399.
Okamoto, T., 1986. Experimental studies of visceral larva migrans with *Toxocara tanuki* Yamaguti, 1941. Jpn. J. Parasitol. 35, 355–364.
Okoshi, S., Usui, M., 1968. Experimental studies on *Toxascaris leonina* VI. Experimental infection of mice, chickens and earthworms with *Toxascaris leonina*, *Toxocara canis* and *Toxocara cati*. Jpn. J. Vet. Sci. 30, 151–166.
Olsen, O.W., Lyons, E.T., 1962. Life cycle of the hookworm, *Uncinaria lucasi* Stiles, of northern fur seals, *Callorhinus ursinus*, on the Pribilof Islands in the Bering Sea. J. Parasitol. 48, 42–43, 2, Sect. 2, Abstract 90 at 37th Annual Meeting ASP.
Ortlepp, M.A., 1922. On the hatching and migration in a mammalian host of larvae of ascarids normally parasitic in cold-blooded vertebrates. J. Trop. Med. Hyg. 15, 1–6.
Pahari, T.K., Sasmal, N.K., 1990a. Experimental infection of mice with Toxocara canis larvae obtained brom Japanese quails. Int. J. Parasitol. 20, 263–264.
Pahari, T.K., Sasmal, N.K., 1990b. Infection of Japanese quail with *Toxocara canis* larvae and establishment of patent infections in pups. Vet. Parasitol. 35, 357–363.
Prociv, P., 1983. Observations on the transmission and development of *Toxocara pteropodis* (Nematoda: Ascaridoidea) in Australia Grey-Headed Flying Fox *Pteropus poliocephalus* (Pteropodidae: Megachiroptera). Z. Parasitenkd. 69, 773–781.
Prociv, P., 1985a. Observations on the prevalence and possible infection source of *Toxocara pteropodis* (Nematoda: Ascaridoidea) in Queensland flying foxes. Aust. Mammal. 8, 319–323.
Prociv, P., 1985b. Observations on *Toxocara pteropodis* infections in mice. J. Helminthol. 59, 267–275.
Prociv, P., 1986. *Toxocara pteropodis*, *T. canis,* and *T. cati* infections in guinea pigs. Trop. Biomed. 3, 97–106.
Prociv, P., Brindley, P.J., 1986a. Oral, parenteral and paratenic infections of mice with *Toxocara pteropodis*. Int. J. Parasitol. 16, 471–474.
Prociv, P., Brindley, P.J., 1986b. Susceptibility of rats to infection with *Toxocara pteropodis*. Z. Parasitenkd. 72, 487–491.
Prociv, P., Mak, J.W., 1987. Experimental *Toxocara pteropodis* infections in the long-tailed macaque, Macaca fascicularis. Trop. Biomed. 4, 37–45.
Prociv, P., Moorhouse, D.E., Mak, J.W., 1986. Toxocariasis—an unlikely cause of Palm Island mystery disease. Med. J. Aust. 145, 14–15.
Ransom, B.H., Foster, W.D., 1920. Observations on the Life History of *Ascaris lumbricoides*. United States Department of Agriculture, Bulletin No. 817. 48 pp.
Redman, W.K., Bryant, J.E., Ahmad, G., 2016. Gastrointestinal helminths of coyotes (*Canis latrans*) from southeast Nebraska and Shenandoah area of Iowa. Vet. World 9, 970–975.
Roberts, F.H.S., 1934. The Large Roundworm of Pigs, Ascaris lumbricoides L., 1758. Its Life History in Queensland, Economic Importance, and Control. Bull. (1), Animal Health Station, Yeerongpilly, Australia, 81 pp.
Roberts, J.A., 1990. The life cycle of *Toxocara vitulorum* in Asian buffalo (*Bubalus bubalis*). Int. J. Parasitol. 20, 833–840.
Roberts, J.A., 1993. *Toxocara vitulorum* in ruminants. Helminthol. Abstr. 62, 151–174.

Santo, J.L.C., Magalhães, N.B., Andrade dos Santos, H., Andrade dos Santos, H., Ribeiro, R.R., Guimarães, M.P., 2012. Parasites of domestic and wild canids in the region of Serra do Cipó National Park, Brazil. Rev. Bras. Parasitol. Vet. 21, 270–277.

Sasmal, N.K., Acharya, S., Laha, R., 2008. Larval migration of *Toxocara canis* in piglets and transfer of larvae from infected porcine tissue to mice. J. Helminthol. 82, 245–249.

Schacher, J.F., 1957. A contribution to the life history and larval morphology of *Toxocara canis*. J. Parasitol. 43, 599–612.

Schnieder, T., Laabs, E.-M., Welz, C., 2011. Larval development of *Toxocara canis* in dogs. Vet. Parasitol. 175, 193–206.

Skryabin, K.I., Schulz, R.S., 1937. Helminthiases of Horned Cattle and Young Bovines, Moscow State Publishing House for Agriculture. (Russian), pp. 610–620.

Smith, M.H., Beaver, P.C., 1953. Persistence and distribution of *Toxocara* larvae in the tissues of children and mice. Pediatrics 12, 491–497.

Smith, J.L., Bowman, D.D., Little, M.D., 1983. Life cycle and development of *Lagochilascaris sprenti* (Nematoda Ascarididae) from opossums (Marsupialia: Didelphidae) in Louisiana. J. Parasitol. 69, 736–745.

Sprent, J.F.A., 1952. On the migratory behavior of the larvae of various Ascaris species in white mice. I. Distribution of larvae in tissues. J. Infect. Dis. 90, 165–176.

Sprent, J.F.A., 1953. On the migratory behavior of the larvae of various *Ascaris* species in white mice. II Longevity. J. Infect. Dis. 92, 114–117.

Sprent, J.F.A., 1956. The life history and development of *Toxocara cati* (Schrank, 1788) in the domestic cat. Parasitology 46, 54–78.

Sprent, J.F.A., 1958. Observations on the development of *Toxocara canis* (Werner, 1782) in the dog. Parasitology 48, 184–209.

Sprent, J.F.A., 1959. The life history and development of Toxascaris leonina (von Linstow 1902) in the dog and cat. Parasitology 49, 330–371.

Sprent, J.F.A., 1972. *Toxocara vajrasthirae* sp. nov. from the hog-badger (*Arctonyx collaris*) of Thailand. Parasitology 65, 491–498.

Sprent, J.F.A., Barrett, M.G., 1964. Large roundworms of dogs and cats: differentiation of *Toxocara canis* and *Toxascaris leonina*. Aust. Vet. J. 40, 166–171.

Stiles, C.W., Hassall, A., 1905. The Determination of Generic Types and a List of Roundworm Genera With Their Original and Type Species. 79USDA Bureau of Animal Industry, Addenda, page 150.

Swerczek, T.W., Nielsen, S.W., Helmboldt, C.F., 1971. Transmammary passage of *Toxocara cati* in the cat. Am. J. Vet. Res. 32, 89–92.

Thomas, L.J., 1937. On the life cycle of *Contracaecum spiculigerum* (Rud.). J. Parasitol. 23, 429–431.

Thust, R., 1966. Elektronenmikroskopische Untersuchungen über den Bau des larvalen Integumentes und zur Häutungsmorphologie von *Ascaris lumbricoides*. Zool. Anz. 177, 411–417.

Tiner, J.D., 1949. Preliminary observations on the life history of Ascaris columnaris. J. Parasitol. 35 (Suppl), 21–22, Abstract from Annual Meeting.

Tiner, J.D., 1952. The migration, distribution in the brain, and growth of ascarid larvae in rodents. J Infect Dis 92, 105–113.

Vizcaychipi, K.A., Rinas, M., Irazu, L., Miyagi, A., Argüelles, C.F., DeMatteo, K.E., 2016. Neotropical zoonotic parasites in bush dogs (*Speothos venaticus*) from upper Paraná Atlantic forests in Misiones, Argentina. Vector Borne Zoonotic Dis. 16, 664–672.

Warren, E.G., 1969. Infections of *Toxocara canis* in dogs fed infected mouse tissues. Parasitology 59, 837–841.

Warren, E.G., 1970a. Observations on the life-cycle of *Toxocara mackerrasae*. Parasitology 60, 239–263.

Warren, E.G., 1970b. Studies on the morphology and taxonomy of the genera *Toxocara* Stiles, 1905 and *Neoascaris* Travassos, 1927. Zool. Anz. 185, 393–442.

Warren, E.G., 1971. Observations on the migration and development of *Toxocara vitulorum* in natural and experimental hosts. Int. J. Parasitol. 1, 85–99.

Warren, E.G., 1972. Two new species of *Toxocara* from viverrid hosts. Parasitology 65, 179–187.

Werner, P.C.F., 1782. Vermium Intestinalium Brevis Expositionis Continuation. S.L. Crusius, Leipzig, p. 28, 2 plates. [In Latin].

Won, K.Y., Kruszon-Moran, D., Schantz, P.M., Jones, J.L., 2008. National seroprevalence and risk factors for zoonotic *Toxocara* spp. infection. Am. J. Trop. Med. Hyg. 79, 552–557.

Wright, W.H., 1935. Observations on the life history of Toxascaris leonina (Nematoda: Ascaridae). Proc. Helminthol. Soc. Wash. 2, 56.

Yoshikawa, M., Nishiofuku, M., Moriya, K., Ouji, Y., Ishizaka, S., Kasahara, K., Mikasa, K., Hirai, T., Mizuno, Y., Ogawa, S., Nakamura, T., Maruyama, H., Akao, N., 2008. A familial case of visceral toxocariasis due to consumption of raw bovine liver. Parasitol. Int. 57, 525–529.

CHAPTER THREE

The anatomy of the third-stage larva of *Toxocara canis* and *Toxocara cati*

Dwight D. Bowman*
Department of Microbiology and Immunology, College of Veterinary Medicine, Cornell University, Ithaca, NY, United States
*Corresponding author: e-mail address: ddb3@cornell.edu

Contents

Abstract

This review describes the morphology and ultrastructure of the third-stage larva of *Toxocara canis*, the larval stage that hatches from the egg and persists in the tissues of various paratenic hosts including infected humans. This larva remains unchanged as it passes from host to host and lives for extended periods in this same body form until it makes its way to the gastro-intestinal tract of its final host. There has been less work on the anatomy and ultrastructure of the larva of *Toxocara cati*, but overall, it appears very similar to that of *T. canis* with the only apparent difference being that the larva is a few microns thinner in diameter. The paper describes the anatomy and ultrastructure of the larva and the various major structures of the various body systems

Advances in Parasitology, Volume 109
ISSN 0065-308X
https://doi.org/10.1016/bs.apar.2020.03.002

including the cuticle, hypodermis, the nervous tissue, oesophagus and the lumen-free intestine, and the large excretory gland cell that fills much of the pseudocoel and which appears to be the source of the components that are recognized immunologically by the infected host. It is suggested that further detailed studies on the larva could provide significant information that would allow a greater understanding of how the larva persists within these hosts and may provide information that would make the larva an excellent link to work on nematode anatomy that would link the work being done with this model system to that of *Caenorhabditis elegans* and the large amount of historical work already performed on adult ascaridoid nematodes.

1. Introduction

The third-stage larvae that hatches from the eggs of either *Toxocara canis* or *Toxocara cati* are the larvae that develop to adults when the final host ingests infective eggs or paratenic hosts. They are also the same larvae that persist in all paratenic hosts for extended periods, e.g., for the life of a mouse or for years in primates. Also, they are the same larvae that can be transferred between paratenic hosts via ingestion in tissues or by inoculation, e.g., subcutaneous, peritoneal, or intravitreal. The larvae that are hatched from eggs can live for many months in simple culture media, i.e., RPMI-1640, for up to a year. Under all these conditions, until they reach the internal milieu of a final host, there is no developmental change. Thus, for a year after completing embryonation to the third stage within the protective eggshell, a year or more in the tissues of a mouse, or several years in those of a pig or a primate, the larvae undergo no recognizable morphologic changes and no apparent increase in cell numbers, and as of yet, there is no indication of any of the cells undergoing replacement by cell division. These larvae persist in the tissues of their hosts homeotherm hosts, and in these hosts can be surrounded by granulomas that often contain eosinophils, but often the larvae remain viable and appear capable of leaving what appears to be a complete granuloma to move to another site or are still alive and infective when the tissues with the granulomas are ingested by another host. Although where the larvae persist in the tissues of their paratenic hosts is less elegant than the nurse-cell arrangement of *Trichinella spiralis*, the larvae of *Toxocara* appear to persist longer in tissues than do those of *T. spiralis* and are less likely to be subjected to calcification by the host than are those of the larvae of *Trichinella* species (Despommier, 1993). Therefore, all the disease caused by the larvae of *Toxocara* in paratenic hosts, including humans, is caused by a single larval type, the unchanging, third-stage larva.

2. Overall morphology

The stage coming out of the egg is the third-stage larva. As described in chapter "History of *Toxocara* and the associated larva migrans" by Bowman for Toxocara and other Ascaridoidean nematodes, the many arguments about whether the larva is a second stage or a third stage seems to finally have reached the consensual conclusion that they actually are third-stage larvae. Images of moulting *Toxocara* larvae showing the two cuticles inside the egg were previously reported by Schacher (1957), Araujo (1972), Brunaska et al. (1995), and if one carefully hatches and examines a number of the larvae from eggs that have recently reached the infective stage the two cuticles will be apparent on some of the larvae. As the larvae stay longer within the eggs and move around within the eggshell, the first-stage cuticle often breaks down before the larva hatches.

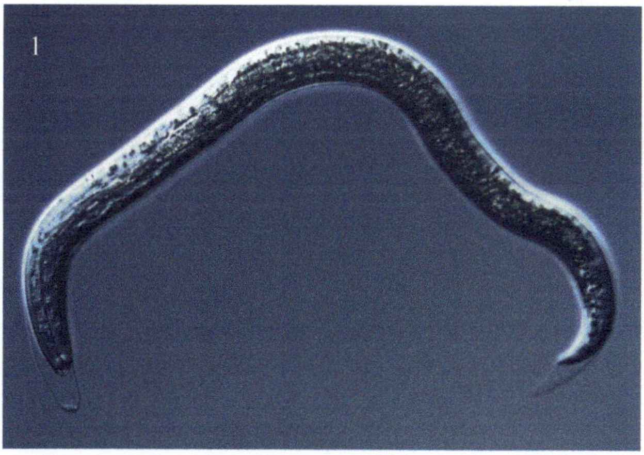

Fig. 1 Physically hatched third-stage larva of *Toxocara canis* showing the sheath that is composed of the second-stage cuticle.

Then, often only a single sheath from the second stage is seen on the hatched larvae as in the artificially hatched larva of *Toxocara canis* shown in Fig. 1; the difficulty in catching larvae bearing the two sheaths is likely what led to the long-misunderstanding as to how many moults occurred within the egg and the numerous descriptions of moulting second- to third-stage larvae in various hosts, they were, often, wishful thinking at best.

Beaver et al. (1952) in the original designation of paediatric visceral larva migrans, illustrated the larva identified as being a larva of *T. canis* or *Toxocara cati* based on a reconstruction of the larva from five serial sections of a larva in liver tissue. Similar eosinophilic granulomatous lesions in children had been previously noted by Perlingiero and György (1947) and Hoeppli et al. (1949) had described lesions in mice with the larvae of *Toxocara canis* in granulomas, but the work of these authors concentrated mainly on the histopathology, not larval morphology. The work by Beaver et al. (1952), clearly showed larva morphology relative to the shape of the head and length and width of the larvae and oesophagus. Ultimately the morphology of *Toxocara canis* and *Toxocara cati* larvae from eggs and paratenic hosts was described by Robert L. Nichols, one of Dr Beaver's students. This work carefully described the larva of *Toxocara canis*, and provided evidence that the larva of *Toxocara cati*, was very similar differing only in maximum body width, and without there being any major morphological or mensurable differences whether the examined larvae were mechanically hatched from infective eggs or recovered from murine tissues, liver, lung, brain, kidney, heart, or skin.

Nichols carefully described the larva and illustrated a heat-killed, third-stage *Toxocara canis* larva pressed from an egg (Fig. 2, fig. 1 Plate I of Nichols, 1956). Overall, the *Toxocara* larvae had a total length of about 410 μm. Nichols described the various organs present in a *Toxocara* larva and how the morphology of histologic sections of *Toxocara* larvae related to the morphology of structures in the whole larva (Fig. 2(1)–(11)). The publication also included an additional three plates of figures showing sections of *T. canis* at almost all levels of the body organized from anterior to posterior, and there are seven sections of *T. cati* from mouse tissues showing similar microanatomy with the difference again being the slightly smaller overall diameter of the larva (Fig. 3).

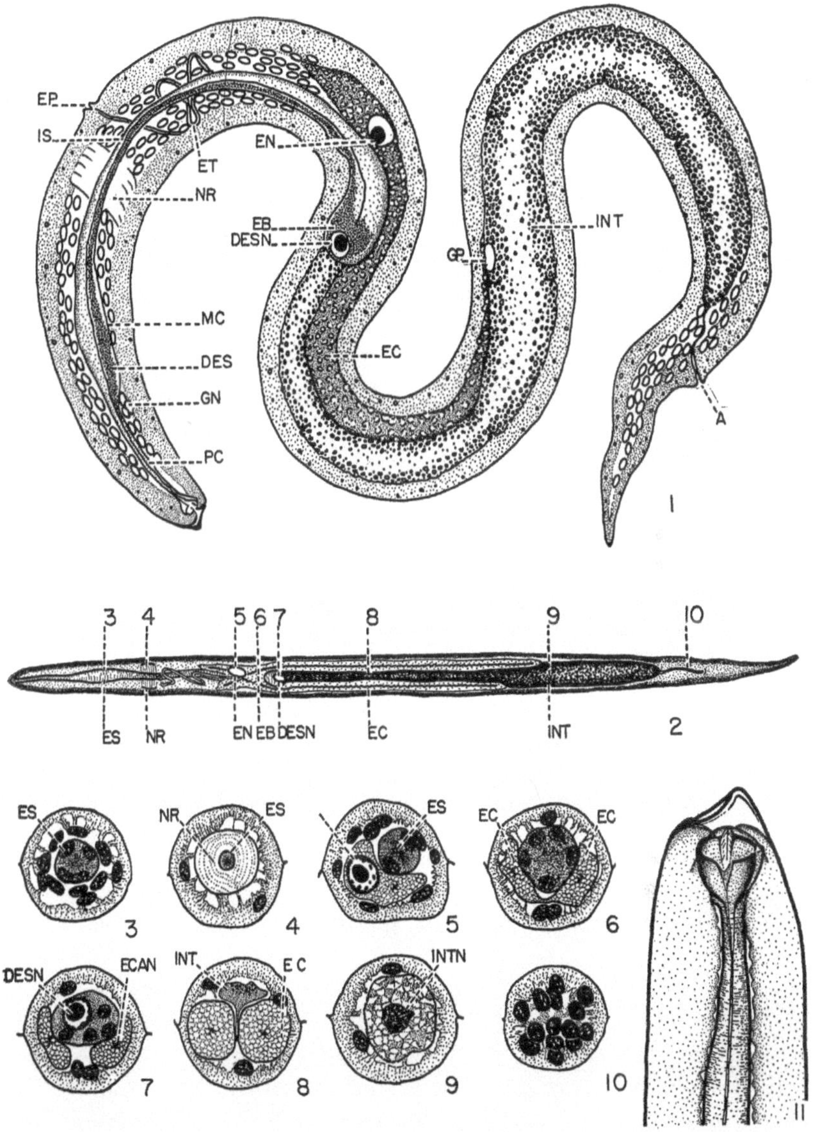

Fig. 2 The legend is as it appeared in the original paper with the exception that the number 2 is added in front of each of the original figure number in the text (All drawings were made with the aid of a camera lucida). (1) Second-stage *Toxocara canis* larva pressed from the egg showing structures evident in lateral view. Heat-killed, unstained (×780). (2) Second-stage *T. canis* larva 4 weeks in mouse brain. Ventral aspect. Heat-killed, unstained (×300). (3)–(10) Transverse sections of a *T. canis* larva 4 weeks in mouse brain at levels indicated in Fig. 2(2) H. and E (×1080). (11) Buccal apparatus and procorpus of a second-stage *T. canis* larva pressed from the egg. Heat-killed, unstained (×1600). Legend for Abbreviations: A, anus; DES, dorsal oesophageal gland; DESN, nucleus of dorsal oesophageal gland; EB, oesophageal bulb; EC, excretory column; ECAN, excretory canaliculus; EN, nucleus of excretory cell; EP, excretory pore; ET, excretory tubule; GN, ganglionic nucleus; GP, genital primordium; INT, intestine; INTN, nucleus of intestinal cell; IS, isthmus; MC, metacorpus; NR, nerve ring; PC, procorpus. *This is Plate 1 from the description by Nichols, R.L., 1956. The etiology of visceral larva migrans. I. Diagnostic morphology of infective second-stage* Toxocara *larvae. J. Parasitol. 42, 349–362.*

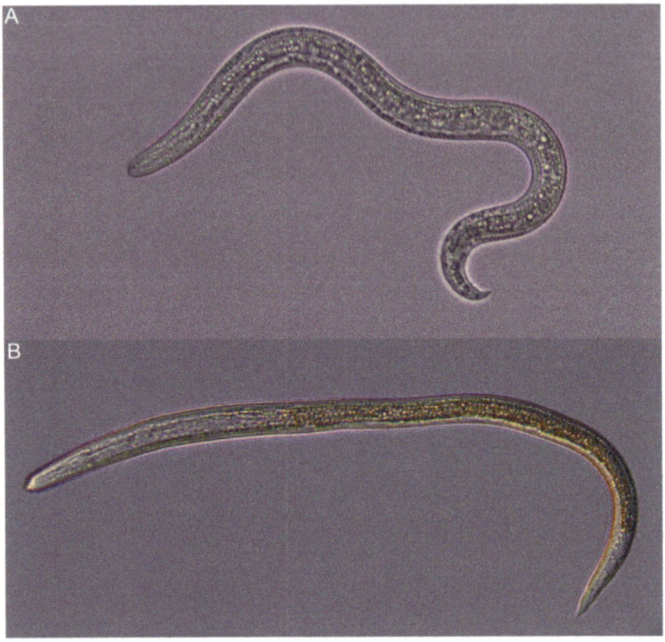

Fig. 3 Living larvae of *Toxocara canis* (A) and *Toxocara cati* (B) taken at the same magnification and fitting the measurements presented by Nichols showing that the *T. canis* larva is slightly broader throughout its length that the larva of *T. cati*.

3. Description of specific tissues

3.1 Hypodermis

The hypodermis is the tissue under the cuticle throughout the length of the worm (Figs 3–8) and is responsible for cuticular regeneration and rearrangement of the cuticle when needed for growth and moulting. The expansions of the hypodermis occur internally at the level of the lateral cords where they support the excretory columns (Fig. 7A and B) and in the ventral and dorsal body portions where they support the associated nerve cords that (Fig. 6B, E, and F). The lateral cords are most pronounced laterally where they occur along the length of the worm under the cuticular lateral alae and appear largest where they support the excretory cell as it travels posteriad along the body (Fig. 2(2) and 2(8)).

3.2 Cuticle

The cuticle is a critical part of the nematodes body plan and life cycle. All nematodes are Ecdysozoans, and all nematodes have a cuticle that is made

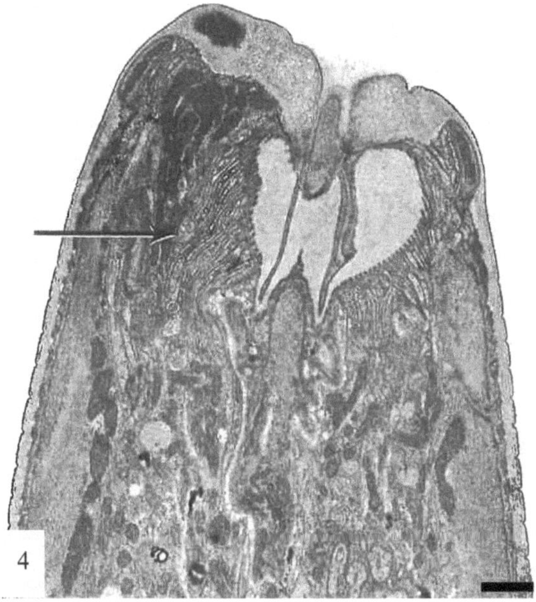

Fig. 4 This is the buccal cavity of a *T. canis* showing that the thickened cuticle in the buccal space. The arrow indicates the lamellar structure that has been suggested to potentially represent a modification of osmoregulation.

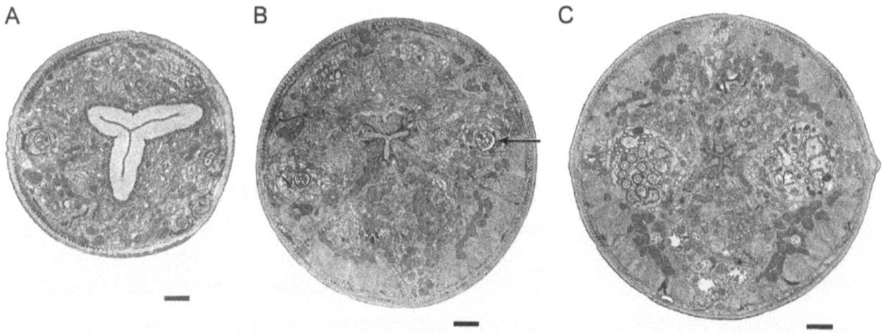

Fig. 5 (A) The most anteriad image showing the thick Y-shaped cuticular lining of the buccal space and vestibule, nerve bundles are evident on the lateral margins. (B) The image is slightly further posteriad and behind the vestibule. Here the cuticular lining of the oesophageal lumen is much thinner. The arrow marks a bundle of sensory neurons that is paired with another bundle that appears slightly lower on the left side of the section. In this image the lamellar network that appears in Figs 4 and 5A are present on the left side of the section and dorsally. At this level there are two muscle cells per quadrant. (C) The columns of nerve tissue on the left and right of the larva are very large and likely represent the neurons the will form the neurons in the papillae and amphids that are present on the anterior end. At this level there are three muscle cells per quadrant. The alae are just becoming salient at this level (Bars = 1 μm; unless otherwise stated, the dorsad of the section is at the top of the image.). *From Bowman, D.D., Oaks, J.A., Grieve, R.B. 1993. Ultrastructure of the infective-stage larva of Toxocara canis (Nematoda: Ascaridoidea). J. Helminthol. Soc. Wash. 60, 183–204.*

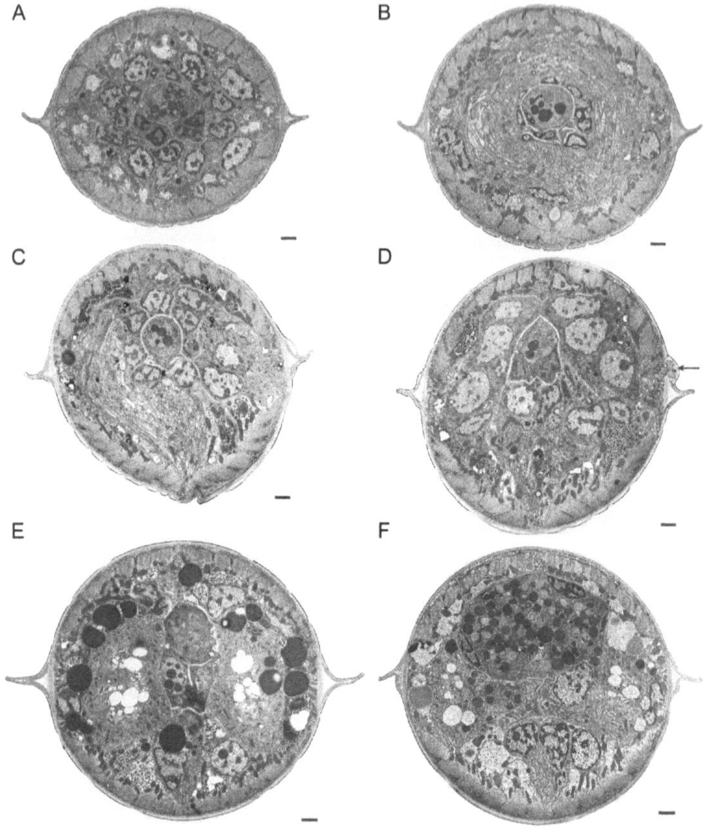

Fig. 6 (A) This section is posterior to the oesophageal metacorpus and anterior to the nerve ring and the forward projecting excretory columns. There are any nuclei here anterior to the bundles of neurons that make up the nerve ring in (B). (B) This is a section through the mass of fibres that make up the nerve ring that contains no nuclei. The alae here are obvious. (C) This is a section just anterior to the opening of the excretory pore that appears at the bottom of the image. There are many nerve fibres entering the ventral nerve cord at this level, but the duct of the excretory gland cell is not in the image. The bum above the ala on the right of the image is the deirid that becomes more obvious in (D). (D) This is a section just posterior to the excretory pore, and sections through the tortuous excretory duct are present. The arrow points to the innervated deirid that appears dorsal to the ala on the right side of the image. There are three muscle cells per quadrant. (E) This image is posterior to the excretory cell nucleus that appears in Fig. 8B. At this level there are two large branches of the excretory on each side of the body and the triradiate lumen of the oesophagus is obvious. (F) This is a transverse section through the larva at the level of the ventriculus at the level of the subventral gland nucleus. The dorsal sector of the oesophagus is enlarged with the contents of the dorsal oesophageal gland. Not that the oesophagus has been displaced dorsally by the excretory cell. The dorsal oesophageal gland nucleus and a subventral oesophageal gland nucleus appears in the longitudinal section shown in Fig. 8A (Bars = 1 μm). *From Bowman D.D., Oaks, J.A., and Grieve, R.B. 1993. Ultrastructure of the infective-stage larva of Toxocara canis (Nematoda: Ascaridoidea). J. Helminthol. Soc. Wash. 60, 183–204.*

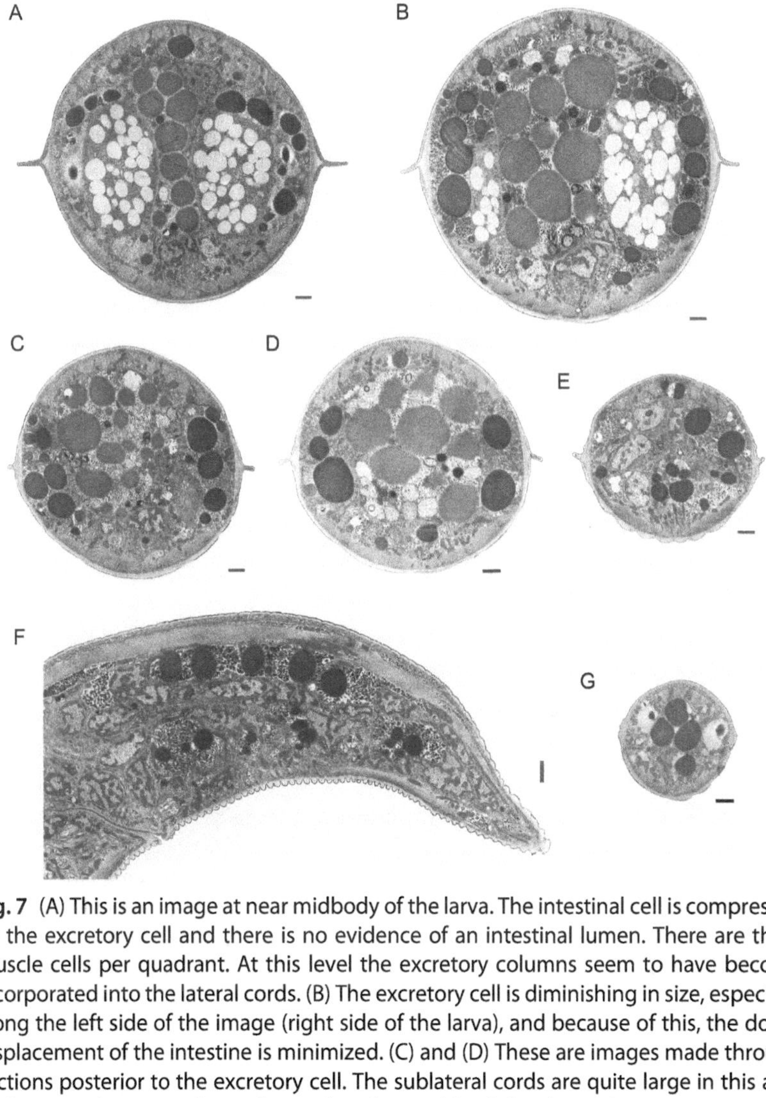

Fig. 7 (A) This is an image at near midbody of the larva. The intestinal cell is compressed by the excretory cell and there is no evidence of an intestinal lumen. There are three muscle cells per quadrant. At this level the excretory columns seem to have become incorporated into the lateral cords. (B) The excretory cell is diminishing in size, especially along the left side of the image (right side of the larva), and because of this, the dorsal displacement of the intestine is minimized. (C) and (D) These are images made through sections posterior to the excretory cell. The sublateral cords are quite large in this area and contain large numbers of mitochondria and lipid droplets. (E) Transverse section posterior to the rectum (shown in F). There is an inward expansion of the lateral cords and nuclei are present in the pseudocoelom. (F) Longitudinal section through the tail showing the relationship of the anus to the tip of the tail and the large number of nuclei around the rectal canal. (G) A section through the body near the tip of the tail. Sections including images of the intestinal tract (Bars = 1 μm). *From Bowman D.D., Oaks, J.A., and Grieve, R.B. 1993. Ultrastructure of the infective-stage larva of Toxocara canis (Nematoda: Ascaridoidea). J. Helminthol. Soc. Wash. 60, 183–204.*

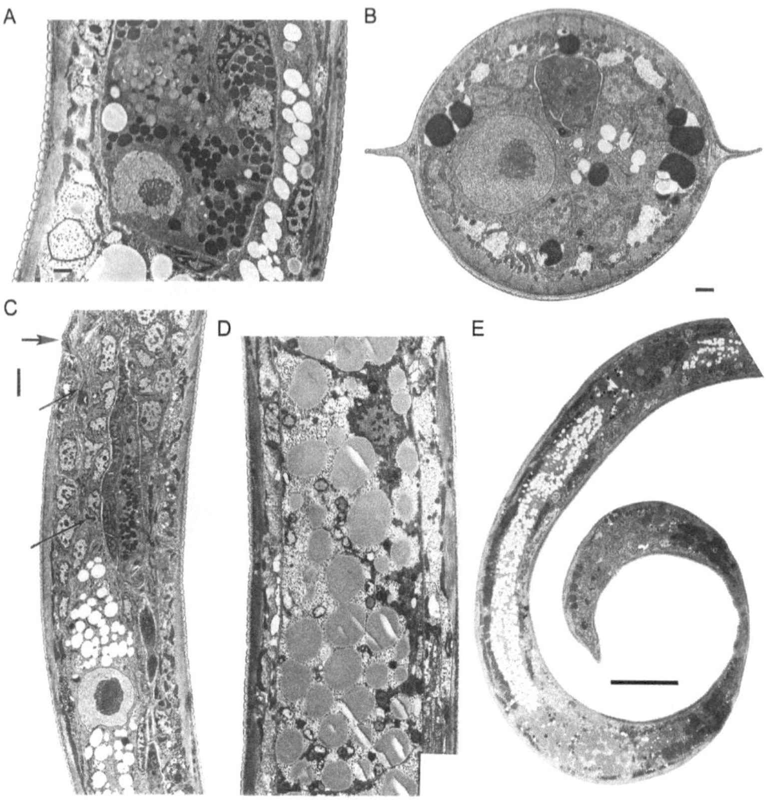

Fig. 8 (A) This is a longitudinal section the ventriculus of the oesophagus with dorsal to the left. The dorsal gland cell nucleus in the third-stage larva is dorsal in location, however, it will migrate to a ventral location as the worm matures (Bar = 1 μm). (B). This is a section of the excretory cell nucleus. It is on the left side of the body, so this would be as though looking from the posterior to the anterior of the work. The oesophagus is distinct and fairly small at this level, and it is clear that at this level the excretory cell commissure occurs on both sides of the body (Bar = 1 μm). (C) Dorsal is to the right. This is a section through the left side of the body of much of a third-stage *T. canis* showing the excretory cell nucleus in the bottom right, the various vesicles contained in the cell anterior and posterior to the nucleus, and the small arrows indicate the tortuous excretory duct, and the larger arrow the excretory pore (Bar = 2 μm). (D) Longitudinal section through an intestinal cell. The large nucleus of this cell can be noted at once end of the cell. Also, in this cell are what appear to be a number of small spheres that suggestive of small nuclei. Dorsal to the left (Bar = 2 μm). (E) This is a longitudinal section through the worm showing the worm from just anterior to the ventriculus to the tip of the tail. The excretory cell is obviously a very large cell compared to the other components of the structures present within the larva. Sections through *Toxocara* larvae in varied orientations as noted individual on the figures. *From Bowman, D.D., Oaks, J.A., Grieve, R.B. 1993. Ultrastructure of the infective-stage larva of Toxocara canis (Nematoda: Ascaridoidea). J. Helminthol. Soc. Wash. 60, 183–204.*

of special forms of collagen. Nematodes on four occasions must replace their cuticles and moult, i.e., undergo ecdysis, where they slough off the old cuticle after the new cuticle is formed. This occurs apparently to allow changes in surface features and body openings. One major difference between the Nematoda and many other Ecdysozoans, e.g., Crustacea, is that nematodes can often grow greatly after they moult (*Toxocara* is a good example because it will grow many centimetres in length after it enters it final external surface as an adult.), but many crustaceans cannot—to grow lobsters have to moult, and after moulting, lay down a new larger cuticle. This may occur several dozen times in their first few years of life.

In the case of the larvae of *T. canis* and *T. cati*, there are no moults in the paratenic host, and thus, one does not need to be concerned with the means by which new cuticle is produced and organized underneath the old cuticle where the changes are taking place. The cuticle does not change structurally on the larva since there are no changes in the external body plan, e.g., no change in body size and no new papillae or sexual openings. The cuticle on the surface of the larvae includes only a few openings, i.e., the three obvious openings are the buccal capsule that leads into the vestibule of the oesophagus, the anus at the end external of the intestinal tract, and the excretory pore that opens the excretory gland to the milieu. There are "openings" for two amphids, one on each side of the buccal opening that will be the amphids on each externo-dorsal surface of two subventral lips of the fourth-stage larvae and adults. Phasmids, which are similar in general structure to amphids, occur near the tips of the tails of fourth-stage and adult *T. canis* and *T. cati* (Schacher, 1957; Sprent, 1956, 1958) Phasmids have also been described on the tails of third-stage larvae of *Toxascaris mystax*, *Baylisascaris procyonis*, *Lagochilascaris sprenti*, and *Hexametra leidyi* (Bowman, 1987).

The buccal capsule (Fig. 4), vestibule, and oesophagus appear in excellent images by Talluri et al. (1986) who describe the muscle cells attached to the oesophageal lining the cuticle at the level of the vestibule that provide for the opening of the vestibule during feeding. Also, the anterior thickened cuticle that is associated with a series of lamellae that are discussed below and serves as the opening to the vestibule of the oesophagus (arrow, Fig. 4, and in Fig. 5A). The lamellar attached to the oesophageal cuticle also fills much of dorsal and lateral fields of the pseudocoel posterior to this site (Fig. 5B). In the slightly more posteriad image at the level of the procorpus (Fig. 5C), the lateral alae are beginning to appear, and they are present here just posterior to the vestibule through the lateral lines of the body from here until after the anus (Figs 6 and 7). The alae are longest at the level of the excretory cell nucleus (Fig. 8B). These laterally projecting "wings" are probably what allow these and other nematode larvae traction to move through tissues since their muscles really only allow undulations to occur dorsal ventrally as the worm moves and it is the probing anterior end of the worm that selects the direction of motion.

3.3 Nervous tissue

The nervous system is difficult to identify in histologic sections of small nematodes that are only a few micrometres in diameter using light microscopy that has a significant resolution of only around 1 μm. Great work was done more than 100 years ago by Goldschmidt in papers published in 1903, 1908, 1909, and 1910 on the nervous system of the adults of *Ascaris suum* and *Parascaris equorum* that led to work by Stretton (1976) and Stretton et al. (1978) and provided a basis for the work leading to that by White et al. (1976) on the nervous system of *Caenorhabditis elegans*. In all the nematodes, it consists of ventral and dorsal nerve cords, with the ventral cord having a greater diameter than the dorsal. Unlike most animal systems, the somatic muscle cells send processes to the bundled nerve cells. Thus, historically, the nervous tissue of the larvae could only be described in a relative general sense relative to locations of visible masses of ganglia.

On the anterior end of the third-stage larva shown by Talluri et al. (1986) the two ventral papillae of what will be the two subventral lips of the mature worms are each towards the front of the protruding ventral cuticle of the buccal cavity that appears as a single structure on the anterior of the worm, and the amphids appear as slits on both lateral sides of the ventral lip material where it joins the dorsal lip that forms the shorter portion of the buccal capsule. It is unclear where or if the lateral papillae that occur on the dorsal lip of the mature worm (Uni and Takada, 1975) occur on the dorsal buccal capsule, i.e., not certain if external or possibly within the buccal space of the third-stage larva. Amphids serve as chemosensory structures, and in the larva, bundles of neurons extend along the lateral cords of the hypodermis in respective subventral sectors from the amphidial opening to the neve ring (Fig. 5A–C). Near the buccal cavity it appears that the nerve bundles have divided and that smaller nerve processes are moving towards the sites of what will ultimately be represented in the fourth-stage larvae and adults as the large pair of papillae near the ventrolateral apex of the dorsal lip, and ventral and dorsolateral area on the subventral lips (Fig. 5A).

As one moves backwards from the anterior end, one can see large numbers of nuclei bunched together around the oesophagus (Fig. 6A) that are anterior to the nerve ring (Fig. 6B) which is composed of nerve fibres. These more or less represent Nichols figures seen in Fig. 2(3) and (4). Just posteriad to the nerve ring is the opening of the excretory pore of the excretory cell (Fig. 6C), followed by even more nuclei that are probably nervous tissue interspersed with the meandering excretory cell canal (Fig. 6D). In this same section, there is a papilla present that is a deirid (Fig. 6D, arrow); Talluri et al. (1986) illustrated the deirid in a scanning electron micrograph image showing it just anterior to the excretory pore and dorsal to the ala as shown in this image. Deirids were also seen by Schacher (1957), who also saw the occasional "post-deirid" in developing *Toxocara*, and Talluri et al. (1986) showed two papillae equivalent to Schacher's post-deirids that they state appeared in pairs on the sides of the worm being located dorsal to the alae at midbody and about one-third posterior to midbody. Fagerholm et al. (1999) described centrids as sensory structures that appeared midbody on fourth-stage *Ascaris suum* larvae and found that the left centrid was situated much more posteriorly on the body that the right centrid. The centrids were also present on the adult *A. suum*, but they were globular appearing in the larva, and appear flattened in the adult.

Slightly further posteriad within the larva, one can see the presence of the two branches of the excretory cell on the two sides of the oesophagus with its expanded subventral oesophageal glands (Fig. 6E) and large numbers of nerve fibres entering the ventral nerve cord. At the level of the ventriculus and the left subventral oesophageal gland nucleus one can see a continued number of nerve fibres and another large bundle of nuclei associated with the neurons in the ventral cord of the larva (Fig. 6F). As one moves further back on the larvae, there were no fortunate sections through additional papillae or phasmids on the third-stage larva (Fig. 7A–G), but it is likely that the phasmid that is present on the adults, as described by Uni and Takada (1975), is present on the tail of the larva near its posterior tip.

3.4 Musculature

This is difficult to appreciate at the level of the light microscope because it is difficult to identify how many muscle cells appear in each quadrant of the body wall. Also, the larvae are too small to allow much differentiation in the stained sections as to layers of cuticle or presence of nervous connections. Nichols did not attempt to determine the number of muscle cells per quadrant. Bowman et al. (1993) reported that the somatic musculature began just posterior to the buccal capsule and extended to near the tip of the tail. The muscle cells are of the meromyarian and platymyarian type. Anteriorly, there are two cells per quadrant (Fig. 5B), and from the nerve ring through the base of the oesophagus, there are three cells per quadrant (Figs 5C and 6). There are usually several bundles of myofibrils per muscle cell (e.g., Fig. 6F). At the beginning of the intestine there are three cells per quadrant (Fig. 7A); in the region of the posterior intestine, there are two cells per quadrant (Fig. 7B–D); and posterior to the anus, there is one cell per quadrant (Fig. 7E–G). The cytoplasmic portions of the muscle cells contain numerous mitochondria and glycogen (e.g., Fig. 6D and E) as well as the muscle cell nucleus (e.g., Fig. 6F).

3.5 Mouth and oesophagus

The oesophagus is about 135 μm long or about one-third the length of the total body (Nichols, 1956). The buccal capsule is cup-shaped and is prolonged anteriorly on the ventral surface of the worm, which thus protrudes further forward than the on the dorsal aspect (Fig. 4). The lumen of the oesophagus is lined with cuticle demarcating the triradiate lumen between the dorsal and two subventral portions. Throughout its length, there are four regions to the oesophagus that make up respectively 15%, 26%, 41%, and 18% of the total oesophageal length; these sections have been identified anteriorly to posteriorly as the slender procorpus, the thicker metacorpus, a slender isthmus, and a terminal bulb that contains the large dorsal oesophageal nucleus that is 4–5 μm in diameter.

The anterior of the buccal cavity was carefully described by Talluri et al. (1986) who examined the lamellar network that occurs in this area of the larva (Fig. 4); these authors make a strong argument that this structure is utilized for the purpose of osmoregulation rather than excretion based on parallels with other osmoregulatory cellular structures seen in crustacea, amphibia, birds, reptiles, and mammals. The ultrastructure of the oesophagus (Bowman et al., 1993; Talluri et al., 1986) shows a thick cuticular lining of the oesophagus lining the triradiate lumen just posterior to the buccal capsule; this cuticle lined triradiate lumen although much thinner persists in the oesophagus throughout its length (Figs 5A and 6A–E), and the images of the intestine posterior to the oesophagus (Fig. 7A–G) support the finding by

Nichols that the intestine has no lumen and is simply a chain of seven contiguous cells without a lumen.

As one moves posteriorly in the sections of the oesophagus, the large dorsal oesophageal gland in the greatest portion of the oesophagus throughout most of its length (Figs 4–6A–F). The ventriculus that becomes more apparent in the developing larva within the final host contains the two subventral glands with their nuclei at the base of oesophagus (Fig. 6F) extend only slightly anteriad into the oesophageal isthmus. The large dorsal gland nucleus that was illustrated by Nichols can be seen on the dorsal side of the ventriculus (Fig. 8A). The relationship of the oesophagus to the excretory cell nucleus is shown in Fig. 8A–C and E.

Talluri et al. (1986) in their examination of the oesophageal gland cells of *T. canis* infective larvae showed that in the larvae the dorsal gland cell emptied into the oesophageal lumen near the anterior and that the two subventral gland cells opened into the oesophagus near the beginning of the ventriculus. Looss (1896) showed nuclear constancy in nematodes relative to radial, marginal, and gland cell nuclei in ascarids. In the case of the adult *Ascaris*, in the oesophagus there are 36 radial nuclei and 12 marginal nuclei, along with, an additional 6 radials and 3 marginals situated near the orifice (Chitwood and Chitwood, 1950). In the infective third-stage larvae, the dorsal gland cell nucleus is dorsal in position and occurs just anterior to the oesophageal-intestinal junction (Fig. 8A). In the ventriculus of the larvae that continue their development in the dog and in the adult *Toxocara*, the dorsal oesophageal gland encircles the oesophageal lumen (Hsü, 1933), and the gland cell nucleus moves to a ventral position within the cell (Sprent, 1956). There are also nerve cell nuclei in the oesophagus. Goldschmidt (1910) found 17 such nuclei, and Hsü (1933) found 18 such nuclei. It is not known whether the number of nuclei in a larval *Toxocara* is the same as the number present in the adult worm.

There has been very little work performed on the material in the oesophageal granules within the oesophagus of *Toxocara* since the work of Drum (1966). In this work, the granules from the oesophagus of adult worms were collected from the homogenized oesophageal tissue of adult worms by washing and ultra-centrifugation. Electron microscopy showed the vesicles to be membrane-bound proteolytic enzymes that were a unique endopeptidase that hydrolyzed peptide bonds or esters containing aromatic amino acid residues. The material from the oesophagus does not seem to be immunogenic or to be secreted by larvae in cultures to any great extent based the fact that the dorsal oesophageal gland tissue does not react with antibodies

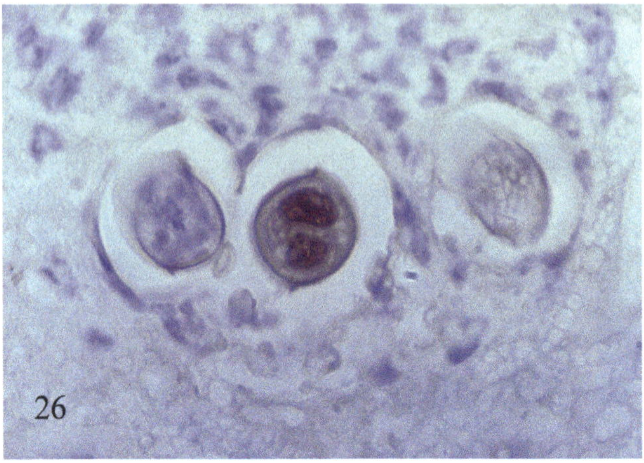

Fig. 9 Section of a larval *T. canis* showing the immunohistochemical staining of antibodies to the excretory-secretory products of cultures of *T. canis* larvae binding to the excretory cell of the larva.

made to excretory secretory materials collected from worms held in culture (Fig. 9, where the section of the worm showing unstained oesophageal tissue appears on the left).

3.6 Intestine

The intestine, as originally described by Nichols (1956), is composed of seven cells and is without an apparent lumen. The lack of a lumen was verified ultrastructurally by Bai et al. (1978), and also no lumen was seen in the study by Bowman et al., 1993 (Figs 7A–G and 8D). In areas where the excretory cell is present, the intestine is compressed by the two columns of this cell and is displaced dorsally (Fig. 7A). The most posteriad intestinal cell ends about 25 μm anterior to the anus, to which it is attached by a thin cuticular tube (Nichols, 1956). Again, if products are leaving larvae via the anus, as with those leaving the oesophagus from the mouth or anus, they are either being excreted or secreted into culture at a minimal level compared to the volume leaving the larva via the excretory pore or are not very antigenic (Fig. 9, with unstained section with intestinal tissue on the right).

3.7 Genital primordium

The genital primordium consists of four cells and occurs on the ventral body wall about two-third of the body length from the anterior end (Nichols, 1956). Sprent (1956) follows the growth of the genital primordium within developing larvae up to fourth-stage larvae. In male worms the primordium divides and grows only posteriorly, while in the female it grows and the posterior portion branches to form the two separate regions of the ovary found in the late fourth-stage larvae and the adult female worms.

3.8 Excretory cell

The largest single structure in a third-stage larval *Toxocara* is the excretory cell which is large in diameter and is of a length that is about 45% of the total body length. The ultrastructure of the excretory cell (or excretory gland cell) of *T. canis* has been described by Kondo et al. (1987) and Vegni-Talluri and Dallai (1989). Overall, the cell is very similar in general morphology and structure to that of the excretory gland cell of *Caenorhabditis elegans*, with the exception that the cell in *C. elegans* is binucleate (Altun and Hall, 2009). Ultrastructurally, the cell in the *Toxocara* larva is characterized by its large size, large nucleus, numerous mitochondria, Golgi bodies, plentiful rough endoplasmic reticula, and its being packed with membrane-bound vesicles throughout.

The excretory cell is about 175 μm long, or about 45% of the larva's total length. It is "H"-shaped with two lateral columns that run to about 35 μm anterior to the base of the oesophagus to about 100 μm posterior to the end of the oesophagus (Figs 2(1) and 8E). Nichols states that the two excretory columns in larvae that have hatched from eggs terminate some 90–100 μm after the end of the oesophagus, but that in larvae recovered from mice as soon as 24 h after infection, the excretory columns are longer, 130–150 μm long, and the excretory canaliculi within the two branches of the cell are more differentiated. Bai et al. (1978) reported that they found no change in size or gross morphology in larvae after 5 or 10 days in mice; however, the authors did state that in the examination of larvae from these mice showed some minimal changes in the excretory cell, the intestine, and in the anterior structure of the buccal capsule. However, the changes presented in their publication are quite difficult to interpret.

The anterior branches of the "H"-shaped excretory cell extend anteriorly to within about 35 μm of the posterior margin of the nerve ring (Figs 2(4), 2(5), and 8E) where it appears laterally on both sides of the oesophagus (Fig. 6E), and from the bridge in the middle of the "H," a tortuous excretory canal travels anteriad (Figs 2(4), 2(5), and 8C small arrows) and opens to the exterior at the excretory pore on the ventral surface of the larva just posterior to the nerve ring (Figs 6C and 8C large arrow).

The nucleus of the excretory cell is on the left side of the worm and is 5–7 μm in diameter, spherical, and has a nucleolus that is around one-third of the nuclear diameter (Fig. 8B and C). As the larvae moult and grow to become adults, the cell is proportionately smaller, but the nucleus will increase in *Toxocara canis* to be greater than 25 μm in diameter. The larvae of other Ascaridoidea potentially causing or potentially causing larval migrans have similar excretory cells with large excretory cell nuclei when recovered from tissues of paratenic hosts: the nuclear diameters are 5 μm in *Toxascaris leonina*, 10 μm in *Lagochilascaris sprenti*, 45 μm in Bay*lisascaris procyonis*, and 120 μm in *Hexametra leidyi* (Bowman, 1987).

3.9 Excretory and secretory products from *Toxocara* larvae

The function of the excretory cell and the contained vesicles has not been fully disclosed, and similarly this is also the case of the free-living *C. elegans* (Altun and Hall, 2009). Again, from the work of Oshima et al. (1963) and De Savigny (1975), it is clear that the larvae produce materials that are recognized immunologically by the host. This excretory gland cell grows and appears to remain active throughout the life of the male and female *Toxocara* and seemingly in all other ascaridoid nematodes. When *T. canis* or *T. cati* larvae are kept at 37 °C in a CO_2 atmosphere, they continue to consistently produce products that serve as diagnostically important antigens for as long as they are in culture (Badley et al., 1987; Lee et al., 2009; Kondo et al., 1987; De Savigny, 1975), and it would seem based on the persistent titres in experimentally infected mice and primates that they also continue to secret these proteins routinely as long as they are alive. In this regard the excretory gland cell appears to be the major source of the soluble material produced by cultured larvae in the diagnosis of toxocariasis as originally proposed by De Savigny (1975). Kondo et al. (1987) showed that the cell was recognized by the FAB fraction of sera from a rabbit infected with 100,000 larvated *T. canis* eggs. Also, monoclonal antibodies that have been generated to the products collected from culture (Bowman et al., 1987) also bind to the material within this cell (Fig. 9).

Other functions of the cell may include a role in the moulting process as suggested by Davey and Sommerville (1974), but since it remains highly active throughout the life of the worm from the time of hatching through the adult stages, this is likely only one of the functions of this cell. Other suggested functions include osmoregulation (Beherenz, 1956), exodigestion (Lee, 1970; Mueller, 1929), acetylcholine inhibition

(Ogilvie and Jones, 1971), protease and substrate secretion to assist in exodigestion related to motility (Bird, 1990; Robertson et al., 1989). Certain monoclonal antibodies that are reactive with the excretory-secretory products are also reactive with the larval surface (Bowman et al., 1987), and component(s) of polyclonal antibody that mediate cellular attachment to larvae in vitro can be removed by preabsorption of the antibody with excretory secretory product (Badley et al., 1987). Whether these antigens are present within the cuticle at deposition or somehow are deposited on the cuticle after creation or by regular secretion from the excretory pore is unknown.

4. Concluding comments

The simple larvae of *T. canis* and *T. cati* are fairly remarkable biological organisms. The requirements for in vitro survival as third-stage larvae requires very little for long-term maintenance, i.e., RPMI 1640 media with salts, amino acids, vitamins, D-glucose, and glutathione. The unchanging larva can live within eggs, RPMI 1640 media, or hosts for years, can enter a paratenic host if eaten while within the eggshell or can be passed from host to host by ingestion of larvae from culture or from or within the tissues of a paratenic host. Also, larvae in paratenic hosts can be passed from one paratenic host to the next as the larvae are ingested and move along the food chain towards the canine or feline final host. The larvae seem to live for years without showing any increase in cell number or loss of cells associated with aging. Although the larva is a third-stage larva, in many ways it behaves in a fashion similar to the second-stage dauer larva of *C. elegans*, i.e., and in the case of *T. canis* and *T. cati*, the dauer state ends when the larvae enters favourable conditions, the intestine of a cat in the case of *T. cati* or a dog in the case of *T. canis*.

One often forgets how much basic information was learned about biology through the general study of nematodes that dealt mainly with the human and swine ascarids, *A. lumbricoides* and *A. suum*, respectively, and the equine ascarid(s) that have been historically been known as *Ascaris megalocep*hala (or *Parascaris equorum* and *Ascaris megalocephala univalens* or *Parascaris univalens*). From the work of the Boveris in their studies of the *A. megalocephala* egg development that followed the cellular division as far as possible within the egg in great detail using the microscopes of the late 1800s and from their work was learned the basis of cell division and the hypothesis that cancer was due to a cell with a certain incorrect chromosome that caused it to undergo continuous growth and cell division (Satzinger, 2008). Work of Van Beneden with *Ascaris megalocephala* provided evidence that two "half" nuclei joined to form the egg and that the chromosome number in somatic cells was constant within each animal and basically provided the world with the evidence for meiosis (Hamoir, 1992). Also, as stated above the work on nervous system of *Ascaris* by Goldschmidt (1903, 1908, 1909, 1910) led to the modern work by Stretton on the neuromuscular system of *Ascaris* (Stretton, 1976; Stretton et al., 1978) and which also culminated in the in-depth examination of the nervous system of *C. elegans* that appeared in a Goldschmidt-like *magnum opus* by White et al. (1976). Other work on *Ascaris* morphology has been performed around the world which includes that of Looss (1896) and Mueller (1929, 1931) on the oesophageal glands of *Ascaris*, and the work of Cram (1925) on the reproduction system of *Ascaris suum*. This is just a short list of the actual work performed on these nematodes and the value of information that it ultimately provided to biology and science in general. It seems that it might be possible to continue the important contributions to the study of biology and parasitology by completing the work that has begun through the further examination of the larva of *Toxocara canis*.

The larva of *T. canis* is fairly ubiquitous on the planet earth, and overall, the eggs are fairly easy to collect from worms harvested from the faeces of treated dogs. Although these worms will not be the same tightly controlled genetic units supplied by *C. elegans*, they should be quite morphologically uniform overall. It seems that it should be possible for *T. canis* as for *C. elegans* to make a complete map of the cells and neurologic connections in the larva from serial microsections and ultrastructural examination. Also, as was shown by the work of the Boveris and others, it should also be possible to map the cellular divisions within the egg of this worm as was done for *Ascaris* and *Parascaris* using modern microscopic and video methods. Finally, it should also be possible to determine when to collect first-stage and second-stage larvae moulting within eggshells such that the entire cellular development and neurologic connections could be pieced together. This would allow an animal parasite to be examined at greater depth and might pave the way for new findings for parasite control and prevention. The *Toxocara canis* genome is now available, and this together with an in-depth description of the cellular morphology of the organism could potentially lead to interesting findings related to a nematode parasite of animals that is also very likely the most common helminth parasite of people on the planet earth.

References

Altun, Z.F., Hall, D.H., 2009. Excretory system. In: Herndon, L.A. (Ed.), WormAtlas. https://doi.org/10.3908/wormatlas.1.17, Last revision: June 4, 2013.

Araujo, P., 1972. Observações pertinenetes ás primeiras ecdises de larvas de Ascaris lumbricoides, A. suum e Toxocara canis. Rev. Inst. Med. Trop. Sao Paulo 14, 83–90.

Badley, J.E., Grieve, R.B., Bowman, D.D., Glickman, L.T., Rockey, J.D., 1987. Analysis of *Toxocara canis* larval excretory-secretory antigens: physiochemical characterization and antibody recognition. J. Parasitol. 73, 593–600.

Bai, S.K., Yun, D.J., Min, D.Y., Lee, K.T., 1978. Ultrastructural changes of Toxocara canis larva in migratory phase. Yonsei J. Med. Sci. 11, 87–100, (in Japanese).

Beaver, P.C., Snyder, C.H., Carrera, G.M., Dent, J.H., Lafferty, J.W., 1952. Chronic eosinophilia due to visceral larva migrans: report of three cases. Pediatrics 9, 7–19.

Beherenz, K.W., 1956. Vergleichende physiologische Untersuchungen iiber die Exkretion parastitischer Nematoden mit Hilfe der Fluoreszenzmikroskopic. Z. Wiss. Zool. 159, 129–164.

Bird, A.F., 1990. Vital staining of glycoprotein secreted by infective third stage larvae of H *Haemonchus contortus* prior to exsheathment. Int. J. Parasitol. 20, 619–624.

Bowman, D.D., 1987. Diagnostic morphology of four larval ascaridoid nematodes that may cause visceral larva migrans. *Toxascaris leonina, Baylisascaris procyonis,* Lagochilascaris sprenti, and Hexametra sprenti. J. Parasitol. 73, 1198–1215.

Bowman, D.D., Mika-Grieve, M., Grieve, R.B., 1987. *Toxocara canis*: monoclonal antibodies to larval excretory-secretory antigens that bind with genus and species specificity to the cuticular surface of infective larvae. Exp. Parasitol. 64, 458–465.

Bowman, D.D., Oaks, J.A., Grieve, R.B., 1993. Ultrastructure of the infective-stage larva of *Toxocara canis* (Nematoda: Ascaridoidea). J. Helminthol. Soc. Wash. 60, 183–204.

Brunaska, M., Dubinsky, P., Reiterova, K., 1995. *Toxocara canis*: ultrastructural aspects of larval moulting in the maturing eggs. Int. J. Parasitol. 25, 683–690.

Chitwood, B.G., Chitwood, M.B., 1950. An Introduction to Nematology. University Park Press, Baltimore, MD, 334 pp.

Cram, E.B., 1925. The egg-producing capacity of *Ascaris lumbricoides*. J. Agric. Res. 30, 977–983.

Davey, K.G., Sommerville, R.G., 1974. Moulting in a parasitic nematode, Phocanema decipiens. VII. The mode of action of the ecdysial hormone. Int. J. Parasitol. 4, 241–259.

De Savigny, D.H., 1975. In vitro maintenance of *Toxocara canis* larvae and a simple method for the production of *Toxocara* ES antigen for use in serodiagnostic tests for visceral larva migrans. J. Parasitol. 61, 781–782.

Despommier, D.D., 1993. *Trichinella spiralis* and the concept of niche. J. Parasitol. 79, 472–482.

Drum, G.E., 1966. The Isolation and Biochemical Properties of the Secretion Granules of the Esophageal Glands of *Toxocara canis* and *Ascaris lumbricoides*. (Ph.D. dissertation) Tulane University, New Orleans, 83 pp.

Fagerholm, H.P., Nansen, P., Roepstorff, A., Bresciani, J., Frandsen, F., Erikaen, L., 1999. Centrids, a pair of asymmetrically arranged sense organs in Ascaris suum (Nematoda, Ascaridoidea). J. Parasitol. 85, 41–47.

Goldschmidt, R.B., 1903. Histologische Untersuchungen an Nematoden. 1. Die Sinnesorgane von Ascaris lumbricoides L. und A. megalocephala Cloqu. vol. 18. Zoologische Jahrbücher. Abteilung für Anatomie und Ontogenie der Tiere, pp. 1–57, plates 1–5.

Goldschmidt, R.B., 1908. Das Nervensystem von *Ascaris lumbricoides* und *megalocephala*. Ein Versuch, in den Aufbau eines einfachen Nervensystems einzudringen. Erster Teil. Z. Wiss. Zool. 90, 73–136.

Goldschmidt, R.B., 1909. Das Nervensystem von *Ascaris lumbricoides* und *megalocephala*. Ein Versuch, in den Aufbau eines einfachen Nervensystems einzudringen. 2. Teil. Z. Wiss. Zool. 92, 306–357.
Goldschmidt, R.B., 1910. Das Nervensystem von *Ascaris lumbricoides* und *megalocephala*. Ein Versuch in den Aufbau eines einfachen Nervensystems einzudringen. III. Teil. In: Festschrift zum sechzigsten Geburtstag Richard Hertwigs. vol. 2. Verlag von Gustav Fischer, Jena, pp. 253–354.
Hamoir, G., 1992. The discovery of meiosis by E. Van Beneden, a breakthrough in the morphological phase of heredity. Int. J. Dev. Biol. 36, 9–15.
Hoeppli, R., Feng, L.C., Li, F., 1949. Histological reactions in the liver of mice due to larvae of different Ascaris species. Peking Nat. Hist. Bull. 18, 119–132.
Hsü, H.F., 1933. Study on the oesophageal glands of parasitic nematoda superfamily Ascaroidea. Chin Med J (Engl) 47, 1247–1288.
Kondo, K., Akao, N., Konishi, Y., Yoshimura, H., Hirose, H., 1987. Immunoelectron microscopic observation of excretory cell of Toxocara canis larva. Jpn. J. Parasitol 36, 187–189.
Lee, D.L., 1970. The fine structure of the excretory system in adult *Nippostrongylus brasiliensis* (Nematoda) and a suggested function for the 'excretory glands'. Tissue Cell 2, 225–231.
Lee, S.-U., Yu, J.-R., Huh, H., 2009. Ultrastructural localization of *Toxocara canis* larval antigen reacted with a seropositive human serum. Korean J. Parasitol. 45, 65–68. https://doi.org/10.3347/kjp.2009.47.1.65.
Looss, A., 1896. Ueber den Bau des Oesophagus bei einigen Ascariden. Zentr. Bakteriol., Parasitenk., Abt. I. 19, 5–13.
Mueller, J.F., 1929. Studies on the microscopical anatomy and physiology of *Ascaris lumbricoides* and *Ascaris megalocephala*. Z. Zellforsch. Mikrosk. Anat. **8**, 362–403, plates 9–13.
Mueller, J.F., 1931. The esophageal glands of *Ascaris*. Z. Zellforsch. Mikrosk. Anat. 12, 436–450, Plates 4–5.
Nichols, R.L., 1956. The etiology of visceral larva migrans. I. Diagnostic morphology of infective second-stage *Toxocara* larvae. J. Parasitol. 42, 349–362.
Ogilvie, B.M., Jones, V.E., 1971. *Nippostrongylus brasiliensis*: a review of immunity and the host/parasite relationship in the rat. Exp. Parasitol. 29, 138–177.
Oshima, T., Nishi, S., Kihata, M., 1963. In vitro cultivation on Toxocara canis larvae with chemically defined media. Jpn. J. Parasitol. 12, 314–315, (in Japanese).
Perlingiero, J.G., György, P., 1947. Report of case with necrosis of liver, pulmonary infiltrations, anemia and ascaris infestation. Am. J. Dis. Child. 73, 34–43.
Robertson, B.D., Bianco, A.T., McKerrow, J.H., Maizels, R.M., 1989. *Toxocara canis*: proteolytic enzymes secreted by the infective larvae in vitro. Exp. Parasitol. 69, 30–36.
Satzinger, H., 2008. Theodor and Marcella Boveri chromosomes and cytoplasm in heredity and development. Nat. Rev. Genet. 9, 231–238.
Schacher, J.F., 1957. A contribution to the life history and larval morphology of *Toxocara canis*. J. Parasitol. 43, 599–612.
Sprent, J.F.A., 1956. The life history and development of Toxocara cati (Schrank, 1788) in the domestic cat. Parasitology 46, 54–78.
Sprent, J.F.A., 1958. Observations on the development of Toxocara canis (Werner, 1782) in the dog. Parasitology 48, 184–209.
Stretton, A.O.W., 1976. Anatomy and development of the somatic musculature of the nematode Ascaris. J. Exp. Biol. 64, 773–788.
Stretton, A.O.W., Fishpool, R.M., Southgate, E., Donmoyer, J.E., Walrond, J.P., Moses, J.E.R., Kass, I.S., 1978. Structure and physiological activity of the motoneurons of the nematode *Ascaris*. Proc. Natl. Acad. Sci. U. S. A. 75, 3493–3497.

Talluri, M.V., Paggi, L., Orecchia, P., Dallai, R., 1986. Fine structure of buccal cavity and esophagus in *Toxocara canis* (Nematoda Ascarididae) infective larvae. J. Ultrastruct. Mol. Struct. Res. 97, 144–157.

Uni, S., Takada, S., 1975. The surface structure of sense organs of *Toxocara cati* (Schrank, 1788) viewed with the scanning electron microscope. Jpn. J. Parasitol. 24, 365–374.

Vegni-Talluri, M., Dallai, R., 1989. Ultrastructure of the excretory-secretory system in Toxocara canis (Nematoda, Ascarididae) infective larvae. Boll. Zool. 56, 285–290.

White, J.G., Southgate, E., Thomson, J.N., Brenner, S., 1976. The structure of the ventral nerve cord of *Caenorhabditis elegans*. Philos. Trans. R. Soc. B 275, 327–348.

CHAPTER FOUR

Visceral larval migrans of *Toxocara canis* and *Toxocara cati* in non-canid and non-felid hosts

Timothy Wu[a], Dwight D. Bowman[b,*]
[a]Department of Biomedical Sciences, Section of Anatomic Pathology, College of Veterinary Medicine, Cornell University, Ithaca, NY, United states
[b]Department of Microbiology and Immunology, College of Veterinary Medicine, Cornell University, Ithaca, NY, United States
*Corrresponding author: e-mail address: ddb3@cornell.edu

Contents

Advances in Parasitology, Volume 109
ISSN 0065-308X
https://doi.org/10.1016/bs.apar.2020.02.001

Abstract

Toxocara canis and *Toxocara cati* are considered the most ubiquitous gastrointestinal helminths in domesticated canids and felids. Ascarid eggs passed in the faeces of canids and felids in a suitable environment may remain infective for years and are capable of infecting not only canids and felids, but a large range of other vertebrate paratenic hosts, including man. Infection with *Toxocara* species also occurs following the ingestion of paratenic hosts containing infective larvae. As infective larvae are incapable of completing their lifecycle in these hosts, they instead travel to different parts of the body, sometimes inducing inflammatory responses, and in some cases remaining entrapped in the body for years. Migration routes depend on the host species; however, nearly all organs may be affected with varying quantities of larval burdens.

1. Introduction

This review characterizes larval survival and persistence in non-canid and non-felid species (with the exception of the domestic cat that has been shown to be susceptible to developing disease from the visceral migration of the larvae of *Toxocara canis*). This review begins with a discussion of the extensive work performed in mice and continues with the presentation on work in other species. It describes the infections in these animals, the changes they induce, and the role they may play in transmission between hosts. While the majority of the information has been generated using *Toxocara canis*, information regarding *Toxocara cati* is discussed where this parasite's involvement has been described.

2. Rodents and lagomorphs

Rodents and lagomorphs have two important roles in toxocariasis, they serve as models of choice for research because the *Toxocara* larvae in the hosts are in a normal host as far as their life cycle is concerned. Also, the murine host is the host animal about which we currently know more than any other on the planet. Some of the other rodents and lagomorphs are used as models because of their larger sizes or because some have been used in the past for specific purposes in laboratory animal science. These other animals, like the mouse, are considered to be potential natural paratenic reservoirs of toxocariasis. Also, since dogs and cats will readily capture and feed on these animals, they also likely play a major role in the epizootiology of the disease in the final hosts in different areas of the world. In spite of these creatures being an important part of the life cycle, the amount of work done on these hosts as reservoirs pales in comparison to the work done on reservoirs hosts, such as those potentially infected with *Borrelia* or other human pathogens such as leishmaniasis or American trypanosomiasis.

Dubinský et al. (1995) examined the small animals, i.e., rodents, Muridae, Arvicolidae, and Gliridae, and shrews (Soridicae). Overall, out of 588 small mammals, 88 (15.1%) were seropositive. Using tissue examination of a subset of 476 of the 588 animals, larvae were recovered from 30 of the examined animals (6.3%), and all these had been had also been found to be seropositive. Hildebransd et al. (2009) in studying rodents from Wroclaw, Poland, found *Toxocara* larvae only in the brains of 4/31 (12.9%) rodents of the species, *Apodemus agrarius*. Krücken et al. (2017) detected *T. canis* in 8 and *T. cati* in 4 in the brains of 257 rodents by PCR, of which 14% were positive by ELISA. Waindok et al. (2019) found no larvae in the brains of 716 rodents that were mainly from the city of Leipzig, Germany. There is unfortunately, very little similar work being performed elsewhere. The serological testing could be applied to a large number of animals fairly economically, and if any dead animals were recovered and larvae discovered, we now have good methods for the molecular identification of the larvae (Marucci et al., 2013). One place small mammal surveillance might have a place would be in control programs to monitor whether the control of parasites in pet dogs and cats is reducing the percentage of reservoir hosts infected.

2.1 Mice

2.1.1 Toxocara canis

Studies conducted on mice have utilized multiple strains, including BALB/c, C57BL/6, C3H/He, DBA/2, NC, and BALB/c nude mice, with a higher rate of larval recovery reported in BALB/c mice (Koizumi and Hayakawa, 1984). Outbred strains seem to be less susceptible than inbred strains, likely due to the ability of outbred strains to more efficiently trap larvae in the liver and thereby prevent systemic circulation (Dunsmore et al., 1983). One of the first papers on the experimental migrations of Ascaridoidean nematodes was that of Hoeppli et al. (1949) that actually occurred before the realization that this was the agent of larval migrans as described by Beaver et al. (1952). Hoeppli et al. (1949) examined the

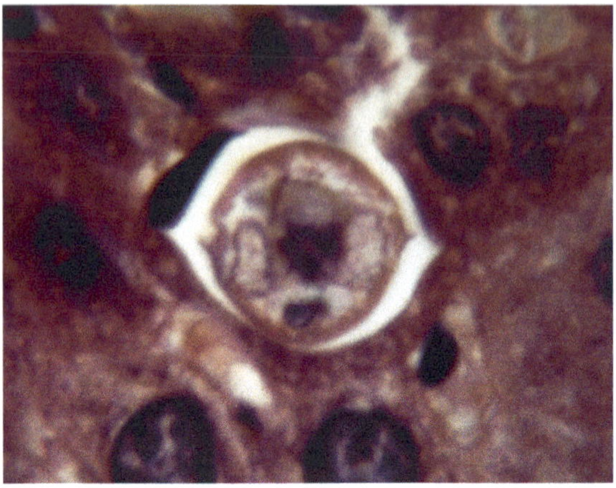

Fig. 1 Mouse liver. Experimentally infected mouse. Third-stage larvae within the hepatic parenchyma is a cross section of a *T. cati* larva, with prominent lateral alae, oesophageal nuclei, and sections through the large excretory cell columns on the lateral sides of the larva (equivalent to the fig. 6 of *T. canis* in section in the publication of Nichols, 1956). H&E stain.

movement of larvae into the liver and the pathology caused by the larvae of *Ascaris lumbricoides*, *Parascaris equorum*, and *Toxocara canis* in mice over the first 10 weeks of infection. They found that after 2 weeks there were almost no larvae of *A. lumbricoides* and *P. equorum* remaining in the liver, but that the larvae of *T. canis* persisted (Fig. 1). They illustrated with excellent photographs the granulomas surrounding the living larvae. These authors stated relative to the work of Fülleborn (1921), who had shown that dogs can be infected by ingesting the larvae encapsulated in organs of other animals, that "A dog therefore which by chance will catch and eat a mouse or rat with encapsulated larvae of *T. canis* in the liver obtained previously by swallowing embryonated eggs from dog's faeces with contaminated food will become infected with *Toxocara canis*".

Toxocara canis has a high degree of infectivity in mice, with 31% of larvae being recovered 60 days after infection in one study (Dissamarn et al., 1968). Larvae hatch in the stomach and reach the small intestine within 2 h, and the colon within 3 h, with a preference for the posterior half of the intestine, especially the ileum. From there, larval migration proceeds between intestinal villi, through the base of the crypts of Lieberkuhn in the intestine, and through the lamina propria and tunica muscularis. Larvae can also penetrate lymphatic vessels, with larvae noted in the mesenteric lymph nodes 2 days post-infection. Additionally, larvae may enter the peritoneal cavity with subsequent invasion of the vascular system, including the hepatic portal vein and central hepatic vein (Abo-Shehada and Herbert, 1984b) (Fig. 1).

Larvae then enter the visceral (hepato-pulmonary) phase, invading the liver within 24 h of infection in one study, and as early as 6 h post-infection in another study (Bisseru, 1969; Chari and Subramanian, 1972). Affected livers may exhibit lymphocytic and neutrophilic inflammation surrounding portal tracts and within the subcapsular region (Bisseru, 1969). Larvae have been noted in the lungs as early as 24 h after infection (Kayes et al., 1987). These larvae are often associated with haemorrhage and aggregates of lymphocytes and neutrophils, with few eosinophils (Bisseru, 1969).

Larvae may be dispersed throughout the musculature and brain by day 7 after infection, and as early as day 2 post-infection, reflecting the end of the visceral phase, and beginning of the myotropic-neurotropic phase (Abo-Shehada and Herbert, 1984a,b; Bisseru, 1969). Interestingly, larvae may prefer the cranial musculature, with a larval burden 3–4 times higher than the number of larvae recovered from the pooled appendicular muscles (Parsons and Grieve, 1990). Muscular lesions may include severe polymyositis, with inflammatory tracks progressing linearly between fibres, and large eosinophilic and granulomatous infiltrates in the connective tissues between fascicles (Kayes and Oaks, 1978).

Larvae are commonly found in the brains of infected mice (Fig. 2). In regard to neural larval migration, Bisseru (1969) postulated that larvae penetrate out of the arteries near the brain surface, where there is subdivision of arteries with a reduction in diameter. A predilection for the cerebellum

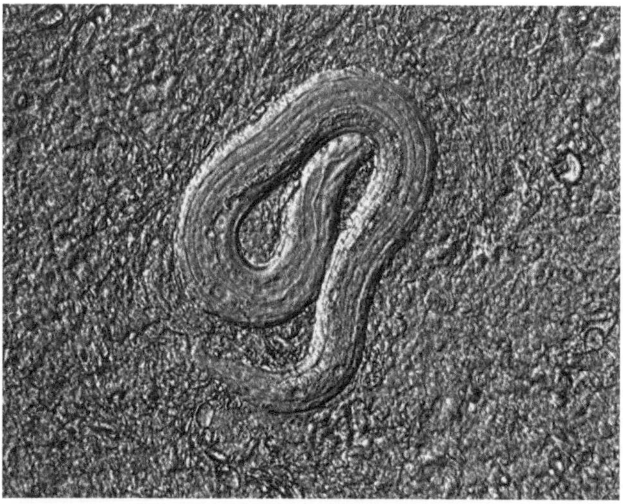

Fig. 2 Mouse brain. *Toxocara canis* larva isolated from mouse brain tissue via squash preparation.

compared to the cerebrum or brainstem has been described (Burren, 1971). Living *Toxocara canis* larvae have been recovered from the brain of experimentally infected mice even 2 years after infection (Sprent, 1953). Previous studies evaluating invasion of the spinal cord in mice recovered motile larvae, accounting for 1.4% of total recovered larvae from the body of the mouse, as early as 1 week post-infection, with persistence in mice spinal cords up to the end of the 4-month study (Olson and Petteway, 1972). Although neurologic signs were not observed in some studies, others have found that infected mice exhibit hyperactivity, as well as elevated shock reaction thresholds, and less avoidance of open fields (Corrêa et al., 2014; Dolinsky et al., 1985; Hay et al., 1986; Sprent, 1953) [*See* chapter "*Toxocara*-induced neural larva migrans (neurotoxocarosis) in rodent model hosts" by Strube et al.]. *Toxocara* larvae are capable of reaching the eye within 3 days of infection, with up to 82% of infected animals exhibiting ocular larval migrans, and a worm burden of up to nine larvae in one eye in one study (Olson, 1976). Both the anterior and posterior chambers can be invaded, though the posterior chamber has been reported to harbour more worms than the anterior (Olson et al., 1970). Aside from these organs, larvae have also been recoverable from the heart, kidneys, spinal cord, salivary glands, spleen, and uterus (Abo-Shehada and Herbert, 1984a,b).

Interestingly, previous studies have shown that repeated infection with *Toxocara canis* larvae results in an acquired immunity in some cases, with granulomatous and eosinophilic inflammation, and fibrosis surrounding increased numbers of entrapped intrahepatic larvae (Nobuaki, 1986). Sensitized mice have less lung pathology compared to control mice, as well as reductions of larval counts in the muscle and brain, presumably due to the delayed migration through the liver (Olson, 1962; Sugane and Oshima, 1983).

Transplacental migration of *T. canis* in paratenic hosts like mice is possible, with larvae found in one-third of mouse pups from infected pregnant mice in one study (Abo-Shehada and Herbert, 1984a,b). Similarly, Lee et al. (1976) found migration to the uterus and placenta by day 9 of pregnancy, and foetal infection by day 11. Transmammary transmission has also been reported, with infection possible even 60 days post-infection (de Souza Aguiar et al., 2015).

2.1.2 *Toxocara cati*

Evaluation of multiple strains of mice have revealed an increased susceptibility of BALB/c mice to *Toxocara cati*, with migration of larvae noted up to 28 days post-infection (Cardillo et al., 2009). Earlier studies of *Toxocara cati* infection in mice revealed findings similar to what has been described in *T. canis* infections, though it has been suggested that *T. cati* eggs hatch faster in the intestine of mice than those of *T. canis* (Cardillo et al., 2009). Indeed, Dubey (1967) found that within 24 h after ingestion of embryonated eggs, hatched larvae had migrated from the intestine to the liver, lungs, and musculature.

Interestingly, there is a tendency of *T. cati* larvae to concentrate in the skeletal muscle, as opposed to *T. canis*, which is typically retained in the brain and liver (Dubey, 1967). Incidence of Intraneural *T. cati* larvae in experimentally infected mice was 8% in one study, and no more than two larvae were found in the brain of a single mouse in another study, representing less than 0.1% of the larvae recovered (Burren, 1971; Dubey, 1967). This is possibly a reflection of the smaller diameter of *Toxocara cati*, which may be narrow enough to pass through the brain capillaries, while *T. canis* is wider and, therefore, penetrates the brain tissue upon encountering sharp bends in the blood vessels at the brain surface (Burren, 1971).

2.2 Rats

2.2.1 *Toxocara canis*

The route of migration in rats infected with *Toxocara canis* is similar to that in mice, with reported larval recovery rates of 42.9% from visceral organs by 3 days post-infection (Lescano et al., 2013). In this study, larvae were found in the musculature and brain by 5 days post-infection, with larval recovery rates of 23.2% and 1.2%, respectively. The peak recovery rate in the brain was at 15 days post-infection, with a recovery rate of 4.5%. At, 60 days after infection, 80.1% of larvae were in the musculature. Previous studies by Burren (1971, 1972) found very few larvae in spinal cords, and no larvae in eyes. Rats infected with *Toxocara canis* may exhibit significant behavioural changes, including increased head dipping and immobility, decreased grooming, and less avoidance of open areas (de Queiroz et al., 2013; Santos et al., 2015).

2.2.2 *Toxocara cati*

Lescano et al. (2013) found that rats infected with *T. cati* exhibited extensive larval migration starting at 3 days post-infection, with reported larval recovery rates of 32.7% and 22.4% in the viscera and musculature, respectively. Neural migration was rare, not exceeding 1.1% of total larval recovery at any timepoint throughout the 60-day study period.

2.3 Gerbils

2.3.1 *Toxocara canis*

Alba-Hurtado et al. (2009) found *T. canis* larvae within the lung and liver of infected gerbils by 12–24 h post-infection, with peak numbers recovered from the lungs between days 3 and 5 post-infection. Larvae were recovered from the musculature at days 10–60 post-infection, and from the brain 20–60 days post-infection. As opposed to mice, most larvae were recovered from the lung instead of the liver.

Gerbils are used as a model for ocular toxocariasis in humans. Alba-Hurtado et al. (2000) found larvae in 90% of gerbil eyes between 0.5- and 60-days post-infection. Furthermore, as opposed to monkeys and guinea pigs, for which ocular changes are usually only present following intravitreal injection of larvae, ocular lesions in gerbils were generated following a single oral inoculation (Takayanagi et al., 1999).

2.3.2 *Toxocara cati*

Akao et al. (2000, 2003) examined both *T. cati* and *T. canis* as they related to ocular larva migrans and cerebellar ataxia in gerbils and rats. Ocular lesions were less common in *T. cati* than in *T. canis* infected gerbils, and *T. canis* was more likely to cause eye lesions to reappear after earlier lesions had cleared. Akao et al. suggested that the larvae in the eye migrate to this site from the brain, which in their studies had greater numbers of *T. canis* than *T. cati* larvae. It was also found that either infection resulted in ataxia in the gerbils and that infection was associated with larvae being present in the cerebellum (Akao et al., 2003).

2.4 Guinea pigs

2.4.1 Toxocara canis *and* Toxocara cati

Prociv (1986) examined the biology of *T. canis* and *T. cati*, along with the bat parasite, *Toxocara pteropodis*, in guinea pigs and found that *T. canis* larvae tended to accumulate in the brains of the guinea pigs, while those of *T. cati* accumulated in the musculature. The *T. pteropodis* larvae did not persist in the guinea pigs for any significant amount of time after infection, all being gone in 7 weeks. A number of other studies, such as those by Sharp and Olson (1962), Ivey (1965), Collins and Ivey (1975), and Wong et al. (1976), were mainly performed to assess the immune response of guinea pigs relative to eosinophilia and hypersensitivity reactions.

2.5 Hamsters

2.5.1 *Toxocara canis*

The larvae of *T. canis* have been shown to undergo a migration pattern in the hamster that is very similar to that which occurs in the mouse. However, hamsters, unlike the other rodents examined, i.e., rats and gerbils, developed granulomata around the larvae that occurred in the cerebellum, but like the other hosts, none in the cerebrum or brainstem (Burren, 1972). Gonçalves dal Silva et al. (2015) have put forth the hamster as an experimental model for toxocariasis, and have presented their significant efforts made in describing the pathology in this host and immunologic advantages of using this host for studying various immunologic, therapeutic, and diagnostics relative to visceral larva migrans.

2.6 Rabbits

2.6.1 Toxocara canis *and* Toxocara cati

Pankavich (1966) and Lautenslager (1972) both examined the migration of *T. canis* and *T. cati* in rabbits with markedly different results; this was probably due to their different methods of larval recovery. Pankavich found that live *T. canis* larvae could be recovered from the lungs, liver, and kidneys of rabbits by 2 days post-infection, and from the brain and musculature by 6 days post-infection, with no larvae being recovered from the spinal cord. The level of *T. canis* larvae within the lungs decreased at 7 days, with no larvae noted in the lungs by the third week post-infection. The liver contained viable larvae throughout the entirety of the 244-day study period. It was also found that of 6 litters totalling 45 kits, there was only one larva each within four kits, three within the liver, and one within the musculature, respectively. Lautenslager examined rabbits for only 40 days after infection and found the majority of *T. canis* larvae encapsulated but viable in the liver, brain, and muscle (Fig. 3).

Pankavich did not examine the musculature and recovered very few *T. cati* larvae from rabbits given infective eggs; the only larvae recovered were a single larva from the lungs 7 days post-infection and three from the liver of another rabbit 28 days post-infection. Lautenslager (1972) examined *T. cati* infected rabbits at 6 and 12 h, daily on days 1–10, and every 5 days thereafter until 40 days post-infection, finding larvae in tissues in high numbers throughout the study. Lautenslager found that the larvae of *T. cati* passed through the liver to the lungs quicker than *T. canis*, and *T. cati* larvae did not remain in either of these organs in any numbers. The migration of *T. canis*

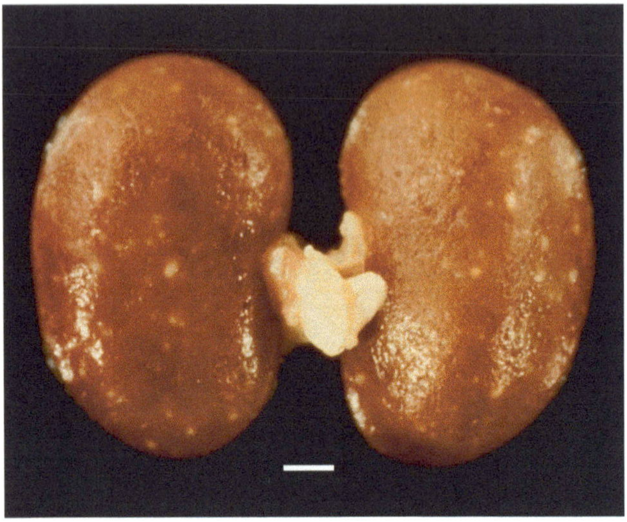

Fig. 3 Rabbit kidney. The cortical surface is covered with dozens of generalized, random, circular, white, raised foci, varying in size from pinpoint to 2 mm in diameter. These nodules are representative of granuloma formation secondary to visceral larva migrans of *T. canis* larvae.

was slightly slower, and many *T. canis* larvae remained in the liver. *T. cati* larvae were found to first enter the musculature by 2 days after infection and the majority of the larvae recovered were in the liver in stable numbers by 15 days after infection. At 40 days after infection, the *T. canis* larval numbers from the musculature were still increasing. Lautenslager also reported that gross lesions occurred in the livers and kidneys of rabbits with larval *T. canis* but not with *T. cati*. Both sets of larvae entered the brain, but *T. canis* remained while *T. cati* seemed to renter the circulation and leave. Both species entered and remained in the eyes of rabbits. *T. canis* larvae, although alive, were often encapsulated within different tissues while those of *T. cati* were not.

3. Artiodactyla

3.1 Pigs

3.1.1 *Toxocara canis*

Sasmal et al. (2008a) found that in piglets fed embryonated eggs, 4.97% of total larvae were recovered from the liver, lungs, heart, kidneys, skeletal muscles, and brain. Larvae were recovered from days 1 to 30 post-infection, with migration to the liver within the first 24h, and other visceral organs within 3 days. Larvae were noted within the muscle by 7 days post-infection, and within the brain by 15 days post-infection. The peak of larval recovery was on day 15 post-infection, with most larvae collected from the liver. Additional studies have revealed a few larvae in the eyes, kidneys, diaphragm, mesenteric lymph nodes, tongue, heart, and small intestinal wall (Taira et al., 2003). By the third day post-infection, pigs infected with *Toxocara canis* develop white spots on the liver that may be up to 3mm in diameter. Ronéus (1963, 1966) thought these spots more conspicuous than those caused by *Ascaris suum* or *Toxocara cati*; Ronéus attributed this to the thicker and more active *T. canis* larva. To verify paratenesis by these larvae, Sasmal et al. (2008a) successfully infected mice by feeding them 5g of liver from the infected piglets.

3.1.2 *Toxocara cati*

Ronéus (1966) found *Toxocara cati* larvae within the liver of pigs by 3 days post-infection. The larvae were associated with white spots on and in the liver parenchyma, histologically appearing as granulation tissue surrounding areas of necrosis and larvae. Larvae were noted within mesenteric lymph nodes by day 3 post-infection, with no associated inflammation. Larvae were noted in the lungs at day 10 post-infection. No larvae were detected in the liver or lungs of pigs by the 63rd day (Ronéus, 1963). Based on morphologic and molecular methods, larvae identified as *Toxocara cati* were recovered from a domestic pig in Italy as part of Trichinella surveillance (Marucci et al., 2013).

3.2 Sheep

3.2.1 *Toxocara canis*

Larval migrans in the sheep is similar to that of other paratenic hosts, with the liver and lungs being the most affected organs (Aldawek et al., 2002). Schaeffler (1960) found that migration appears to be influenced by the age of the sheep, with hardly any migration beyond the liver in yearlings, while very young lambs exhibited migration to mesenteric lymph nodes, pancreas, heart, lungs, kidney, brain, and muscles as early as 4 days post-infection. Larvae remained alive without apparent decrease in numbers for the entirety of the study, lasting 12 weeks in yearlings and 8 weeks in lambs.

3.3 Goats

3.3.1 *Toxocara canis*

The migratory pathway of larvae in goats is much the same as in other mammals. Sinha (1969), in evaluating 24 goats for *Toxocara canis* migration, noted larvae were in the liver as early as 1 day post-infection and remained within the liver throughout the entirety of the 64-day study. Larvae were recovered from the lungs by 3 days post-infection. Migration to the brain occurred at 6 days post-infection, with a few cases where larvae were recovered from the spinal cord beginning at 24 days post-infection. Larvae were not recovered from the heart, spleen, shoulder, or musculature (Sinha, 1969).

3.4 Cattle

3.4.1 *Toxocara canis*

Fitzgerald and Mansfield (1970) reported that young calves fed embryonated eggs had recoverable larvae in the liver, lungs, and mesentery starting 3 days post-infection. Larvae were recovered from the kidneys at 5 days post-infection, and the brain at 11 days post-infection. Attempts to recover larvae from muscle tissue were not made in this study.

4. Non-human primates

4.1 Toxocara canis

Larvae are able to live in large numbers within the tissues of non-human primates for a long time, with reported survival times of up to 9–10 years (Beaver, 1962). A study investigating larval migration in nine macaques inoculated with embryonated eggs found considerable numbers of viable larvae in the viscera and central nervous system in three out of nine macaques. Gross findings consisted of granuloma formation and focal tissue destruction caused by migrating larvae in the liver, lungs, kidneys, pancreas, heart, diaphragm, central nervous system, and eyes. Tomimura et al. (1976) found larvae not only within the cerebrum, but also within the spinal cord. Ocular larval migrans was examined in the eyes of primates using the intra-vitreal inoculation of larvae hatched experimentally from infective eggs (Watzke et al., 1984).

5. AVES

5.1 Chickens

5.1.1 *Toxocara canis*

In a study lasting 142 days, Galvin (1964) found that living larvae could be recovered from chicken tissues throughout the study and that about 30% of the larvae were still present at the study's termination. At termination, almost all larvae were recovered from the liver, although in the first days of the infection, larvae were found in the lungs. Throughout the infections, occasionally a single or very few larvae were found on different days in kidney, brain, viscera (heart, spleen, and pancreas), and muscle. The majority of recovered larvae were alive and active. The only evidence of disease in infected chickens were a few subcapsular and intraparenchymal cysts in the liver beginning 6 days after infection. Okoshi and Usui (1968) also found the majority of larvae of *T. canis* in the livers of chickens 90 days after infection with none at that time in the muscles or other tissues. Tsvetaeva et al. (1979) reported that larvae of *T. canis* survived in chickens up to 45 months with some of the larvae being within parasitic granulomas. Mossalam et al. (1972) found larvae subcapsularly within chicken livers at 10, 20, and 30 days post-infection, with necrosis, eosinophils, and lymphocytes, and the lungs contained larvae surrounded by lymphocytes and eosinophils by day 10 post-infection, with granulation tissue noted at day 20 post-infection. Okoshi and Usui (1968) found that larvae from mice and chickens recovered from chicken tissues were orally infective to mice. Also, they found that larvae recovered from earthworms were infective to mice and chickens, and the larva could be further passed from the infected chicken to mice.

5.1.2 *Toxocara cati*

Okoshi and Usui (1968) and Taira et al. (2011) found that *Toxocara cati* larvae behaved much differently than those of *T. canis* in chickens. In the case of *T. cati*, the larvae rapidly passed through the liver and then lungs with the majority then being found in the musculature where they remained viable. The larvae were predominantly in the liver by day 1 post-infection, the lungs 2–3 days post-infection, rare larvae were detected in the brain by 2 days post-infection, and in the muscles from 7 days post-infection and onward. Larvae were still detected within muscle tissue at 176 days post-infection. These larvae were still infective when inoculated into mice, highlighting the zoonotic potential of poultry meat as a causative agent of human toxocariasis. Taira et al. (2011) reported ocular larval migrans at all timepoints through 176 days post-infection. Taira et al. (2011) also were able to infect mice orally with larvae recovered from chicken tissue. In the earthworm work of Okoshi and Usui (1968), the larvae from earthworms did not infect chickens.

5.2 Pigeon (*Columba livia domestica*)

5.2.1 Toxocara canis

Galvin (1964) found the major difference between *Toxocara* in chickens and pigeons to be that at 142 days after infection, 30% of inoculated larvae were recovered from chickens and only 18% from pigeons. The major lesions seen were in the liver where the majority of larvae were found. The lesions were worse in the pigeons than in the chickens, and by 3 months after infection granulomatous lesions were visible and up to 0.8 mm in diameter. The larvae in the granulomas histologically all appeared alive at the time of collection and fixation.

5.3 Japanese quail (*Coturnix japonica*)

5.3.1 Toxocara canis

Japanese Quail have been examined as to their ability to become infected with larvae and the distribution of larvae in their tissues and the ability of these larvae to infect dogs (Pahari and Sasmal, 1990a), the ability to infect quail by feeding them earthworms containing larvae (Pahari and Sasmal, 1991), and the transmission of larvae from quail to mice (Pahari and Sasmal, 1990b). In quail given infective eggs, the larvae were found mainly in the livers. After 50 larvae harvested from quails 30 days after infection were fed to mice, the mice were examined 6 and 12 days after infection and the greatest numbers of larvae recovered at 6- and 12-days post-infection were in the muscles (Pahari and Sasmal, 1990b). Maruyama et al. (1994) in a similar study gave 500 larvae from quail to each of 50 mice and examined the mice at different times from 6 h to 120 after inoculation; living larvae were found in all mice with the majority being in the liver and brain, but the muscle of the carcass was not examined with the total percentage of recovered larvae being somewhere around 20% on day 120. Pahari and Sasmal (1991) found that the larvae persisted in earthworms less than 20 days; however, having fed quail each three earthworms that had been exposed to infective eggs in soil, quail were infected but only six or so larvae were recovered from each quail fed the earthworms with larvae, but again the carcass was not examined. When three young dogs were given around 400 larvae each, the dogs developed patent infections with an average infection rate of about 22% with a mean of 87 adult worms per dog 40 days after infection (Pahari and Sasmal, 1990a).

6. Incidental finding of *Toxocara* larvae in naturally infected mammalian and avian hosts

Toxocara larvae were found in a Rook (*Corvus frugilegus*) in a survey monitoring birds of the family Corvidae for trichinosis in the Ferrara, Parma and Piacenza provinces of Italy. A digest of the tissues of a *C. frugilegus* revealed a larva of *Toxocara* that was shown morphologically and by PCR followed by sequencing to be a larva of *Toxocara*, and perhaps *Toxocara cati* (Garbarino et al., 2013). Based on the fact that the other work done in avian hosts shows that *T. canis* tends to stay in the liver in birds, it seems that this may be a *T. cati* larva since they appear more likely to be in the muscle tissues.

Marucci also working on trichinosis surveillance has found a number of cases where *Toxocara* larvae have been found in tissues, and they have a molecular method that can distinguish between *T. canis* and *T. cati*. The only animal positive for *T. canis* was a Badger (*Meles meles*); there were seven animals that were found infected with *T. cati*: three Hooded Crows (*Corvus cornix*); two Common Kestrels (*Falco tinnunculus*); a Hen Harrier (*Circus cyaneus*); a Rough Legged Buzzard (*Buteo lagopus*); and a domestic pig.

7. Reptiles

Merdivenci and Sezen (1965) demonstrated that tortoises bear some degree of resistance to *Toxocara canis*, which could be reduced by increasing the ambient temperature to an extent unusual for the species. In this study, tortoises infected with embryonated eggs and placed in 24–26 °C tanks did not have any larval migration in the liver or lungs, while those housed in 37 °C tanks did contain intrahepatic larvae.

8. Invertebrates

8.1 Earthworms

8.1.1 Toxocara canis *and* Toxocara cati

Sprent (1956) found the larvae of *Toxocara cati* in earthworms and cockroaches and not in beetle larvae or woodlice. Experimental infection of earthworms (*Eisenia foetida*) with *Toxocara canis* and *Toxocara cati* revealed larvae throughout the anterior, middle, and posterior part of the body in both cases. Larvae extracted from earthworms have also been found capable of infecting mice (Okoshi and Usui, 1968; Pahari and Sasmal, 1990b). Henson (1975) showed that the African night crawler, *Eudrilus eugeniae*, could be infected and maintain larval *T. canis* for at least 30 days.

8.2 Snails

8.2.1 *Toxocara cati*

Cardillo et al. (2016) found *Toxocara cati* larvae in land snails (*Rumina decollate*) collected in open spaces of a Buenos Aires city hospital. They found that 25% of sampled snails that were pooled (three snails per pool) prior to pepsin digestion were positive, and the larvae were identified both morphologically and by molecular methods.

8.3 Cockroaches

8.3.1 *Toxocara canis*

Experimental infections of cockroaches (*Periplaneta americana*) found that these insects were able to harbour viable eggs and larvae from days 1 to 5 post-infection, with eggs and larvae found in rectal contents but not in tissues of cockroaches, though somatic migration has been previously reported in infected cockroaches (Sasmal et al., 2008b; Sprent, 1956). Puppies infected with cockroach faeces developed patent infections of *Toxocara canis*, with eggs and larvae appearing in pup faeces at 38 days post-infection, and adult worms recovered at necropsy from the proximal part of the duodenum (Sasmal et al., 2008b).

9. The domestic cat (*Felis catus*) as a paratenic host

9.1 Toxocara canis

After the discovery of a naturally infected cat with severe disease that was expected to be due to *Toxocara canis* from the size of the larvae seen in

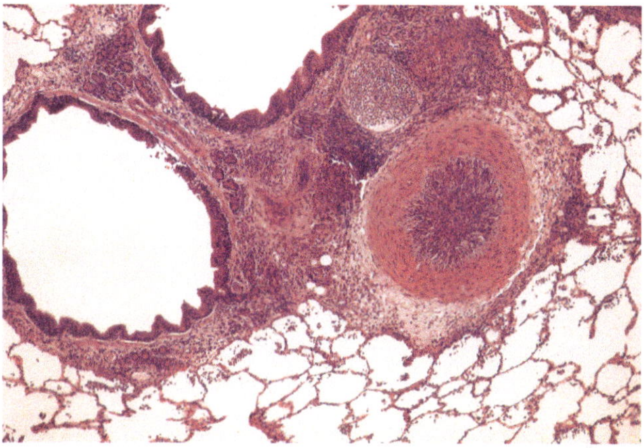

Fig. 4 Cat lung. The artery lumen is filled with eosinophils, and the tunica media is hypertrophied. The tunica adventitia is expanded by edea. The surrounding connective tissue is infiltrated by a dense population of eosinophils, occasionally forming vague nodules. H&E stain.

histological sections (the larvae are slightly wider than those of *T. cati* (Parsons et al., 1988), the disease was reproduced in cats experimentally. In the reproduced disease, the lesions were as striking as those in the naturally infected animal (Parsons et al., 1989); however, the infected cats with *Toxocara canis* did not exhibit any clinical signs aside from a mild cough and sinusitis in one cat. The major necropsy findings were hepatomegaly and pleuropneumonia with multifocal, white to grey nodules within the liver, lungs, and kidneys, with live larvae recovered from liver nodules. Histologic findings included eosinophilic granulomas within the liver, and variably severe, eosinophilic arteritis and bronchiolitis with medial hypertrophy and hyperplasia of the pulmonary arteries (Fig. 4). The bone marrow exhibited marked eosinophilic hyperplasia. There were no eye lesions noted. Additional affected areas included the heart, skeletal muscles, lymph nodes, pancreas, and brain, which had variable levels of granulomatous to eosinophilic inflammation (Fig. 5).

10. Human infections from the ingestion of paratenic hosts

Most larva migrans cases are seen in children 1–5 years of age and are acquired by ingestion of infective eggs in contaminated soil (Dissamarn et al., 1968; Glickman and Summers, 1983). Other cases may by acquired through

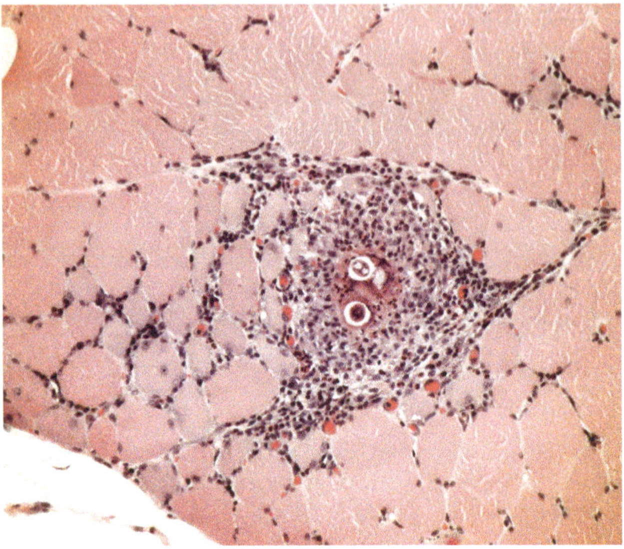

Fig. 5 Cat quadriceps. There are two sections of a *T. canis* larva within the muscle, surrounded by a dense population of eosinophils and macrophages, which extend between myofibres multifocally. H&E stain.

the ingestion of raw or poorly cooked infected meat, especially the liver, of animals which once served as paratenic hosts (Beaver, 1966). Indeed, the first suggestion of larval migrans from the ingestion of raw liver was made by Whitby in 1928 as discussed by Beaver (1956) who wrote—including a quote by Whitby: "It has not been shown that the eosinophilia associated with raw liver diets was due to larval nematode infections acquired from the liver, but it is possible that Whitby (1928) was closer to the truth than he thought when he stated, 'The eosinophilic reaction with liver treatment is probably well known to those who have had opportunities of studying numbers of cases, but those unaware of the phenomenon are not unlikely to suspect that parasites derived from the raw liver have been implanted in the patient'".

There have been multiple cases of visceral larval migrans in humans following the ingestion of raw liver and raw meat product. Sources have included raw liver from chickens (Morimatsu et al., 2006; Park et al., 2010) and duck (Hoffmeister et al., 2007); another case was associated with the ingestion of raw chicken meat where the patient developed pulmonary toxocariasis (Fujii et al., 2011). Another avian source of infection was ostrich liver, where the patient developed eosinophilic meningitis

(Noh et al., 2012). Raw cattle liver and some mammalian meat items have on occasion also been a source of infection. Finsterer et al. (2010) reported a case of human neurotoxocariasis in a patient who ingested raw goat meat. Yang et al. (2014) reported on ocular larva migrans occurring in five cases in men who had ingested various combinations of raw cow liver, minced raw beef, deer blood, and raw rabbit liver. Kim et al. (2013) also had reported a case of ocular toxocariasis in a man who had had a history of eating raw cow liver during the month prior to presentation. Yoshikawa et al. (2008) reported on a familial case of visceral toxocariasis in the liver and lungs of three family members who regularly ingested raw cow liver. Lim et al. (2009) reported on a case of pulmonary toxocariasis in a 14-year-old patient that initially masqueraded as metastatic tumour nodules in this patent who had osteosarcoma and had frequently ingested raw cow liver. Park et al. (2012) also reported on cases of toxocariasis masquerading as liver and lung metastases in patients with gastrointestinal cancer where all five patients had eaten thick slices of raw bovine liver weekly, and Hisamatsu et al. (2008) reported on a case in a patient who often ate raw beef liver where toxocariasis showed migratory nodular shadows with halos on follow up after the patient had nodular shadows found on the left lung at a routine checkup who was then checked serologically and treated with albendazole. Enko et al. (2009) reported on a case of fulminant eosinophilic myocarditis where the patient had eaten raw deer meat before presentation; the patient was shown to have severe interstitial edema with moderate myocardial necrosis. Abe et al. (2002) had also reported on a case of myocarditis and larval toxocariasis in a patient who had consumed raw meat (type not recorded) prior to admission. Mitamura et al. (2007) reported on a case in a 21 year-old woman with low grade fever, dry cough, polyarthralgia, and general fatigue who was then found by computed tomography to have multiple small nodules in both lung fields, and had the habit of eating raw meat and cattle liver. The woman also had a high serologic titre, and responded to anthelminthic therapy.

Choi et al. (2008) examined eosinophilia and the ingestion of raw meat and liver in Korea utilizing 120 patients who had reported to a hospital clinic for eosinophilia of unknown aetiology and volunteered for the study. Of these patients, 86.7% were positive serologically for *Toxocara*, and it was decided that 92.3% were confidently diagnosed with toxocariasis since they were not found to have any other causes for their increased eosinophil counts; there were 24 excluded patients since they were serologically positive for other parasites, i.e., *Clonorchis sinensis*, *Paragonimus westermani*, sparganosis, and cysticercosis. Among those positive for toxocariasis, 87.5% had a history of recently eating raw cow liver, while only 25% of seronegative patients had recently eaten raw cow liver. In the 28 patients that ate raw cow liver ≥4 times a year, the seropositive rate was 96.4%, and of the 45 who had eaten cow liver in the last 6 months, the seropositive rate was 95.6%. Twenty one patients also ate raw liver from other animals: pig (7), dog (4), goat (3), chicken (3), rabbit (2), duck (1), and goose (1), and 19 patients drank blood of animals including deer, goat, duck, cow, pig, or mud turtle.

Visceral larva migrans has also been associated with ingestion of earthworms in one case, with associated pulmonary nodules, hypereosinophilia, and hypergammaglobulinemia (Cianferoni et al., 2006). Fellrath and Magnaval (2014) reported a case of severe neurologic, ocular and pulmonary disease associated with toxocariasis after the ingestion of live slugs; this patient had a long-standing history of eating two or three slugs daily as an alternative therapy of gastroesophageal reflux. These authors also cite two previous cases where toxocariasis occurred in patients who ate raw snails as a remedy for gastric ulcers. One occurred in Catalonia (Romeu et al., 1991) and one in Italy (Caldera et al., 2013). These authors suggested that the snails likely had infective *Toxocara* eggs within their digestive tract or present in the snail mucous, but the work of Cardillo et al. (2016) had not yet been published.

11. Conclusion

Toxocariasis is an omnipresent parasite that can utilize many different pathways to make its way back to its final host. The larvae can pass from host to host, although unlike with *Toxoplasma gondii*, since there is no multiplication in each host, it would seemingly dwindle with each host and ultimately fade away. Fortunately, there are only a few helminth parasites that cause fulminant disease in hosts when there is an immunologic dysfunction or intervention, and fortunately, *Toxocara* is not one of these agents. At the same time, the question remains how many cases of visceral and ocular larva migrans are too many, and how important is the prevention of this and visceral disease. Until we have a *Toxocara* free island or colony, we are unlikely to know if there is a benefit to man and beast being without this companion.

References

Abe, K., Shimokawa, H., Kubota, T., Nawa, Y., Takeshita, A., 2002. Myocarditis associated with visceral larva migrans due to *Toxocara canis*. Intern. Med. 41, 706–708.

Abo-Shehada, M.N., Herbert, I.V., 1984a. The migration of larval *Toxocara canis* in mice I. Migration through the intestine in primary infections. Vet. Parasitol. 17, 65–73.

Abo-Shehada, M.N., Herbert, I.V., 1984b. The migration of larval *Toxocara canis* in mice II. Post-intestinal migration in primary infections. Vet. Parasitol. 17, 75–83.

Akao, N., Takayanagi, T.H., Suzuki, R., Tsukidate, S., Fujita, K., 2000. Ocular larva migrans caused by *Toxocara cati* in Mongolian gerbils and a comparison of ophthalmologic findings with those produced by *T. canis*. J. Parasitol. 89, 1133–1135.

Akao, N., Tomoda, M., Hayashi, E., Suzuki, R., Shimizu-Suganuma, M., Shichinohe, K., Fujita, K., 2003. Cerebellar ataxia due to *Toxocara* infection in Mongolian gerbil, *Meriones unguiculatus*. Vet. Parasitol. 113, 229–237.

Alba-Hurtado, F., Tortora, P.J.L., Tsutsumi, V., Ortega-Pierres, M.G., 2000. Histopathological investigation of experimental ocular toxocariasis in gerbils. Int. J. Parasitol. 30, 143–147.

Alba-Hurtado, F., Munoz-Guzman, M.A., Valdivia-Anda, G., Tortora, J.L., Ortega-Pierres, M.G., 2009. *Toxocara canis*: larval migration dynamics, detection of antibody reactivity to larval excretory–secretory antigens and clinical findings during experimental infection of gerbils (*Meriones unguiculatus*). Exp. Parasitol. 122, 1–5.

Aldawek, A.M., Levkut, M., Revajova, V., Kolodzieyski, L., Sevelkova, Z., Dubinsky, P., 2002. Larval toxocarosis in sheep: the immunohistochemical characterization of lesions in some affected organs. Vet. Parasitol. 105, 207–214.

Beaver, P.C., 1956. Larva migrans. Exp. Parasitol. 5, 587–621.

Beaver, P.C., 1962. Toxocarosis (visceral larva migrans) in relation to tropical eosinophilia. Bull. Soc. Pathol. Exot. 55, 555–576.

Beaver, P.C., 1966. Zoonoses, with particular reference to parasites of veterinary importance. In: Soulsby, E.J.L. (Ed.), Biology of Parasites. Academic Press, New York, NY, pp. 215–227.

Beaver, P.C., Snyder, C.H., Carrera, G.M., Dent, J.H., Lafferty, J.W., 1952. Chronic eosinophilia due to visceral larva migrans. Report of three cases. Pediatrics 9, 7–19.

Bisseru, B., 1969. Studies on the liver, lung, brain and blood of experimental animals infected with *Toxocara canis*. J. Helminthol. 43, 267–272.

Burren, C., 1971. The distribution of *Toxocara* larvae in the central nervous system of the mouse. Trans. R. Soc. Trop. Med. Hyg. 65, 450–453.

Burren, C., 1972. The distribution of *Toxocara canis* larvae in the central nervous system of rodents. Trans. R. Soc. Trop. Med. Hyg. 66, 937–942.

Caldera, F., Burlone, M.E., Genchi, C., Prisi, M., Bartoli, E., 2013. *Toxocara* encephalitis presenting with autonomous nervous system involvement. Infection 41, 691–694.

Cardillo, N., Prous, C.G., Krivokapich, S., Pittaro, M., Ercole, M., Perez, M., Pasqualetti, M., Fariña, F., Rosa, A., Gatti, G., Ribicich, M., 2009. Experimental infection with *Toxocara cati* in BALB/c mice, migratory behaviour and pathological changes. Zoonoses Public Health 56, 198–205.

Cardillo, N., Gonzales Prous, C., Krivokapick, S., Pittaro, M., Ercole, M., Perez, M., Pasqualetti, M., Fariña, F., Rosa, A., Gatti, G., Ribicich, M., 2016. First report of Toxocara cati in the domestic land snail Rumina decollate. Rev. Argent. Microbiol. 48, 206–209.

Chari, S., Subramanian, G., 1972. Histopathological and histochemical changes following invasion of mice by *Toxocara canis* (Werner, 1782). Indian J. Anim. Sci. 42, 957–960.

Choi, D., Lim, J.H., Choi, D.C., 2008. Toxocariasis and ingestion of raw cow liver in patients with eosinophilia. Korean J. Parasitol. 46, 139–143.

Cianferoni, A., Schneider, L., Schantz, P.M., Brown, D., Fox, L.M., 2006. Visceral larva migrans associated with earthworm ingestion: clinical evolution in an adolescent patient. Pediatrics 117, e336–e339.

Collins, R.F., Ivey, M.H., 1975. Specificity and sensitivity of skin test reactions to extracts of Toxocara canis and Ascaris suum II. Homologous 48-hour passive cutaneous anaphylaxis tests with sera from infected Guinea pigs. Am. J. Trop. Med. Hyg. 24, 460–464.

Corrêa, F.M., Chieffi, P.P., Lescano, S.A.Z., do Santo, S.V., 2014. Behavioral and memory changes in Mus musculus coinfected by *Toxocara canis* and *Toxoplasma gondii*. Rev. Inst. Med. Trop. Sao Paulo 56, 353–356.

de Queiroz, M.L., Viel, T.A., Papa, C.H.G., Lescano, S.A.Z., Chieffi, P.P., 2013. Behavioral changes in *Rattus norvegicus* coinfected by *Toxocara canis* and *Toxoplasma gondii*. Rev. Inst. Med. Trop. Sao Paulo 55, 51–53.

de Souza Aguiar, P., Furtado, R.D., da Costa de Avila, L.F., de Lima Telmo, P., Rodrigues Martins, L.H., Aires Berne, M.E., Almeida da Silva, P.E., Scaini, C.J., 2015. Transmammary infection in BALB/c mice with chronic toxocariasis. Parasitol. Int. 64, 145–147.

Dissamarn, R., Chai-Anan, P., Thirapat, K., Aranyakananda, P., Sri-Vorant, P., Chitrakorn, P., 1968. The infectivity of *Toxocara canis* larva in experimental animals. J. Med. Assoc. Thai. 51, 173–177.

Dolinsky, Z.S., Hardy, C.A., Burright, R.G., Donovick, P.J., 1985. The progression of behavioral and pathological effects of the parasite *Toxocara canis* in the mouse. Physiol. Behav. 35, 33–42.

Dubey, J.P., 1967. Migration of *Toxocara cati* larvae in mice. Trop. Geogr. Med. 20, 172–176.

Dubinský, P., Havasiová-Reiterová, K., Peťko, B., Horvorka, I., Tomašovičová, O., 1995. Role of small mammals in the epidemiology of toxocariasis. Parasitology 110, 187–193.

Dunsmore, J., Thompson, R.C.A., Bates, I.A., 1983. The accumulation of *Toxocara canis* larvae in the brains of mice. Int. J. Parasitol. 13, 517–521.

Enko, K., Tada, T., Ohgo, K.O., Nagase, S., Nakamura, K., Ohta, K., Ichiba, S., Ujike, Y., Nawa, Y., Maruyam, H., Ohe, T., Kusano, K.F., 2009. Fulminant eosinophilic myocarditis associated with visceral larva migrans caused by *Toxocara canis* infections. Circ. J. 73, 1344–1348.

Fellrath, J.-M., Magnaval, J.-F., 2014. Toxocariasis after slug ingestion characterized by severe neurologic, ocular, and pulmonary involvement. Open Forum Infect. Dis. 1, ofu063. https://doi.org/10.1093/ofid/ofu063.

Finsterer, J., Kallab, V., Auer, H., 2010. Neurotoxocariasis associated with lower motor neuron disease. Report of one case. Rev. Med. Chil. 138, 483–486.

Fitzgerald, P., Mansfield, M., 1970. Visceral larva migrans (*Toxocara canis*) in calves. Am. J. Vet. Res. 31, 561–565.

Fujii, Y., Matak, H., Koreeda, Y., Kawabata, T., Hamada, M., Hakashioya, J., Tomiyama, Y., Kawabata, M., 2011. A case of pulmonary toxocariasis successfully treated with ivermectin. (in Japanese). J. Jpn. Respir. Soc. 49, 399–403.

Fülleborn, F., 1921. Askarisinfektion durch Verzehren eingekapselter Larven und über gelungene intrauterine Askarisinfektion. Arch. Schiffs Trop. Hyg. 25, 367–375. (In German).

Galvin, T.J., 1964. Experimental *Toxocara canis* infections in chickens and pigeons. J. Parasitol. 50, 124–127.

Garbarino, C., Rubini, S., Merialdi, G., Merenda, M., Bolobnesi, E., Licata, E., Genchi, D., Marucci, G., Pozio, E., 2013. In: Rilevamento di larve di *Toxocara* spp. in muscoli di corvidi sottoposti a digestione artificiale per la ricerca di *Trichinella* spp. XV Congresso Nazionale Società Italiana di Diagnostica di Laboratorio Veterinaria. Monreale (PA), 23–25 October, pp. 259–260.

Glickman, L., Summers, B., 1983. Experimental *Toxocara canis* infection in cynomolgus macaques (*Macaca fascicularis*). Am. J. Vet. Res. 44, 2347–2354.

Gonçalves dal Silva, A.M., Chieffi, P.P., Ferreira da Silva, W.L., Kanshiro, E.H.Y., Rubinsky-Elefant, G., Cunha-Neto, E., Mairena, E.C., De Brito, T., 2015. The hamster (*Mesocricetus auratus*) as an experimental model of toxocariasis: histopathological, immunohistochemical, and immunoelectron microscopic findings. Parasitol. Res. 114, 809–821.

Hay, J., Arnott, M.A., Aitken, P.O., Kendall, A.T., 1986. Experimental toxocariasis and hyperactivity in mice. Z. Parasitenkd. 72, 115–120.

Henson, R.N., 1975. Experimental infection of the African night crawler *Eudrilus eugenieae* (Kinberg) with the common dog ascarid *Toxocara canis* (Werner). Tex. J. Sci. 26, 598–599.

Hildebransd, J., Zalesny, G., Okulewicz, A., Baaszkiewicz, K., 2009. Preliminary studies on the zoonotic importance of rodents as a reservoir of toxocariasis from recreation grounds in Wroclaw (Poland). Helminthologia 46, 80–84.

Hisamatsu, Y., Ishii, H., Kai, N., Amemiya, Y., Otani, S., Morinaga, R., Shirai, R., Umeki, K., Tokimatsu, I., Hiramatsu, K., Kadota, J.-I., 2008. Case of toxocariasis showing migratory nodular shadows with halos. J. Jpn. Res. Soc. 46, 1343–3490. (in Japanese).

Hoeppli, R., Feng, L.C., Li, F., 1949. Histological reactions in the liver of mice due to larvae of different *Ascaris* species. Peking Nat. Hist. Bull. 18, 119–312.

Hoffmeister, B., Glaeser, S., Flick, H., Pornschlegel, S., Suttorp, N., Bergmann, F., 2007. Cerebral toxocariasis after consumption of raw duck liver. Am. J. Trop. Med. Hyg. 76, 600–602.

Ivey, M.H., 1965. Immediate hypersensitivity and serological responses in guinea Pigs infected with *Toxocara canis* or *Trichinella spiralis*. Am. J. Trop. Med. Hyg. 14, 1044–1051.

Kayes, S., Oaks, J.A., 1978. Development of the granulomatous response in murine toxocariasis. Initial events. Am. J. Pathol. 93, 277–294.

Kayes, S.G., Jones, R.E., Omholt, P.E., 1987. Use of bronchoalveolar lavage to compare local pulmonary immunity with the systemic immune response of *Toxocara canis*-infected mice. Infect. Immun. 55, 2132–2136.

Kim, Y.J., Moon, C.H., Chang, J.H., 2013. Toxocariasis of the optic disc. J. Neuro-Ophthalmol. 33, 151–152.

Koizumi, T., Hayakawa, J.-I., 1984. Mouse strain difference in visceral larva migrans of *Toxocara canis*. Exp. Anim. 33, 291–295.

Krücken, J., Blümke, J., Maaz, D., Demeler, J., Ramüunke, S., Antolová, D., Schaper, R., Samson-Himmelstjerna, G. von, 2017. Small rodents as paratenic or intermediate hosts of carnivore parsites in Berlin, Germany. PLoS ONE 12, e0172829.

Lautenslager, J.P., 1972. *Toxocara* Visceral Larva Migrans in Rabbits. PhD Thesis, University of Guelph, Canada, ON, p. 133.

Lee, K.-T., Min, H.-K., Soh, C.-T., 1976. Transplacental migration of *Toxocara canis* larvae in experimentally infected mice. J. Parasitol. 62, 460–465.

Lescano, S.A.Z., Santos, S.V., Queiroz, M.S., Castro, J.M., Chieffi, P.P., 2013. Migration routes of *Toxocara canis* and *Toxocara cati* in tissues of experimentally infected *Rattus norvegicus*. Neotrop. Helminthol. 7, 149–153.

Lim, Y.-H., Kim, J.H., Oh, S.H., Jeon, S.C., Koh, H.C., Lee, Y.-H., 2009. Pulmonary toxocariasis masquerading as metastatic tumor nodules in a child with osteosarcoma. Pediatr. Blood Cancer 53, 1343–1345.

Nichols, R.L., 1956. The etiology of visceral larva migrans: I. Diagnostic morphology of the infective second-stage *Toxocara* larvae. J. Parasitol. 42, 349–362.

Marucci, G., Interisano, M., La Rosa, G., Pozio, E., 2013. Molecular identification of nematode larvae different from those of the *Trichinella* genus detected by muscle digestion. Vet. Parasitol. 194, 117–120.

Maruyama, S., Yamamoto, K., Katusube, Y., 1994. Infectivity of *Toxocara canis* larvae from Japanese quails to mice. J. Vet. Med. Sci. 56, 399–401.

Merdivenci, A., Sezen, Y., 1965. The resistance of tortoises, *Testudo graeca* L., against *Toxocara canis* infection. Parasitol. Res. 25, 387–392.

Mitamura, M., Fukuoka, Y., Haruta, Y., Korarada, S., Tada, Y., Nagasawa, K., 2007. J. Jpn. Assoc. Infect. Dis. 81, 305–308.

Morimatsu, Y., et al., 2006. A familial case of visceral larva migrans after ingestion of raw chicken livers: appearance of specific antibody in bronchoalveolar lavage fluid of the patients. Am. J. Trop. Med. Hyg. 75, 303–306.

Mossalam, I., Atallah, O.A., Hosney, Z., 1972. Experimental studies on visceral larva migrans of *Toxocara canis* in laboratory animals. Acta Vet. Acad. Sci. Hung. 22, 71–80.

Nobuaki, A., 1986. An immunopathological study of the liver of mice infected with *Toxocara canis*. Jpn. J. Parasitol. 35, 135–140.

Noh, Y., Hong, S.T., Yun, J.Y., Park, H.-K., Oh, J.-H., Kim, Y.-E., Jeon, B.-S., 2012. Meningitis by *Toxocara canis* after ingestion of raw ostrich liver. J. Korean Med. Sci. 27, 1105–1108.

Okoshi, S., Usui, M., 1968. Experimental studies on *Toxascaris leonina*. VI. Experimental infection of mice, chickens and earthworms with *Toxascaris leonina*, *Toxocara canis* and *Toxocara cati*. Jpn. J. Vet. Sci. 30, 151–166.

Olson, L.J., 1962. Organ distribution of *Toxocara cams* larvae in normal mice and in mice previously infected with *Toxocara*, *Ascaris* or *Trichinella*. Tex. Rep. Biol. Med. 20, 651–657.

Olson, L.J., 1976. Ocular toxocariasis in mice: distribution of larvae and lesions. Int. J. Parasitol. 6, 247–251.

Olson, L.J., Izzat, N.N., Petteway, M.B., Reinhart, J.A., 1970. Ocular toxocariasis in mice. Am. J. Trop. Med. Hyg. 19, 238–243.

Olson, L.J., Petteway, M.B., 1972. Invasion of the spinal cord of mice by *Toxocara canis*. J. Parasitol. 56, 413–414.

Pahari, T.K., Sasmal, N.K., 1990a. Infection of Japanese quail with *Toxocara canis* larvae and establishment of patent infection in pups. Vet. Parasitol. 35, 357–364.

Pahari, T.K., Sasmal, N.K., 1990b. Experimental infection of mice with *Toxocara canis* larvae obtained from Japanese quails. Int. J. Parasitol. 20, 263–264.

Pahari, T.K., Sasmal, N.K., 1991. Experimental infection of Japanese quail with *Toxocara canis* larvae through earthworms. Vet. Parasitol. 39, 337–340.

Pankavich, J.A., 1966. The Distribution, Migration, and Development of *Toxocara canis*, *Toxascaris leonina*, and *Toxocara cati* in the Rabbit. PhD Thesis, New York University, New York, NY. 125 pp.

Park, M.S., Ahn, Y.-J., Moon, K.-R., 2010. Familial case of visceral larval migrans of *Toxocara canis* after ingestion of raw chicken liver. Korean J. Pediatr. Gastroenterol. Nutr. 13, 70–74.

Park, S., Kim, Y.S., Kim, Y.J., Kyung, S.Y., Park, J.-W., Jeong, S.H., Lee, S.Y., 2012. Toxocariasis masquerading as liver and lung metastatic nodules in patents with gastrointestinal cancer: clinicopathologic study of five cases. Dig. Dis. Sci. 57, 155–160.

Parsons, J.C., Grieve, R.B., 1990. Kinetics of liver trapping of infective larvae in murine toxocariasis. J. Parasitol. 76, 529–536.

Parsons, J.C., Bowman, D.D., Gillette, D.M., Grieve, R.B., 1988. Disseminated granulomatous disease in a cat caused by larvae of *Toxocara canis*. J. Comp. Pathol. 99, 343–346.

Parsons, J.C., Bowman, D.D., Grieve, R.B., 1989. Pathological and haematological responses of cats experimentally infected with *Toxocara canis* larvae. Int. J. Parasitol. 19, 479–488.

Prociv, P., 1986. *Toxocara pteropodis*, *T. canis* and *T. cati* infections in guinea pigs. Trop. Biomed. 3, 97–106.

Romeu, J., Roig, J., Bada, J.L., Riera, C., Muñoz, C., 1991. Adult human toxocariasis acquired by eating raw snails. J. Infect. Dis. 164, 483.

Ronéus, O., 1963. Parasitic liver lesions in swine, experimentally produced by visceral larva migrans of *Toxocara cati*. Acta Vet. Scand. 4, 170–196.

Ronéus, O., 1966. Studies on the aetiology and pathogenesis of white spots in the liver of pigs. Acta Vet. Scand. 7 (Suppl. 16). 137 pp.

Santos, S.V., Moura, J.V.L., Lescano, S.A.Z., Castro, J.M., Ribeiro, M.C.S.A., Chieffi, P.P., 2015. Behavioural changes and muscle strength in Rattus norvegicus experimentally infected with *Toxocara cati* and *T. canis*. J. Helminthol. 89, 465–470.

Sasmal, N.K., Acharya, S., Laha, R., 2008a. Larval migration of *Toxocara canis* in piglets and transfer of larvae from infected porcine tissue to mice. J. Helminthol. 82, 245–249.

Sasmal, N.K., Pahari, T.K., Laha, R., 2008b. Experimental infection of the cockroach *Periplaneta americana* with *Toxocara canis* and the establishment of patent infections in pups. J. Helminthol. 82, 97–100.

Schaeffler, W.F., 1960. Experimental infection of sheep with the dog ascarid, *Toxocara canis*. J. Parasitol. 46, 17 (5; Sect. 2) Abstract 45. Annual Meeting of the American Society of parasitologists, Los Angeles, California, USA.

Sharp, A.D., Olson, L.J., 1962. Responses in *Toxocara-*, *Ascaris-*, and *Trichinella*-infected Guinea pigs to homologous and heterologous challenge. J. Parasitol. 48, 362–367.

Sinha, B.N., 1969. The migratory behaviour of the larvae of *Toxocara canis* (Werner 1782) in Spanish goats. Southwest. Vet. 23, 37–41. Fall 1969.

Sprent, J.F.A., 1953. On the migratory behaviour of the larvae of various ascaris species in white mice: II longevity. J. Infect. Dis. 92, 114–117.

Sprent, J.F.A., 1956. The life history and development of *Toxocara cati* (Schrank 1788) in the domestic cat. Parasitology 46 (1–2), 54–78.

Sugane, K., Oshima, T., 1983. Trapping of large numbers of larvae in the livers of *Toxocara canis*-reinfected mice. J. Helminthol. 57, 95–99.

Taira, K., Saeed, I., Lind, P., Murrell, K.D., Kapel, C.M.O., 2003. Population dynamics of *Toxocara canis* in pigs receiving a single or multiple infection. Parasitology 127, 593–602.

Taira, K., Saitoh, Y., Kapel, C.M.O., 2011. *Toxocara cati* larvae persist and retain high infectivity in muscles of experimentally infected chickens. Vet. Parasitol. 180, 287–291.

Takayanagi, T.H., Akao, N., Suzuki, R., Tomoda, M., Tsukidate, S., Fujita, K., 1999. New animal model for human ocular toxocariasis: ophthalmoscopic observation. Br. J. Ophthalmol. 83, 967–972.

Tomimura, T., Yokota, M., Takiguchi, H., 1976. Experimental visceral larva migrans in monkeys. I. Clinical, hematological, biochemical and gross pathological observations on monkeys inoculated with embryonated eggs of the dog ascarid, *Toxocara canis*. Nihon Juigaku Zasshi 38, 533–548.

Tsvetaeva, N.P., Sosipatrova, L.A., Smirnov, A.G., 1979. Pathological changes in chicks infected with *Toxocara canis*. Veterinariya, Moscow 10, 75–77.

Waindok, P., Özbakiş-Beceriklisoy, G., Juneck-Erfurth, E., Springer, A., Pfeffer, M., Lischik, M., Stube, C., 2019. Parasites in brains of wild rodents (Arvicolinae and Murinae) in the city of Leipzig, Germany. Int. J. Parasitol. Parasites Wildl. 10, 211–217.

Watzke, R.C., Oaks, J.A., Folk, J.C., 1984. *Toxocara canis* infection of the eye: correlation of clinical observations with developing pathology in the primate model. Arch. Ophthalmol. 102, 282–291.

Whitby, L.E.H., 1928. Leucocytic changes resulting from the treatment of pernicious anemia with liver. Lancet 1, 285–286.

Wong, H.S.W., Embil, J.A., Ozere, R.L., 1976. *Ascaris suum* and *Toxocara canis*: egg extract antigens in Guinea pigs and the macrophage migration inhibition test. Exp. Parasitol. 40, 421–426.

Yang, H.K., Woo, S.J., Hwang, J.M., 2014. *Toxocara* optic neuropathy after ingestion of raw meat products. Optom. Vis. Sci. 91, e267–e273.

Yoshikawa, M., Nishiofuku, M., Moriya, K., Ouji, Y., Ishizaka, S., Kasahara, K., Mikas, K.-I., Hirai, T., Mizuno, Y., Ogawa, S., Nakamura, T., Maruyama, H., Akao, N., 2008. A familial case of visceral toxocariasis due to consumption of raw bovine liver. Parasitol. Int. 57, 525–529.

CHAPTER FIVE

Toxocara "omics" and the promises it holds for medicine and veterinary medicine

Wen-Bin Zheng[a,b], Yang Zou[b], Xing-Quan Zhu[b,c,*], Guo-Hua Liu[a,*]

[a]Hunan Provincial Key Laboratory of Protein Engineering in Animal Vaccines, College of Veterinary Medicine, Hunan Agricultural University, Changsha, China
[b]State Key Laboratory of Veterinary Etiological Biology, Key Laboratory of Veterinary Parasitology of Gansu Province, Lanzhou Veterinary Research Institute, Chinese Academy of Agricultural Sciences, Lanzhou, China
[c]Jiangsu Co-innovation Center for the Prevention and Control of Important Animal Infectious Diseases and Zoonoses, Yangzhou University College of Veterinary Medicine, Yangzhou, China
*Corresponding authors: e-mail address: xingquanzhu1@hotmail.com; liuguohua5202008@163.com

Contents

Abstract

Toxocariasis is one of the most neglected worldwide zoonoses that is caused by larval nematode parasites of the genus *Toxocara*, *Toxocara canis*, and to a lesser extent, *Toxocara cati*, whose migration mechanism is still largely unknown. Fortunately, some advanced tools have been employed, such as genomics, transcriptomics, and proteomics, to better understand the molecular biology and regulatory mechanisms of *Toxocara*. Using genomics and transcriptomics, we can identify a large number of genes that participate in the development of *Toxocara* and the interaction of parasites and

Advances in Parasitology, Volume 109
ISSN 0065-308X
https://doi.org/10.1016/bs.apar.2020.01.002

their hosts and can predict the functions of unknown genes by comparing them with other relevant species. Using proteomics, we can identify somatic proteins and excretory and secretory (ES) proteins that perform specific biological functions in tissue degradation, pathogen invasion, immune evasion or modulation. These "omics" techniques also can contribute enormously to the development of new drugs, vaccines and diagnostic tools for toxocariasis. In a word, by utilizing "omics", we can better understand the *Toxocara* and toxocariasis. In this review, we summarized the representative achievements in *Toxocara* and the interaction between *Toxocara* spp. and their hosts based on expressed sequence tags (ESTs), microarray gene expression, next-generation sequencing (NGS) technologies and liquid chromatography-tandem mass spectrometry (LC-MS/MS), hoping to better understand the molecular biology of *Toxocara*, and contribute to new progress in the application areas of new drugs, vaccines and diagnostic tool for toxocariasis in the future.

1. Introduction

Toxocariasis caused by *Toxocara canis* from canids and, to a lesser level, *Toxocara cati* from felids, is an important parasitic disease of humans, causing visceral larva migrans (VLM), ocular toxocariasis (OT), neurotoxocariasis (NT) and covert toxocariasis (CT) in many countries and territories (Chen et al., 2018; Ma et al., 2018; Rostami et al., 2019). *Toxocara* has a perfect life cycle in definitive hosts and can survive for a long time in paratenic hosts, such as rodents, humans and other animals (Strube et al., 2013). The female worm that is in the intestines of definitive hosts can excrete a large number of eggs into the environment, with 21% prevalence of *Toxocara* eggs in soil samples in public places all over the word (Fakhri et al., 2018), which ensures *Toxocara* to tenaciously survive and endlessly reproduce in complex environments.

Gene families that modulate host immune responses and regulate parasite development, as well as protein families that are potential targets for drug development were identified and analyzed by large-scale genome comparison of worms, accelerating the search for new interventions (International Helminth Genomes Consortium, 2019). In the past 10 years, enormous advances have been acquired in "omics" studies of parasites (Chuan et al., 2010; Cwiklinski and Dalton, 2018; Stoltzfus et al., 2017). The advent and integration of "omics" technologies could provide a unique opportunity for global investigations of parasites, allowing the systems biology of parasites to be explored (Bourgard et al., 2018; Cwiklinski and Dalton, 2018). Moreover, WormBase ParaSite (http://parasite.wormbase.org/) and the

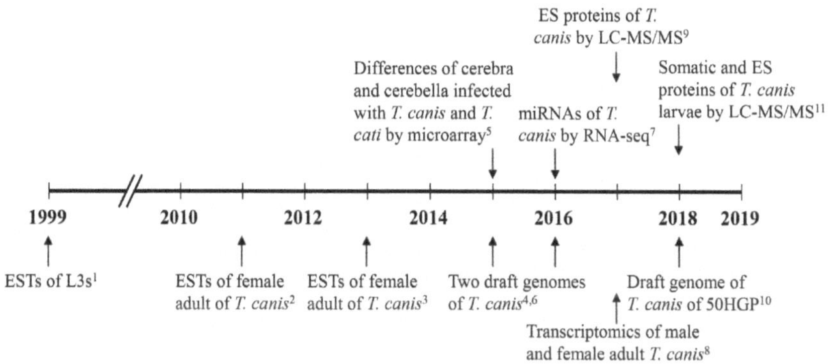

Fig. 1 Schematic presentation of major *Toxocara* "omics" advances detailed over time. The principal references are denoted by numbers as follows: (1) Tetteh et al., 1999; (2) Zhou et al., 2011; (3) Kim et al., 2013; (4) Zhu et al., 2015; (5) Janecek et al., 2015; (6) Kong et al., 2016; (7) Ma et al., 2016; (8) Zhou et al. (2017); (9) Sperotto et al., 2017; (10) 50HGP, https://www.sanger.ac.uk/science/collaboration/50hgp; (11) da Silva et al., 2018.

50 helminth genomes project (50HGP; https://www.sanger.ac.uk/science/collaboration/50hgp) promote the development of comparative genomics and will undoubtedly contribute to the further exploration of a number of parasites (Howe et al., 2016).

The completion of the first *T. canis* draft genome is a landmark in *Toxocara* research, providing potential global insight into the molecular biology of the genus *Toxocara* (Zhu et al., 2015). The application of transcriptomics and proteomics techniques has also greatly accelerated the research progress in *Toxocara*. Information provided by "omics" projects not only can augment the understanding of *Toxocara* biology and pathogenesis, but also can enormously contribute to the development of new drugs, vaccines and diagnostic tools. In this review, we summarize the representative achievements in *Toxocara* and the interaction between *Toxocara*-host utilizing "omics" technologies (Fig. 1), hoping to better understand the molecular biology of *Toxocara* and contribute to the application areas of diagnosis, treatment, prevention and control in toxocariasis in the future.

2. Characteristics of the *T. canis* genome

The genome of *T. canis* has been explored extensively (Gasser et al., 2016; Kong et al., 2016; Zhu et al., 2015). These studies allowed the assemblage of the *T. canis* genome at the scaffold level (Table 1), however, draft genomes of other *Toxocara* species are not yet available for comparisons.

Table 1 Outline of genome assembly and annotation in the three available draft genomes of *Toxocara canis*.

BioSample	SAMN02905866	SAMN04961616	SAMEA1034752
Release date	2014/12/18	2016/7/6	2018/11/28
BioProject	PRJNA248777	PRJNA320963	PRJEB533
Assembly	GCA_000803305.1	GCA_001680135.1	GCA_900622545.1
WGS	JPKZ01	LYYD01	UYWY01
Genome coverage	246x	317x	163x
Size (bp)	317,115,901	341,776,187	299,788,016
Genome GC content (%)	40.0	39.3	38.7
Level	Scaffold	Scaffold	Scaffold
Number of scaffolds	22,857	10,853	29,185
Scaffold N50	375,067	108,950	31,192
Contig N50	18,797	9977	15,449
Number of genes	18,596	20,178	20,264
Number of proteins	1859	22,358	20,220
Mean gene length (bp)	8416	6055	5678
Mean exon number per gene	7.4	7.1	5.9

The genome size of *T. canis* is similar to those of *Ascaris lumbricoides* (316.975 Mb provided by 50HGP) and *A. suum* (272.783 Mb, Jex et al., 2011; 298.028 Mb, Wang et al., 2017a).

Zhu et al. (2015) found that 67.5% (n = 12,559) predicted genes of *T. canis* had a homologue either in *A. suum* (n = 11,658; 62.7%), *B. malayi* (n = 8395; 45.1%), *C. elegans* (n = 9002; 48.4%), or *P. pacificus* (n = 7968; 42.8%), as well as, a total of 5918 genes were mutual among all 5 species and 6037 genes were exclusive for *T. canis*. 78.4% (n = 14,583) of *T. canis* genes were annotated, revealing at least 127 GTPases, 268 ion channels, 273 receptors, 355 transcription factors, 373 peptidases, 408 phosphatases, 458 kinases, 530 transporters and 870 *T. canis* excretory and secretory (TES) proteins (Gasser et al., 2016; Zhu et al., 2015).

Kong et al. (2016) found that 72.47% ($n=16{,}203$) predicted genes of *T. canis* had a homologue either in *A. suum* ($n=14{,}620$; 65.3%), *B. malayi* ($n=12{,}454$; 55.7%), *C. elegans* ($n=12{,}476$; 55.8%), or *Trichinella spiralis* ($n=10{,}042$; 44.9%), as well as, a total of 8798 protein sequences that were mutual among all 5 species and 6155 protein sequences that were exclusive for *T. canis*. 2299 domains were found from 22,358 protein sequences and the correlation coefficient between *T. canis* and *C. elegans* was 0.6984, but it was 0.917 between *T. canis* and *A. suum* utilizing the upper 50 domains (Kong et al., 2016). There are 127 enzymes-related KEGG pathway in *T. canis*, including the mucin type O-glycan biosynthesis pathway that is a common pathway in nematodes (Staudacher, 2015). Proteins sequences for T-cell and B-cell regulation (e.g. E3 ubiquitin-protein ligase cbl-b and antigen T-cell receptor, zeta chain) and protective against stress (HSP 70, HSP 90, macrophage migration inhibitory factor and superkiller viralicidic activity 2-like 2) were found (Kong et al., 2016). The new genes of endoprotease bli-4, cuticle collagen domain protein and cuticle protein isoform b-like were identified, which are components of cuticle (Kong et al., 2016; Page et al., 2014). Mucin protein coding sequence of mucin 12Ea and polymorphic mucin variant C6/1/40r2.1 were also found (Kong et al., 2016), which may protect the intestinal mucosa epithelial cells of *T. canis* by forming its mucoid coat. Ryanodine receptor calcium release channels and tropomodulin-family proteins were identified (Kong et al., 2016), which may participate in the migration of *T. canis* in hosts by contributing to muscle contraction of *T. canis*.

3. Transcriptomics

3.1 Analysis of neurotoxocarosis in mice caused by *T. canis* and *T. cati* infection by microarray gene expression

Janecek et al. (2015) discovered 2304 differentially transcribed genes (DTGs) from cerebra and 1954 DTGs from cerebella in female mice at 42 days after *T. canis* infection, revealing larger alterations in cerebra than that in cerebella infected with *T. canis*. Only 113 DTGs were identified from cerebra and 760 DTGs were detected from cerebella in female mice at 42 days after *T. cati* infection, showing greater alterations in cerebella than that in cerebra infected with *T. cati*. These results once again confirmed previous research that *T. canis* prefer to settle in cerebrum; while *T. cati* larvae prefer to settle in cerebellum at 42 days post infection (Janecek et al., 2014).

No significantly enriched biological modules were clustered based on up-regulated DTGs in cerebra infected with *T. cati*; whereas, up-regulated DTGs in cerebella infected with *T. cati*, as well as in cerebra and cerebella infected with *T. canis*, were predominantly classified to immune and defence responses, especially "defence/inflammatory response" (Janecek et al., 2015), by which hosts could resist larvae infection. The host reactions mediated by *T. cati* larvae infection seemed to be weaker, which may due to fewer *T. cati* larvae reaching the brain, especially the murine cerebrum (Janecek et al., 2014). For down-regulated DTGs, they mainly related to "sensory organ development" in cerebra infected with *T. cati*; whereas, it is remarkable that the DTGs were associated with "lipid/cholesterol biosynthetic process" in cerebra and cerebella infected with *T. canis* (Janecek et al., 2015).

The brain cholesterol plays an important role in the myelin sheaths of neurons, and the alterations in the myelin membrane can cause neurodegeneration (Bjorkhem and Meaney, 2004). The nerve fibre demyelination and the neurological symptoms could be due to the disturbances of cholesterol concentration or the down-regulation of key genes of cholesterol synthesis caused by strong influence of signal transduction in *T. canis* infection (Bjorkhem and Meaney, 2004; Epe et al., 1994). The up-regulation of apolipoprotein D has been found in patients with schizophrenia or Alzheimer's disease (AD) in the dorsolateral prefrontal cortex and in rodents after traumatic brain injury (Janecek et al., 2015). The up-regulation of apolipoproteins, such as apolipoprotein D, identified from mice cerebra and cerebella after *T. canis* infection (Janecek et al., 2015), may play an important role in lipid biosynthetic pathways.

No gene was enriched in "cholesterol synthesis" in cerebra or cerebella infected with *T. cati*, and down-regulated DTGs were associated with "sensory organ development" in cerebra and "regulation of transcription" in cerebella (Janecek et al., 2015). Enrichment score of "axonogenesis" was lower in cerebella with only three genes (Isl2, Myh10 and Hoxa1) (Janecek et al., 2015), indicating a less important role in pathogenesis. Among them, the down-regulation of Myh10, which is a biomarker for AD, can cause change of the subcellular localization of amyloid precursor protein (APP) (Massone et al., 2007).

3.2 mRNA expression of *T. canis*

3.2.1 Analysis of gene expression by expressed sequence tags (ESTs)

Before the NGS strategy was applied in *Toxocara*, gene expression of *T. canis* has been explored by EST strategy (Kim et al., 2013; Tetteh et al., 1999; Zhou et al., 2011).

Tetteh et al. (1999) sequenced 261 clones from the arrested stage larvae cultured *in vitro* for 6 months, which identified 128 distinct gene products with only three known genes of *T. canis* (including 60S ribosomal protein L3, mucin 1 and phosphatidylethanolamine-binding protein) and 47 novel genes. The abundant transcripts that had homologues were discussed, such as C-type lectin (TES-32), mucin 1 (TES-120), phosphatidylethanolamine-binding protein (TES-26), protein synthesis and modification factors, glycolysis, respiration, and other metabolic enzymes. Tetteh et al. (1999) found that there were relatively few housekeeping genes and no genes related to cell replication or reproduction, showing a pattern that was consistent with the developmental arrest of *T. canis*. This study was the first attempt toward a comprehensive gene catalogue of *T. canis*, providing a springboard for subsequent researches.

Zhou et al. (2011) sequenced 218 clones from adult female *T. canis*, obtaining 215 high-quality ESTs and 79 unigenes. Among the 79 unigenes, 77.22% had a homologue in the NR protein database, with 52 "known genes", 4 "putative genes" and 5 "unknown genes". Among the 215 high-quality ESTs, 34.42% ($n=74$) participated in cell defence/immunity, 13.95% ($n=30$) participated in metabolism, 6.98% ($n=15$) participated in cell signalling/communication, 3.26% ($n=7$) participated in cell structure, and 2.79% ($n=6$) participated in reproduction. Zhou et al. (2011) identified 19 immune-related genes from 73 ESTs, such as immunosuppressive ovarian message (IOM) protein, C-type lectin and lysozyme. Among them, IOM protein with 32 ESTs were the largest group in *T. canis*. The domains of chitin-binding domain type 2 (ChtBD2), C-type lectin or carbohydrate-recognition (CLECT), papain family cysteine protease (Pept_C1) and von Willebrand factor type A (VWA) were predicted in some immune-related unigenes by SMART (Zhou et al., 2011).

Kim et al. (2013) sequenced 7949 clones from adult female *T. canis,* obtaining 808 contigs and 1262 singletons. They found that *T. canis* was quite similar to some parasitic nematodes by gene functional annotation analysis, such as *T. leonine*, but different from the free-living nematode *C. elegans*. In cellular component category, the genes number of *T. canis* localized in "cells" and "organelle" were more than that in *C. elegans*, but it was opposite in "membrane". In the biological process category, the number of *T. canis* genes localized in "cellular process", "developmental process", "metabolic process" and "multicellular organismal process" were more than that in *C. elegans*, but it was the opposite in "single-organism process category". In the molecular function category, the number of *T. canis* genes localized in "binding", "catalytic activity proteins" and "structural molecule activity" were more than that in *C. elegans*, but it was the opposite in "electron carrier activity", suggesting that *T. canis* have a simpler metabolic system than free-living nematodes (Kim et al., 2013).

3.2.2 Analysis of mRNA expression by RNA-seq

Zhu et al. (2015) identified the gut-, stage- and gender-enriched mRNA profiles of *T. canis* by RNA-seq. Genes of the intestinal tract were related to fatty acid elongation, molecular uptake, and degradation through lysosomes, protein digestion, the metabolism of xenobiotic metabolism, as well as the transportation of amino acids, drugs, lipids and sugars, which are associated with the functions of digestion, absorption and detoxification in the gut of *T. canis*.

Compared with the L3 of *T. canis*, the pathways of ABC transporters, carbon metabolism, lysosome activity, xenobiotic metabolism, and DNA replication/repair were enriched in the adult stage of *T. canis* (Zhu et al., 2015), probably linking to the processes of digestion and reproduction. Meanwhile, the pathways of cuticle formation and/or shedding and neuronal signalling were mainly enriched in the L3 stage, including col-121, dpy-5 and sqt-1 (Abete-Luzi and Eisenmann, 2018; Peixoto et al., 2000; Thacker et al., 2006). The homologue genes which were associated with regulating dauer-like signalling pathway were up-regulated (such as daf-9, daf-12, osm-3 and osm-6) or down-regulated (two paralogs of mek-2) in L3s (Crook, 2014; Daniels et al., 2000), which supported the hypothesis that L3s can become "dauer larvae" in tissue granulomas and culture medium.

Zhu et al. (2015) identified 3760 genes in female and male adult *T. canis*, with 26% having no homologues in any other organisms. In female adult *T. canis*, the genes of signal transduction pathways were found, mainly involved in acetylcholine receptors, neuroactive GABA glycine, and G protein-coupled receptors linked to embryogenesis and germ cell proliferation (Zhu et al., 2015). Moreover, genes that linked to egg laying, eggshell synthesis in oogenesis, oocyte maturation and embryonic development, and vulva development, were identified in female adults of *T. canis* (Zhu et al., 2015). In male adult *T. canis*, the genes inferred to be associated with energy metabolism, epinephrine-like hormone regulation (octopamine and tyramine), protein degradation and spermatogenesis were identified (Zhu et al., 2015). The genes of proteasome-related enzyme groups and kinases were identified in male adult *T. canis*, such as protein-serine/threonine and -tyrosine kinases that were linked to sperm and spermatogenesis. Genes linked to the 26S proteasome and recycling of ubiquitin moieties were identified in male-enriched profiles, which participate in the germline development and spermatogenesis of *T. canis* (Zhu et al., 2015).

Zhou et al. (2017) analyzed the mRNA profiles in female and male adult *T. canis* by RNA-seq, showing 321 exclusively transcribed genes in female *T. canis* and 1467 exclusively transcribed genes in male *T. canis*, of which 26 and 90 genes may participate in reproductive processes, such as gamete generation, germ cell development and mating. A total of 51 and 145 up-regulated mRNAs were identified in female and male *T. canis*, respectively, which participated in the embryonic morphogenesis and development, moulting and nematode development (Zhou et al., 2017). ALG-1 was identified, which participate in miRNA silencing pathway (Kotagama et al., 2019). Nine genes (ALG-5, ALG-6, CSR-1, NRDE-3, RdRP-1, RdRP-3, WAGO-1, WAGO-2 and WAGO-3) were predicted to participate in *endo*-siRNAs pathways by homology searching (Zhou et al., 2017). However, 43 essential effector genes were found to be associated with the RNAi pathway in the study of Zhu et al. (2015). The absence of PIWI-related proteins, such as argonaute proteins, verified that no gene was involved in piRNA pathways in *T. canis*, which is unambiguously supported in other clade III parasites (Hoogstrate et al., 2014; Sarkies et al., 2015; Wang et al., 2011).

3.2.3 Analysis of microRNA expression by RNA-seq

Ma et al. (2016) identified 560 (555 known and 5 novel) and 619 (617 known and 2 novel) miRNAs by RNA-seq in male and female adult *T. canis*, respectively. Among all known miRNAs in male *T. canis*, miR-51-3p and miR-3070-2-3p had higher expression with more than a million reads, whereas, miR-279b-3p (451,632 reads), miR-71c-5p (340,196 reads), miR-71 (339,285 reads) and miR-265 (231,054 reads) had higher expression in the female *T. canis*. In addition, all novel miRNAs in male and female *T. canis* had lower expression, with the exception of novel_Tc-miR-47 (with 5888 reads) in the male *T. canis*. No piRNA sequence was found in both male and female *T. canis* (Ma et al., 2016).

Ma et al. (2016) found that 218 and 255 of those identified miRNAs were exclusively expressed in male and female adult *T. canis*, respectively. Among them, 213 known and 5 novel miRNAs can target 10,815 and 44 genes in male *T. canis*, respectively, which could participate in the biological processes of embryonic morphogenesis and hemidesmosome assembly, as well as the pathways of adherens junction, biotin metabolism, basal transcription factors, focal adhesion, protein digestion/absorption, proteasome, spliceosomes, ribosome, the PI3K/Akt signalling and ubiquitin-mediated proteolysis, moreover, 223 known and 2 novel miRNAs can target 9076 and 73 genes in the female, respectively, which could be associated with the processes of embryonic morphogenesis, regulation of cell division, hemidesmosome assembly, RNA polyadenylation and nucleus organization, and the pathways of biotin metabolism, proteasome and spliceosomes (Ma et al., 2016).

A total of 52 differentially expressed miRNAs participate in developmental and reproductive processes by GO annotation analysis, among which, miR-2305 and miR-6090 were associated with meiosis and the development of embryos/larvae (Ma et al., 2016). 60 miRNAs may participate in immune responses in the host, as well as mucin type O-glycan biosynthesis and vesicular transport in *T. canis* (Staudacher, 2015). 42 miRNAs were considered to be excreted or secreted by *T. canis* larvae, which could participate in the interaction between *T. canis* and the hosts by modulating host immune-related genes, such as lectins, mucins and other enzymes (Buck et al., 2014; Maizels, 2013; Twu and Johnson, 2014; Zheng et al., 2013).

35 miRNAs were predicted to target cytochrome P450, ABC transporter and multidrug resistance-associated protein genes, which could regulate drug target genes and/or drug resistance (Britton et al., 2014; Devaney et al., 2010; Lalaouna et al., 2014); however, no miRNA was associated with nicotinic acetylcholine receptors genes, ligand-gated ion channels genes or P-glycoprotein-encoding genes that play important roles in anthelminthic resistance (Prichard and Roulet, 2007; Rao et al., 2009; Williamson et al., 2009). In addition, 83 miRNAs may participate in ion channels, kinases, receptors, signalling molecules and transcription factors, suggesting that these miRNAs could be linked to the pathway of basal calcium signalling and the phosphatidylinositol signalling system in *T. canis* (Ma et al., 2016).

4. Proteomics

4.1 Analysis of excretory and secretory (ES) proteins of *Toxocara canis* larvae by LC-MS/MS

Sperotto et al. (2017) identified 19 ES proteins from the *T. canis* larvae by LC-MS/MS utilizing stained bands. Among them, six were 26-kDa secreted antigens. TES-32 was the glycosylated protein primarily released by *T. canis* cultivated *in vitro*, with a carbohydrate recognition domain that is similar to that of mammalian cells (Loukas et al., 1999). TES-32 can inhibit host immune responses by competitive inhibition of lectin to interfere with adhesion and cell signalling during inflammatory processes in hosts infected with parasites (Loukas et al., 2000). TES-120 can help *T. canis* in defence against the cellular immune system of hosts (Maizels, 2007; Maizels et al., 1993). The majority of the 19 proteins were enriched in binding functions, such as organic cyclic compound binding, inorganic ion binding and protein binding (Sperotto et al., 2017).

da Silva et al. (2018) discovered 64 ES proteins from the *T. canis* larvae by LC-MS/MS. Among them, TES-26, a homologue to the phosphatidylethanolamine-binding protein family, is anchored in the plasma membrane and participate in the transport of cell signalling and lipids (Gems et al., 1995; Maizels et al., 2000). This protein may participate in the interaction between the parasite and Toll-like receptors of APCs (da Silva et al., 2018). Recombinant TES-26 is a potential diagnostic candidate antigen for human toxocariasis (Varghese et al., 2017). Zhu et al. (2015) predicted that there are at least 14 peptidases in *T. canis* ES proteins, which participate in tissue degradation, migration and immune evasion/modulation, and have the potential to become targets for vaccines or drugs. But these proteins were not found in ES proteins of *T. canis* larvae in the two proteomics studies (da Silva et al., 2018; Sperotto et al., 2017).

4.2 Analysis of somatic proteins of *Toxocara canis* larvae by LC-MS/MS

da Silva et al. (2018) identified 582 larval extract proteins by LC-MS/MS, such as calreticulin, cystatin, arginase and cathepsins-B, -L, -Z with the function of immunoregulation. Cathepsins can play roles in regulating host immunity, causing the proteolytic degradation of MHC-II invariant chain (Williamson et al., 2003). Allergenic proteins (polyprotein ABA-1 and OV-17), HSPs (HSP β-1, HSP-12.2, HSP 70, HSP 75 KDa and HSP 90-α), superoxide dismutase and galectin were identified in the larval extract (da Silva et al., 2018). HSPs are important immunomodulatory molecules that play crucial roles in parasite survival (Perez-Morales and Espinoza, 2015). Proteins that participate in energy metabolism process were identified (e.g. 2,3 bisphosphoglycerate, glucose-6-phosphate, hexokinase, phosphoenolpyruvate carboxykinase and phosphoglycerate mutase activity), which contribute to the mechanisms of migration, evasion and survival of *T. canis* in the host (da Silva et al., 2018). Some calcium-binding proteins were also identified, such as calreticulin, annexin, calumenin-A and calnexin, which were also described in the study of Zhu et al. (2015). Helminth annexins are important in the regulation of coagulation, inflammation and intracellular calcium signalling, as well as, in the formation and regulation of ion channels (Cross et al., 2016; Hofmann et al., 2010), thus, annexins are valuable vaccine candidates for preventing *Toxocara* infections. Calreticulins help parasites evade hosts' immune response by participate in cellular Ca^{2+} homeostasis and immune regulation, binding to C1q and inactivating lysis mediated by the classical complement pathway (Ferreira et al., 2004). Some metallopeptidases, such as neprilysin, aminopeptidase, macrophage migration inhibitory factor-like protein, neuroserpin and leukotriene, were identified in the larval extract (da Silva et al., 2018).

da Silva et al. (2018) identified macrophage migration inhibitory factor (MIF)-like protein in both ES proteins and larval extract proteins, which mediates innate and adaptive immune responses and can control the inflammatory response and decrease the production of IL-1β, IL-12p40 and TNF-α (Park et al., 2009; Stavitsky et al., 2003; Wang et al., 2017b). A recent study has shown that recombination Tg-MIF protein is a potential vaccine candidate against toxoplasmosis (Liu et al., 2019). Transthyretin-like protein 46 was found in both ES proteins and larval extract proteins (da Silva et al., 2018), which contributes to the transport of vitamin A and retinoic acid in parasites (Eneqvist et al., 2003; Vercauteren et al., 2003). C-Type lectins were identified in both ES proteins and larval extract proteins of *T. canis* (da Silva et al., 2018). Galectin is another kind of lectin found in both ES proteins and larval extract proteins of *T. canis* and many other nematodes, which can control cell adhesion and modulate cellular immune response, and participate in apoptosis, immune regulation, inflammatory reaction and tumour genesis (Turner et al., 2008).

Superoxide dismutase (in ES proteins and larval extract proteins) and glutathione s-transferase (in larval extract proteins) were found on the *T. canis* surface (da Silva et al., 2018), which contribute to *T. canis* escaping from the host immune responses and neutralizes attack by reactive oxygen species (Joachim and Ruttkowski, 2011; Zelck and Von Janowsky, 2004).

Serine/threonine protein kinase and protein-tyrosine phosphatase were also identified in larval extract proteins (da Silva et al., 2018), which was consistent with previous studies (Ma et al., 2014; Zhu et al., 2015). These enzymes were associated with apoptosis, cell division, exocytosis, neurological activity, cell signalling, ion channel electrophysiology and signal transduction receptors (Forrester et al., 2004; Hoppe et al., 2010;

Hu et al., 2007; Klumpp and Krieglstein, 2002). Serine/threonine protein kinase participates in reproduction by regulating spermatogenesis, and it may be a novel target for drugs and vaccines against *T. canis* (Ma et al., 2015).

5. Conclusions and future perspective

5.1 Research status of *Toxocara* "omics"

The progress of genomic exploration provided critical resources for deciphering *Toxocara* from global molecular level; transcriptomics and proteomics analyses have identified many genes and proteins that participate in the development of the parasite and the interaction of *Toxocara*-hosts; microarray gene expression analysis has revealed major differences in neurotoxocarosis caused by *T. canis* and *T. cati*, providing a promising foundation to evaluate the particular pathogenetic mechanisms and to discover possible therapeutic targets. Bioinformatics analyses based on these "omics" have provided opportunities to explore the CAP proteins in *T. canis* and discover new interventions against toxocariasis (Stroehlein et al., 2016), and have also revealed specific dauer-like signalling pathway components that regulate the development and migration of *T. canis* in the mammalian host (Ma et al., 2019b). The genes acquired by "omics" have been further explored by RNAi, such as serine/threonine protein phosphatase 1 and Aquaporin 1 (Ma et al., 2015, 2019a). These studies can provide better understanding of the development, metabolism and heredity of *Toxocara*, and can identify many valuable genes and proteins that will contribute to new progress in the application areas of drugs, vaccines and diagnostic tool.

5.2 Prospects of the application of new technologies in *Toxocara* research

An important objective of biological research is to elucidate the particular functions of genes in the growth, development and disease of organisms. CRISPR/Cas9 technology, as the most effective method of gene editing, was first applied to *C. elegans* in 2013, and since then, the targeting efficiency has been continuously enhanced (Au et al., 2019). The combination of genome-wide CRISPR/Cas9 screening and NGS have been applied to human cells and *Toxoplasma gondii*, which can contribute to rapidly identify genes in a variety of biological processes and enable the explorations of metabolic needs, drug-resistance mechanisms, and host specificity of pathogens. The development and application of CRISPR/Cas9 in *Toxocara* can quickly and accurately explore the biological functions of genes identified by "omics" and will certainly bring the *Toxocara* research to a higher level. Stage-specific post-translational modification and DNA methylation can provide insight into the features and regulatory factors in *Toxocara* development. The researches of interaction between *Toxocara* and hosts based on the "omics" can directly explore the influence and mechanism of host immunity and inflammatory response against *Toxocara*, as well as the development and immune evasion mechanism of *Toxocara* in the host.

5.3 Challenges and inadequacies of *Toxocara* research

For *Toxocara*, (i) the biological functions of many genes and proteins still remain unknown, especially those genes that do not have homology; (ii) the research mainly focuses on the L3s and adults of *Toxocara*, with little attention to the L4s; (iii) *Toxocara* has not yet been shown to develop from larva to adult within *in vitro* cultures, so, the culture methods need to be improved. For studying *Toxocara*-host interactions; (iv) the different migration of *Toxocara* in definitive and paratenic hosts is still not entirely clear. For disease diagnosis; (v) there are many similar proteins in different parasitic nematodes, so, misdiagnoses are common, especially in the case of serological diagnosis. *T. canis* and *T. cati* infections cannot be distinguished in the pig model by Western blotting using ES proteins, even under the ideal setting that the infection dose and infection time are known (Poulsen et al., 2015).

5.4 Future directions of *Toxocara* research

Soil-transmitted helminths (STHs) still threaten humans worldwide (Schulz et al., 2018). Although specific measures have been taken for controlling them, infections with STHs persist, with 1.79 billion, 1.65 billion and 1.5 billion people being infected in 2005, in 2015 and in 2018, respectively (GBD 2015 Disease and Injury Incidence and Prevalence Collaborators, 2016; World Health Organization, 2018). As one of the major STHs, tremendous advances made on the "omics" of *Toxocara* and the availability of massive "omics" data have provided solid foundation and invaluable resources for fundamental studies of the physiology, developmental biology, and pathogenesis of *Toxocara*, as well as the interaction between *Toxocara* and their hosts. Progress on *Toxocara* "omics" has also held promises for medicine and veterinary medicine, particularly in the areas of better diagnostic methods, effective vaccines, and effective drugs.

Acknowledgements

This work was supported by the Planned Programme of Hunan Province Science and Technology Innovation (grant no. 2018RS3085), the Elite Program of Chinese Academy of Agricultural Sciences and the Agricultural Science and Technology Innovation Program (ASTIP) (grant no. CAAS-ASTIP-2016-LVRI-03).

References

Abete-Luzi, P., Eisenmann, D.M., 2018. Regulation of *C. elegans* L4 cuticle collagen genes by the heterochronic protein LIN-29. Genesis 56, 1–8. https://doi.org/10.1002/dvg.23106.

Au, V., Li-Leger, E., Raymant, G., Flibotte, S., Chen, G., Martin, K., Fernando, L., Doell, C., Rosell, F.I., Wang, S., Edgley, M.L., Rougvie, A.E., Hutter, H., Moerman, D.G., 2019. CRISPR/Cas9 methodology for the generation of knockout deletions in *Caenorhabditis elegans*. G3 (Bethesda) 9, 135–144. https://doi.org/10.1534/g3.118.200778.

Bjorkhem, I., Meaney, S., 2004. Brain cholesterol: long secret life behind a barrier. Arterioscler. Thromb. Vasc. Biol. 24, 806–815. https://doi.org/10.1161/01.ATV.0000120374.59826.1b.

Bourgard, C., Albrecht, L., Kayano, A., Sunnerhagen, P., Costa, F.T.M., 2018. *Plasmodium vivax* biology: insights provided by genomics, transcriptomics and proteomics. Front. Cell. Infect. Microbiol. 8, 34. https://doi.org/10.3389/fcimb.2018.00034.

Britton, C., Winter, A.D., Gillan, V., Devaney, E., 2014. microRNAs of parasitic helminths—identification, characterization and potential as drug targets. Int. J. Parasitol. Drugs Drug Resist. 24, 85–94. https://doi.org/10.1016/j.ijpddr.2014.03.001.

Buck, A.H., Coakley, G., Simbari, F., McSorley, H.J., Quintana, J.F., Le Bihan, T., Kumar, S., Abreu-Goodger, C., Lear, M., Harcus, Y., Ceroni, A., Babayan, S.A., Blaxter, M., Ivens, A., Maizels, R.M., 2014. Exosomes secreted by nematode parasites transfer small RNAs to mammalian cells and modulate innate immunity. Nat. Commun. 5, 5488. https://doi.org/10.1038/ncomms6488.

Chen, J., Liu, Q., Liu, G.H., Zheng, W.B., Hong, S.J., Sugiyama, H., Zhu, X.Q., Elsheikha, H.M., 2018. Toxocariasis: a silent threat with a progressive public health impact. Infect. Dis. Poverty 7, 59. https://doi.org/10.1186/s40249-018-0437-0.

Chuan, J., Feng, Z., Brindley, P.J., McManus, D.P., Han, Z., Jianxin, P., Hu, W., 2010. Our wormy world genomics, proteomics and transcriptomics in east and southeast Asia. Adv. Parasitol. 73, 327–371. https://doi.org/10.1016/s0065-308x(10)73011-6.

Crook, M., 2014. The dauer hypothesis and the evolution of parasitism: 20 years on and still going strong. Int. J. Parasitol. 44, 1–8. https://doi.org/10.1016/j.ijpara.2013.08.004.

Cross, M., Klepzig, E., Dallaston, M., Young, N.D., Bailey, U.M., Mason, L., Jones, M.K., Gasser, R.B., Hofmann, A., 2016. Exploring the molecular mechanisms of parasite-host interactions with a view towards new therapeutics and vaccines. Postepy Biochem. 62, 370–376.

Cwiklinski, K., Dalton, J.P., 2018. Advances in *fasciola hepatica* research using 'omics' technologies. Int. J. Parasitol. 48, 321–331. https://doi.org/10.1016/j.ijpara.2017.12.001.

da Silva, M.B., Urrego, A.J., Oviedo, Y., Cooper, P.J., Pacheco, L.G.C., Pinheiro, C.S., Ferreira, F., Briza, P., Alcantara-Neves, N.M., 2018. The somatic proteins of *Toxocara canis* larvae and excretory-secretory products revealed by proteomics. Vet. Parasitol. 259, 25–34. https://doi.org/10.1016/j.vetpar.2018.06.015.

Daniels, S.A., Ailion, M., Thomas, J.H., Sengupta, P., 2000. Egl-4 acts through a transforming growth factor-beta/SMAD pathway in *Caenorhabditis elegans* to regulate multiple neuronal circuits in response to sensory cues. Genetics 156, 123–141.

Devaney, E., Winter, A.D., Britton, C., 2010. microRNAs: a role in drug resistance in parasitic nematodes? Trends Parasitol. 26, 428–433. https://doi.org/10.1016/j.pt.2010.05.003.

Eneqvist, T., Lundberg, E., Nilsson, L., Abagyan, R., Sauer-Eriksson, A.E., 2003. The transthyretin-related protein family. Eur. J. Biochem. 270, 518–532. https://doi.org/10.1046/j.1432-1033.2003.03408.x.

Epe, C., Sabel, T., Schnieder, T., Stoye, M., 1994. The behavior and pathogenicity of *Toxocara canis* larvae in mice of different strains. Parasitol. Res. 80, 691–695. https://doi.org/10.1007/BF00932955.

Fakhri, Y., Gasser, R.B., Rostami, A., Fan, C.K., Ghasemi, S.M., Javanian, M., Bayani, M., Armoon, B., Moradi, B., 2018. *Toxocara* eggs in public places worldwide—a systematic review and meta-analysis. Environ. Pollut. 242, 1467–1475. https://doi.org/10.1016/j.envpol.2018.07.087.

Ferreira, V., Molina, M.C., Valck, C., Rojas, A., Aguilar, L., Ramírez, G., Schwaeble, W., Ferreira, A., 2004. Role of calreticulin from parasites in its interaction with vertebrate hosts. Mol. Immunol. 40, 1279–1291. https://doi.org/10.1016/j.molimm.2003.11.018.

Forrester, S.G., Warfel, P.W., Pearce, E.J., 2004. Tegumental expression of a novel type II receptor serine/threonine kinase (SmRK2) in *Schistosoma mansoni*. Mol. Biochem. Parasitol. 136, 149–156. https://doi.org/10.1016/j.molbiopara.2004.03.007.

Gasser, R.B., Korhonen, P.K., Zhu, X.Q., Young, N.D., 2016. Harnessing the *Toxocara* genome to underpin Toxocariasis research and new interventions. Adv. Parasitol. 91, 87–110. https://doi.org/10.1016/bs.apar.2015.12.001.

GBD 2015 Disease and Injury Incidence and Prevalence Collaborators, 2016. Global, regional, and national incidence, prevalence, and years lived with disability for 310 diseases and injuries, 1990–2015: a systematic analysis for the Global Burden of Disease Study 2015. Lancet 388, 1545–1602. https://doi.org/10.1016/S0140-6736(16)31678-6.

Gems, D., Ferguson, C.J., Robertson, B.D., Nieves, R., Page, A.P., Blaxter, M.L., Maizels, R.M., 1995. An abundant, trans-spliced mRNA from *Toxocara canis* infective larvae encodes a 26-kDa protein with homology to phosphatidylethanolamine-binding proteins. J. Biol. Chem. 270, 18517–18522. https://doi.org/10.1074/jbc.270.31.18517.

Hofmann, A., Osman, A., Leow, C.Y., Driguez, P., McManus, D.P., Jones, M.K., 2010. Parasite annexins—new molecules with potential for drug and vaccine development. Bioessays 32, 967–976. https://doi.org/10.1002/bies.200900195.

Hoogstrate, S.W., Volkers, R.J., Sterken, M.G., Kammenga, J.E., Snoek, L.B., 2014. Nematode endogenous small RNA pathways. Worm 3, e28234. https://doi.org/10.4161/worm.28234.

Hoppe, P.E., Chau, J., Flanagan, K.A., Reedy, A.R., Schriefer, L.A., 2010. *Caenorhabditis elegans* unc-82 encodes a serine/threonine kinase important for myosin filament organization in muscle during growth. Genetics 184, 79–90. https://doi.org/10.1534/genetics.109.110189.

Howe, K.L., Bolt, B.J., Cain, S., Chan, J., Chen, W.J., Davis, P., Done, J., Down, T., Gao, S., Grove, C., Harris, T.W., Kishore, R., Lee, R., Lomax, J., Li, Y., Muller, H.M., Nakamura, C., Nuin, P., Paulini, M., Raciti, D., Schindelman, G., Stanley, E., Tuli, M.A., Van Auken, K., Wang, D., Wang, X., Williams, G., Wright, A., Yook, K., Berriman, M., Kersey, P., Schedl, T., Stein, L., Sternberg, P.W., 2016. WormBase 2016: expanding to enable helminth genomic research. Nucleic Acids Res. 44, D774–D780. https://doi.org/10.1093/nar/gkv1217.

Hu, M., Abs, E.L.O.Y.G., Campbell, B.E., Boag, P.R., Nisbet, A.J., Beveridge, I., Gasser, R.B., 2007. *Trichostrongylus vitrinus* (Nematoda: Strongylida): molecular characterization and transcriptional analysis of Tv-stp-1, a serine/threonine phosphatase gene. Exp. Parasitol. 117, 22–34. https://doi.org/10.1016/j.exppara.2007.03.008.

International Helminth Genomes Consortium, 2019. Comparative genomics of the major parasitic worms. Nat. Genet. 51, 163–174. https://doi.org/10.1038/s41588-018-0262-1.

Janecek, E., Beineke, A., Schnieder, T., Strube, C., 2014. Neurotoxocarosis: marked preference of *Toxocara canis* for the cerebrum and *T. cati* for the cerebellum in the paratenic model host mouse. Parasit. Vectors 7, 194. https://doi.org/10.1186/1756-3305-7-194.

Janecek, E., Wilk, E., Schughart, K., Geffers, R., Strube, C., 2015. Microarray gene expression analysis reveals major differences between *Toxocara canis* and *Toxocara cati* neurotoxocarosis and involvement of *T. canis* in lipid biosynthetic processes. Int. J. Parasitol. 45, 495–503. https://doi.org/10.1016/j.ijpara.2015.02.009.

Jex, A.R., Liu, S., Li, B., Young, N.D., Hall, R.S., Li, Y., Yang, L., Zeng, N., Xu, X., Xiong, Z., Chen, F., Wu, X., Zhang, G., Fang, X., Kang, Y., Anderson, G.A., Harris, T.W., Campbell, B.E., Vlaminck, J., Wang, T., Cantacessi, C., Schwarz, E.M., Ranganathan, S., Geldhof, P., Nejsum, P., Sternberg, P.W., Yang, H., Wang, J., Wang, J., Gasser, R.B., 2011. *Ascaris suum* draft genome. Nature 479, 529–533. https://doi.org/10.1038/nature10553.

Joachim, A., Ruttkowski, B., 2011. Prostaglandin D (2) synthesis in *Oesophagostomum dentatum* is mediated by cytosolic glutathione S-transferase. Exp. Parasitol. 127, 604–606. https://doi.org/10.1016/j.exppara.2010.10.020.

Kim, K.U., Park, S.K., Kang, S.A., Park, M.K., Cho, M.K., Jung, H.J., Kim, K.Y., Yu, H.S., 2013. Comparison of functional gene annotation of *Toxascaris leonina* and *Toxocara canis* using CLC genomics workbench. Korean J. Parasitol. 51, 525–530. https://doi.org/10.3347/kjp.2013.51.5.525.

Klumpp, S., Krieglstein, J., 2002. Serine/threonine protein phosphatases in apoptosis. Curr. Opin. Pharmacol. 2, 458–462. https://doi.org/10.1016/S1471-4892(02)00176-5.

Kong, J., Won, J., Yoon, J., Lee, U., Kim, J.I., Huh, S., 2016. Draft genome of *Toxocara canis*, a pathogen responsible for visceral larva migrans. Korean J. Parasitol. 54, 751–758. https://doi.org/10.3347/kjp.2016.54.6.751.

Kotagama, K., Schorr, A.L., Steber, H.S., Mangone, M., 2019. ALG-1 influences accurate mRNA splicing patterns in the *Caenorhabditis elegans* intestine and body muscle tissues by modulating splicing factor activities. Genetics 212, 931–951. https://doi.org/10.1534/genetics.119.302223.

Lalaouna, D., Eyraud, A., Chabelskaya, S., Felden, B., Massé, E., 2014. Regulatory RNAs involved in bacterial antibiotic resistance. PLoS Pathog. 28, e1004299. https://doi.org/10.1371/journal.ppat.1004299.

Liu, K., Wen, H., Cai, H., Wu, M., An, R., Chu, D., Yu, L., Shen, J., Chen, L., Du, J., 2019. Protective effect against toxoplasmosis in BALB/c mice vaccinated with *Toxoplasma gondii* macrophage migration inhibitory factor. Front. Microbiol. 10, 813. https://doi.org/10.3389/fmicb.2019.00813.

Loukas, A., Mullin, N.P., Tetteh, K.K., Moens, L., Maizels, R.M., 1999. A novel C-type lectin secreted by a tissue-dwelling parasitic nematode. Curr. Biol. 9, 825–828. https://doi.org/10.1016/s0960-9822(99)80366-2.

Loukas, A., Doedens, A., Hintz, M., Maizels, R.M., 2000. Identification of a new C-type lectin, TES-70, secreted by infective larvae of *Toxocara canis*, which binds to host ligands. Parasitology 121, 545–554. https://doi.org/10.1017/s0031182099006721.

Ma, G.X., Zhou, R.Q., Hu, S.J., Huang, H.C., Zhu, T., Xia, Q.Y., 2014. Molecular characterization and functional analysis of serine/threonine protein phosphatase of *Toxocara canis*. Exp. Parasitol. 141, 55–61. https://doi.org/10.1016/j.exppara.2014.03.019.

Ma, G.X., Zhou, R.Q., Song, Z.H., Zhu, H.H., Zhou, Z.Y., Zeng, Y.Q., 2015. Molecular mechanism of serine/threonine protein phosphatase 1 (PP1cα-PP1r7) in spermatogenesis of *Toxocara canis*. Acta Trop. 149, 148–154. https://doi.org/10.1016/j.actatropica.2015.05.026.

Ma, G., Luo, Y., Zhu, H., Luo, Y., Korhonen, P.K., Young, N.D., Gasser, R.B., Zhou, R., 2016. MicroRNAs of *Toxocara canis* and their predicted functional roles. Parasit. Vectors 9, 229. https://doi.org/10.1186/s13071-016-1508-3.

Ma, G., Holland, C.V., Wang, T., Hofmann, A., Fan, C.K., Maizels, R.M., Hotez, P.J., Gasser, R.B., 2018. Human toxocariasis. Lancet Infect. Dis. 18, e14–e24. https://doi.org/10.1016/s1473-3099(17)30331-6.

Ma, G., Jiang, A., Luo, Y., Luo, Y., Huang, H., Zhou, R., 2019a. Aquaporin 1 is located on the intestinal basolateral membrane in *Toxocara canis* and might play a role in drug uptake. Parasit. Vectors 12, 243. https://doi.org/10.1186/s13071-019-3500-1.

Ma, G., Wang, T., Korhonen, P.K., Nie, S., Reid, G.E., Stroehlein, A.J., Koehler, A.V., Chang, B.C.H., Hofmann, A., Young, N.D., Gasser, R.B., 2019b. Comparative bioinformatic analysis suggests that specific dauer-like signalling pathway components regulate *Toxocara canis* development and migration in the mammalian host. Parasit. Vectors 12, 32. https://doi.org/10.1186/s13071-018-3265-y.

Maizels, R., 2007. Regulation of the immune system in metazoan parasite infections. Novartis Found. Symp. 281, 192. https://doi.org/10.1002/9780470062128.ch16.

Maizels, R.M., 2013. *Toxocara canis*: molecular basis of immune recognition and evasion. Vet. Parasitol. 193, 365–374. https://doi.org/10.1016/j.vetpar.2012.12.032.

Maizels, R.M., Bundy, D.A., Selkirk, M.E., Smith, D.F., Anderson, R.M., 1993. Immunological modulation and evasion by helminth parasites in human populations. Nature 365, 797–805. https://doi.org/10.1038/365797a0.

Maizels, R.M., Tetteh, K.K., Loukas, A., 2000. *Toxocara canis*: genes expressed by the arrested infective larval stage of a parasitic nematode. Int. J. Parasitol. 30, 495–508. https://doi.org/10.1016/s0020-7519(00)00022-9.

Massone, S., Argellati, F., Passalacqua, M., Armirotti, A., Melone, L., d'Abramo, C., Marinari, U.M., Domenicotti, C., Pronzato, M.A., Ricciarelli, R., 2007. Downregulation of myosin II-B by siRNA alters the subcellular localization of the amyloid precursor protein and increases amyloid-beta deposition in N2a cells. Biochem. Biophys. Res. Commun. 362, 633–638. https://doi.org/10.1016/j.bbrc.2007.08.061.

Page, A.P., Stepek, G., Winter, A.D., Pertab, D., 2014. Enzymology of the nematode cuticle: a potential drug target? Int. J. Parasitol. Drugs Drug Resist. 4, 133–141. https://doi.org/10.1016/j.ijpddr.2014.05.003.

Park, S.K., Cho, M.K., Park, H.K., Lee, K.H., Lee, S.J., Choi, S.H., Ock, M.S., Jeong, H.J., Lee, M.H., Yu, H.S., 2009. Macrophage migration inhibitory factor homologs of anisakis simplex suppress Th2 response in allergic airway inflammation model via CD4+CD25+Foxp3+ T cell recruitment. J. Immunol. 182, 6907–6914. https://doi.org/10.4049/jimmunol.0803533.

Peixoto, C.A., Alves, L.C., de Melo, J.V., de Souza, W., 2000. Ultrastructural analyses of the *Caenorhabditis elegans* sqt-1(sc13) left roller mutant. J. Parasitol. 86, 269–274. https://doi.org/10.1645/0022-3395(2000)086[0269:uaotce]2.0.co;2.

Perez-Morales, D., Espinoza, B., 2015. The role of small heat shock proteins in parasites. Cell Stress Chaperones 20, 767–780. https://doi.org/10.1007/s12192-015-0607-y.

Poulsen, C.S., Skov, S., Yoshida, A., Skallerup, P., Maruyama, H., Thamsborg, S.M., Nejsum, P., 2015. Differential serodiagnostics of *Toxocara canis* and *Toxocara cati*—is it possible? Parasite Immunol. 37, 204–207. https://doi.org/10.1111/pim.12181.

Prichard, R.K., Roulet, A., 2007. ABC transporters and beta-tubulin in macrocyclic lactone resistance: prospects for marker development. Parasitology 134, 1123–1132. https://doi.org/10.1017/s0031182007000091.

Rao, V.T., Siddiqui, S.Z., Prichard, R.K., Forrester, S.G., 2009. A dopamine-gated ion channel (HcGGR3*) from *Haemonchus contortus* is expressed in the cervical papillae and is associated with macrocyclic lactone resistance. Mol. Biochem. Parasitol. 166, 54–61. https://doi.org/10.1016/j.molbiopara.2009.02.011.

Rostami, A., Ma, G., Wang, T., Koehler, A.V., Hofmann, A., Chang, B.C.H., Macpherson, C.N., Gasser, R.B., 2019. Human toxocariasis—a look at a neglected disease through an epidemiological 'prism. Infect. Genet. Evol. 74, 104002. https://doi.org/10.1016/j.meegid.2019.104002.

Sarkies, P., Selkirk, M.E., Jones, J.T., Blok, V., Boothby, T., Goldstein, B., Hanelt, B., Ardila-Garcia, A., Fast, N.M., Schiffer, P.M., Kraus, C., Taylor, M.J., Koutsovoulos, G., Blaxter, M.L., Miska, E.A., 2015. Ancient and novel small RNA pathways compensate for the loss of piRNAs in multiple independent nematode lineages. PLoS Biol. 13, e1002061. https://doi.org/10.1371/journal.pbio.1002061.

Schulz, J.D., Moser, W., Hurlimann, E., Keiser, J., 2018. Preventive chemotherapy in the fight against soil-transmitted helminthiasis: achievements and limitations. Trends Parasitol. 34, 590–602. https://doi.org/10.1016/j.pt.2018.04.008.

Sperotto, R.L., Kremer, F.S., Aires Berne, M.E., Costa de Avila, L.F., da Silva Pinto, L., Monteiro, K.M., Caumo, K.S., Ferreira, H.B., Berne, N., Borsuk, S., 2017. Proteomic analysis of *Toxocara canis* excretory and secretory (TES) proteins. Mol. Biochem. Parasitol. 211, 39–47. https://doi.org/10.1016/j.molbiopara.2016.09.002.

Staudacher, E., 2015. Mucin-type O-glycosylation in invertebrates. Molecules 20, 10622–10640. https://doi.org/10.3390/molecules200610622.

Stavitsky, A.B., Metz, C., Liu, S., Xianli, J., Bucala, R., 2003. Blockade of macrophage migration inhibitory factor (MIF) in *Schistosoma japonicum*-infected mice results in an increased adult worm burden and reduced fecundity. Parasite Immunol. 25, 369–374. https://doi.org/10.1046/j.1365-3024.2003.00641.x.

Stoltzfus, J.D., Pilgrim, A.A., Herbert, D.R., 2017. Perusal of parasitic nematode "omics" in the post-genomic era. Mol. Biochem. Parasitol. 215, 11–22. https://doi.org/10.1016/j.molbiopara.2016.11.003.

Stroehlein, A.J., Young, N.D., Hall, R.S., Korhonen, P.K., Hofmann, A., Sternberg, P.W., Jabbar, A., Gasser, R.B., 2016. CAP protein superfamily members in *Toxocara canis*. Parasit. Vectors 9, 360. https://doi.org/10.1186/s13071-016-1642-y.

Strube, C., Heuer, L., Janecek, E., 2013. *Toxocara* spp. infections in paratenic hosts. Vet. Parasitol. 193, 375–389. https://doi.org/10.1016/j.vetpar.2012.12.033.

Tetteh, K.K., Loukas, A., Tripp, C., Maizels, R.M., 1999. Identification of abundantly expressed novel and conserved genes from the infective larval stage of *Toxocara canis* by an expressed sequence tag strategy. Infect. Immun. 67, 4771–4779.

Thacker, C., Sheps, J.A., Rose, A.M., 2006. *Caenorhabditis elegans* dpy-5 is a cuticle procollagen processed by a proprotein convertase. Cell. Mol. Life Sci. 63, 1193–1204. https://doi.org/10.1007/s00018-006-6012-z.

Turner, D.G., Wildblood, L.A., Inglis, N.F., Jones, D.G., 2008. Characterization of a galectin-like activity from the parasitic nematode, *Haemonchus contortus*, which modulates ovine eosinophil migration in vitro. Vet. Immunol. Immunopathol. 122, 138–145. https://doi.org/10.1016/j.vetimm.2007.11.002.

Twu, O., Johnson, P.J., 2014. Parasite extracellular vesicles: mediators of intercellular communication. PLoS Pathog. 10, e1004289. https://doi.org/10.1371/journal.ppat.1004289.

Varghese, A., Raina, O.K., Chandra, D., Mirdha, B.R., Kelawala, N.H., Solanki, J.B., Kumar, N., Ravindran, R., Arun, A., Rialch, A., Lalrinkima, H., Kelawala, R.N., Samanta, S., 2017. Sero-detection of *Toxocara canis* infection in human with *T. canis* recombinant arginine kinase, cathepsin L-1 and TES-26 antigens. Acta Parasitol. 62, 775–778. https://doi.org/10.1515/ap-2017-0093.

Vercauteren, I., Geldhof, P., Peelaers, I., Claerebout, E., Berx, G., Vercruysse, J., 2003. Identification of excretory-secretory products of larval and adult *Ostertagia ostertagi* by immunoscreening of cDNA libraries. Mol. Biochem. Parasitol. 126, 201–208. https://doi.org/10.1016/s0166-6851(02)00274-8.

Wang, J., Czech, B., Crunk, A., Wallace, A., Mitreva, M., Hannon, G.J., Davis, R.E., 2011. Deep small RNA sequencing from the nematode *Ascaris* reveals conservation, functional diversification, and novel developmental profiles. Genome Res. 21, 1462–1477. https://doi.org/10.1101/gr.121426.111.

Wang, J., Gao, S., Mostovoy, Y., Kang, Y., Zagoskin, M., Sun, Y., Zhang, B., White, L.K., Easton, A., Nutman, T.B., Kwok, P.Y., Hu, S., Nielsen, M.K., Davis, R.E., 2017a. Comparative genome analysis of programmed DNA elimination in nematodes. Genome Res. 27, 2001–2014. https://doi.org/10.1101/gr.225730.117.

Wang, Y., Lu, M., Wang, S., Ehsan, M., Yan, R., Song, X., Xu, L., Li, X., 2017b. Characterization of a secreted macrophage migration inhibitory factor homologue of the parasitic nematode *Haemonchus contortus* acting at the parasite-host cell interface. Oncotarget 8, 40052–40064. https://doi.org/10.18632/oncotarget.16675.

Williamson, A.L., Brindley, P.J., Loukas, A., 2003. Hookworm cathepsin D aspartic proteases: contributing roles in the host-specific degradation of serum proteins and skin macromolecules. Parasitology 126, 179–185. https://doi.org/10.1017/s0031182002002706.

Williamson, S.M., Robertson, A.P., Brown, L., Williams, T., Woods, D.J., Martin, R.J., Sattelle, D.B., Wolstenholme, A.J., 2009. The nicotinic acetylcholine receptors of the parasitic nematode Ascaris suum: formation of two distinct drug targets by varying the relative expression levels of two subunits. PLoS Pathog. 5, e1000517. https://doi.org/10.1371/journal.ppat.1000517.

World Health Organization, 2018. Soil-transmitted helminth infections. http://www.who.int/news-room/fact-sheets/detail/soil-transmitted-helminth-infections.

Zelck, U.E., Von Janowsky, B., 2004. Antioxidant enzymes in intramolluscan *Schistosoma mansoni* and ROS-induced changes in expression. Parasitology 128, 493–501. https://doi.org/10.1017/s0031182004004895.

Zheng, Y., Cai, X., Bradley, J.E., 2013. MicroRNAs in parasites and parasite infection. RNA Biol. 10, 371–379. https://doi.org/10.4161/rna.23716.

Zhou, R., Xia, Q., Huang, H., Lai, M., Wang, Z., 2011. Construction of a cDNA library from female adult of *Toxocara canis*, and analysis of EST and immune-related genes expressions. Exp. Parasitol. 129, 120–126. https://doi.org/10.1016/j.exppara.2011.07.005.

Zhou, R.Q., Ma, G.X., Korhonen, P.K., Luo, Y.L., Zhu, H.H., Luo, Y.F., Gasser, R.B., Xia, Q.Y., 2017. Comparative transcriptomic analyses of male and female adult *Toxocara canis*. Gene 600, 85–89. https://doi.org/10.1016/j.gene.2016.11.024.

Zhu, X.Q., Korhonen, P.K., Cai, H., Young, N.D., Nejsum, P., von Samson-Himmelstjerna, G., Boag, P.R., Tan, P., Li, Q., Min, J., Yang, Y., Wang, X., Fang, X., Hall, R.S., Hofmann, A., Sternberg, P.W., Jex, A.R., Gasser, R.B., 2015. Genetic blueprint of the zoonotic pathogen *Toxocara canis*. Nat. Commun. 6, 6145. https://doi.org/10.1038/ncomms7145.

PART II

The effects of infection, host response to infection, diagnosis, and treatment of people

CHAPTER SIX

Toxocariasis and the clinical spectrum

H. Auer*, J. Walochnik
Medical Parasitology, Institute of Specific Prophylaxis and Tropical Medicine, Center of Pathophysiology, Infectiology and Immunology, Medical University Vienna, Vienna, Austria
*Corresponding author: e-mail address: herbert.auer@meduniwien.ac.at

Contents

Abstract

Toxocara canis and *T. cati* are among the most widely distributed helminthic species in the world with a high zoonotic impact. Millions of people are infected[a] and hundreds of thousands are suffering from toxocarosis, a disease encompassing four different entities: larva migrans visceralis (VLM) syndrome, ocular larva migrans (OLM) syndrome, covert toxocarosis (covT), common toxocarosis (comT) and neurotoxocarosis (NT). *Toxocara* infections in humans may remain clinically inapparent but may also induce severe diseases. This contribution gives a synoptic overview of the most important historical, clinical, diagnostic and therapeutical aspects of toxocarosis in humans.

[a] Due to the fact that *Toxocara* spp. do not multiply in humans (and also not in other non-natural hosts, e.g., poultry, rabbits), the correct terminology would be "infestation", but the term "infection" is so much more common in daily medical-linguistic usage, that it is also used throughout this contribution (Aspöck and Walochnik 2002).

Advances in Parasitology, Volume 109
ISSN 0065-308X
https://doi.org/10.1016/bs.apar.2020.01.005

1. Historical aspects

Roundworms as parasites of dogs and cats have been known to mankind presumably since the domestication of dogs and cats, 15,000–20,000 and 8000–10,000 years ago, respectively. They emerge in the scientific literature more than 200 years ago. The original description of *T. canis* dates back to 1782, when the German parasitologist, Paul Christian Friedrich Werner, described this parasite as *Lumbricus canis*. The Australian biologist and helminthologist Thomas Harvey Johnston eventually transferred it to the newly established genus *Toxocara* (in: Stiles, 1905), *T. cati* was originally described as *Ascaris cati* by the German botanist Franz de Paula von Schrank (1788) and assigned to the genus *Toxocara* by the French parasitologist Brumpt (1927). However, the medical relevance of *T. canis* was not recognized before the midst of the 20th century (Beaver et al., 1952), that of *T. cati* a few years later. Today, we also know other species of the family Ascarididae accidentally causing disease in humans: *Ascaris suum* (the large roundworm of pigs), *Baylisascaris procyonis* (the roundworm of the racoon, *Procyon lotor*) and *Lagochilascaris minor* (roundworm of various wild mammals). *Parascaris equorum* (the roundworm of horses and other equine mammals) (Coombs and Crompton, 1991), *Toxascaris leonina, Toxocara pteropodis* and *T. vitulorum,* formerly considered as human parasites, have been classified as unconfirmed human parasites by Ashford (2001) (Table 1).

Even though Chandler (1925), Fülleborn (1921), and Schwartz (1932) already mentioned migrating ascarid larvae in different human tissues during the first third of the 20th century, the presumably first human case of a larva migrans visceralis was described by Perlingiero and György (1947), when they took care of a 2-year-old boy suffering from fever, loss of weight, vomiting, coughing, diarrhoea, hepatomegaly and eosinophilia in the General Hospital of Philadelphia. The clinical status of the patient improved substantially after he had vomited an adult male *Ascaris lumbricoides*: Thus, the symptoms were attributed to this parasite. Five years later, Beaver et al. (1952) reported on three children suffering from hepatomegaly, anaemia and eosinophilia and as a *Toxocara canis* larva was detected in the liver biopsy of one of the children the disease was designated visceralis larva migrans-syndrome (VLM) (Nichols, 1956). Interestingly, the first case reports of putative *Toxocara cati* infections in humans date back more than 100 years earlier, namely to 1824 (Pickells, 1824) and 1839 (O'Brien, 1839), both from Ireland and to 1963 from England (Cobbold, 1863).

Table 1 Overview about the roundworm species (family Ascarididae) causing a larva migrans syndrome.

Species	Natural host	Geographic distribution	Form of disease	Organ involvement	Medical relevance	Author
Ascaris suum Goeze 1782	Pig	Worldwide	Visceral, cerebral	Liver, lung, CNS	Presumably millions of people infected worldwide and ten thousands suffering from Ascaris suum ascaridiosis (larva migrans syndrome)	Petithory et al. (1994), Izumikawa et al. (2011), and Schneider et al. (2015)
Baylisascaris procyonis (Stefanski and Zarnowski, 1951)	Racoon	Americas, Europe Asia	Visceral, neural, ocular (diffuse unilateral subacute neuroretinitis/DUSN)	Lung, CNS, eye	Very rare but associated with severe or fatal neurological disease	Gavin et al. (2005) and Kazacos et al. (2013)
Lagochilascaris minor Leiper, 1909	Wild mammals	Central, South America, Trinidad and Tobago	Cutaneous visceral, cerebral	Neck, middle ear, mastoid, tonsils, nasal sinuses, lungs, sacral region, eyeballs, dental alveoli, meninges	More than 100 cases registered worldwide	Aquino et al. (2018) and Campos et al. (2017)
Parascaris equorum (Goeze, 1782) Yorke & Maplestone, 1926	Equids	Worldwide	Visceral	Lung	Not confirmed	Coombs and Crompton (1991) and Ashford (2001)

Continued

Table 1 Overview about the roundworm species (family Ascarididae) causing a larva migrans syndrome.—cont'd

Species	Natural host	Geographic distribution	Form of disease	Organ involvement	Medical relevance	Author
Toxascaris leonina (von Linstow, 1902) Leiper, 1907	Felids, canids	Worldwide	Unknown	Adult worm detected in the small intestine of man	Not confirmed	Leiper (1907), Coombs and Crompton (1991), and Ashford (2001)
Toxocara canis (Werner, 1782) Johnston, 1916 *Toxocara cati* (Schrank, 1788) Brumpt, 1927	Canids, felids	Worldwide	Visceral, ocular, cerebral	Nearly all organs	Millions of people infected worldwide and thousands suffering from toxocarosis	Beaver et al. (1952), Wilder (1950), Glickman and Schantz (1981), Bass et al. (1983), Taylor et al. (1987), Magnaval et al. (1994), Magnaval et al. (2001a,b), Finsterer and Auer (2007), and Deshayes et al. (2016)
Toxocara pteropodis Baylis, 1936	Bats	Oceania	Visceral (?)	Unknown	Not confirmed	Prociv (1989), Coombs and Crompton (1991), and Ashford (2001)
Toxocara vitulorum (Goeze, 1782) Travassos, 1927	Ruminants	Worldwide	Visceral (?)	Unknown	Not confirmed	van Gorp et al. (1987), Coombs and Crompton (1991), and Ashford (2001)

Since Wilder (1950), we know a second clinical syndrome of human toxocarosis, the "Ocular Larva Migrans-Syndrome" (OLM): she discovered nematode larvae (hookworms) in 24 out of 46 enucleated eyes of children operated due to suspected retinoblastoma. In fact, in at least four of these 24 "retinoblastoma" eyes, stage 3 larvae of *T. canis* were identified retrospectively by the Institute of Pathology of the Walter Reed Army Medical Centre in Washington DC (Nichols, 1956).

In the 1950s, based on the seminal and, particularly experimental, studies by Beaver et al. (1952), Dent and Carrera (1953) and Nichols et al. (1956), the identification and differentiation of nematode larvae (*Toxocara, Ascaris,* hookworms) in human tissues (liver, lung, brain) reached a professional level and an essential improvement of species diagnosis. Also, in the 1950s, Sprent and English (1958) established the medical and public health relevance of roundworms of dogs and cats.

Although millions of people all over the world are infected by *Toxocara* spp. and hundred thousands have been or are suffering from (the different forms) of toxocarosis or at least feel impaired in their well-being, and although toxocarosis gains increasing relevance in public health (Chen et al., 2018), this helminthozoonosis still represents a severely neglected disease. Only very rarely, it is included into differential diagnostics, particularly in Central Europe and other "highly developed" countries, which is mainly due to the ignorance of the medical staff.

2. Terminological aspects

Before discussing the clinical spectrum of *Toxocara* infections and toxocarosis in detail, a few terminological aspects should be taken into consideration:

1. Based on the guidelines of the "Council for International Organizations for Medical Sciences (CIOMS/WHO, 1987)" and due to the "standardized nomenclature for parasitic diseases (SNOAPAD)" formulated by Kassai et al. (1988) the term "toxocarosis" should be preferred to "toxocariasis".
2. "Toxocarosis" (or formerly toxocariasis) is a clinical term and should be used for the disease (e.g. symptoms, pathological laboratory results) caused by larvae of *Toxocara canis* or *T. cati*.
3. Thus, we should be aware of the fact, that there is a great difference between a (clinically asymptomatic) *Toxocara* infection, on one hand and the clinically manifest disease "toxocarosis", on the other. The sole

detection of specific anti-*Toxocara* antibodies in a clinically healthy person (e.g. found within serological screening studies) is not sufficient to use the term "toxocarosis". Correspondingly, laboratory animals experimentally infected with *Toxocara* eggs do also not necessarily suffer from the disease toxocarosis, but can "only" have a *Toxocara* infection. All in all, we should be careful when choosing between the terms "toxocaral infection" and "toxocarosis".

3. *Toxocara canis* and *T. cati*

Even though *T. cati* was discussed as potential human parasite already in the midst of the 19th century (Cobbold, 1863; O'Brien, 1839; Pickells, 1824)—much earlier than *T. canis*—, these early reports did not consider it as causative agent of a larva migrans syndrome and the medical relevance of *T. cati* seems to be altogether lower compared to *T. canis*. The high levels of *T. cati* infections in cat populations worldwide (summarized, e.g., by Fisher, 2003), and the high environmental contamination with *T. cati* eggs, holding a high risk of infection for humans, are in stark contrast to the few conclusive reports on its clinical relevance and course of disease (Eberhard and Alfano, 1998; Sakai et al., 1998; Shimokawa et al., 1982; Sick and Hennerici, 2014). In fact, we still do not know, if the clinical course of *T. cati* infections differs (substantially?) from that of *T. canis*. This clearly needs further efforts in research.

4. Clinical aspects

Toxocara canis and *T. cati* are among the most prevalent parasitic helminths with zoonotic impact, but we also know that presumably most infections of humans are never diagnosed due to the fact that the majority of infections remain without clinical symptoms. On the other hand, a considerably high number of infected individuals (possibly several hundred thousand) suffer from this zoonosis. Today, we differentiate between the "classical" VLM and the OLM syndrome, and—at least—three further syndromes: covert toxocarosis (CovT), common toxocarosis (ComT) and neurotoxocarosis or cerebral toxocarosis (NT). While the VLM and the OLM syndrome are clinically distinguishable from each other very easily, the attribution of patients to covert or common toxocarosis instead of VLM is hampered by the potentially diffuse clinical picture (Smith et al., 2009).

Nevertheless, based on the case history and by careful consideration and reflection of all available clinical data and laboratory findings (including serological results evaluated by an experienced parasitologist) the differentiation between the four (traditional) forms of toxocarosis should be feasible. On the other hand, the clinical spectrum of visceral toxocarosis itself may be highly pleomorphic, so that the VLM syndrome has been divided into subforms depending on the (main) symptoms and organs involved in the disease (e.g. cutaneous toxocarosis, cardiac toxocarosis etc.).

4.1 The visceral larva migrans (VLM syndrome or visceral toxocarosis)

"Classical" VLM is characterized particularly by anorexia, abdominal pain, fever, hepatomegaly and recurring cough; leucocytosis, eosinophilia and, occasionally, hypergammaglobulinemia may be additional indicators for a VLM syndrome (Despommier, 2003; Gillespie, 1993; Glickman, 1993; Macpherson, 2013; Magnaval et al., 2001a,b). The "typical" VLM patient has been described as 2–7 years old, geophageous (Pica syndrome) and with close contact to pet animals (Glickman and Schantz, 1981). However, based on our own experiences, we know today, that (1) not only children but also adults of up to more than 80 years old may suffer from toxocarosis (Auer and Aspöck, 2004), that (2) no direct contact with pet animals is necessary to acquire the infection, and that (3) also oral ingestion of undercooked meat (e.g. poultry, hares, even snails), contaminated with *Toxocara* larvae, may lead to infection. We assume that the environmental contamination with *Toxocara* eggs and their airborne distribution has to be considered as one of the most important sources of infection (Auer and Aspöck, 1995, 2004; Deutz et al., 1998).

4.1.1 Visceral toxocarosis and cutaneous manifestations

It is evident, that skin manifestations may be involved in VLM; numerous reports confirm this fact (transient rash, urticaria, chronic prurigo, pruritus, atopic dermatitis, non-atopic eczema), and also seroepidemiologic studies support that patients suffering from "unclear skin conditions" are not rarely positive for anti-*Toxocara* antibodies (Ehrhard and Kernbaum, 1979; Gavignet et al., 2008; Humbert et al., 2000; Ismail and Khalafallah, 2005; Ronellenfitsch et al., 2007; Wolfrom et al., 1995). However, the causative relationship between *Toxocara* infections and skin manifestations are still unresolved and should be clarified.

4.1.2 Visceral toxocarosis and cardiac manifestations

Without any doubt, cardiac manifestations represent a special form of VLM, which is convincingly demonstrated by numerous case reports (Abe et al., 2002; Enko et al., 2009; Friedman and Herveda, 1960; Kim et al., 2012; Vargo et al., 1977), a carefully review (Kuenzli et al., 2016) and also by our own observations during the past 30 years (Auer, not published so far). The clinical spectrum encompasses asymptomatic, oligo- as well as severely symptomatic patients suffering from myocarditis, endocarditis, pericarditis up to cardiac tamponade, endocardial thrombosis and heart failure (Kuenzli et al., 2016).

4.1.3 Visceral toxocarosis and asthma

An association between *Toxocara* infection and asthma has been assumed and discussed for decades, but remains unclear (Desowitz et al., 1981), although several studies indicate causal connections between larval migration and asthmatic symptoms (Aghaei et al., 2018; Buijs et al., 1994, 1995; Pinelli and Aranzamendi, 2012; Sharghi et al., 2001). However, a serological screening of 191 patients (living in and near Vienna) of varying atopy status and degree of bronchial activity, demonstrated that the *Toxocara* seroprevalence among patients with bronchial hyperreactivity or atopy was not higher than in the normal population (Zacharasiewicz et al., 2000).

4.1.4 Visceral toxocarosis and the rheumatic complex

Toxocara infections are often associated with clinical pictures (rheumatoid arthritis, chronic arthritis, reactive arthritis) belonging to the rheumatic complex; however, no convincing causal explanation of this association has been found so far (Bellanger et al., 2011; Chiardola et al., 2008; Dromer et al., 1993; Jimenez-Balderas et al., 2012; Kinceková et al., 1997; Kraus et al., 1995; van Linthoudt et al., 1990; Viola et al., 2016).

4.1.5 Visceral toxocarosis and other manifestations

Besides the "classical" VLM symptoms, cases with other clinical manifestations have also been observed: patients diagnosed with hypereosinophilia syndrome, patients suffering from peritonitis, mimicking a lymphoma and others (Arslan et al., 2019; Bachmeyer et al., 2003; Merdin et al., 2016).

In summary, due to the fact that the clinical spectrum of the VLM syndrome is so complex and extremely pleomorphic, the term "VLM syndrome" may be supplemented by "sensu lato", if toxocarosis in general is under discussion.

4.2 The ocular larva migrans (OLM syndrome or ocular toxocarosis)

The ocular larva migrans (OLM) syndrome is particularly a syndrome of older children and adults and appears as unilateral loss of vision, occasionally combined with strabismus (Dinning et al., 1988). Invasion of *Toxocara* larvae into the retina can lead to the formation of a granuloma inducing distorted vision, heterotopia and ablatio of the macula (Gillespie, 1993; Good et al., 2004; Shields, 1984; Small et al., 1989). The OLM syndrome is not uncommonly also observed in uveitis-patients (Barisani-Asenbauer et al., 2012; Shields, 1984; Stewart et al., 2005). Further complications encompass diffuse endophthalmitis or papillitis with or without glaucoma due to migrating or dying larvae. In young children, OLM syndrome must be differentiated from retinoblastoma (Despommier and Karapelou, 1987). The good news is that the tests for retinoblastoma are getting better all the time (Ghiam et al., 2019), and it is now rare that the misdiagnosis of ocular larva migrans as retinoblastoma will lead to an unnecessary enucleation.

4.3 The inapparent and covert toxocarosis (CovT)

In 1983, Bass et al. suggested to add a new entity of toxocarosis, which they called *inapparent toxocarosis* (*IT*), characterized by clinically more or less inapparent or mild symptoms with or without eosinophilia. Finally, Taylor et al. (1987) established a further category, termed *covert toxocarosis-syndrome (CovT) for a group of* children from Ireland suffering from coughing, abdominal pain, headaches and wheezing with or without eosinophilia. Additional symptoms, including behaviour disturbances (sleep disturbances, irritability and being "cranky") were observed. The first CT case in Austria was documented in 1998 (Varga et al., 1998).

4.4 The common toxocarosis (ComT)

The clinical picture of *common toxocarosis* (*ComT*) was observed the first time during the course of a "case control study" in adults in La Reunion, characterized by weakness, pruritus, eczema, respiratory problems and abdominal pain, sometimes accompanied by eosinophilia and elevated IgE levels (Magnaval et al., 1994).

4.5 The neurotoxocarosis (NT or cerebral toxocarosis)

The invasion of *Toxocara* larvae into the brain and the spinal cord may result in a further disease entity, namely neurotoxocarosis or cerebral toxocarosis (NT)

(Deshayes et al., 2016; Finsterer and Auer, 2007; Janecek et al., 2017; Magnaval et al., 2001a,b). Although only around 20 NT cases have been reported between 1950 and 2000, we have knowledge that NT is much more prevalent than commonly assumed. The clinical spectrum of NT comprises diverse symptoms (e.g. headache, fever, weakness, epileptic seizures, meningitis, encephalitis, myelitis, cerebral vasculitis, paraparesis) (Caldera et al., 2013; Finsterer and Auer, 2007; Ruttinger and Hadidi, 1991; Singer et al., 2011) and, very rarely, Bell's Palsy (Bachtiar et al., 2012). Additionally, there is increasing evidence that *Toxocara* infections may cause epileptic seizures (Fan et al., 2015), neurodegenerative disorders (Fan et al., 2015; Luna et al., 2018) and impaired cognitive development of children (Holland and Hamilton, 2013; Stewart et al., 2005). The pathological impact of *Toxocara* infections of the brain has been demonstrated convincingly by experimental studies in laboratory animals (Fan et al., 2015; Heuer et al., 2015; Strube et al., 2013).

5. Co-infections

Although our knowledge on the clinical manifestations of toxocarosis has increased considerably over the past decades, the medical relevance of co-infections with viruses, bacteria and other parasites, including their interferences with each other, and with *Toxocara* in particular, is rather unresolved and under-investigated so far. Fact is, that numerous cases of co-infections in humans with *Toxocara* and other parasites (e.g. with *Toxoplasma gondii, Plasmodium falciparum, Echinococcus granulosus*) (cited in Jones et al., 2008; Kamuyu et al., 2014; Macpherson, 2013), have been published, but essentially nothing is known of their interactions.

Based on our experience, obtained during the past years, we know, that patients infected with *Borrelia* spp. or even suffering from borreliosis, are not rarely co-infected with larvae of *Toxocara* spp. or *Ascaris suum* or both: between July 2014 and December 2015, 38, 236 and 44 out of 318 "borreliosis patients" (185 ♂, 133 ♀, age range: <1 to >90, tested by *Toxocara* excretory/secretory (TES) ELISA and TES-immunoblot and *Ascaris suum* immunoblot), had specific antibodies against *Toxocara canis, Ascaris suum* and both species, respectively, (Auer and Aspöck, 2006; Auer and Obiltschnig, 2019; Schneider and Auer, 2016). A considerable number of these patients did not improve significantly when treated with antibiotics against *Borrelia*, but recovered rapidly under or after anthelminthic treatment with albendazole (Auer and Obiltschnig, 2019). However, the causal connections between *Borrelia* infections and infections with larvae of *Toxocara* spp. remain to be elucidated. The diverse aspects of co-infections certainly require more research.

6. Diagnostic aspects

The definitive diagnosis of a *Toxocara* infection or a toxocarosis can basically only be achieved by direct detection methods, e.g., histological or immunohistological detection of larvae or larval metabolic products, respectively (Auer and Aspöck, 2006) or detection of specific *Toxocara* DNA in the tissues of the liver (Kirchner and Altmann, 1987), brain (Hill et al., 1985), lung, eyes (Neafie and Connor, 1976) or large intestine (Auer and Aspöck, 2006). Considering the fact that the likelihood of obtaining an appropriate biopsy from a patient is rather low, nearing zero, such tests seem unsuited for routine diagnostics (Auer and Aspöck, 1998; Jacobs et al., 1997).

Thus, the diagnosis "toxocarosis" is only feasible by considering clinical symptoms, as well as anamnestic (geographic, behavioural and medical history) and laboratory diagnostic data (differential blood counts, immunoglobulin levels, liver function, inflammatory signs), including additional findings by imaging techniques, and, particularly, by serological tests (using TES antigen). However, the essential precondition is that physicians be aware of the existence of *Toxocara* and include toxocarosis in their differential lists.

There is no doubt that the detection of specific antibodies against TES antigen represents the most important diagnostic tool for diagnosing *Toxocara* infections (de Savigny 1975; de Savigny et al., 1979). TES antigen is used all over the world, is well-characterized at the protein and nucleic acid levels (Maizels et al., 1984; Yamasaki et al., 2000), can be used in ELISA as well as immunoblot tests (Magnaval et al., 1991), and is characterized by high sensitivity and specificity (Jacquier et al., 1991; Pollard, 1979; Speiser and Gottstein, 1984). The serological discrimination between *T. canis* and *T. cati* is not possible by TES-ELISA or TES-immunoblot, but is also not necessary under clinical aspects. Patients suffering from OLM sometimes show only very weak or even negative antibody titres (Petithory et al., 1994; Schantz et al., 1979). Thus, in cases of suspected OLM syndrome, we use both, not only the TES-ELISA but also the slightly more sensitive TES-immunoblot, thereby significantly increasing the sensitivity of our serology (Auer and Aspöck, 2006). The detection of other antibody classes than

IgG (IgE, IgA) and the detection of circulating antigen by antibody capture ELISAs has provided no essential improvements in diagnostics. In contrast, the detection of "eosinophil cationic proteins" (ECP) in the serum of toxocarosis patients has been reported to enable the differentiation between recent and latent infection (Magnaval et al., 2001a,b).

The detection of specific *Toxocara* DNA (ribosomal ITS-2 region), established by Jacobs et al. (1997), (and also available in our laboratory) enables the differentiation between *T. canis* and *T. cati*; however, biopsy specimens are necessary, thus this tool is redundant in routine diagnostics.

7. Therapeutical aspects

The treatment of toxocarosis still represents an unresolved problem. The main question is, if a patient should be treated at all, because *Toxocara* infections are considered self-limiting infections. A pragmatic approach is to treat only patients suffering from (severe) toxocarosis (e.g. acute VLM) (Magnaval et al., 1994). OLM and NT patients can receive symptomatic treatment (e.g. with corticosteroids, anticonvulsants) or a combination of symptomatic and anthelminthic treatments (Barisani-Asenbauer et al., 2001; Dietrich et al., 1998). Anthelminthic treatment of patients diagnosed with "covert or common toxocarosis" is only indicated if patients suffer from the infection. Serologically positive but healthy persons should never be treated anthelminthically.

The spectrum of anthelminthics utilized encompasses the benzimidazoles, thiabendazole, mebendazole and albendazole, as well as diethylcarbamacine (DEC). Due to negative side effects (allergic reactions) of DEC, the non-availability of thiabendazole in many countries and the limited resorption of mebendazole, albendazole remains the drug of choice (Magnaval, 1995, 1998; Magnaval and Charlet, 1987; Stürchler et al., 1989). Although, albendazole is not considered an optimal anthelminthic, it is widely used. A Japanese study on long-term administration of albendazole reported an efficacy rate of up to 80% (in *Toxocara* as well as in *Ascaris suum* infected patients suffering from VLM syndrome) (Hombu et al., 2019). However, international guidelines on the treatment of toxocarosis are lacking so far.

Toxocara spp. and the various clinical appearances induced by them have been and are still fascinating and exciting topics of medical and scientific research. Although our level on knowledge about epidemiology, nosology and diagnostics has enormously increased since the 1950s considerable gaps on the immunological mechanisms of onset or non-onset of the disease "toxocarosis" still exist. Hopefully, these gaps will be closed with ambitious efforts in the near future—perhaps by means of new laboratory technologies.

References

Abe, K., Shimokawa, H., Kubota, T., Nawa, Y., Takeshita, A., 2002. Myocarditis associated with visceral larva migrans due to Toxocara canis. Intern. Med. 41 (9), 706–708. https://doi.org/10.2169/internalmedicine.41.706.

Aghaei, S., Riahi, S.M., Rostami, A., Mohammadzadeh, I., Javanian, M., Tohidi, E., Foroutan, M., Esmaeili Dooki, M., 2018. Toxocara spp. infection and risk of childhood asthma: a systematic review and meta-analysis. Acta Trop. 182, 298–304. https://doi.org/10.1016/j.actatropica.2018.03.022. Epub 2018 Mar 21.

Aquino, R.T., Magliari, M.E., Vital Filho, J., Silva, M.A., Lima, C.A., Rocha, A.J., Silva, C.J., Rewin, J.A., Nahas, T.R., Chieffi, P.P., 2018. Lagochilascariasis leading to severe involvement of ocular globes, ears and meningen. Rev. Inst. Med. Trop. Sao Paulo 50 (6), 355–358. https://doi.org/10.1590/s0036-46652008000600009.

Arslan, F., Baysal, N.B., Aslan, A., Ates, B.C., Vahaboglu, H., 2019. Toxocara related peritonitis: a case report and review of literature. Parasitol. Int. 73, 101950. https://doi.org/10.1016/j.parint.2019.101950.

Ashford, R.W., 2001. Current usage of nomenclature for parasitic diseases, with special reference to those involving arthropods. Med. Vet. Entomol. 15, 121–125.

Aspöck, H., Walochnik, J., 2002. Was Sind Parasiten? vol. 6. Denisia, pp. 1–12.

Auer, H., Aspöck, H., 1995. Toxokarose in Österreich—Epidemiologie, Diagnostik und Therapie. Mitt. Österr. Ges. Tropenmed. Parasitol. 17, 61–70.

Auer, H., Aspöck, H., 1998. Die Toxokarose-Forschung in Österreich—Ergebnisse, Probleme, Herausforderungen. Mitt. Österr. Ges. Tropenmed. Parasitol. 20, 17–28.

Auer, H., Aspöck, H., 2004. Nosologie und Epidemiologie der Toxokarose des Menschen—die aktuelle situation in Österreich. Wien. Klin. Wochenschr. 116 (Suppl. 4), 7–18.

Auer, H., Aspöck, H., 2006. Diagnostik der Toxocara-Infestationen und der Toxokarose. J. Lab. Med. 30 (1), 1–12.

Auer, H., Obiltschnig, A., 2019. Ascaris suum and the larva migrans viceralis syndrome in Austria. Unpublished Data.

Bachmeyer, C., Lamarque, G., Morariu, R., Molina, T., Bourée, P., Delmer, A., 2003. Visceral larva migrans mimicking lymphoma. Chest 123, 1296–1297.

Bachtiar, A., Auer, H., Finsterer, J., 2012. Paralisis de Bell y dolor facial asociados con infección por Toxocara sp. Rev. Chilena Infectol. 29 (5), 551–553. https://doi.org/10.4067/S0716-10182012000600015.

Barisani-Asenbauer, T., Maca, S.M., Hauff, W., Kaminski, S.L., Domanovits, H., Auer, H., 2001. Treatment of ocular toxocariasis with albendazole. J. Ocul. Pharmacol. Ther. 17, 287–294. https://doi.org/10.1089/108076801750295317.

Barisani-Asenbauer, T., Maca, S.M., Mejdoubi, L., Emminger, W., Machold, K., Auer, H., 2012. Uveitis—a rare disease often associated with systemic diseases and infections—a systematic review of 2619 patients. Orphanet J. Rare Dis. 29 (7), 57. https://doi.org/10.1186/1750-1172-7-57.

Bass, J.L., Mehta, K.A., Glickman, L.T., Blocker, R., Eppes, B.M., 1983. Asymptomatic toxocariasis in children: a prospective study and a treatment trial. Clin. Pediatr. 26, 441–446. https://doi.org/10.1177/000992288702600902.

Beaver, P.C., Snyder, H.C., Carrera, C.M., Dent, J.H., Lafferty, J.W., 1952. Chronic eosinophilia due to visceral larva migrans. Pediatrics 9, 7–19.

Bellanger, A.P., Bamoulid, J., Millon, L., Chalopin, J.M., Humbert, P., 2011. Rheumatoid purpura associated with toxocariasis. Can. Fam. Physician 57 (12), 1413–1414.

Brumpt, E.J., 1927. Précis de Parasitologie. Librairie de l'lAcadémie de Médecine, Paris, pp. 1–1452.

Buijs, J., Lokhorst, W.H., Robinson, J., Nijkamp, F.P., 1994. Toxocara canis-induced murine pulmonary inflammation: analysis of cells and proteins in lung tissue and bronchoalveolar lavage fluid. Parasite Immunol. 16, 1–9.

Buijs, J., Egbers, M.W.M.C., Nijkamp, F.P., 1995. Toxocara canis-induced airway eosinophilia and tracheal hyporeactivity in guinea pigs and mice. Eur. J. Pharmacol. 293, 207–215. https://doi.org/10.1164/ajrccm.151.3.7881685.

Caldera, F., Burlone, M.E., Genchi, C., Pirisi, M., Bartoli, E., 2013. Toxocara encephalitis presenting with autonomous nervous system involvement. Infection 41 (3), 691–694. https://doi.org/10.1007/s15010-012-0342-6.

Campos, D.M.B., Barbosa, A.P., Oliveira, J.A., Tavares, G.G., Cravo, P.V.L., Ostermayer, A.L., 2017. Human lagochilascariasis—a rare helminthic disease. PLoS Negl. Trop. Dis. 11 (6), e0005510. https://doi.org/10.1371/journal. Pntd.0005510. eCollection 2017 Jun.

Chandler, A.C., 1925. The helminthic parasites of cats in Calcutta and the relation of cats to human helminthic infections. Indian J. Med. Res. 13, 213–228.

Chen, J., Liu, Q., Liu, G.H., Zheng, W.B., Hong, S.J., Sugiyama, H., Zhu, X.Q., Elsheikha, H.M., 2018. Toxocariasis: a silent threat with a progressive public health impact. Infect. Dis. Poverty 7 (1), 59. https://doi.org/10.1186/s40249-018-0437-0.

Chiardola, F., Schneeberger, E.E., Citera, G., Rosemffet, G.M., Kuo, L., Santillan, G., Maldonado-Cocco, J.A., 2008. Prevalence and clinical significance of eosinophilia in patients with rheumatoid arthritis in Argentina. J. Clin. Rheumatol. 14 (4), 211–213. https://doi.org/10.1097/RHU.0b013e31817738ce.

CIOMS/WHO, 1987. International Nomenclature of Diseases. vol. 2. Council for International Organizations of Medical Sciences & World Health Organization, Geneva. 4.

Cobbold, T.S., 1863. On the occurrence of Ascaris mystax in the human subject. Lancet 81, 31–34.

Coombs, I., Crompton, D.W.T., 1991. A Guide to Human Helminths. Taylor and Francis, London, New York, Philadelphia, 196 pp.

de Savigny, D.H., 1975. In vitro maintenance of Toxocara canis larvae and a simple method for the production of Toxocara ES antigens for use in serodiagnostic tests for visceral larva migrans. J. Parasitol. 61, 781–782.

de Savigny, D.H., Voller, A., Woodruff, A.W., 1979. Toxocariasis: serological diagnosis by enzyme immunoassay. J. Clin. Pathol. 32 (3), 284–288. https://doi.org/10.1136/jcp.32.3.284.

Dent, J.H., Carrera, G.M., 1953. Eosinophilia in childhood caused by visceral larva migrans. J. La. State Med. Soc. 105 (7), 275–280.

Deshayes, S., Bonhomme, J., de La Blanchardière, A., 2016. Neurotoxocariasis: a systematic literature review. Infection 44 (5), 565–574. https://doi.org/10.1007/s15010-016-0889-8. Epub 2016 Mar 23.

Desowitz, R.S., Rudoy, R., Barnwell, J.W., 1981. Antibodies to canine helminth parasites in asthmatic and nonasthmatic children. Int. Arch. Allergy Appl. Immunol. 65 (4), 361–366. https://doi.org/10.1159/000232777.

Despommier, D.D., 2003. Toxocariasis: clinical aspects, epidemiology, medical ecology, and molecular aspects. Clin. Microbiol. Rev. 16, 265–272. https://doi.org/10.1128/cmr.16.2.265-272.2003.

Despommier, D.D., Karapelou, J., 1987. Parasite Life Cycles. Springer Verlag, New York, pp. 1–127.

Deutz, A., Fuchs, K., Auer, H., Kerbl, U., Aspoeck, H., Koefer, J., 1998. Toxocara-infestations in Austria: a study on the risk of infection of farmers, slaughterhouse staff, hunters and veterinarians. Parasitol. Res. 97, 390–394. https://doi.org/10.1007/s00436-005-1469-5n.

Dietrich, A., Auer, H., Tittl, M., Barisani-Asenbauer, T., 1998. Okuläre Toxokarose in Österreich. Dtsch. Med. Wochenschr. 123, 626–630. https://doi.org/10.1055/s-2007-1024030.

Dinning, W.J., Gillespie, S.H., Cooling, R.J., Maizels, R.M., 1988. Toxocariasis: a practical approach to management of ocular disease. Eye (Lond.) 2, 580–582. https://doi.org/10.1038/eye.1988.108.

Dromer, C., Constantin, A., Amar, J., Caulier, M., Billey, T., Chamontin, B., Magnaval, J.F., Fournié, B., 1993. Rheumatologic aspects of toxocariasis (visceral Larva migrans). Apropos of 2 cases. Rev. Rhum. Ed Fr. 60 (9), 621–624.

Eberhard, M.L., Alfano, E., 1998. Adult Toxocara cati infections in U.S. children: report of four cases. Am. J. Trop. Med. Hyg. 59 (3), 404–406. https://doi.org/10.4269/ajtmh.1998.59.404.

Ehrhard, T., Kernbaum, S., 1979. Toxocara canis et toxocarose humaine. Bull. Inst. Pasteur 77, 225–287.

Enko, K.E., Tada, T., Ohgo, K.O., Nagase, S., Nakamura, K., Ohta, K., Ichiba, S., Ujike, Y., Nawa, Y., Maruyama, H., Ohe, T., Kusano, K.F., 2009. Fulminant eosinophilic myocarditis associated with visceral larva migrans caused by Toxocara canis infection. Circ. J. 73 (7), 1344–1348. Epub 2008 Dec 27.

Fan, C.K., Holland, C.V., Loxton, K., Barghouth, U., 2015. Cerebral toxocariasis: silent progression to neurodegenerative disorders? Clin. Microbiol. Rev. 28 (3), 663–686. https://doi.org/10.1128/CMR.00106-14.

Finsterer, J., Auer, H., 2007. Neurotoxocarosis. Rev. Inst. Med. Trop. Sao Paulo 49 (5), 279–287. https://doi.org/10.1590/s0036-46652007000050000.

Fisher, M., 2003. Toxocara cati: an underestimated zoonotic agent. Trends Parasitol. 19, 167–170.

Friedman, S., Herveda, A.R., 1960. Severe myocarditits with recovery in a child with visceral larva migrans. J. Pediatr. 56 (1), 91–96. https://doi.org/10.1016/s0022-3476(60)80292-2.

Fülleborn, F., 1921. Askarisinfektion durch Verzehren eingekapselter Larven und übergelungene intrauterine Askarisinfektion. Arch. Schiffs-u. Tropen-Hyg. 25, 367–375.

Gavignet, B., Piarroux, R., Aubin, F., Millon, L., Humbert, P., 2008. Cutaneous manifestations of human toxocariasis. J. Am. Acad. Dermatol. 59 (6), 1031–1042. https://doi.org/10.1016/j.jaad.2008.06.031.

Gavin, P.J., Kazacos, K.R., Shulman, S.T., 2005. Baylisascariasis. Clin. Microbiol. Rev. 18 (4), 703–718. https://doi.org/10.1128/CMR.18.4.703-718.2005.

Ghiam, B.K., Xu, L., Berry, J.L., 2019. Aqueous humor markers in retinoblaostoma, a review. Transl. Vis. Sci. Technol. 8 (2), 13. https://doi.org/10.1167/tvst.8.2.13.

Gillespie, S.H., 1993. The clinical spectrum of human toxocariasis. In: Lewis, J.W., Maizels, R.M. (Eds.), Toxocara and Toxocariasis. Institute of Biology and British Society for Parasitology, pp. 55–61.

Glickman, L.T., 1993. The epidemiology of human toxocariasis. In: Lewis, J.W., Maizels, R.M. (Eds.), Toxocara and Toxocariasis. Institute of Biology and British Society for Parasitology, pp. 2–10.

Glickman, L.T., Schantz, P.M., 1981. Epidemiology and pathogenesis of zoonotic toxocariasis. Epidemiol. Rev. 3, 30–50. https://doi.org/10.1093/oxfordjournals.epirev.a036235.

Good, B., Holland, C.V., Taylor, R.H., Larragy, J., Moriarty, P., O'Regan, M., 2004. Ocular toxocariasis in schoolchildren. Clin. Infect. Dis. 39, 173–178. https://doi.org/10.1086/421492.
Heuer, L., Haendel, S., Beineke, A., Strube, C., 2015. Effects of Toxocara larvae on brain cell survival by in vitro model assessment. Parasitology 142 (10), 1326–1334. https://doi.org/10.1017/S0031182015000694.
Hill, I.R., Denham, D.A., Scholtz, C.L., 1985. Toxocara canis larvae in the brain of a British child. Trans. R. Soc. Trop. Med. Hyg. 79 (3), 351–354. https://doi.org/10.1016/0035-9203(85)90378-5.
Holland, C.V., Hamilton, C.M., 2013. The significance of cerebral toxocariasis: a model system for exploring the link between brain involvement, behaviour and the immune response. J. Exp. Biol. 216 (Pt. 1), 78–83. https://doi.org/10.1242/jeb.074120.
Hombu, A., Yoshida, A., Kikuchi, T., Nagayasu, E., Kuroki, M., Maruyama, H., 2019. Treatment of larva migrans syndrome with long-term administration of albendazole. J. Microbiol. Immunol. Infect. 52 (1), 100–105. https://doi.org/10.1016/j.jmii 2017.07.002. Epub 2017 Jul 14.
Humbert, P., Niezborola, M., Salembier, R., Aubin, F., Piarroux, R., Buchet, S., Barale, T., 2000. Skin manifestations associated with toxocariasis: a case control study. Dermatology 201, 230–234. https://doi.org/10.1159/000018493.
Ismail, M., Khalafallah, O., 2005. Toxocara canis and chronic urticaria in Egyptian patients. J. Egypt. Soc. Parasitol. 35 (3), 833–840.
Izumikawa, K., Kohno, Y., Izumikawa, K., Hara, K., Hayashi, H., Maruyama, H., Kohno, S., 2011. Eosinophilic pneumonia due to visceral larva migrans possibly caused by Ascaris suum: a case report and review of recent literatures. Jpn. J. Infect. Dis. 64 (5), 428–432.
Jacobs, D.E., Xingquan, Z., Gasser, R., Chilton, N.B., 1997. PCR-based methods for the identification of potentially zoonotic ascaridoid parasites of the dog, fox and cat. Acta Trop. 68 (2), 191–200.
Jacquier, P., Gottstein, B., Stingelin, Y., Eckert, J., 1991. Immunodiagnosis of toxocarosis in humans: evaluation of a new enzyme-linked immunosorbent assay kit. J. Clin. Microbiol. 29 (9), 1831–1835.
Janecek, E., Waindok, P., Bankstahl, M., Strube, C., 2017. Abnormal neurobehaviour and impaired memory function as a consequence of Toxocara canis- as well as Toxocara cati-induced neurotoxocarosis. PLoS Negl. Trop. Dis. 11 (5), e0005594. https://doi.org/10.1371/journal.pntd.0005594.
Jimenez-Balderas, F.J., Camargo-Coronel, A., Gargia-Jaimes, J., Zonana-Nacach, A., Alcantara-Anguianoi, I., Carrillo-Becerril, L., Tapia-Romero, R., Gonzalez, T.S., Villalobos-Gomez, F., Martinez-Hernandez, S., Ventura-Juarez, J., Jimenez-Balderas, E.A., Méndez-Samperio, P., De-la-Rosa-Arana, J.L., 2012. A study on parasites in Mexican rheumatic disease patients. J. Egypt. Soc. Parasitol. 42 (2), 271–280.
Jones, J.L., Kruszon-Moran, D., Won, K., Wilson, M., Schantz, P.M., 2008. Toxoplasma gondii and Toxocara spp. co-infection. Am. J. Trop. Med. Hyg. 78 (1), 35–39.
Kamuyu, G., Bottomley, C., Mageto, J., Lowe, B., Wilkins, P.P., Noh, J.C., Nutman, T.B., Ngugi, A.K., Odhiambo, R., Wagner, R.G., Kakooza-Mwesige, A., Owusu-Agyei, S., Ae-Ngibise, K., Masanja, H., Osier, F.H., Odermatt, P., Newton, C.R., 2014. Study of epidemiology of epilepsy in demographic sites (SEEDS) group. Exposure to multiple parasites is associated with the prevalence of active convulsive epilepsy in sub-Saharan Africa. PLoS Negl. Trop. Dis. 8 (5), e2908. https://doi.org/10.1371/journal.pntd.0002908.
Kassai, T., Cordero del Campillo, M., Euzeby, J., Gaafar, S., Hiepe, T., Homonas, C.A., 1988. Standardized nomenclature of animal parasitic diseases (SNOAPAD). Vet. Parasitol. 29, 299–326.

Kazacos, K.R., Jelicks, L.A., Tanowit, H.B., 2013. Baylisascaris larva migrans. Handb. Clin. Neurol. 114, 251–262. https://doi.org/10.1016/B978-0-444-53490-3.00020-0.

Kim, J.H., Chung, W.B., Chang, K.Y., Ko, S.Y., Park, M.H., Sa, Y.K., Choi, Y.S., Park, C.S., Lee, M.Y., 2012. Eosinophilic myocarditis associated with visceral larva migrans caused by Toxocara canis infection. J. Cardiovasc. Ultrason. 20 (3), 150–153. https://doi.org/10.4250/jcu.2012.20.3.150.

Kinceková, J., Dubinský, P., Filka, J., Vargová, V., 1997. Toxocara infections in childhood in relation to reactive arthritis. Epidemiol. Mikrobiol. Imunol. 46 (1), 39–41.

Kirchner, T., Altmann, H.W., 1987. Parasitic larva as a cause of circumscribed liver lesions. Morphology and differential diagnosis. Pathologe 8 (1), 31–36.

Kraus, A., Valencia, X., Cabral, A.R., de la Vega, G., 1995. Visceral larva migrans mimicking rheumatic diseases. J. Rheumatol. 22, 497–500.

Kuenzli, E., Neumayr, A., Chaney, M., Blum, J., 2016. Toxocariasis-associated cardiac diseases—a systematic review of the literature. Acta Trop. 154, 107–120. https://doi.org/10.1016/j.actatropica.2015.11.003.

Leiper, R.T., 1907. Two ne genera of nematodes ocasionally parasitic in man. Br. Med. J. 1, 1296–1298.

Luna, J., Cicero, C.E., Rateau, G., Quattrocchi, G., Marin, B., Bruno, E., Dalmay, F., Druet-Cabanac, M., Nicoletti, A., Preux, P.M., 2018. Updated evidence of the association between toxocariasis and epilepsy: systematic review and meta-analysis. PLoS Negl. Trop. Dis. 12 (7), e0006665. https://doi.org/10.1371/journal.pntd.0006665.

Macpherson, C.N.L., 2013. The epidemiology and public health importance of toxocariasis: a zoonosis of global importance. Int. J. Parasitol. 43 (12–13), 999–1008. https://doi.org/10.1016/j.ijpara.2013.07.004.

Magnaval, J.F., 1995. Comparative efficacy of diethylcarbamacine and mebendazole for the treatment of human toxocariasis. Parasitology 110, 529–533.

Magnaval, J.F., 1998. Apparent weak effiocacy of ivermectin for treatment of human toxocariasis. Antimicrob. Agents Chemother. 42, 2770.

Magnaval, J.P., Charlet, J.P., 1987. Efficacité comparée du thiabendazole et du mébendazole dans le traitment de la toxocarose. Therapie 42, 541–544.

Magnaval, J.F., Fabre, R., Maurières, P., Charlet, J.P., de Larrard, B., 1991. Application of the Western blotting procedure for the immunodiagnosis of human toxocariasis. Parasitol. Res. 77 (8), 697–702.

Magnaval, J.F., Glickman, L.T., Dorchies, P., 1994. La toxocarose, une zoonose helminthique majeure. Rev. Med. Vet. 145, 611–627.

Magnaval, J.F., Berry, A., Fabre, R., Morassin, N.B., 2001a. Eosinophil cationic protein as a possible marker of active human Toxocara infection. Allergy 56, 1096–1099. https://doi.org/10.3347/kjp.2001.39.1.1.

Magnaval, J.F., Glickman, L.T., Dorchies, P., Morassin, B., 2001b. Highlights of human toxocariasis. Korean J. Parasitol. 1, 1–11.

Maizels, R.M., de Savigny, D., Ogilvie, B.M., 1984. Characterization of surface and excretory-secretory antigens of Toxocara canis infective larvae. Parasite Immunol. 6 (1), 23–37.

Merdin, A., Ogur, E., Çiçek Kolak, Ç., Avcı Merdin, F., 2016. A rare cause of hyper-eosinophilia: a case report. Turkiye Parazitol. Derg. 40 (2), 114–116. https://doi.org/10.5152/tpd.2016.4211.

Neafie, R.C., Connor, D.H., 1976. Visceral larva migrans. In: Binord, C.H., Connor, D.H. (Eds.), Pathology of Tropical and Extraordinary Diseases. Armed Forces Institute of Pathology, Washington, DC, pp. 433–436.

Nichols, R.L., 1956. The etiology of visceral larva migrans. I. Diagnostic morphology of infective second stage larvae. J. Parasitol. 42, 349–362.

Nichols, R.L., Beaver, P.C., Carrera, G.M., Staggers, R.J., 1956. Visceral larva migrans: with a case report. Am. J. Pathol. 32, 777–803.
O'Brien, B., 1839. On an Undescribed Species of Human Intestinal Worms. vol. 1. Dublin Med. Press, pp. 103–104.
Perlingiero, J.G., György, P., 1947. Chronic eosinphilia. Report of a case with necrosis of the liver, pulmonary infiltrations, anemia and ascaris infection. Am. J. Dis. Child. 73, 34–43.
Petithory, J.C., Beddok, A., Quedoc, M., 1994. Ascaridiasis zoonoses: visceral larva migrans syndrome. Bull. Acad. Natl. Med. 178 (4), 635–647.
Pickells, W., 1824. Case of a young woman who has discharged and continuous to discharge, from her stomach, a number of insects in different stages of their existence. Tr. Ass. King's and Queen's Coll. Phys. Ireland 4, 189–214.
Pinelli, E., Aranzamendi, C., 2012. Toxocara infection and its association with allergic manifestations. Endocr. Metab. Immune Disord. Drug Targets 12 (1), 33–44.
Pollard, Z.F., 1979. Ocular Toxocara in siblings of two families. Diagnosis confirmed by ELISA test. Arch. Ophthalmol. 97 (12), 2319–2320. https://doi.org/10.1001/archopht.1979.01020020535004.
Prociv, P., 1989. Toxocara pteropodis and visceral larva migrans. Parasitol. Today 5, 106–109. https://doi.org/10.1016/0169-4758(89)90047-1.
Ronellenfitsch, U., Bircher, A., Hatz, C., Blum, J., 2007. Parasiten als Ursache von Urtikaria. Hautarzt 58, 133–141. https://doi.org/10.1007/s00105-006-1174-z.
Ruttinger, P., Hadidi, H., 1991. MRI in cerebral toxocaral disease. J. Neurol. Neurosurg. Psychiatry 54, 361–362. https://doi.org/10.1136/jnnp.54.4.361.
Sakai, R., Kawashima, H., Shibui, H., Kamata, K., Kambara, C., Matsuoka, H., 1998. Toxocara cati-induced ocular toxocarisais. Arch. Ophthalmol. 116, 1686–1687.
Schantz, P.M., Meyer, D., Glickman, L.T., 1979. Clinical, serologic, and epidemiologic characteristics of ocular toxocariasis. Am. J. Trop. Med. Hyg. 28 (1), 24–28. https://doi.org/10.4269/ajtmh.1979.28.24.
Schneider, R., Auer, H., 2016. Incidence of Ascaris suum-specific antibodies in Austrian patients with suspected larva migrans visceralis (VLM) syndrome. Parasitol. Res. 115 (3), 1213–1219. https://doi.org/10.1007/s00436-015-4857-5. Epub 2015 Dec 5.
Schneider, R., Obwaller, A., Auer, H., 2015. Immunoblot for the detection of Ascaris suum-specific antibodies in patients with visceral larva migrans (VLM) syndrome. Parasitol. Res. 114, 305–310. https://doi.org/10.1007/s00436-014-4196-y.
Schrank, F.P., 1788. Verzeichnisse der bisher hinlänglich bekannten Eingeweidewürmer nebst einer Abhandlung über ihre Artverwandtschaft. Johann Baptist Strobl, München, pp. 1–116.
Schwartz, B., 1932. Some parasites of dogs and cats transmissible to human beings and domesticated animals. Vet. Alumni Quart., Ohio State Univ. 20, 5.
Sharghi, N., Schantz, P.M., Caramico, L., Ballas, K., Teague, B.A., Hotez, P.J., 2001. Environmental exposure to Toxocara as a possible risk factor for asthma: a clinic-based case-control study. Clin. Infect. Dis. 32 (7), E111–E116. Epub 2001 Mar 19.
Shields, J.A., 1984. Ocular toxocariasis. A review. Surv. Ophthalmol. 28, 361–381.
Shimokawa, H., Nakashima, T., Akagi, K., Omae, T., Tsuji, M., 1982. Visceral larva migrans by Toxocara cati. Fukuoka Igaku Zasshi 73 (1), 64–69.
Sick, C., Hennerici, M.G., 2014. Expect the unexpected: a case of eosinophilic meningitis in toxocariasis. Case Rep. Neurol. 6, 259–263. https://doi.org/10.1159/00036906.
Singer, O.C., Conrad, F., Jahnke, K., Hattingen, E., Auer, H., Steinmetz, H., 2011. Severe meningoencephalomyelitis due to CNS-Toxocarosis. J. Neurol. 258 (4), 696–698. https://doi.org/10.1007/s00415-010-5807-x.

Small, K.W., McCuen, B.W., de Juan Jr., E., Machemer, R., 1989. Surgical management of retinal traction caused by toxocariasis. J. Ophthalmol. 108 (1), 10–14. https://doi.org/10.1016/s0002-9394(14)73253-2.
Smith, H., Holland, C., Taylor, M., Magnaval, J.F., Schantz, P.M., Maizels, R., 2009. How common is human toxocariasis? Towards standardizing our knowledge. Cell Trends Parasitol. 25 (4), 182–188. https://doi.org/10.1016/.pt.2009.01.006.
Speiser, F., Gottstein, B., 1984. A collaborative study on larval excretory/secretory antigens of Toxocara canis for the immunodiagnosis of human toxocariasis with ELISA. Acta Trop. 41 (4), 361–372.
Sprent, J.F.A., English, P.B., 1958. The large roundworms of dogs and cats—a public health problem. Aust. Vet. J. Parasitol. 48, 16–171.
Stewart, J.M., Cubillan, L.D.P., Cunningham, E.T., 2005. Prevalence, clinical features, and causes of vision loss among patients with ocular toxocariasis. Retina 25, 1005–1013.
Stiles, C.W., 1905. The determination of generic types, and a list of roundworm genera with their original and type species. In: Stiles, C.W., Hassall, A. (Eds.), Bulletin 79. Bureau of Animal Industry, United States Department of Agriculture, pp. 1–150.
Strube, C., Heuer, L., Janecek, E., 2013. Toxocara spp. infections in paratenic hosts. Vet. Parasitol. 193 (4), 375–389. https://doi.org/10.1016/j.vetpar.2012.12.033.
Stürchler, D., Schubarth, P., Gualzata, M., Gottstein, B., Oettli, A., 1989. Thiabendazole vs. Albendazole in treatment of toxocariasis. Ann. Trop. Med. Parasitol. 83, 473–476. https://doi.org/10.1080/00034983.1989.11812374.
Taylor, M.R., Keane, C.T., O'Connor, P., Girdwood, R.A.W., Smith, H., 1987. Clinical features of covert toxocarosis. Scand. J. Infect. Dis. 19, 693–696. https://doi.org/10.3109/0036554870911720.
van Gorp, K., Mangelschots, M., Brandt, J., 1987. Toxocara vitulorum: a possible agent of larva migrans in humans? In: Geerts, S., Kumar, V., Brandt, J. (Eds.), Helminth Zoonoses. Martinus Nijhoff Publishers, pp. 159–166.
van Linthoudt, D., Mean, A.P., Favre, R., Ott, H., 1990. Arthritis of the hip associated with infantile toxocariasis. Schweiz. Rundsch. Med. Prax. 79 (36), 1022–1024.
Varga, E.M., Auer, H., Zach, M., 1998. Toxocariasis in a 5-year-old boy manifesting as bronchial asthma and behavioral disorder. Klin. Padiatr. 210 (3), 128–131. https://doi.org/10.1055/s-2008-1043864.
Vargo, T.A., Singer, D.B., Gillatte, P.C., Fernbach, D.J., 1977. Myocarditis due to visceral larva migrans. J. Pediatr. 90 (2), 322–323. https://doi.org/10.1016/s0022-3476(77)80666-5.
Viola, G.R., Giacomin, M.F., França, C.M., Sallum, A.M., Jacob, C.M., Silva, C.A., 2016. Chronic polyarthritis as isolated manifestation of toxocariasis. Rev. Bras. Reumatol. Engl. Ed. 56 (2), 185–187. https://doi.org/10.1016/j.rbre.2014.07.005.
Werner, P.C.F., 1782. Vermium Intestinalium Praesertim Taeniae Humanae, Brevis Expositionis, Continuatio. Lipsiae, pp. 1–28.
Wilder, H.C., 1950. Nematode endophthalmitis. Trans. Am. Acad. Ophthalmol. Otolaryngol. 55, 99–109.
Wolfrom, E., Chene, G., Boisseau, H., Beylot, C., Geniaux, M., Taieb, A., 1995. Chronic urticaria and Toxocara canis. Lancet 345, 196. https://doi.org/10.1016/s0140-6736(95)90202-3.
Yamasaki, H., Araki, K., Lim, P.K., Zasmy, N., Mak, J.W., Taib, R., Aoki, T., 2000. Development of a highly specific recombinant Toxocara canis second-stage larva excretory-secretory antigen for immunodiagnosis of human toxocariasis. J. Clin. Microbiol. 38 (4), 1409–1413.
Zacharasiewicz, A., Auer, H., Brath, H., Stohlhofer, B., Frank, W., Aspöck, H., Zwick, H., 2000. Toxocara and bronchial hyperreactivity-results of a seroprevalence study. Wien. Klin. Wochenschr. 112 (21), 922–926.

Further reading

Dent, J.H., Despommier, D.D., Gwadz, R.G., Hotez, P.J., 1995. Parasitic Diseases. Springer-Verlag, New York, pp. 1–647.

Pawlowski, Z., 2001. Toxocariasis in humans: clinical expression and treatment dilemma. J. Helminthol. 75, 299–305.

Schnieder, T., Laabs, E.M., Welz, C., 2011. Larval development of Toxocara canis in dogs. Vet. Parasitol. 175 (3–4), 193–206. https://doi.org/10.1016/j.vetpar.2010.10.027.

CHAPTER SEVEN

Serodiagnostic methods for diagnosing larval toxocariasis

Rahmah Noordin*, Muhammad Hafiznur Yunus, Siti Naqiuyah Tan Farrizam, Norsyahida Arifin
Institute for Research in Molecular Medicine, Universiti Sains Malaysia, Gelugor, Pulau Pinang, Malaysia
*Corresponding author: e-mail address: rahmah8485@gmail.com

Contents

Abstract

Toxocariasis is a human infection primarily caused by larvae of *Toxocara canis* from dogs, and also by *T. cati* from cats. Children have a more significant risk of acquiring the infection due to their closer contact with pets, and greater chances of ingesting soil. Diagnosis of toxocariasis is based on clinical, epidemiological, and serological data. Indirect IgG ELISA is a widely used serodiagnostic method for toxocariasis, with native *T. canis* TES most commonly used as the antigen. Western blots, using the same antigen, can be used to confirm positive ELISA findings to reduce false-positive results. Improvements in *Toxocara* serodiagnosis include the use of recombinant TES antigens, simpler and more rapid assay formats, and IgG4 subclass detection. Also, incorporation of recombinant *T. cati* TES protein increases the diagnostic sensitivity. Development of antigen detection tests using polyclonal and monoclonal antibodies, nanobodies, or aptamers can complement the antibody detection assays, and enhance the effectiveness of the serodiagnosis.

Advances in Parasitology, Volume 109
ISSN 0065-308X
https://doi.org/10.1016/bs.apar.2020.01.003

1. Introduction

Toxocariasis is a significant zoonotic disease caused by infection with the larvae of *Toxocara canis* and *T. cati*, two major roundworms found in dogs and cats, respectively. Unfortunately, these two animals are also the favourite companion animals of humans. The rise in the number of feral and stray populations in addition to the complexity of infection sources of *Toxocara* spp. contribute to the high prevalence of toxocariasis in both developing and developed countries (Fialho and Correa, 2016). According to population-based reports, seroprevalence of *Toxocara* infections ranged from 2.5% in urban Europe to 85% in rural tropics (Cassenote et al., 2014; Macpherson, 2013; Pinelli et al., 2011; Smith et al., 2009; Stensvold et al., 2009; Won et al., 2008).

Environmental contamination spreads the infection to humans through ingestion of embryonated/larvated *Toxocara* eggs in soil or contaminated food, or by ingestion of encapsulated larvae in improperly cooked meat (Chen et al., 2018). Children have a higher incidence of seropositivity, partly due to their more significant risk of accidentally ingesting soil and their closer contact with pets. Although patients infected with toxocariasis may suffer from a systemic syndrome known as visceral larva migrans (VLM), neurological or eye manifestations (ocular larval migrans or OLM), clinicians often have difficulty in diagnosing toxocariasis cases due to the common signs and symptoms that often resemble other helminthic infections, allergic reactions, and asthma. The non-standardized clinical definition of the disease and the vague presenting symptoms make the diagnosis of toxocariasis a major challenge. Furthermore, most patients are asymptomatic and may be left undiagnosed and untreated. Thus, the real global burden of toxocariasis is probably underestimated. The disease has been aptly listed as one of the five most neglected diseases by the Centers for Disease Control (CDC), USA (Moreira et al., 2014).

Diagnosis of *Toxocara* infection requires a high index of suspicion. It is primarily based on clinical, epidemiological, and laboratory data, including serology, radiological imaging, eosinophilia, and IgE level (Fillaux and Magnaval, 2013). A definitive test to detect *Toxocara* infection is by biopsy examination to locate the larvae in infected tissues or body fluids such as cerebrospinal or ocular fluid. However, this method is somewhat "controversial" because it is invasive, insensitive, and time-consuming (Pawlowski, 2001; Rubinsky-Elefant et al., 2010). The *Toxocara* larvae can be difficult to distinguish from the larvae of other ascarids due to their morphological similarities, especially when only parts of the larvae or larval debris is in the tissues (Chen et al., 2012). Although DNA amplification increases diagnostic sensitivity and specificity, using the invasive biopsy method remains an issue. As stated above the clinical diagnosis may be inconclusive, and laboratory abnormalities, such as blood eosinophilia, are indecisive since they may be due to other parasitic infections. Sound clinical knowledge and careful assessment of epidemiological data (such as contact with dogs or cats, consumption of raw meat, and geophagia) are required, as well as support from accurate laboratory tests.

2. The role and relevance of serodiagnosis

Diagnosis of toxocariasis is considered as highly probable if elevated serum anti-*Toxocara* antibodies are detected, in combination with symptoms, elevated eosinophil count, and no reasonable alternative diagnosis. However, if there is documented seroconversion, the diagnosis can be considered as definitive (Van Den Broucke et al., 2015). Over the years, numerous serological assays have been developed to detect *Toxocara* infections, with enzyme-linked immunosorbent assays (ELISA) being the assay of choice for disease detection, mapping seroprevalence and epidemiological studies across the world. However, in cases of chronic pruriginous skin disorders, there is evidence that immunoblot shows better sensitivity in detecting toxocariasis seropositivity (Bellanger et al., 2010). These methods mostly detect the presence of anti-*Toxocara* IgG antibody in human serum samples. Meanwhile, research on immunoassay targeting IgE against *Toxocara* TES has also been getting more attention as of late. This is particularly true especially in patients with a significant level of specific IgE, the titer decreased after anti-helminthic therapy, thus IgE TES-ELISA has been used in treatment monitoring (Fillaux and Magnaval, 2013). The serodiagnostic method was much improved in the mid-1970s after de Savigny and co-workers created a breakthrough with the development of an in vitro culture method for *T. canis* infective-stage larvae hatched in vitro from eggs that allowed mass production of *T. canis* excretory-secretory (TES) antigen (de Savigny, 1975; Oshima et al., 1963). In combination with ELISA, the use of TES antigen has remarkably improved the sensitivity and specificity of toxocariasis serodiagnosis when compared to the earlier techniques that used somatic antigens derived from embryonated eggs or adult worms.

Researchers have explored new techniques, assay formats, and better-quality antigens to increase the assay's diagnostic sensitivity and specificity. To date, indirect IgG-based ELISA is considered an effective method to diagnose human toxocariasis. In comparison to the plate ELISA, Bojanich et al. (2012) demonstrated that a dot-ELISA exhibited better stability, could be produced at a lower cost, and was easier to perform without the need of specialized equipment, making it a suitable assay for epidemiological surveillance of toxocariasis in developing countries. Western blotting is also commonly used for diagnosis, often to 'confirm' ELISA results, and to diagnose toxocariasis in patients with chronic urticaria. Other more recent serodiagnostic techniques include lateral flow rapid tests and microfluidic immunosensors. Table 1 lists serodiagnostic methods that have been used in the past two decades for the diagnosis of human toxocariasis.

3. Serodiagnostic assays: Enzyme-linked immunosorbent assay (ELISA)

3.1 Antibody detection ELISA

Early efforts at developing *Toxocara* serodiagnostic methods were based on the utilization of homologous and heterologous antigens derived from extracts of adult worms and eggs of *T. canis* (Smith and Noordin, 2006). They were used in assays despite being highly cross-reactive with *Ascaris* and other parasites (Maizels et al., 1987). Subsequently, the introduction of the in vitro cultivation system to produce TES antigen (de Savigny, 1975), in conjunction with ELISA, had tremendously enhanced the development of serodiagnostic tools with improved performance.

ELISA is a well-known technique based on the detection of antigen-antibody interactions. A specific antigen is bound to a solid phase, and the antibody is detected from a liquid sample, usually serum or plasma. An enzyme conjugated to a secondary antibody is then bound to the antigen-antibody complex, followed by the addition of a substrate to give a colour change upon reaction with the enzyme. A spectrophotometer quantitatively reads the colour strength as an optical density value.

The first ELISA that utilized TES was reported to show improved serodiagnosis of toxocariasis with a sensitivity of 78% and specificity of 92% (Glickman et al., 1978). Indirect ELISA and dot-ELISA were two formats that have been frequently described in the literature (Rudzinska et al., 2017). There are several commercial IgG-TES-ELISA kits on the market, including Toxocara IgG ELISA (IgG) (Cypress Diagnostics, Belgium), *Toxocara canis*

Table 1 Serological assays reported for diagnosis of toxocariasis.
(A) Antibody detection

Technique	Antigen	Type of assay	Performance	References
Indirect ELISA	TES-58 and TES-68	IgM	Sensitivity: 100% Specificity: 100%	Peixoto et al. (2011)
		IgG	Sensitivity: 100% Specificity: 71%	Peixoto et al. (2011)
	TCLA	IgG	Sensitivity: 92.2% Specificity: 86.6%	Jin et al. (2013)
	dTES	IgG	Sensitivity: 100% Specificity: 100%	Roldan et al. (2015)
	Native TES	IgG	Sensitivity: 50% Specificity: 73%	Watthanakulpanich et al. (2008)
	Pre-coated TES antigen	IgG	Sensitivity: 97.1% Specificity: 36%	Noordin et al. (2005)
	Native TES	IgG1	Sensitivity: 60% Specificity: 76%	Watthanakulpanich et al. (2008)
		IgG2	Sensitivity: 98% Specificity: 71%	Watthanakulpanich et al. (2008)
		IgG3	Sensitivity: 78% Specificity: 81%	Watthanakulpanich et al. (2008)
		IgG4	Sensitivity: 45.7% Specificity: 78.6%	Watthanakulpanich et al. (2008)
	Pre-coated TES antigen	IgG4	Sensitivity: 50% Specificity: 73%	Noordin et al. (2005)
	rTES-26, rTES-30, rTES-120	IgG4	Sensitivity: 80–93 Specificity: 92–96%	Norhaida et al. (2008) and Mohamad et al. (2009)
Dot-ELISA	Native TES	IgG	Sensitivity: 100% Specificity: 95%	Roldan et al. (2006)
Western blot	TES-Ag	IgG	Sensitivity: Not specified Specificity: 23–35 bands of TES-Ag (100%)	Smith et al. (2009) and Macpherson (2013)
	d-TES	IgG	No cross-reactivity	Roldan et al. (2015)
Immunochromatographic lateral flow	rTES-26, rTES-30, rTES-120	IgG, IgG4	Sensitivity: 85.7–93.1% Specificity: 90.1–100%	Lim et al. (2015) and Yunus et al. (2018)

(B) Antigen detection

Technique	Capture antibody (coated on plate)	Detector antibody	Limit of detection	Reference
Sandwich ELISA	Antibody to *T. canis* native TES	Rabbit anti-TES-HRP	78 ng mL^{-1}	Luo et al. (1999)
	mAb to *T. canis* native TES mAb to *T. cati* native TES	Rabbit anti-TES-HRP Rabbit anti-TES-HRP	4 ng mL^{-1} 5 ng mL^{-1}	Yokoi et al. (2002) and Zibaei et al. (2010)
	PoAb to *T. canis* native TES	mAb to *T. canis* native TES and goat anti-mouse- HRP	440 pg mL^{-1}	Rodríguez-Caballero et al. (2015)
	Biotinylated-bivalent Nb to *T. canis* native TES	Nb-HRP	0.650 ng mL^{-1}	Morales-Yanez et al. (2019)
Microfluidic fluorescent immunosensor	TES-3-AP-SNs	IgG-CdSe-ZnS QDs	0.12 ng mL^{-1}	Medawar et al. (2017)
Electrochemical biosensor	Biotinylated-bivalent Nb to *T. canis* native TES	Nb-HRP	10 pg mL^{-1} 30 ng mL^{-1}	Morales-Yanez et al. (2019)

TES, *Toxocara canis* excretory and secretory antigens; dTES, deglycosylated TES antigens; rTES, recombinant TES antigens; WB, Western blot; TCLA, *T. canis* larvae antigen; PoAb, polyclonal antibodies; mAb, monoclonal antibodies; Nb, nanobodies; AP-SNs, aminopropyl-functionalised silica nanoparticles; CdSe-ZnS QDs, cadmium selenide zinc sulphide quantum dots; HRP, horseradish peroxidase.

ELISA kit (Bordier Affinity Products SA, Switzerland), and NovaLisa *Toxocara* IgG ELISA (NovaTec Immunodiagnostica GmbH, Dietzenbach, Germany). Their reported diagnostic sensitivities and specificities ranged from 91% to 97%, and 86% to 96%, respectively (Choi et al., 2008; Fillaux and Magnaval, 2013; Jacquier et al., 1991; Jin et al., 2013; Smith and Noordin, 2006).

Notably, most of these commercial kits are IgG assays which contribute to the non-uniformity of detecting toxocariasis due to IgG being a long-lasting antibody that does not discriminate past and recent infections. A significant issue with IgG ELISA is the cross-reactivity problems with other parasitoses such as filariasis, strongyloidiasis, trichinellosis, and ascariasis, suggesting that this assay may be less relevant for use in areas where polyparasitism is endemic (Jacquier et al., 1991; Lynch et al., 1988). In this regard, the diagnostic potential of IgG subclasses for serodiagnosis of toxocariasis have been investigated. *Toxocara*-specific IgG2 and IgG3 were reported to achieve increased sensitivity and specificity (Watthanakulpanich et al., 2008). Meanwhile, an ELISA based on *Toxocara*-specific IgG4 detection was reported to improve the diagnostic specificity, thus significantly reducing the cross-reactivity issues faced when using native antigen. However, it showed a reduction in diagnostic sensitivity as compared to the standard IgG ELISA (Noordin et al., 2005; Smith and Noordin, 2006; Watthanakulpanich et al., 2008). Nevertheless, an IgG4-ELISA using recombinant proteins (rTES-120 and rTES-30) was reported to achieve 100% sensitivity and specificity of $\geq$92% (Mohamad et al., 2009). In another development, an IgG ELISA using deglycosylated TES was reported to show 100% diagnostic sensitivity and specificity (Roldan et al., 2015) and IgE-TES ELISA is more valuable for monitoring post-treatment (Fillaux and Magnaval, 2013).

3.2 Antigen detection ELISA

The inability of IgG ELISAs to differentiate between current and resolved infections calls for the development of an antigen detection assay. Such an assay may enable detection of antigens circulated by the dormant *Toxocara* larvae that remain metabolically active in the human body (de Savigny, 1975).

An antigen-capture ELISA utilizes antibody bound to a stationary phase that binds the circulating antigen released by the parasite (Robertson et al., 1988). The capture antibody may be in the form of polyclonal or monoclonal antibody. With a polyclonal antibody, the antigen-antibody interaction occurs on one or more epitopes of the given antigen, while the interaction of antigen to a monoclonal antibody occurs on one specific epitope of the antigen (Lipman et al., 2005). Early attempts in detecting circulating TES antigen using polyclonal antibody in human serum samples (Luo et al., 1999) showed unsatisfactory diagnostic sensitivity which may be attributed to the low larval burden (Gillespie et al., 1993; Robertson et al., 1988). The use of a polyclonal antibody is also confounded by cross-reactivity problems (Gillespie et al., 1993; Robertson et al., 1988). The application of monoclonal antibody offers the potential of increased diagnostic performance. Studies have shown increased specificity of sandwich ELISAs utilizing monoclonal antibodies when used on multi-parasitized serum samples (Ishiyamna et al., 2009; Zibaei et al., 2010).

The detection limits of circulating TES antigen were found to be $440\,\mathrm{pg\,mL^{-1}}$ to $78\,\mathrm{ng\,mL^{-1}}$ (Gillespie et al., 1993; Ishiyamna et al., 2009; Robertson et al., 1988; Rodríguez-Caballero et al., 2015; Zibaei et al., 2010). The antigen detection ELISA is thus useful in distinguishing between current and past infection, as the presence of the antigen in an antibody-positive patient shows an ongoing or active infection. Furthermore, in patients with inactive infection, circulating TES antigen was undetectable (Gillespie et al., 1993). Nevertheless, the sensitivity of an antigen detection test would be expected to be lower than an antibody detection test; thus, the former (antigen detection test) is expected to complement, but not replace the latter.

Recently, a study reported on the use of nanobodies to detect TES antigen (Morales-Yanez et al., 2019). Nanobodies are naturally occurring antibodies composed of heavy chains with a comprehensive antigen-binding range that can be easily engineered, thus suitable for application in an antigen detection assay (Dmitriev et al., 2016; Helma et al., 2015; Morales-Yanez et al., 2019). The study demonstrated the use of three nanobodies that were specific towards TES components of *T. canis* using immunoblots; and a limit of detection of $0.650\,\mathrm{ng\,mL^{-1}}$ in a sandwich ELISA. The application of nanobodies seemed to offer an opportunity to develop a promising serodiagnostic tool for toxocariasis.

4. Western blot

Frequently, the initial serological findings are confirmed by performing a Western blot to avoid false-positive results and to evaluate cross-reactions with other infective agents (Ma et al., 2018). Unlike the

ELISA, the Western blot is an immunoblotting technique that can qualitatively detect antibodies specific to the antigen, where the results can be visualized as bands using a chromogenic or chemiluminescence substrate, with the latter observed on an X-ray film. Earlier studies used serum from infected rabbits, and humans (primarily with OLM) tested with native TES antigen. The Western blots revealed multiple protein bands of low molecular weights, i.e., 24, 28, 30, and 35 kDa, and three protein bands at high molecular weights, i.e., 132, 147 and 200 kDa (Fillaux and Magnaval, 2013; Magnaval et al., 1991). The three protein bands of low molecular weights were reported to be *Toxocara*-specific (Fillaux and Magnaval, 2013; Magnaval et al., 1991; Park et al., 2000), this was later confirmed by subsequent studies that described the same banding patterns (Morales et al., 2002; Roldán and Espinoza, 2009; Zarnowska and Jastrzebska, 1994). When compared to commercial TES-ELISA kits, an in-house Western blot was found to have a 55% higher diagnostic sensitivity (Courtade et al., 1995; Fillaux and Magnaval, 2013; Gueglio et al., 1994). A commonly reported commercial Western blot kit is *Toxocara* WB-IgG (LDBIO Diagnostics, Lyon, France); however, its diagnostic performance varies in different studies (Artinyan et al., 2014; Despreaux et al., 2016; Lotsch et al., 2016; Macpherson, 2013).

Similar to the ELISA, the diagnostic performance of Western blot is dependent on the type of antigen (e.g. larval lysate, native TES, deglycosylated TES, or recombinant TES) and the type of secondary antibody (e.g. total IgG, IgG subclasses, or IgM) used. Cross-reactivity may still be seen with a Western blot assay; furthermore, the technique requires trained personnel.

5. *Toxocara* excretory-secretory antigens

5.1 Native TES antigen

Prior to the use of TES antigen in diagnosis, most assays for human toxocariasis used antigens obtained from water-soluble, somatic antigens of *T. canis* embryonated eggs, infective larvae or adult worms which have low sensitivity and high rate of cross-reactivity to other ascarids (Girdwood et al., 1978; Smith et al., 1982). Native TES contains a mixture of highly immunogenic glycoproteins, thus making it highly sensitive. The use of TES antigen has also significantly increased the diagnostic assay specificity (Magnaval et al., 2001). It is now a standard immunodiagnostic reagent and is widely used for serodiagnosis of human toxocariasis.

To prepare native TES antigen, briefly, non-embryonated eggs are isolated from *Toxocara* adult worms obtained from the animal host. The eggs are embryonated and hatched to release the larvae. The larvae are then cultivated in a defined culture medium to produce the TES. Thus, the amount of antigen produced depends on the number of larvae (de Savigny, 1975; Elefant et al., 2006; Thomas et al., 2016). The method has been improved to enhance the production of TES and achieve higher larval purity (Alcantara-Neves et al., 2008; Ponce-Macotela et al., 2011; Sperotto et al., 2017; Thomas et al., 2016).

TES antigens are secretions of a complex set of glycoproteins by *Toxocara* larvae which can be characterized as mucins, lectins, and other TES products (Dlugosz et al., 2015; Holland and Smith, 2006). *Toxocara* mucins are composed of separate segments, a glycosylated and a non-glycosylated domains (Gems et al., 1995; Maizels et al., 2000); they typically migrate at molecular mass of approximately 120 kDa on SDS-PAGE gel, hence named as TES-120; and do not correspond to the actual molecular mass (~40–45 kDa) due to the heavy glycosylation (Loukas et al., 2000). Five distinct mucins have been discovered, i.e., MUC-1, MUC-2, MUC-3, MUC-4, and MUC-5, for which the first three are the most dominant mucins, corresponding to the surface coat mucins (Gems and Maizels, 1996; Loukas et al., 2000). Meanwhile, MUC-4 seems to be less important due to the discrepancy in the sequence against the surface coat glycoproteins of the family mucins and MUC-5 is less likely to be identified as *Toxocara* mucin (Doedens et al., 2001).

Toxocara lectins, on the other hand, are TES glycoprotein, which is known as C-type lectin (CTL). They have significant roles as diagnostic markers in an infection (Dodd and Drickamer, 2001) and have a clear functional interaction between host and parasite during the infection (Loukas et al., 1999). CTL-1 or TES-32/30 is one of the most prominent larval proteins with significant diagnostic value. The other well-researched TES products are TES-26 (PEB-1), which is known as the most functioning phosphatidylethanolamine-binding protein (Gems et al., 1995), TES-400, TES-45, and TES-55.

5.2 Recombinant TES antigen

In recent years, efforts have been focused on producing recombinant TES antigens that can improve serodiagnosis of toxocariasis, as a substitution for native TES antigen. Thus far, four recombinant TES proteins have been reported to be of good diagnostic potential, i.e., rTES-26, rTES-30, rTES-120, and *T. cati* rTES-120. Being antigens that are produced in a highly purified and standardized manner, the use of recombinant TES antigen has reduced cross-reactions with other parasitic diseases, thus increased the assay diagnostic specificity (Mohamad et al., 2009; Wickramasinghe et al., 2008; Yamasaki et al., 2000; Yunus et al., 2018). A study to investigate the diagnostic potential of the three recombinant *T. canis* antigens was conducted using various immunoglobulin classes, i.e., IgM, IgE, IgG, and the subclasses. The study revealed significant increases in the specificity of ELISAs when IgG4 antibody was used in the assays. Although the sensitivity of rTES-26 was lower than rTES-30 and rTES-120, its specificity was the highest. The combined use of these three recombinant antigens increased the diagnostic sensitivity compared to the use of single recombinant antigens (Mohamad et al., 2009; Yunus et al., 2018).

6. Role of *Toxocara cati* in serodiagnosis

T. canis has been regarded as the main source of human infection. The importance of *T. cati* as an aetiologic agent of toxocariasis in humans has been underestimated, despite its high prevalence in cat populations as reported in France (Fromont et al., 2001), Denmark (Heilskov, 2002), Brazil (Labarthe et al., 2004), and the Netherlands (Robben et al., 2004). Moreover, sandboxes and garden soil are more often polluted with *T. cati* than *T. canis eggs*, (Jansen et al., 1993; Overgaauw and Knapen, 2008) thus highlighting the risk of *T. cati* infections to humans.

A high degree of homology between TES antigen from both species has been reported (Fillaux and Magnaval, 2013; Hogarth-Scott et al., 1969). However, they are not the same as shown by several studies (Kennedy et al., 1987; Zahabiun et al., 2015). In the study by Kennedy et al. (1987), seven of eight monoclonal antibodies against *T. canis* reacted to both *T. canis* and *T. cati* antigens, however, one monoclonal antibody (MoAb Tcn-2) only reacted to *T. canis* and not to *T. cati* antigen. The result implied that despite the high homology between the two antigens, there might be important differences between them and thus is likely that some cases of *T. cati* infection may be missed by tests using only *T. canis* antigen.

Several studies have reported human toxocariasis caused by *T. cati*. Petithory et al. (1993) reported that 3 out of 10 OLM patients showed a higher reaction to *T. cati* antigen than *T. canis* antigen through a mini-Ouchterlony test. In other case studies, it was reported that the antibody titers of OLM patients showed a greater reaction with *T. cati* antigen compared to *T. canis* antigen, therefore suggesting that OLM is often caused by *T. cati* (Sakai et al., 1998; Zibaei et al., 2014). *T. cati* infection was also reported in a liver biopsy from a VLM patient who showed the presence of the larvae and the serum was strongly positive in an Ouchterlony test using *T. cati* antigen (Shimokawa et al., 1982). ELISAs and Western blots utilizing *T. cati* TES antigen on some patients produced better sensitivity as compared to using *T. canis* TES antigen (Zibaei et al., 2016). These findings suggest that toxocariasis infection caused by *T. cati* may be missed in some cases if only *T. canis* diagnostic reagent were used in the serodiagnosis.

A study of native *T. cati* TES showed seven protein bands at molecular masses of 20, 28, 32, 42, 50, 70, and 150 kDa. The fractions at 42 and 50 kDa were found to be highly antigenic; thus, they may be useful for serodiagnosis (Zibaei et al., 2016). Thus far, there is only one recombinant protein reported for *T. cati*, i.e., rTES-120 (Zahabiun et al., 2015). In a Western blot study, the diagnostic performance of *T. cati* rTES-120 was compared to its *T. canis* homologue, and it showed an increased diagnostic sensitivity when results from both species are considered.

7. Challenges in serodiagnosis of toxocariasis

Since the first reported incidence of toxocariasis in 1950, poor understanding of the global and public health impact of the infection remains, possibly due to insufficient awareness as well as lack of clinical and laboratory diagnostic efficacy to detect *Toxocara* infection. The known limitation of *Toxocara* antigen-based assay is the significant cross-reactivity with other helminths such as *A. lumbricoides* particularly in the area with polyparasitism (Fillaux and Magnaval, 2013). In order to reduce cross-reactivity with other infections, one study proposed an extra step of serum absorption with either extract of non-homologous parasite, i.e., *A. suum* (Camargo et al., 1992; Elefant et al., 2006) or use of an antigen panel of extracts from nematodes, cestodes, and protozoa (Lynch et al., 1988). This step, however, is rather cumbersome (Fillaux and Magnaval, 2013) and although it helps to enhance diagnostic specificity, it causes a reduction in the diagnostic sensitivity (Zhan et al., 2015).

TES-based ELISAs are considered as the standard method for diagnosis of toxocariasis; however, it is still far from being an excellent reference standard due to some weaknesses. Lack of confirmatory serological test makes the development of new diagnostic methods a challenge since researchers usually must rely on and compare their new finding with the results from the TES-ELISA. Besides, the production of TES antigen being laborious and time-consuming, and the production is limited due to difficulty in obtaining adult worms for larval cultivation. In some regions, the availability of TES-ELISA is an issue. Mendonça et al. (2013) reported that many areas in Brazil could not access ELISA kits due to their high cost, despite the high seroprevalence of toxocariasis in the country. In the United States, ELISA for serodiagnosis of parasitic disease is not widely available since it is an uncommon diagnosis made by physicians and the *Toxocara* antigen is also not easily accessible (Hotez and Wilkins, 2009). The use of recombinant antigens would be able to address some of the above challenges.

Serological tests detecting anti-*Toxocara* antibodies may have less value in the case of OLM and neurotoxocariasis. In some cases, the serum of OLM patients may repeatedly produce negative results due to the low serum antibody response (Smith et al., 2009). Low larval load present in the infected area may cause very low titers of antibody responses, and in some cases, it may be even undetectable (Magnaval et al., 2002; Sharkey and McKay, 1993). As for neurotoxocariasis cases, it has been reported that the ELISA gave a false-negative result when tested on CSF of a patient clinically diagnosed with toxocariasis (Xinou et al., 2003).

Lack of knowledge by physicians of the infection has also contributed to the misdiagnosis or underdiagnosis of the infection. A study among 2684 paediatricians in the United States revealed that 85% of the assessed paediatricians admitted not to have current knowledge about toxocariasis (Woodhall et al., 2017). Some of them (29%) did not even include *Toxocara* diagnosis in the list of presumptive diagnosis when assessing patients.

8. Advances in serological diagnosis of toxocariasis

ELISA and Western blot kits are expensive for developing countries and not cost-effective for single samples. They also require a skilled technician and a reliable cold chain transport. Rapid lateral flow immunoassay is a promising approach for serodiagnosis in low resource settings and has been used for the diagnosis of many helminthic and protozoan diseases. It is a simpler and more convenient method that does not require sophisticated equipment and provide visual results in less than 30 minutes (Momcilovic et al., 2019). A prototype rapid test called iToxocara utilizes rTES-30 antigen, and an evaluation study of its performance showed 85.7% diagnostic sensitivity and 90.1% specificity (Lim et al., 2015). However, only serum or plasma can only be used as samples, and lysed blood cells can interfere with the binding of antigen to antibody. A recent report by Yunus et al. (2018) was on a laboratory prototype of a lateral flow IgG4 rapid test utilizing three recombinant *T. canis* antigens (rTES-26, rTES-30 and rTES-120) with a sensitivity of 93.1% and 100% specificity.

The development of analytical devices that enable digitalization and quantification of biological reactions offers opportunities for more advanced developments in the disease diagnosis, with objective, reliable, and rapid results. One study described the application of microfluidic immunosensor using laser-induced fluorescence (LIF) incorporated with TES antigen coupled to silica nanoparticles to detect IgG anti-*T. canis* antibodies which have a limit of detection of $0.12\,ng\,mL^{-1}$ (Medawar et al., 2017). In another recent study, nanobodies (Nbs) were utilized in an electrochemical magneto-sensor and showed an improved diagnostic sensitivity of 10-fold as compared to ELISA (Francisco Morales-Yánez et al., 2018; Morales-Yanez et al., 2019). The analytical sensitivity of the sensor was $15\,pg\,mL^{-1}$ in serum spiked with TES antigen, and no cross-reactivity was observed with antigens from other nematode infections.

9. Way forward for serodiagnosis of toxocariasis

Laboratory diagnosis, coupled with clinical findings and patient history, is essential in the diagnosis of human toxocariasis. Although native TES-based ELISA offers better specificity compared to other forms of native antigen, it still has the potential to cross-react with other helminth infections when used in developing tropical areas with polyparasitism. Innumerable studies have documented the use of recombinant antigens to replace the TES antigen to counter the specificity issue. As mentioned earlier, the most commonly reported recombinant antigens used for human toxocariasis studies are rTES-26, rTES-30/-32, and rTES-120. The use of more than one recombinant antigen would be useful and increases the diagnostic performance of the serodiagnostic test (Mohamad et al., 2009; Yunus et al., 2018; Zahabiun et al., 2015). Since ruling out a single antigen could reduce the performance of the assay, it may be useful to include all the recombinant antigens as a diagnostic panel or as a chimeric antigen (Mohamad et al., 2009; Yunus et al., 2018). The use of a chimeric antigen has been examined in several other parasitic infections and has shown promising results. For example, a genetically engineered recombinant chimeric plasmid containing epitopes of six *Toxoplasma gondii* gene products, i.e., MIC2, MIC3, M2AP, GRA3, GRA7, and SAG1 had been successfully produced to replace the use of tachyzoite extract in serological assays (Beghetto et al., 2006).

A recent report described several abundant novel larval transcripts from *T. canis*, i.e., ANT-3, ANT-5, ANT-30, and ANT-34. Antibodies produced against the corresponding recombinant proteins did not react with the native parasite antigen; however, antibodies to two of them were detected in patient sera, which suggest that they are expressed by the parasite post-infection (Callister et al., 2008). The diagnostic value of these proteins should be further studied.

As described earlier, there is also a need for the development of diagnostic tools that include *T. cati* recombinant antigen, combined with *T. canis* recombinant antigens to enable detection of infections caused by both species. The role of other species in *Toxocara* genus in causing human infection needs to be elucidated. *T. malaysiensis* was discovered in Malaysian domestic cats, and several studies have reported that the worm is a distinct species from *T. canis* and *T. cati*, but the genome is similar to *T. cati* (Gibbons et al., 2001). The early hypothesis suggested that *T. malaysiensis* is also a zoonotic parasite (Li et al., 2006); thus, it may have a significant public health impact. The species was also reported in China (Li et al., 2006) and Vietnam (Le et al., 2016). *T. vitulorum*, a parasite of cattle and water buffalo, showed evidence of somatic migration of the larva in experimental animals (Omar and Barriga, 1991). Macpherson (2013) also hypothesized that repeated human infection by *T. vitulorum* might lead to disease. However, more data is needed to determine whether the migrating larvae persist in human tissues. Also further studies on contributions of all *Toxocara* species infecting humans are essential to uncover unique antigens or antibody response that may be of diagnostic potential and may help in developing serodiagnostic assays that can detect all species and/or differentiate the infecting species.

Use of synthetic peptides is one of the most recent strategies used in many research fields. They can be produced as identical copies of the protein either by recombinant protein synthesis or through chemical peptide synthesis. The antigenic epitopes of the known *Toxocara* protein can be predicted, and peptides synthesized and tested for their diagnostic potential. Using bioinformatics and modelling, a novel synthetic protein was designed comprising immunodominant B cell epitopes of *T. canis* TES-26, TES-30, and TES-120 that was predicted to be useful for diagnosis for human toxocariasis (Ebrahimi et al., 2019). Synthetic peptides have been used to detect antigens of other parasites such as *T. gondii* (Bastos et al., 2016; Dai et al., 2012),

Strongyloides (Feliciano et al., 2016), *Fasciola hepatica* (Noya et al., 2016) and *Trypanosoma cruzi* (Houghton et al., 2002). Thus, this promising approach should also be applied in the development of a better serodiagnostic assay for toxocariasis.

Development of aptamers that bind *Toxocara* proteins of diagnostic importance is another interesting approach worth pursuing. In combination with other reagents, it can be used to develop better antigen detection tests. Also, recombinant *Toxocara* monoclonal antibodies can be used for the same purpose, and for quality control of commercial kits. In conclusion, despite the improvements made in serodiagnosis of toxocariasis, there are still many gaps that can be filled, thus providing exciting opportunities for further research.

Acknowledgement

We would like to acknowledge the contributions from Universiti Sains Malaysia RU grant No. 1001/CIPPM/8012202 and the Ministry of Education, through the Higher Centre of Excellence (HICoE) grant No. 311/CIPPM/4401005.

References

Alcantara-Neves, N.M., Dos Santos, A.B., Mendonca, L.R., Figueiredo, C.A., Pontes-de-Carvalho, L., 2008. An improved method to obtain antigen-excreting Toxocara canis larvae. Exp. Parasitol. 119, 349–351.

Artinyan, E., Uysal, H.K., Akgul, O., Altiparmak, S., Oner, Y.A., 2014. Research on Toxocara canis antibodies obtained from patients with eosinophilia. Indian J. Med. Microbiol. 32, 383–386.

Bastos, L.M., Macedo Jr., A.G., Silva, M.V., Santiago, F.M., Ramos, E.L., Santos, F.A., Pirovani, C.P., Goulart, L.R., Mineo, T.W., Mineo, J.R., 2016. Toxoplasma gondii-derived synthetic peptides containing B- and T-cell Epitopes from GRA2 protein are able to enhance mice survival in a model of experimental toxoplasmosis. Front. Cell. Infect. Microbiol. 6, 59.

Beghetto, E., Spadoni, A., Bruno, L., Buffolano, W., Gargano, N., 2006. Chimeric antigens of Toxoplasma gondii: toward standardization of toxoplasmosis serodiagnosis using recombinant products. J. Clin. Microbiol. 44, 2133–2140.

Bellanger, A.-P., Humbert, P., Gavignet, B., Deschaseaux, A.D., Barisien, C., Roussel, S., Millon, L., Aubin, F., Piarroux, R., 2010. Comparative assessment of enzyme-linked immunosorbent assay and Western blot for the diagnosis of toxocariasis in patients with skin disorders. Br. J. Dermatol. 162, 80–82.

Bojanich, M.V., Marino, G.L., López, M.Á., Alonso, J.M., 2012. An evaluation of the dot-ELISA procedure as a diagnostic test in an area with a high prevalence of human *Toxocara canis* infection. Mem. Inst. Oswaldo Cruz 107, 194–197.

Callister, D.M., Winter, A.D., Page, A.P., Maizels, R.M., 2008. Four abundant novel transcript genes from Toxocara canis with unrelated coding sequences share untranslated region tracts implicated in the control of gene expression. Mol. Biochem. Parasitol. 162, 60–70.

Camargo, E.D., Nakamura, P.M., Vaz, A.J., da Silva, M.V., Chieffi, P.P., de Melo, E.O., 1992. Standardization of dot-ELISA for the serological diagnosis of toxocariasis and comparison of the assay with ELISA. Rev. Inst. Med. Trop. Sao Paulo 34, 55–60.

Cassenote, A.J., Lima, A.R., Pinto Neto, J.M., Rubinsky-Elefant, G., 2014. Seroprevalence and modifiable risk factors for Toxocara spp. in Brazilian schoolchildren. PLoS Negl. Trop. Dis. 8, e2830.

Chen, J., Zhou, D.H., Nisbet, A.J., Xu, M.J., Huang, S.Y., Li, M.W., Wang, C.R., Zhu, X.Q., 2012. Advances in molecular identification, taxonomy, genetic variation and diagnosis of Toxocara spp. Infect. Genet. Evol. 12, 1344–1348.

Chen, J., Liu, Q., Liu, G.H., Zheng, W.B., Hong, S.J., Sugiyama, H., Zhu, X.Q., Elsheikha, H.M., 2018. Toxocariasis: a silent threat with a progressive public health impact. Infect. Dis. Poverty 7, 59.

Choi, D., Lim, J.H., Choi, D.C., Paik, S.W., Kim, S.H., Huh, S., 2008. Toxocariasis and ingestion of raw cow liver in patients with eosinophilia. Korean J. Parasitol. 46, 139–143.

Courtade, H., Recco, P., Magnaval, J.F., Charlet, J.P., Seguela, J.P., 1995. Etude comparative de deux tests Elisa toxocara vis à vis du Western-blot. Bull. Soc. Fr. Parasitol. 13, 37–53.

Dai, J., Jiang, M., Wang, Y., Qu, L., Gong, R., Si, J., 2012. Evaluation of a recombinant multiepitope peptide for serodiagnosis of Toxoplasma gondii infection. Clin. Vaccine Immunol. 19, 338–342.

de Savigny, D.H., 1975. In vitro maintenance of Toxocara canis larvae and a simple method for the production of Toxocara ES antigen for use in serodiagnostic tests for visceral larva migrans. J. Parasitol. 61, 781–782.

Despreaux, R., Fardeau, C., Touhami, S., Brasnu, E., Champion, E., Paris, L., Touitou, V., Bodaghi, B., Lehoang, P., 2016. Ocular Toxocariasis: clinical features and long-term visual outcomes in adult patients. Am. J. Ophthalmol. 166, 162–168.

Dlugosz, E., Wasyl, K., Klockiewicz, M., Wisniewski, M., 2015. Toxocara canis mucins among other excretory-secretory antigens induce in vitro secretion of cytokines by mouse splenocytes. Parasitol. Res. 114, 3365–3371.

Dmitriev, O.Y., Lutsenko, S., Muyldermans, S., 2016. Nanobodies as probes for protein dynamics in vitro and in cells. J. Biol. Chem. 291, 3767–3775.

Dodd, R.B., Drickamer, K., 2001. Lectin-like proteins in model organisms: implications for evolution of carbohydrate-binding activity. Glycobiology 11, 71R–79R.

Doedens, A., Loukas, A., Maizels, R.M., 2001. A cDNA encoding Tc-MUC-5, a mucin from Toxocara canis larvae identified by expression screening. Acta Trop. 79, 211–217.

Ebrahimi, M., Seyyedtabaei, S.J., Ranjbar, M.M., Tahvildar-Biderouni, F., Javadi-Mamaghani, A., 2019. Designing and modeling of multi-epitope proteins for diagnosis of Toxocara canis infection. Int. J. Pept. Res. Ther. 1–10. https://doi.org/10.1007/s10989-019-09940-1.

Elefant, G.R., Shimizu, S.H., Sanchez, M.C., Jacob, C.M., Ferreira, A.W., 2006. A serological follow-up of toxocariasis patients after chemotherapy based on the detection of IgG, IgA, and IgE antibodies by enzyme-linked immunosorbent assay. J. Clin. Lab. Anal. 20, 164–172.

Feliciano, N.D., Ribeiro, V.S., Gonzaga, H.T., Santos, F.A., Fujimura, P.T., Goulart, L.R., Costa-Cruz, J.M., 2016. Short epitope-based synthetic peptides for serodiagnosis of human strongyloidiasis. Immunol. Lett. 172, 89–93.

Fialho, P.M., Correa, C.R., 2016. A systematic review of Toxocariasis: a neglected but high-prevalence disease in Brazil. Am. J. Trop. Med. Hyg. 94, 1193–1199.

Fillaux, J., Magnaval, J.F., 2013. Laboratory diagnosis of human toxocariasis. Vet. Parasitol. 193, 327–336.

Francisco Morales-Yánez, T.S., Marie, H., Idalia, S., Karolien, D.W., Katja, P., Serge, M., 2018. Ultrasensitive detection of *Toxocara canis* excretory secretory antigens by a nanobody electrochemical magnetosensor assay. Am. J. Trop. Med. Hyg. 99, 238.

Fromont, E., Morvilliers, L., Artois, M., Pontier, D., 2001. Parasite richness and abundance in insular and mainland feral cats: insularity or density? Parasitology 123, 143–151.

Gems, D., Maizels, R.M., 1996. An abundantly expressed mucin-like protein from Toxocara canis infective larvae: the precursor of the larval surface coat glycoproteins. Proc. Natl. Acad. Sci. U. S. A. 93, 1665–1670.

Gems, D., Ferguson, C.J., Robertson, B.D., Nieves, R., Page, A.P., Blaxter, M.L., Maizels, R.M., 1995. An abundant, trans-spliced mRNA from Toxocara canis infective larvae encodes a 26-kDa protein with homology to phosphatidylethanolamine-binding proteins. J. Biol. Chem. 270, 18517–18522.

Gibbons, L.M., Jacobs, D.E., Sani, R.A., 2001. Toxocara malaysiensis n. sp. (Nematoda: Ascaridoidea) from the domestic cat (Felis catus Linnaeus, 1758). J. Parasitol. 87, 660–665.

Gillespie, S.H., Bidwell, D., Voller, A., Robertson, B.D., Maizels, R.M., 1993. Diagnosis of human toxocariasis by antigen capture enzyme linked immunosorbent assay. J. Clin. Pathol. 46, 551–554.

Girdwood, R.W.A., Smith, H.V., Bruce, R.G., Quinn, R., 1978. Human *Toxocara* infection in west of Scotland. Lancet 311, 1318.

Glickman, L., Schantz, P., Dombroske, R., Cypess, R., 1978. Evaluation of serodiagnostic tests for visceral larva migrans. Am. J. Trop. Med. Hyg. 27, 492–498.

Gueglio, B., de Gentile, L., Nguyen, J.M., Achard, J., Chabasse, D., Marjolet, M., 1994. Epidemiologic approach to human toxocariasis in western France. Parasitol. Res. 80, 531–536.

Heilskov, L., 2002. Prevalence of intestinal Toxocara cati infections in cats from a rural area in Denmark. Dansk Veterinaertidsskrift 85, 6–11.

Helma, J., Cardoso, M.C., Muyldermans, S., Leonhardt, H., 2015. Nanobodies and recombinant binders in cell biology. J. Cell Biol. 209, 633–644.

Hogarth-Scott, R.S., Johansson, S.G.O., Bennich, H., 1969. Antibodies to *Toxocara* in the sera of visceral larva migran: the significance raised levels of IgE. Clin. Exp. Immunol. 5, 619–625.

Holland, C., Smith, H.V., 2006. Toxocara: The Enigmatic Parasite. CABI.

Hotez, P.J., Wilkins, P.P., 2009. Toxocariasis: America's most common neglected infection of poverty and a helminthiasis of global importance? PLoS Negl. Trop. Dis. 3, e400.

Houghton, R.L., Benson, D.R., Reynolds, L.D., Mcneill, P.D., Sleath, P.R., Lodes, M.J., Skeiky, Y.A.W., Leiby, D.A., Badaro, R., Reed, S.G., 2002. A multi-epitope synthetic peptide and recombinant protein for the detection of antibodies to *Trypanosoma cruzi* in radioimmunoprecipitation-confirmed and consensus-positive sera. J Infect Dis 179, 1226–1234.

Ishiyamna, S., Ono, K., Rai, S.K., Uga, S., 2009. Method for detecting circulating Toxocara canis antigen and its application in human serum samples. Nepal Med. Coll. J. 11, 9–13.

Jacquier, P., Gottstein, B., Stingelin, Y., Eckert, J., 1991. Immunodiagnosis of toxocarosis in humans: evaluation of a new enzyme-linked immunosorbent assay kit. J. Clin. Microbiol. 29, 1831–1835.

Jansen, J., van Knapen, F., Schreurs, M., van Wijngaarden, T., 1993. Toxocara ova in parks and sand-boxes in the city of Utrecht. Tijdschr. Diergeneeskd. 118, 611–614.

Jin, Y., Shen, C., Huh, S., Sohn, W.M., Choi, M.H., Hong, S.T., 2013. Serodiagnosis of toxocariasis by ELISA using crude antigen of Toxocara canis larvae. Korean J. Parasitol. 51, 433–439.

Kennedy, M.W., Maizels, R.M., Meghji, M., Young, L., Qureshi, F., Smith, H.V., 1987. Species-specific and common epitopes on the secreted and surface antigens of Toxocava cati and Toxocara canis infective larvae. Parasite Immunol. 9, 407–420.

Labarthe, N., Serrao, M.L., Ferreira, A.M., Almeida, N.K., Guerrero, J., 2004. A survey of gastrointestinal helminths in cats of the metropolitan region of Rio de Janeiro, Brazil. Vet. Parasitol. 123, 133–139.

Le, T.H., Anh, N.T., Nguyen, K.T., Nguyen, N.T., Thuy Do, T.T., Gasser, R.B., 2016. Toxocara malaysiensis infection in domestic cats in Vietnam—an emerging zoonotic issue? Infect. Genet. Evol. 37, 94–98.

Li, M.W., Zhu, X.Q., Gasser, R.B., Lin, R.Q., Sani, R.A., Lun, Z.R., Jacobs, D.E., 2006. The occurrence of Toxocara malaysiensis in cats in China, confirmed by sequence-based analyses of ribosomal DNA. Parasitol. Res. 99, 554–557.

Lim, P.K., Yamasaki, H., Mak, J.W., Wong, S.F., Chong, C.W., Yap, I.K., Ambu, S., Kumarasamy, V., 2015. Field evaluation of a rapid diagnostic test to detect antibodies in human toxocariasis. Acta Trop. 148, 32–37.

Lipman, N.S., Jackson, L.R., Trudel, L.J., Weis-Garcia, F., 2005. Monoclonal versus polyclonal antibodies: distinguishing characteristics, applications, and information resources. ILAR J. 46, 258–268.

Lotsch, F., Obermuller, M., Mischlinger, J., Mombo-Ngoma, G., Groger, M., Adegnika, A.A., Agnandji, S.T., Schneider, R., Auer, H., Ramharter, M., 2016. Seroprevalence of Toxocara spp. in a rural population in central African Gabon. Parasitol. Int. 65, 632–634.

Loukas, A., Mullin, N.P., Tetteh, K.K., Moens, L., Maizels, R.M., 1999. A novel C-type lectin secreted by a tissue-dwelling parasitic nematode. Curr. Biol. 9, 825–828.

Loukas, A., Hintz, M., Linder, D., Mullin, N.P., Parkinson, J., Tetteh, K.K., Maizels, R.M., 2000. A family of secreted mucins from the parasitic nematode Toxocara canis bears diverse mucin domains but shares similar flanking six-cysteine repeat motifs. J. Biol. Chem. 275, 39600–39607.

Luo, Z.J., Wang, G.X., Yang, C.I., Lou, C.H., Cheng, S.W., Liao, L., 1999. Detection of circulating antigens and antibodies in Toxocara canis infection among children in Chengdu, China. J. Parasitol. 85, 252–256.

Lynch, N.R., Wilkes, L.K., Hodgen, A.N., Turner, K.J., 1988. Specificity of *Toxocara* ELISA in tropical populations. Parasite Immunol. 10, 323–337.

Ma, G., Holland, C.V., Wang, T., Hofmann, A., Fan, C.-K., Maizels, R.M., Hotez, P.J., Gasser, R.B., 2018. Human toxocariasis. Lancet Infect. Dis. 18, e14–e24.

Macpherson, C.N., 2013. The epidemiology and public health importance of toxocariasis: a zoonosis of global importance. Int. J. Parasitol. 43, 999–1008.

Magnaval, J.F., Fabre, R., Maurières, P., Charlet, J.P., de Larrard, B., 1991. Application of the Western blotting procedure for the immunodiagnosis of human toxocariasis. Parasitol. Res. 77, 697–702.

Magnaval, J.F., Glickman, L.T., Dorchies, P., Morassin, B., 2001. Highlights of human toxocariasis. Korean J. Parasitol. 39, 1–11.

Magnaval, J.F., Malard, L., Morassin, B., Fabre, R., 2002. Immunodiagnosis of ocular toxocariasis using Western-blot for the detection of specific anti-Toxocara IgG and CAP for the measurement of specific anti-Toxocara IgE. J. Helminthol. 76, 335–339.

Maizels, R.M., Kennedy, M.W., Meghji, M., Robertson, B.D., Smith, H.V., 1987. Shared carbohydrate epitopes on distinct surface and secreted antigens of the parasitic nematode Toxocara canis. J. Immunol. 139, 207–214.

Maizels, R.M., Tetteh, K.K., Loukas, A., 2000. Toxocara canis: genes expressed by the arrested infective larval stage of a parasitic nematode. Int. J. Parasitol. 30, 495–508.

Medawar, V., Messina, G.A., Fernández-Baldo, M., Raba, J., Pereira, S.V., 2017. Fluorescent immunosensor using AP-SNs and QDs for quantitation of IgG anti-Toxocara canis. Microchem. J. 130, 436–441.

Mendonça, L.R., Figueiredo, C.A., Esquivel, R., Fiaccone, R.L., Pontes-de-Carvalho, L., Cooper, P., Barreto, M.L., Alcantara-Neves, N.M., 2013. Seroprevalence and risk factors for *Toxocara* infection in children from an urban large setting in Northeast Brazil. Acta Trop. 128, 90–95.

Mohamad, S., Azmi, N.C., Noordin, R., 2009. Development and evaluation of a sensitive and specific assay for diagnosis of human toxocariasis by use of three recombinant antigens (TES-26, TES-30USM, and TES-120). J. Clin. Microbiol. 47, 1712–1717.

Momcilovic, S., Cantacessi, C., Arsic-Arsenijevic, V., Otranto, D., Tasic-Otasevic, S., 2019. Rapid diagnosis of parasitic diseases: current scenario and future needs. Clin. Microbiol. Infect. 25, 290–309.

Morales, O.L., López, M.C., Nicholls, R.B., Agudelo, C., 2002. Identification of Toxocara canis antigens by western blot in experimentally infected rabbits. Rev. Inst. Med. Trop. Sao Paulo 44, 213–216.

Morales-Yanez, F.J., Sariego, I., Vincke, C., Hassanzadeh-Ghassabeh, G., Polman, K., Muyldermans, S., 2019. An innovative approach in the detection of Toxocara canis excretory/secretory antigens using specific nanobodies. Int. J. Parasitol. 49, 635–645.

Moreira, G.M., Telmo Pde, L., Mendonca, M., Moreira, A.N., Mcbride, A.J., Scaini, C.J., Conceicao, F.R., 2014. Human toxocariasis: current advances in diagnostics, treatment, and interventions. Trends Parasitol. 30, 456–464.

Noordin, R., Smith, H.V., Mohamad, S., Maizels, R.M., Fong, M.Y., 2005. Comparison of IgG-ELISA and IgG4-ELISA for Toxocara serodiagnosis. Acta Trop. 93, 57–62.

Norhaida, A., Suharni, M., Liza Sharmini, A.T., Tuda, J., Rahmah, N., 2008. rTES-30USM: cloning via assembly PCR, expression, and evaluation of usefulness in the detection of toxocariasis. Ann. Trop. Med. Parasitol. 102, 151–160.

Noya, V., Brossard, N., Berasain, P., Rodriguez, E., Chiale, C., Mazal, D., Carmona, C., Freire, T., 2016. A mucin-like peptide from Fasciola hepatica induces parasite-specific Th1-type cell immunity. Parasitol. Res. 115, 1053–1063.

Omar, H.M., Barriga, O.O., 1991. Biology and pathophysiology of Toxocara vitulorum infections in a rabbit model. Vet. Parasitol. 40, 257–266.

Oshima, T., Nishi, S., Kihata, M., 1963. *In-vitro* cultivation on *Toxocara canis* larvae with chemically defined media. Jpn. J. Parasitol. 12 (Suppl. 1), 314.

Overgaauw, P.A., Knapen, F.V., 2008. Toxocarosis, an important zoonosis. EJCAP 18, 259–266.

Park, S.P., Park, I., Park, H.Y., Lee, S.U., Huh, S., Magnaval, J.F., 2000. Five cases of ocular toxocariasis confirmed by serology. Korean J. Parasitol. 38, 267–273.

Pawlowski, Z., 2001. Toxocariasis in humans: clinical expression and treatment dilemma. J. Helminthol. 75, 299–305.

Peixoto, P.L., Nascimento, E., de Miranda, R.R.C., Araújo, R.N., Cançado, G.G.L., Rocha, R.L., Fujiwara, R.L., 2011. Identification of candidate antigens from adult stages of Toxocara canis for the serodiagnosis of human toxocariasis. Mem. Inst. Oswaldo Cruz 106, 200–206.

Petithory, J.C., Chaumeil, C., Liotet, S., Rosseau, M., Bisognani, C., 1993. Immunological studies on ocular larva migrans. In: Lewis, J.W., Maizels, R.M. (Eds.), Toxocara and Toxocariasis: Clinical, Epidemiological and Molecular Perspectives. The British Society for Parasitology with the Institute of Biology. 81–89.

Pinelli, E., Herremans, T., Harms, M.G., Hoek, D., Kortbeek, L.M., 2011. Toxocara and Ascaris seropositivity among patients suspected of visceral and ocular larva migrans in the Netherlands: trends from 1998 to 2009. Eur. J. Clin. Microbiol. Infect. Dis. 30, 873–879.

Ponce-Macotela, M., Rodriguez-Caballero, A., Peralta-Abarca, G.E., Martinez-Gordillo, M.N., 2011. A simplified method for hatching and isolating Toxocara canis larvae to facilitate excretory-secretory antigen collection in vitro. Vet. Parasitol. 175, 382–385.

Robben, S.R., le Nobel, W.E., Döpfer, D., Hendrikx, W.M., Boersema, J.H., Fransen, F., Eysker, M.E., 2004. Infections with helminths and/or protozoa in cats in animal shelters in the Netherlands. Tijdschr. Diergeneeskd. 129, 2–6.

Robertson, B.D., Burkot, T.R., Gillespie, S.H., Kennedy, M.W., Wambai, Z., Maizels, R.M., 1988. Detection of circulating parasite antigen and specific antibody in *Toxocara canis* infections. Clin. Exp. Immunol. 74, 236–241.

Rodríguez-Caballero, A., Martínez-Gordillo, M.N., Medina-Flores, Y., Medina-Escutia, M.E., Meza-Lucas, A., Correa, D., Caballero-Salazar, S., Ponce-Macotela, M., 2015. Successful capture of Toxocara canis larva antigens from human serum samples. Parasit. Vectors 8, 264.

Roldán, W.H., Espinoza, Y.A., 2009. Evaluation of an enzyme-linked immuno-electrotransfer blot test for the confirmatory serodiagnosis of human toxocariasis. Mem. Inst. Oswaldo Cruz 104, 411–418.

Roldan, W.H., Cornejo, W., Espinoza, Y., 2006. Evaluation of the dot enzyme-linked immunosorbent assay in comparison with standard ELISA for the immunodiagnosis of human toxocariasis. Mem. Inst. Oswaldo Cruz 10, 71–74.

Roldan, W.H., Elefant, G.R., Ferreira, A.W., 2015. Deglycosylation of Toxocara excretory-secretory antigens improves the specificity of the serodiagnosis for human toxocariasis. Parasite Immunol. 37, 557–567.

Rubinsky-Elefant, G., Hirata, C.E., Yamamoto, J.H., Ferreira, M.U., 2010. Human toxocariasis: diagnosis, worldwide seroprevalences and clinical expression of the systemic and ocular forms. Ann. Trop. Med. Parasitol. 104, 3–23.

Rudzinska, M., Kowalewska, B., Sikorska, K., 2017. Clinical usefulness of Western blotting and ELISA avidity for the diagnosis of human toxocariasis. Parasite Immunol. 39, 1–6.

Sakai, R., Kawashima, H., Shibui, H., Kamata, K., Kambara, C., Matsuoka, H., 1998. Toxocara cati–induced ocular Toxocariasis. Arch. Ophthalmol. 116, 1686–1687.

Sharkey, J.A., McKay, P.S., 1993. Ocular toxocariasis in a patient with repeatedly negative ELISA titre to Toxocara canis. Br. J. Ophthalmol. 77, 253–254.

Shimokawa, H., Nakashima, T., Akagi, K., Omae, T., Tsuji, M., 1982. Visceral larva migrans by Toxocara cati. Fukuoka Igaku Zasshi. 73, 64–69.

Smith, H., Noordin, R., 2006. Diagnostic limitations and future trends in the serodiagnosis of human toxocariasis. In: Holland, C.V., Smith, H.V. (Eds.), Toxocara: The Enigma Parasite. CABI Publishing. p. 113.

Smith, H.V., Quinn, R., Bruce, R.G., Girdwood, R.W.A., 1982. Development of the serological response in rabbits infected with *Toxocara canis* and *Toxascaris leonina*. Trans. R. Soc. Trop. Med. Hyg. 76, 89–94.

Smith, H., Holland, C., Taylor, M., Magnaval, J.F., Schantz, P., Maizels, R., 2009. How common is human toxocariasis? Towards standardizing our knowledge. Trends Parasitol. 25, 182–188.

Sperotto, R.L., Kremer, F.S., Aires Berne, M.E., Costa de Avila, L.F., da Silva Pinto, L., Monteiro, K.M., Caumo, K.S., Ferreira, H.B., Berne, N., Borsuk, S., 2017. Proteomic analysis of Toxocara canis excretory and secretory (TES) proteins. Mol. Biochem. Parasitol. 211, 39–47.

Stensvold, C.R., Skov, J., Moller, L.N., Jensen, P.M., Kapel, C.M., Petersen, E., Nielsen, H.V., 2009. Seroprevalence of human toxocariasis in Denmark. Clin. Vaccine Immunol. 16, 1372–1373.

Thomas, D., Jeyathilakan, N., Abdul Basith, S., Senthilkumar, T.M., 2016. In vitro production of Toxocara canis excretory-secretory (TES) antigen. J. Parasit. Dis. 40, 1038–1043.

Van Den Broucke, S., Kanobana, K., Polman, K., Soentjens, P., Vekemans, M., Theunissen, C., Vlieghe, E., Van Esbroeck, M., Jacobs, J., Van Den Enden, E., Van Den Ende, J., Van Gompel, A., Clerinx, J., Bottieau, E., 2015. Toxocariasis diagnosed in international travelers at the Institute of Tropical Medicine, Antwerp, Belgium, from 2000 to 2013. PLoS Negl. Trop. Dis. 9, e0003559.

Watthanakulpanich, D., Smith, H.V., Hobbs, G., Whalley, A.J., Billington, D., 2008. Application of Toxocara canis excretory-secretory antigens and IgG subclass antibodies (IgG1-4) in serodiagnostic assays of human toxocariasis. Acta Trop. 106, 90–95.

Wickramasinghe, S., Yatawara, L., Nagataki, M., Takamoto, M., Watanabe, Y., Rajapakse, R.P., Uda, K., Suzuki, T., Agatsuma, T., 2008. Development of a highly sensitive IgG-ELISA based on recombinant arginine kinase of Toxocara canis for serodiagnosis of visceral larva migrans in the murine model. Parasitol. Res. 103, 853–858.

Won, K.Y., Kruszon-Moran, D., Schantz, P.M., Jones, J.L., 2008. National seroprevalence and risk factors for zoonotic Toxocara spp. infection. Am. J. Trop. Med. Hyg. 79, 552–557.

Woodhall, D.M., Garcia, A.P., Shapiro, C.A., Wray, S.L., Shane, A.L., Mani, C.S., Stimpert, K.K., Fox, L.M., Montgomery, S.P., 2017. Assessment of U.S. pediatrician knowledge of toxocariasis. Am. J. Trop. Med. Hyg. 97, 1243–1246.

Xinou, E., Lefkopoulos, A., Gelagoti, M., Drevelegas, A., Diakou, A., Milonas, I., Dimitriadis, A.S., 2003. CT and MR imaging findings in cerebral toxocaral disease. AJNR Am. J. Neuroradiol. 24, 714–718.

Yamasaki, H., Araki, K., Lim, P.K.C., Zasmy, N., Mak, J.W., Taib, R., Aoki, T., 2000. Development of a highly specific recombinant *Toxocara canis* second-stage larva excretory-secretory antigen for immunodiagnosis of human toxocariasis. J. Clin. Microbiol. 38, 1409–1413.

Yokoi, K., Kobayashi, F., Sakai, J., Usui, M., Tsuji, M., 2002. Sandwich ELISA detection of excretory-secretory antigens of *Toxocara canis* larvae using a specific monoclonal antibody. Southeast Asian J. Trop. Med. Public Health 33, 33–37.

Yunus, M.H., Tan Farrizam, S.N., Abdul Karim, I.Z., Noordin, R., 2018. A lateral flow rapid test for human toxocariasis developed using three Toxocara canis recombinant antigens. Am. J. Trop. Med. Hyg. 98, 32–38.

Zahabiun, F., Sadjjadi, S.M., Yunus, M.H., Rahumatullah, A., Moghaddam, M.H., Saidin, S., Noordin, R., 2015. Production of Toxocara cati TES-120 recombinant antigen and comparison with its T. canis homolog for serodiagnosis of toxocariasis. Am. J. Trop. Med. Hyg. 93, 319–325.

Zarnowska, H., Jastrzebska, M., 1994. Excretory-secretory larval antigens of Toxocara canis: physico-chemical characteristics and specificity assayed by Western blot technique. Acta Parasitol. 39, 41–45.

Zhan, B., Ajmera, R., Geiger, S.M., Gonçalves, M.T.P., Liu, Z., Wei, J., Wilkins, P.P., Fujiwara, R., Gazzinelli-Guimaraes, P.H., Bottazzi, M.E., Hotez, P., 2015. Identification of immunodominant antigens for the laboratory diagnosis of toxocariasis. Trop. Med. Int. Health 20, 1787–1796.

Zibaei, M., Sadjjadi, S.M., Ishiyama, S., Sarkari, B., Uga, S., 2010. Production of monoclonal antibody against Toxocara cati second-stage larvae and its application for the detection of circulating antigens. Hybridoma (Larchmt) 29, 217–220.

Zibaei, M., Sadjjadi, S.M., Jahadi-Hosseini, S.H., 2014. Toxocara cati larvae in the eye of a child: a case report. Asian Pac. J. Trop. Biomed. 4, S53–S55.

Zibaei, M., Sadjjadi, S.M., Sarkari, B., Uga, S., 2016. Evaluation of Toxocara cati excretory-secretory larval antigens in serodiagnosis of human toxocariasis. J. Clin. Lab. Anal. 30, 248–253.

CHAPTER EIGHT

Clinical pathology of larval toxocariasis

Katarzyna Mazur-Melewska*, Anna Mania, Wojciech Sluzewski, Magdalena Figlerowicz
Department of Infectious Diseases and Child Neurology, Karol Marcinkowski University of Medical Sciences, Poznań, Poland
*Corresponding author: e-mail address: katarzynamelewska@ump.edu.pl

Contents

Abstract

Human toxocariasis is a worldwide helminth zoonosis caused by roundworms of the genus *Toxocara*. Toxocariasis is the most common helminth infection in many countries. Disease caused by *Toxocara* can be classified into five clinical forms: generalised, neurological, ocular, covert, and asymptomatic. The clinical pathology of toxocariasis largely depends on the form of infection, the intensity of the infection, the larvae localisation, and the age of the host.

Because histological and molecular examination of toxocariasis is limited by difficulties in obtaining material to analyse, clinical diagnosis is often based on nonspecific tests, such as the detection of eosinophilia and hyperimmunoglobulinemia E (Hyper-IgE). Specific analysis uses an initial ELISA test to detect anti-*Toxocara* IgG and requires confirmation for all positive results via Western blot. This strategy does not distinguish between actual and recent infections, making the monitoring of disease a challenge for clinicians. Additional research will be required to distinguish active disease from the presence of recent infection.

Human toxocariasis is a worldwide helminth zoonosis caused by roundworms of the genus *Toxocara*, including mainly two species, i.e., *T. canis* and *T. cati* (Hotez and Wilkins, 2009; Schantz, 1989). The disease was first described in the 1950s. Current data indicates that toxocariasis is the most common worm infection in many countries and that its global importance may be significantly underestimated (Ma et al., 2018; Macpherson, 2013).

Advances in Parasitology, Volume 109
ISSN 0065-308X
https://doi.org/10.1016/bs.apar.2020.01.004

Toxocariasis occurs in five clinical forms: generalised (visceral larvae migrans syndrome, VLM), neurological (neurological larvae migrans syndrome, NLM), ocular (ocular larvae migrans syndrome, OLM), covert, and asymptomatic. Classic VLM manifests as inflammation and enlargement of the peripheral lymph nodes, liver, and spleen. The NLM form of the disease is usually asymptomatic, although there may be clinical symptoms ranging from eosinophilic meningoencephalitis to mild neurological deficiencies. OLM is a localised eye infection with progressive ocular damage. The covert form presents nonspecifically, with clinical symptoms that include lymphadenopathy, dermatological disorders (commonly urticaria), arthralgia, and asthma. Asymptomatic infection is diagnosed when eosinophilia and *Toxocara sp.* antibodies are suddenly detected in a child without the typical symptoms of infection (Despommier, 2003). The clinical form of the disease depends on the efficiency of the immune system, the intensity of the infestation, the localisation of the larvae, the age of the host, and the history of reinfection (Mazur-Melewska et al., 2012).

The diagnosis of parasite infection (especially in fully symptomatic forms) is often a challenge for clinicians. In many situations, such diagnoses require concurrent differentiation procedures, which include taking a clinical history and performing a combination of laboratory investigations.

1. Clinical history

Properly taken, a history about the course of illness is the first step in the diagnosis of toxocariasis. First, the clinician should ask about classic, but nonspecific, symptoms of parasite infection such as the occurrence of headaches, stomach aches, arthralgia, skin lesions, chronic cough and strabismus. Second, there are crucial facts like whether the patient had contact with domestic animals, had consumed of raw vegetables or uncooked meat, or whether the patient had travelled to tropical areas. In children, particular habits, like geophagia, nail-biting, poor personal hygiene, and close contact with puppies, as well as lack of parental supervision, increase the risk of infection (Gawor et al., 2014; Mazur-Melewska et al., 2012).

2. Laboratory diagnosis

2.1 Nonspecific tests

2.1.1 Hyperleukocytosis

The first parameter which can suggest toxocariasis is hyperleukocytosis. With respect to intensive infection, especially in cases of VLM, the number of general leukocytes detected is massive and can measure between 30,000 and 60,000 cells/mm^3 (Chen et al., 2018; Fillaux and Magnaval, 2013). In these cases, it can be quite common for the patient to be placed under haematological observation.

2.1.2 Eosinophilia

Through the precise analysis of peripheral blood cells, elevated levels of leukocytes can be identified as eosinophils (Altcheh et al., 2003; Fillaux and Magnaval, 2013). Their number is proportional to tissue eosinophilia, which comprises the local reaction to the migration of larvae, and the antigens that remain after their presence, within internal organs (Meeusen and Balic, 2000). Many cases reported in the literature suggest that such a situation is seen in the acute phase of toxocariasis when the eosinophils migrate with peripheral blood flow from bone marrow to tissues inflamed by larvae. In chronic infection, chemotactic stimulation is reduced, and the migration of eosinophils presenting as peripheral blood eosinophilia is diminished (Carvalho and Rocha, 2011).

Some authors have demonstrated an association between the form of toxocariasis and number of eosinophils detected, suggesting that eosinophil counts above 2000–3000 cells/mm^3 can be connected with VLM and lower values (in the range of 400 cells/mm^3) is more commonly observed in covert and asymptomatic cases (Yoon et al., 2018). In contrast, patients developing isolated OLM present with eosinophil counts that appear normal. This can be explained to low larval antibodies in the blood of these patients (Fillaux and Magnaval, 2013) due to a disease process that can be caused even by a single parasite. The patients who present combined forms, such as both VLM and OLM manifesting at the same time, develop an increased eosinophil counts in the blood that is typical of that seen in visceral forms (Yoon et al., 2018). The prevalence of toxocariasis is quite high among those patients diagnosed with eosinophilia of unknown origin, and the assessment for *Toxocara* infection is recommended for this group (Kim et al., 2017). The positive correlation between the eosinophil count after and before treatment has been confirmed, making the number of leukocytes and eosinophils the most significant marker monitoring the effects of therapy (Wiśniewska-Ligier et al., 2012).

2.1.3 Cytological characteristics of other body fluids

NLM is not frequently diagnosed based on non-specific clinical symptoms like headache, seizures, or paresthesia. The neurotoxocariasis diagnosis is based on cerebrospinal fluid (CSF) examination, which presents as pleocytosis with eosinophilia and a high titre of anti-*Toxocara* antibodies. The clinical improvement after anthelmintic therapy, decreasing the number of eosinophils in CSF are the positive markers of the effectivity of therapy (Deshayes et al., 2016; Nicoletti, 2013). Eosinophils in the aqueous or vitreous humour during OLM have also been reported; however, the phenomenon has only been minimally investigated (Fillaux and Magnaval, 2013; Nicoletti, 2013). Pulmonary involvement may result in eosinophilia that is detectable in bronchoalveolar lavage (BAL) fluid. One case of marked pulmonary infiltration had levels of eosinophils at 64% in the analysis of BAL fluid (Roig et al., 1992).

2.1.4 Total serum immunoglobulin level

The elevation of total serum immunoglobulin E (IgE) concentration during *Toxocara* infection was first described by Hogarth-Scott et al. (1969). In these studies, a 10- to 15-fold increase of IgE was observed in the serum of VLM patients. During the following years, serum hyperimmunoglobulinemia measures were also performed in patients with pulmonary infiltration and OLM. It was also confirmed that the level of IgE can correlate with the level of activity of toxocariasis and can be a good marker for evaluating the efficiency of treatment (Mazur-Melewska et al., 2015; Obwaller et al., 1998). In experimental murine toxocariasis models, the development of eosinophilia in *T. canis*-infected mice was accompanied by the release of a prominent level of serum IgE between weeks 2 and 21, with a peak at week 6 (Elsheikha et al., 2008). The elevation of antigen-specific and nonspecific IgE confirmed that the host response is regulated by Th2 immunity and the production of the cytokines IL-4, IL-5 and IL-13 by CD4(+) cells (Mazur-Melewska et al., 2014; Nutman, 2015).

The mechanism of regulation is not fully understood. Some data suggest the protective activity of IgE against intestinal nematode infections. In fact, immunoglobulin E specifically, is positively correlated with resistance to infection. This effect is generated by interactions between IgE and cells that express the high-affinity IgE receptor (FcεRI). The binding of parasite-specific IgE and antigen to FcεRI receptors, in combination with the activation of effector cells (macrophages and basophils), can result in the production and release of biologically active mediators that favour parasite expulsion (Mukai et al., 2016). Another hypothesis which suggests a mechanism for the elimination of parasites is antibody-dependent cellular cytotoxicity (ADCC) via IgE and/or IgG receptors. Classically, nematode infections are characterised by the production of large amounts of nonspecific IgE.

The parasite-specific IgE molecules can only be detected at the later stages of primary infection, or after multiple infections. Pritchard (1993) proposed a hypothesis stating that the nonspecific IgE is used to compete with parasite-specific IgE for receptor binding sites, which could interfere with the ability of IgE-mediated immunity to expel the parasites.

Others have suggested the concentration of total serum IgG showed an association with seropositivity for toxocariasis (Despommier, 2003; Fillaux and Magnaval, 2013); however, no correlation was found between IgG concentration and the form of infection or patients age (Mazur-Melewska et al., 2012, 2015).

2.1.5 Markers of inflammation

Laboratory markers of inflammation such as elevated sedimentation rate and positive C-reactive protein tests have been occasionally reported during the course of VLM syndrome (8). Additionally, the occurrence of mild anaemia has been reported. In OLM/CLM and covert toxocariasis, these abnormalities are very uncommon. Magnaval et al. (2001) reported that only 11% of patients with a covert form of the disease presented with elevated sedimentation rates.

Toxocara infection induces a polarised TH2 response, typically reflected in the secretion of cytokines that are involved in the activation of mast cells, eosinophils, and macrophages and the secretion of high levels of IgE. In experimental analysis using mice infected by *Toxocara* larvae, the authors confirmed the activation of the TH2 response through the observation of significant increases in cytokines such as IL-4, IL-5, IL-13, and IL-33, in addition to increases in the levels of IL-6 and IL-17. No significant elevation of IL-10, TNF-α, or IFN-γ levels were observed (Resende et al., 2015). The infection was confirmed by morphological analysis, which showed that larval migration through the organs of the mice had moved from the liver in the first 24 h of infection, later reaching the lungs on the third day and the brain after fifth day of infection. Peripheral leukocytosis with early neutrophilia and dominant eosinophilia were remarkable during the infection (Resende et al., 2015). Analysis of cytokines, which was performed by authors in children with serologically and radiologically confirmed VLM, also showed an elevation in the concentrations of IL-1a, IL-4, IL-6, and IL-10; however, the significance of the observed increases of IL-1a and IL-6 were borderline. Furthermore, IFN production was not elevated. The authors found a positive correlation between eosinophil counts, total IgE level, and the production of IL-4 and IL-6 in children with VLM.

IL-10, and IL-1 did not correlate, however, with eosinophil counts and the total IgE levels (Mazur-Melewska et al., 2014). Nagy et al., who analysed patients with toxocariasis-associated lung inflammation manifested by chronic cough, also showed that levels of protective proinflammatory cytokines (IL-6, IFN-gamma and IL-13) were elevated simultaneous with increases in anti-inflammatory IL-10 (Nagy et al., 2012).

In summary, *Toxocara* infection involves the production of Th2 cytokines, including IL-4, IL-5 and IL-13, and is associated with elevated counts of peripheral blood eosinophils and increased expression of their degranulation products. The production of IFN-γ by peripheral leukocytes is not prominent in toxocariasis, but IL-10 production may be increased in some infected individuals (Zibaei et al., 2019).

2.2 Specific examination

2.2.1 Histology

The definitive diagnosis of a helminth infection is based on macroscopic or microscopic observation of the parasite. This larval nematode can be found in cerebrospinal fluid and ocular fluids, where it can be motile (de Souza and Nakashima, 1995; Eberhardt et al., 2005). Human toxocariasis can be confirmed by histopathological examination, directed by the morphological identification of third-stage larval forms present in affected tissue including the brain, liver, eyes or lungs (Hill et al., 1985; Kirchner and Altmann, 1987). In patients with OLM, mobile larvae under the can be observed using ophthalmoscopy (Watthanakulpanich, 2010). *Toxocara canis and cati* larvae identified through morphological examination exhibit characteristic anatomy and on average, they are 0.4 mm in length, 0.02 mm in breadth, and the length of the oesophagus is about 30 percent of the total larval body length (Nichols, 1956).

Traditional morphological examination presents many limitations. First, the test is time-consuming and difficult to perform. Further, biopsies are only possible for localised toxocariasis, not covert forms of the disease. Additionally, larvae are very small and difficult to locate if they migrate, as occurs in VLM forms of the disease. The morphological methods are not objective, because their reliability is dependent on researcher experience.

2.2.2 Molecular techniques

The histopathological examination can be supplemented by molecular techniques, such as polymerase chain reaction (PCR) amplification, DNA hybridisation and restriction fragment length polymorphism or sequencing of *Toxocara* ribosomal DNA. These tests are used to identify genetic variations between *Toxocara* nematodes (Chen et al., 2012; Domżał et al., 2008; Tian and O'Hagan, 2015). The ability of researchers to detect parasite DNA in the brain, liver, lungs and blood of experimentally infected mice has been demonstrated. The disease was identified by PCR within 48 h after infection, while ELISA test required 14 days after inoculation for the appearance of serological conversion (Moura et al., 2018). The use of *Toxocara* PCR testing in human toxocariasis is still under investigation.

2.2.3 Serological methods

Using a combination of diagnostic methods, both histological and molecular, relies on the ability of researchers to obtain human tissue for analysis. The biopsy is possible in localised toxocariasis, not in the covert form of the disease. Additionally, larvae are very small and difficult to locate if they migrate in VLM form. The surgical excision of the parasite itself or granulomas surrounding the nematode body is not practical for most clinicians. Therefore, diagnosis is commonly based on clinical and serologic diagnosis (Mohamad et al., 2009). In fact, the diagnosis of human toxocariasis depends on the detection of the *Toxocara* excretory-secretion (TES) IgG antibodies in the blood of patients (Watthanakulpanich, 2010). The use of TES antigens harvested from larvae provides the highest level of sensitivity and specificity compared to antigens taken from the adult forms of the parasite (Roldán et al., 2017). The level and the type of antibodies will not distinguish between acute and chronic infection, however (Fillaux and Magnaval, 2013).

Specific IgM and IgA antibodies, which are used to predict the presence of many viral diseases, persist and do not facilitate predictions of time of infection. Roldán et al. (2017) documented that IgM-TES tests are not very specific with regard to *Toxocara* infection. Using ELISA tests they confirmed anti-*Toxocara* IgM in 91.4% of patients with toxocariasis, 76% in patients with other helminth infections, and 45.3% in healthy individuals. Using a Western-Blot (WB) test with specific IgM-TES antibodies showed that the antibody was present in 94.8% of sera taken from patients with toxocariasis, 65.3% in sera from patients with other helminth infections, and 41% in the sera of healthy individuals (Roldán et al., 2017).

In the early 90s it was suggested that IgE-TES ELISA was the most useful serodiagnostic test because it does not detect isohemagglutinins. In practise, the IgE-TES ELISA test, with a cut-off point of 20 units (TU/L), presented a specificity of 89.8%, and produced a sensitivity of only 53.2%. In the same test, about 20% of patients had negative, undetectable levels of IgE-TES. The significant titers of IgE-TES were seen primarily in people with a history of allergies (43). In fact, the test is used in some clinical settings to monitor the effectiveness of anthelmintics therapy, because even though antibodies are persistent, their levels decrease after successive treatments in atopic patients (Gawor et al., 2014; Magnaval et al., 2001, 2006).

For these reasons, clinical diagnoses are based on the detection specific, anti-*Toxocara* IgG (IgG-TES) in patients with blood eosinophilia. The combination of both types of tests enhance the probability of reaching a proper diagnosis, because the false-positive tests are possible in patients with the other helminth zoonosis, especially ascaridiosis (Smith et al., 2009). The sensitivity of IgG-TES ELISA test was evaluated, and it was determined that the test was 92.3% effective with an 89.6% specificity (Norhaida et al., 2008). One practical problem is that IgG often persists in the blood for years, a response that does not allow for the establishment of active and persistent infection or reinfection. Unfortunately, it also makes monitoring the effectiveness of treatment difficult (Dziemian et al., 2008; Ma et al., 2018).

The Western-blotting procedure for the detection of IgG-TES was established in the late 1980s by Magnaval et al. (1991). In subsequent studies, the specificity of WB was confirmed, but the value of the test is limited by the time and cost required to perform the test. Fully symptomatic VLM, common toxocariasis with eosinophilia and high concentrations of IgE can be initially diagnosed using IgG-TES ELISA. To follow good laboratory practise procedures, all positive ELISA results, especially when impacting clinical discussions regarding non-specific disease symptoms, a "grey-zone" ELISA test WB should be used to improve the sensitivity and specificity of diagnosis (Fillaux and Magnaval, 2013; Magnaval et al., 1991). In addition to assisting in the diagnosis of *Toxoplasma* infection, measuring IgG avidity can assist in the differentiation between recent and distant toxocariasis. In Poland, Dziemian et al. (2008) presented results indicating that IgG-TES avidity increases from a low index typically seen in early infection to the higher values in prospective analyses made repeatedly over the period of 3–12 months. The therapy, which was administered after making a diagnosis, didn't have an influence on avidity, an observation that was opposite to what was observed in the analysis of *Toxoplasma* antibodies. This concept has very promising clinical implications, but validation studies are needed.

3. Conclusion

The actual diagnostic strategy applied to identify toxocariasis is based on the initial detection of TES-IgG using ELISA and relies on the confirmation of antibodies via WB. The procedure is easier in patients with eosinophilia and those with high concentrations of IgE in blood samples, in other words, in VLM or common clinical form. The method used for immunodiagnosis has is limited by its ability to sufficiently distinguish active and chronic toxocariasis. Further research is needed to improve and eliminate this problem.

References

Altcheh, J., Nallar, M., Conca, M., Biancardi, M., Freilij, H., 2003. Toxocariasis: aspectos clínicos y de laboratorio en 54 pacientes. An. Pediatr. 58 (5), 425–431.

Carvalho, E., Rocha, R., 2011. Toxocariasis: visceral larva migrans in children. J. Pediatr. (Rio J) 87 (2), 100–110.

Chen, J., Zhou, D., Nisbet, A.J., Xu, M., Huang, S., Li, M., Wang, C., Zhu, X., 2012. Advances in molecular identification, taxonomy, genetic variation and diagnosis of Toxocara spp. Infect. Genet. Evol. 12 (7), 1344–1348.

Chen, J., Liu, Q., Liu, G., Zheng, W., Hong, S., Sugiyama, H., Zhu, X., Elsheikha, H., 2018. Toxocariasis: a silent threat with a progressive public health impact. Infect. Dis. Poverty 7 (1), 59. https://doi.org/10.1186/s40249-018-0437-0.

de Souza, E., Nakashima, Y., 1995. Diffuse unilateral subacute neuroretinitis. Ophthalmology 102 (8), 1183–1186.

Deshayes, S., Bonhomme, J., de La Blanchardière, A., 2016. Neurotoxocariasis: a systematic literature review. Infection 44 (5), 565–574. https://doi.org/10.1007/s15010-016-0889-8.

Despommier, D., 2003. Toxocariasis: clinical aspects, epidemiology, medical ecology, and molecular aspects. Clin. Microbiol. Rev. 16 (2), 265–272.

Domżał, D., Talar-Wojnarowska, R., Niedworok, M., Małecka-Panas, E., 2008. Diagnosis of toxocarosis using methods of molecular biology. Prz. Gastroenterol. 3 (5), 227–231.

Dziemian, E., Żarnowska, H., Kołodziej-Sobocinska, M., Machnicka, B., 2008. Determination of the relative avidity of the specific IgG antibodies in human toxocariasis. Parasite Immunol. 30, 187–190.

Eberhardt, O., Bialek, R., Nägele, T., Dichgans, J., 2005. Eosinophilic meningomyelitis in toxocariasis: case report and review of the literature. Clin. Neurol. Neurosurg. 107 (5), 432–438.

Elsheikha, H.M., El-Beshbishi, S.N., El-Shazly, A.M., Hafez, A.O., Morsy, T.A., 2008. Kinetics of eosinophilia and IgE production in experimental murine toxocariasis. J. Egypt. Soc. Parasitol. 38 (1), 53–64.

Fillaux, J., Magnaval, J., 2013. Laboratory diagnosis of human toxocariasis. Vet. Parasitol. 193 (4), 327–336.

Gawor, J., Borecka, A., Marczyńska, M., Dobosz, S., Żarnowska-Prymek, H., 2014. Risk of human toxocarosis in Poland due to Toxocara infection of dogs and cats. Acta Parasitol. 60 (1), 99–104. https://doi.org/10.1515/ap-2015-0012.

Hill, I.R., Denham, D.A., Scholtz, C.L., 1985. *Toxocara canis* larvae in the brain of a British child. Trans. R. Soc. Trop. Med. Hyg. 79 (3), 351–354.

Hogarth-Scott, R.S., Johansson, S.G., Bennich, H., 1969. Antibodies to Toxocara in the sera of visceral larva migrans patients: the significance of raised levels of IgE. Clin. Exp. Immunol. 5 (6), 619–625.

Hotez, P.J., Wilkins, P.P., 2009. Toxocariasis: America's most common neglected infection of poverty and a helminthiasis of global importance? PLoS Negl. Trop. Dis. 3 (3), e400. https://doi.org/10.1371/journal.pntd.0000400.

Kim, H., Seo, J., Lee, J., Choi, B., Park, S., 2017. Evaluation of the prevalence and clinical impact of toxocariasis in patients with eosinophilia of unknown origin. Korean J. Intern. Med. 32 (3), 523–529.

Kirchner, T., Altmann, H.W., 1987. Parasitenlarven als Ursache umschriebener Leberherde. Morphologie und Differentialdiagnose. Pathologe 8, 31–36.

Ma, G., Holland, C., Wang, T., Hofmann, A., Fan, C., Maizels, R., Hotez, P., Gasser, R., 2018. Human toxocariasis. Lancet Infect. Dis. 18 (1), e14–e24.

Macpherson, C., 2013. The epidemiology and public health importance of toxocariasis: a zoonosis of global importance. Int. J. Parasitol. 43 (12 – 13), 999–1008.

Magnaval, J.F., Fabre, R., Maurieres, P., Charlet, J.P., de Larrard, B., 1991. Application of the western blotting procedure for the immunodiagnosis of human toxocariasis. Parasitol. Res. 77, 697–702.

Magnaval, J.F., Glickman, L.T., Dorchies, P., Morassin, B., 2001. Highlights of human toxocariasis. Korean J. Parasitol. 39 (1), 1–11. https://doi.org/10.3347/kjp.2001.39.1.1.

Magnaval, J., Faufingue, J., Morassin, B., Fabre, R., 2006. Eosinophil cationic protein, specific IgE and IgG4 in human toxocariasis. J. Helminthol. 80 (4), 417–423. https://doi.org/10.1017/JOH2006369.

Mazur-Melewska, K., Mania, A., Figlerowicz, M., Kemnitz, P., Służewski, W., Michalak, M., 2012. The influence of age on a clinical presentation of Toxocara spp. infection in children. Ann. Agric. Environ. Med. 19 (2), 233–236.

Mazur-Melewska, K., Jończyk, K., Modlińska-Cwalińska, A., Figlerowicz, M., Służewski, W., 2014. Visceral larva migrans syndrome: analysis of serum cytokine levels in children with hepatic lesions confirmed in radiological findings. Parasite Immunol. 36 (12), 668–673.

Mazur-Melewska, K., Jonczyk-Potoczna, K., Kemnitz, P., Mania, A., Figlerowicz, M., Służewski, W., 2015. Toksokaroza płucna u dzieci. Pneumonol. Alergol. Pol. 83 (4), 250–255.

Meeusen, E., Balic, A., 2000. Do eosinophils have a role in the killing of helminth parasites? Parasitol. Today 16 (3), 95–101.

Mohamad, S., Azmi, N., Noordin, R., 2009. Development and evaluation of a sensitive and specific assay for diagnosis of human toxocariasis by use of three recombinant antigens (TES-26, TES-30USM, and TES-120). J. Clin. Microbiol. 47 (6), 1712–1717.

Moura, M.Q., Macedo, M.R., Terto, W.D., Avila, L.F., Leite, F.P., Scaini, C.J., Pinto, N.B., Capella, G.D., Strothmann, A.L., Villela, M.M., Berne, M.E., 2018. Detection of Toxocara canis DNA in tissues of experimentally infected mice. Acta Trop. 187 (11), 51–56.

Mukai, K., Tsai, M., Starkl, P., Marichal, T., Galli, S., 2016. IgE and mast cells in host defense against parasites and venoms. Semin. Immunopathol. 38 (5), 581–603.

Nagy, D., Bede, O., Danka, J., SzÉnási, Z., Sipka, S., 2012. Analysis of serum cytokine levels in children with chronic cough associated with Toxocara canis infection. Parasite Immunol. 34 (12), 581–588.

Nichols, R.L., 1956. The etiology of visceral larva migrans. I. Diagnostic morphology of infective second-stage Toxocara larvae. J. Parasitol. 42 (4), 349–362.

Nicoletti, A., 2013. Toxocariasis. In: Handbook of Clinical Neurology, vol. 114. Elsevier, pp. 217–228.

Norhaida, A., Suharni, M., Liza Sharmini, A.T., Tuda, J., Rahmah, N., 2008. rTES-30USM: cloning via assembly PCR, expression, and evaluation of usefulness in the detection of toxocariasis. Ann. Trop. Med. Parasitol. 102 (2), 151–160. https://doi.org/10.1179/136485908X252250.

Nutman, T., 2015. Looking beyond the induction of Th2 responses to explain immunomodulation by helminths. Parasite Immunol. 37 (6), 304–313.

Obwaller, A., Jensen-Jarolim, E., Auer, H., Huber, A., Kraft, D., Aspock, H., 1998. Toxocara infestations in humans: symptomatic course of toxocarosis correlates significantly with levels of IgE/anti-IgE immune complexes. Parasite Immunol. 20 (7), 311–317.

Pritchard, D., 1993. Immunity to helminths: is too much IgE parasite- rather than host-protective? Parasite Immunol. 15 (1), 5–9.

Resende, N., Gazzinelli-Guimarães, P., Barbosa, F., Oliveira, L., Nogueira, D., Gazzinelli-Guimarães, A., Gonçalves, M., Amorim, C., Oliveira, F., Caliari, M., Rachid, M., Volpato, G., Bueno, L., Geiger, S., Fujiwara, R., 2015. New insights into the immunopathology of early Toxocara canis infection in mice. Parasit. Vectors 8 (1), 354–365.

Roig, J., Romeu, J., Riera, C., Texido, A., Domingo, C., Morera, J., 1992. Acute eosinophilic pneumonia due to toxocariasis with bronchoalveolar lavage findings. Chest 102 (1), 294–296.

Roldán, W.H., Elefan, G.R., Ferreira, A.W., 2017. Immunoglobulin M antibodies are not specific for serodiagnosis of human toxocariasis. Parasite Immunol. 39, e12447. https://doi.org/10.1111/pim.12447.

Schantz, P.M., 1989. *Toxocara* larva migrans now. Am. J. Trop. Med. Hyg. 41 (Suppl. 3 Pt. 4), 21–34.

Smith, H., Holland, C., Taylor, M., Magnaval, J.F., Schantz, P., Maizels, R., 2009. How common is human toxocariasis? Towards standardizing our knowledge. Trends Parasitol. 25, 182–188.

Tian, J.X., O'Hagan, S., 2015. Toxocara polymerase chain reaction on ocular fluids in bilateral granulomatous chorioretinitis. Int. Med. Case Rep. J. 8, 107–110. https://doi.org/10.2147/IMCRJ.S84185.

Watthanakulpanich, D., 2010. Diagnostic trends of human toxocariasis. Trop. Med. Parasitol. 33 (1), 44–52.

Wiśniewska-Ligier, M., Woźniakowska-Gęsicka, T., Sobolewska-Dryjańska, J., Markiewicz-Jóźwiak, A., Wieczorek, M., 2012. Analysis of the course and treatment of toxocariasis in children—a long-term observation. Parasitol. Res. 110 (6), 2363–2371. https://doi.org/10.1007/s00436-011-2772-y.

Yoon, S., Baek, S., Park, S., Shin, B., Kwon, H., Cho, Y., Moon, H., Kim, T., 2018. Clinical course and treatment outcomes of toxocariasis-related eosinophilic disorder. Medicine 97 (37), e12361.

Zibaei, M., Shayesteh, Z., Moradi, N., Bahadory, S., 2019. Human Toxocara infection: allergy and immune responses. Anti-Inflammatory Anti-Allergy Agents Med. Chem. 18, 82–91. https://doi.org/10.2174/1871523018666181210115840.

CHAPTER NINE

Imaging of toxocariasis

Christoph F. Dietrich[a,*], Carmen Cretu[b], Yi Dong[c]
[a]Department of Internal Medicine (DAIM), Kliniken Hirslanden Beau Site, Salem und Permanence, Bern, Switzerland
[b]Department of Parasitology, Carol Davila University of Medicine and Pharmacy, Colentina Clinical Hospital, Bucharest, Romania
[c]Department of Ultrasound, Zhongshan Hospital, Fudan University, Shanghai, China
*Corresponding author: e-mail address: christoph.dietrich@ckbm.de

Contents

Abstract

Several imaging modalities have now been employed to visualize the manifestations of larval *Toxocara* infection in hepatic, neurologic, ocular, renal, and other anatomical sites. This report reviews the usefulness and value of these individual imaging methods in diagnosis and follow-up of the different cases causing eosinophilic (granulomatous) infiltrations the liver, lungs, brain, heart, and eyes. Imaging provides a means of assisting in diagnosis and management in this infection where diagnosis by biopsy is often unlikely to capture an actual larva for the purpose of making a definitive diagnosis on the basis of larval morphology or DNA detection.

Advances in Parasitology, Volume 109
ISSN 0065-308X
https://doi.org/10.1016/bs.apar.2020.03.001

1. Introduction

Imaging of parasitic diseases has recently increased in importance due to worldwide migrations in general and of refugees in particular. For these reasons, diseases rarely observed in the Western World have gained importance in daily practice. In addition to the imaging features of recently published reports on hydatid diseases (Brunetti et al., 2018; Dietrich and Hocke, 2011; Dietrich et al., 2009, 2016a,b, 2018), ascariasis (Dietrich et al., 2017; Dong et al., 2018), schistosomiasis (Richter et al., 2016a,b), fasciolosis (Dietrich et al., 2015) and the other liver flukes *Clonorchis* and *Opisthorchis* (Dietrich et al., 2014) and filariosis (Dietrich et al., 2019), and herewith, we summarize the imaging and especially ultrasound features of the round worm infection toxocariasis.

Many organs can be involved but most often the liver and brain. Since humans are not primary hosts of these organisms, the ingested eggs or larvae can only evolve into migrating larvae, which are released into the small bowel. From there, these larvae enter the portal venous system through the intestinal walls and migrate systemically to infect and cause eosinophilic (granulomatous) infiltrations the liver, lungs, brain, heart, and eyes (Laroia et al., 2016).

2. Imaging

Imaging of the most prominent manifestations of hepatic *Toxocara* infections can be done using ultrasound (US), contrast enhanced ultrasound (CEUS), contrast enhanced computed tomography (ceCT), contrast enhanced magnetic resonance imaging (ceMRI) and positron emission tomography (PET). US and CEUS have been established for many organs (Claudon et al., 2013a,b). Cerebral manifestations are generally examined using CT and MRI (Ishibashi et al., 1992; Jain et al., 1994; Zachariah et al., 1994), whereas ocular manifestations can be diagnosed using US, CEUS, ceCT and ceMRI. For imaging of cerebral manifestations US and CEUS are not applied. The lung is generally examined using CT and the value of ultrasound has not been examined so far. With all the imaging methods mentioned, toxocariasis can present as symptomatic disease or an incidental finding without clinical symptoms. The imaging features are mainly explained by the direct inflammatory granulomatous process and the surrounding inflammatory reaction and immunological activity.

2.1 Liver

The liver is the visceral organ most commonly affected in VLM. The typical hepatic granulomas have multinucleated giant cells and epithelioid cells surrounding necrotic debris or amorphous eosinophilic material (Rubinsky-Elefant et al., 2010). Liver abscess formation is a rare condition associated with *Toxocara* infection. It is still a matter of debate whether liver abscess results from severe parasitic infection or whether human toxocariasis is a predisposing cause of pyogenic liver abscess formation. Liver resection is the only treatment option when sepsis fails to respond to conservative treatment (Treska et al., 2011).

On CT or MR imaging, hepatic lesions are seen as multiple, ill-defined, oval lesions that measure 1.0–1.5 cm in diameter. Sometimes, the lesion may be angular or trapezoidal. On sonography, the lesions appear as multiple, small, oval hypoechoic lesions in the liver parenchyma. The lesions differ from metastatic nodules is as much as they have fuzzy margins, are uniform in size, non-spherical in shape and are best seen on portal venous phase. On follow-up imaging, the lesions may improve, or sometimes a change positions, reflecting migration of larva in the liver, supporting the phenomenon of visceral larva migrans (Lim, 2008).

As has been reported, more than one third of patients with toxocariasis exhibited organ involvement, particularly hepatic involvement (Yoon et al., 2018). The liver is an important site for controlling the migration of *Toxocara* larvae (liver entrapment); dissemination occurs via the bloodborne route (Overgaauw, 1997). The typical ultrasound features of hepatic toxocariasis are hepatomegaly with or without ill-defined small (typically <10 mm) hypoechoic focal liver lesions, which typically appear 8–10 weeks post infection, and perihepatic lymphadenopathy as a sign of hepatic inflammation (Baldisserotto et al., 1999; Lim, 2008; Sakai et al., 2006). A so-called "bean sign" has been reported within such a focal liver lesion (FLL) characterized as a central echo or echoline (Ha et al., 2016). In the first month after infection ultrasound is often negative (Lim, 2008). In more chronic stages, the hypoechoic FLL are surrounded by a hyperechoic reaction, which may be observed for years. Phlegmonous inflammation and abscess formation are rarely observed and require prompt diagnosis to exclude neoplasia and other threatening inflammatory diseases, e.g., tuberculosis, amebiasis, and the so-called "pseudo-inflammatory liver tumour" (Kabaalioglu et al., 2005). Urgent treatment is required in patients with abscess formation (Fig. 1).

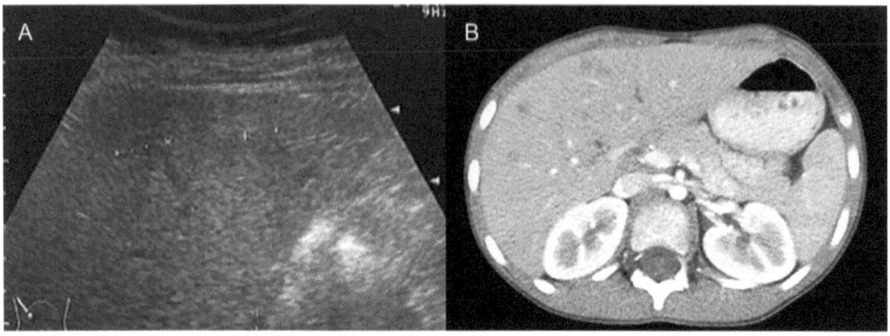

Fig. 1 Toxocariasis of the liver. B-mode ultrasound image showed small slightly hypoechogenic focal liver lesions peripherally located in the right lobe of liver (A). The finding was confirmed by computed tomography as hypodense FLL in the right liver lobe (B).

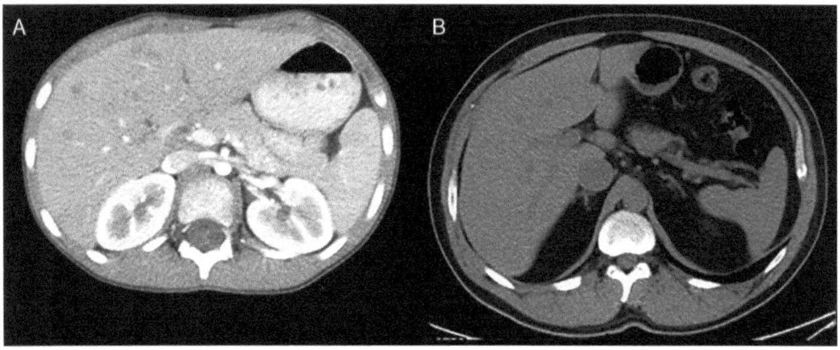

Fig. 2 Diffuse liver granulomas toxocariasis. CT scan showed diffused hypodense focal liver lesions in the liver (A). MRI showed the corresponding hypointense FLL (B).

Diagnosis of hepatic toxocariasis can be difficult, when liver lesions present as multiple hypoechoic lesions with regular borders (Fig. 2). These sonographic findings are non-specific and cannot be used to differentiate the lesions from other types of granuloma, inflammatory lesions or infarction (Coskun and Akinci, 2013) (Fig. 3).

Contrast enhancement profiles with *Toxocara* focal liver lesions are similar to fasciolosis, and may be best seen in the portal venous and sinusoidal phase with contrast enhanced ultrasound (CEUS), computed tomography (ceCT) and magnetic resonance imaging (ceMRI) (Chang et al., 2006; Sarda and Kannan, 1992). Since the lesions are hypoenhancing in the portal venous and sinusoidal phases, they might be confused with metastases.

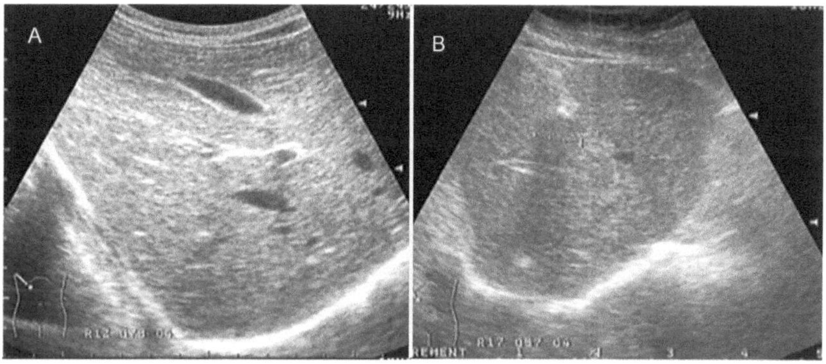

Fig. 3 Focal liver granulomas toxocariasis. A recently formulated toxocariasis granuloma (A). B-mode ultrasound scan showed an ill-defined hypoechoic lesion located in the right liver lobe. An old toxocariasis granuloma. B-mode ultrasound showed a hypoechoic lesion with posterior shadow (B).

Visceral larva migrans (VLM), caused by the dog and cat roundworms *Toxocara canis* and *Toxocara cati*, respectively, has emerged as a significant cause of eosinophilic liver abscess. Differentiation of eosinophilic liver abscess associated with toxocariasis from metastasis or primary liver malignancy is sometimes difficult. Previous studies demonstrated the radiologic resolution of eosinophilic liver abscess associated with toxocariasis being accelerated with albendazole treatment, because treatment can lead to sever hypersensitivity reactions (Overgaauw, 1997). Hence, the inconvenience associated with long-term follow-up and unnecessary concerns from patients can be eliminated with albendazole treatment (Jang et al., 2015). A high degree of clinical suspicion for hepatic VLM should be considered in a patient with a history of ingestion of soil, i.e., a child with pika, raw food in the past, presenting severe eosinophilia and a variety of symptoms which reflect high numbers of larvae (Overgaauw, 1997). Symptom remission, eosinophilia remission, and complete radiological resolution of lesions can be complete with surgery (Park et al., 2018). VLM manifests in the liver as eosinophilic granulomas. This pathological entity is a lesser known presentation of parasitic liver abscesses. Eosinophilic abscesses or granulomas are necrotizing lesions seen in the liver. They appear as ill-defined, conglomerating, and sometimes discrete focal lesions, with imaging features resembling nonspecific abscesses or mimicking cystic/liquefied mass lesions. These lesions may sometimes gradually change shape and positions on successive imaging, which is consistent with the presentation of migratory larva disease (Lim, 2008).

On MR images, toxocariasis presents as single or multiple, small, oval lesions scattered in the liver parenchyma (Azuma et al., 2002). On unenhanced MR images, the lesions are of faint low-signal intensity on T1-weighted images and of faint high signal intensity on T2-weighted images, with poorly defined margins. The lesions differ from metastatic nodules in that they have fuzzy margins, are uniform in size, have a non-spherical shape and are best seen on portal venous phase. On follow-up imaging, the lesions may improve, or sometimes may change positions reflecting migration of larvae in the liver, consistent with the phenomenon of visceral larva migrans (Lim, 2008).

Larvae do not migrate continuously but tend to rest periodically before continuing their migration. During such periods of reduced movement, the larvae induce an immunologically mediated inflammatory response (Smith, 1993), may produce granulomatous reactions in the viscera, which can be recognized by ultrasound, MRI or CT scans as masses within the abdomen (Ghoroobi et al., 2017). The larvae migrate to the liver from the digestive system through the portal vein, as VLM, where antigens from the parasites induce local allergic reactions in the liver. Clinical symptoms of eosinophilic granuloma of the liver (EGL) by VLM include fever, abdominal discomfort, general fatigue, and/or cough. Most reports documented that EGL are caused by VLM. However, parasites are not always demonstrable by serological, histopathological, or immunochemical examinations. When acting as allergens to induce type I responses, microscopic agents other than parasites in the intestinal tract could induce eosinophilic inflammation in the liver (Yamamoto et al., 2015).

In imaging, EGL by VLM appears as a macroscopic nodule, rather than microscopic diffuse inflammation. Imaging series show solitary or plural nodules with irregular shapes, these lesions are usually oval or elongated, and are sometimes angulated or trapezoid rather than round, with ill-defined margins. Conventional grey scale ultrasound might show a single, hypoechoic lesion with irregular margins in the liver, and Doppler ultrasound may reveal abundant arterial flow signals around the lesion, but no blood flow signal is detected within the lesion. CT can depict a lesion of low density on plain imaging, and a hypodense lesion with rim enhancement in both early and late phases of dynamic enhanced CT. MRI may show a hypointense lesion on T1-weighted imaging, and a hyperintense lesion on T2-weighted imaging, also a lesion of low intensity with rim enhancement in the early phase of Gd-EOB-DTPA MRI and defective uptake in the late phase. On PET-CT, those lesion might show slightly high standardized uptake value (SUV)

(Yamamoto et al., 2015). A unique characteristic feature of these abscesses on noncontrast MRI study is the presence of a hyperintense rim on T1-weighted sequences, with corresponding diffusion restriction on echo planar imaging (Laroia et al., 2016).

2.2 Pancreas

There is no literature about pancreatic toxocariasis in human beings.

2.3 Spleen

There is no literature about splenic toxocariasis in human beings. However, we have observed one case with diffuse toxocariasis of the spleen (Fig. 4).

2.4 Kidney

The first case of *Toxocara* eosinophilic ascites after combined pancreas and kidney transplantation was reported in recent years (Schaffellner et al., 2010). In some areas, toxocariasis should not be missed in the differential diagnosis of renal diseases especially in those who do not respond to traditional management (Nada et al., 1996).

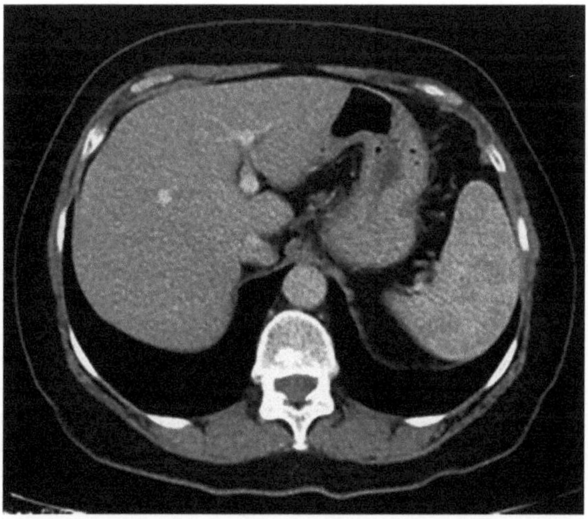

Fig. 4 Diffuse spleen toxocariasis. Inhomogeneous hypodense lesion with unclear margin located in the spleen.

2.5 Other abdominal, retroperitoneal and pelvic organs, lymph nodes and structures reported in the literature

Visceral larva migrans (VLM) most commonly occurs as a febrile disease of childhood particularly affecting children between 1 and 7 years of age. Pulmonary, dermatological, hepatic, lymphatic, cardiac, rheumatological and neurological manifestations may occur (Kabaalioglu et al., 2005).

In one case, a large retroperitoneal toxocariasis mass that involved the right liver lobe, bladder, ileocecal valve, small and large intestines was reported (Ghoroobi et al., 2017).

2.6 Musculoskeletal (skin)

An impairment on the muscular strength was observed in rats infected with *Toxocara canis* 30 days after inoculation (Chieffi et al., 2009).

2.7 Neurotoxocariasis

Toxocara canis larvae can cross the blood-brain barrier leading to neurotoxocariasis (Sanchez et al., 2018). To date, CNS infestation of *T. canis* larvae in humans is thought to be rare, even if in animal models, including primates, larvae often migrate to the brain (Graeff-Teixeira et al., 2009).

The diagnosis of neurotoxocariasis is challenging because there is no distinct clinical syndrome. Neurotoxocariasis is not a frequent diagnosis probably due to the non-specific nature of its symptoms, as well as the lack of confirmatory diagnostic tests (Sanchez et al., 2018). The clinical presentation consists of a wide spectrum of neurological manifestations, from meningitis, encephalitis, and myelitis, to cerebral vasculitis, however, asymptomatic infection is probably common (Fan et al., 2015).

Diagnosis of neurotoxocariasis is based on the presence of a high titre of anti-*Toxocara* antibody in the cerebrospinal fluid or in the serum, presence of eosinophilia in the serum or cerebrospinal fluid, and clinical and radiological improvement after anthelmintic therapy; however, universally accepted diagnostic criteria are lacking (Sanchez et al., 2018).

A variety of brain imaging findings have been reported in relation to neurotoxocariasis, mainly including CT and MRI. MRI findings in this large population were all suggestive, but none of them can be considered specific to neurotoxocariosis, and most of these findings can be seen in many other infectious or inflammatory conditions (Bachli et al., 2004; Choi et al., 2013; Feske et al., 2015; Gorgulu et al., 2006; Kwon, 2015; Moiyadi et al., 2007; Singer et al., 2011; Xinou et al., 2003). MRI findings include single or multiple subcortical, cortical or white matter hyperintense lesions, best visualized on FLAIR and T2-weighted imaging, usually isointense or hypointense on T1 (Fig. 5). These imaging findings are suggestive but not specific to neurotoxocariasis. A definitive diagnosis is made by serology on CSF, or rarely histological confirmation (Deshayes et al., 2016). Diagnostic imaging examinations found hypodense lesions in cerebral scanner sequences and hyperintense lesions in cerebral MRI T2-weighted sequences in 65 and 57% of encephalitis cases respectively, and in 92% of myelitis cases in medullary MRI T2-weighted sequences (Deshayes et al., 2016). A diagnosis of neurotoxocariasis is also supported by clinical and MRI improvement after specific anthelmintic treatment (Sick and Hennerici, 2014).

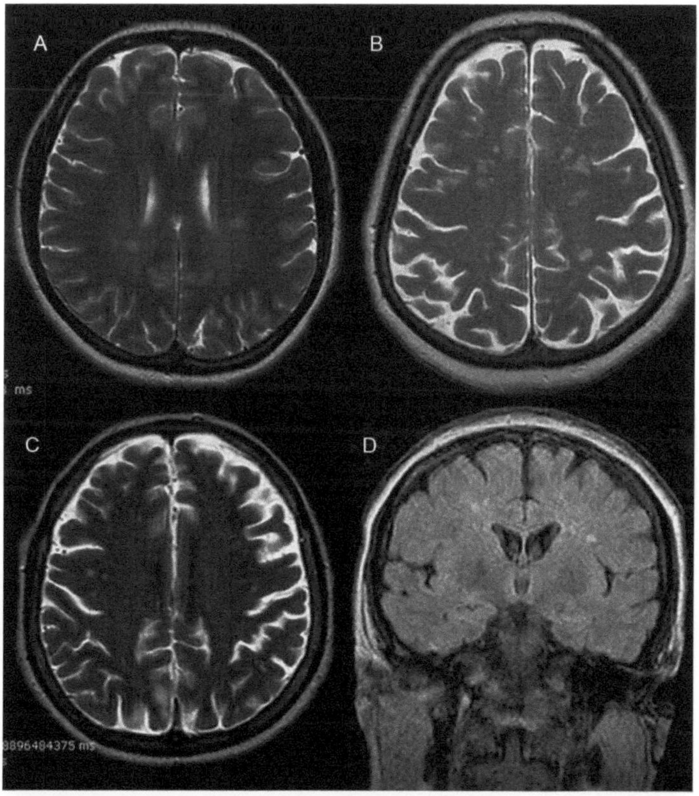

Fig. 5 Brain toxocariasis on MRI (A). Multiple subcortical located white matter hyperintense lesions which were best visualized on FLAIR (B) and T2-weighted imaging (C). The lesions were isointense on T1-weighted images (D).

Diagnostic imaging examinations often identified abnormalities with an abnormal brain CT in 65.2% of cases, an abnormal brain MRI in 57.4% of cases and an abnormal medullary MRI in 91.5% of cases (Deshayes et al., 2016). In cases with symptoms of encephalitis, brain CT might reveal multiple subcortical, cortical or white matter circumscribed hypodense lesions (Fig. 6). When performed, brain MRI showed hypointense lesions on T1-weighted sequences and hyperintense on T2-weighted sequences, with a homogenous enhancement after the administration of contrast agents (Deshayes et al., 2016).

When utilized in cases of cerebral toxocariasis, MRI often reveals the presence of a granulomatous process leading to reversible single or multiple ring-enhancing lesions. However, ring-enhancing lesions are a common finding that can be related to different disease processes such as infective, neoplastic, and inflammatory conditions (Sanchez et al., 2018). These imaging findings are suggestive but not specific to neurotoxocariasis (Fig. 6).

2.8 Ocular toxocariasis

Ocular toxocariasis (OT), first described by Wilder in 1950, is a zoonotic parasitic infection mainly caused by the intraocular invasion by a third-stage larva of *Toxocara canis* or *Toxocara cati*, usually presenting as a severe unilateral intraocular inflammatory response in a child or young adult, which is an important cause of blindness in this population (Chen et al., 2018a,b). The approach of *Toxocara* larvae to the eye remains unclear. Possible approaches

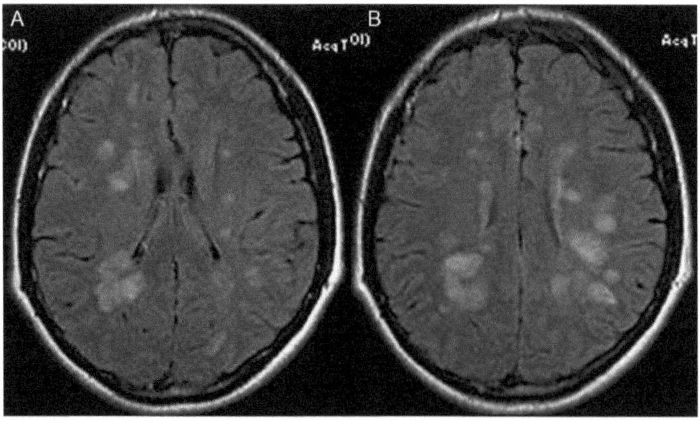

Fig. 6 Brain toxocariasis on CT. Brain CT might find multiple subcortical (A), cortical or white matter circumscribed hypodense lesions (B).

include the pathways from the (1) internal carotid artery to the ophthalmic artery, central retinal artery or posterior ciliary artery, (2) cerebrum to the optic nerve and (3) cerebrospinal fluid cavity of the cerebrum to the choroid (Padhi et al., 2014). The eye is affected often in those with covert or common toxocariasis, where symptoms remain mild and non-specific. Unfortunately, although OT is relatively uncommon, the majority of cases occur in children (Woodhall et al., 2014).

Relative to the public health importance of toxocariasis, in the United States, the average age of OT patients is 8–16 years (Woodhall et al., 2014). Based on a survey of ophthalmologists in Alabama, the prevalence of OT was estimated to be 1 case/1000 persons (Maetz et al., 1987), and Good et al. reported a similar prevalence among children in Ireland in 2004 (Good et al., 2004). In OT patients, inflammation caused by *Toxocara* larvae can cause severe, irreversible ophthalmologic injury, such as retinal detachment or formation of a subretinal granulomatous mass or scar; unilateral permanent vision loss develops in many OT patients (Woodhall et al., 2014). The main ocular manifestations of OT include leukocoria, strabismus, intraocular granulomas, vitreous strands, retinal folds and vitritis. Laboratory abnormalities are less likely to be found in OT patients. In addition to clinical history, systemic evaluation and serology, ultrasound aids diagnosis of ocular toxocariasis, especially with regard to media opacities (Morais et al., 2012).

Common diagnostic approaches of OT include slit-lamp biomicroscopy, funduscopy, immunological tests and imaging (Fig. 7). OT is classified into three main clinical types by Wilkinson and Welch, that is, peripheral granulomas accounting for 50–64%, posterior pole granulomas accounting for 25–36%, and endophthalmitis accounting for less than 25% according to various reports (Arevalo et al., 2013).

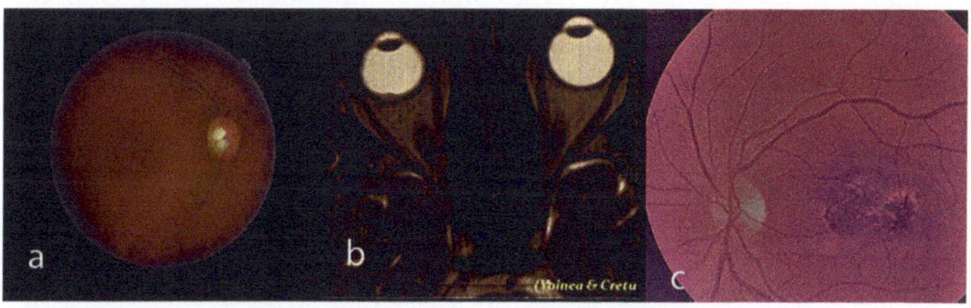

Fig. 7 Common diagnostic approaches of ocular toxocariasis include slit-lamp biomicroscopy (A), funduscopy (B) and imageological examinations (C).

Three patterns of ocular toxocariasis on ultrasound have been reported, including peripheral or posterior pole granulomas and chronic endophthalmitis. The most consistent ultrasound finding in the eye was a high-reflectivity retinal mass, located in the posterior pole or periphery, which may be calcified, and which has as its main characteristic the adherence of vitreous membranes. A vitreal fold is a characteristic sign. Secondary cataracts, glaucoma and retinal detachment are the most serious complications (Arevalo et al., 2013).

However, conventional ultrasound or CDI are not suitable for detailed pathological detection of the anterior segment because of their limited spatial resolution (Chen et al., 2018a,b). The utilization of ultrasound biomicroscopy (UBM) verifies the existence of the combined subtype (with both peripheral and posterior pole granulomas) and improves the detection rate of peripheral granulomas, which is of great importance to the diagnosis and differential diagnosis of OT. UBM seems to be a valuable and reliable diagnostic technique for the evaluation of patients with ocular toxocariasis (Chen et al., 2018a,b; Liu et al., 2017). While using a very high- or a high-frequency transducer (18 and 70 MHz), small linear hyperechoic and hyper-refringent subepidermal and intrafollicular structures suggestive of fragments of larvae, hypoechoic dermal and hypodermal tunnels that match with dilatation of lymphatic ducts, and inflammatory dermal and hypodermal ultrasound signs can support the diagnosis (Ogueta et al., 2019) (Figs 8 and 9).

2.9 Chest imaging

Toxocariasis has become a frequent cause of eosinophilic lung disease, and its prevalence has increased (Park et al., 2014). Pulmonary toxocariasis is usually asymptomatic or it only causes non-specific mild symptoms such as a cough or chest pain. The most common pulmonary symptoms in our review were cough and dyspnea, and the most common finding on chest imaging was bilateral pulmonary nodules (Bouree et al., 1997; Ranasuriya et al., 2014). Pulmonary involvement occurs in 20–85% of patients of visceral larva migrans (Sakai et al., 2006). Kwon et al. reported a prevalence of 68% toxocariasis in patients with eosinophilia, and 24% had lung invasion (Kwon et al., 2006).

Pulmonary toxocariasis manifests as multiple lesions in four radiologic patterns with a subpleural and lower lung zone predominance on initial and follow-up chest CT scans. A linear opacity may be one of many clues

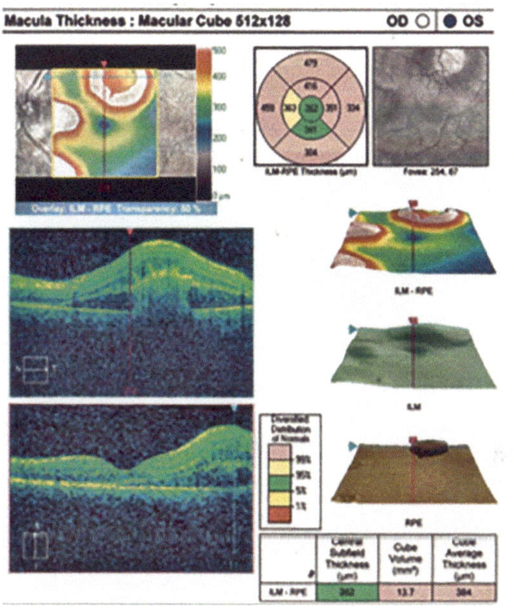

Fig. 8 The utilization of ultrasound biomicroscopy verifies the existence of the combined subtype, including peripheral granulomas. It improves the detection rate of peripheral granulomas, which is of great importance to the diagnosis and differential diagnosis of ocular toxocariasis.

in the diagnosis of pulmonary toxocariasis on CT (Lee et al., 2015). When transient and migratory pulmonary infiltrates on chest CT scans are associated with blood eosinophilia and *Toxocara* seropositivity, clinicians should consider asymptomatic toxocariasis as a cause of unexplained new pulmonary infiltrates in countries with dietary habits of raw meat intake (Kang et al., 2013).

Radiological studies may be helpful in patients with suspected toxocariasis. Even without clinical symptoms, common chest CT abnormalities may be observed, such as nodules, nodules with a GGO halo, and focal GGO. Therefore, if these findings are detected at chest CT within an appropriate clinical setting, such as eating raw meat, playing in soil or a play area where dogs or cats may have defecated routinely or playing in soil in an area with puppies that have not been kept free of infection by their owners, travelling to developing countries, clinicians would be advised to check the *Toxocara* IgG levels, regardless of the presence or absence of any clinical symptoms (Hur et al., 2014).

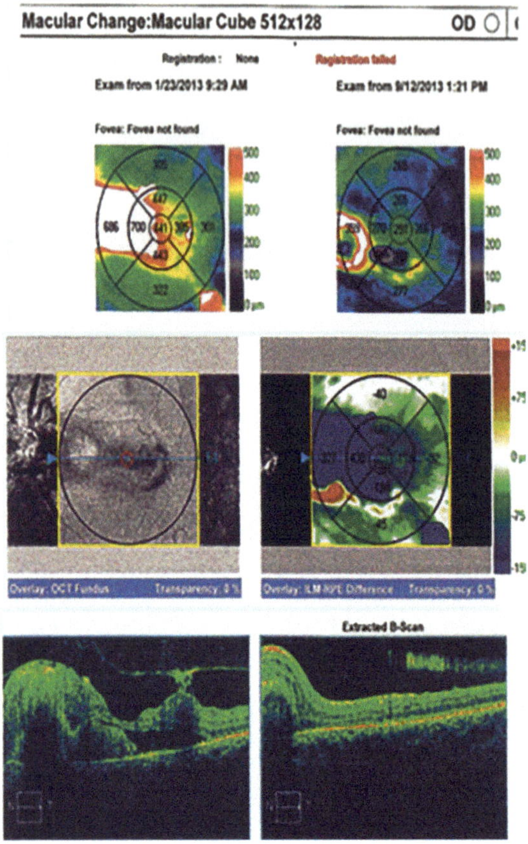

Fig. 9 The utilization of ultrasound biomicroscopy verifies the existence of the combined subtype, including posterior pole granulomas. It improves the detection rate of peripheral granulomas, which is of great importance to the diagnosis and differential diagnosis of ocular toxocariasis.

Chest X-ray and CT typically reveal bilateral peribronchial infiltration, but more widespread parenchymal infiltrates can be seen, more often in the lower parts of the lung (Huntley et al., 1965; Shrand, 1964; Snyder, 1961). Chest X-ray can also show migratory lung infiltrates (Fig. 10A); Loeffler syndrome, infiltrative pneumonia, bronchopneumonia, pleural effusion, atelectasis (Jeanfaivre et al., 1996).

The chest computed tomography (CT) findings of toxocariasis have been described in several articles (Hur et al., 2014; Kang et al., 2013; Sakai et al., 2006; Yoon et al., 2009). CT may demonstrate ill-defined

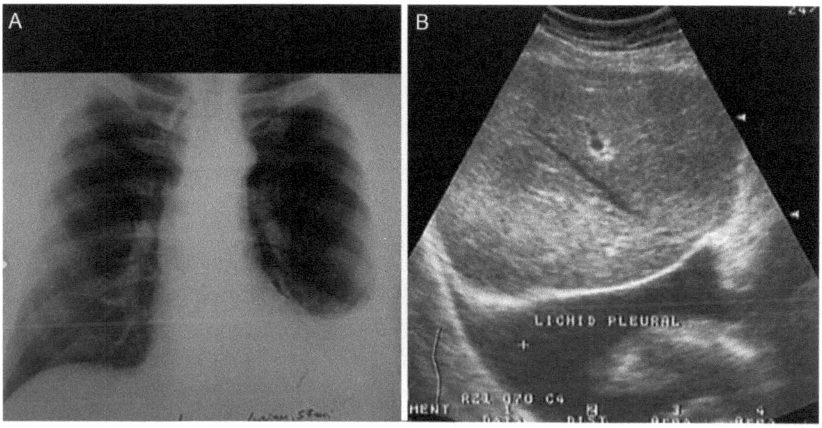

Fig. 10 (A) Chest X-ray showed bilateral peribronchial infiltration of lung toxocariasis, more often in the lower parts of the lung. (B) B-mode ultrasound scan showed pleural effusion of lung toxocariasis. Subpleural anechoic area indicated the pleural effusion on B-mode ultrasound.

subpleural nodules mimicking metastatic disease (Anderson et al., 2006; Ota et al., 2009), as well as, ground-glass and linear opacities (Lee et al., 2015). Various eosinophilic lung diseases might show similar findings to those of toxocariasis and so there is still considerable overlap in CT findings (Bouchard et al., 1994). Pulmonary toxocariasis manifests as multiple lesions in four radiologic patterns with a subpleural and lower lung zone predominance on initial and follow-up chest CT scans. A linear opacity may be one of many clues in the diagnosis of pulmonary toxocariasis on CT (Lee et al., 2015).

The most common chest CT findings in toxocariasis cases are multiple bilateral ill-defined ground-glass opacity (GGO) with or without a solid portion (Ranasuriya et al., 2014; Sakai et al., 2006; Yoon et al., 2009) (Fig. 11). In patients with eosinophilia, a nodule with a GGO halo was significantly more frequent. Other CT findings did not show a statistically significant relationship with serological markers (Lee et al., 2015).

The radiologic findings of pulmonary toxocariasis could be categorized into four patterns: GGOs with or without a solid portion, solid nodules, patchy consolidations, and focal linear opacity (Lee et al., 2015). The pulmonary lesions predominantly involve the subpleural area and almost always involve the lower lung zone. This distribution may be explained by larval migration from the peritoneal space to the lung via the pleural cavity

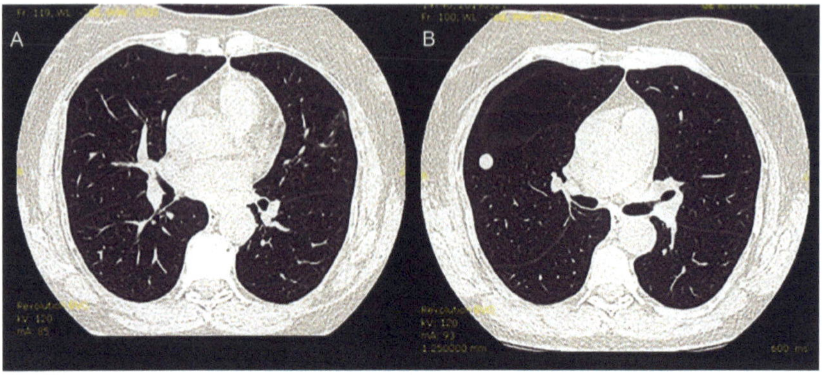

Fig. 11 The most common chest CT findings in lung toxocariasis cases are multiple bilateral ill-defined subpleural ground-glass opacity with (A) or without a solid portion (B).

(Lee et al., 2015). Pleural effusion and pericardial effusions may be seen in the context of pulmonary and cardiac involvement respectively.

Follow-up CT is frequently used to confirm transience or improvement of pulmonary lesions in pulmonary toxocariasis, an awareness of the temporal changes in imaging findings is required to understand the disease course and evaluate treatment options (Lee et al., 2015).

2.10 Differential diagnosis

For patients with liver involvement, the differential diagnosis includes all kinds of febrile and afebrile eosinophilic diseases and in rare circumstances metastatic diseases. Serology allows differentiation from other eosinophilic syndromes caused by other tissue migrating larvae, such as *Fasciola* spp., *Paragonimus* spp., schistosomes, *Ascaris* spp., *Trichinella spiralis*, filariae, *Ancylostoma* spp., *Strongyloides stercoralis*, which may have similar clinical and imaging features (Jacob et al., 1994; Seon et al., 2015).

In the case of OT, toxoplasmosis and other parasitic ocular infections, CMV, bartonellosis, tuberculosis (Field et al., 2010) and other granulomatous diseases (Paul et al., 2009) should be considered, especially in immune-compromised patients with AIDS related neoplastic diseases. Retinoblastoma should be considered in children, when biochemistry and blood cell analysis of ocular fluid clarify the diagnosis.

The differential diagnosis in patients with pulmonary symptoms includes parasitic diseases with transpulmonary migration including ascariasis, hook worms and strongyloides larvae, all of which may be detected on stool examination (Nicoletti, 2013). Allergic bronchopulmonary aspergillosis may have similar symptoms but takes a more chronic disease. In the case of hepatic involvement with periportal fibrosis and eosinophilia, schistosomiasis should be considered—we refer to recently published reviews (Richter et al., 2016a,b).

Johkoh et al. (2000) reported that various eosinophilic lung diseases showed similar findings to those of toxocariasis, so there was still considerable overlap in these findings (Hansell et al., 2008). The radiologic features of pulmonary toxocariasis overlap with those of other roundworm (*Ascaris* species) and hookworm (*Ancylostoma* and *Necator* species) infections in that they manifest as diffuse transient pulmonary opacities. Previous studies have shown that the most common imaging finding of pulmonary ascariasis is nodules with a GGO halo in the peripheral lung, which is similar to pulmonary toxocariasis (Okada et al., 2007; Sakai et al., 2006). In addition, pulmonary paragonimiasis may mimic pulmonary toxocariasis because both may show a focal consolidation pattern. However, pleuroparenchymal paragonimiasis is somewhat different from pulmonary toxocariasis in that paragonimiasis more commonly manifests as patchy consolidation, pleural effusion, pneumothoraces, and worm cysts (Woodhall et al., 2014) (Fig. 10B).

2.11 Interventional imaging (biopsy, drainage)

Direct diagnosis of *Toxocara* infection is not easy, because patients do not excrete parasite material such as eggs or larvae, while migrating larvae are not easily found in biopsy material. The diagnosis of toxocariasis and *Toxocara* infection in paratenic or accidental hosts can be made by histopathological examination (Ma et al., 2018). Sampling tissue biopsies or fluid samples is invasive and can be impractical, so diagnosis of *Toxocara* infection and toxocariasis in human beings has relied on the use of serological and immunological techniques (Roldan et al., 2015).

3. Conclusion

Diagnostic imaging has improved remarkably in the last several decades, and it is likely to continue to increase in terms of resolution, clarity, and ease of use. It can now provide information on larval localization and the extent of disease in different organs of infected patients. New methods can now also reveal images of superb quality in the eye and in different rodent model systems. Perhaps, a day may come where with appropriate labels and improved resolution and penetrance that the application of "micro-imaging" systems may allow the conclusive diagnoses of larval infection without the need of biopsies and will allow real-time examination of the effects of treatment.

Acknowledgement

We acknowledge the advice from Robert Akpata, French National Institute of Health and Medical Research (INSERM).

References

Anderson, A., Fordham, L.A., Bula, M.L., Blatt, J., 2006. Visceral larval migrans masquerading as metastatic disease in a toddler with Wilms tumor. Pediatr. Radiol. 36, 265–267.

Arevalo, J.F., Espinoza, J.V., Arevalo, F.A., 2013. Ocular toxocariasis. J. Pediatr. Ophthalmol. Strabismus 50, 76–86.

Azuma, K., Yashiro, N., Kinoshita, T., Yoshigi, J., Ihara, N., 2002. Hepatic involvement of visceral larva migrans due to *Toxocara canis*: a case report—CT and MR findings. Radiat. Med. 20, 89–92.

Bachli, H., Minet, J.C., Gratzl, O., 2004. Cerebral toxocariasis: a possible cause of epileptic seizure in children. Childs Nerv. Syst. 20, 468–472.

Baldisserotto, M., Conchin, C.F., Soares, M.G., Araujo, M.A., Kramer, B., 1999. Ultrasound findings in children with toxocariasis: report on 18 cases. Pediatr. Radiol. 29, 316–319.

Bouchard, O., Arbib, F., Paramelle, B., Brambilla, C., 1994. Acute eosinophilic pneumonia and the larva migrans syndrome: apropos of a case in an adult. Rev. Mal. Respir. 11, 593–595.

Bouree, P., Grimault, E., Fromentin, J., Tandjaoui-Lambiotte, H., Tazi, A., Battesti, J.P., 1997. Visceral larva migrans in adults with severe pulmonary manifestations. Presse Med. 26, 70–72.

Brunetti, E., Tamarozzi, F., Macpherson, C., Filice, C., Piontek, M.S., Kabaalioglu, A., Dong, Y., Atkinson, N., Richter, J., Schreiber-Dietrich, D., Dietrich, C.F., 2018. Ultrasound and cystic echinococcosis. Ultrasound Int. Open 4, E70–E78.

Chang, S., Lim, J.H., Choi, D., Park, C.K., Kwon, N.H., Cho, S.Y., Choi, D.C., 2006. Hepatic visceral larva migrans of *Toxocara canis*: CT and sonographic findings. Am. J. Roentgenol. 187, W622–W629.

Chen, Q., Gu, J., Jiang, R., Zhou, M., Chang, Q., 2018a. Role of ultrasound biomicroscopy in diagnosis of ocular toxocariasis. Br. J. Ophthalmol. 102, 642–646.

Chen, J., Liu, Q., Liu, G.H., Zheng, W.B., Hong, S.J., Sugiyama, H., Zhu, X.Q., Elsheikha, H.M., 2018b. Toxocariasis: a silent threat with a progressive public health impact. Infect. Dis. Poverty 7, 59.

Chieffi, P.P., Aquino, R.T., Paschoalotti, M.A., Ribeiro, M.C., Nasello, A.G., 2009. Muscular strength decrease in *Rattus norvegicus* experimentally infected by *Toxocara canis*. Rev. Inst. Med. Trop. Sao Paulo 51, 73–75.

Choi, J.H., Cho, J.W., Lee, J.H., Lee, S.W., Kim, H.J., Choi, K.D., 2013. Obstructive hydrocephalus due to CNS toxocariasis. J. Neurol. Sci. 329, 59–61.

Claudon, M., Dietrich, C.F., Choi, B.I., Cosgrove, D.O., Kudo, M., Nolsoe, C.P., Piscaglia, F., Wilson, S.R., Barr, R.G., Chammas, M.C., Chaubal, N.G., Chen, M.H., Clevert, D.A., Correas, J.M., Ding, H., Forsberg, F., Fowlkes, J.B., Gibson, R.N., Goldberg, B.B., Lassau, N., Leen, E.L., Mattrey, R.F., Moriyasu, F., Solbiati, L., Weskott, H.P., Xu, H.X., 2013a. Guidelines and good clinical practice recommendations for Contrast Enhanced Ultrasound (CEUS) in the liver—update 2012: a WFUMB-EFSUMB initiative in cooperation with representatives of AFSUMB, AIUM, ASUM, FLAUS and ICUS. Ultrasound Med. Biol. 39, 187–210.

Claudon, M., Dietrich, C.F., Choi, B.I., Cosgrove, D.O., Kudo, M., Nolsoe, C.P., Piscaglia, F., Wilson, S.R., Barr, R.G., Chammas, M.C., Chaubal, N.G., Chen, M.H., Clevert, D.A., Correas, J.M., Ding, H., Forsberg, F., Fowlkes, J.B., Gibson, R.N., Goldberg, B.B., Lassau, N., Leen, E.L., Mattrey, R.F., Moriyasu, F., Solbiati, L., Weskott, H.P., Xu, H.X., 2013b. Guidelines and good clinical practice recommendations for contrast enhanced ultrasound (CEUS) in the liver—update 2012: a WFUMB-EFSUMB initiative in cooperation with representatives of AFSUMB, AIUM, ASUM, FLAUS and ICUS. Ultraschall. Med. 34, 11–29.

Coskun, F., Akinci, E., 2013. Hepatic toxocariasis: a rare cause of right upper abdominal pain in the emergency department. Türk. Parazitol. Derg. 37, 151–153.

Deshayes, S., Bonhomme, J., de La Blanchardiere, A., 2016. Neurotoxocariasis: a systematic literature review. Infection 44, 565–574.

Dietrich, C.F., Hocke, M., 2011. Interventionelle Therapie der Echinokokkose. In: Dietrich, C.F., Nurnberg, D. (Eds.), Interventionelle Sonographie. Thieme Verlag, pp. 240–256.

Dietrich, C.F., Mueller, G., Beyer-Enke, S., 2009. Cysts in the cyst pattern. Z. Gastroenterol. 47, 1203–1207.

Dietrich, C.F., Lembcke, B., Jenssen, C., Hocke, M., Ignee, A., Hollerweger, A., 2014. Intestinal ultrasound in rare gastrointestinal diseases, update, part 1. Ultraschall. Med. 35, 400–421.

Dietrich, C.F., Kabaalioglu, A., Brunetti, E., Richter, J., 2015. Fasciolosis. Z. Gastroenterol. 53, 285–290.

Dietrich, C.F., Lorentzen, T., Appelbaum, L., Buscarini, E., Cantisani, V., Correas, J.M., Cui, X.W., D'Onofrio, M., Gilja, O.H., Hocke, M., Ignee, A., Jenssen, C., Kabaalioğlu, A., Leen, E., Nicolau, C., Nolsøe, C.P., Radzina, M., Serra, C., Sidhu, P.S., Sparchez, Z., Piscaglia, F., 2016a. EFSUMB guidelines on interventional ultrasound (INVUS), part III—abdominal treatment procedures (long version). Ultraschall. Med. 37, E1–E32.

Dietrich, C.F., Lorentzen, T., Appelbaum, L., Buscarini, E., Cantisani, V., Correas, J.M., Cui, X.W., D'Onofrio, M., Gilja, O.H., Hocke, M., Ignee, A., Jenssen, C., Kabaalioğlu, A., Leen, E., Nicolau, C., Nolsøe, C.P., Radzina, M., Serra, C., Sidhu, P.S., Sparchez, Z., Piscaglia, F., 2016b. EFSUMB guidelines on interventional ultrasound (INVUS), part III—abdominal treatment procedures (short version). Ultraschall. Med. 37, 27–45.

Dietrich, C.F., Sharma, M., Chaubal, N., Dong, Y., Cui, X.W., Schindler-Piontek, M., Richter, J., Radzina, M., Sandouk, F., Kucharzik, T., Schreiber-Dietrich, D., 2017. Ascariasis imaging: pictorial essay. Z. Gastroenterol. 55, 479–489.

Dietrich, C.F., Atkinson, N.S.S., Lee, W.J., Kling, K., Neumayr, A., Braden, B., Richter, J., Akpata, R., Southisavath, P., Schreiber-Dietrich, D., Dong, Y., 2018. Never seen before? Opisthorchiasis and Clonorchiasis. Z. Gastroenterol. 56, 13–1520.

Dietrich, C.F., Chaubal, N., Hoerauf, A., Kling, K., Piontek, M.S., Steffgen, L., Mand, S., Dong, Y., 2019. Review of dancing parasites in lymphatic filariasis. Ultrasound Int. Open 5, E65–E74.

Dong, Y., Mao, F., Cao, J., Zhang, Q., Yang, D., Wang, W.P., Dietrich, C.F., 2018. Differential diagnosis of gallbladder ascariasis debris: the added value of contrast enhanced ultrasound with high frequency transducer. Med. Ultrason. 20, 413–419.

Fan, C.K., Holland, C.V., Loxton, K., Barghouth, U., 2015. Cerebral toxocariasis: silent progression to neurodegenerative disorders? Clin. Microbiol. Rev. 28, 663–686.

Feske, S.K., Goldberg, M., Dudzinski, D.M., Gonzalez, R.G., Kovach, A.E., 2015. CASE RECORDS of the MASSACHUSETTS GENERAL HOSPITAL. Case 29-2015. A 38-year-old pregnant woman with headache and visual symptoms. N. Engl. J. Med. 373, 1154–1164.

Field, V., Gautret, P., Schlagenhauf, P., Burchard, G.D., Caumes, E., Jensenius, M., Castelli, F., Gkrania-Klotsas, E., Weld, L., Lopez-Velez, R., de Vries, P., von Sonnenburg, F., Loutan, L., Parola, P., EuroTravNet Network, 2010. Travel and migration associated infectious diseases morbidity in Europe, 2008. BMC Infect. Dis. 10, 330.

Ghoroobi, J., Mohajerzadeh, L., Khoddami, M., Mirshemirani, A., Sadeghian, N., Mahdavi, A., Hatefi, S., 2017. Abdominal mass secondary to human toxocariasis. APSP J. Case Rep. 8, 4.

Good, B., Holland, C.V., Taylor, M.R.H., Larragy, J., Moriarty, P., O'Regan, M., 2004. Ocular toxocariasis in schoolchildren. Clin. Infect. Dis. 39, 173–178.

Gorgulu, A., Albayrak, B.S., Gorgulu, E., Tural, O., 2006. Postoperative cerebral abscess formation caused by *Toxocara canis* in a meningioma cavity. J. Neurooncol 77, 325–326.

Graeff-Teixeira, C., da Silva, A.C., Yoshimura, K., 2009. Update on eosinophilic meningoencephalitis and its clinical relevance. Clin. Microbiol. Rev. 22, 322–348.

Ha, K.H., Song, J.E., Kim, B.S., Lee, C.H., 2016. Clinical characteristics and progression of liver abscess caused by toxocara. World J. Hepatol. 8, 757–761.

Hansell, D.M., Bankier, A.A., MacMahon, H., McLoud, T.C., Muller, N.L., Remy, J., 2008. Fleischner Society: glossary of terms for thoracic imaging. Radiology 246, 697–722.

Huntley, C.C., Costas, M.C., Lyerly, A., 1965. Visceral larva migrans syndrome: clinical characteristics and immunologic studies in 51 patients. Pediatrics 36, 523–536.

Hur, J.H., Lee, I.J., Kim, J.H., Kim, D.G., Hwang, H.J., Koh, S.H., Lee, K., 2014. Chest CT findings of toxocariasis: correlation with laboratory results. Clin. Radiol. 69, e285–e290.

Ishibashi, H., Shimamura, R., Hirata, Y., Kudo, J., Onizuka, H., 1992. Hepatic granuloma in toxocaral infection: role of ultrasonography in hypereosinophilia. J. Clin. Ultrasound 20, 204–210.

Jacob, C.M., Pastorino, A.C., Peres, B.A., Mello, E.O., Okay, Y., Oselka, G.W., 1994. Clinical and laboratorial features of visceral toxocariasis in infancy. Rev. Inst. Med. Trop. Sao Paulo 36, 19–26.

Jain, R., Sawhney, S., Bhargava, D.K., Panda, S.K., Berry, M., 1994. Hepatic granulomas due to visceral larva migrans in adults: appearance on US and MRI. Abdom. Imaging 19, 253–256.

Jang, E.Y., Choi, M.S., Gwak, G.Y., Koh, K.C., Paik, S.W., Lee, J.H., Paik, Y.H., Yoo, B.C., 2015. Enhanced resolution of eosinophilic liver abscess associated with toxocariasis by albendazole treatment. Korean J. Gastroenterol. 65, 222–228.

Jeanfaivre, T., Cimon, B., Tolstuchow, N., de Gentile, L., Chabasse, D., Tuchais, E., 1996. Pleural effusion and toxocariasis. Thorax 51, 106–107.

Johkoh, T., Muller, N.L., Akira, M., Ichikado, K., Suga, M., Ando, M., Toshinaga, T., Kiyama, T., Mihara, N., Honda, O., Tomiyama, N., Nakamura, H., 2000. Eosinophilic lung diseases: diagnostic accuracy of thin-section CT in 111 patients. Radiology 216, 773–780.

Kabaalioglu, A., Ceken, K., Alimoglu, E., Saba, R., Apaydin, A., 2005. Hepatic toxocariasis: US, CT and MRI findings. Ultraschall. Med. 26, 329–332.

Kang, Y.R., Kim, S.A., Jeon, K., Koh, W.J., Suh, G.Y., Chung, M.P., Kim, H., Kwon, O.J., Kang, E.S., Um, S.W., 2013. Toxocariasis as a cause of new pulmonary infiltrates. Int. J. Tuberc. Lung Dis. 17, 412–417.

Kwon, H.H., 2015. Toxocariasis: a rare cause of multiple cerebral infarction. Infect. Chemother. 47, 137–141.

Kwon, N.H., Oh, M.J., Lee, S.P., Lee, B.J., Choi, D.C., 2006. The prevalence and diagnostic value of toxocariasis in unknown eosinophilia. Ann. Hematol. 85, 233–238.

Laroia, S.T., Rastogi, A., Bihari, C., Bhadoria, A.S., Sarin, S.K., 2016. Hepatic visceral larva migrans, a resilient entity on imaging: experience from a tertiary liver center. Trop. Parasitol. 6, 56–68.

Lee, K.H., Kim, T.J., Lee, K.W., 2015. Pulmonary toxocariasis: initial and follow-up CT findings in 63 patients. Am. J. Roentgenol. 204, 1203–1211.

Lim, J.H., 2008. Toxocariasis of the liver: visceral larva migrans. Abdom. Imaging 33, 151–156.

Liu, J., Li, S., Deng, G., Yang, W., Chen, W., Lu, H., 2017. Ultrasound biomicroscopic imaging in paediatric ocular toxocariasis. Br. J. Ophthalmol. 101, 1514–1517.

Ma, G., Holland, C.V., Wang, T., Hofmann, A., Fan, C.K., Maizels, R.M., Hotez, P.J., Gasser, R.B., 2018. Human toxocariasis. Lancet Infect. Dis. 18, e14–e24.

Maetz, H.M., Kleinstein, R.N., Federico, D., Wayne, J., 1987. Estimated prevalence of ocular toxoplasmosis and toxocariasis in Alabama. J. Infect. Dis. 156, 414.

Moiyadi, A., Mahadevan, A., Anandh, B., Shivashankar, R.S., Chickabasavaiah, Y.T., Shankar, S.K., 2007. Visceral larva migrans presenting as multiple intracranial and intraspinal abscesses. Neuropathology 27, 371–374.

Morais, F.B., Maciel, A.L., Arantes, T.E., Muccioli, C., Allemann, N., 2012. Ultrasonographic findings in ocular toxocariasis. Arq. Bras. Oftalmol. 75, 43–47.

Nada, S.M., Abazza, B.E., Mahmoud, L.A., Habeeb, Y.S., Hussein, H.F., Amer, O.T., 1996. Toxocariasis as a cause of renal disease in children in Sharkia Governorate, Egypt. J. Egypt. Soc. Parasitol. 26, 709–717.

Nicoletti, A., 2013. Toxocariasis. Handbook of Clinical Neurology 114, 217–228.

Ogueta, I., Navajas-Galimany, L., Concha-Rogazy, M., Alvarez-Veliz, S., Vera-Kellet, C., Gonzalez-Bombardiere, S., Wortsman, X., 2019. Very high- and high-frequency ultrasound features of cutaneous larva migrans. J. Ultrasound Med. 38, 3349–3358.

Okada, F., Ono, A., Ando, Y., Yotsumoto, S., Yotsumoto, S., Tanoue, S., Matsumoto, S., Wakisaka, M., Mori, H., 2007. Pulmonary computed tomography findings of visceral larva migrans caused by *Ascaris suum*. J. Comput. Assist. Tomogr. 31, 402–408.

Ota, K.V., Dimaras, H., Heon, E., Babyn, P.S., Yau, Y.C., Read, S., Budning, A., Gallie, B.L., Chan, H.S., 2009. Toxocariasis mimicking liver, lung, and spinal cord metastases from retinoblastoma. Pediatr. Infect. Dis. J. 28, 252–254.

Overgaauw, P.A.M., 1997. Aspects of *Toxocara* epidemiology: human toxocarosis. Crit. Rev. Microbiol. 23, 215–231.

Padhi, T.R., Das, S., Sharma, S., Rath, S., Rath, S., Tripathy, D., Panda, K.G., Basu, S., Besirli, C.G., 2014. Ocular parasitoses: a comprehensive review. Surv. Ophthalmol. 62, 161–189.

Park, B.M., Jeong, S.O., Park, H.S., Jung, S.S., Kim, S.Y., Kim, J.O., Lee, J.E., 2014. Differences in the clinical and radiological characteristics of lung-involved toxocariasis between toxocariasis with eosinophilia and those without eosinophilia. J. Thorac. Dis. 6, 1757–1764.

Park, K.Y., Park, H.K., Hwang, H.S., Ryu, J.S., Lee, K.G., Jang, K.S., 2018. Space occupying lesion in the liver caused by hepatic visceral larva migrans: a case report. Am. J. Trop. Med. Hyg. 99, 1602–1605.

Paul, M., Stefaniak, J., Twardosz-Pawlik, H., Pecold, K., 2009. The co-occurrence of *Toxocara* ocular and visceral larva migrans syndrome: a case series. Cases J. 2, 6881.

Ranasuriya, G., Mian, A., Boujaoude, Z., Tsigrelis, C., 2014. Pulmonary toxocariasis: a case report and literature review. Infection 42, 575–578.

Richter, J., Azoulay, D., Dong, Y., Holtfreter, M.C., Akpata, R., Calderaro, J., El-Scheich, T., Breuer, M., Neumayr, A., Hatz, C., Kircheis, G., Botelho, M.C., Dietrich, C.F., 2016a. Ultrasonography of gallbladder abnormalities due to schistosomiasis. Parasitol. Res. 115, 2917–2924.

Richter, J., Botelho, M.C., Holtfreter, M.C., Akpata, R., El Scheich, T., Neumayr, A., Brunetti, E., Hatz, C., Dong, Y., Dietrich, C.F., 2016b. Ultrasound assessment of schistosomiasis. Z. Gastroenterol. 54, 653–660.

Roldan, W.H., Elefant, G.R., Ferreira, A.W., 2015. Deglycosylation of Toxocara excretory-secretory antigens improves the specificity of the serodiagnosis for human toxocariasis. Parasite Immunol. 37, 557–567.

Rubinsky-Elefant, G., Hirata, C.E., Yamamoto, J.H., Ferreira, M.U., 2010. Human toxocariasis: diagnosis, worldwide seroprevalences and clinical expression of the systemic and ocular forms. Ann. Trop. Med. Parasitol. 104, 3–23.

Sakai, S., Shida, Y., Takahashi, N., Yabuuchi, H., Soeda, H., Okafuji, T., Hatakenaka, M., Honda, H., 2006. Pulmonary lesions associated with visceral larva migrans due to *Ascaris suum* or *Toxocara canis*: imaging of six cases. Am. J. Roentgenol. 186, 1697–1702.

Sanchez, S.S., Garcia, H.H., Nicoletti, A., 2018. Clinical and magnetic resonance imaging findings of neurotoxocariasis. Front. Neurol. 9, 53.

Sarda, A.K., Kannan, R., 1992. Visceral larva migrans masquerading as liver secondaries. J. Indian Med. Assoc. 90, 302.

Schaffellner, S., Wagner, D., Sereinigg, M., Jakoby, E., Kniepeiss, D., Stiegler, P., Valentin, T., Iberer, F., Tscheliessnigg, K.H., 2010. First case of *Toxocara* eosinophilic ascites after combined pancreas and kidney transplantation. Am. J. Transplant. 10, 2727.

Seon, H.J., Kim, Y.I., Lee, J.H., Kim, S.H., Kim, Y.H., 2015. Differential chest computed tomography findings of pulmonary parasite infestation between the paragonimiasis and nonparagonimiatic parasite infestation. J. Comput. Assist. Tomogr. 39, 956–961.

Shrand, H., 1964. Visceral larva migrans. *Toxocara* canis infection. Lancet 1, 1357–1359.

Sick, C., Hennerici, M.G., 2014. Expect the unexpected: a case of isolated eosinophilic meningitis in toxocariasis. Case Rep. Neurol. 6, 259–263.

Singer, O.C., Conrad, F., Jahnke, K., Hattingen, E., Auer, H., Steinmetz, H., 2011. Severe meningoencephalomyelitis due to CNS-Toxocarosis. J. Neurol. 258, 696–698.

Smith, H.V., 1993. Antibody reactivity in human toxocariasis. In: Lewis, J.W., Maizels, R.M. (Eds.), *Toxocara* and Toxocariasis, Clinical, Epidemiological and Molecular Perspectives. British Society for Parasitology and Institute of Biology, England, pp. 91–109.

Snyder, C.H., 1961. Visceral larva migrans—ten years' experience. Pediatrics 28, 85–91.

Treska, V., Sutnar, A., Mukensnabl, P., Manakova, T., Sedlacek, D., Mirka, H., Ferda, J., 2011. Liver abscess in human toxocariasis. Bratisl. Lek. Listy 112, 644–647.

Woodhall, D.M., Eberhard, M.L., Parise, M.E., 2014. Neglected parasitic infections in the United States: toxocariasis. Am. J. Trop. Med. Hyg. 90, 810–813.

Xinou, E., Lefkopoulos, A., Gelagoti, M., Drevelegas, A., Diakou, A., Milonas, I., Dimitriadis, A.S., 2003. CT and MR imaging findings in cerebral toxocaral disease. Am. J. Neuroradiol. 24, 714–718.

Yamamoto, T., Miyazaki, T., Kurashima, Y., Ohata, K., Okawa, M., Tanaka, S., Uenishi, T., Miyaji, K., Fukumoto, N., 2015. Solitary hepatic eosinophilic granuloma accompanied by eosinophilia without parasitosis: report of a case. Int. Surg. 100, 1011–1017.

Yoon, Y.S., Lee, C.H., Kang, Y.A., Kwon, S.Y., Yoon, H.I., Lee, J.H., Lee, C.T., 2009. Impact of toxocariasis in patients with unexplained patchy pulmonary infiltrate in Korea. J. Korean Med. Sci. 24, 40–45.

Yoon, S.Y., Baek, S., Park, S.Y., Shin, B., Kwon, H.S., Cho, Y.S., Moon, H.B., Kim, T.B., 2018. Clinical course and treatment outcomes of toxocariasis-related eosinophilic disorder. Medicine (Baltimore) 97, e12361.

Zachariah, S.B., Zachariah, B., Varghese, R., 1994. Neuroimaging studies of cerebral "visceral larva migrans" syndrome. J. Neuroimaging 4, 39–40.

Further reading

Despommier, D., 2003. Toxocariasis: clinical aspects, epidemiology, medical ecology, and molecular aspects. Clin. Microbiol. Rev. 16, 265–272.

McManus, R., Hamilton, C.M., Holland, C.V., 2018. Toxocara spp. In: Rose, J.B., Jiménez-Cisneros, B. (Eds.), Global Water Pathogens Project. Michigan State University, UNESCO, East Lansing, MI. http://www.waterpathogens.org. Robertson, L (eds) Part 4 Helminths, http://www.waterpathogens.org/book/toxocara.

CHAPTER TEN

Toxocara-induced neural *larva migrans* (neurotoxocarosis) in rodent model hosts

Christina Strube[a,*], Patrick Waindok[a], Marie-Kristin Raulf[a,b], Andrea Springer[a]

[a]Institute for Parasitology, Centre for Infection Medicine, University of Veterinary Medicine Hannover, Hanover, Germany

[b]Immunology Unit & Research Centre for Emerging Infections and Zoonoses, University of Veterinary Medicine Hannover, Hanover, Germany

[*]Corresponding author: e-mail address: christina.strube@tiho-hannover.de

Contents

Abstract

Neural *larva migrans* (NLM), or neurotoxocarosis, induced by *Toxocara canis* or *Toxocara cati* results from migrating and persisting larvae in the central nervous system of paratenic hosts, including humans. As the diagnosis of NLM in humans is not straightforward, most knowledge on the disease is derived from only a few published clinical cases. To improve our understanding of human NLM, studies on the pathogenesis and clinical symptoms in laboratory animal model systems are indispensable, and rodents have been accepted as the most appropriate model organisms for NLM. As research has mostly focused on neuroinvasive *T. canis*-larvae, information regarding the pathogenesis of *T. cati*-induced NLM remains scarce. This review summarises the current state of

Advances in Parasitology, Volume 109
ISSN 0065-308X
https://doi.org/10.1016/bs.apar.2020.01.006

knowledge on neuroinvasion by both *T. canis* and *T. cati* in different rodent model hosts, the resulting behavioural changes, and histopathological alterations during the course of NLM as well as the potential molecular pathogenic mechanisms.

1. Introduction

The syndrome of neural *larva migrans* (NLM) is induced by the accumulation and persistence of nematode larvae in the central nervous system (CNS). Besides *Baylisascaris procyonis*, the raccoon roundworm, two zoonotic species of *Toxocara* roundworms play a prominent role in induction of NLM (Fan et al., 2015; Finsterer and Auer, 2007). These are the dog and cat roundworms, *Toxocara canis* and *Toxocara cati*, respectively, which are frequently occurring intestinal parasites of canids and felids with a worldwide distribution. Migration and persistence of *Toxocara*-larvae in paratenic hosts, including humans, is responsible for one of the most common zoonotic infections worldwide that can result in the signs and symptoms associated with the general conditions known as visceral *larva migrans* (Rubinsky-Elefant et al., 2010). In those cases with neuroinvasion, the associated *Toxocara*-larvae cause NLM, which is also known as neurotoxocarosis or cerebral toxocarosis. Clinical cases of NLM in humans are associated with encephalitis, myelitis, cerebral vasculitis, eosinophilic meningoencephalitis, optic neuritis, and other neurologic inflammatory diseases, and affected patients may suffer from headache, oversensitivity to light, weakness and confusion (Eberhardt et al., 2005; Fan et al., 2015; Finsterer and Auer, 2007; Moreira-Silva et al., 2004). Neurodegenerative and neuropsychiatric disorders as well as various cognitive deficits have also been described as a consequence of NLM (El-Sayed and Ismail, 2012; Fan et al., 2015; Richartz and Buchkremer, 2002; Walsh and Haseeb, 2012). Furthermore, cerebral *Toxocara* infection is controversially discussed as a cause of epilepsy, schizophrenia and Alzheimer's disease (Celik et al., 2013; Fan et al., 2015; Kamuyu et al., 2014; Kaplan et al., 2008). However, due to the cryptic nature of the cerebral infection, diagnosis remains challenging. Thus, the number of reported NLM cases is small and probably underestimated. Most knowledge on NLM is derived from only few clinical cases or studies correlating seropositivity against *Toxocara* with neurological disorders, as reviewed by Fan et al. (2015). In order to achieve a deeper understanding of behavioural and pathological implications of NLM, laboratory animal model systems are a necessity (Fan et al., 2015). The impact of *Toxocara*-larvae on paratenic hosts has been studied in a variety of animal models, including experimental infections of mice, rats, gerbils, pigs, primates and avian species (Strube et al., 2013). While most of these paratenic hosts exhibit a comparable somatic migration of *Toxocara*-larvae, rodents seem to be the most appropriate model organisms for NLM (Boes and Helwigh, 2000; Strube et al., 2013). Nevertheless, larval migration patterns and neuropathogenicity of *Toxocara* may differ between different rodent species and strains (Cox and Holland, 2001a; Epe et al., 1994; Hamilton et al., 2006), resulting in potentially conflicting conclusions. Furthermore, as *T. canis* is assumed to be the causative agent of most human NLM cases, the majority of experimental NLM studies have focused on this species, while the pathogenesis of *T. cati*-induced NLM has only been marginally studied to date (Fisher, 2003; Fukae et al., 2012; Smith et al., 2009). This review intends to provide a comprehensive overview of the neuro-invasiveness of *T. canis*-larvae as well as *T. cati*-larvae in different rodent species and strains, the resulting neurobehavioural changes and progression of histopathological alterations during the course of NLM, as well as the underlying molecular pathogenic mechanisms.

2. Larval migration to cerebral tissues

Somatic migration of *Toxocara*-larvae in paratenic hosts may be divided into three phases. The acute phase of infection, equivalent to the hepato-pulmonary phase, encompasses the period from infection to approximately day 14 *post infection* (pi), when larvae penetrate the intestinal wall and migrate via the circulatory system to the liver and the lungs and further to somatic tissues. The progressive migration and accumulation of larvae in somatic tissues at the beginning of the myotropic-neurotropic phase indicates the subacute phase of infection, which lasts approximately until day 28 pi. This phase is characterised by the onset of behavioural alterations and, in case of NLM, by inflammatory reactions in the brain of infected paratenic hosts. The chronic stage of infection starts approximately at day 28 pi and is accompanied by progressive behavioural and pathological effects. In this phase, larvae resume their migration throughout the entire body to species-dependent predilection sites, where the larvae may persist as the infective stage for months to years (Abo-Shehada et al., 1984; Janecek et al., 2014; Sprent, 1952). Table 1 summarises the maximum recovery rates of neurotropic *T. canis*- and *T. cati*-larvae in different rodent

Table 1 Overview of the mean maximum recovery of neurotropic *Toxocara canis*- and *T. cati*-larvae in different rodent species and strains.

			Inoculation dose	Maximum recovery in the CNS (% of the inoculation dose)			
Rodent species	Strain	*Toxocara* species	(infective eggs)	Acute phase	Subacute phase	Chronic phase	References
Mouse (*Mus musculus*)							
Inbred							
	n.d.	*T. canis*	500	8.6	8.8	10.6	Min (1982)
	BALB/c	*T. canis*	5	n.d.	n.d.	3.2	Fonseca et al. (2017)
			50	n.d.	n.d.	6.0	
			500	n.d.	n.d.	2.6	
	BALB/c	*T. canis*	6	33.3	33.3	66.7	Ollero et al. (2008)
			12	41.7	91.7	108.3	
			50	6.0	22.0	28.0	
			100	12.0	7.0	17.0	
			200	24.5	30.0	23.0	
			1000	9.1	9.1	9.5	
			4×50[a]	n.d.	n.d.	39.0	
			4×250[a]	n.d.	n.d.	34.9	

	BALB/c	*T. canis*	1000[b]	n.d.	6.7	14.7	Epe et al. (1994)
	BALB/c	*T. canis*	1000	n.d.	n.d.	13.6	Pinelli et al. (2005)
	BALB/c	*T. canis*	2000	10.3	17.6	18.6	Hamilton et al. (2006)
	BALB/c	*T. cati*	1000	0.4	0.2	1.9	Cardillo et al. (2009)
	BALB/c	*T. cati*	2000	0.3	0.3	1.2	Janecek et al. (2014)
	C57BL6/J	*T. canis*	5	n.d.	n.d.	6.6	Havasiová-Reiterová et al. (1995)
			7	n.d.	n.d.	14.3	
			1000	n.d.	n.d.	10.2	
	C57BL/6J	*T. canis*	1000	4.5	n.d.	9.0	Dunsmore et al. (1983)
	C57BL/6J	*T. canis*	1000	9.9	14.2	16.4	Dvorožňáková et al. (2003)
	C57BL6/J	*T. canis*	1000[b]	n.d.	7.7	11.0	Epe et al. (1994)
	C57BL/6J	*T. canis*	2000	7.1	18.6	19.1	Hamilton et al. (2006)
	C57BL/6J	*T. canis*	2000	1.7	0.9	1.8	Janecek et al. (2014)
	C57BL6/J	*T. cati*	5	n.d.	n.d.	4.0	Havasiová-Reiterová et al. (1995)
			7	n.d.	n.d.	2.3	
			500	n.d.	n.d.	0.1	
	C57BL/6J	*T. cati*	1000	0.4	0.2	0.2	Hrckova et al. (2001)

Continued

Table 1 Overview of the mean maximum recovery of neurotropic *Toxocara canis*- and *T. cati*-larvae in different rodent species and strains.—cont'd

Rodent species	Strain	*Toxocara* species	Inoculation dose (infective eggs)	Maximum recovery in the CNS (% of the inoculation dose) Acute phase	Subacute phase	Chronic phase	References
	C57BL/6J	*T. cati*	2000	0.2	0.4	0.5	Janecek et al. (2014)
	NIH	*T. canis*	100	n.d.	n.d.	3.2	Holland and Cox (2001)
			1000	n.d.	n.d.	1.1	
			3000	n.d.	n.d.	1.3	
			4 × 250[a]	n.d.	n.d.	0.4	
	NIH	*T. canis*	2000	8.2	9.4	14.4	Hamilton et al. (2006)
	C3H/He	*T. canis*	1000[b]	n.d.	9.5	9.6	Epe et al. (1994)
	C3H/He	*T. canis*	2000	9.8	12.3	18.1	Hamilton et al. (2006)
	CBA/Ca	*T. canis*	2000	9.5	18.3	19.0	Hamilton et al. (2006)
	DBA/2	*T. canis*	1000[b]	n.d.	12.1	8.1	Epe et al. (1994)
	A/J	*T. canis*	2000	10.6	10.8	14.7	Hamilton et al. (2006)
	SWR	*T. canis*	2000	4.7	12.1	11.9	Hamilton et al. (2006)

Outbred							
	HaM/ICR	*T. canis*	200	3.5	10.5	12.5	Kayes and Oaks (1976)
			600	2.3	7.0	9.7	
			1000	5.3	6.4	6.4	
	ICR	*T. canis*	250	0.1	0.3	2.0	Liao et al. (2008)
	LACA	*T. canis*	100	n.d.	n.d.	4.4	Holland and Cox (2001)
			1000	n.d.	n.d.	5.9	
			3000	n.d.	n.d.	6.1	
			4×250[a]	n.d.	n.d.	3.5	
	LACA	*T. canis*	2000	n.d.	n.d.	3.3	Cox and Holland (1998)
	CD1	*T. canis*	500	2.3	4.8	n.d.	Abdel-Hameed (1984)
	CD1	*T. canis*	1000	1.3	n.d.	2.7	Good et al. (2001)
			3000	1.6	n.d.	2.2	
	Canberra	*T. canis*	1000	3.0	2.8	4.9	Dunsmore et al. (1983)
			5000	3.1	3.6	5.6	
	Swiss albino	*T. canis*	1000	n.d.	6.5	10.6	Eid et al. (2015)

Continued

Table 1 Overview of the mean maximum recovery of neurotropic *Toxocara canis*- and *T. cati*-larvae in different rodent species and strains.—cont'd

Rodent species	Strain	*Toxocara* species	Inoculation dose (infective eggs)	Maximum recovery in the CNS (% of the inoculation dose)			References
				Acute phase	Subacute phase	Chronic phase	
	Swiss albino	*T. canis*	1000	n.d.	6.3	10.3	Othman et al. (2010)
	NMRI	*T. canis*	1000[b]	n.d.	7.1	3.8	Epe et al. (1994)
Rat (*Rattus norvegicus*)							
	Cheek-Jones	*T. canis*	20,000	n.d.	0.4	n.d.	Olson and Rose (1966)
	n.d.	*T. canis*	300	0.1	0.4	0.9	Santos et al. (2017)
	Wistar	*T. canis*	500	1.7	4.5	3.9	Lescano et al. (2004)
	Wistar	*T. canis*	3000	0.3[c]	0.2[c]	0.1[c]	Burren (1972)
	Wistar	*T. cati*	300	1.1	0.5	1.1	Santos et al. (2009)
	Wistar	*T. cati*	1000	0.0[d]	0.0	0.0	Taira et al. (2013)
	Wistar	*T. cati*	2500	0.0	n.d.	0.1	Zibaei et al. (2010)

Gerbil (*Meriones unguiculatus*)						
	T. canis	1000	n.d.	n.d.	n.d.	Alba-Hurtado et al. (2009)
	T. canis	1000	3.1	n.d.	n.d.	Cho et al. (2007)
	T. canis	2000	0.3	1.2	1.4	Burren (1972)
	T. cati	240	0.0	0.0	1.3	Zibaei et al. (2010)
Golden hamster (*Mesocricetus auratus*)						
	T. canis	2000	0.8[c]	1.3[c]	1.8[c]	Burren (1972)
Guinea pig (*Cavia porcellus*)						
	T. canis	2500	0.5	0.0	n.d.	Olson and Schulz (1963)

[a]Inoculation occurred weekly over a period of 28 days.
[b]Rodents were infected with 1000 hatched infective larvae instead of infective eggs.
[c]Recovery rates refer to 50mg cerebral tissue.
[d]Larval recovery rate in relation to infection dose is 0.02%.
Days post infection (pi) were categorised as acute (days 0–13 pi), subacute (days 14–27 pi) and chronic (starting day 28 pi) phase of infection.
n.d., not determined.
If more than one investigation per phase of infection was assessed, the mean of the highest recovery rate during the respective phase of infection was used for calculating the frequency of larval recovery in relation to the initial inoculation dose.

species and strains in relation to the initial inoculation dose during the three phases of infection, i.e., acute (0–13 days pi), subacute (14–27 days pi) and chronic (starting day 28 pi). If more than one investigation per phase of infection was assessed, the mean of the highest recovery rate during the respective phase of infection was used for calculating the frequency of larval recovery in relation to the initial inoculation dose. Relation to total recovery of larvae was not calculated as this value was not reported in all of the studies.

2.1 Neuroinvasion in mice

Mice (*Mus musculus*) have frequently been used as model organisms investigating larval migration patterns as well as behavioural and pathological changes provoked by neuroinvasive *Toxocara*-larvae. Cerebral larval counts are highly dependent on the day post infection, the laboratory mouse strain, and the inoculation dose (Cox and Holland, 1998; Havasiová-Reiterová et al., 1995; Kayes and Oaks, 1976; Ollero et al., 2008). The first *T. canis*-larvae reach the brain as early as 2 days pi (Janecek et al., 2014). As studies differ in examined mouse strains, the choice of different study days pi and varying time intervals between investigations (which could not all be taken into account in Table 1), the temporal accumulation remains contradictory. Dvorožňáková et al. (2003) and Cardillo et al. (2009) described a relatively constant recovery of *T. canis*- and *T. cati*-larvae throughout the study period after the first neuroinvasion, while others reported a peak of cerebral larval recovery rates at the beginning of the chronic phase of infection (Epe et al., 1994; Min, 1982). However, the overall trend given in Table 1 comprises a continuous accumulation of *Toxocara*-larvae in the brain during the course of infection. Nevertheless, a comprehensive study at days 2, 7, 14, 21, 28, 35, 42 and 98 pi during the three phases of infection conducted by Janecek et al. (2014) led to the hypothesis that neuroinvasion occurs in a biphasic pattern. Based on the ratio of larval numbers recovered from the brains to larval numbers recovered from the whole carcasses, the first cerebral migration peaked at day 7 pi during the hepato-pulmonary phase while it decreased from day 14 to day 28 pi. A second cerebral migration peak was observed at the beginning of the chronic phase (day 35 pi), and lasted until the end of the study at day 98 pi (Janecek et al., 2014).

The pathology of NLM varies in different experimental mouse strains, e.g., inbred strains, such as BALB/c and C57BL/6J, and outbred strains, like Swiss albino and LACA. Inbred BALB/c mice exhibit a distinct susceptibility to *T. canis*-infections, wherefore this mouse strain has been established as a suitable model for toxocarosis in several studies (Strube et al., 2013). Moreover, *T. canis*-larvae exhibit a high neuro-affinity in BALB/c mice. The brain recovery rates of *T. canis*-larvae in the chronic phase of infection varied between 9.5% and 18.6% of the total inoculation dose when mice were infected with 1000 or more embryonated eggs (Epe et al., 1994; Hamilton et al., 2006; Ollero et al., 2008; Pinelli et al., 2005). Further, inbred C57BL/6J mice are commonly used in experimental studies on NLM. The high neuro-affinity of *T. canis* in C57BL/6J mice is reflected by cerebral larval recovery rates of up to 19.1% of the initial inoculation dose (Dvorožňáková et al., 2003; Epe et al., 1994; Hamilton et al., 2006; Havasiová-Reiterová et al., 1995). Interestingly, some studies determined low cerebral recovery rates of 1.8% and 9.0% of the initial inoculation dose in C57BL/6J mice, but in relation to the overall number of recovered larvae, a total of 57.5% and 87.5% of larvae, respectively, migrated to cerebral tissues (Dunsmore et al., 1983; Janecek et al., 2014). Albeit BALB/c and C57BL/6J are the most commonly used mouse strains in NLM research, neuroinvasion and accumulation of *T. canis*-larvae have been described for a variety of other inbred strains. In these strains, cerebral larval recovery rates ranged between 1.1% and 18.1% of the initial inoculation dose (Epe et al., 1994; Hamilton et al., 2006; Holland and Cox, 2001).

The neuroinvasion of *Toxocara*-larvae is also described in outbred mouse strains as more larvae accumulated in the CNS than in other organs such as the liver or the lungs, even though most larvae were recovered from the remaining carcass excluding the aforementioned organs (Wade and Georgi, 1987). But contrarily to inbred mouse strains, outbred strains seem to be less susceptible to neuroinvasive *Toxocara*-larvae. Cerebral larval burdens in LACA mice ranged between 6.1% and 7.3% of the inoculation dose (Cox and Holland, 1998; Holland and Cox, 2001), while a maximum recovery rate of 10.5% was detected in Swiss albino mice (Eid et al., 2015). Further studies with other outbred strains also described rather low cerebral recovery rates of 2.0% and 10.3% (Abdel-Hameed, 1984; Dunsmore et al., 1983; Good et al., 2001; Kayes and Oaks, 1976; Liao et al., 2008). Various immunological differences between inbred and outbred mice are well-documented, and in case of toxocarosis, outbred strains may exhibit a greater ability to trap larvae during the hepato-pulmonary phase and prevent systemic circulation (Dunsmore et al., 1983; Tuttle et al., 2018).

In contrast to *T. canis*, only a few studies deal with the somatic migration behaviour of *T. cati*-larvae in mice. While *T. canis*-larvae exhibit a strong neuro-affinity and mainly accumulate in the cerebrum, *T. cati*-larvae display a lower neuro-affinity, as the majority can be recovered from muscle tissue, and mainly migrate to the cerebellum upon neuro-infection (Cardillo et al., 2009; Havasiová-Reiterová et al., 1995; Hrckova et al., 2001; Janecek et al., 2014). BALB/c mice seem to be more susceptible to neuroinvasive *T. cati*-larvae than C57BL/6J mice, as 1.2–1.9% of the initial inoculation dose were recovered from BALB/c mouse brains (Cardillo et al., 2009; Janecek et al., 2014) in comparison to only 0.2–0.5% from C57BL/6J mouse brains (Havasiová-Reiterová et al., 1995; Hrckova et al., 2001; Janecek et al., 2014).

The inoculum size seems to have no major impact on the neuro-affinity of migrating larvae. Even low inoculation doses of *T. canis* and *T. cati* entail similar distributions in murine organs and the number of larvae in the brain increases proportional to the inoculation dose (Camparoto et al., 2008; Good et al., 2001; Havasiová-Reiterová et al., 1995; Ollero et al., 2008). However, it remains unclear if multiple infections with *Toxocara*-larvae result in higher cerebral burdens. In a study with LACA and NIH mice, more *T. canis* larvae were recovered from brains after a single dose of 1000 infective eggs compared to the same inoculation dose administered over 28 days (250 infective eggs per week) (Holland and Cox, 2001). In BALB/c mice, similar multiple infection doses resulted in a higher number of larvae reaching the brain (Ollero et al., 2008). Furthermore, Kolbeková et al. (2011) revealed that neuroinvasion in pre-infected BALB/c mice started as early as 6h after reinfection compared to 60h after primary infection.

2.2 Neuroinvasion in other rodent species

Mice are the most widely used animal models for NLM, but rats (*Rattus norvegicus*) are also considered as potential paratenic hosts and have been used in NLM research (Strube et al., 2013). Burren (1972) detected *T. canis*-larvae in brains of 11 of 12 infected Wistar rats and Olson and Rose (1966) recovered an average of 3.0% of the inoculation dose from the brain of Cheek-Jones albino rats during the second and third week of infection. In a comprehensive investigation of *T. canis* larval migration in Wistar rats, between 1.3% and 4.5% of the initial inoculation dose were recovered from cerebral tissues, with highest neuroinvasion in the subacute phase (Lescano et al., 2004). Analogous to the previously observed migration routes in mice, *T. cati*-larvae seem to exhibit a lower neuro-affinity in rats than larvae of *T. canis*. A maximum of 1.1% of the inoculation dose was recovered by

Santos et al. (2009) in brains of *T. cati*-infected Wistar rats, while Zibaei et al. (2010) detected only 0.1% of the inoculation dose in the brains of two Wistar rats. Furthermore, upon experimental infection of 42 Wistar rats, only one larva, i.e., 0.02% of the inoculation dose, was recovered in the brain of one animal, whereas all other recovered larvae were found in other tissues (Taira et al., 2013).

Neuroinvasion of *Toxocara* has also been described in Mongolian gerbils (*Meriones unguiculatus*). For instance, neuro-affinity in gerbils was confirmed by Alba-Hurtado et al. (2009), who detected a higher number of *T. canis*-larvae per gram brain mass (52 and 50 larvae, respectively) than in other tissues. In comparison to other neuroinvasive nematode larvae, e.g., *Baylisascaris procyonis* and *B. transfuga*, cerebral larvae counts in gerbils were highest for *T. canis* (3.1%) (Cho et al., 2007). Even though Burren (1972) recovered 1.4% of *T. canis*-larvae in brains of gerbils in the chronic phase of infection compared to 0.1% in brains of rats, recovery rates of nearly 20.0% have been reported for mice inoculated with comparable amounts of embryonated eggs (cf. Table 1). As in mice and rats, *T. canis* and *T. cati* seem to exhibit a divergent migration pattern in gerbils. Considerably more *T. canis*- than *T. cati*-larvae were recovered from gerbil brains by Akao et al. (2000). Furthermore, Zibaei et al. (2010) detected a maximum of 3 *T. cati*-larvae in brains of gerbils (equivalent to 1.3% of the inoculation dose), while recovery rates were higher for other body tissues. Overall, data on NLM in gerbils offers little insight into general relationships and room for interpretation as the number of studies and sample sizes is rather low.

Neuroinvasion of *T. canis*-larvae has also been detected in brains of hamsters (*Mesocricetus auratus*) and guinea pigs (*Cavia porcellus*). However, since only less than half of the infected hamsters displayed a similar larval migration pattern as described for mice and rats (Burren, 1972) and *Toxocara*-larvae could not be recovered from the carcasses of infected guinea pigs beyond the acute phase of infection (Olson and Schulz, 1963), these rodent species do not seem to be suitable models for NLM.

3. Behavioural alterations observed in *Toxocara*-infected rodents

Knowledge regarding the impact of *Toxocara* infection on the cognitive development of humans is limited to few clinical case reports and population-based studies examining the relationship between neuropsychological parameters and *Toxocara*-seropositivity (Erickson et al., 2015; Holland and Hamilton, 2013; Jarosz et al., 2010; Walsh and Haseeb, 2012). In contrast, experimental work on rodents as model organisms has fuelled the hypothesis that cerebral *Toxocara* infection might lead to deficits in memory and learning as well as behavioural alterations.

3.1 Neurobehavioural changes in *Toxocara*-infected mice

Neurobehavioural phenotyping of *T. canis*-infected inbred and outbred mice has revealed neurological and motoric dysfunctions such as tumbling motions, ataxia, disturbed balance and impaired righting reflexes. These alterations mainly started in the subacute phase of infection and progressively increased in severity during the course of infection. In addition, infected mice were less active and spent less time climbing and grooming than uninfected mice (Cox and Holland, 1998; Dolinsky et al., 1985; Hamilton et al., 2006; Holland and Cox, 2001; Janecek et al., 2017). Further, *T. canis*-infected mice were less inquisitive as well as less explorative in novel situations. They showed reduced levels of aggressive behaviour and increased levels of flight and defensive behaviours. In the elevated plus maze test, which is used to assess anxiety vs. exploratory behaviour in rodents by allowing them to choose between open and enclosed arms of a maze (Pellow et al., 1985; Rodgers and Johnson, 1995), *Toxocara*-infected mice spent more time in exposed areas, indicating a reduced level of anxiety (Cox and Holland, 1998; Holland and Cox, 2001).

Overall, similar behavioural alterations have been observed in both outbred and inbred mouse strains, however, differences have been noted for some behaviours. While mobility was decreased in *Toxocara*-infected inbred NIH mice, the reverse was true for outbred LACA mice (Cox and Holland, 2001a,b). Interestingly, *T. canis*-infection appears to be associated with hyperactivity in an outbred strain of albino mice (Hay et al., 1986).

The impairment of learning and memory during *T. canis*-infection is illustrated for example by the water task paradigm, in which infected mice generally took longer to find the previously learned location of a water source compared to uninfected control mice, even though the observed differences were not statistically significant (Cox and Holland, 2001b; Hamilton et al., 2006). Furthermore, *T. canis*-induced memory impairments were illustrated by the continuously increasing time to find a food reward in a maze, with an increasing number of entries into dead end arms (illustrated in Supplementary material in the online version at https://doi.org/10.1016/bs.apar.2020.01.006) (Janecek et al., 2017). The magnitude of behavioural alterations seems to be correlated to the number of larvae in the brain. Abnormal social behaviour, like reduced aggressiveness, was more pronounced in LACA mice harbouring high numbers of *T. canis* in the brain, while low larval numbers lead rather to more risky behaviour (Cox and Holland, 1998, 2001a).

As behavioural data in the frame of *T. cati*-induced NLM is scarce, Janecek et al. (2017) investigated behavioural outcomes of both *T. canis*- and *T. cati*-infection in mice. The most salient characteristics in *T. cati*- compared to *T. canis*-infected C57BL/6J mice were a delayed onset of and less severe behavioural changes. Memory impairments as well as the reduction in exploratory behaviour occurred later during the course of infection. Furthermore, *T. cati*-infected mice displayed reduced fear- and flight-related reactions rather than motoric and neurological disorders (Janecek et al., 2017). Studies concerning the impact of *T. cati*-infection on the behaviour of outbred mouse strains or the correlation of the cerebral larval burden with behavioural changes have not been published to date.

3.2 Neurobehavioural changes in other rodents infected with *Toxocara*

Similar to mice, *T. canis*-infected rats showed an impaired body position and gait as well as a decrease in grooming and exploration behaviour compared to their uninfected counterparts (Al-Hassnawi and Al-Quraishi, 2013, 2014; Chieffi et al., 2009; Queiroz et al., 2013). Furthermore, spatial locomotion and general activity were either not affected or even increased in *T. canis*-infected rats (Al-Hassnawi and Al-Quraishi, 2014; Chieffi et al., 2010; Queiroz et al., 2013). Furthermore, the elevated plus-maze apparatus indicated a higher degree of anxiety during infection (Chieffi et al., 2010). The ability of learning and memory, tested via a Hebb and Williams maze, was impaired as of the subacute phase of infection (Olson and Rose, 1966). Santos et al. (2015) compared behavioural changes and muscle strength between rats experimentally infected with *T. canis* and *T. cati* during the course of infection. *T. cati*-infected rats did not differ from the uninfected control group in the elevated plus maze test and exhibited similar locomotor activity (Santos et al., 2015). Noteworthy, muscle strength of both infection groups was reduced as early as day 5 pi in both infection groups, but *T. cati*-infected rats showed a greater decrease in muscle strength in the chronic phase of infection than *T. canis*-infected rats (Santos et al., 2015). This difference may be due to the fact that *T. cati*-larvae mainly accumulate in muscle tissue of rats (Santos et al., 2009), as also shown for mice (Janecek et al., 2014).

In general, mice and rats have been the most widely used model organisms in studies on the aetiology, pathophysiology and pharmacology of neuropsychiatric diseases for well over a century (Ellenbroek and Youn, 2016). Thus, experimental research regarding NLM has focused on these two rodent species, and data on *Toxocara*-induced behavioural changes in other rodents, like hamsters or guinea pigs, are missing. Nevertheless, *T. canis*-infected gerbils developed neurological abnormalities like an unsteady gait and circular movements (Alba-Hurtado et al., 2009). Akao et al. (2003) observed behavioural abnormalities in 46% of *T. canis*-infected and in 71% of *T. cati*-infected gerbils, including a swinging gait, circular movements, paraplegia of the hind limbs and urinary incontinence (Akao et al., 2003). Notably, *T. cati*-infected gerbils showed a delayed onset of behavioural alterations, similar to the previously described findings in mice (Janecek et al., 2017).

4. *Toxocara*-induced histopathological alterations

4.1 Histopathological changes in *Toxocara*-infected mouse brains

The neuroinvasion of migrating *Toxocara*-larvae results in parenchymal damage accompanied by haemorrhagic lesions in the brain, which are visible macroscopically (Fig. 1) and microscopically from day 7 pi on (Cardillo et al., 2009; Heuer et al., 2015a; Janecek et al., 2014; Springer et al., 2019).

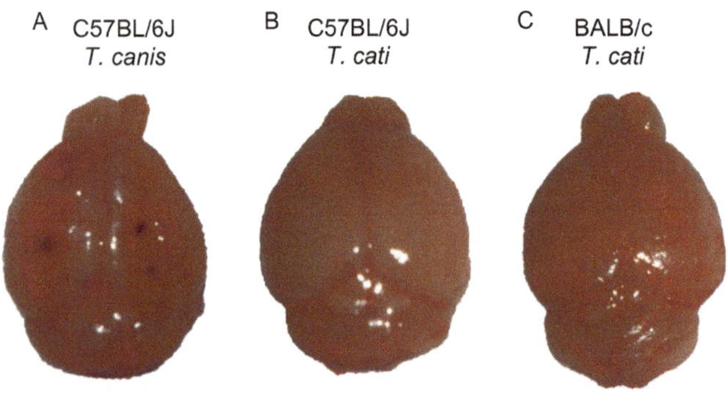

Fig. 1 Haemorrhagic lesions in the brains of a (A) *T. canis*-infected C57BL/6J mouse, (B) *T. cati*-infected C57BL/6J mouse and (C) *T. cati*-infected BALB/c mouse on day 7 pi (Institute for Parasitology, University of Veterinary Medicine Hannover, archive).

Subsequently, neurodegenerative processes and demyelination are frequently observed histopathological hallmarks of NLM in rodents (Dolinsky et al., 1985; Epe et al., 1994; Heuer et al., 2015a; Janecek et al., 2014; Springer et al., 2019).

In *T. canis*-infected inbred mouse strains, demyelination, focal malacia, mixed-cell infiltration as well as congestion and neuronal necrosis have been described (Epe et al., 1994; Fonseca et al., 2017). Noteworthy, these changes were delayed and less severe in brains of BALB/c mice than in other mouse strains (C3H, C57BL/6J, DBA and NMRI) examined by Epe et al. (1994). Further neurodegenerative lesions described in *T. canis*-infected C57BL/6J mice include focal accumulation of gitter cells, i.e., microglial phagocytic cells containing degenerating myelin (Fig. 2A), and the presence of swollen

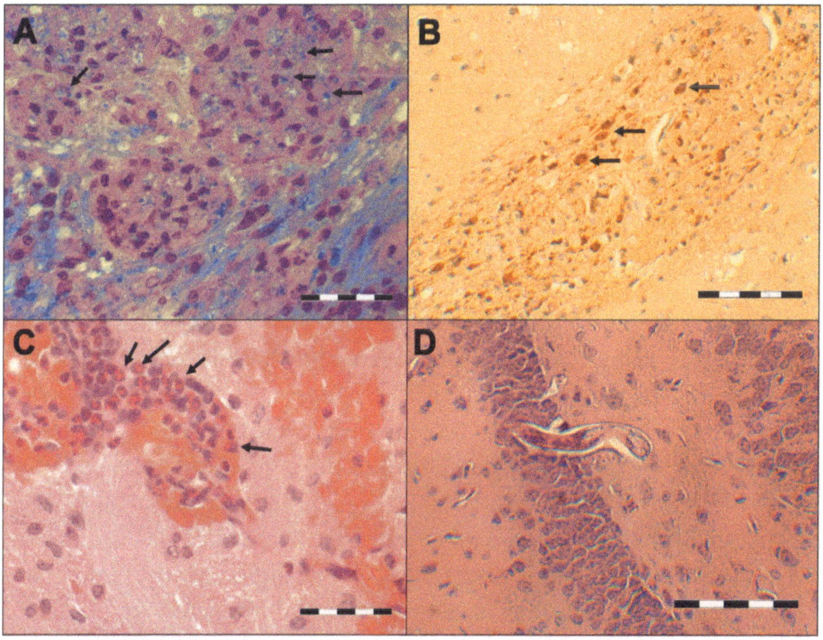

Fig. 2 Histopathological alterations due to NLM in C57BL/6J mice. (A) Gitter cells with blue inclusions of myelin (arrows), illustrating myelinophagia. Luxol fast blue stain, *T. canis*-infection, day 42 pi. Scale bar represents 50 μm. (B) Accumulation of β-APP (arrows) indicating axonal damage, immunohistochemistry, *T. canis*-infection day 70 pi. Scale bar represents 100 μm. (C) Haemorrhage with infiltration of eosinophilic granulocytes (arrows). Haematoxylin-eosin stain, *T. cati*-infection, day 14 pi. Scale bar represents 50 μm. (D) *T. canis*-larva in the hippocampus. Haematoxylin-eosin stain, day 14 pi. Scale bar represents 100 μm (Institute for Parasitology, University of Veterinary Medicine Hannover, archive).

axons, so-called spheroids, along with cholesterol crystals, indicating axonal damage (Heuer et al., 2015a; Janecek et al., 2014; Springer et al., 2019). Axonal damage was further confirmed by immunohistochemical detection of axonal β-amyloid precursor protein (β-APP) accumulation as early as day 7 pi (Fig. 2B) (Heuer et al., 2015a; Liao et al., 2008; Springer et al., 2019). Such intra-axonal β-APP accumulation is an established marker for early axonopathies and represents the main feature of diffuse axonal injuries (Blennow et al., 2012). The depletion of neurite outgrowth inhibitor-A (NOGO-A)-positive cells confirmed the loss of mature, myelinated oligodendrocytes (Heuer et al., 2015a). Demyelination was also evident on the molecular level by transcription and expression patterns of myelin marker genes, including the major myelin proteins myelin basic protein (Mbp) and proteolipid protein (Plp), and minor components of myelin such as 2′,3′-cyclic nucleotide 3′-phosphodiesterase (Cnp), myelin-associated glycoprotein (Mag) and myelin oligodendrocyte glycoprotein (Mog). Both *T. canis*- and *T. cati*-infected mice showed enhanced transcription of Cnp and Mog at the early onset of disease (day 28 pi). Upon severe demyelination at later time points (day 120 pi), transcription of Mbp was decreased in cerebra and cerebella of *T. canis*-infected mice. Interestingly, increased CNPase protein expression indicated the concurrent onset of remyelination (Heuer et al., 2015a).

As compared to *T. canis*-infected mice, neurodegenerative changes and structural damage in *T. cati*-infected mice were noted later during the course of infection, appeared less severe and were mainly located in the cerebellum (Heuer et al., 2015a, Janecek et al., 2014, Springer et al., 2019). These results reflect the tropism of *T. canis* to the cerebrum, while larvae of *T. cati* are less neuroinvasive and preferentially migrate to the cerebellum (Janecek et al., 2014). In contrast, brain parts affected by neurodegeneration in *T. canis*-infected mice included cerebral fibre tracts like the corpus callosum, fornix and anterior commissure (Springer et al., 2019). Especially the fornix plays an important role regarding memory function (Aggleton et al., 1992; Buckley et al., 2004), thus, the observed histopathological lesions in these fibre tracts may explain the severe memory impairments in *T. canis*-infected mice (Janecek et al., 2017; Springer et al., 2019).

Although eosinophilic meningitis is a well-described consequence of human NLM, Kolbeková et al. (2011) observed leukostasis in brain vessels of *T. canis*-infected BALB/c mice only occasionally, while absence of inflammatory reactions and leukocytic infiltration was described in several other studies (Cardillo et al., 2009; Eid et al., 2015; Epe et al., 1994;

Liao et al., 2008; Othman et al., 2010). These results, in some way, may be dependent on the investigated mouse strain as Springer et al. (2019) detected eosinophilic meningitis and perivascular lymphocytic cuffs involving eosinophilic and neutrophilic granulocytes in the cerebrum as well as the cerebellum of *T. canis*- and *T. cati*-infected C57BL/6 mice (Fig. 2C).

A common observation in many studies was that the *Toxocara*-larvae themselves were scattered throughout the parenchyma of the brain, but neither trapped by inflammatory cells nor encapsulated into granulomas (Fig. 2D) (Akao et al., 2003; Cardillo et al., 2009; Dunsmore et al., 1983; Eid et al., 2015; Epe et al., 1994; Janecek et al., 2014; Kolbeková et al., 2011; Olson and Rose, 1966; Othman et al., 2010). It remains to be clarified whether this immunological non-reactivity against larvae is mediated by shedding of the larval glycocalyx, thereby hindering antibody recognition of larvae through the host, or an active manipulation of the hosts' immune response by TES-AG, which might mimic host tissue antigenic components to escape immune recognition (Maizels, 2013).

4.2 Histopathological changes in brains of other rodents infected with *Toxocara*

Concerning rats, the only published study on histopathological changes during NLM showed that no significant immunological reactivity was noted around neuroinvasive larvae (Olson and Rose, 1966). In Mongolian gerbils, *T. canis*- as well as *T. cati*-infection is characterised by severe degenerative changes, including the loss of Purkinje cells, nerve fibres and nerve sheaths, but these are limited to the cerebellum. As in mice and rats, no inflammatory cell infiltrations could be observed in the immediate surroundings of larvae or in the brain parenchyma of both infection groups (Akao et al., 2003). Thus, this seems to be a common observation across different rodent species.

4.3 Neuroinflammatory processes during NLM

To investigate the pathogenic impact of *Toxocara*-larvae and their products on central nervous cell lines, Heuer et al. (2015b) co-cultured murine CAD cells, which differentiate into a primary neuron-like phenotype, as well as microglial BV-2 and oligodendrocytal BO-1 cells and murine brain slices with viable *T. canis*- and *T. cati*-larvae for 5 and 6 days, respectively. While the survival of differentiated CAD cells was impaired, the viability of oligodendrocytal and microglial cells as well as brain slices was not influenced by larval presence. In contrast, cultured murine astrocytes treated with *T. canis* TES-AG showed morphological changes, resulting in apoptosis (Chou and Fan, 2018; Hsiao et al., 2013). Overall, these results indicate that cytotoxic effects of larvae alone are not sufficient to explain the extensive neurodegeneration observed *in vivo*, and that immune-mediated mechanisms likely play an important role.

Using whole genome microarray expression analysis, Janecek et al. (2015) identified a plethora of differentially transcribed genes (DTGs) in brains of *T. canis*- and *T. cati*-infected C57BL/6J mice at day 42 pi. In cerebra and cerebella of *T. canis*-infected mice, a total of 2304 and 1954 DTGs were found, respectively. Annotation by the Gene Ontology database associated most up-regulated DTGs with the term immune response, especially with defence/inflammatory response, while most down-regulated DTGs were associated with lipid/cholesterol biosynthetic processes (Janecek et al., 2015). Reactions in *T. cati*-infected brains were less severe, as only 113 and 760 differentially transcribed genes were determined in cerebra and cerebella, respectively.

In *T. canis*- as well as *T. cati*-infected C57BL/6J mice, microglia/macrophage activation was observed in affected brain areas but it remains unknown whether microglia are activated via the classical (M1 phenotype) or the alternative pathway (M2 state) (Springer et al., 2019). Microglia of the M1 state secrete different pro-inflammatory cytokines, such as interleukin (IL)-1β, IL-6 and tumour necrosis factor-α (TNF-α), which are potentially neurotoxic substances that may exacerbate neurodegeneration when excessively secreted, a process termed reactive microgliosis (Lull and Block, 2010; Subramaniam and Federoff, 2017). In contrast, alternatively activated M2 are associated with immunoregulation and tissue repair (Subramaniam and Federoff, 2017). Beside microglia activation, elevated glial fibrillary acidic protein (GFAP)-expression has been detected by immunohistochemistry, providing evidence for astrocytic activation and reactive astrogliosis in the cerebral parenchyma (Eid et al., 2015; Liao et al., 2008; Othman et al., 2010). Furthermore, *T. canis*-infection causes an elevated expression of inducible nitric oxide synthase (iNOS) in glial cells, which can have detrimental effects on the brain if produced in excess (Boje, 1996; Gargili et al., 2004; Liao et al., 2008; Othman et al., 2010).

Neuroinflammatory processes are initiated by potent pro-inflammatory cytokines, e.g., TNF-α, interferon (IFN)-γ and IL-6, but excessive or inappropriate neuroinflammatory reactions may be detrimental for cerebral tissues. Therefore, these reactions are usually balanced and regulated by anti-inflammatory and neuroprotective mediators. Helminth infections commonly induce a strong type 2 response, which is characterised, for example, by the secretion of the anti-inflammatory cytokines IL-4, IL-5 and IL-13 (Gause et al., 2003; Pulendran and Artis, 2012). Table 2 summarises studies on inflammation-related mediators in the brains of *Toxocara*-infected mice. Hamilton et al. (2008) investigated the cerebral expression of the cytokines IL-5, IL-10 and IFN-γ in *T. canis*-infected inbred BALB/c and NIH mice in relation to corresponding levels in uninfected controls. Levels of pro-inflammatory IFN-γ were highly increased in the acute phase of infection, but declined thereafter, while levels of anti-inflammatory IL-10 were increased in infected BALB/c and NIH mice from the end of the acute to the beginning of the chronic phase of infection. The mRNA levels of anti-inflammatory IL-5 fluctuated during the course of infection in both mouse strains, reaching a peak in infected BALB/c mice at the beginning of the chronic phase of infection (Hamilton et al., 2008). A continuous increase of IL-5 mRNA transcription was also noted in outbred Swiss albino mice (Eid et al., 2015). Beside IL-5, *T. canis*-infection in Swiss albino mice led to significantly elevated transcription rates of IL-6 and TNF-α (Othman et al., 2010). The expression of transforming growth factor (TGF)-β1 markedly declined in brains of outbred ICR mice during the chronic phase of infection but, interestingly, corresponding proteins remained abundantly present at that time (Liao et al., 2008). Waindok and Strube (2019) quantified cytokine and chemokine concentrations by multiplex bead array assay in *Toxocara*-infected C57BL/6J mice, revealing discrepancies in the patterns of assessed metabolite concentrations and mRNA transcription rates described in other studies. Even though a transcriptional upregulation for IFN-γ and TNF-α has been shown in brains of *T. canis*-infected mice (Eid et al., 2015; Hamilton et al., 2008; Othman et al., 2010), concentrations of pro-inflammatory cytokines including IFN-γ, TNF-α, IL-1α, IL-1β and IL-6 were not elevated during *T. canis*- and *T. cati*-induced NLM (Waindok and Strube, 2019). Instead, IL-4 and IL-5 concentrations were increased in cerebra of *T. canis*-infected mice in the acute and subacute phase of infection and declined with the beginning of the chronic phase, while this pattern was absent in *T. cati*-infected mice (Waindok and Strube, 2019).

Further important signalling mediators are chemokines, which play key roles in phagocytosis, apoptosis and leukocyte extravasation as well as cytokine secretion during neuroinflammatory processes (Cartier et al., 2005). Levels of pro-inflammatory macrophage inflammatory protein (MIP)-1α (CCL3), but not MIP-1β (CCL4) and monocyte chemotactic protein

Table 2 Overview of studies investigating *Toxocara*-induced alterations of inflammatory mediators in brains of infected mice as models for paratenic hosts.

Annotation	*Toxocara* spp.	Mouse strain	Analytes	Method	References
Neuro-transmitters	*T. canis*	Swiss albino	GABA, glutamate, dopamine, noradrenaline, serotonin	Reverse-phase HPLC, spectrofluorometry	Othman et al. (2010)
Brain injury-associated biomarkers	*T. canis*	BALB/c	LPx, SOD, NADPH-d	Immunohistochemistry	Gargili et al. (2004)
	T. canis	BALB/c; NIH	iNOS	Semi-quantitative RT-PCR	Hamilton et al. (2008)
	T. canis	ICR	GFAP, NF-L, tTG, AβPP, S100B, TGF-β1	RT-PCR	Liao et al. (2008)
			GFAP, NF-L, tTG, AβPP, S100B, TGF-β1, tau, UPS	Western blot and ELISA	
			GFAP	Immunohistochemistry	
	T. canis	Swiss albino	iNOS, GFAP	Immunohistochemistry	Othman et al. (2010)
	T. canis	Swiss albino	GFAP	Immunohistochemistry	Eid et al. (2015)
Cytokines	*T. canis*	BALB/c; NIH	IL-5, IL-10, IFN-γ	Semi-quantitative RT-PCR	Hamilton et al. (2008)
	T. canis	Swiss albino	IL-5	Semi-quantitative RT-PCR	Eid et al. (2015)
	T. canis	Swiss albino	IL-6, TNF-α	Semi-quantitative RT-PCR	Othman et al. (2010)
	T. canis, *T. cati*	C57BL/6J	G-CSF, GM-CSF, IFN-γ, IL-1α, IL-1β, IL-2, IL-3, IL-4, IL-5, IL-6, IL-9, IL-10, IL-12, IL-13, IL-17, TNF-α	Multiplex bead array assay	Waindok and Strube (2019)
Chemokines	*T. canis*, *T. cati*	C57BL/6J	eotaxin (CCL11), KC (CXCL1), MCP-1 (CCL2), MIP-1α (CCL3), MIP-1β (CCL4), RANTES (CCL5)	Multiplex bead array assay	Waindok and Strube (2019)
Oxylipins	*T. canis*, *T. cati*	C57BL/6J	Miscellaneous, e.g., prostanoids, leukotrienes, HETEs, NPD1, 13-HODE, 9-HODE	Liquid chromatography electrospray-ionisation-tandem mass spectrometry	Waindok et al. (2019)

(MCP)-1 (CCL2) were consistently increased in cerebra and cerebella of *T. canis*-infected as well as the cerebella of *T. cati*-infected C57BL/6J mice. The same pattern was detected for anti-inflammatory eotaxin (CCL11), which is suggested to act cooperatively with IL-5 in regulating blood and tissue eosinophilia (Collins et al., 1995; Mould et al., 1997). Concentrations of RANTES ("Regulated upon activation normal T cell expressed and presumably secreted"; CCL5) were almost exclusively affected in cerebella of both infection groups during the subacute and chronic phase of NLM (Waindok and Strube, 2019).

In addition to cyto- and chemokines, bioactive regulatory lipids (also called oxylipins, e.g. octadecanoids, eicosanoids and docosanoids) are involved in the complex molecular signalling network during infection and inflammation (Dennis and Norris, 2015; Yang et al., 2011). In accordance with cytokine concentrations, pro-inflammatory oxylipins such as prostanoids showed little alterations during the course of infection, while potentially anti-inflammatory oxylipins peaked in the subacute phase of infection and declined gradually during the chronic phase in *T. canis*- as well as *T. cati*-infected C57BL/6J mice (Waindok et al., 2019). Furthermore, the ratio of 13-hydroxyoctadecadienoic acid (HODE) to 9-HODE, a proposed biomarker for the immunological status of an active infection (Tam, 2013; Tam et al., 2013), was clearly shifted towards an anti-inflammatory immune response in *Toxocara*-infected mice, particularly in the subacute and at the beginning of the chronic phase of infection (Waindok et al., 2019). Similarly, neuroprotectin (NPD) 1, a major bioactive effector with anti-inflammatory and neuroprotective properties (Schwab et al., 2007; Serhan, 2006; Serhan and Petasis, 2011) was detected primarily in the subacute and at the beginning of the chronic phase of infection, but was below the detection level in brains of the uninfected control group (Waindok et al., 2019).

Apart from inflammatory mediators such as cyto- and chemokines as well as oxylipins, neuroinvasion of *T. canis* also affects neurotransmitter patterns. Levels of GABA, dopamine and serotonin progressively declined during the course of infection in Swiss albino mice, while levels of glutamate and norepinephrine showed the inverse pattern (Othman et al., 2010). These neurotransmitters may participate in neuroinflammatory reactions. Excessive secretion of cerebral norepinephrine, for instance, can result in elevated levels of pro-inflammatory cytokines such as IL-1β and IL-6 (Johnson et al., 2005), while serotonin is considered a neuromodulator regulating, among others, mood and behaviour (Lucki, 1998).

5. Conclusions and open questions

Rodents are considered as appropriate models for NLM as they present similar clinical symptoms and neuropathological alterations as humans. However, potential confounding variables such as the genetic background of the animals, inoculation dose and duration of infection need to be taken into account when drawing conclusions from rodent models and comparing data from different studies. The neuro-affinity of migrating larvae clearly differs between rodent species and strains; and inbred mice seem to have the highest susceptibility towards neuroinvasive *Toxocara*-larvae. In mice as the best-studied rodent model, migratory routes of *T. canis* and *T. cati* appear to be similar, but *T. canis* exhibits a higher CNS affinity and a preference for the cerebrum. Various neurological and locomotor as well as sensorimotor dysfunctions have been described due to infection with *T. canis* in inbred and outbred mice, along with a reduced level of aggressiveness and anxiety. In addition, learning and memory impairment during *T. canis*-infection has been documented in different mouse strains with different methodologies. In contrast to *T. canis*, *T. cati*-infection rather resulted in reduced fear- and flight-related reactions instead of motoric and neurological disorders, and memory impairment was less severe. Nevertheless, behavioural testing is strongly dependent on various confounding parameters, therefore, refinement and standardisation of behavioural testing in NLM research would be desirable. Pathological alterations in cerebral tissues of rodents mainly included haemorrhages, necrosis and axonal injuries as well as gliosis, demyelination and malacia as well as infiltration of eosinophilic granulocytes in cerebral tissues—a hallmark of NLM in humans. It remains unknown why neuroinvasive *Toxocara*-larvae are not trapped by inflammatory cells or encapsulated into granulomas in the brain. Further research is needed to investigate the immunopathological mechanisms leading to neurodegeneration in detail and to identify potential parasite-induced immunomodulatory effects. So far, the cerebral immune response during murine *Toxocara* infection has been characterised as predominantly anti-inflammatory. Even though transcription rates of pro-inflammatory signalling molecules were increased in several studies, the actual metabolite concentrations only changed marginally. Instead, a variety of inflammation-related signalling molecules of the cytokine, chemokine and oxylipin family with anti-inflammatory properties were found to be increased, especially in the subacute and at the beginning of the chronic phase of infection. Nevertheless, further in depth analyses are required to elucidate the interplay of these signalling molecules and further players in the pathogenesis of *T. canis*- and *T. cati*-induced NLM.

References

Abdel-Hameed, A.A., 1984. Effects of benzimidazole anthelmintics on the survival and migratory behavior of *Toxocara canis* larvae in the mouse. Am. J. Vet. Res. 45, 1430–1433.

Abo-Shehada, M.N., Al-Zubaidy, B.A., Herbert, I.V., 1984. The migration of larval *Toxocara canis* in mice. I. Migration through the intestine in primary infections. Vet. Parasitol. 17, 65–73.

Aggleton, J.P., Keith, A.B., Rawlins, J.N., Hunt, P.R., Sahgal, A., 1992. Removal of the hippocampus and transection of the fornix produce comparable deficits on delayed non-matching to position by rats. Behav. Brain Res. 52, 61–71.

Akao, N., Takayanagi, T.H., Suzuki, R., Tsukidate, S., Fujita, K., 2000. Ocular larva migrans caused by *Toxocara cati* in Mongolian gerbils and a comparison of ophthalmologic findings with those produced by *T. canis*. J. Parasitol. 86, 1133–1135.

Akao, N., Tomoda, M., Hayashi, E., Suzuki, R., Shimizu-Suganuma, M., Shichinohe, K., Fujita, K., 2003. Cerebellar ataxia due to *Toxocara* infection in Mongolian gerbils, *Meriones unguiculatus*. Vet. Parasitol. 113, 229–237.

Alba-Hurtado, F., Munoz-Guzman, M.A., Valdivia-Anda, G., Tortora, J.L., Ortega-Pierres, M.G., 2009. *Toxocara canis*: larval migration dynamics, detection of antibody reactivity to larval excretory-secretory antigens and clinical findings during experimental infection of gerbils (*Meriones unguiculatus*). Exp. Parasitol. 122, 1–5.

Al-Hassnawi, A.T.S., Al-Quraishi, M.A., 2013. The effects of *Toxocara canis* infection with and without red light on the levels of melatonin hormone and cytokines peripherial blood of albino rat. J. Nat. Sci. Res. 3, 178–186.

Al-Hassnawi, A.T.S., Al-Quraishi, M.A., 2014. The effect of experimental *Toxocara canis* infection on behavior manipulating in albino rats. J. Univ. Babylon Pure Appl. Sci. 22, 2389–2395.

Blennow, K., Hardy, J., Zetterberg, H., 2012. The neuropathology and neurobiology of traumatic brain injury. Neuron 76, 886–899.

Boes, J., Helwigh, A.B., 2000. Animal models of intestinal nematode infections of humans. Parasitology 121, 97–111.

Boje, K.M., 1996. Inhibition of nitric oxide synthase attenuates blood-brain barrier disruption during experimental meningitis. Brain Res. 720, 75–83.

Buckley, M.J., Charles, D.P., Browning, P.G., Gaffan, D., 2004. Learning and retrieval of concurrently presented spatial discrimination tasks: role of the fornix. Behav. Neurosci. 118, 138–149.

Burren, C.H., 1972. The distribution of *Toxocara canis* larvae in the central nervous system of rodents. Trans. R. Soc. Trop. Med. Hyg. 66, 937–942.

Camparoto, M.L., Fulan, B., Colli, C.M., Paludo, M.L., Falavigna-Guilherme, A.L., Fernandez, M.A., 2008. Initial stage of development and migratory behavior of *Toxocara canis* larvae in BALB/c mouse experimental model. Genet. Mol. Res. 7, 444–450.

Cardillo, N., Rosa, A., Ribicich, M., Lopez, C., Sommerfelt, I., 2009. Experimental infection with *Toxocara cati* in BALB/c mice, migratory behaviour and pathological changes. Zoonoses Public Health 56, 198–205.

Cartier, L., Hartley, O., Dubois-Dauphin, M., Krause, K.H., 2005. Chemokine receptors in the central nervous system: role in brain inflammation and neurodegenerative diseases. Brain Res. Brain Res. Rev. 48, 16–42.

Celik, T., Kaplan, Y., Atas, E., Oztuna, D., Berilgen, S., 2013. *Toxocara* seroprevalence in patients with idiopathic Parkinson's disease: chance association or coincidence? Biomed. Res. Int. 2013, 685196.
Chieffi, P.P., Aquino, R.T., Paschoalotti, M.A., Ribeiro, M.C., Nasello, A.G., 2009. Muscular strength decrease in *Rattus norvegicus* experimentally infected by *Toxocara canis*. Rev. Inst. Med. Trop. Sao Paulo 51, 73–75.
Chieffi, P.P., Aquino, R.T., Pasqualotti, M.A., Ribeiro, M.C., Nasello, A.G., 2010. Behavioral changes in *Rattus norvegicus* experimentally infected by *Toxocara canis* larvae. Rev. Inst. Med. Trop. Sao Paulo 52, 243–246.
Cho, S., Egami, M., Ohnuki, H., Saito, Y., Chinone, S., Shichinohe, K., Suganuma, M., Akao, N., 2007. Migration behaviour and pathogenesis of five ascarid nematode species in the Mongolian gerbil *Meriones unguiculatus*. J. Helminthol. 81, 43–47.
Chou, C.M., Fan, C.K., 2018. Significant apoptosis rather autophagy predominates in astrocytes caused by *Toxocara canis* larval excretory-secretory antigens. J. Microbiol. Immunol. Infect. https://doi.org/10.1016/j.jmii.2018.06.006, in press.
Collins, P.D., Marleau, S., Griffiths-Johnson, D.A., Jose, P.J., Williams, T.J., 1995. Cooperation between interleukin-5 and the chemokine eotaxin to induce eosinophil accumulation in vivo. J. Exp. Med. 182, 1169–1174.
Cox, D.M., Holland, C.V., 1998. The relationship between numbers of larvae recovered from the brain of *Toxocara canis*-infected mice and social behaviour and anxiety in the host. Parasitology 116, 579–594.
Cox, D.M., Holland, C.V., 2001a. Influence of mouse strain, infective dose and larval burden in the brain on activity in *Toxocara*-infected mice. J. Helminthol. 75, 23–32.
Cox, D.M., Holland, C.V., 2001b. Relationship between three intensity levels of *Toxocara canis* larvae in the brain and effects on exploration, anxiety, learning and memory in the murine host. J. Helminthol. 75, 33–41.
Dennis, E.A., Norris, P.C., 2015. Eicosanoid storm in infection and inflammation. Nat. Rev. Immunol. 15, 511–523.
Dolinsky, Z.S., Hardy, C.A., Burright, R.G., Donovick, P.J., 1985. The progression of behavioral and pathological effects of the parasite *Toxocara canis* in the mouse. Physiol. Behav. 35, 33–42.
Dunsmore, J.D., Thompson, R.C., Bates, I.A., 1983. The accumulation of *Toxocara canis* larvae in the brains of mice. Int. J. Parasitol. 13, 517–521.
Dvorožňáková, E., Borošková, Z., Tomašovicová, O., 2003. Changes in CD4+ and CD8+ T cells after immunomodulation of *Toxocara canis* infected mice. Helminthologica 40, 1–7.
Eberhardt, O., Bialek, R., Nagele, T., Dichgans, J., 2005. Eosinophilic meningomyelitis in toxocariasis: case report and review of the literature. Clin. Neurol. Neurosurg. 107, 432–438.
Eid, M.M., El-Kowrany, S.I., Othman, A.A., El Gendy, D.I., Saied, E.M., 2015. Immunopathological changes in the brain of immunosuppressed mice experimentally infected with *Toxocara canis*. Korean J. Parasitol. 53, 51–58.
Ellenbroek, B., Youn, J., 2016. Rodent models in neuroscience research: is it a rat race? Dis. Model. Mech. 9, 1079–1087.
El-Sayed, N.M., Ismail, K.A., 2012. Relationship between *Toxocara canis* infection and schizophrenia. Rawal. Med. J. 37, 155–161.
Epe, C., Sabel, T., Schnieder, T., Stoye, M., 1994. The behavior and pathogenicity of *Toxacara canis* larvae in mice of different strains. Parasitol. Res. 80, 691–695.
Erickson, L.D., Gale, S.D., Berrett, A., Brown, B.L., Hedges, D.W., 2015. Association between toxocariasis and cognitive function in young to middle-aged adults. Folia Parasitol. (Praha) 62, 048.

Fan, C.K., Holland, C.V., Loxton, K., Barghouth, U., 2015. Cerebral toxocariasis: silent progression to neurodegenerative disorders? Clin. Microbiol. Rev. 28, 663–686.

Finsterer, J., Auer, H., 2007. Neurotoxocarosis. Rev. Inst. Med. Trop. Sao Paulo 49, 279–287.

Fisher, M., 2003. *Toxocara cati*: an underestimated zoonotic agent. Trends Parasitol. 19, 167–170.

Fonseca, G.R.E., Santos, S.V.D., Chieffi, P.P., Paula, F.M., Gryschek, R.C.B., Lescano, S.A.Z., 2017. Experimental toxocariasis in BALB/c mice: relationship between parasite inoculum and the IgG immune response. Mem. Inst. Oswaldo Cruz 112, 382–386.

Fukae, J., Kawanabe, T., Akao, N., Kado, M., Tokoro, M., Yokoyama, K., Hattori, N., 2012. Longitudinal myelitis caused by visceral larva migrans associated with *Toxocara cati* infection: case report. Clin. Neurol. Neurosurg. 114, 1091–1094.

Gargili, A., Demirci, C., Kandil, A., Cetinkaya, H., Atukeren, P., Gumustas, M.K., 2004. In vivo inhibition of inducible nitric oxide and evaluation of the brain tissue damage induced by *Toxocara canis* larvae in experimentally infected mice. Chin. J. Physiol. 47, 189–196.

Gause, W.C., Urban Jr., J.F., Stadecker, M.J., 2003. The immune response to parasitic helminths: insights from murine models. Trends Immunol. 24, 269–277.

Good, B., Holland, C.V., Stafford, P., 2001. The influence of inoculum size and time post-infection on the number and position of *Toxocara canis* larvae recovered from the brains of outbred CD1 mice. J. Helminthol. 75, 175–181.

Hamilton, C.M., Stafford, P., Pinelli, E., Holland, C.V., 2006. A murine model for cerebral toxocariasis: characterization of host susceptibility and behaviour. Parasitology 132, 791–801.

Hamilton, C.M., Brandes, S., Holland, C.V., Pinelli, E., 2008. Cytokine expression in the brains of *Toxocara canis*-infected mice. Parasite Immunol. 30, 181–185.

Havasiová-Reiterová, K., Tomašovicová, O., Dubinský, P., 1995. Effect of various doses of infective *Toxocara canis* and *Toxocara cati* eggs on the humoral response and distribution of larvae in mice. Parasitol. Res. 81, 13–17.

Hay, J., Arnott, M.A., Aitken, P.P., Kendall, A.T., 1986. Experimental toxocariasis and hyperactivity in mice. Z. Parasitenkd. 72, 115–120.

Heuer, L., Beyerbach, M., Luhder, F., Beineke, A., Strube, C., 2015a. Neurotoxocarosis alters myelin protein gene transcription and expression. Parasitol. Res. 114, 2175–2186.

Heuer, L., Haendel, S., Beineke, A., Strube, C., 2015b. Effects of *Toxocara* larvae on brain cell survival by in vitro model assessment. Parasitology 142, 1326–1334.

Holland, C.V., Cox, D.M., 2001. *Toxocara* in the mouse: a model for parasite-altered host behaviour? J. Helminthol. 75, 125–135.

Holland, C.V., Hamilton, C.M., 2013. The significance of cerebral toxocariasis: a model system for exploring the link between brain involvement, behaviour and the immune response. J. Exp. Biol. 216, 78–83.

Hrckova, G., Velebný, S., Tomasovicova, O.G., Medvedóvá, M., Pajerský, A., 2001. Pathomorphological changes in mice infected with *Toxocara cati* following administration of fenbendazole and glucan. Acta Parasitol. 46, 313–320.

Hsiao, W.W., Liao, H.S., Lin, H.H., Lee, Y.L., Fan, C.K., Liao, C.W., Lin, P.Y., Hwu, E.T., Chang, C.S., 2013. Biophysical analysis of astrocytes apoptosis triggered by larval E/S antigen from cerebral toxocarosis-causing pathogen *Toxocara canis*. Anal. Sci. 29, 885–892.

Janecek, E., Beineke, A., Schnieder, T., Strube, C., 2014. Neurotoxocarosis: marked preference of *Toxocara canis* for the cerebrum and *T. cati* for the cerebellum in the paratenic model host mouse. Parasit. Vectors 7, 194.

Janecek, E., Wilk, E., Schughart, K., Geffers, R., Strube, C., 2015. Microarray gene expression analysis reveals major differences between *Toxocara canis* and *Toxocara cati* neurotoxocarosis and involvement of *T. canis* in lipid biosynthetic processes. Int. J. Parasitol. 45, 495–503.

Janecek, E., Waindok, P., Bankstahl, M., Strube, C., 2017. Abnormal neurobehaviour and impaired memory function as a consequence of *Toxocara canis*- as well as *Toxocara cati*-induced neurotoxocarosis. PLoS Negl. Trop. Dis. 11, e0005594.

Jarosz, W., Mizgajska-Wiktor, H., Kirwan, P., Konarski, J., Rychlicki, W., Wawrzyniak, G., 2010. Developmental age, physical fitness and *Toxocara* seroprevalence amongst lower-secondary students living in rural areas contaminated with *Toxocara* eggs. Parasitology 137, 53–63.

Johnson, J.D., Campisi, J., Sharkey, C.M., Kennedy, S.L., Nickerson, M., Greenwood, B.N., Fleshner, M., 2005. Catecholamines mediate stress-induced increases in peripheral and central inflammatory cytokines. Neuroscience 135, 1295–1307.

Kamuyu, G., Bottomley, C., Mageto, J., Lowe, B., Wilkins, P.P., Noh, J.C., Nutman, T.B., Ngugi, A.K., Odhiambo, R., Wagner, R.G., Kakooza-Mwesige, A., Owusu-Agyei, S., Ae-Ngibise, K., Masanja, H., Osier, F.H., Odermatt, P., Newton, C.R., Study of Epidemiology of Epilepsy in Demographic Sites Group, 2014. Exposure to multiple parasites is associated with the prevalence of active convulsive epilepsy in sub-Saharan Africa. PLoS Negl. Trop. Dis. 8, e2908.

Kaplan, M., Kalkan, A., Kuk, S., Demirdag, K., Ozden, M., Kilic, S.S., 2008. *Toxocara* seroprevalence in schizophrenic patients in Turkey. Yonsei Med. J. 49, 224–229.

Kayes, S.G., Oaks, J.A., 1976. Effect of inoculum size and length of infection on the distribution of *Toxocara canis* larvae in the mouse. Am. J. Trop. Med. Hyg. 25, 573–580.

Kolbeková, P., Větvička, D., Svoboda, J., Skírnisson, K., Leissová, M., Syrůček, M., Marečková, H., Kolářová, L., 2011. *Toxocara canis* larvae reinfecting BALB/c mice exhibit accelerated speed of migration to the host CNS. Parasitol. Res. 109, 1267–1278.

Lescano, S.Z., Queiroz, M.L., Chieffi, P.P., 2004. Larval recovery of *Toxocara canis* in organs and tissues of experimentally infected *Rattus norvegicus*. Mem. Inst. Oswaldo Cruz 99, 627–628.

Liao, C.W., Fan, C.K., Kao, T.C., Ji, D.D., Su, K.E., Lin, Y.H., Cho, W.L., 2008. Brain injury-associated biomarkers of TGF-beta1, S100B, GFAP, NF-L, tTG, AbetaPP, and tau were concomitantly enhanced and the UPS was impaired during acute brain injury caused by *Toxocara canis* in mice. BMC Infect. Dis. 8, 84.

Lucki, I., 1998. The spectrum of behaviors influenced by serotonin. Biol. Psychiatry 44, 151–162.

Lull, M.E., Block, M.L., 2010. Microglial activation and chronic neurodegeneration. Neurotherapeutics 7, 354–365.

Maizels, R.M., 2013. *Toxocara canis*: molecular basis of immune recognition and evasion. Vet. Parasitol. 193, 365–374.

Min, H.K., 1982. Migratory behavior of *Toxocara canis* lavae in the brain of mice with special reference to distribution. Ewha Med. J. 5, 201–206.

Moreira-Silva, S.F., Rodrigues, M.G., Pimenta, J.L., Gomes, C.P., Freire, L.H., Pereira, F.E., 2004. Toxocariasis of the central nervous system: with report of two cases. Rev. Soc. Bras. Med. Trop. 37, 169–174.

Mould, A.W., Matthaei, K.I., Young, I.G., Foster, P.S., 1997. Relationship between interleukin-5 and eotaxin in regulating blood and tissue eosinophilia in mice. J. Clin. Invest. 99, 1064–1071.

Ollero, M.D., Fenoy, S., Cuéllar, C., Guillén, J.L., del Aguila, C., 2008. Experimental toxocariosis in BALB/c mice: effect of the inoculation dose on brain and eye involvement. Acta Trop. 105, 124–130.

Olson, L.J., Rose, J.E., 1966. Effect of *Toxocara canis* infection on the ability of white rats to solve maze problems. Exp. Parasitol. 19, 77–84.

Olson, L.J., Schulz, C.W., 1963. Nematode induced hypersenistivity reactions in Guinea pigs: onset of eosinophilia and positive Schultz-Dale following graded infections with *Toxocara canis*. Ann. N. Y. Acad. Sci. 113, 440–455.

Othman, A.A., Abdel-Aleem, G.A., Saied, E.M., Mayah, W.W., Elatrash, A.M., 2010. Biochemical and immunopathological changes in experimental neurotoxocariasis. Mol. Biochem. Parasitol. 172, 1–8.

Pellow, S., Chopin, P., File, S.E., Briley, M., 1985. Validation of open: closed arm entries in an elevated plus-maze as a measure of anxiety in the rat. J. Neurosci. Methods 14, 149–167.

Pinelli, E., Withagen, C., Fonville, M., Verlaan, A., Dormans, J., van Loveren, H., Nicoll, G., Maizels, R.M., van der Giessen, J., 2005. Persistent airway hyper-responsiveness and inflammation in *Toxocara canis*-infected BALB/c mice. Clin. Exp. Allergy 35, 826–832.

Pulendran, B., Artis, D., 2012. New paradigms in type 2 immunity. Science 337, 431–435.

Queiroz, M.L., Viel, T.A., Papa, C.H., Lescano, S.A., Chieffi, P.P., 2013. Behavioral changes in *Rattus norvegicus* coinfected by *Toxocara canis* and *Toxoplasma gondii*. Rev. Inst. Med. Trop. Sao Paulo 55, 51–53.

Richartz, E., Buchkremer, G., 2002. Zerebrale Toxokariasis: seltene Ursache kognitiver Störungen. Ein Beitrag zur Differenzialdiagnostik der Demenz [Cerebral toxocariasis: a rare cause of cognitive disorders. A contribution to differential dementia diagnosis]. Nervenarzt 73, 458–462.

Rodgers, R.J., Johnson, N.J., 1995. Factor analysis of spatiotemporal and ethological measures in the murine elevated plus-maze test of anxiety. Pharmacol. Biochem. Behav. 52, 297–303.

Rubinsky-Elefant, G., Hirata, C.E., Yamamoto, J.H., Ferreira, M.U., 2010. Human toxocariasis: diagnosis, worldwide seroprevalences and clinical expression of the systemic and ocular forms. Ann. Trop. Med. Parasitol. 104, 3–23.

Santos, S.V., Lescano, S.Z., Castro, J.M., Chieffi, P.P., 2009. Larval recovery of *Toxocara cati* in experimentally infected *Rattus norvegicus* and analysis of the rat as potential reservoir for this ascarid. Mem. Inst. Oswaldo Cruz 104, 933–934.

Santos, S.V., Moura, J.V., Lescano, S.A., Castro, J.M., Ribeiro, M.C., Chieffi, P.P., 2015. Behavioural changes and muscle strength in *Rattus norvegicus* experimentally infected with *Toxocara cati* and *T. canis*. J. Helminthol. 89, 465–470.

Santos, S.V.D., Santos, F.H.Y., Lescano, S.A.Z., Santos, D.M.D., Tiago, E.D.S., Fonseca, G.R.E., Ribeiro, M., Chieffi, P.P., 2017. Migration pattern of *Toxocara canis* larvae in experimentally infected male and female *Rattus norvegicus*. Rev. Soc. Bras. Med. Trop. 50, 698–700.

Schwab, J.M., Chiang, N., Arita, M., Serhan, C.N., 2007. Resolvin E1 and protectin D1 activate inflammation-resolution programmes. Nature 447, 869–874.

Serhan, C.N., 2006. Novel chemical mediators in the resolution of inflammation: resolvins and protectins. Anesthesiol. Clin. 24, 341–364.

Serhan, C.N., Petasis, N.A., 2011. Resolvins and protectins in inflammation resolution. Chem. Rev. 111, 5922–5943.

Smith, H., Holland, C., Taylor, M., Magnaval, J.F., Schantz, P., Maizels, R., 2009. How common is human toxocariasis? Towards standardizing our knowledge. Trends Parasitol. 25, 182–188.

Sprent, J.F., 1952. On the migratory behavior of the larvae of various *Ascaris* species in white mice. I. Distribution of larvae in tissues. J Infect Dis 90, 165–176.

Springer, A., Heuer, L., Janecek-Erfurth, E., Beineke, A., Strube, C., 2019. Histopathological characterization of *Toxocara canis*- and *T. cati*-induced neurotoxocarosis in the mouse model. Parasitol. Res. 118, 2591–2600.

Strube, C., Heuer, L., Janecek, E., 2013. Toxocara spp. infections in paratenic hosts. Parasitology 193, 375–389.

Subramaniam, S.R., Federoff, H.J., 2017. Targeting microglial activation states as a therapeutic avenue in Parkinson's disease. Front. Aging Neurosci. 9, 176.

Taira, K., Yanagida, T., Akazawa, N., Saitoh, Y., 2013. High infectivity of *Toxocara cati* larvae from muscles of experimentally infected rats. Vet. Parasitol. 196, 397–400.

Tam, V.C., 2013. Lipidomic profiling of bioactive lipids by mass spectrometry during microbial infections. Semin. Immunol. 25, 240–248.

Tam, V.C., Quehenberger, O., Oshansky, C.M., Suen, R., Armando, A.M., Treuting, P.M., Thomas, P.G., Dennis, E.A., Aderem, A., 2013. Lipidomic profiling of influenza infection identifies mediators that induce and resolve inflammation. Cell 154, 213–227.

Tuttle, A.H., Philip, V.M., Chesler, E.J., Mogil, J.S., 2018. Comparing phenotypic variation between inbred and outbred mice. Nat. Methods 15, 994–996.

Wade, S.E., Georgi, J.R., 1987. Radiolabeling and autoradiographic tracing of *Toxocara canis* larvae in male mice. J. Parasitol. 73, 116–120.

Waindok, P., Strube, C., 2019. Neuroinvasion of *Toxocara canis*- and *T. cati*-larvae mediates dynamic changes in brain cytokine and chemokine profile. J. Neuroinflammation 16, 147.

Waindok, P., Janecek-Erfurth, E., Lindenwald, D., Wilk, E., Schughart, K., Geffers, R., Balas, L., Durand, T., Rund, K.M., Schebb, N.H., Strube, C., 2019. Multiplex profiling of inflammation-related bioactive lipid mediators in *Toxocara canis*- and *Toxocara* cati-induced neurotoxocarosis. PLoS Negl. Trop. Dis. 13, e0007706.

Walsh, M.G., Haseeb, M.A., 2012. Reduced cognitive function in children with toxocariasis in a nationally representative sample of the United States. Int. J. Parasitol. 42, 1159–1163.

Yang, J., Dong, H., Hammock, B.D., 2011. Profiling the regulatory lipids: another systemic way to unveil the biological mystery. Curr. Opin. Lipidol. 22, 197–203.

Zibaei, M., Sadjjadi, S.M., Uga, S., 2010. Experimental *Toxocara cati* infection in gerbils and rats. Korean J. Parasitol. 48, 331–333.

CHAPTER ELEVEN

Neurotoxocariasis

Alessandra Nicoletti*
Department G.F. Ingrassia, Section of Neurosciences, University of Catania, Catania, Italy
*Corresponding author: e-mail address: anicolet@unict.it

Contents

Abstract

Human toxocariasis, caused by larvae of the *Toxocara* spp., is one of the most prevalent zoonosis with a worldwide distribution. *Toxocara* larvae can cross the blood-brain barrier, invading the central nervous system (CNS), leading to neurotoxocariasis. The clinical presentation consists of a wide spectrum of neurological manifestations such as meningitis, encephalitis, myelitis and cerebral vasculitis, but asymptomatic CNS infection is common. Despite the high seroprevalence, neurotoxocariasis is thought to be rare, even if in many animal models larvae usually migrate to the brain. Indeed, diagnosis of neurotoxocariasis is rarely considered, and the exact prevalence of CNS involvement is still unknown. Diagnosis of neurotoxocariasis is generally based on the detection of specific antibodies to *Toxocara* excretory-secretory antigens by ELISA in CSF or serum, and clinical and radiological improvement after anthelmintic therapy, but definitive diagnosis is given by histological confirmation, which is rarely available. Treatment is based on anti-helminthic drugs, commonly albendazole, generally administered with concomitant corticosteroids coverage.

At the population level, serological studies suggest an association between *Toxocara* infections and epilepsy, as well as with other neurodegenerative and psychiatric disorders. Nonetheless the possible role of *Toxocara* spp. in the pathogenesis of these disorders is still matter of debate.

Advances in Parasitology, Volume 109
ISSN 0065-308X
https://doi.org/10.1016/bs.apar.2020.01.007

1. Introduction

Human toxocariasis is a neglected parasitic zoonosis mainly caused by larvae of *Toxocara canis* or *Toxocara cati*, which are intestinal ascarid nematodes of canids and felids, respectively.

Toxocariasis is one of the most prevalent zoonosis worldwide, even if the parasite tends to be more prevalent in tropical settings with seroprevalence that reaches up to 80–90%, while in Western countries seroprevalence ranges from 35% to 42% in rural areas and from 2% to 5% in urban areas (Fan et al., 2015). Adult worms of *Toxocara* spp. live in the small intestines of various wild or domestic definitive hosts. Infected definitive hosts, such as dogs and cats, excrete eggs in the faeces, which then contaminate the environment where under suitable conditions (humidity and temperature) remain infective for several months or even years. Eggs containing infective third-stage larvae are accidentally ingested by human beings from contaminated raw vegetables, from contaminated soil, from eating undercooked or raw meats of infected paratenic hosts, and through direct contact with pets (Ma et al., 2018). Ingested eggs develop into juvenile larvae that cross the small intestine and migrate to any organ through the circulatory system, resulting in a multisystemic inflammatory tissue reaction. Visceral larva migrans (VLM) and ocular larva migrans (OLM) are the most common clinical manifestations, even if most infections remain undiagnosed due to the asymptomatic, mild or nonspecific clinical nature of the infection (Ma et al., 2018; Nicoletti, 2013). *Toxocara* larvae can cross the blood-brain barrier, invading the central nervous system (CNS), leading to neurotoxocariasis. Neurotoxocariasis (NT) in humans was first described by Beautyman and Woolf in 1951 in an autopsy study of a child who died of poliomyelitis, in whom a larva was found in the left thalamus (Beautyman and Woolf, 1951). Thereafter several autopsy studies described the presence of *T. canis* in the leptomeninges, in both the grey and white matter of the cerebrum, the cerebellum, and the spinal cord. Pathogenesis of NT is complex and probably due to the interaction of several factors such as host genetic factors, the number of ingested ova, and previous exposure to the parasite.

Neurological manifestations of NT consist of a wide spectrum of clinical presentation, but asymptomatic CNS infection is common. According to recent reviews, approximately 100 cases of neurotoxocariasis have been reported in the literature since 1956 (Deshayes et al., 2016; Fan et al., 2015; Sánchez et al., 2018). Diagnosis of NT is based on the presence of a high titre of anti-*Toxocara* antibodies in cerebrospinal fluid (CSF), presence of eosinophilia in serum or CSF or in serum, neuroimages, and clinical and radiological improvement after anthelmintic therapy, but definitive diagnosis is possible only by histological confirmation that is rarely available (Finsterer and Auer, 2007; Nicoletti, 2013).

Human NT is thought to be rare even though in many animal models, such as rodents, pig and primates, *Toxocara* larvae usually migrate to the brain. Animal models serve as a comparison to human toxocariasis. According to the literature on toxocariasis in pigs, considered a useful animal model due to a similar immunological response as well as many physiological and biochemical similarities, *Toxocara* larvae can be recovered in the brain on days 10–21 post-infection, but they totally disappeared after 126 days (Strube et al., 2013). As a matter of fact, despite the high *Toxocara* seroprevalence, NT is rarely taken into account in clinical settings, thus the exact prevalence of CNS involvement in toxocariasis is still unknown and information on the impact of NT is lacking.

2. Clinical manifestations

Neurological manifestation of NT includes meningitis, encephalitis, myelitis and cerebral vasculitis. Clinical manifestations are not specific but rather reflect the location of the lesions in the nervous system. NT mainly occurs in adult men (about 75% of cases reported in literature were men with a mean age of 42.5 ± 15.5) (Sánchez et al., 2018), contrary to VLM that is more frequently reported in childhood (Ma et al., 2018). Regarding the geographical distribution the largest number of cases with encephalic localisation have been reported from Europe followed by the Americas while just few cases have been described in Asia. Conversely the majority of cases with spinal cord involvement have been reported from Asia (Fan et al., 2015). Concomitant liver or lung involvement has been rarely described (Deshayes et al., 2016; Sánchez et al., 2018).

2.1 Myelitis

Isolated myelitis represents the most common presentation of NT occurring in about 70% of cases (Deshayes et al., 2016; Fan et al., 2015; Sánchez et al., 2018). Clinical manifestations include sensory and motor disturbances, predominantly involving the lower limbs and often accompanied by autonomic dysfunction. Nonetheless it should be noted that the majority of *Toxocara* myelitis (56 cases, about half of all cases of NT reported in literature) were reported in three different case series (Jabbour et al., 2011; Lee et al., 2009, 2010). Overall, about 60% of the published cases were diagnosed in Korea and Japan, while only a few were in Western countries (Deshayes et al., 2016; Fan et al., 2015; Sánchez et al., 2018). Actually, the diagnosis has been confirmed by biopsy in just one patient; while for more than 40% of cases, it was supported only by the detection of specific serum antibodies to *Toxocara* excretory-secretory antigens detected by ELISA and confirmed by Western Blot (WB) in only a few patients (Sánchez et al., 2018). Almost all patients were treated with anti-helminthic drugs, generally accompanied with corticosteroids, and for the majority, a clinical and radiological improvement was reported.

2.2 Cerebral toxocariasis

Encephalic localisation has been reported in about 30% of patients with different presentations such as meningitis, encephalitis, meningoencephalitis, encephalomyelitis, and meningoencephalomyelitis, but cerebral abscesses have been also described in a few cases. Encephalic/meningeal toxocariasis involvement is associated with a wide range of clinical manifestations including headache, seizures, focal deficits, confusional state, and cognitive impairment, with or without fever (Deshayes et al., 2016; Fan et al., 2015; Sánchez et al., 2018). A case of obstructive hydrocephalus due to toxocariasis was reported in a 46-year-old man who developed headache, diplopia, and visual deficits (Choi et al., 2013). Cerebral vasculitis due to NT was also observed. Vasculitis represents a rare and severe presentation that manifests with headache, cognitive impairment, and acute ischemic events (Sánchez et al., 2018). The diagnosis of cerebral toxocariasis was confirmed by biopsy just in six cases, but for the majority it was supported by the detection of antibody to *T. canis* in CSF. Also, in case with this syndrome, almost all cases were treated with anti-helminthic drugs, almost always in combination with corticosteroids, and for the majority, a clinical and radiological improvement was reported.

3. Toxocariasis and other neuropsychiatric disorders

Several epidemiological studies have suggested a possible association between *Toxocara* seropositivity and different neurological disorders (Fan et al., 2015). Early reports demonstrated high *Toxocara* seropositivity among people with epilepsy (PWE) (Critchley et al., 1982; Woodruff et al., 1966). Following these preliminary observations, several case-controls studies and two meta-analyses have been carried out suggesting a possible role of toxocariasis in the incidence of epilepsy (Luna et al., 2018). In particular, a recent meta-analysis including 4740 subjects from 11 case-control studies carried out in 13 countries reported a significant positive association between epilepsy and *Toxocara* spp. seropositivity with a pooled OR of 1.69 (95% CI 1.42–2.01) (Luna et al., 2018). However, even if epidemiological studies provide the most reliable evidence of association, this does not necessarily imply causation. As a matter of fact, due to the lack of evidence supporting a direct epileptogenic role, the role of exposition to *Toxocara* spp. and the subsequent development of epilepsy is still a matter of debate, even if different mechanisms could be involved. In a few cases reported in literature, epileptic seizures are probably due to the presence of granulomatous reactions induced by *Toxocara* larvae, generally associated with the presence of typical ring-enhancing lesions o MRI (Sánchez et al., 2018; Wagner and Newton, 2009). On the other hand, experimental studies carried out in animal models have showed that the presence of *Toxocara* larvae in the brain increases the permeability of the blood-brain barrier, and the production of proinflammatory cytokines leading to neuronal damage (Fan et al., 2015). Similar physiopathological mechanisms have been hypothesised to play a major role in the epileptogenesis due to neurocysticercosis (Nash et al., 2015) suggesting that the two parasites may share a common epileptogenic pathway. Finally, there is growing evidence that autoantibodies against neuronal elements may play a role in some types of epilepsy. Clues of the autoimmune nature of epilepsy came from the presence of antibodies to a major excitatory neurotransmitter in the CNS (Levite, 2002). Toxocariasis produces a marked immune response including autoantibody production; however, it is unclear as to the relation of these immune mechanisms to epileptogenesis (Obwaller et al., 2004).

Furthermore, some case-control studies suggest a higher *Toxocara* seroprevalence among subjects affected by schizophrenia as well as other psychiatric conditions with respect to control subjects. Even if these data suggest a possible pathogenetic role of *Toxocara* in psychiatric disorders, due to the retrospective nature of these studies a reverse causality cannot be excluded; thus, it is possible that psychiatric patients have a higher risk of infection due to abnormal behavioural changes, such as poor hygiene as well as a propensity to eat inappropriate things (Fan et al., 2015).

Several experimental and epidemiological studies demonstrated an association between CNS inflammation and cognitive impairment, particularly in Alzheimer's disease where CNS inflammation seem to be implicated in the development of amyloid plaques. On this ground a possible role of toxocariasis on the development of cognitive impairment has been hypothesised, even if to date few clinical or population-based studies have been performed. Depressive symptoms, mental confusion and cognitive impairment have been described in subjects with NT (Deshayes et al., 2016) and some case-control studies in children population suggests poor performance among seropositive subjects. A recent large, population-based study, including a sample of 3949 children living in the United States, reported statistically lower cognitive scores among seropositive children (Walsh and Haseeb, 2012). Nonetheless longitudinal data are needed to elucidate the actual relationship between diminished cognitive function and toxocariasis (Fan et al., 2015).

4. Diagnosis of neurotoxocariasis

Diagnosis of neurotoxocariasis is generally based on the detection of specific antibodies to *Toxocara* excretory-secretory antigens by ELISA in CSF or serum, presence of serum or CSF eosinophilia, and clinical and radiological improvement after anthelmintic therapy (Finsterer and Auer, 2007; Nicoletti, 2013). However, definitive diagnosis is provided only by histological confirmation or by the PCR detection of *Toxocara* spp. DNA in samples from affected tissues, both rarely available. Thus serological or immunological methods alone do not allow for an unequivocal diagnosis of infection (Fan et al., 2015; Ma et al., 2018). Presence of serum or CSF eosinophilia support the diagnosis of NT and represent an important finding, because generally clinicians tend to look for eosinophilia as a basis to suspect a parasitic infection. Nonetheless it should be noted that serum eosinophilia was reported only in about 65% of patients, while the presence of CSF pleocytosis was present just in 40% of patients (Sánchez et al., 2018). Their absence thus does not exclude CNS *Toxocara* involvement. Increased serum IgE levels were almost always positive, but this finding was reported in less than 50% of the cases (Sánchez et al., 2018).

4.1 Serological assay

The standard serological test is an ELISA based on secretory-excretory antigens (TES) from *Toxocara canis* infective-stage larvae hatched *in vitro* from eggs (de Savigny et al., 1979). These antigens are a mixture of several glycoproteins that have Th2 type immune response with high levels of interleukin (IL) 4 and IL5. ELISA for the detection of specific IgG antibodies to TES in serum has a sensitivity of 78% and a specificity of 92% for the diagnosis of VLM, although cross-reactions with other nematode infections (e.g., *Ascaris lumbricoides*, filariasis or strongyloidiasis) reduce its specificity, particularly in tropical areas (Fillaux and Magnaval, 2013). Indeed, cross-reactivity between the higher molecular weight components of TES (>32 kDa) with antibodies from other nematode infections occurs, thus TES-ELISA remains problematic in areas of endemic polyparasitism. Furthermore, as for any antibody test, a positive IgG ELISA cannot distinguish between past and current infection, although decreasing antibody titres after antihelminthic treatment or following clinical remission are highly suggestive of the diagnosis (Ma et al., 2018). The use of fractionated native TES in the western blot (WB) assay overcomes the issues with cross-reactions to other nematodes in ELISA assays because the low molecular weight bands (24–32 kDa) are specific for *Toxocara* infection (Magnaval et al., 1991). Unfortunately, WB is more expensive and labour-intensive than ELISA, and thus screening with the indirect TES–IgG–ELISA, followed by confirmation with the TES-WB, is considered a more effective approach (Ma et al., 2018).

Recombinant antigens have also been developed showing in general an increased sensitivity and specificity with respect to TES, even if performance of these new assays must be fully validated (Fan et al., 2015; Ma et al., 2018). The detection of IgG subclasses has been found to be more effective for immunodiagnosis of *Toxocara* spp. infection. IgG2 antibodies specific to the glycan of *Toxocara* excretory-secretory antigens yields the highest sensitivity, though at a reduced specificity, while the use of IgG4 significantly increases specificity. IgG4 may reflect prolonged antigenic stimulation, thus, this antibody subclass could be useful for monitoring larval viability before and after treatment (Fan et al., 2015).

4.2 Neuroimaging

Neuroimaging supports the diagnosis of NT, and MRI and CT scans have been performed in all cases reported in the literature. Furthermore the radiological improvement after anthelmintic therapy is considered one of the main criteria for the diagnosis of NT.

With MRI, spinal toxocariasis is characterised by swelling and enlargement of the involved spinal segment and hyperintensity on T2 and FLAIR sequences with focal nodular enhancement after gadolinium injection (Fig. 1). The enhancing area is generally smaller than the affected area with

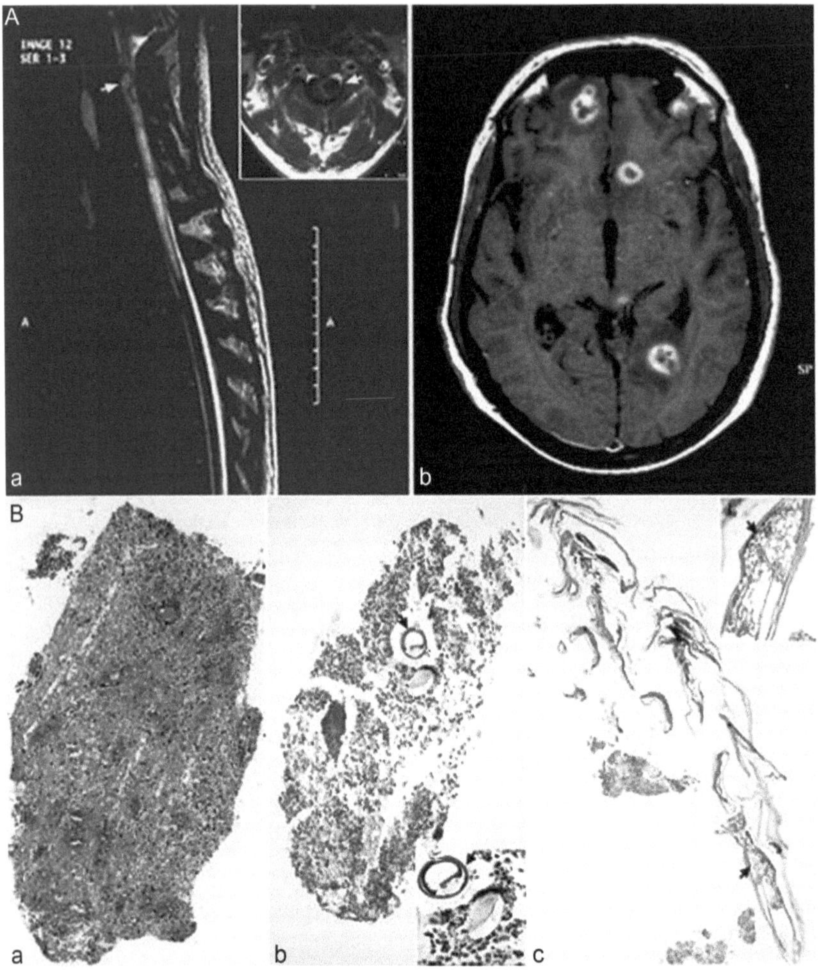

Fig. 1 (A) MRI findings. (a) T2-weighted sagital image of spine showing hyperintense lesion (arrow) with extensive perilesional edema in high cervical cord. (b) T1-weighted axial post-contrast image of brain shows multiple ring-enhancing lesions in bilateral frontoparietal deep white matter with nodular enhancement of the wall seen in left frontal lesion (Moiyadi et al., 2007). (B) Histologic findings. Small fragments of inflamed gliotic tissue from the cord (a) and necrotic purulent material (b) were included in the resected tissue. Within the necrotic material, longitudinally sectioned larvae of Toxocara were identifiable (c). Fragments of lateral alae lined by outer cuticle (b: inset, arrows) and cross-sections of excretory columns (c: inset, arrows) were dispersed within the purulent exudate (Moiyadi et al., 2007).

a tendency to involve the posterior-lateral areas of the cord. Lesions varied in size; they were almost always singular and located at the thoracic and cervical levels (Sánchez et al., 2018).

Also, MRI findings of cerebral toxocariasis are not specific, showing single or multiple subcortical, cortical, or white matter hyperintense lesions on FLAIR and T2WI. These lesions are generally isointense or hypointense in T1WI and hypodense on cerebral CT scan. Homogeneous or punctuate enhancement after gadolinium injection has been reported, and in few cases, single or multiple ring-enhancing lesions were described (Fig. 1). Focal meningeal contrast enhancement has been also described in a few patients (Sánchez et al., 2018).

Imaging of vasculitis generally shows ischemic lesions that can be also demonstrated in the acute phase by diffusion-weighted imaging sequences. MRI angiography and angiography can be useful to demonstrate stenoses or occlusion of the encephalic arteries, but these have been performed in just a few cases (Sánchez et al., 2018).

4.3 Histopathological examination

Histopathological examination generally shows a granulomatous inflammatory response containing large numbers of eosinophils and neutrophils in the parenchyma with perivascular lymphocytic infiltrate (Fig. 1). *Toxocara* larvae were detected in only two cases. The absence of larvae can be explained by the fact that the larvae are not permanently trapped by the reaction of the host but rather can escape, migrate, and trigger other inflammatory foci (Sánchez et al., 2018).

5. Treatment

Due to the lack of controlled studies treatment of NT is still controversial. Different anti-helminthic drugs (thiabendazole, mebendazole, albendazole and diethylcarbamazine) have been commonly used in patients with NT, with albendazole being the drug most commonly administered (Sánchez et al., 2018). Albendazole, in fact, has proven effective in the treatment of some neuro-helminthiases such as cysticercosis and hydatidosis and it is recommended also for the treatment of NT because it crosses the blood-brain barrier, shows a better pharmacological profile, and is better tolerated than mebendazole and diethylcarbamazine (Nicoletti, 2013). Albendazole is generally administered at a dosage of 800 mg per day in adults, or 15 mg/kg/day in children. Nonetheless there is no consensus regarding the dosage as well as the treatment duration that should continue between 21 and 28 days or until complete resolution of the clinical symptoms and normalisation of the MRI, even if it sometimes needs to be repeated (Deshayes et al., 2016).

Although there is no consensus concerning the utility of corticosteroids in the treatment of NT in the majority of cases (about 90%), anti-helminthic drugs have been administered in combination with corticosteroids, while some cases of myelitis (about 15%) have been treated with corticosteroids alone. With the exception of a few cases, after treatment, almost all patients improved clinically and radiologically, but an improvement was also reported for those cases with the spinal cord involvement treated with corticosteroids alone (Sánchez et al., 2018).

6. Conclusion

Although *Toxocara* is one of the most prevalent helminthiases worldwide, diagnosis of NT is rarely considered in many clinical settings, and the number of cases tends to be underestimated.

To date diagnosis is generally based on the following findings: blood and/or CSF eosinophilia, high titre of anti-*Toxocara* antibodies in blood and CSF, hypodense lesions on brain CTs and/or hyperintense lesions on T2-weighted brain or spine MRIs, and above all the clinical and/or radiological improvement after anthelmintic therapy (Deshayes et al., 2016). Nonetheless it should be underlined that none of these findings are specific and each one has a limited diagnostic value. Indeed, due to the lack of a confirmatory test for most of the cases reported in literature the diagnosis of NT can be considered only presumptive.

In particular, the presence of serum eosinophilia and CSF pleocytosis is not a rule (Sánchez et al., 2018), thus the diagnosis of NT should be considered also in their absence. Furthermore, blood eosinophilia is common for patients who have lived in tropical areas, due to common antigenic determinants between different tropical nematodes and *Toxocara* spp. (Deshayes et al., 2016).

Neuroimaging, as reported, is not specific and the serological test commonly used (ELISA) has low specificity. In particular MRI findings related to the spinal cord involvement, the most common presentation of NT, are indistinguishable from other inflammatory and infective myelitis. Furthermore, almost all cases of NT reported in literature have been treated with anti-helminthic drugs in association with corticosteroids and the majority of inflammatory myelopathy such as, autoimmune myelopathy (e.g., aquaporin-4-IgG seropositive neuromyelitis optica, multiple sclerosis, paraneoplastic myelopathies) (Flanagan, 2016) are responsive to corticosteroids treatment. Thus, the clinical and radiological improvement, considered an important criterion for the diagnosis of NT and reported in almost all cases, could not be univocally attributable to the anti-helminthic drugs. For this reason, a comprehensive CSF evaluation (e.g., presence of autoantibodies, anti-AQP4-IgG, paraneoplastic autoantibodies, invective agents) should always be performed and the exclusion of other diagnosis is mandatory. Actually, in about 40% of cases diagnosed as *Toxocara* myelitis, the diagnosis is supported only by the presence of serum antibodies detected by ELISA. However, seroprevalence in the general population is high also in western countries, thus seropositivity does not necessarily implicate a CNS involvement, mainly in endemic areas. Consequently, the detection of anti-*Toxocara* antibodies in CSF is fundamental. Nonetheless, also in the case of cerebral toxocariasis, the diagnosis can be difficult. Spinal epidural lipomatosis (SEL0), for example, is a common MRI finding that can be related to different disease processes. In particular in *T. solium* endemic areas, where there is often also a high *Toxocara* seroprevalence reported in the general population, the presence of a SEL and its resolution after cysticidal drug therapy is considered to be major criteria for the diagnosis of neurocysticercosis (Del Brutto et al., 2017), even in the presence of negative serological tests for antibodies to *T. solium*. In this scenario a possible diagnosis of NT cannot be entirely ruled out.

On the other hand, when evaluated, increased serum IgE levels were almost always found, thus this might represent a valuable support for the diagnosis. As reported IgG4 may reflect prolonged antigenic stimulation, thus the monitoring of this antibody subclass after treatment could also provide reliable evidence of *Toxocara* infection (Fan et al., 2015).

In conclusion, due to the lack of widely accepted, standard diagnostic criteria, there is a great variability in case definitions, diagnostic procedures, and diagnostic certainty for NT. The pathogenetic mechanisms related to the passage of *Toxocara* larvae through the CNS are not entirely understood and the development of a standardised diagnostic work-up as well as standardised and validated diagnostic criteria is an essential requirement to improve our knowledge and to evaluate the real impact of NT. Considering the high seroprevalence, detection of anti-*Toxocara* antibodies in CSF should be part of the diagnostic work-up in all cases of myelitis, encephalitis, encephalomyelitis, at least in patients with unknown aetiology.

Nonetheless, due to the lack of awareness regarding this neglected parasitic disease and its possible etiological role in neurological disorders, diagnosis of NT is rarely considered and anti-*Toxocara* antibodies levels in CSF are almost never determined. Large multicentre studies including cases of myelitis, encephalitis and encephalomyelitis with unknown aetiology should be performed using standardised diagnostic criteria in order to evaluate the real impact of NT.

References

Beautyman, W., Woolf, A.L., 1951. An ascaris larva in the brain in association with acute anterior poliomyelitis. J. Pathol. Bacteriol. 63, 635–647.

Choi, J.H., Cho, J.W., Lee, J.H., Lee, S.W., Kim, H.J., Choi, K.D., 2013. Obstructive hydrocephalus due to CNS toxocariasis. J. Neurol. Sci. 329, 59–61.

Critchley, E.M., Vakil, S.D., Hutchinson, D.N., Taylor, P., 1982. Toxoplasma, toxocara, and epilepsy. Epilepsia 23, 315–321.

de Savigny, D.H., Voller, A., Woodruff, A.W., 1979. Toxocariasis: serological diagnosis by enzyme immunoassay. J. Clin. Pathol. 32, 284–288.

Del Brutto, O.H., Nash, T.E., White, A.C., Rajshekhar, V., Wilkins, P.P., Singh, G., Vasquez, C.M., Salgado, P., Gilman, R.H., Garcia, H.H., 2017. Revised diagnostic criteria for neurocysticercosis. J. Neurol. Sci. 371, 202–210.

Deshayes, S., Bonhomme, J., de La Blanchardière, A., 2016. Neurotoxocariasis: a systematic literature review. Infection 44, 565–574.

Fan, C.K., Holland, C.V., Loxton, K., Barghouth, U., 2015. Cerebral toxocariasis: silent progression to neurodegenerative disorders? Clin. Microbiol. Rev. 28, 663–686.

Fillaux, J., Magnaval, J.F., 2013. Laboratory diagnosis of human toxocariasis. Vet. Parasitol. 193, 327–336.

Finsterer, J., Auer, H., 2007. Neurotoxocariosis. Rev. Inst. Med. Trop. Sao Paulo 49, 279–287.

Flanagan, E.P., 2016. Autoimmune myelopathies. Handb. Clin. Neurol. 133, 327–351.

Jabbour, R.A., Kanj, S.S., Sawaya, R.A., Awar, G.N., Hourani, M.H., Atweh, S.F., 2011. *Toxocara canis* myelitis: clinical features, magnetic resonance imaging (MRI) findings, and treatment outcome in 17 patients. Medicine (Baltimore). 90, 337–343.

Lee, J.Y., Kim, B.J., Lee, S.P., Jeung, Y.J., Oh, M.J., Park, M.S., Paeng, J.W., Lee, B.J., Choi, D.C., 2009. Toxocariasis might be an important cause of atopic myelitis in Korea. J. Korean Med. Sci. 24, 1024–1030.

Lee, I.H., Kim, S.T., Oh, D.K., Kim, H.J., Kim, K.H., Jeon, P., Byun, H.S., 2010. MRI findings of spinal visceral larva migrans of *Toxocara canis*. Eur. J. Radiol. 75, 236–240.

Levite, M., 2002. Autoimmune epilepsy. Nat. Immunol. 3, 500.

Luna, J., Cicero, C.E., Rateau, G., Quattrocchi, G., Marin, B., Bruno, E., Dalmay, F., Druet-Cabanac, M., Nicoletti, A., Preux, P.M., 2018. Updated evidence of the association between toxocariasis and epilepsy: systematic review and meta-analysis. PLoS Negl. Trop. Dis. 12, e0006665.

Ma, G., Holland, C.V., Wang, T., Hofmann, A., Fan, C.K., Maizels, R.M., Hotez, P.J., Gasser, R.B., 2018. Human toxocariasis. Lancet Infect. Dis. 18, e14–e24.

Magnaval, J.F., Fabre, R., Maurieres, P., Charlet, J.P., de Larrard, B., 1991. Application of the western blotting procedure for the immunodiagnosis of human toxocariasis. Parasitol. Res. 77, 697–702.

Moiyadi, A., Mahadevan, A., Anandh, B., Shivashankar, R.S., Chickabasavaiah, Y.T., Shankar, S.K., 2007. Visceral larva migrans presenting as multiple intracranial and intraspinal abscesses. Neuropathology 27, 371–374.

Nash, T.E., Mahanty, S., Loeb, J.A., Theodore, W.H., Friedman, A., Sander, J.W., Singh, G., Cavalheiro, E., Del Brutto, O.H., Takayanagui, O.M., Fleury, A., Verastegui, M., Preux, P.M., Montano, S., Pretell, E.J., White, A.C., Gonzales, A.E., Gilman, R.H., Garcia, H.H., 2015. Neurocysticercosis: a natural human model of epileptogenesis. Epilepsia 56, 177–183.

Nicoletti, A., 2013. Toxocariasis. Handb. Clin. Neurol. 114, 217–228.

Obwaller, A., Duchêne, M., Walochnik, J., Wiedermann, G., Auer, H., AspoÈck, H., 2004. Association of autoantibodies against small nuclear ribonucleoproteins (snRNPs) with symptomatic *Toxocara canis* infestation. Parasite Immunol. 26, 327–333.

Sánchez, S.S., García, H.H., Nicoletti, A., 2018. Clinical and magnetic resonance imaging findings of neurotoxocariasis. Front. Neurol. 9, 53.

Strube, C., Heuer, L., Janecek, E., 2013. *Toxocara* spp. infections in paratenic hosts. Vet. Parasitol. 193, 375–389.

Wagner, R.G., Newton, C.R., 2009. Do helminths cause epilepsy? Parasite Immunol. 31, 697–705.

Walsh, M.G., Haseeb, M.A., 2012. Reduced cognitive function in children with toxocariasis in a nationally representative sample of the United States. Int. J. Parasitol. 42, 1159–1163.

Woodruff, A.W., Bisseru, B., Bowe, J.C., 1966. Infection with animal helminths as a factor in causing poliomyelitis and epilepsy. Br. Med. J. 1, 1576–1579.

Further reading

Feske, S.K., Goldberg, M., Dudzinski, D.M., Gonzalez, R.G., Kovach, A.E., 2015. Case records of the Massachusetts General Hospital. Case 29-2015. A 38-year-old pregnant woman with headache and visual symptoms. N. Engl. J. Med. 373, 1154–1164.

Kazek, B., Jamroz, E., Mandera, M., Bierzyńska-Macyszyn, G., Kluczewska, E., Marszał, E., 2006. The cerebral form of toxocarosis in a seven-year-old patient. Folia Neuropathol. 44, 72–76.

Park, C.W., Choe, W.J., Chun, Y.I., 2012. Eosinophilic myelitis in the cervical cord mimicking intramedullary cord tumor. J. Korean Neurosurg. Soc. 52, 410–413.

CHAPTER TWELVE

Pathogenesis of cerebral toxocariasis and neurodegenerative diseases

Chia-Kwung Fan*
Department of Molecular Parasitology and Tropical Diseases, School of Medicine, College of Medicine, Taipei Medical University, Taipei, Taiwan
Research Center of International Tropical Medicine, College of Medicine, Taipei Medical University, Taipei, Taiwan
Tropical Medicine Division, International PhD Program in Medicine, College of Medicine, Taipei Medical University, Taipei, Taiwan
*Corresponding author: e-mail address: tedfan@tmu.edu.tw

Contents

Abstract

Toxocara canis belongs to one of zoonotic parasites that commonly infects canines worldwide, and its eggs in host faeces may contaminate the food, water, soil and their fur as well as the larvae entrapped in the granuloma can infect paratenic hosts including mice and humans. Survivability of *T. canis* embryonated eggs under moist, cool conditions may be as long as 2–4 years or more. In paratenic hosts such as mice and humans, *T. canis* L3 larvae neither moult, grow, nor replicate and will wander through a number of internal organs in humans so as to cause Th2-dominant pathology in various internal organs as leading to neurotoxocariasis (NT), ocular toxocariasis (OT), or visceral larva migrans (VLM). Although the systemic immune response to *T. canis* has been widely reported, the immune response in the brain has received little attention.

Advances in Parasitology, Volume 109
ISSN 0065-308X
https://doi.org/10.1016/bs.apar.2020.01.008

Differential cytokine expression and other brain injury-associated biomarkers or neurodegeneration-associated factors have been observed in infected versus uninfected outbred and inbred mice. Preliminary data have also suggested a possible link between significant memory impairment and cytokine production associated with *T. canis* infection in the hippocampus which has been long recognised as being responsible for learning and memory functions. Notably, it remains an enigma concerning cerebral invasion by *T. canis* larvae rarely induces a recognisable neurological syndrome or its involvement in neuropathological disorders in humans. Exploration of the relationship between host and parasite in the brain may elucidate the cryptic symptoms of human cerebral toxocariasis, with patients presenting with mental retardation, epilepsy, neurodegeneration and other central nervous system (CNS) disorders.

1. Introduction

Toxocara canis and *Toxocara cati*, zoonotic parasites, belong to the genus of *Toxocara* whose definitive host is the dogs and foxes for *T. canis* and cats for *T. cati*, respectively. The adult worms predominately parasitize the upper digestive tract of the final hosts (Fan et al., 2015). The final hosts ingest food or water contaminated by infective *Toxocara* eggs, larvae hatch from the eggs in the small intestine then penetrate the gut wall, and are transported to the liver and lungs via the blood circulation. Subsequently, the larvae undergo a further migration by the tracheal route to mature to adulthood in the small intestine. Patent infections can develop in dogs and cats of all ages through accidental ingestion of eggs or via consumption of larvae within tissues of paratenic hosts, e.g., lambs or chickens. In general, patent infections occur in dogs 4–5 weeks after infection and in cats 8 weeks after infection. In addition, puppies, unlike kittens, may be infected by the transplacental route (Overgaauw and van Knapen, 2013; Sprent, 1956).

The adult female worm may produce up to 200,000 unembryonated eggs per day, releasing them to the environment via the dog's faeces which can become infectious in soil under appropriate conditions after an incubation period of 2–5 weeks, depending on both temperature and humidity (Despommier, 2003; Glickman and Schantz, 1981). Different diagnostic methods employed and dog populations, e.g., stray or domestic dogs, age of dogs or geographic variation, urban or rural areas, as well as, high or low-income countries and a country's climate will influence the infection rate. The prevalence of infection in dogs with adult *Toxocara* worms ranging from 1.4% in UK to 51% in Nigeria have been documented (Batchelor et al., 2008; Sowemimo, 2007); nevertheless, the prevalence in most of the dog studies has been recorded between 10% and 30% (Rubel et al., 2003). However, studies in the UK and Denmark showed a 91% prevalence in feral farm cats and 79% in stray cats, respectively, but between 15% and 60% was reported in most of the studies (Fisher, 2003; Takeuchi-Storm et al., 2015). A recent study from Japan (Macuheggs et al., 2013) indicated that in samples from 34 sandpits taken in the Tokyo metropolitan area, 41.2% (14/34 samples) were contaminated with *T. cati* eggs as examined by PCR analysis. *T. cati* may play a more important role in human toxocariasis than previously recognised; for example, a number of studies suggest that *T. cati* is the causative agent of ocular toxocariasis (OT) (Fisher, 2003). Therefore, the high prevalence of *Toxocara* together with the high fecundity of *Toxocara* and the increased number of pet animals in Western countries, can explain why soil in parks, playgrounds, and other public places may be highly contaminated by *Toxocara* eggs, posing serious hazards to human health (Fakhri et al., 2018). Moreover, *Toxocara* eggs are very resistant to physical and chemical agents, and they may survive well for 6–12 months during the winter under several factors, e.g., temperature, light, humidity, pH and so on; and it is noteworthy that under moist and cool conditions, its survivability may be as long as 2–4 years or more (Azam et al., 2012). Of particular note, a study conducted by Fan et al. (2003) utilising 2% formalin-preserved *T. canis* embryonated eggs kept at 4 °C for at least 14 months to inoculate ICR outbred mice and found larvae recovered from the liver and brain at 469 days post-infection were still alive. Furthermore, these larvae could cause various degrees of Th2-related granulomatous inflammatory injuries to internal organs, e.g., the liver and lungs, reflecting its pathogenicity and infectivity might be retained even after long-term storage in 2% formalin.

2. Human toxocariasis and common serodiagnostic assay

Humans can acquire such an infection through accidental consumption of embryonated eggs contaminating soils, raw fruits or vegetables (Fan et al., 2015; Ma et al., 2018); however, to a lesser extent, humans can also become infected by ingesting larvae via raw or undercooked meat or giblets from paratenic hosts, e.g., chickens, cows, ducks, deer, pigs, sheep, rabbits or ostriches (Hoffmeister et al., 2007; Jabbour et al., 2011; Lee et al., 2010; Noh et al., 2012). When ingested, larvae may emerge from the swallowed eggs then penetrate through the submucosa of the small intestine and further migrate to various internal organs through the circulatory system, resulting in a multi-systemic inflammatory reaction in various internal organs causing visceral larva migrans (VLM) or invading the eyes may cause ocular toxocariasis (OT), and most frequently, as "covert toxocariasis" in children experiencing fever, headache, behavioural and sleep disturbances, cough, anorexia, abdominal pain, hepatomegaly, nausea and vomiting, and as "common toxocariasis" in adults who may show weakness, pruritus, rash, breathing difficulties and abdominal pain. The latter two syndromes are defined solely by serum conversion and unspecific symptoms (Fan et al., 2015; Ma et al., 2018). However, once the larvae have invaded and are persisting in the central nervous system (CNS), they may cause neurotoxocarosis (NT) (Fan et al., 2015; Ma et al., 2018); thus, potentially leading to meningitis, encephalitis, myelitis, cerebral vasculitis or behavioural disorders (Deshayes et al., 2016; Fan et al., 2015). Furthermore, when *T. canis* larval invade the brain, they may cause cerebral toxocariasis (CT) which can result in behavioural alterations, memory impairment and cognitive dysfunctions and is additionally controversially discussed as a cause of neuropsychological disturbances like dementia or depression (Fan et al., 2015; Moiyadi et al., 2007). When humans are infected by *T. canis*, the invading larvae will remain its current form with no further growth or development making diagnosis difficult (Holland and Hamilton, 2013). Currently, diagnosis in the context of investigative and clinical practice predominantly relies on immunological techniques. *T. canis* larval excretory-secretory antigens-based ELISA (TcES-ELISA) or the utilisation of fractionated, TcES antigens in western blotting (TcES-WB) is most commonly utilised immunological techniques, although nowadays recombinant antigens used for both serological methods, proven more specific than TcES, have also been produced (Yamasaki et al., 2000; Yunus et al., 2018). However, in subtropical and tropical regions where polyparasitism is endemic, employing TcES-WB, rather than TcES-ELISA, to make a diagnosis of *T. canis* infection by detection of IgG reactivity to fractionated bands at 24–32 kDa has been reportedly to reach reasonable and acceptable sensitivity (95%) and specificity (95%) and also may greatly reduce antigenic cross-reactivity (Fillaux and Magnaval, 2013; Smith et al., 2009).

3. Seroepidemiology study of *Toxocara* spp. infection in humans

Worldwide seroepidemiological surveys as assessed by IgG antibody levels have shown that human toxocariasis is one of the most common helminthiases in the world. In Western industrial countries, e.g., USA and UK, the seroprevalence varies between 2% and 5% in urban areas, reaches 15–20% in semi-rural zones such as residential outskirts of large cities, and peaks at 35–42% in rural areas (Magnaval et al., 2001). For example, even in the USA, *Toxocara* sp. infection is reportedly one of the important childhood zoonotic infections and occurs more frequently in populations with lower socioeconomic status and African Americans (Barry et al., 2013). In contrast, comparatively higher seroprevalences have been reported from developing countries, ranging from 93% in La Reunion, 86.8% in Marshall Island, 81% in Nepal, 63.2% in Indonesia, 58% in Malaysia, 44.6% in Swaziland, 36% in Brazil and 53.2% in Nigeria (Fan et al., 2015; Sowemimo et al., 2017). However, variation in detection methods (ELISA or WB), cut-off titers and by the general difficulty in exploring the relationships between titers, infection and clinical disease hinders a valid comparison of seroprevalence data between countries (Smith et al., 2009). Noteworthy, those seroprevalence data indicates that exposure to *T. canis* infection is quite common and because of the potential to contribute to significant disease, should not be ignored (Ma et al., 2018). Thus, it appears that cases of CT tend to be underestimated due to non-specific clinical signs. Moreover, most cases of human CT are assumed to be caused by *T. canis* larvae and most studies concerning toxocariasis and CT have focused on *T. canis* as the major causative agent. Noteworthy, *T. cati* larvae may cause human toxocariasis that have been recently reported as important causative agent that can't be ignored since they show similar visceral larval migration patterns to *T. canis* larvae despite *T. canis* exhibits a stronger preference in invading the cerebrum, while *T. cati* larvae prefer invading the cerebellum as investigated using mice. Therefore, *T. cati* should not be neglected as a causative pathogen for CT in humans (Waindok and Strube, 2019).

4. Global human cerebral toxocariasis cases with various neurological disorders (1985–2019)

Signs related to the larval migration in the brain may cause severe neurological diseases such as meningitis, encephalitis or cerebral vasculitis, but usually relating to relatively non-specific clinical signs, e.g., headaches and fever (Fan et al., 2015; Ma et al., 2018). Moreover, there has been discussion in the literature about possible associations between CT and neurodegenerative disorders, including seizure, schizophrenia, cognitive deficits, idiopathic Parkinson's disease and/or dementia (Fan et al., 2015; Ma et al., 2018). Since the accuracy of various diagnostic approaches for the detection of CT cases has improved greatly over the last 35 years, CT cases are thought to be greatly increased. In order to determine how many CT cases were reported during the period from January 1985 to August 2019, we searched reports with brain involvement due to *T. canis* infection from PubMed, and 28 patients with various neurological manifestations have been recorded, including 6 cases of eosinophilic meningoencephalitis, 6 cases of seizure (Fig. 1), 5 cases of cerebral vasculitis (Fig. 2), 3 cases of

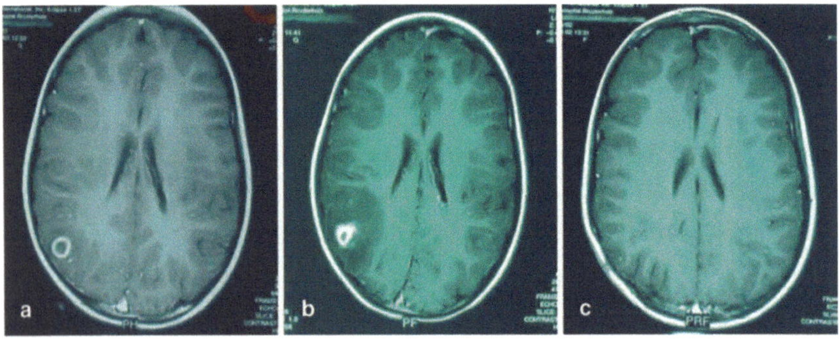

Fig. 1 (A–C) Toxocariasis lesion of right parietal in an 11-year-old girl. (A) Axial post-contrast T1-weighted MRI scan shows a thin ring enhancement without edema. (B) Axial MRI scan 6 weeks later shows a thick diffuse with ring enhancement and perifocal edema. (C) Postoperative axial MRI scan (1 year later) shows no pathological gadolinium enhancement. *Reuse permission from Springer Nature, Licence No. 4686600619802.*

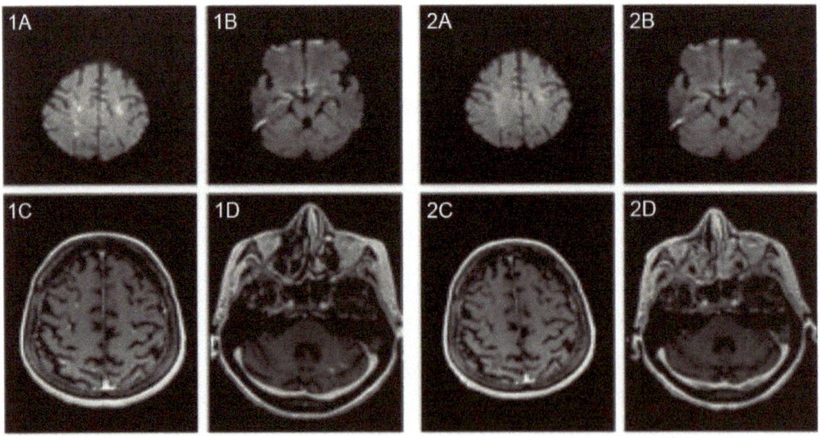

Fig. 2 Cerebral magnetic resonance imaging of the patient on admission (1) and at follow-up at 4 months (2) with hyper-intense lesions in diffusion weighted images in the cerebrum and cerebellum (A and B) and multiple contrast enhancing cortical and cerebellar lesions (C and D) with improvement after 4 months. *Reuse permission from John Wiley and Sons, Licence No. 4686601493568.*

eosinophilic meningitis, 2 cases of eosinophilic encephalitis, 2 cases of cognitive impairment, and 1 case each for eosinophilic encephalitis, fibrotic arachnoidea, bilateral subdural hematoma with a small subarachnoid haemorrhage, cerebral meningoradiculitis and multiple cerebral infarction (Table 1). Further analysis of the number of CT cases revealed Europe had the highest number with 19 cases and 3 cases occurred in each of Asia, North America and South America. These patients were predominantly adults. The average age was 35.2 ± 22.4 years, of which females (38.8 ± 24.4 years) were older than male patients (30.7 ± 21.1 years). As shown in Table 1, 35.7% (10/28) and 32.1% (9/28) of CT cases had eosinophilia detected in blood and CSF, respectively, emphasising the importance of eosinophilia as a diagnostic references for CT (Hotez and Wilkins, 2009). Moreover, most CT cases can be detected by medical imaging techniques including computed tomography and magnetic resonance imaging (MRI) which is able to detect and localise lesions caused by migrating *Toxocara* spp. larvae in brain tissues, thus supporting a tentative diagnosis of CT (Rüttinger and Hadidi, 1991). In addition, MRI has better sensitivity in revealing granulomas appearing as hyper-intense areas on T2-weighted images, primarily located cortically or subcortically in brain areas (Jabbour et al., 2011). Altogether, although cerebral injury cases caused by *T. canis* is increased, it remains an enigma that the exact frequency of toxocariasis with cerebral involvement is currently unknown and our knowledge about the impact on the neuropsychology in humans remains sorely lacking (Holland and Hamilton, 2013). Moreover, asymptomatic CT is probably the common occurrence in CT cases which causes it to remain undiagnosed and underestimated (Sánchez et al., 2018).

5. Cerebral toxocariasis and immunopathogenesis

Magnaval et al. intended to characterise a recognisable cerebral syndrome associated with *Toxocara* infection among French adults, and they concluded that migration of *Toxocara* larvae in the brain does not induce a recognisable neurological syndrome but is correlated with several risk factors, e.g., exposure to dogs, rural residence and dementia based on a case-control study (Magnaval et al., 1997). Although Worley et al. failed to establish a relationship between *Toxocara* seropositivity and cognitive abnormalities in young children after controlling for social class in two American studies (Worley et al., 1984), Marmor et al., on the contrary, suggested a role for toxocariasis in subtle effects on cognition (Marmor et al., 1987). In a Polish study, Jarosz et al. focused on the relationship

Table 1 Neurological manifestations in cerebral toxocariasis cases from January 1985 to August 2019.

Number	Neurological manifestations and patient's age	Diagnostic findings	Medication	Country	References
1	Cerebral vasculitis; 66-year-old woman	11% eosinophil in CSF; anti-*T. canis* IgG antibody in the blood and CSF (ELISA, WB)	Improved spontaneously without any anthelmintic treatment	France	Hamidou et al. (2002)
2	Cerebral vasculitis; 75-year-old woman	50% eosinophils in blood; MRI; anti-*T. canis* IgG antibody in the blood and CSF (ELISA, WB)	Albendazole + dexamethason	Austria	Helbok et al. (2007)
3	Cerebral vasculitis; 45-year-old man	Anti-*T. canis* IgE antibody in the blood and CSF (ELISA); Cerebral angiography	Unknown	France	Lompo et al. (2012)
4	Cerebral vasculitis; 49-year-old man	Anti-*T. canis* IgE antibody in the blood and CSF (ELISA)	Anthelmintic treatment	France	Lompo et al. (2012)
5	Eosinophilic meningitis; 11-year-old girl	30% eosinophil in CSF; anti-*T. canis* IgG antibody in the blood (ELISA)	Diethylcarbamazine	Britain	Gould et al. (1985)
6	Eosinophilic meningitis; 17-year-old boy	75% eosinophils in CSF; MRI; anti-*T. canis* IgG antibody in the blood and CSF (ELISA)	Albendazole	Korea	Noh et al. (2012)
7	Eosinophilic meningitis; 54-year-old man	CT; anti-*T. canis* IgG antibody in the blood (WB) + Toxocara DNA in CSF	Albendazole + corticosteroids	Italy	Caldera et al. (2013)

8	Eosinophilic encephalitis; 48-year-old woman	57% eosinophils in blood; MRI; CT; indirect immunofluorescence test; IQ of 90 reduced to 55 (WIP)	Diethylcarbamazine + Fenbendazole + prednisone	Germany	Sommer et al. (1994)
9	Eosinophilic meningoencephalitis; 18-year-old man	Eosinophilia in blood; CT; anti-*T. canis* IgG antibody in the blood (ELISA)	Thiabendazole + dexamethasone	Brazil	Barra et al. (1996)
10	Eosinophilic meningoencephalitis; 2-year-old boy	58% eosinophils in CSF; MRI; anti-*T. canis* IgG antibody in the blood and CSF (ELISA)	Albendazole + dexamethasone	Brazil	Vidal et al. (2003)
11	Eosinophilic meningoencephalitis; 54-year-old woman	36% eosinophils in CSF; CT; MRI; anti-*T. canis* IgG antibody in the blood and CSF (ELISA)	Albendazole + methylprednisolone	Greece	Xinou et al. (2003)
12	Eosinophilic meningoencephalitis; 5-year-old girl	57% eosinophils in CSF; MRI; anti-*T. canis* IgG antibody in the blood and CSF (ELISA)	Albendazole	Brazil	Moreira-Silva et al. (2004)
13	Eosinophilic meningoencephalitis; 45-year-old man	70% eosinophils in blood; CT	Albendazole + prednisolone	France	Mrissa et al. (2005)
14	Eosinophilic meningoencephalitis; 54-year-old woman	10% eosinophils in CSF; anti-*T. canis* IgG antibody in the blood and CSF (ELISA)	Albendazole + methylprednisolone	USA	Keller et al. (2008)

Continued

Table 1 Neurological manifestations in cerebral toxocariasis cases from January 1985 to August 2019.—Cont'd

Number	Neurological manifestations and patient's age	Diagnostic findings	Medication	Country	References
15	Bilateral subdural hematoma and a small subarachnoid haemorrhage; 2.5-year-old infant autopsy	*NA	*NA	Britain	Hill et al. (1985)
16	Fibrotic arachnoidea; 53-year-old woman	Granulomatous mass with *Toxocara* larva identified by histopathology	Surgery	Italy	Villano et al. (1992)
17	Cerebral meningoradiculitis	Eosinophilia in the CSF; anti-*T. canis* IgG antibody in the blood and CSF (Immunodiagnostic)	Unclear	France	Robinson et al. (2002)
18	Seizure; 1-year-old boy	58% eosinophils in blood; CT; anti-*T. canis* IgG antibody in the blood (ELISA)	Thiabendazole + prednisolone	USA	Fortenberry et al. (1991)
19	Seizure; 26-year-old woman	6% eosinophils in blood; CT; Cranial MRI; anti-*T. canis* IgG antibody in the blood (ELISA)	Diethylcarbamazine	Germany	Rüttinger and Hadidi (1991)
20	Epileptic seizure; 7-year-old girl	9% eosinophils in blood; CT scan and MRI; *T. canis* larva identified in histological section	Mebendazole	Poland	Kazek et al. (2006)
21	Seizures; 13-year-old girl	CT scan, MRI, Histopathology	Albendazole	India	Jarosz et al. (2010)

22	Epileptic seizure; 11-year-old girl	9.5% eosinophils in blood; CT scan, MRI; anti-*T. canis* IgG antibody in the blood (ELISA)	Albendazole	Switzerland	Bachli et al. (2004)
23	Cognitive impairments and dementia; 65-year-old woman	Eosinophilia in CSF; CT; EEG; anti-*T. canis* IgG antibody in the CSF (ELISA)	Albendazole	Germany	Richaratz and Buchkremer (2002)
24	Cognitive impairments; 45-year-old man	Normal eosinophils in CSF; MRI; anti-*T. canis* IgG antibody in the blood and CSF (WB)	Albendazole + prednisolone	Germany	Scheid et al. (2008)
25	Encephalitis/brain abscess; 56-year-old woman	Normal eosinophils in blood; MRI; anti-*T. canis* IgG antibody in the blood and CSF (WB)	Albendazole	Turkey	Erdem Kivrak et al. (2014)
26	Multiple cerebral infarction; 39-year-old man	27.0% eosinophils in blood; MRI; anti-*T. canis* IgG antibody in the blood (ELISA)	Albendazole + prednisolone	Korea	Kwon (2015)
27	Juvenile myoclonic epilepsy; 19-year-old man	10.0% eosinophils in blood; MRI; anti-*T. canis* IgG antibody in the blood (ELISA)	Albendazole + valproic acid	Germany	Emmer et al. (2015)
28	Reversible cerebral vasoconstriction or vasculitis; A 38-year-old pregnant woman	33.0% eosinophils in blood; MRI; anti-*T. canis* IgG antibody in the blood (ELISA)	Albendazole + prednisolone	USA	Feske et al. (2015)

*NA, not available.

between *Toxocara* seropositivity and developmental age and physical fitness in over 200 children aged 14–16 years in a rural Polish village found that seropositive boys had significantly lower end-of-year grades than their sero-negative counterparts, providing an explanation that behavioural factors such as spending more time in playing outdoors rather than studying increased the frequently of exposing themselves to *Toxocara* infection (Jarosz et al., 2010). From these studies mentioned above, there is clearly a paucity of studies that provide evidence for the role of *Toxocara* in cognitive deficits in humans.

Since the studies concerning assessment of humoral and cellular immune response from CSF or brain of clinical CT patients are rare, mice have been utilised as a useful model for human *Toxocara* infection studies. Murine models have at least three excellent advantages as models for studying CT. Firstly, wild mice are known to be naturally infected with *Toxocara* (Dubinský et al., 1995); secondly, there is experimental evidence for larval accumulation over time (Dunsmore et al., 1983); and thirdly, mice with different genetic backgrounds, e.g., outbred or inbred, differ in their capacity to harbour larvae in the brain, suggesting the influence of host genetics and immunity on cerebral infection (Cox and Holland, 2001; Skerrett and Holland, 1997). Mice therefore, represent useful model systems to explore the impact of *Toxocara* on brain biology and behaviour, and provide possible insights into human CT.

Helminth infection induces a polarised Th2 response, typically various interleukins (IL), e.g., IL-4, IL-5 and IL-13 cytokines, that are involved in the activation of mast cells, eosinophils, and macrophages as well as high levels of IgE response. Triggering of the Th2 response normally may coincide with downmodulation of the Th1 inflammatory response along with reduced tumour necrosis factor alpha (TNF-α), interferon gamma (IFN-γ) and IL-17 expressions (Maizels, 2013). However, helminth parasites can evade the host immune system, e.g., by the activation of regulatory T cells that induce the production of downregulating cytokines, such as IL-10 and transforming growth factor beta (TGF-β) (Allen and Maizels, 2011). In the immunopathogenesis in toxocariasis, a careful balance among pro-, anti-inflammatory, and regulatory responses to *Toxocara* spp. are normally orchestrated by the immune system and have been confirmed by substantial studies, indirectly reflecting the immune systems often unsuccessful attempts to eradicate the long surviving larvae in paratenic hosts (Allen and Maizels, 2011; Fan et al., 2013; Maizels, 2013). Moreover, *T. canis* larvae do not reproduce in the mammalian paratenic host, and the long-term survival

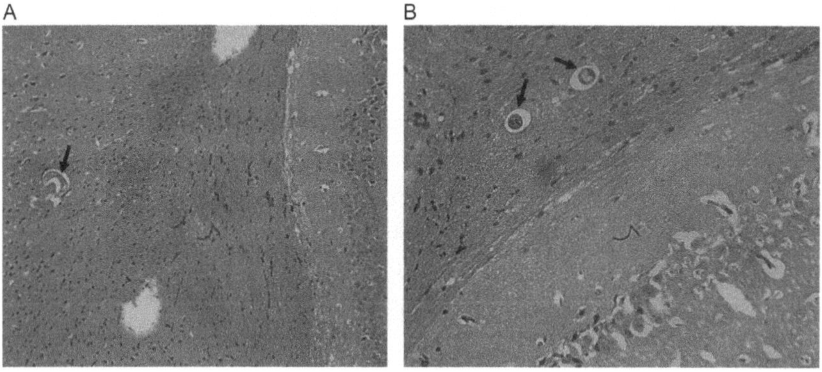

Fig. 3 Larval section of *Toxocara canis* found in the brain with no leukocyte infiltration from mice inoculated with a single dose of 250 embryonated eggs at (A) 8 weeks and (B) 12 weeks post-infection by pathological assessment with HE stains at 200 × magnification. Arrow indicates larval sections.

of larvae in the host may trigger systematic Th2 immune responses due to the multicellular nature of helminth that differ from immune responses to microbial pathogens (Maizels, 2013). However, most of the pathological studies on the brains of mice invaded by *T. canis* L3 larvae do not show any infiltrated leukocytes (Fig. 3), and most of the studies suggest that this is due to the brain per se being protected from host damage from invading pathogens and self-induced immune attacks (Holland and Hamilton, 2013).

It has been hypothesized that the symptoms or impairments may be relevant to the unclear mechanism of cytokines-or IL-causing inflammation during the *T. canis* larval invasion in the brain. In the study of Waindok and Strube (2019), they employed C57Bl/6J mice as paratenic host models to analyse 23 different cytokines and chemokines expressed during the course of *T. canis*-induced CT at six different time points at days 7, 14, 28, 42, 70 and 98 post-infection (pi) and found brain-body mass ratios of *T. canis*-infected mice were significantly lower than those of the uninfected control group at day 14 pi, and also at day 28 pi. Moreover, the study also showed a continuous decrease of pro-inflammatory cytokine concentrations, including TNF-α, IFN-γ, GM-CSF and IL-6, in the cerebrum over the course of infection. Additionally, *T. canis*-induced CT was characterised by significantly elevated levels of anti-inflammatory IL-4 and IL-5 in the cerebrum in the acute and subacute phase of the disease. The high neural affinity of *T. canis* led to a prominent increase of eotaxin and MIP-1α in the cerebrum. Their study provides valuable insights into key regulatory mechanisms of *Toxocara* species in paratenic hosts and the cerebral cyto-/chemokine milieu is shifted to a predominantly anti-inflammatory immune response during CT, possibly enabling both survival of the parasite and the neuro-infected paratenic host. Alteration of eotaxin and MIP-1α concentrations are congruent with the high neural affinity of *T. canis* and species-specific tropism of *T. canis* to the cerebrum.

T. canis L3 invading the human/mouse brain may result in symptoms such as motor impairments, as well as, behavioural alterations, memory impairment and cognitive dysfunctions, and in addition, a controversial cause of neuropsychological disturbances like seizure, schizophrenia, cognitive deficits or dementia (Fan et al., 2015; Holland and Hamilton, 2013).

5.1 Seizure

A seizure is a paroxysmal event due to an excessive, hypersynchronous signalling from CNS neurons or neuronal networks. This abnormal electrical activity causes a range of clinical/behavioural manifestations, such as, dramatic convulsions. Recent advances in experimental neuroscience have revealed that inflammation can facilitate seizures or sustain seizure activity. Two hypotheses have been linked to seizures. In the epileptic brain, neuroinflammation can exacerbate seizures or increase their frequency by directly effecting neurovascular and glial function. Moreover, the effects of systemic inflammation can be mediated or facilitated damage to the blood-brain barrier (BBB) by activation of circulating leukocytes and the release of molecular mediators that increase vascular permeability. In a study of the BBB related to CT, Liao et al. (2008b) evaluated the BBB permeability and BBB injury as assessed by the cerebral Evans blue (EB) concentration as well as by pathological changes and glial fibrillary acidic protein (GFAP) expression in *T. canis*-infected mice monitored from 3 days (dpi) to 8 weeks post-infection (wpi). They found that BBB permeability increased as evidenced by a significantly elevated EB concentration in brains of infected mice. BBB injury appeared due to enhanced GFAP protein and mRNA expressions from 4 to 8 wpi. Leukocytes might have been unrelated to BBB impairment because there was no inflammatory cell infiltration despite *T. canis* larvae having invaded the brain; whereas markedly elevated substance P (SP) protein and NK-1R mRNA expressions concomitant with enhanced claudin-5 expression seemed to be associated with persistent BBB impairment in this experimental CT model. Their study may provide a clue to further support the possible mechanism of seizures occurred to the CT due to persistent BBB impairment.

5.2 Schizophrenia

Schizophrenia is a severe, disabling mental disorder characterised by a range of clinical features such as positive and negative symptoms that can have a devastating impact on patients, their family, and society including the patients' health related quality of life (Brisch et al., 2014). The prevalence of schizophrenia has been estimated to be 1% of the adult population, developing in late adolescence or early adulthood lasting throughout their lifetime (Barch and Ceasar, 2012). Schizophrenia can cause cognitive deficits which may affect working memory, episodic memory, language and executive function, attention inhibition, processing speed, and sensory processing (Fabiani et al., 2013). The presence of *T. canis* larvae in the CNS may cause neurological and psychiatric disorders that could contribute to schizophrenia, but this association has received little attention in comparison to *Toxoplasma* (Carlsson and Lindqvist, 1963). The "original dopamine hypothesis" developed by Carlsson and Lindqvist (1963) states that alterations in dopamine (DP) results in schizophrenic symptoms. DP is produced in various structures of the brain including the substantia nigra, striatum, prefrontal cortex, ventral tegmental region, and hippocampus of the brain (Shen et al., 2012). Increased sub-cortical release of DP can cause the positive symptoms of schizophrenia, which include hallucinations and delusions. This is thought to be due to a disturbed cortical pathway through the nucleus accumbens resulting in an augmentation of D2 receptor activation. Decreased D1 receptor activation in the prefrontal cortex and decreased activity of the nucleus caudatus is thought to cause the negative symptoms of schizophrenia, which include anhedonia (i.e., inability to experience pleasure from enjoyable activities or social interactions), lack of motivation (Pogarell et al., 2012). The "revised dopamine hypothesis" proposes DP hyperactivity in the mesolimbic areas, particularly in the hippocampus, and DP hypoactivity in the prefrontal cortex in schizophrenia patients (Dickson and Briggs, 2013).

In a murine model, Othman et al. (2010) found that DP levels were significantly decreased over time in the brains of mice infected with *Toxocara*. In contrast, unpublished data indicating enhanced expressions of tyrosine hydroxylase (TH), which is capable of catalysing the conversion of the amino acid L-tyrosine to L-3,4-dihydroxy-phenylalanine (L-DOPA), a precursor for DP, was detected in the brains of *Toxocara*-infected ICR outbred mice (C.K. Fan et al., unpublished data). TH is present in the CNS, peripheral sympathetic neurons and the adrenal medulla. Substantial studies have indicated that alterations of TH activity may be involved in disorders such as schizophrenia (Kaplan et al., 2008). However, the role of the DP system as implicated in a schizophrenia disorder in CT remains to be elucidated comprehensively.

5.3 Cognitive deficits

Substantial studies have indicated that CNS inflammation is correlated with the cognitive dysfunction in a number of neurological diseases, e.g., Alzheimer's dementia, because CNS inflammation has been confirmed to be implicated in the development of amyloid neuritic plaques, one of the hallmarks of Alzheimer's disease (AD) (Gorelick, 2010). The impact of *T. canis* infection on cognitive development in humans is sorely lacking, with very few clinical or population-based studies having examined the relationship between *T. canis* seropositivity and neuropsychological parameters (Jarosz et al., 2010). Some clinical studies have described various cognitive deficits associated with infection including lack of developmental progress and speech, depressive symptoms and cognitive deficits possibly indicative of dementia, mental confusion and cognitive impairment, slowed cognitive information processing, impairments of short term and working memory spans, and mental fluency (Salvador et al., 2010).

At the population level, the first report was by Worley et al. (1984) who found an association between *T. canis* seropositivity and poor reading achievement, distractibility and lower intelligence in kindergarten children but the effects of social class were not considered in the analysis. Later, Marmor et al. (1987) undertook neuropsychological tests on children aged 1–15 years and found significant cognitive deficits in *T. canis* seropositive children compared with seronegative controls when adjusted for race, socioeconomic status and blood lead concentrations. Thereafter, Nelson et al. (1996) evaluated cognitive function in children aged 1–4 years and identified lower mental development scores and IQ levels in *T. canis* seropositive children, however, blood lead levels, which have been linked with cognitive impairment, were not assessed in these subjects.

In a significant advance, Walsh and Haseeb (2012), utilised data from the third National Health and Nutrition Examination Survey (1988–1994) to assess a large nationally representative sample of children (3949 subjects) living in the USA. The authors reported statistically lower cognitive scores on both the Wechsler Intelligence Scale for Children-Revised (WISC-R) and the Wide Range Achievement Test-Revised (WRAT-R) in seropositive children compared with seronegative children independent of socioeconomic status, rural residence, gender, ethnicity, cytomegalovirus infection and lead levels in blood. Nevertheless, establishing an etiological relationship between toxocariasis and diminished cognitive function warrants further comprehensive investigation.

Data from murine models on the relationship between *T. canis* infection, learning and memory may be particularly relevant to human infection (Fan et al., 2015; Holland and Hamilton, 2013). Cox and Holland (2001) utilised a novel environment containing a water-finding apparatus to test the ability of mice to remember the location of the resource, specifically measuring time to enter the alcove, find the water tube and drink from it. In outbred LACA mice, those with moderate to high levels of larvae in the brain showed a relative time latency compared with mice with zero to low larval load. Additionally, BALB/c mice infected with *Toxocara* took a statistically significantly longer time to find and drink from the tube than both control BALB/c mice and infected NIH mice, suggesting a degree of memory impairment. Additionally, studies have shown that memory impairment may be attributable to the location of the larval invasion in the brain, specifically, the telencephalon and the cerebellum, which are both areas of the brain associated with learning, memory, and the coordination and control of voluntary movement (Hamilton et al., 2006).

5.4 Idiopathic Parkinson disease

The idiopathic form of Parkinson disease (IPD) is one of the most common neurodegenerative disorders characterised by a progressive loss of dopaminergic (DA) neurons in the substantia nigra, leading to several clinical motor symptoms including rigidity, akinesia, and resting tremor. The molecular pathways resulting in these clinical alterations may be due to environmental factors or genetic influence, or a combination of both resulting in neuronal degeneration (Shulman et al., 2011). Oxidative stress, mitochondrial abnormalities, neuroinflammatory processes, cytokines, a rise in intracytoplasmic free calcium, excitatory amino acids and apoptotic processes have been implicated in the pathologic mechanism of the neurologic degeneration seen in IPD. Recently, both microglial and infiltrated peripheral immune cells and their neurotoxic products including pro-inflammatory cytokines, reactive oxygen species, and nitric oxide were implicated in the initiation of neuroinflammation responsible for the pathogenesis of IPD. The relationship between infectious agents and IPD remains unclear, although a few studies have indicated a possible role for infectious agents, e.g., influenza virus has been implicated in the pathogenesis of IPD (Tufekci et al., 2011).

T. canis larval invasion into the brain may cause neurological and psychiatric disorders that may include IPD; however, the relationship between *T. canis* infection and IPD has received little attention. The primary symptoms of IPD result from greatly reduced activity of DP-secreting cells caused by cell death in substantia nigra, specifically in the region of the pars compacta thus possibly leading to insufficient production of DP in certain neurons within parts of the midbrain (Shulman et al., 2011). Çelik et al. (2013) found that although seroprevalence of *T. canis* in patients with IPD (6.0%) was higher than that in the control groups (0%); no statistical difference was found. In a murine model, Othman et al. (2010) demonstrated a significant increase in gene expression of nitric oxide and pro-inflammatory cytokines in the brains of *Toxocara*-infected mice, especially in the chronic stage. Although pro-inflammatory cytokines can be neuro-protective, a sustained or overstimulated increase can result in deleterious effects on neurons. Particularly, when compared to uninfected mice, *T. canis*-infected mice showed significantly lower levels of GABA, DP, monoamines, and serotonin. As discussed in section Schizophrenia, our previous study found, in contrast, that DP expression increased in the brains of *Toxocara*-infected outbred ICR mice inoculated with a single dose of 250 *T. canis* infective eggs (Fan et al., unpublished data). This difference in DP expression between two animal studies warrants further investigation to further elucidate the possibility of DP-related IPD occurring in CT.

5.5 Dementia

The causes of dementia, a decline in cognitive function severe enough to affect social or occupational functioning, are complex and may be due to AD or vascular dementia (Sun et al., 2014). Pathogenesis of dementia is postulated to be very similar to that of cognitive dysfunction, indicating CNS inflammation is implicated in this neurodegenerative disease due to the development of amyloid neuritic plaques (Gorelick, 2010).

T. canis seroprevalence has been found to be higher among various patient groups with neuropsychiatric disorders, e.g., seizure, cognitive deficits, IPD and schizophrenia compared to control groups (Kamuyu et al., 2014; Walsh and Haseeb, 2012); however, clinical cases concerning the status of *T. canis* infection among dementia patient are rare. In Table 1, only one CT case who exhibited dementia and depression was reported by

Richaratz and Buchkremer (2002). In this case, a 65-year-old woman presenting with a long history of depression and cognitive decline was found to have eosinophilia and antibodies reactive against *T. canis* antigen in her CSF. The infection was possibly attributable to her occupation as a shepherd with a high frequency of close contact with dogs. Her cognitive deficits improved with albendazole. Nevertheless, *T. canis*-causing dementia cases are rarely reported and may be overlooked due to the fact that most human cases with CT do not present with significantly clinical neurological signs as a consequence of light parasitic burdens, and in addition, the longevity of *T. canis* larvae resident in the internal organs including the brain (Holland and Hamilton, 2013); therefore, a more comprehensive investigation of the link between CT and dementia is required.

6. A hypothesis: Cerebral toxocariasis may develop to Alzheimer's disease silently

Using the mouse model to study the impact of *Toxocara* infection behaviour, infected mice appear to be less active and explorative, less responsive to novelty, and less aversive to open areas and predator stimuli than uninfected animals. The abnormal behavioural changes are likely to be related to the location of *T. canis* larval invasion in the brain, the immune response directed against *T. canis* larvae and more importantly due to pathological effects rather than parasite-altered host behaviour. Experimental work in mice has established evidence that may have implications for human health. This includes differences in the number of larvae recovered from the brains of genetically different inbred mice infected with the same inoculum, patterns in cerebral larval distribution, behavioural alterations being dose-dependent, cerebral infection leading to deficits in learning and memory and infection inducing an inflammatory cerebral immune response (Holland and Hamilton, 2013). Chronic exposure to pro-inflammatory cytokines including IL-1β, IL-6, and TNF-α that promote neural injuries, may exacerbate the neurodegenerative progression and compromise vulnerable neurons (González et al., 2014). Our knowledge of the systemic immune response to *T. canis* greatly exceeds that of the immune response in the brain. Experiments conducted by Hamilton et al. (2008) showed that the cerebral immune response of *T. canis*-infected BALB/c mice exhibited significantly higher levels of mRNA for various cytokines including IL-5, IL-10, and IFN-γ and inducible nitric oxide synthase (iNOS) than *T. canis*-infected NIH mice, particularly on days 35 and 42 post-infection, and these responses are in accordance with observed behavioural alterations and memory impairment. Dantzer et al. (2008) proposed a term called "sickness behaviour" that was triggered by pro-inflammatory cytokines involved in an array of behavioural symptoms, e.g., decreased exploration, reduced learning and memory, and depressed locomotor activity. Additionally, they reported increased IL-1β levels were linked to learning and memory impairment, elucidating the interference of increased cytokine production with hippocampal-dependent memory storage. Moreover, Liao et al. (2008a) observed enhanced increases in several brain injury-associated biomarkers (BIABs) including TGF-β1 (transforming growth factor β1), GFAP (glial fibrillary acidic protein), NF-L (neurofilament light chain), S100B, AβPP (β-amyloid precursor proteins), TG 2 (tissue transglutaminases) and p-tau in brains of ICR outbred mice inoculated with a single dose of 250 *T. canis* infective eggs. In addition, these authors also assessed blood-brain barrier (BBB) impairment through cerebral Evans blue (EB) concentration, pathological changes and GFAP expression in a similar experiment and concluded that abnormal BBB permeability and cerebral injury increased with the duration of infection but not the numbers of larvae in the brain (Liao et al., 2008b). Liao et al. (2008a), meanwhile, also indicated that enhanced BIABs expressions, which may be deleterious to the brain, can be attributed to UPS (ubiquitin proteasome system) dysfunction that is unable to degrade unwanted, misfolded, or damaged proteins, which can potentially form toxic aggregates in the brain of *T. canis*-infected mice. It has been hypothesized that elevated ubiquitin conjugates leading to intracellular deposits of aggregated protein found in many sporadic and hereditary neurodegenerative diseases, suggestive of a link between UPS dysfunction and pathogenesis, such as the case of Alzheimer's disease (AD) (Wang and Saunders, 2014). Therefore, cerebral infection by *T. canis* may increase the risk of developing neurodegenerative disease such as AD.

A further study focuses on the hippocampus which has long been recognised as being responsible for learning and memory functions, being *Toxocaral* invasion of this site may cause neuroinflammatory and neurodegenerative disorders. Results indicated there was an insignificant difference in learning and memory function between the experimental mice and uninfected control mice, which was assessed by pathological changes, expressions of neurodegeneration-associated factors (NDAFs), including TGF-β1, S100B, GFAP, TG2, claudin-5, substance P (SP) and IL-1β, and the UPS function as well as associated cognitive behaviour in ICR mice orally inoculated with a high (1000 eggs), medium (500 eggs) or low-dose (250 eggs) of *T. canis* embryonated eggs during a 20-week investigation, possibly because the site where *T. canis* larvae invaded was the surrounding area but not the hippocampus per se. Nevertheless, enhanced expressions of NDAFs, persistent UPS impairment and excess Aβ42 accumulation concomitantly emerged in the hippocampus of the experimental mice at 8, 16, and 20 wpi. We thus postulate that progressive CT may still progress into neurodegeneration due to enhanced NDAFs expressions, persistent UPS impairment and excess Aβ accumulation in the hippocampus (Chou et al., 2017). In addition, whether the excretory-secretory antigens (TcES Ag) secreted from *T. canis* larvae might have the cytotoxic effects on astrocytes was also assessed by apoptosis and autophagy expression. The results showed TcES Ag treatment reduced astrocytes viability and caused morphological changes. Expressions of autophagy associated proteins including Beclin 1, phosphor-mTOR and LC3-II was not significantly

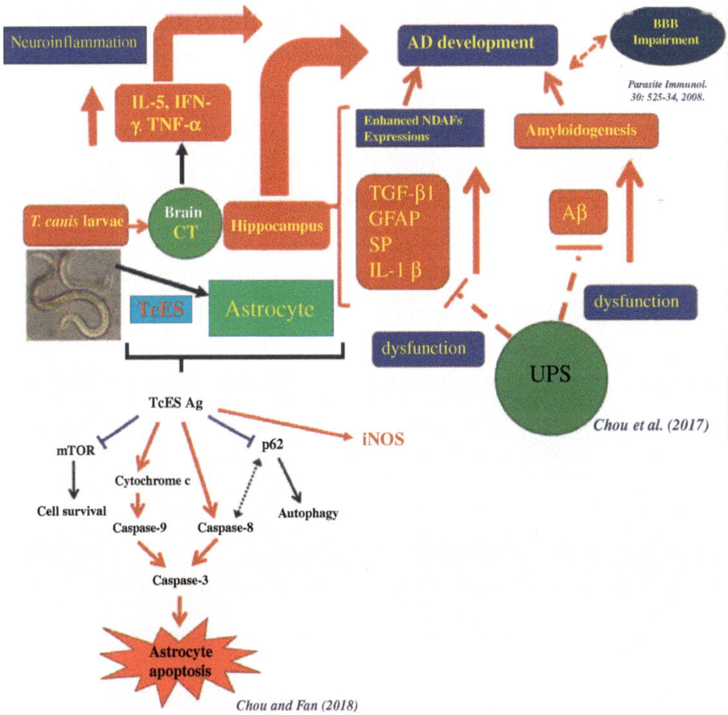

Fig. 4 Hypothesis illustration: Cerebral toxocariasis may progress to Alzheimer's disease owing to neuroinflammation, blood-brain barrier dysfunction, enhanced neurodegeneration-associated factors (NDAFs) expression, aberrant amyloidogenesis, ubiquitin proteasome system impairment and significant astrocytic apoptosis. *Reuse permission from Elsevier, Licence No. 4686621130892.*

changed; however, p62 as well as the cell survival protein, mTOR, was concomitantly decreased in TcES Ag treatment. Significantly accelerated cleaved caspase-3 and cytochrome *c* expression as well as enhanced caspase-9 and caspase-8 activation were found in astrocytes stimulated by TcES Ag. Caspase-3 activity and apoptotic cells numbers were also increased as detected by fluorescence microscopy. It can be concluded that TcES Ag may trigger astrocytes apoptosis predominantly through intrinsic and extrinsic pathways rather autophagy, revealing a novel role of astrocytes in the pathogenesis of CT (Chou and Fan, 2018). Furthermore, Othman et al. (2010) demonstrated increased levels of pro-inflammatory cytokines including IL-6, TNF-α, and iNOS, significant disturbances in neurotransmitters, and enhanced expression of GFAP in *T. canis*-infected mice brain were more apparent in the chronic stage of infection. Of particular importance was their novel observation that the normal pattern of neurotransmitters, e.g., GABA, dopamine, and serotonin, were disrupted as a result of *T. canis* infection. Since changes in neurotransmitter patterns have been linked to various clinical manifestations in humans, including seizures, behavioural disturbances, and enhanced pro-inflammatory cytokine expressions, this may provide an explanation of the behavioural and cognitive impairments seen in cerebral toxocariasis. Illustration of the hypothesis that cerebral toxocariasis may progress to Alzheimer's disease due to neuroinflammation, blood-brain barrier dysfunction, enhanced neurodegeneration-associated factors (NDAFs) expression, amyloidogenesis, ubiquitin proteasome system impairment and astrocyte apoptosis that can be seen in Fig. 4.

References

Allen, J.E., Maizels, R.M., 2011. Diversity and dialogue in immunity to helminths. Nat. Rev. Immunol. 11, 375–388.

Azam, D., Ukpai, O.M., Said, A., Abd-Allah, G.A., Morgan, E.R., 2012. Temperature and the development and survival of infective canis larvae. Parasitol. Res. 110, 649–656.

Bachli, H., Minet, J.C., Gratzl, O., 2004. Cerebral toxocariasis: a possible cause of epileptic seizure in children. Childs Nerv. Syst. 63, 301–387.

Barch, D.M., Ceasar, A., 2012. Cognition in schizophrenia: core psychological and neural mechanisms. Trends Cogn. Sci. 16, 27–34.

Barra, L.A., dos Santos, W.F., Chieffi, P.P., Bedaque, E.A., Salles, P.S., Capitão, C.G., Vianna, S., Hanna, R., Pedretti Júnior, L., 1996. Visceral larva migrans: a mixed form of presentation in an adult. The clinical and laboratory aspects. Rev. Soc. Bras. Med. Trop. 29, 373–376.

Barry, M.A., Weatherhead, J.E., Hotez, P.J., Woc-Colburn, L., 2013. Childhood parasitic infections endemic to the United States. Pediatr. Clin. N. Am. 60, 471–485.

Batchelor, D.J., Tzannes, S., Graham, P.A., Wastling, J.M., Pinchbeck, G.L., German, A.J., 2008. Detection of endoparasites with zoonotic potential in dogs with gastrointestinal disease in the UK. Transbound. Emerg. Dis. 55, 99–104.

Brisch, R., Saniotis, A., Wolf, R., Bielau, H., Bernstein, H.G., Steiner, J., Bogerts, B., Braun, A.K., Jankowski, Z., Kumaritlake, J., Henneberg, M., Gos, T., 2014. The role of dopamine in schizophrenia from a neurobiological and evolutionary perspective: old fashioned, but still in vogue. Front. Psych. 5, 47.

Caldera, F., Burlone, M.E., Genchi, C., Pirisi, M., Bartoli, E., 2013. *Toxocara* encephalitis presenting with autonomous nervous system involvement. Infection 41, 691–694.

Carlsson, A., Lindqvist, M., 1963. Effect of chlorpromazine or haloperidolon formation of 3-methoxytyramine and normetanephrine in mouse brain. Acta Pharmacol. Toxicol. 20, 140–144.

Çelik, T., Kaplan, Y., Ataş, E., Öztuna, D., Berilgen, S., 2013. *Toxocara* seroprevalence in patients with idiopathic Parkinson's disease: chance association or coincidence? Biomed. Res. Int. 2013, 685196.

Chou, C.M., Fan, C.K., 2018. Significant apoptosis rather autophagy predominates in astrocytes caused by *Toxocara canis* larval excretory-secretory antigens. J. Microbiol. Immunol. Infect. pii: S1684-1182(18)30223-8.

Chou, C.M., Lee, Y.L., Liao, C.W., Huang, Y.C., Fan, C.K., 2017. Enhanced expressions of neurodegeneration-associated factors, UPS impairment, and excess Aβ accumulation in the hippocampus of mice with persistent cerebral toxocariasis. Parasit. Vectors 10, 620.

Cox, D.M., Holland, C.V., 2001. Relationship between three intensity levels of *Toxocara canis* larvae in the brain and effects on exploration, anxiety, learning and memory in the murine host. J. Helminthol. 75, 33–41.

Dantzer, R., O'Connor, J.C., Freund, G.G., Johnson, R.W., Kelley, K.W., 2008. From inflammation to sickness and depression: when the immune system subjugates the brain. Nat. Rev. Neurosci. 9, 46–56.

Deshayes, S., Bonhomme, J., de La Blanchardière, A., 2016. Neurotoxocariasis: a systematic literature review. Infection 44, 565–574.

Despommier, D., 2003. Toxocariasis: clinical aspects, epidemiology, medical ecology, and molecular aspects. Clin. Microbiol. Rev. 16, 265–272.

Dickson, P.W., Briggs, G.D., 2013. Tyrosine hydroxylase: regulation by feedback inhibition and phosphorylation. Adv. Pharmacol. 68, 13–21.

Dubinský, P., Havasiová-Reiterová, K., Petko, B., Hovorka, I., Tomasovicová, O., 1995. Role of small mammals in the epidemiology of toxocariasis. Parasitology 110, 187–193.

Dunsmore, J.D., Thompson, R.C.A., Bates, I.A., 1983. The accumulation of *Toxocara canis* larvae in the brains of mice. Int. J. Parasitol. 13, 517–521.

Emmer, A., Surov, A., Kornhuber, M.E., 2015. Incidental cerebral toxocarosis as confirmed by cerebrospinal fluid cytology. Am. J. Med. 128, e35–e36.

Erdem Kivrak, E., Sıpahi, O.R., Korkmaz, M., Işikgöz Taşbakan, M., Pullukçu, H., Arda, B., Yamazhan, T., Ulusoy, S., 2014. A rarely seen cause of brain abscess: neurotoxocariasis. Mikrobiyol. Bul. 48, 507–511.

Fabiani, S., Pinto, B., Bruschi, F., 2013. Toxoplasmosis and neuropsychiatric diseases: can serological studies establish a clear relationship? Neurol. Sci. 34, 417–425.

Fakhri, Y., Gasser, R.B., Rostami, A., Fan, C.K., Ghasemi, S.M., Javanian, M., Bayani, M., Armoon, B., Moradi, B., 2018. *Toxocara* eggs in public places worldwide—a systematic review and meta-analysis. Environ. Pollut. 242, 1467–1475.

Fan, C.K., Lin, Y.H., Du, W.Y., Su, K.E., 2003. Infectivity and pathogenicity of 14-month-cultured embryonated eggs of *Toxocara canis* in mice. Vet. Parasitol. 113, 145–155.

Fan, C.K., Liao, C.W., Cheng, Y.C., 2013. Factors affecting disease manifestation of toxocarosis in humans: genetics and environment. Vet. Parasitol. 193, 342–352.

Fan, C.K., Holland, C.V., Loxton, K., Barghouth, U., 2015. Cerebral toxocariasis: silent progression to neurodegenerative disorders? Clin. Microbiol. Rev. 28, 663–686.

Feske, S.K., Goldberg, M., Dudzinski, D.M., Gonzalez, R.G., Keggsch, A.E., 2015. A 38-year-old pregnant woman with headache and visual symptoms. N. Engl. J. Med. 373, 1154–1164.

Fillaux, J., Magnaval, J.F., 2013. Laboratory diagnosis of human toxocariasis. Vet. Parasitol. 193, 327–336.

Fisher, M., 2003. *Toxocara cati*: an underestimated zoonotic agent. Trends Parasitol. 19, 167–170.

Fortenberry, J.D., Kenney, R.D., Younger, J., 1991. Visceral larval migrans producing static encephalopathy in an infant. Pediatr. Infect. Dis. J. 10, 403–406.

Glickman, L.T., Schantz, P.M., 1981. Epidemiology and pathogenesis of zoonotic toxocariasis. Epidemiol. Rev. 3, 230–250.

González, H., Elgueta, D., Montoya, A., Pacheco, R., 2014. Neuroimmune regulation of microglial activity involved in neuroinflammation and neurodegenerative diseases. J. Neuroimmunol. 274, 1–13.

Gorelick, P.B., 2010. Role of inflammation in cognitive impairment: results of observational epidemiological studies and clinical trials. Ann. N. Y. Acad. Sci. 1207, 155–162.

Gould, I.M., Newell, S., Green, S.H., George, R.H., 1985. Toxocariasis and eosinophilic meningitis. Br. Med. J. 291, 1239–1240.

Hamidou, M.A., Fradet, G., Kadi, A.M., Robin, A., Moreau, A., Magnaval, J.F., 2002. Systemic vasculitis with lymphocytic temporal arteritis and *Toxocara canis* infection. Arch. Intern. Med. 162, 1521–1524.

Hamilton, C.M., Stafford, P., Pinelli, E., Holland, C.V., 2006. A murine model for cerebral toxocariasis: characterization of host susceptibility and behaviour. Parasitology 132, 791–801.

Hamilton, C.M., Brandes, S., Holland, C.V., Pinelli, E., 2008. Cytokine expression in the brains of *Toxocara canis*-infected mice. Parasite Immunol. 30, 181–185.

Helbok, R., Brenneis, C., Engelhardt, K., Beer, R., Lackner, P., Brössner, G., Pfausler, B., Schmutzhard, E., 2007. A rare case of *Toxocara canis* cerebral vasculitis. Eur. J. Neurol. 14, e49.

Hill, I.R., Denham, D.A., Scholtz, C.L., 1985. *Toxocara canis* larvae in the brain of a British child. Trans. R. Soc. Trop. Med. Hyg. 79, 351–354.

Hoffmeister, B., Glaeser, S., Flick, H., Pornschlegel, S., Suttorp, N., Bergmann, F., 2007. Cerebral toxocariasis after consumption of raw duck liver. Am. J. Trop. Med. Hyg. 76, 600–602.

Holland, C.V., Hamilton, C.M., 2013. The significance of cerebral toxocariasis: a model system for exploring the link between brain involvement, behaviour and the immune response. J. Exp. Biol. 216, 78–783.

Hotez, P.J., Wilkins, P.P., 2009. Toxocariasis: America's most common neglected infection of poverty and a helminthiasis of global importance? PLoS Negl. Trop. Dis. 3, e400.

Jabbour, R.A., Kanj, S.S., Sawaya, R.A., Awar, G.N., Hourani, M.H., Atweh, S.F., 2011. *Toxocara canis* myelitis: clinical features, magnetic resonance imaging (MRI) findings, and treatment outcome in 17 patients. Medicine 90, 337–343.

Jarosz, W., Mizgajska-Wiktor, H., Kirwan, P., Konarski, J., Rychlicki, W., Wawrzyniak, G., 2010. Developmental age, physical fitness and *Toxocara* seroprevalence amongst lower-secondary students living in rural areas contaminated with *Toxocara* eggs. Parasitology 137, 53–63.

Kamuyu, G., Bottomley, C., Mageto, J., Lowe, B., Wilkins, P.P., Noh, J.C., Nutman, T.B., Ngugi, A.K., Odhiambo, R., Wagner, R.G., Kakooza-Mwesige, A., Owusu-Agyei, S., Ae-Ngibise, K., Masanja, H., Osier, F.H., Odermatt, P., Newton, C.R., 2014. Study of epidemiology of epilepsy in demographic sites (SEEDS) group. Exposure to multiple parasites is associated with the prevalence of active convulsive epilepsy in sub-Saharan Africa. PLoS Negl. Trop. Dis. 8, e2908.

Kaplan, M., Kalkan, A., Kuk, S., Demirdag, K., Ozden, M., Kilic, S.S., 2008. *Toxocara* seroprevalence in schizophrenic patients in Turkey. Yonsei Med. J. 49, 224–229.

Kazek, B., Jamroz, E., Mandera, M., Bierzyńska-Macyszyn, G., Kluczewska, E., Marszał, E., 2006. The cerebral form of toxocarosis in a seven-year-old patient. Folia Neuropathol. 44, 72–76.

Keller, M., Pavia, A.T., Byington, C.L., 2008. Possible intrafamilial transmission of *Toxocara* causing eosinophilic meningitis in an infant. Pediatr. Infect. Dis. J. 27, 849–850.

Kwon, H.H., 2015. Toxocariasis: a rare cause of multiple cerebral infarction. Infect. Chemother. 47, 137–141.

Lee, I.H., Kim, S.T., Oh, D.K., Kim, H.J., Kim, K.H., Jeon, P., Byun, H.S., 2010. MRI findings of spinal visceral larva migrans of *Toxocara canis*. Eur. J. Radiol. 75, 236–240.

Liao, C.W., Fan, C.K., Kao, T.C., Ji, D.D., Su, K.E., Lin, Y.H., Cho, W.L., 2008a. Brain injury-associated biomarkers of TGF-beta1, S100B, GFAP, NF-L, tTG, AbetaPP, and tau were concomitantly enhanced and the UPS was impaired during acute brain injury caused by *Toxocara canis* in mice. BMC Infect. Dis. 8, 84.

Liao, C.W., Cho, W.L., Kao, T.C., Su, K.E., Lin, Y.H., Fan, C.K., 2008b. Blood-brain barrier impairment with enhanced SP, NK-1R, GFAP and claudin-5 expressions in experimental cerebral toxocariasis. Parasite Immunol. 30, 525–534.

Lompo, L.D., Kamdem, F.K., Revenco, E., Allibert, R., Medeiros, E., Vuillier, F., Moulin, T., 2012. *Toxocara canis* cerebral vasculitis revealed by iterative strokes. Rev. Neurol. (Paris) 168, 533–537.

Ma, G., Holland, C.V., Wang, T., Hofmann, A., Fan, C.K., Maizels, R.M., Hotez, P.J., Gasser, R.B., 2018. Human toxocariasis. Lancet Infect. Dis. 18, e14–e24.

Macuheggs, K., Akao, N., Fujinami, Y., Kumagai, T., Ohta, N., 2013. Contamination, distribution and pathogenicity of *Toxocara canis* and *T. cati* eggs from sandpits in Tokyo, Japan. J. Helminthol. 87, 271–276.

Magnaval, J.F., Galindo, V., Glickman, L.T., Clanet, M., 1997. Human *Toxocara* infection of the central nervous system and neurological disorders: a case control study. Parasitology 115, 537–543.

Magnaval, J.F., Glickman, L.T., Dorchies, P., Morassin, B., 2001. Highlights of human toxocariasis. Korean J. Parasitol. 39, 1–11.

Maizels, R.M., 2013. *Toxocara canis*: molecular basis of immune recognition and evasion. Vet. Parasitol. 193, 365–374.

Marmor, M., Glickman, L., Shofer, F., Faich, L.A., Rosenberg, C., Cornblatt, B., Friedman, S., 1987. *Toxocara canis* infection of children: epidemiologic and neuropsychologic findings. Am. J. Public Health 77, 554–559.

Moiyadi, A., Mahadevan, A., Anandh, B., Shivashankar, R.S., Chickabasavaiah, Y.T., Shankar, S.K., 2007. Visceral larva migrans presenting as multiple intracranial and intraspinal abscesses. Neuropathology 27, 371–374.

Moreira-Silva, S.F., Rodrigues, M.G., Pimenta, J.L., Gomes, C.P., Freire, L.H., Pereira, F.E., 2004. Toxocariasis of the central nervous system: with report of two cases. Rev. Soc. Bras. Med. Trop. 37, 169–174.

Mrissa, R., Battikh, R., Ben Abdelhafidh, N., Jemli, B., Azzouz, O., Zaouali, J., Louzir, B., M'sadek, F., Ben Abdallah, N., Gargouri, S., Yedeas, M., Othmani, S., 2005. *Toxocara canis* encephalitis: case report. Rev. Med. Interne 26, 829–832.

Nelson, S., Greene, T., Ernhart, C.B., 1996. *Toxocara canis* infection in preschool age children: risk factors and the cognitive development of preschool children. Neurotoxicol. Teratol. 18, 167–174.

Noh, Y., Hong, S.T., Yun, J.Y., Park, H.K., Oh, J.H., Kim, Y.E., Jeon, B.S., 2012. Meningitis by *Toxocara canis* after ingestion of raw ostrich liver. J. Korean Med. Sci. 27, 1105–1108.

Othman, A.A., Abdel-Aleem, G.A., Saied, E.M., Mayah, W.W., Elatrash, A.M., 2010. Biochemical and immunopathological changes in experimental neurotoxocariasis. Mol. Biochem. Parasitol. 172, 1–8.

Overgaauw, P.A., van Knapen, F., 2013. Veterinary and public health aspects of *Toxocara* spp. Vet. Parasitol. 193, 398–403.

Pogarell, O., Koch, W., Karch, S., Dehning, S., Müller, N., Tatsch, K., Poepperl, G., Möller, H.J., 2012. Dopaminergic neurotransmission in patients with schizophrenia in relation to positive and negative symptoms. Pharmacopsychiatry 45, S36–S41.

Richaratz, E., Buchkremer, G., 2002. Cerebral toxocariasis: a rare cause of cognitive disorders. A contribution to differential dementia diagnosis. Nervenarzt 73, 458–462.

Robinson, A., Tannier, C., Magnaval, J.F., 2002. *Toxocara canis* meningoradiculitis. Rev. Neurol. 158, 351–353.

Rubel, D., Zunino, G., Santillán, G., Wisnivesky, C., 2003. Epidemiology of *Toxocara canis* in the dog population from two areas of different socioeconomic status, Greater Buenos Aires, Argentina. Vet. Parasitol. 115, 275–286.

Rüttinger, P., Hadidi, H., 1991. MRI in cerebral toxocaral disease. J. Neurol. Neurosurg. Psychiatry 54, 361–362.

Salvador, S., Ribeiro, R., Winckler, M.I., Ohlweiler, L., Riesgo, R., 2010. Pediatric neurotoxocariasis with concomitant cerebral, cerebellar, and peripheral nervous system involvement: case report and review of the literature. J. Pediatr. 86, 531–534.

Sánchez, S.S., García, H.H., Nicoletti, A., 2018. Clinical and magnetic resonance imaging findings of neurotoxocariasis. Front. Neurol. 9, 53.

Scheid, R., Tina Jentzsch, R., Schroeter, M.L., 2008. Cognitive dysfunction, urinary retention, and a lesion in the thalamus–beware of possible toxocariasis of the central nervous system. Clin. Neurol. Neurosurg. 110, 1054–1057.

Shen, L.H., Liao, M.H., Tseng, Y.C., 2012. Recent advances in imaging of dopaminergic neurons for evaluation of neuropsychiatric disorders. J. Biomed. Biotechnol. 2012, 259349.

Shulman, J.M., De Jager, P.L., Feany, M.B., 2011. Parkinson's disease: genetics and pathogenesis. Annu. Rev. Pathol. 6, 193–222.

Skerrett, H., Holland, C.V., 1997. Variation in the larval recovery of *Toxocara canis* from the murine brain: implications for behavioural studies. J. Helminthol. 71, 253–255.

Smith, H., Holland, C., Taylor, M., Magnaval, J.F., Schantz, P., Maizels, R., 2009. How common is human toxocariasis? Towards standardizing our knowledge. Trends Parasitol. 25, 182–188.

Sommer, C., Ringelstein, E.B., Biniek, R., Glöckner, W.M., 1994. Adult *Toxocara canis* encephalitis. J. Neurol. Neurosurg. Psychiatry 57, 229–231.

Sowemimo, O.A., 2007. Prevalence and intensity of *Toxocara canis* (Werner, 1782) in dogs and its potential public health significance in Ile-Ife, Nigeria. J. Helminthol. 81, 433–438.

Sowemimo, O.A., Lee, Y.L., Asaolu, S.O., Chuang, T.W., Akinwale, O.P., Badejoko, B.O., Gyang, V.P., Nwafor, T., Henry, E., Fan, C.K., 2017. Seroepidemiological study and associated risk factors of *Toxocara canis* infection among preschool children in Osun State, Nigeria. Acta Trop. 173, 85–89.

Sprent, J.F.A., 1956. The life history and development of *Toxocara cati* (Shrank 1788) in the domestic cat. Parasitology 46, 54–78.

Sun, Y., Lee, H.J., Yang, S.C., Chen, T.F., Lin, K.N., Lin, C.C., Wang, P.N., Tang, L.Y., Chiu, M.J., 2014. A nationwide survey of mild cognitive impairment and dementia, including very mild dementia, in Taiwan. PLoS One 9, e100303.

Takeuchi-Storm, N., Mejer, H., Al-Sabi, M.N.S., Olsen, C.S., Thamsborg, S.M., Enemark, H.L., 2015. Gastrointestinal parasites of cats in Denmark assessed by necropsy and concentration McMaster technique. Vet. Parasitol. 214, 327–332.

Tufekci, K.U., Genc, S., Genc, K., 2011. The endotoxin-induced neuroinflammation model of Parkinson's disease. Parkinsons Dis. 2011, 487450.

Vidal, J.E., Sztajnbok, J., Seguro, A.C., 2003. Eosinophilic meningoencephalitis due to *Toxocara canis*: case report and review of the literature. Am. J. Trop. Med. Hyg. 69, 341–343.

Villano, M., Cerillo, A., Narciso, N., Vizioli, L., Del Basso De Caro, M., 1992. A rare case of *Toxocara canis* arachnoidea. J. Neurosurg. Sci. 36, 67–69.

Waindok, P., Strube, C., 2019. Neuroinvasion of *Toxocara canis*- and *T. cati*-larvae mediates dynamic changes in brain cytokine and chemokine profile. J. Neuroinflammation 16, 147.

Walsh, M.G., Haseeb, M.A., 2012. Reduced cognitive function in children with toxocariasis in a nationally representative sample of the United States. Int. J. Parasitol. 42, 1159–1163.

Wang, H., Saunders, A.J., 2014. The role of ubiquitin-proteasome in the metabolism of amyloid precursor protein (APP): implications for novel therapeutic strategies for Alzheimer's disease. Discov. Med. 18, 41–50.

Worley, G., Green, J.A., Frothingham, T.E., Sturner, R.A., Walls, K.W., Pakalnis, V.A., Ellis Jr., G.S., 1984. *Toxocara canis* infection: clinical and epidemiological associations with seropositivity in kindergarten children. J. Infect. Dis. 149, 591–597.

Xinou, E., Lefkopoulos, A., Gelagoti, M., Drevelegas, A., Diakou, A., Milonas, I., Dimitriadis, A.S., 2003. CT and MR imaging findings in cerebral toxocaral disease. Am. J. Neuroradiol. 24, 714–718.

Yamasaki, H., Araki, K., Lim, P.K., Zasmy, N., Mak, J.W., Taib, R., Aoki, T., 2000. Development of a highly specific recombinant *Toxocara canis* second-stage larva excretory-secretory antigen for immunodiagnosis of human toxocariasis. J. Clin. Microbiol. 38, 1409–1413.

Yunus, M.H., Tan Farrizam, S.N., Abdul Karim, I.Z., Noordin, R., 2018. A lateral flow rapid test for human toxocariasis developed using three *Toxocara canis* recombinant antigens. Am. J. Trop. Med. Hyg. 98, 32–38.

Further reading

Anthony, R.M., Rutitzky, L.I., Urban, J.F., Stadecker, M.J., Gause, W.C., 2007. Protective immune mechanisms in helminth infection. Nat. Rev. Immunol. 7, 975–987.

Cox, D.M., Holland, C.V., 1998. The relationship between numbers of larvae recovered from the brain of *Toxocara canis*-infected mice and social behaviour and anxiety in the host. Parasitology 116, 579–594.

Dupas, B., Barrier, J., Barre, P., 1986. Detection of *Toxocara* by computed tomography. Br. J. Radiol. 59, 518–519.

Rostami, A., Ma, G., Wang, T., Koehler, A.V., Hofmann, A., Chang, B.C.H., Macpherson, C.N., Gasser, R.B., 2019. Human toxocariasis—a look at a neglected disease through an epidemiological 'prism'. Infect. Genet. Evol. 74, 104002.

CHAPTER THIRTEEN

Neurocognitive and neuropsychiatric effects of toxocariasis

Shawn D. Gale[a,b,*], Dawson W. Hedges[a,b]

[a]Department of Psychology, Brigham Young University, Provo, UT, United States
[b]The Neuroscience Centre, Brigham Young University, Provo, UT, United States
*Corresponding author: e-mail address: shawn_gale@byu.edu

Contents

Abstract

Caused by the neuroinvasive nematodes *Toxocara canis* and *Toxocara cati*, human toxocariasis has a worldwide distribution with seroprevalence in humans associated with low socioeconomic status and low educational attainment. Third-stage *Toxocara* larvae can invade human tissues, including the brain and spine, where they can result in encephalitis, meningitis, and inflammation. *Toxocara* infection in animal models has been associated with cognitive and behavioural changes. In humans, preliminary cross-sectional research suggests that *Toxocara* seropositivity is associated with worse cognitive function in children and adults. Additional preliminary cross-sectional findings suggest associations between *Toxocara* seropositivity and neuropsychiatric function, including schizophrenia and neurologic conditions such as epilepsy. Given the widespread distribution of human toxocariasis and early evidence suggesting that it can be associated with cognitive and neuropsychiatric function in humans, additional research regarding the effects of toxocariasis on the human brain is required.

Advances in Parasitology, Volume 109
ISSN 0065-308X
https://doi.org/10.1016/bs.apar.2020.01.009

1. Introduction

Caused by the closely related nematodes *Toxocara canis* and *Toxocara cati* that infect the definitive hosts dogs and cats, respectively, throughout much of the world (Holland and Hamilton, 2013), human toxocariasis can have a variety of manifestations in humans including common or covert toxocariasis (Ma et al., 2018), visceral larval migrans, ocular larval migrans, and neurotoxocariasis (Deshayes et al., 2016). Because humans are a paratenic host for *Toxocara canis* and *Toxocara cati*, the nematode is unable to mature in humans (Ma et al., 2018); however, third-stage *Toxocara* larvae from eggs ingested from the environment and larvae ingested from inadequately cooked meat of other paratenic hosts can invade human tissues including the brain (Holland and Hamilton, 2013). Considered a neglected parasitic infection (Hotez and Wilkins, 2009; Woodhall and Fiore, 2014), human toxocariasis has a worldwide distribution with a seroprevalence that varies widely (Rostami et al., 2019; Rubinsky-Elefant et al., 2010), ranging from 2.4% in Denmark (Stensvold et al., 2009) through 5.1% in the United States (Berrett et al., 2017) and 51% in South Korea (Lee et al., 2015) to as high as 80% in some regions of Africa (Lotsch et al., 2017) and over 90% in La Réunion France (Macpherson, 2013). Moreover, some findings suggest that the seroprevalence of toxocariasis might become higher due to its increasing geographic distribution, increasing urban density, and increasing numbers of untreated and/or stray dogs and cats (Macpherson, 2013). In humans, *Toxocara* seroprevalence varies according to age, sex, educational attainment, and socioeconomic status, with low educational attainment and socioeconomic standing associated with comparatively higher seroprevalences (Berrett et al., 2017), although there are aspects of the epidemiology of *Toxocara* that are still not fully understood (Holland, 2017), such as the effects of differences in sampling and detection methods and the inability to definitively discriminate between species *Toxocara canis* and *Toxocara cati*. In addition, a better understanding of the differences between common toxocariasis and neurotoxocariasis is needed (Ma et al., 2018).

At least in part because of the propensity for migrating *Toxocara* third-stage larvae to invade the brain (Holland and Hamilton, 2013), where they can result in inflammatory changes, human neurotoxocariasis can result in myelitis, encephalitis, and meningitis (Deshayes et al., 2016), and toxocariasis has been associated with cognitive deficits in children (Marmor et al., 1987; Walsh and Haseeb, 2012) and adults (Erickson et al., 2015). Preliminary findings also suggest a possible association between toxocariasis and multiple sclerosis (Sondergaard and Theorell, 2004), and there is evidence of neurodegenerative-related pathology such as beta-amyloid in mouse models of cerebral toxocariasis (Chou et al., 2017). Based on *Toxocara* involvement in the human brain and evidence that it can adversely affect brain function, we provide in this chapter a review of the association between toxocariasis from both *Toxocara canis* and *Toxocara cati* and cognitive and neuropsychiatric function in animal models and in humans, including both children and adults.

We searched the National Library of Medicine's PubMed to identify potential articles in English for inclusion in this review. In particular, we included articles from both animal models and human studies that contained data about *Toxocara* infection in animal models and seropositivity and seroprevalence in humans and associated cognitive and neuropsychiatric findings. We used the search terms "(*Toxocara canis* OR *Toxocara cati* OR toxocariasis OR neurotoxocariasis) AND (cognit* OR cognitive OR memory OR attention OR language OR neuropsychological OR reasoning OR IQ OR "reaction time")" to search for cognitive aspects of toxocariasis. We also carried out a search with the following terms, "(Toxocariasis OR *Toxocara* OR *Toxocara canis* OR *Toxocara cati* OR neurotoxocariasis) AND (psych* OR dementia OR schizophrenia OR mood OR mental OR "mental illness" Or Alzheimer's OR anxiety OR depression)." We also searched through the reference sections of articles we reviewed and otherwise conducted hand searches for additional articles. Although detection of anti-*Toxocara* antibodies in the cerebral spinal fluid aids in the diagnosis of neurotoxocariasis (Ma et al., 2018), few studies investigating associations between toxocariasis and cognitive and neuropsychiatric function include clinical evidence of anti-*Toxocara* antibodies in cerebral spinal fluid. As such, we included articles looking at associations between cognitive and neuropsychiatric function and a diagnosis of toxocariasis based on seropositivity alone in the absence of any corroborating clinical evidence or findings in cerebral spinal fluid. In addition, because most assays do not distinguish between *Toxocara canis* and *Toxocara cati* (Ma et al., 2018), the articles from human studies we reviewed could include seropositivity from either *Toxocara canis* or *Toxocara cati* or both.

2. Cognition and behaviour in animal models of toxocariasis

Prior research has investigated associations between infection with *Toxocara* and cognition and behaviour in animal models. In a mouse model, both *Toxocara canis* and *Toxocara cati* infection were associated with memory deficits and less exploratory behaviour with greater deficits in the group infected with *Toxocara canis* compared to the group infected with *Toxocara cati* (Janecek et al., 2017). Similarly, another study also suggested possible memory impairment in mice infected with *Toxocara* (Hamilton et al., 2006). In contrast, another study did not find statistically significant differences between mice infected with *Toxocara canis* and uninfected mice in spatial learning based on performance in the Morris Water Maze task. The authors also reported in this study that they did not find *Toxocara canis* larvae in the hippocampus, which they speculated could account for their not finding significant differences between the two groups in spatial memory (Chou et al., 2017).

Despite not finding statistically significant differences in spatial learning between mice infected with *Toxoplasma canis* and uninfected mice, Chou et al. (2017) reported increased amyloid beta in the hippocampus and increased expression of other factors associated with neurodegeneration in mice infected with *Toxocara canis* compared to uninfected mice and suggested that neurotoxocariasis could be associated with Alzheimer's disease.

Some of the behavioural and changes associated with *Toxocara* infection in animal models ultimately could facilitate *Toxocara* transmission via predation (Chieffi et al., 2010). For example, Cox and Holland (2001) studied the intensity of *Toxocara infection* and found exploration behaviour was impaired in the highest intensity group, a behavioural change that potentially could result in increased vulnerability to predation. Relatedly, the decreased anxiety in open spaces associated with *Toxocara* infection could also increase the risk of predation. Finally, Cox and Holland (2001) also observed that more time was required to find water in the moderate- and high-intensity groups and thought that this might represent memory impairment. Not all studies have found the same results (Correa et al., 2014), however, a pilot study found similar behavioural changes in rats infected with *Toxocara*, but the effect was not present in animals coinfected with another parasite, *Toxoplasma gondii* (Queiroz et al., 2013). One study described the changes in mice infected with *Toxocara* as having impairments "… in orienting and processing information from their environment" (Dolinsky et al., 1985).

Toxocara infection in animals is also associated with other alternations in behaviour. In a mouse model, mice infected with *Toxocara cati* had less response to a sudden noise and less flight behaviour than uninfected mice (Janecek et al., 2017). In this study, the mice infected with *Toxocara canis* had stereotypical circling, whereas the mice infected with *Toxocara cati* did not (Janecek et al., 2017), a finding suggesting that in mice *Toxocara canis* might result in more severe behavioural changes than does *Toxocara cati*. Prior studies have also suggested behavioural changes in mice infected with *Toxocara* including aspects of social behaviour, depending on parasitic load, activity levels, and aggression (Strube et al., 2013).

Overall, animal models suggest the possibility that infection with *Toxocara* could result in adverse cognitive and behavioural changes. The degree to which any of these observed behavioural changes might also occur in humans seropositive for *Toxocara* is unclear.

3. Cognitive and neuropsychiatric function in human toxocariasis

A systematic literature review of neurotoxocariasis, which would presumably be the most likely diagnosis associated with *Toxocara* infection to be associated with cognitive or behavioural impairments, published in 2016 found a total of 100 published case reports of neurotoxocariasis (Deshayes et al., 2016). Forty-seven percent of these cases had evidence of encephalitis, 33% had focal deficits, 23% had confusion, 14% had seizures, and 11% had cognitive disorders. Cognitive disorders and cognitive impairment are not necessarily the same; it is possible to have impairments in cognitive function that do not result in an obvious cognitive disorder, such as a dementia like Alzheimer's disease, and cognitive impairment might be underdiagnosed without comprehensive neurocognitive testing as was done by Scheid et al. (2008), who evaluated multiple cognitive domains and also assessed psychological symptoms in a case of toxocariasis.

Given the widespread distribution and evidence of brain involvement in human toxocariasis, there is surprisingly little information about associations between *Toxocara* seropositivity and cognitive function. Despite the comparatively few studies looking at the effects of neurotoxocariasis on human cognition, however, several case reports and studies suggest that neurotoxocariasis is associated with cognitive deficits in humans. In an early study of 333 children aged 5–7 years, there was no association between cognitive function and *Toxocara* seropositivity in the children in the models that controlled for potentially confounding variables (Worley et al., 1984). In contrast, another early but larger study consisting of 4652 children aged one to 15 years matched for lead levels (Marmor et al., 1987) found small differences in cognitive function between seronegative and seropositive

Toxocara children in adjusted models, with the seropositive children having worse cognition than the seronegative children. Similarly, Nelson et al. (1996) found that children seropositive for toxocariasis had worse cognitive function than seronegative children. Utilising a large dataset collected by the Centres for Disease Control in the United States, the Third National Health and Nutrition Examination Survey (NHANES; 1988–94), Walsh and Haseeb (2012) found evidence of reduced cognitive function in children seropositive for *Toxocara*. The nationally representative sample included 688 children who were *Toxocara* seropositive and 3261 who were seronegative. The assay utilised did not distinguish between *T. canis* and *T. cati*. The average age of the children in the seropositive group was 11.6 years and 10.9 years in the seronegative group. Measures of cognitive function were related to math and reading skills as well as a measure of attention (digit span) and a measure of non-verbal reasoning and visual-spatial organisation (block design). The analyses controlled for gender, ethnicity, income level, another measure of socioeconomic status (household income relative to poverty threshold), urban versus rural residence, infection with cytomegalovirus, and lead levels in the blood.

In a study similar to that of Walsh and Haseeb (2012), Erickson et al. (2015) used the NHANES III dataset to determine if seropositivity for *Toxocara* was related to cognitive function in young to middle-aged adults. This study included 4279 adults aged 21–59 years, used similar control variables to those that Walsh and Haseeb (2012) used, and found that *Toxocara* seropositivity was associated with slower information processing speed. The NHANES III data from that time period suggested a weighted prevalence of 16%, while an updated study using NHANES data collected more recently in the 2011–12 and 2013–14 cycles, found a much lower prevalence of 5.1% in a sample ranging in age from 6 to over 80 years (Berrett et al., 2017).

As is the case with cognition, there is only limited information available about any associations between neurotoxocariasis and neuropsychiatric diseases (Alvarado-Esquivel, 2013). A small study of inpatients with a variety psychiatric disorders compared to controls in Mexico found that the inpatients had a higher seroprevalence of *Toxocara* compared to the controls, although only 4.7% of the patients had IgG antibodies to *Toxocara* and there were no differences between patients and controls in the males. The author acknowledged that while infection with *Toxocara* could cause neuropsychiatric disease, it was also possible that psychiatric disease could be a predisposing factor for infection with *Toxocara* (Alvarado-Esquivel, 2013). Similarly, Cong et al. (2014) found a higher seroprevalence (16.40%) in psychiatric patients whose diagnoses ranged from mood disorders to dementia and schizophrenia, compared to healthy individuals (13.07%) in Shandong Province, Eastern China. A study in Iran found a higher seroprevalence of *Toxocara* in patients diagnosed with schizophrenia (14%) compared to matched healthy controls (4.3%) (Khademvatan et al., 2014). The authors suggested that the lack of self-care and poor hygiene among those with schizophrenia likely increased their risk for *Toxocara* infection. Of note, they did not find a higher prevalence of toxoplasmosis in those with schizophrenia, in contrast to other findings showing an association between toxoplasmosis and schizophrenia (Yolken et al., 2009). In similar studies, the seroprevalence of toxocariasis was higher in people with schizophrenia than in controls in a study from Turkey (Kaplan et al., 2008) and in one from Egypt (El-Sayed and Ismail, 2012). However, not all studies have found a higher *Toxocara* seroprevalence among those diagnosed with schizophrenia (Alvarado-Esquivel et al., 2014). Finally, limited work has investigated associations between self-violence including suicide attempts and *Toxocara* seropositivity, as there have been with other parasitic infections (Pedersen et al., 2012). In one study, however, there was no association was between *Toxocara* infection and suicide attempts in a group of psychiatric outpatients in Mexico (Alvarado-Esquivel et al., 2015).

While not a neuropsychiatric illness, epilepsy is often associated with changes in behaviour, mood, and cognition (Helmstaedter and Witt, 2017). There have been observations of a higher seroprevalence of *Toxocara* (19.85%) in those with epilepsy compared to healthy controls (1.38%) but no difference in seroprevalence of toxoplasmosis (Allahdin et al., 2015). While there are conflicting findings between studies on the association between epilepsy and toxocariasis, a recent systematic review and meta-analysis demonstrated an association between seropositivity of *Toxocara* and epilepsy, with an odds ratio of 1.69 (Luna et al., 2018). To put this into context, neurocysticercosis, which is infection with the tapeworm *Taenia solium*, accounts for a high amount of epilepsy cases, particularly outside of the United States (Degiorgio et al., 2004), with an odds ratio of neurocysticercosis and associated epilepsy estimated at 2.7 (Debacq et al., 2017).

4. Conclusions

Toxocariasis remains a neglected disease (Hotez and Wilkins, 2009), and its associations with human cognition and behaviour are likely even more neglected. Despite the overall lack of research investigating associations between human toxocariasis and cognition and neuropsychiatric function, many of the available research findings suggest that toxocariasis is indeed associated with cognitive and neuropsychiatric function. Although the findings are not completely consistent, most of the animal models suggest that toxocariasis is associated with both deficits in cognition and behavioural changes, with toxocariasis appearing to affect memory, learning, and startle behaviour. While relatively few studies have investigated associations between toxocariasis and cognitive and neuropsychiatric function in humans, the majority of the few available studies have found negative associations between toxocariasis and cognitive function.

Several biologically plausible and not mutually exclusive mechanisms underlying the putative association between cognitive dysfunction and toxocariasis and between neuropsychiatric function and toxocariasis exist. Animal models and clinical cases of human neurotoxocariasis demonstrate the physically destructive effects of the parasite on brain tissue, which results in the presence of biomarkers typically associated with acute brain injury (Liao et al., 2008b). Further, the immunological response to toxocariasis including proinflammatory cytokines and the effects of toxocariasis on chemokines, could contribute to brain dysfunction (Waindok and Strube, 2019). In addition, mouse models show neurodegenerative changes associated with cerebral toxocariasis, including amyloid beta accumulation and enhanced expression of the ubiquitin-proteasome system (Chou et al., 2017), which suggest also a possible association with Alzheimer's disease. Toxocariasis is also associated with neurotransmitter changes and with blood-brain barrier impairment (Liao et al., 2008a; Othman et al., 2010), which could be part of a pathway towards cognitive dysfunction. Because *Toxocara* third-stage larvae can enter the lung (Ma et al., 2018), lung dysfunction including pulmonary fibrosis and asthma is associated with *Toxocara* (Ma et al., 2018); the resulting compromise in respiratory function and change in blood oxygen could be independently associated with some of the cognitive and neuropsychiatric findings associated with toxocariasis. Development of neurologic disease associated with toxocariasis, such as epilepsy, in those infected with toxocariasis (Luna et al., 2018) could be associated with cognitive dysfunction. Finally, the potential effects of any of the changes associated with toxocariasis could affect the developing brain. For example, *Toxocara* infection has been associated with both stunting and poor nutrition (Grantham-McGregor et al., 2007; Stephensen, 1999), which may affect brain development and function. Neuroinflammation likely affects synaptic expression and brain development (Mottahedin et al., 2017). In a longitudinal study, any helminth infection between ages 1 and 2 years was associated with later cognitive impairments (Blouin et al., 2018).

5. Future directions

Because of the widespread worldwide distribution of human toxocariasis and evidence indicating associations between toxocariasis and cognition and neuropsychiatric function, future research needs to continue to investigate the effects of human toxocariasis on human cognition and neuropsychiatric function in a variety of samples from different regions of the world. There are still large deficiencies in knowledge about the effects of toxocariasis on human cognition and behaviour and about the toll that it might take on human cognitive capital and neuropsychiatric function. Similarly, additional research to take into account demographic and medical variables that might protect against or be risk factors for cognitive and neuropsychiatric dysfunction associated with toxocariasis. In addition to the considerable deficiencies in knowledge about the epidemiology and pathophysiology of toxocariasis (Ma et al., 2018; Rostami et al., 2019) are substantial gaps in knowledge about the effects of toxocariasis on human cognition and neuropsychiatric function (Rostami et al., 2019).

Acknowledgement

We thank Ollie Fegter for her assistance with database searches and acquisition of relevant journal articles.

References

Allahdin, S., Khademvatan, S., Rafiei, A., Momen, A., Rafiei, R., 2015. Frequency of Toxoplasma and Toxocara sp. antibodies in epileptic patients, in South Western Iran. Iran. J. Child Neurol. 9, 32–40.

Alvarado-Esquivel, C., 2013. Toxocara infection in psychiatric inpatients: a case control seroprevalence study. PLoS One 8, e62606.

Alvarado-Esquivel, C., Hernandez-Tinoco, J., Sanchez-Anguiano, L.F., Cisneros-Martinez, J.A., 2014. Low seroprevalence of Toxocara infection in schizophrenic inpatients in Durango, Mexico: a case control study. Int. J. Biomed. Sci. 10, 269–271.

Alvarado-Esquivel, C., Hernandez-Tinoco, J., Sanchez-Anguiano, L.F., 2015. Lack of association between Toxocara exposure and suicide attempts in psychiatric patients. J. Parasitol. Res. 2015, 608604.

Berrett, A.N., Erickson, L.D., Gale, S.D., Stone, A., Brown, B.L., Hedges, D.W., 2017. Toxocara seroprevalence and associated risk factors in the United States. Am. J. Trop. Med. Hyg. 97, 1846–1850.

Blouin, B., Casapia, M., Joseph, L., Gyorkos, T.W., 2018. A longitudinal cohort study of soil-transmitted helminth infections during the second year of life and associations with reduced long-term cognitive and verbal abilities. PLoS Negl. Trop. Dis. 12, e0006688.
Chieffi, P.P., Aquino, R.T., Pasqualotti, M.A., Ribeiro, M.C., Nasello, A.G., 2010. Behavioral changes in Rattus norvegicus experimentally infected by Toxocara canis larvae. Rev. Inst. Med. Trop. Sao Paulo 52, 243–246.
Chou, C.M., Lee, Y.L., Liao, C.W., Huang, Y.C., Fan, C.K., 2017. Enhanced expressions of neurodegeneration-associated factors, UPS impairment, and excess Abeta accumulation in the hippocampus of mice with persistent cerebral toxocariasis. Parasit. Vectors 10, 620.
Cong, W., Zhang, X.X., Zhou, N., Yu, C.Z., Chen, J., Wang, X.Y., Li, B., Qian, A.D., Zhu, X.Q., 2014. Toxocara seroprevalence among clinically healthy individuals, pregnant women and psychiatric patients and associated risk factors in Shandong Province, Eastern China. PLoS Negl. Trop. Dis. 8, e3082.
Correa, F.M., Chieffi, P.P., Lescano, S.A., Santos, S.V., 2014. Behavioral and memory changes in Mus musculus coinfected by *Toxocara canis* and *Toxoplasma gondii*. Rev. Inst. Med. Trop. Sao Paulo 56, 353–356.
Cox, D.M., Holland, C.V., 2001. Relationship between three intensity levels of *Toxocara canis* larvae in the brain and effects on exploration, anxiety, learning and memory in the murine host. J. Helminthol. 75, 33–41.
Debacq, G., Moyano, L.M., Garcia, H.H., Boumediene, F., Marin, B., Ngoungou, E.B., Preux, P.M., 2017. Systematic review and meta-analysis estimating association of cysticercosis and neurocysticercosis with epilepsy. PLoS Negl. Trop. Dis. 11, e0005153.
Degiorgio, C.M., Medina, M.T., Duron, R., Zee, C., Escueta, S.P., 2004. Neurocysticercosis. Epilepsy Curr. 4, 107–111.
Deshayes, S., Bonhomme, J., De La Blanchardiere, A., 2016. Neurotoxocariasis: a systematic literature review. Infection 44, 565–574.
Dolinsky, Z.S., Hardy, C.A., Burright, R.G., Donovick, P.J., 1985. The progression of behavioral and pathological effects of the parasite *Toxocara canis* in the mouse. Physiol. Behav. 35, 33–42.
El-Sayed, N.M., Ismail, K.A., 2012. Relationship between *Toxocara canis* infection and schizophrenia. Rawal Med. J. 37, 155–161.
Erickson, L.D., Gale, S.D., Berrett, A., Brown, B.L., Hedges, D.W., 2015. Association between toxocariasis and cognitive function in young to middle-aged adults. Folia Parasitol. 62, 048.
Grantham-McGregor, S., Cheung, Y.B., Cueto, S., Glewwe, P., Richter, L., Strupp, B., International Child Development Steering Group, 2007. Developmental potential in the first 5 years for children in developing countries. Lancet 369, 60–70.
Hamilton, C.M., Stafford, P., Pinelli, E., Holland, C.V., 2006. A murine model for cerebral toxocariasis: characterization of host susceptibility and behaviour. Parasitology 132, 791–801.
Helmstaedter, C., Witt, J.A., 2017. How neuropsychology can improve the care of individual patients with epilepsy. Looking back and into the future. Seizure 44, 113–120.
Holland, C.V., 2017. Knowledge gaps in the epidemiology of Toxocara: the enigma remains. Parasitology 144, 81–94.
Holland, C.V., Hamilton, C.M., 2013. The significance of cerebral toxocariasis: a model system for exploring the link between brain involvement, behaviour and the immune response. J. Exp. Biol. 216, 78–83.
Hotez, P.J., Wilkins, P.P., 2009. Toxocariasis: America's most common neglected infection of poverty and a helminthiasis of global importance? PLoS Negl. Trop. Dis. 3, e400.
Janecek, E., Waindok, P., Bankstahl, M., Strube, C., 2017. Abnormal neurobehaviour and impaired memory function as a consequence of Toxocara canis- as well as Toxocara cati-induced neurotoxocarosis. PLoS Negl. Trop. Dis. 11, e0005594.

Kaplan, M., Kalkan, A., Kuk, S., Demirdag, K., Ozden, M., Kilic, S.S., 2008. Toxocara seroprevalence in schizophrenic patients in Turkey. Yonsei Med. J. 49, 224–229.
Khademvatan, S., Khajeddin, N., Izadi, S., Yousefi, E., 2014. Investigation of anti-Toxocara and anti-toxoplasma antibodies in patients with schizophrenia disorder. Schizophr. Res. Treatment 2014, 230349.
Lee, J.Y., Yang, M.H., Hwang, J.H., Kang, M., Paeng, J.W., Yune, S., Lee, B.J., Choi, D.C., 2015. The prevalence of toxocariasis and diagnostic value of serologic tests in asymptomatic Korean adults. Allergy Asthma Immunol. Res. 7, 467–475.
Liao, C.W., Cho, W.L., Kao, T.C., Su, K.E., Lin, Y.H., Fan, C.K., 2008a. Blood-brain barrier impairment with enhanced SP, NK-1R, GFAP and claudin-5 expressions in experimental cerebral toxocariasis. Parasite Immunol. 30, 525–534.
Liao, C.W., Fan, C.K., Kao, T.C., Ji, D.D., Su, K.E., Lin, Y.H., Cho, W.L., 2008b. Brain injury-associated biomarkers of TGF-beta1, S100B, GFAP, NF-L, tTG, AbetaPP, and tau were concomitantly enhanced and the UPS was impaired during acute brain injury caused by *Toxocara canis* in mice. BMC Infect. Dis. 8, 84.
Lotsch, F., Vingerling, R., Spijker, R., Grobusch, M.P., 2017. Toxocariasis in humans in Africa—a systematic review. Travel Med. Infect. Dis. 20, 15–25.
Luna, J., Cicero, C.E., Rateau, G., Quattrocchi, G., Marin, B., Bruno, E., Dalmay, F., Druet-Cabanac, M., Nicoletti, A., Preux, P.M., 2018. Updated evidence of the association between toxocariasis and epilepsy: systematic review and meta-analysis. PLoS Negl. Trop. Dis. 12, e0006665.
Ma, G., Holland, C.V., Wang, T., Hofmann, A., Fan, C.K., Maizels, R.M., Hotez, P.J., Gasser, R.B., 2018. Human toxocariasis. Lancet Infect. Dis. 18, e14–e24.
Macpherson, C.N., 2013. The epidemiology and public health importance of toxocariasis: a zoonosis of global importance. Int. J. Parasitol. 43, 999–1008.
Marmor, M., Glickman, L., Shofer, F., Faich, L.A., Rosenberg, C., Cornblatt, B., Friedman, S., 1987. *Toxocara canis* infection of children: epidemiologic and neuropsychologic findings. Am. J. Public Health 77, 554–559.
Mottahedin, A., Ardalan, M., Chumak, T., Riebe, I., Ek, J., Mallard, C., 2017. Effect of neuroinflammation on synaptic organization and function in the developing brain: implications for neurodevelopmental and neurodegenerative disorders. Front. Cell. Neurosci. 11, 190.
Nelson, S., Greene, T., Ernhart, C.B., 1996. *Toxocara canis* infection in preschool age children: risk factors and the cognitive development of preschool children. Neurotoxicol. Teratol. 18, 167–174.
Othman, A.A., Abdel-Aleem, G.A., Saied, E.M., Mayah, W.W., Elatrash, A.M., 2010. Biochemical and immunopathological changes in experimental neurotoxocariasis. Mol. Biochem. Parasitol. 172, 1–8.
Pedersen, M.G., Mortensen, P.B., Norgaard-Pedersen, B., Postolache, T.T., 2012. *Toxoplasma gondii* infection and self-directed violence in mothers. Arch. Gen. Psychiatry 69, 1123–1130.
Queiroz, M.L., Viel, T.A., Papa, C.H., Lescano, S.A., Chieffi, P.P., 2013. Behavioral changes in Rattus norvegicus coinfected by *Toxocara canis* and *Toxoplasma gondii*. Rev. Inst. Med. Trop. Sao Paulo 55, 51–53.
Rostami, A., Ma, G., Wang, T., Koehler, A.V., Hofmann, A., Chang, B.C.H., Macpherson, C.N., Gasser, R.B., 2019. Human toxocariasis—a look at a neglected disease through an epidemiological 'prism'. Infect. Genet. Evol. 74, 104002.
Rubinsky-Elefant, G., Hirata, C.E., Yamamoto, J.H., Ferreira, M.U., 2010. Human toxocariasis: diagnosis, worldwide seroprevalences and clinical expression of the systemic and ocular forms. Ann. Trop. Med. Parasitol. 104, 3–23.
Scheid, R., Tina Jentzsch, R., Schroeter, M.L., 2008. Cognitive dysfunction, urinary retention, and a lesion in the thalamus—beware of possible toxocariasis of the central nervous system. Clin. Neurol. Neurosurg. 110, 1054–1057.

Sondergaard, H.P., Theorell, T., 2004. A putative role for Toxocara species in the aetiology of multiple sclerosis. Med. Hypotheses 63, 59–61.

Stensvold, C.R., Skov, J., Moller, L.N., Jensen, P.M., Kapel, C.M., Petersen, E., Nielsen, H.V., 2009. Seroprevalence of human toxocariasis in Denmark. Clin. Vaccine Immunol. 16, 1372–1373.

Stephensen, C.B., 1999. Burden of infection on growth failure. J. Nutr. 129, 534S–538S.

Strube, C., Heuer, L., Janecek, E., 2013. Toxocara spp. infections in paratenic hosts. Vet. Parasitol. 193, 375–389.

Waindok, P., Strube, C., 2019. Neuroinvasion of *Toxocara canis*- and *T. cati*-larvae mediates dynamic changes in brain cytokine and chemokine profile. J. Neuroinflammation 16, 147.

Walsh, M.G., Haseeb, M.A., 2012. Reduced cognitive function in children with toxocariasis in a nationally representative sample of the United States. Int. J. Parasitol. 42, 1159–1163.

Woodhall, D.M., Fiore, A.E., 2014. Toxocariasis: a review for pediatricians. J. Pediatric Infect. Dis. Soc. 3, 154–159.

Worley, G., Green, J.A., Frothingham, T.E., Sturner, R.A., Walls, K.W., Pakalnis, V.A., Ellis Jr., G.S., 1984. *Toxocara canis* infection: clinical and epidemiological associations with seropositivity in kindergarten children. J. Infect. Dis. 149, 591–597.

Yolken, R.H., Dickerson, F.B., Fuller Torrey, E., 2009. Toxoplasma and schizophrenia. Parasite Immunol. 31, 706–715.

PART III

Epidemiology

CHAPTER FOURTEEN

Global and regional seroprevalence estimates for human toxocariasis: A call for action

Guangxu Ma[a], Ali Rostami[b], Tao Wang[a], Andreas Hofmann[a], Peter J. Hotez[c,d,e], Robin B. Gasser[a,*]

[a]Department of Veterinary Biosciences, Melbourne Veterinary School, Faculty of Veterinary and Agricultural Sciences, The University of Melbourne, Parkville, VIC, Australia
[b]Infectious Diseases and Tropical Medicine Research Center, Health Research Institute, Babol University of Medical Sciences, Babol, Iran
[c]Texas Children's Hospital Center for Vaccine Development, Departments of Pediatrics and Molecular Virology & Microbiology, National School of Tropical Medicine, Baylor College of Medicine, Houston, TX, United States
[d]Department of Biology, Baylor University, Waco, TX, United States
[e]Hagler Institute for Advanced Studies at Texas A&M University, College Station, TX, United States
*Corresponding author: e-mail address: robinbg@unimelb.edu.au

Contents

Abstract

Human toxocariasis is a parasitic disease transmitted usually from dogs and/or cats that are infected with *Toxocara* species, and can be associated with a range of allergic, neurological and/or visual disorders. Recent epidemiological research has estimated that ~1.4 billion people worldwide, particularly in subtropical and tropical regions, are infected with, or exposed to *Toxocara* species, indicating that human toxocariasis is a neglected tropical disease. Here, we review recent research efforts, consider risk factors, discuss limitations in current seroprevalence estimates, and propose some future research directions towards improved awareness, surveillance, prevention and control of this neglected disease.

Advances in Parasitology, Volume 109
ISSN 0065-308X
https://doi.org/10.1016/bs.apar.2020.01.011

1. Introduction

Human toxocariasis is a parasitic disease of global importance (Ma et al., 2018; Rostami et al., 2019a). This disease is caused by infection with larvae of species of *Toxocara*, particularly *T. canis* (dog roundworm) and/or *T. cati* (cat roundworm) (Strube et al., 2013). Infection is transmitted to humans via the faecal-oral route, and usually occurs following the accidental ingestion of infective eggs from contaminated water, food or soil (Manini et al., 2012), or following the consumption of undercooked viscera and meat containing infective larvae (Morimatsu et al., 2006; Yoshikawa et al., 2008). Young children and owners of dogs or cats are more likely to be infected (Fisher, 2003; Macpherson, 2013; Won et al., 2008). Human toxocariasis is also considered a poverty-related neglected disease, arising in both urban and rural areas where stray dogs and cats are prevalent. Although most people infected with *Toxocara* are asymptomatic, clinical syndromes can develop in some individuals, depending on the larval burden and the immune response induced. These syndromes include visceral larva migrans (VLM), ocular larva migrans (OLM), neurotoxocariasis (NT) and covert/common toxocariasis (CT) (see Ma et al., 2018), and can associate with allergic, neurological and/or visual disorders (Cooper, 2008; Fan et al., 2015; Gavignet et al., 2008; Mohammadzadeh et al., 2018; Woodhall et al., 2012), or cognitive and intellectual deficits in children (Hotez, 2014; Walsh and Haseeb, 2012).

Recent studies have investigated the prevalence of *Toxocara* infection in dogs and cats worldwide (see Rostami et al., 2020a,b in this issue), and the contamination of soil with *Toxocara* eggs, particularly in countries in the Western Pacific, Africa and South-East Asia regions (Fakhri et al., 2018). The widespread distribution of *Toxocara* eggs indicates a significant global risk factor for *Toxocara* infection in humans. Apart from the nationwide investigations of human toxocariasis in the United States (Liu et al., 2018; Won et al., 2008), up-to-date large-scale epidemiological studies are still lacking for most other countries (Ma et al., 2018; Rostami et al., 2019a). Major knowledge gaps remain in the epidemiology of human toxocariasis at the global, regional and national levels (Holland, 2017; Ma et al., 2018), and prevention or control campaigns are absent.

The diagnosis of human toxocariasis can be presumed based on clinical signs (e.g., VLM and/or OLM), and supported by results from blood tests (e.g., eosinophilia and anti-*Toxocara* antibodies) or the detection of

Toxocara DNA in tissues or body fluid samples from affected patients (Fillaux and Magnaval, 2013; Moreira et al., 2014; Smith and Noordin, 2006). Despite some limitations, the approach of detecting anti-*Toxocara* serum antibodies has been widely employed to detect humans infected with, or exposed to *Toxocara* spp., and to estimate the seroprevalence in human populations. Specifically, serological techniques, such as enzyme-linked immunosorbent assays (ELISAs) and Western blot (WB) analysis, have been commonly used for seroprevalence surveys of human toxocariasis (Fillaux and Magnaval, 2013; Ma et al., 2018). Although numerous investigations have been conducted to estimate the prevalence of anti-*Toxocara* serum antibodies in humans, until recently there was no systematic review or meta-analysis of published information and data. Here, we summarise recent studies conducted to estimate the anti-*Toxocara* seroprevalence and establish risk factors for *Toxocara* infection in humans worldwide, discuss possible limitations of seroprevalence estimates, and propose areas of future research of toxocariasis. A comprehensive understanding of the *Toxocara* infection or exposure in humans worldwide is likely to advance our knowledge of the epidemiology of human toxocariasis, raising public awareness of this neglected parasitic disease.

2. Worldwide and WHO regional prevalence estimates

When the first diagnosis of human toxocariasis was made (Wilder, 1950), there were major gaps in our knowledge of the epidemiology of this disease (Holland, 2017; Smith et al., 2009). Almost 70 years later, there are still areas with a substantial lack of information.

Recently, Ma et al. (2018) appraised and summarised 106 nationwide or regional studies of the prevalence of anti-*Toxocara* serum antibodies in humans (without clinical signs of toxocariasis). This work revealed a particularly high prevalence (>80%) of humans infected with or exposed to *Toxocara* species in some tropical and subtropical countries/regions (e.g., Indonesia, Kashmir, Marshall Islands, Nepal and Nigeria). Seropositive humans were reported to be common in countries including Brazil, China, India and Iran, and some industrialised countries such as Japan, the United Kingdom and the United States (Ma et al., 2018). Published surveys of anti-*Toxocara* serum antibodies indicated that tens of millions of people are likely exposed to or infected with *Toxocara* spp. (reviewed by Ma et al., 2018), suggesting the neglected nature of toxocariasis. However, there is still a lack of information on the global, regional and national levels.

To address this limitation, Rostami et al. (2019a) conducted the first systematic review and meta-analysis of all publicly accessible literature on anti-*Toxocara* seroprevalence in humans. In this study, 253 datasets representing 265,327 participants from 71 countries were selected, appraised and analysed. The results indicated a global seroprevalence of 19% (95% confidence interval [CI] 16.6–21.4%) (Rostami et al., 2019a). Extrapolating to the global population (2016), ~1.4 billion individuals worldwide were estimated to be infected with or exposed to *Toxocara* species (Rostami et al., 2019a). Although the heterogeneity ($I^2=99.6\%$, $P<0.001$) of these datasets required that information and data needed to be interpreted with caution, the seroprevalence estimates for human toxocariasis appeared to be robust.

The estimated seroprevalence of human toxocariasis varied greatly among geographical regions defined by WHO (Rostami et al., 2019a). The prevalence rates of human toxocariasis were estimated at 38%, 34%, 24%, 23%, 11%, and 8% in the African, South-East Asia, Western Pacific regions, the Americas, Europe, and the Eastern Mediterranean region, respectively (Fig. 1). In the North and South Americas, the seroprevalences were estimated at 13% and 28%, respectively. Population-based estimations suggested that the highest burdens (~664 million individuals) of human toxocariasis were in South-East Asia region (e.g., India, Indonesia and Nepal), and the lowest (~54 million) in the Eastern Mediterranean region (Rostami et al., 2019a). The findings suggested environmental, socioecological and genetic effects on the seroprevalence of human toxocariasis.

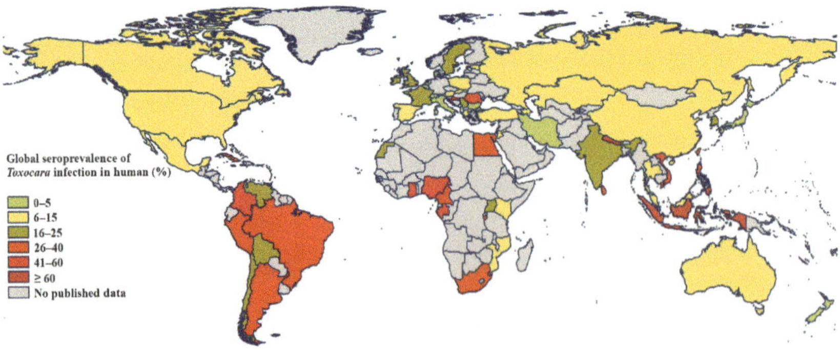

Fig. 1 Seroprevalence estimates for *Toxocara* infection or exposure in humans worldwide.

Shown in Table 1 is a comparison of the prevalence estimates for *Toxocara* infection(s) of dogs, cats and humans, listing also the most highly prevalent regions globally (Rostami et al., 2019a,b; see Rostami et al., 2020a,b in this issue). In brief, Africa emerges as the region with the highest overall prevalence of *Toxocara* infection or exposure, suggesting that toxocariasis

Table 1 A summary of global, regional and national prevalence estimates for *Toxocara* infection in dogs and cats, soil contamination by *Toxocara* eggs in public areas, and *Toxocara* infection or exposure in humans.

WHO-region / Country	Prevalence of *Toxocara* infection in dogs % (95% CI)[a]	Prevalence of *Toxocara* infection in cats % (95% CI)[b]	Soil contamination by *Toxocara* eggs % (95% CI)[c]	Seroprevalence of *Toxocara* infection or exposure in humans % (95% CI)[d]
Global	**11 (11 − 12)**	**17 (16–18)**	**21 (16–27)**	**19 (17–21)**
Africa	**19 (14–24)**	**43 (28–58)**	**27 (11–47)**	**38 (26–51)**
Nigeria	17 (10–25)	50 (44–55)	24 (7–47)	44 (19–72)
Kenya	N/A	23 (16–33)	25 (16–38)	8 (4–12)
South-East Asian	**12 (7–18)**	**15 (10–20)**	**21 (3–49)**	**34 (20–49)**
India	13 (6–22)	30 (1–60)	12 (7–19)	20 (10–32)
Thailand	5 (4–8)	12 (6–17)	8 (3–10)	6 (4–9)
Western Pacific	**6 (3–10)**	**17 (15–20)**	**35 (15–58)**	**24 (16–34)**
China	39 (31–47)	15 (11–18)	75 (74–75)	15 (12–18)
Malaysia	7 (0–33)	11 (8–13)	38 (0–91)	15 (5–29)
Japan	2 (0–3)	11 (7–15)	46 (5–91)	4 (2–5)
Australia	4 (2–6)	8 (5–12)	0 (0–1)	7 (5–9)
South America	**11 (8–15)**	**13 (8–17)**	**25 (18–33)**	**28 (23–33)**
Brazil	9 (6–13)	9 (6–12)	30 (21–39)	28 (21–35)
Argentina	12 (10–15)	36 (31–40)	8 (0–25)	35 (26–45)
Venezuela	11 (9–14)	N/A	29 (19–40)	18 (13–24)
North America	**11 (11–12)**	**18 (15–21)**	**13 (8–23)**	**13 (10–16)**
Canada	7 (3–12)	15 (9–20)	33 (19–49)	6 (3–11)
USA	5 (3–6)	20 (16–25)	12 (4–23)	9 (6–13)
Mexico	7 (3–13)	25 (7–42)	25 (23–27)	15 (8–22)

Continued

Table 1 A summary of global, regional and national prevalence estimates for *Toxocara* infection in dogs and cats, soil contamination by *Toxocara* eggs in public areas, and *Toxocara* infection or exposure in humans.—Cont'd

WHO-region / Country	Prevalence of *Toxocara* infection in dogs % (95% CI)[a]	Prevalence of *Toxocara* infection in cats % (95% CI)[b]	Soil contamination by *Toxocara* eggs % (95% CI)[c]	Seroprevalence of *Toxocara* infection or exposure in humans % (95% CI)[d]
Europe	**11 (9–13)**	**18 (16–20)**	**18 (14–22)**	**11 (9–13)**
Spain	8 (3–14)	20 (14–26)	7 (5–8)	4 (3–13)
Turkey	13 (6–21)	20 (16–24)	16 (11–23)	7 (3–12)
Poland	11 (3–24)	28 (9–47)	20 (14–26)	16 (10–23)
Italy	9 (6–11)	20 (14–27)	15 (12–19)	4 (3–7)
France	8 (4–12)	40 (15–66)	38 (21–58)	18 (11–25)
Russia	9 (0–44)	3 (1–5)	23 (13–36)	7 (0–30)
Romania	17 (15–19)	23 (20–26)	22 (11–37)	42 (38–47)
Ireland	57 (52–61)	42 (35–50)	13 (9–17)	29 (28–31)
United Kingdom	4 (2–9)	19 (9–28)	6 (4–9)	24 (21–26)
Belgium	13 (6–23)	14 (8–21)	10 (5–17)	6 (5–6)
Slovakia	19 (10–30)	N/A	12 (8–16)	15 (11–18)
Middle East and North Africa	**19 (14–26)**	**22 (15–28)**	**18 (14–24)**	**8 (5–12)**
Iran	16 (9–23)	26 (15–37)	20 (13–29)	6 (3–9)
Egypt	14 (4–28)	8 (5–12)	13 (7–20)	32 (10–60)
Jordan	1 (0–4)	N/A	15 (11–21)	11 (9–13)

[a]Rostami et al. (2020b).
[b]Rostami et al. (2020a).
[c]Fakhri et al. (2018).
[d]Rostami et al. (2019a).
Abbreviations: WHO, World Health Organisation; N/A, data not available.

represents an important 'One Health' issue in this region. South-East Asia and South America also represent prominent areas of *Toxocara* seroprevalence and exposure. In this context, it also highlights how human toxocariasis might be considered, alongside ascariasis, trichuriasis, hookworm infection, and strongyloidiasis, as a major soil-transmitted helminth disease in Africa, Asia and the Americas.

3. Geographical and climatic factors

Environmental conditions (e.g., temperature, moisture and precipitation) play roles in the embryonation of *Toxocara* eggs (Azam et al., 2012; Gamboa, 2005; Keegan and Holland, 2013) and, thus, might influence the transmission of infection. In dogs and cats, *Toxocara* infection has been reported in >60 and 51 countries, respectively (see Rostami et al., 2020a,b in this issue), implying a broad distribution of infective eggs in public areas (21%; 95% CI 16–27%) (Fakhri et al., 2018; Lee et al., 2010), and essentially a transmission reservoir for human toxocariasis. However, there was no comprehensive evidence or report to link environmental factors and the distribution of *Toxocara* eggs in the environment to the prevalence of human toxocariasis.

Rostami et al. (2019a) explored these aspects using a meta-regression analysis of geographically classified datasets, revealing a significant negative correlation between increasing geographical latitude and seroprevalence of *Toxocara* infection or exposure (coefficient = −0.005, P-value < 0.001). The geographical prevalence of *Toxocara* infection or exposure was found to be in accord with the distribution of *Toxocara* eggs in public places worldwide (Table 1; Fakhri et al., 2018). By contrast, positive correlations were indicated between the relative humidity (coefficient = 0.005, P-value < 0.001), mean temperature (coefficient = 0.01; P-value < 0.001), precipitation rates (coefficient = 0.0001, P-value < 0.001) and the prevalence of *Toxocara* infection or exposure (Rostami et al., 2019a). Interestingly, high levels of contamination of soil with *Toxocara* eggs and a high risk of human toxocariasis appear to exist in areas of low latitude (0°–30°) and high environmental humidity. In addition, high seroprevalence rates were estimated in countries with an annual mean temperature of 25–30 °C, such as Colombia (47%), Gabon (60%), Indonesia (63%) and the Philippines (67%) (Rostami et al., 2019a).

4. Socio-demographic variables and risk factors

Apart from geographical and climatic factors, socio-demographic variables (e.g., socioecological and genetic factors) also associate with the prevalence of human toxocariasis (Ma et al., 2018). Meta-regression analysis (Rostami et al., 2019a) showed clear negative correlations between the income level (coefficient = −0.082; P-value < 0.001) or the human development index of a country (coefficient = −0.084; *P*-value < 0.001) and the anti-*Toxocara* seroprevalence. Interestingly, time-dependent meta-regression analysis of epidemiological studies did not show a significant change in seroprevalence of human toxocariasis over the past decades (1980–2019) (Rostami et al., 2019a).

Knowledge of the distribution of *Toxocara* species and anti-*Toxocara* seroprevalence in humans could help identify major risk factors for toxocariasis. Indeed, recent analyses have revealed that factors such as age and sex, dog and cat ownership (e.g., deworming and faecal management), behaviour and habits (e.g., hygiene, drinking raw water and eating raw/undercooked viscera) and profession (e.g., hunter and veterinarian) are likely determinants of human toxocariasis (Alvarado-Esquivel et al., 2015; Bojanich et al., 2015; Cong et al., 2014; Dantas-Torres and Otranto, 2014; Mattos et al., 2016). In Rostami et al. (2019a), some of these factors were highly ranked, such as being young (odds ratio: 1.9) or male (odds ratio: 1.3); having contact with soil (odds ratio: 2.1); consuming untreated water (odds ratio: 2.0) or raw meat or viscera (odds ratio: 1.6); having contact with dogs (odds ratio: 1.7) or cats (odds ratio: 1.6); and living in a rural area (odds ratio: 1.8).

Soil and water contaminated with *Toxocara* eggs might represent a significant source of *Toxocara* infection to humans. During urbanisation throughout the world in the past decades, the numbers of dogs and cats have increased substantially in many countries (Greene, 2012). The activities of these animals (including defaecation) in public places, such as beaches, parks and children's playgrounds, likely increase the dispersal of *Toxocara* eggs (Bojanich et al., 2015; Otero et al., 2018). The higher anti-*Toxocara* seroprevalence estimates found in children compared with adults (Rostami et al., 2019a) might relate to a more frequent ingestion of infective eggs from contaminated soil/sand or from animals (Holland et al., 1995; Hotez and Wilkins, 2009; Ma et al., 2018). In addition, veterinarians and some groups of people living in rural areas are more likely to be infected by *Toxocara* species, which can be explained by activities such as hunting and the handling of, or close contact with dogs and/or cats (Lee et al., 2015; Ma et al., 2018; Mattos et al., 2016; Rubinsky-Elefant et al., 2008; Won et al., 2008).

5. Diagnostic approach: Effect on prevalence estimates

The principal approach used for the diagnosis of *Toxocara* infection or exposure in humans is serology. Usually, ELISA and WB analysis

(Fillaux and Magnaval, 2013; Smith and Noordin, 2006) are employed. These techniques rely on the use of *T. canis* excretory and secretory antigens (TES) to bind specific immunoglobulins (IgM and IgG) or specific IgG subclasses (IgG1, IgG2, IgG3 and/or IgG4) (Fillaux and Magnaval, 2013; Smith and Noordin, 2006). Although these techniques have been widely employed in previous epidemiological studies of human toxocariasis (reviewed by Ma et al., 2018; Rostami et al., 2019a, b), some may have limitations that can affect their performance in an epidemiological setting and the interpretation of test results.

Diagnostic specificity and sensitivity of a serological assay can have a significant impact on seroprevalence estimates (Moreira et al., 2014; Smith and Noordin, 2006). Particularly ELISAs using different TES antigens to detect total IgG or specific IgG subclasses varied markedly in specificity and sensitivity (cf. Ma et al., 2018). Considering potential cross-reactivity with antigens from other helminths (e.g., *Ascaris*, *Strongyloides* and/or *Trichinella* species), WB analysis is commonly recommended to confirm ELISA test-positive results, particularly in tropical climatic regions where polyparasitism is common (Fillaux and Magnaval, 2013; Smith and Noordin, 2006). However, a recent analysis indicated that the prevalence of anti-*T. canis* serum antibodies estimated by WB analysis (28%) was higher than that estimated (19%) using ELISA (Rostami et al., 2019a), although this finding needs to be interpreted with caution, because of the bias in the numbers of samples tested by ELISA ($n=240$) vs WB analysis ($n=10$), and an inadequate description of some of the test protocols employed in published studies (cf. Rostami et al., 2019a).

Given the variables in serological investigations, including diagnostic specificity and sensitivity as well as cut-off values for seropositivity, some prevalence estimates can be inaccurate. Therefore, large-scale and standardised epidemiological studies employing ELISA, WB analysis or a combination of the two techniques are required to evaluate the effects of specificity and sensitivity on the seroprevalence estimations. Importantly, an optimised approach (e.g., ELISA plus WB analysis) using a standard operating procedure (e.g., dilution of serum; blocking agent used; recombinant TES; crude or purified secondary antibody conjugate; incubation temperatures and times; indicator system employed; data collection and interpretation) should be established for the laboratory diagnosis of human toxocariasis in future epidemiological studies, to achieve confident global and regional seroprevalence estimates.

6. Prevalence estimates: Possible limitations and future focus

Despite the availability of the first seroprevalence estimates for *Toxocara* infection or exposure in human populations worldwide, there are still considerable gaps in our knowledge and understanding of human toxocariasis. These gaps relate mainly to limitations in data availability or accuracy, and geographical coverage.

First, apart from Austria, Denmark, Japan, Malaysia, Sweden and the United States, nationwide datasets are mostly lacking for other countries (Ma et al., 2018). Moreover, although there are several investigations in densely populated countries, such as China and India (cf. Ma et al., 2018), regional datasets are not sufficiently comprehensive for nationwide estimations. In addition, often small numbers of serum samples were tested, and limited information on socio-demography and risk factors, such as age, sex, physical and clinical status, education, profession, living conditions and pet ownership was available. These issues could lead to inaccurate seroprevalence estimates.

Second, it is difficult to discriminate active infection from past exposure to *Toxocara*. Although ELISA and WB analysis were commonly used in the previous epidemiological studies, neither the detection of immunoglobulin class (IgA, IgE, IgG or IgM) nor the detection of immunoglobulin subclass (IgG4) using these techniques can distinguish current from past *Toxocara* infection in humans (Fillaux and Magnaval, 2013). Clinical symptoms of human toxocariasis, an elevated level of blood eosinophil cationic protein and IgG antibody avidity can be observed in an active infection (Fillaux and Magnaval, 2013; Ma et al., 2018), but such information is mostly lacking from published studies. Modified (e.g., glycosylated and di-*O*-methylated) TES antigens appeared to be promising to achieve higher specificity and sensitivity in assays (Elefant et al., 2016; Roldán et al., 2015), but still need detailed evaluations in well-controlled and larger-scale epidemiological investigations.

Third, differentiation of infections with different species of *Toxocara* is not possible using serological methods. Poulsen et al. (2015) attempted to differentiate *T. canis* from *T. cati* infections in a pig model using WB analysis, but failed to find any protein that could be used as a diagnostic marker. Importantly, pronounced heterogenic protein patterns were observed in individual hosts infected with *T. cati* ($n=7$) (Poulsen et al., 2015).

Although such work has not been validated in a larger-scale study, it does raise issues about choosing a cut-off for seropositivity and interpreting seroprevalence estimates. Clearly, more attention should be paid to the possible impact of such variations on prevalence estimates.

Fourth, the current seroprevalence estimates cannot be used to indicate the prevalence of toxocariasis-associated chronic disease, including allergic or neurological disorders. Although systematic reviews and meta-analyses have revealed significant associations between the presence of anti-*Toxocara* antibodies and asthma (Aghaei et al., 2018; Li et al., 2014) and epilepsy (Luna et al., 2018; Quattrocchi et al., 2012), there are still very few studies in these areas. In addition, whether seropositivity reflects active disease vs past exposure/infection still needs to be resolved, unless new antigen or nucleic acid detection-based methods emerge. Another key question relates to the chronology of asthma, as the seroconversion from *Toxocara* spp. infection is unclear (Fialho et al., 2018). We also need to better understand how *Toxoplasma* plays a role in neurological disorders and whether *Toxocara* contributes to such disorders, as *Toxocara* and *Toxoplasma* co-infections appear to be common in humans (Celik et al., 2013; Jones et al., 2008; Liu et al., 2019). Without addressing such questions, clear links between anti-*Toxocara* prevalence and neurological diseases, including cognitive delays, remain elusive.

7. Concluding remarks

The high seroprevalence estimates for human toxocariasis worldwide (mean of ~19%) and in selected countries (up to 44%) call for well-designed epidemiological studies as well as surveillance and prevention programs. Although mass drug administration (MDA) programs have been implemented to reduce the burden of some neglected tropical diseases (NTDs), including soil-transmitted helminthiasis (Lo et al., 2017), this is not the case for human toxocariasis. Indeed, to our knowledge, there has been no effort to implement strategic monitoring, reporting, prevention and/or control programs for toxocariasis in countries that now seem to need them most. For example, might African and some South-East Asian countries, where the prevalence of toxocariasis is greatest, benefit from MDA programs targeting this disease alongside other major soil-transmitted helminthiases? Dogs and cats infected with *Toxocara* as well as soil and water contaminated with *Toxocara* eggs are pronounced sources of human infection and/or disease (Ma et al., 2018; Overgaauw and van Knapen, 2013;

Rostami et al., 2019b), but there are no systematic programs to monitor and prevent toxocariasis. Given the public health importance of human toxocariasis, we believe, based on the evidence reviewed here, that this is a neglected disease that needs to be tackled in numerous underprivileged countries using a 'One Health' approach (cf. Ma et al., 2018).

Yet another consideration is the finding of toxocariasis in urban settings and the fact that in the coming decades it is expected that the human population will become increasingly urbanised (Hotez, 2017). With the anticipated formation and expansion of new mega-cities in Africa and Asia, it will be interesting to see whether toxocariasis emerges as potentially the most widely prevalent human helminthiasis (Hotez, 2018).

The massive seroprevalences in places like the Marshall Islands (up to 87%), St. Lucia (87%) and La Reunion (93%) (Fu et al., 2014; Magnaval et al., 1994; Thompson et al., 1986) reinforce the need to make people in these locations aware of the possible impact of toxocariasis, life cycle of *T. canis* and *T. cati* and the risks factors (e.g., contacting with soil, drinking untreated water, raising dogs and cats, being young and living in rural areas) associated with human toxocariasis (Smith et al., 2009). Knowledge about faecal management and hygiene is also critical for effective intervention (Ma et al., 2018; Rostami et al., 2019b). In addition, aspects of the epidemiology, clinical syndromes and the technical limitations of diagnosis of human toxocariasis (VLM, OLM, NT and CT) should be emphasised to medical practitioners in these areas.

Clearly, improved diagnostic tools are needed to more reliably record the prevalence of human toxocariasis. Although the global seroprevalence was estimated, the prediction was based on the presence of anti-*Toxocara* antibodies in people without clinical manifestation of disease. ELISA and WB analysis techniques cannot provide information regarding the phase of infection, which also significantly hinders further exploration of *Toxocara* infection-associated complications (e.g., allergic and neurologic disorders). Species-specific diagnostic tools are required for a better understanding of human toxocariasis and related diseases. Despite the many advantages of polymerase chain reaction (PCR)-based molecular techniques over current serological methods in distinguishing species, sampling tissue or fluid from humans is invasive and clearly impractical for large-scale investigations. Although challenging, a comprehensive biological understanding of *Toxocara* spp. at the molecular level might pave the way to new diagnostic markers, such as secreted antigens and/or circulating microRNAs from the parasites (cf. Gasser et al., 2016; Ma et al., 2016; Zhu et al., 2015).

In conclusion, the present chapter reinforces the notion that human toxocariasis is a neglected disease, particularly in tropical and subtropical regions of the world. We believe that this disease should receive more attention by WHO and government health authorities than presently is the case, and that there should be a concerted effort globally to reduce *Toxocara* exposure and infection in underprivileged communities where seroprevalence is high and the disease burden likely to be substantial.

Acknowledgements

The authors thank researchers in this field for their efforts and contributions. R.B.G. thanks the Australian Research Council, the National Health and Medical Research Council of Australia, Melbourne Water Corporation and Yourgene Health for support.

References

Aghaei, S., Riahi, S.M., Rostami, A., Mohammadzadeh, I., Javanian, M., Tohidi, E., Foroutan, M., Esmaeili Dooki, M., 2018. *Toxocara* spp. infection and risk of childhood asthma: a systematic review and meta-analysis. Acta Trop. 182, 298–304.

Alvarado-Esquivel, C., Hernández-Tinoco, J., Sánchez-Anguiano, L.F., Ramos-Nevárez, A., Cerrillo-Soto, S.M., Guido-Arreola, C.A., Saenz-Soto, L., 2015. Detection of IgG against *Toxocara* in sera of employees of meat industry. Int. J. Biomed. Sci. 11, 152–156.

Azam, D., Ukpai, O.M., Said, A., Abd-Allah, G.A., Morgan, E.R., 2012. Temperature and the development and survival of infective *Toxocara canis* larvae. Parasitol. Res. 110, 649–656.

Bojanich, M.V., Alonso, J.M., Caraballo, N.A., Itatí Schöller, M., López Mde, L., García, L.M., Basualdo, J.Á., 2015. Assessment of the presence of *Toxocara eggs* in soils of an arid area in central-western Argentina. Rev. Inst. Med. Trop. Sao Paulo 57, 73–76.

Celik, T., Kaplan, Y., Atas, E., Oztuna, D., Berilgen, S., 2013. *Toxocara* seroprevalence in patients with idiopathic Parkinson's disease: chance association or coincidence? Biomed. Res. Int. 2013, 685196.

Cong, W., Zhang, X.X., Zhou, N., Yu, C.Z., Chen, J., Wang, X.Y., Li, B., Qian, A.D., Zhu, X.Q., 2014. *Toxocara* seroprevalence among clinically healthy individuals, pregnant women and psychiatric patients and associated risk factors in Shandong Province, Eastern China. PLoS Negl. Trop. Dis. 8, e3082.

Cooper, P.J., 2008. *Toxocara canis* infection: an important and neglected environmental risk factor for asthma? Clin. Exp. Allergy 38, 551–553.

Dantas-Torres, F., Otranto, D., 2014. Dogs, cats, parasites, and humans in Brazil: opening the black box. Parasit. Vectors 7, 22.

Elefant, G., Roldán, W.H., Seeböck, A., Kosma, P., 2016. Evaluation of a di-O-methylated glycan as a potential antigenic target for the serodiagnosis of human toxocariasis. Parasite Immunol. 38, 236–243.

Fakhri, Y., Gasser, R.B., Rostami, A., Fan, C.K., Ghasemi, S.M., Javanian, M., Bayani, M., Armoon, B., Moradi, B., 2018. *Toxocara* eggs in public places worldwide—a systematic review and meta-analysis. Environ. Pollut. 242, 1467–1475.

Fan, C.K., Holland, C.V., Loxton, K., Barghouth, U., 2015. Cerebral toxocariasis: silent progression to neurodegenerative disorders? Clin. Microbiol. Rev. 28, 663–686.

Fialho, P.M.M., Correa, C.R.S., Lescano, S.Z., 2018. Asthma and seroconversion from *Toxocara* spp. infection: which comes first? Biomed. Res. Int. 2018 4280792.

Fillaux, J., Magnaval, J.F., 2013. Laboratory diagnosis of human toxocariasis. Vet. Parasitol. 193, 327–336.

Fisher, M., 2003. *Toxocara cati*: an underestimated zoonotic agent. Trends Parasitol. 19, 167–170.

Fu, C.J., Chuang, T.W., Lin, H.S., Wu, C.H., Liu, Y.C., Langinlur, M.K., Lu, M.Y., Hsiao, W.W., Fan, C.K., 2014. Seroepidemiology of *Toxocara canis* infection among primary schoolchildren in the capital area of the Republic of the Marshall Islands. BMC Infect. Dis. 14, 261.

Gamboa, M., 2005. Effects of temperature and humidity on the development of eggs of *Toxocara canis* under laboratory conditions. J. Helminthol. 79, 327–331.

Gasser, R.B., Korhonen, P.K., Zhu, X.Q., Young, N.D., 2016. Harnessing the *Toxocara* genome to underpin toxocariasis research and new interventions. Adv. Parasitol. 91, 87–110.

Gavignet, B., Piarroux, R., Aubin, F., Millon, L., Humbert, P., 2008. Cutaneous manifestations of human toxocariasis. J. Am. Acad. Dermatol. 59, 1031–1042.

Greene, C.E., 2012. Infectious Diseases of the Dog and Cat, fourth ed. Elsevier Saunders, St Louis, MO, ISBN: 9781416061304, p. 2012.

Holland, C.V., 2017. Knowledge gaps in the epidemiology of *Toxocara*: the enigma remains. Parasitology 144, 81–94.

Holland, C., O'lorcain, P., Taylor, M., Kelly, A., 1995. Sero-epidemiology of toxocariasis in school children. Parasitology 110, 535–545.

Hotez, P.J., 2014. Neglected infections of poverty in the United States and their effects on the brain. JAMA Psychiat. 71, 1099–1100.

Hotez, P.J., 2017. Global urbanization and the neglected tropical diseases. PLoS Negl. Trop. Dis. 11, e0005308.

Hotez, P.J., 2018. Human parasitology and parasitic diseases: heading towards 2050. Adv. Parasitol. 100, 29–38.

Hotez, P.J., Wilkins, P.P., 2009. Toxocariasis: America's most common neglected infection of poverty and a helminthiasis of global importance? PLoS Negl. Trop. Dis. 3, e400.

Jones, J.L., Kruszon-Moran, D., Won, K., Wilson, M., Schantz, P.M., 2008. *Toxoplasma gondii* and *Toxocara* spp. co-infection. Am. J. Trop. Med. Hyg. 78, 35–39.

Keegan, J.D., Holland, C., 2013. A comparison of *Toxocara canis* embryonation under controlled conditions in soil and hair. J. Helminthol. 87, 78–84.

Lee, A.C., Schantz, P.M., Kazacos, K.R., Montgomery, S.P., Bowman, D.D., 2010. Epidemiologic and zoonotic aspects of ascarid infections in dogs and cats. Trends Parasitol. 26, 155–161.

Lee, J.Y., Yang, M.H., Hwang, J.H., Kang, M., Paeng, J.W., Yune, S., Lee, B.J., Choi, D.C., 2015. The prevalence of toxocariasis and diagnostic value of serologic tests in asymptomatic Korean adults. Allergy, Asthma Immunol. Res. 7, 467–475.

Li, L., Gao, W., Yang, X., Wu, D., Bi, H., Zhang, S., Huang, M., Yao, X., 2014. Asthma and toxocariasis. Ann. Allergy Asthma Immunol. 113, 187–192.

Liu, E.W., Chastain, H.M., Shin, S.H., Wiegand, R.E., Kruszon-Moran, D., Handali, S., Jones, J.L., 2018. Seroprevalence of antibodies to *Toxocara* species in the United States and associated risk factor, 2011–2014. Clin. Infect. Dis. 66, 2016–2212.

Liu, E.W., Elder, E.S., Rivera, H.N., Kruszon-Moran, D., Handali, S., Jones, J.L., 2019. Concurrent seroprevalence of antibodies to *Toxoplasma gondii* and *Toxocara* species in the United States, 2011–2014. Clin. Infect. Dis. 68, 712–713.

Lo, N.C., Addiss, D.G., Hotez, P.J., King, C.H., Stothard, J.R., Evans, D.S., Colley, D.G., Lin, W., Coulibaly, J.T., Bustinduy, A.L., Raso, G., Bendavid, E., Bogoch, I.I., Fenwick, A., Savioli, L., Molyneux, D., Utzinger, J., Andrews, J.R., 2017. A call to strengthen the global strategy against schistosomiasis and soil-transmitted helminthiasis: the time is now. Lancet Infect. Dis. 17, e64–e69.

Luna, J., Cicero, C.E., Rateau, G., Quattrocchi, G., Marin, B., Bruno, E., Dalmay, F., Druet-Cabanac, M., Nicoletti, A., Preux, P.M., 2018. Updated evidence of the association between toxocariasis and epilepsy: systematic review and meta-analysis. PLoS Negl. Trop. Dis. 12, e0006665.

Ma, G., Luo, Y., Zhu, H., Luo, Y., Korhonen, P.K., Young, N.D., Gasser, R.B., Zhou, R., 2016. MicroRNAs of *Toxocara canis* and their predicted functional roles. Parasit. Vectors 9, 229.

Ma, G., Holland, C.V., Wang, T., Hofmann, A., Fan, C.K., Maizels, R.M., Hotez, P.J., Gasser, R.B., 2018. Human toxocariasis. Lancet Infect. Dis. 18, e14–e24.

Macpherson, C.N., 2013. The epidemiology and public health importance of toxocariasis: a zoonosis of global importance. Int. J. Parasitol. 43, 999–1008.

Magnaval, J.F., Michault, A., Calon, N., Charlet, J.P., 1994. Epidemiology of human toxocariasis in La Réunion. Trans. R. Soc. Trop. Med. Hyg. 88, 531–533.

Manini, M.P., Marchioro, A.A., Colli, C.M., Nishi, L., Falavigna-Guilherme, A.L., 2012. Association between contamination of public squares and seropositivity for *Toxocara* spp. in children. Vet. Parasitol. 188, 48–52.

Mattos, G.T., Santos, P.C., Telmo, P.L., Berne, M.E., Scaini, C.J., 2016. Human toxocariasis: prevalence and factors associated with biosafety in research laboratories. Am. J. Trop. Med. Hyg. 95, 1428–1431.

Mohammadzadeh, I., Riahi, S.M., Saber, V., Darvish, S., Amrovani, M., Arefkhah, N., Rostami, A., 2018. The relationship between *Toxocara* species seropositivity and allergic skin disorders: a systematic review and meta-analysis. Trans. R. Soc. Trop. Med. Hyg. 112, 529–537.

Moreira, G.M., Telmo Pde, L., Mendonça, M., Moreira, A.N., McBride, A.J., Scaini, C.J., Conceição, F.R., 2014. Human toxocariasis: current advances in diagnostics, treatment, and interventions. Trends Parasitol. 30, 456–464.

Morimatsu, Y., Akao, N., Akiyoshi, H., Kawazu, T., Okabe, Y., Aizawa, H., 2006. A familial case of visceral larva migrans after ingestion of raw chicken livers: appearance of specific antibody in bronchoalveolar lavage fluid of the patients. Am. J. Trop. Med. Hyg. 75, 303–306.

Otero, D., Alho, A.M., Nijsse, R., Roelfsema, J., Overgaauw, P., de Carvalho, L.M., 2018. Environmental contamination with *Toxocara* spp. eggs in public parks and playground sandpits of Greater Lisbon, Portugal. J. Infect. Public Health 11, 94–98.

Overgaauw, P.A., van Knapen, F., 2013. Veterinary and public health aspects of *Toxocara* spp. Vet. Parasitol. 193, 398–403.

Poulsen, C.S., Skov, S., Yoshida, A., Skallerup, P., Maruyama, H., Thamsborg, S.M., Nejsum, P., 2015. Differential serodiagnostics of *Toxocara canis* and *Toxocara cati*—is it possible? Parasite Immunol. 37, 204–207.

Quattrocchi, G., Nicoletti, A., Marin, B., Bruno, E., Druet-Cabanac, M., Preux, P.M., 2012. Toxocariasis and epilepsy: systematic review and meta-analysis. PLoS Negl. Trop. Dis. 6, e1775.

Roldán, W.H., Elefant, G.R., Ferreira, A.W., 2015. Deglycosylation of *Toxocara* excretory-secretory antigens improves the specificity of the serodiagnosis for human toxocariasis. Parasite Immunol. 37, 557–567.

Rostami, A., Riahi, S.M., Holland, C.V., Taghipour, A., Khalili Fomeshi, M., Fakhri, Y., Omrani, V.F., Hotez, P.J., Gasser, R.B., 2019a. Seroprevalence estimates of toxocariasis in people worldwide: a systematic review and meta-analysis. PLoS Negl. Trop. Dis. 13, e0007809.

Rostami, A., Ma, G., Wang, T., Koehler, A.V., Hofmann, A., Chang, B.C., Macpherson, C.N., Gasser, R.B., 2019b. Human toxocariasis—a look at a neglected disease through an epidemiological 'prism'. Infect. Genet. Evol. 74, 104002.

Rostami, A., Kish, M.S., Ma, G., Wang, T., Ebrahimi, M., Fakhri, Y., Mirjalali, H., Hofmann, A., Macpherson, C.N., Hotez, P.J., Gasser, R.B., 2020a. Global prevalence of *Toxocara* infection in cats. In: Advances in Parasitology. Vol. 109. pp. 615–639. Chapter 30—This Special Issue.

Rostami, A., Riahi, S.M., Hofmann, A., Ma, G., Wang, T., Behniafar, H., Taghipour, A., Fakhri, Y., Spotin, A., Chang, B.C.H., Macpherson, C.N., Hotez, P.J., Gasser, R.B., 2020b. Global prevalence of *Toxocara* infection in dogs. In: Advances in Parasitology. Vol. 109. pp. 561–583. Chapter 28—This Special Issue.

Rubinsky-Elefant, G., da Silva-Nunes, M., Malafronte, R.S., Muniz, P.T., Ferreira, M.U., 2008. Human toxocariasis in rural Brazilian Amazonia: seroprevalence, risk factors, and spatial distribution. Am. J. Trop. Med. Hyg. 79, 93–98.

Smith, H., Noordin, R., 2006. Diagnostic limitations and future trends in the serodiagnosis of human toxocariasis. In: Holland, C.V., Smith, H.V. (Eds.), *Toxocara*: The Enigmatic Parasite. In: vol. 2006. CABI, Wallingford, pp. 89–112.

Smith, H., Holland, C., Taylor, M., Magnaval, J.F., Schantz, P., Maizels, R., 2009. How common is human toxocariasis? Towards standardizing our knowledge. Trends Parasitol. 25, 182–188.

Strube, C., Heuer, L., Janecek, E., 2013. *Toxocara* spp. infections in paratenic hosts. Vet. Parasitol. 193, 375–389.

Thompson, D.E., Bundy, D.A., Cooper, E.S., Schantz, P.M., 1986. Epidemiological characteristics of *Toxocara canis* zoonotic infection of children in a Caribbean community. Bull. World Health Organ. 64, 283–290.

Walsh, M.G., Haseeb, M., 2012. Reduced cognitive function in children with toxocariasis in a nationally representative sample of the United States. Int. J. Parasitol. 42, 1159–1163.

Wilder, H.C., 1950. Nematode endophthalmitis. Trans. Am. Acad. Ophthalmol. Otolaryngol. 55, 99–109.

Won, K.Y., Kruszon-Moran, D., Schantz, P.M., Jones, J.L., 2008. National seroprevalence and risk factors for zoonotic *Toxocara* spp. infection. Am. J. Trop. Med. Hyg. 79, 552–557.

Woodhall, D., Starr, M.C., Montgomery, S.P., Jones, J.L., Lum, F., Read, R.W., Moorthy, R.S., 2012. Ocular toxocariasis: epidemiologic, anatomic, and therapeutic variations based on a survey of ophthalmic subspecialists. Ophthalmology 119, 1211–1217.

Yoshikawa, M., Nishiofuku, M., Moriya, K., Ouji, Y., Ishizaka, S., Kasahara, K., Mikasa, K., Hirai, T., Mizuno, Y., Ogawa, S., Nakamura, T., Maruyama, H., Akao, N., 2008. A familial case of visceral toxocariasis due to consumption of raw bovine liver. Parasitol. Int. 57, 525–529.

Zhu, X.Q., Korhonen, P.K., Cai, H., Young, N.D., Nejsum, P., Samson-Himmelstjerna, V.G., Boag, P.R., Tan, P., Li, Q., Min, J., Yang, Y., Wang, X., Fang, X., Hall, R.S., Hofmann, A., Sternberg, P.W., Jex, A.R., Gasser, R.B., 2015. Genetic blueprint of the zoonotic pathogen *Toxocara canis*. Nat. Commun. 6, 6145.

CHAPTER FIFTEEN

Toxocara seroprevalence in Canada—Climate, environment and culture

Richard S. Bradbury*, Indu S. Panicker
School of Health and Life Sciences, Federation University Australia, Berwick, VIC, Australia
*Corresponding author: e-mail address: rbradbury@federation.edu.au

Contents

Abstract

Human infection with larvae of canine and feline roundworms belonging to the genus *Toxocara* can lead to devastating visceral, neural or ocular larvae migrans disease. However, such overt disease represents a fraction of cases. Far more common is covert toxocariasis, a less severe, but clinically symptomatic form of disease, and those who are exposed to infective larvae and seroconvert, but appear to be asymptomatic.

Canada represents a unique epidemiological environment for *Toxocara* infection and exposure. Although the freezing conditions of the vast Arctic Tundra region of the North are thought unlikely to support the lifecycle of *Toxocara* spp., exposure and seroconversion does occur in people belonging to Inuit communities of this region. Further south, in the sub-Arctic of northern Quebec and Saskatchewan, there is a higher seroprevalence in many Canadian First Nations communities. The epidemiology of these infections is different to that seen in the non-Indigenous communities of the Humid Continental region. Poverty and climate play a major part in the risk of *Toxocara* seropositive status in Canada, but other factors such as unique cultural practices, population density of humans and reservoir hosts, and contact with wildlife are also factors in exposure and subsequent seroconversion in Canadian communities.

This review discusses previous *Toxocara* seroprevalence studies performed in Canada, summarizes the data for domestic and wild animal reservoir hosts of *Toxocara canis*, *Toxocara cati*, *Toxocara vitulorum* and the closely related helminth, *Toxascaris leonina*. It also discusses how the unique and varied aspects of climate, culture and environment impacts human *Toxocara* exposure in Canada.

Advances in Parasitology, Volume 109
ISSN 0065-308X
https://doi.org/10.1016/bs.apar.2020.03.003

1. Introduction

Toxocariasis was first reported in Canada in 1957 by Mckee (1957), who described two cases of visceral larva migrans syndrome consistent with *Toxocara canis* infection. One year later, Wong and Laxdal reported a third clinically identified case (Wong and Laxdal, 1958). It was not until 1974 that a histologically confirmed case of *Toxocara* larva migrans was reported in Canada. This involved a rapidly fatal infection in an 18 month old boy, where larvae morphologically consistent with *Toxocara* spp. were found upon autopsy in the child's liver, heart and brain (Mikhael et al., 1974).

There is limited data on the true prevalence of overt toxocariasis in Canada, and no accurate statistics on the prevalence of covert toxocariasis. Fanning et al. found 18 cases of visceral larva migrans and three cases of ocular larva migrans reported in records between 1952 and 1978 from one Toronto hospital (Fanning et al., 1981). A further single case of ocular larva migrans from Toronto was described by Ota et al. (2009). A recent study reviewed hospital discharge records in all Canadian provinces, except Quebec, for records of toxocariasis. This study estimated that there were 0.010 cases of toxocariasis requiring hospitalization per 100,000 of population per year (Schurer et al., 2016). Overt toxocariasis patients were most commonly from low income urban core neighbourhoods, consistent with seroprevalence data from the United States (Schurer et al., 2016). However, this data is likely an underestimate of true overt *Toxocara* infections due to under-reporting and under-diagnosis (Schurer et al., 2016). Furthermore, the more insidious clinical manifestations of the far more common condition of covert toxocariasis in seropositive individuals will not lead to hospitalization and would not have been detected by this study (Schurer et al., 2016).

Although Canada is also an industrialized country in North America, culturally and economically similar to the United States of America, the status of *Toxocara* and toxocariasis in this nation is remarkably different to that of the Canadian's southern neighbours. Firstly, the environmental differences, in particular the vast expanse of Canada and its harsh northern winters decrease the intensity of exposure to *Toxocara* larvae. In the Canadian Arctic, where the majority of people are Inuit and temperatures are below freezing for much of the year, the duration of transmission of *Toxocara* will be much shorter than in the warmer southern regions of Canada. As a consequence of the great differences in human and wildlife population densities, cultural practices and climate between the northern and southern regions of

Canada, the epidemiology of infection and exposure between these two regions differs markedly. The combined factors of environmental and cultural diversity, plus the low population density and abundance of potential wildlife reservoirs combine to make Canada a unique epidemiological environment for toxocariasis in humans.

2. *Toxocara* seroprevalence studies in Canada

No large-scale nationwide serosurvey of *Toxocara* antibody prevalence in the general Canadian population has ever been performed. An early serosurvey by Viens (1977) included 943 "normal" people in Montreal, Quebec using an immunofluorescence antibody test (IFAT). A provincial serosurvey of children using an in-house second stage larval secretory antigen ELISA occurred in Nova Scotia (Embil et al., 1988). All other *Toxocara* seroprevalence surveys conducted in Canada have been focused on Canadian First Nations and Inuit communities or select groups such as veterinary clinic workers and people with asthma or epilepsy (Table 1). The absence of a general nationwide urban, rural and remote population survey makes comparison of the Canadian data with population studies in other countries problematic. It also makes it difficult to determine the significance of data generated in the many surveys in Indigenous communities, as there is no background prevalence rate with which to compare these results. The seroprevalences of between 10.0% and 19.5% found in two early Canadian studies (Embil et al., 1988; Tanner et al., 1987) are possibly falsely elevated and incomparable to more recent seroprevalence studies due to the poor specificity of early *Toxocara* ELISA techniques. All results from recent (since 2004) Canadian surveillance studies are comparable, having employed a standardized commercial TES ELISA test kits (produced by In Vitro Diagnostics of Carlsbad, California) and reporting seroprevalences ranging between 0.6% and 13.4% (Table 1).

The prevalence of antibodies to *Toxocara* spp. in Canada declines with increasing northerly latitudes. This phenomenon of lower seroprevalence with increasing latitude is also seen in surveys of the Inuit people of the Canadian Arctic regions. For example, a survey of an Inuit community living in Nunavik, northern Quebec (latitude 55.3°) found an average seroprevalence between 1.7% and 5.5% (Messier et al., 2012). By comparison, at latitudes with an Arctic Tundra climate, the *Toxocara* seroprevalence in Inuit people sampled was between 0.9% and 1.9% (Goyette et al., 2014). Clearly, the frozen nature of northern Canada provides some protection to the people of that region from exposure to *Toxocara* larvae.

Table 1 Human Toxocara IgG antibody seroprevalence surveys in Canada.

Year/s of sample collection	Participant group (age range)	Region	Latitude	Köppen climate type[a]	Laboratory method	Number of samples tested (n)	Sero-prevalence (%)	References
1975	Asthmatic children	Montreal, Quebec	45.5°	Humid Continental	IFAT	50	22.0	Viens (1977)
1975	Epileptic children	Montreal, Quebec	45.5°	Humid Continental	IFAT	43	16.0	Viens (1977)
1975	Children with eosinophilia	Montreal, Quebec	45.5°	Humid Continental	IFAT	102	41.0	Viens (1977)
1975	Epileptic adults	Montreal, Quebec	45.5°	Humid Continental	IFAT	63	20.0	Viens (1977)
1975	"Normal persons"	Montreal, Quebec	45.5°	Humid Continental	IFAT	940	4.5	Viens (1977)
1980's	Inuit (all ages)[b]	Northern Quebec	55.3–62.4°	Arctic Tundra & Sub-Arctic	TCLA ELISA	759	11.0	Tanner et al. (1987)
1980's	First nations (all ages)[b]	Northern Quebec	50.4–53.7°	Sub-Arctic	TCLA ELISA	436	10.0	Tanner et al. (1987)
1981	Veterinary personnel (adults)	Toronto, Ontario	43.7°	Humid Continental	TES ELISA	113	8.8	Yang et al. (1982)
1981	Hospital inpatients (adults)	Toronto, Ontario	43.7°	Humid Continental	TES ELISA	114	9.6	Yang et al. (1982)

1982–1984	Children (<1–15 years)	Halifax (urban), Nova Scotia	44.6°	Humid Continental	TCSE ELISA	449	14.0	Embil et al. (1988)
1982–1984	Children (<1–15 years)	Rural Nova Scotia	43.6–47.0	Humid Continental	TCSE ELISA	524	19.5	Embil et al. (1988)
1983–1986	Inuit (all ages)[b]	Kuujjuaq, Quebec	58.1°	Sub-Arctic	ns "ELISA"	nd[c]	7.0	Curtis et al. (1988)
1983–1986	Inuit (all ages)[b]	Salluit, Quebec	62.1°	Arctic Tundra	ns "ELISA"	nd[c]	20.0	Curtis et al. (1988)
2004	Inuit (18–74 years)	Nunavik region, Quebec	55.3–62.0°	Sub-Arctic	TES ELISA	917	3.9	Messier et al. (2012)
2005	Cree (adults)[d]	Mistissini, Quebec	50.4°	Sub-Arctic	TES ELISA	48	4.2	Lévesque et al. (2007)
2007	Cree (≥15 years)	Wemindji, Quebec	53.0°	Sub-Arctic	TES ELISA	140	1.4	Campagna et al. (2011)
2007	Cree (≥15 years)	Eastmain, Quebec	52.2°	Sub-Arctic	TES ELISA	111	5.4	Campagna et al. (2011)
2008	Cree (all ages)	Waskaganish, Quebec	51.4°	Sub-Arctic	TES ELISA	265	9.9	Sampasa-Kanyinga et al. (2012)
2008	Cree (all ages)	Chisasibi, Quebec	53.8°	Sub-Arctic	TES ELISA	163	0.6	Sampasa-Kanyinga et al. (2012)

Continued

Table 1 Human Toxocara IgG antibody seroprevalence surveys in Canada.—cont'd

Year/s of sample collection	Participant group (age range)	Region	Latitude	Köppen climate type[a]	Laboratory method	Number of samples tested (n)	Sero-prevalence (%)	References
2007–2008	Inuit (≥18 years)	Inuvialuit Settlement Region, North West Territories	66.5–70.0°	Arctic Tundra	TES ELISA	362	1.1	Goyette et al. (2014)
2007–2008	Inuit (≥18 years)	Nunavut	70.3–83.1°	Arctic Tundra	TES ELISA	1923	1.9	Goyette et al. (2014)
2007–2008	Inuit (≥18 years)	Nunatsiavut, Labrador & Newfoundland	59.7–64.3°	Arctic Tundra & Sub-arctic	TES ELISA	310	0.9	Goyette et al. (2014)
2010–2011	Dene (adults)	Northern Saskatchewan	54.0–59.0°	Sub-Arctic	TES ELISA	201	13.4	Schurer et al. (2013)
2011	Saulteaux (>4 years)	Southern Saskatchewan	50.7–52.2°	Humid Continental	TES ELISA	113	4.4	Schurer et al. (2014)

[a]Köppen climate data from Government of Canada (2016).
[b]Hospital patients and outpatients.
[c]Combined number of samples from both Kuujjuaq and Salluit was 264.
[d]Specifically hunters, trappers and their spouses.
IFAT, *Toxocara canis* crude third stage larvae immunofluorescence antibody test; TCLA, *Toxocara canis* crude third stage larval antigen prepared from embryonated eggs; TCSE, *Toxocara canis* second stage larval secretory antigen; TES, *Toxocara canis* excretory/secretory antigen; nd, no data.

3. *Toxocara* seroprevalence in Inuit people of the frozen north

The Arctic Canadian North is characterized by extended periods of temperatures below freezing. The Arctic Tundra climate region includes the Arctic Circle above latitude 66.0°, but extends below into latitudes between 55° and 60° at various points (Government of Canada, 2016). This climate region is characterized by extended periods of temperatures below freezing. It also boasts a very low human population density when compared to the warmer southern regions of Canada (Statistics Canada, 2016). Those people who do live in this region are overwhelmingly Inuit in ethnicity (Statistics Canada, 2019). An early seroprevalence survey in Salluit, an Inuit community on the northern coast of Quebec found a surprisingly high seroprevalence of 20% (Curtis et al., 1988); however, the authors suggested that this high prevalence might be attributable to cross-reaction of their ELISA technique with another helminth infections (Curtis et al., 1988). The only recent survey of Inuit communities in the Arctic Tundra climate region, using a specific commercial TES ELISA kit, found that *Toxocara* seroprevalence rates were low (between 0.9% and 1.9%; Table 1) (Goyette et al., 2014). The associations of latitude and the degree of *Toxocara* exposure in this region are driven by a combination of factors including climate, culture, population density and the abundance of wildlife reservoirs.

Exposure to *Toxocara* larvae requires ingestion of larvated eggs or hypobiotic larvae in raw or undercooked meat of a paratenic host (Ma et al., 2018). Specific cultural practices undertaken by some Inuit people risk exposure via these methods. However, due to the extreme cold of the Arctic regions and very short warm season, periods of time in which such exposure may occur are limited. With regard to exposure to eggs, many Inuit people will hunt or trap wolves and the entrails of these hunted animals are often left near houses, increasing the potential for exposure to *Toxocara* eggs by children and domestic animals (Khan, 2001). While such practices should lead to high *Toxocara* seroprevalences in this group, the cold temperatures of the Canadian frozen north are protective as *Toxocara* eggs do not survive long periods in these conditions (Jenkins et al., 2013). The importance of climate in lowering *Toxocara* exposure rates in northern Canada is that the season of the year in which shed eggs may reach viability is very limited. Temperatures as low as −2 °C will arrest the development of unembryonated *Toxocara* eggs, but will not make them unviable, with embryonation observed upon return to higher temperatures after at least 6 weeks (Azam et al., 2012). Therefore, it is possible that eggs shed in the environment may become viable during the short warm periods in these latitudes, but such periods are brief. Embryonated *Toxocara* eggs have been shown to retain viability for up to 34 days at −20 °C (O'Lorcain, 1995), but it is generally accepted that the long term freezing temperatures of the Arctic region render eggs unviable (Jenkins et al., 2013). The cold effect limits the length of time that humans are exposed to viable, embryonated eggs from their immediate environment, with that limited time period increasing incrementally as latitude increases.

Another cultural practice of some Inuit people is the eating of raw meat and the offal of hunted animals (Curtis et al., 1988; Khan, 2001). This uncooked game meat is usually stored outdoors prior to consumption (Curtis et al., 1988) and domestic dogs are often fed wild game meat (Salb et al., 2008), including known *Toxocara* paratenic hosts such as rabbits and rodents (Ma et al., 2018; Salb et al., 2008). Under normal circumstances, such activity would lead to increased exposure to *Toxocara* larvae from the meat of paratenic hosts. Freezing renders both *T. canis* and *Toxocara cati* larvae unviable, but cooling to lower temperatures (0 °C–4 °C) does not eliminate viable larvae (Dutra et al., 2013; Taira et al., 2012). Indeed, in one study, hunting was negatively associated with *Toxocara* infection. The same study did find an association of consumption of marine mammal meat with the presence of antibodies to *Toxocara* spp. (Goyette et al., 2014). This was suggested as being due to contamination of meat with *Toxocara* eggs from domestic dogs in the hunting camps rather than due to marine mammals acting as paratenic hosts (Goyette et al., 2014).

The harsh environment and sparse population of the Arctic Circle region limits the number of definitive hosts depositing viable eggs in the environment. While some potential wildlife host species such as the arctic fox (*Vulpes lagopus*) and arctic wolf (*Canis lupus arctos*) are found in these very northerly regions, the population density of wild canids is generally lower than would be expected in the warmer south. Although Inuit people keep working dogs and pet dogs, the lower population density of humans in these regions and the cold climate makes the intensity of environmental contamination from domestic dog sources less likely than would be seen in a built up urban environment with a higher population density of domestic dogs and cats and warmer climate. Indeed, *T. canis* infection prevalence in domestic dogs incrementally decreases with higher latitudes in Canada (Table 2),

Table 2 Surveys of Toxocara spp.in domestic animals, dogs and cats in Canada.

Year	Source	Species	Region	Laboratory method/s	Number of samples tested (*n*)	Prevalence (%)	References
1949	Dogs	*Toxocara canis*	St. Hyacinthe, QC	$ZnSO_4$-C	155	52.6	Choquette and Gelinas (1950)
1949	Dogs	*Toxascaris leonina*	St. Hyacinthe, QC	$ZnSO_4$-C	155	10.5	Choquette and Gelinas (1950)
1971	Dogs	*Toxocara canis*	Central SK	SSF-C	48	19.7	Unruh et al. (1973)
1971	Dogs	*Toxascaris leonina*	Central SK	SSF-C	48	20.6	Unruh et al. (1973)
1971	Dogs	*Toxocara canis*	Central SK	SSF-C	254	3.9	Unruh et al. (1973)
1971	Dogs	*Toxascaris leonina*	Central SK	SSF-C	254	3.5	Unruh et al. (1973)
1971	Dogs	*Toxocara canis*	Northern AB	SSF-C	272	0.0	Unruh et al. (1973)
1971	Dogs	*Toxascaris leonina*	Northern AB	SSF-C	272	25.5	Unruh et al. (1973)
1971	Dogs	*Toxocara canis*	NT	SSF-C	327	0.3	Unruh et al. (1973)
1971	Dogs	*Toxascaris leonina*	NT	SSF-C	327	22.9	Unruh et al. (1973)
1971–1972	Dogs (stray)	*Toxocara canis*	Halifax, NS	NaCl-P	474	26.6	Malloy and Embil (1978)
1971–1972	Dogs (stray)	*Toxascaris leonina*	Halifax, NS	NaCl-P	474	1.3	Malloy and Embil (1978)

Continued

Table 2 Surveys of Toxocara spp.in domestic animals, dogs and cats in Canada.—cont'd

Year	Source	Species	Region	Laboratory method/s	Number of samples tested (*n*)	Prevalence (%)	References
1971–1972	Dogs (stray)	*Toxocara cati*	Halifax, NS	NaCl-P	299	25.1	Malloy and Embil (1978)
1971–1972	Dogs (stray)	*Toxascaris leonina*	Halifax, NS	NaCl-P	299	0.3	Malloy and Embil (1978)
1974	Dogs	*Toxocara canis*	Montreal, QC	FEA	332	34.0	Ghadiran et al. (1976), Viens (1977)
1974	Dogs	*Toxascaris leonina*	Montreal, QC	FEA	332	11.4	Ghadiran et al. (1976), Viens (1977)
1975	Dogs (stray)	*Toxocara canis*	Montreal, QC	$ZnSO_4$ + FEA	239	43.5	Seah et al. (1975)
1977	Dogs	*Toxocara canis*	Montreal, QC	FEA	332	34.0	Viens (1977)
1977	Dogs	*Toxascaris leonina*	Montreal, QC	FEA	332	11.4	Viens (1977)
1983–1986	Dogs	*Toxascaris leonina*	Northern QC	SSF-C	94	40.0	Curtis et al. (1988)
1998–2008	Cats	*Toxocara cati*	Southern SK	SSF-C	635	4.7	Hoopes et al. (2013)
1998–2008	Cats	*Toxascaris leonina*	Southern SK	SSF-C	635	0.2	Hoopes et al. (2013)
1999	Cats	*Toxocara cati*	Saskatoon, SK	Nec	52	17.3	Pomroy (1999)
2006	Dogs	*Toxocara spp*	Northern Canada	SSF-C	129	79.0	Salb et al. (2008)

2006	Dogs	*Toxocara canis*	PE	$ZnSO_4$-C	209	11.8	Uehlinger et al. (2013)
2007	Dogs	*Toxocara canis*	Coastal BC	SSF-C	75	4.0	Bryan et al. (2011)
2007	Dogs	*Toxascaris leonina*	Coastal BC	SSF-C	75	1.0	Bryan et al. (2011)
2008–2009	Dogs	*Toxocara canis*	Saskatoon, SK	SSF-C	457	0.2	Gaunt and Carr (2011)
2008–2009	Dogs	*Toxascaris leonina*	Saskatoon, SK	SSF-C	457	0.7	Gaunt and Carr (2011)
2008–2009	Dogs	*Toxocara canis*	Calgary, AB	$ZnSO_4$-C	619	2.1	Joffe et al. (2011)
2008–2009	Dogs	*Toxascaris leonina*	Calgary, AB	$ZnSO_4$-C	619	1.3	Joffe et al. (2011)
2008–2009	Cats	*Toxocara cati*	Calgary, AB	$ZnSO_4$-C	153	6.5	Joffe et al. (2011)
2009	Cats (shelter)	*Toxocara cati*	National	SSF-C	636	16.5	Villeneuve et al. (2015)
2009	Cats (shelter)	*Toxascaris leonina*	National	SSF-C	636	3.0	Villeneuve et al. (2015)
2009	Cats (feral)	*Toxocara cati*	PE	$ZnSO_4$-C	78	34.0	Stojanovic and Foley (2011)
2009–2010	Dogs (shelter)	*Toxocara canis*	National	SSF-C	1086	12.7	Villeneuve et al. (2015)
2010–2011	Dogs	*Toxocara*	Northern SK	SSF-C	195	4.1	Schurer et al. (2013)
2010–2011	Dogs	*Toxascaris*	Northern SK	SSF-C	195	8.2	Schurer et al. (2013)
2011–2013	Dogs	*Toxocara canis*	Southeastern, SK	SSF-C-S	51	11.6	Schurer et al. (2014)

Continued

Table 2 Surveys of Toxocara spp.in domestic animals, dogs and cats in Canada.—cont'd

Year	Source	Species	Region	Laboratory method/s	Number of samples tested (*n*)	Prevalence (%)	References
2011–2013	Dogs	*Toxascaris leonina*	Southeastern, SK	SSF-C-S	51	15.7	Schurer et al. (2014)
2015	Cats (rural)	*Toxocara*	AB	SSF-C	27	15.0	Hoopes et al. (2015)
2015	Cats (rural)	*Toxascaris*	AB	SSF-C	27	4.0	Hoopes et al. (2015)
2015	Cats (stray and pet)	*Toxocara*	SK	SSF-C	192	0.8	Hoopes et al. (2015)
2015	Cats (stray and pet)	*Toxascaris*	SK	SSF-C	192	0.0	Hoopes et al. (2015)
2020	Dogs (pet)	*Toxocara canis*	PE	$ZnSO_4$-C	15,016	2.4	Morandi et al. (2020)
2020	Cats (pet)	*Toxocara cati*	PE	$ZnSO_4$-C	2391	3.2	Morandi et al. (2020)

Nec, necropsy; FEA, formalin-ether/ethyl acetate sedimentation; NaCl-P, saturated salt passive flotation; SSF-C, saturated sucrose centrifugal flotation; SSF-C-S, saturated sucrose double centrifugal flotation modified Stoll counts; $ZnSO_4$-C, zinc sulphate centrifugal flotation.

AB, Alberta; BC, British Columbia; MB, Manitoba; NT, Northwest Territories; PE, Prince Edward Island; QC, Quebec; SK, Saskatchewan.

and has not been reported from dogs residing north of latitude 63° (Jenkins et al., 2013). The colder temperatures in northern regions also limit the degree of outside play and geophagia by children (Campagna, 2009), which is a primary risk factor for *Toxocara* exposure (Hamilton, 1996). Thus, the Frozen North of Canada provides a protection to the Inuit people against *Toxocara* infection. This is further supported by the two to fourfold higher seroprevalence (3.9%) seen in one Inuit community at the more southerly latitudes in Nunavik, Quebec (Messier et al., 2012). Both historical data and current projections indicate a warming climate in northern Canada (Campagna et al., 2011), which will potentially extend the periods of time in which exposure to viable *Toxocara* eggs and larvae may occur, and may subsequently increase *Toxocara* seroprevalence in this region.

4. *Toxocara* seroprevalence in first nations and Inuit people of the sub-arctic

Between latitudes 50.0° and 66.0° is the Canadian sub-arctic. Long and very cold winters are interspersed with short but sustained warmer periods in the summer months. As noted in the previous section, this effect of climate greatly impacts the period of time that viable *Toxocara* eggs are present in the environment and increases the likelihood of exposure for those living in this region.

The earliest *Toxocara* antibody serosurveys of Indigenous Canadians were carried out among hospitalized and outpatients from First Nations and Inuit communities of northern Quebec (Curtis et al., 1988; Tanner et al., 1987). In both cases, sera from in-patients and out-patients from local hospitals were surveyed. This region has a mostly sub-Arctic climate, but this transforms into an Arctic Tundra climate on its northern-most coastlines (Government of Canada, 2016). Tanner et al.'s survey found that the overall seroprevalence of *Toxocara* antibodies between First Nations and Inuit peoples was comparable, and seroprevalence increased with age, as seen in many other *Toxocara* seroprevalence surveys. These authors did note an unusually high seroprevalence of up to 40% in the Arctic Tundra climate Inuit village of Povungnituk (Tanner et al., 1987). The authors expressed surprise at this finding, given that *Toxocara* eggs should not survive the Arctic winter. Two possible reasons for this anomaly were proposed. The first was that *T. canis* imported with dogs from more southerly regions had infected the community. The second intriguing suggestion was that these people were developing antibodies against *Toxascaris leonina*, a parasite of dogs and wild canids similar to *T. canis*, and that these were cross-reacting in the crude larval antigen ELISA test employed for this study (Tanner et al., 1987). Curtis et al. only surveyed subjects from one sub-Arctic Inuit community (Kuujjuaq) and found an unusually high seroprevalence for such communities of 7.0% (Curtis et al., 1988). Unfortunately, this report did not describe the type of antigen used in their *Toxocara* ELISA test, nor how it was prepared (Curtis et al., 1988). Therefore the relative specificity of these results cannot be determined in comparison with more recent serosurveys from the same region, which have all used a commercial TES ELISA technique (Campagna et al., 2011; Sampasa-Kanyinga et al., 2012).

A survey of an Inuit community in the sub-Arctic Nunavik region of northern Quebec demonstrated a higher seroprevalence than that found in Inuit people from the Arctic Tundra climate Nunavut and North West Territories. Fourteen communities were sampled around both the Hudson Bay and Ungava Bay regions (Messier et al., 2012). The results from both sites differed markedly, with those in the Hudson Bay region having a seroprevalence of 5.5%, while those in Ungava Bay region had only a 1.7% seroprevalence. This difference reached significance ($P = 0.002$) (Messier et al., 2012). Low numbers of positives meant that statistically valid information regarding risk factors could not be determined in many cases, but seroprevalence did appear to increase with age (Messier et al., 2012). There was also a marked discrepancy in overall seroprevalence among those who had only an elementary school education (5.5%) compared to those who had attended secondary school (3.3%) (Messier et al., 2012), though it should be considered that this may also be a factor of age with much older residents less likely to have been required to attend secondary education. Indeed, the odds ratio (O.R.) of those aged 50–74 being seropositive was a startling 17.4 (Messier et al., 2012). Increasing *Toxocara* antibody status with age is a commonly observed phenomena in affected communities, resulting from a combination of increased opportunity for exposure over time and the lasting duration of *Toxocara* IgG antibodies. The reasons for the discrepancy in average seroprevalence between the westerly Hudson Bay and easterly Ungava Bay was not elucidated.

Adult *Toxocara* seroprevalence study have been conducted in four Cree First Nation communities of central Quebec (Campagna et al., 2011; Lévesque et al., 2007; Sampasa-Kanyinga et al., 2012). Seroprevalence rates varied between 0.6% and 9.9% (Table 1). These *Toxocara* antibody seroprevalence rates are quite low in comparison to that seen using the same method in the general community of the United States between 1988 and 1994

(13.9% seroprevalence; (Won et al., 2008). However, in three of these communities, over 30% of seropositive people had eosinophilia and one had unexplained transient abdominal pain (Campagna et al., 2011; Sampasa-Kanyinga et al., 2012). These results demonstrate that many of those people who are infected in these communities are exposed to sufficiently high larval loads resulting in detectable signs and symptoms. The other two serosurveys performed in the southern half of Canada were in Saskatchewan, involving testing of adults and children of the Saulteaux First Nation and adults of Dene First Nation community (Schurer et al., 2013, 2014).

A relatively high prevalence of *Toxocara* seropositivity of 9.9% in a Cree community living in Waskaganish, in the western portion of James Bay, Quebec was at odds with much lower seroprevalences found in nearby Cree communities (Sampasa-Kanyinga et al., 2012). The authors found that seroprevalence was not associated with dog ownership, but the handling of Caribou in the higher seroprevalence community was associated with seropositivity, though there was a limited sample to draw inference from for this finding (Sampasa-Kanyinga et al., 2012). No other potential causes of this unusually high seroprevalence were identified.

Another comparably high seroprevalence (13.4%) was detected in adults of a Dene First Nation people community surveyed in a sub-Arctic climate region of northern Saskatchewan (Schurer et al., 2013). In this community, *Toxocara* antibody positive status was significantly associated with being between ages 5–17 (O.R. 3.4) and feeding pets a non-commercial pet food diet (O.R. 15). The authors correctly note that feeding pets non-commercial food may correlate with poverty, an established risk factor for toxocariasis in Canada and elsewhere (Schurer et al., 2013, 2016). Despite this, feeding dogs and cats potentially infected paratenic hosts would increase the likelihood of their immediate home environment being heavily contaminated with *Toxocara* eggs. Furthermore, feeding pets with non-commercial food may also correlate with lowered rates of anthelmintic administration by owners. That dogs in Canadian First Nations communities are often of younger ages, which leads to greater susceptibility to intestinal *T. canis* infection, and are rarely dewormed has been discussed by other authors (Jenkins et al., 2011). The authors of this study noted that the seroprevalence in both of the surveyed Saskatchewan communities (Schurer et al., 2013, 2014) was equivalent or much lower than that seen in a nationwide study in the United States using an equivalent test methodology (Won et al., 2008). It was suggested that the colder climate of Saskatchewan, where winter temperatures are routinely between −20 and −30 °C, combined with the habit of domestic dogs to defecate in the bush, away from human dwellings would lead to lower seroprevalences (Schurer et al., 2013).

5. *Toxocara* seroprevalence in the people of humid continental Canada

A serosurvey of a Saulteaux First Nation community living in a Humid Continental region of southern Saskatchewan found a seroprevalence of *Toxocara* antibodies of only 4.4% (Schurer et al., 2014). Despite this relatively low seroprevalence, several risk factors were identified. Dog ownership and feeding raw meat to domestic dogs were not identified as significant risk factors (Schurer et al., 2014). Children between the ages of 11 and 17 years had increased seroprevalence compared to younger children (Schurer et al., 2014), attributable to increased opportunity for exposure with increasing age and the lasting nature of IgG antibodies. Most interestingly, having a previous history of dog bite was positively correlated with *Toxocara* antibody positive status in this survey. As the life cycle of *T. canis* does not involve biting, it was suggested as more likely that this simply reflected increased close contact with dogs in seropositive people (Schurer et al., 2014).

Few *Toxocara* serosurveys of predominantly non-Indigenous Canadian population groups have been conducted. The first was a study of children with eosinophilia, asthmatic children, children and adults with epilepsy and the general population in Montreal, Quebec using an IFAT. The difference in seroprevalence between "normal" controls in the general population and those with specific disease was marked. The control group of 943 normal Montreal residents were found to have a low (4.5%) seroprevalence. In contrast, the seroprevalences of *Toxocara* IgG antibodies in adults and children with epilepsy and children with asthma were up five times higher, while children with eosinophilia were found to have a profound 10-fold higher seroprevalence (41.0%) (Table 1). This study is one of several to have suggested a positive association between asthma, epilepsy and *Toxocara* antibody positive status (Li et al., 2014; Quattrocchi et al., 2012).

A survey of 113 veterinary clinic personnel in Toronto, including veterinarians, laboratory technicians, kennel workers, nurses, clerks, drivers and students, found an 8.8% seroprevalence of *Toxocara* antibodies. This was almost identical to the 9.0% seroprevalence in a control group of 114 in-patients at a Toronto hospital for adults. Data on seroprevalence in relation to years of employment at a veterinary clinic was inconclusive.

Dog ownership, age, sex and occupational exposure were not associated with higher antibody positive status in either the veterinary workers or controls (Yang et al., 1982).

Another study was of rural and urban children in Nova Scotia in the early 1980's (Embil et al., 1988). Some broad risk factors for toxocariasis in Nova Scotia were identified. Boys had a higher seroprevalence than girls (15.0% vs 12.9%) and children from rural areas had much higher seroprevalence (19.5%) than those from the city of Halifax (14.0%). Having a household dog and living in a rural area was positively associated with seropositivity ($P=0.010$), as was being in the older (7–15 years) age cohort of rural children ($P=0.005$), indeed over one quarter of older cohort rural children were seropositive. These two risk factors may have been associated, as older children and rural children were significantly more likely to have a household dog ($P<0.01$ and $P<0.001$, respectively). The trend towards higher seroprevalence in older children from rural areas was not reflected in their urban counterparts ($P=0.88$) (Embil et al., 1988).

The seroprevalence of *Toxocara* antibodies in both rural and urban Nova Scotia children was much higher than was seen in children from the United States using the same method on serum samples collected nationwide in the early 1970's (Herrmann et al., 1985). An explanatory factor for this anomaly is poverty, an acknowledged risk factor for *Toxocara* seropositivity (Liu et al., 2017). Nova Scotia has one of the lowest gross domestic products of any of the populated Canadian provinces (Statistics Canada, 2020). It should also be noted that overall incomes are lower in rural Canada than in urban areas (Rupnik et al., 2001) and that the rural poor in Canada have less access to health education, healthcare and other services than their urban counterparts (DesMeules et al., 2006). The very high prevalences of *Toxocara* antibodies reported in this Nova Scotia study may be a factor of the specificity of the in-house ELISA test employed. A repeat sampling of rural and urban Canadians living in the Humid Continental climate region and employing a modern high-specificity *Toxocara* recombinant antigen serological test is indicated.

Another potential risk in rural Canada is exposure to *Toxocara* spp. from working dogs, domestic dogs, wildlife and agricultural animals. The high rates of *Toxocara* intestinal infection in wild canids and felids (Table 3) not only provides a direct exposure risk to humans interacting with the Canadian wilderness, but also an increased risk of intestinal infection in their hunting and working dogs. While *T. canis* and *T. cati* remain the primary known causes of toxocariasis in humans, the related ascarid species,

Table 3 Surveys of *Toxocara* and *Toxascaris* spp.in agricultural animals, wild animals and the environment in Canada.

Year	Source	Species	Region	Laboratory method/s	Number tested (*n*)	Prevalence of *Toxocara* or *Toxascaris* eggs (%)	References
1974	Public parks	*Toxocara* sp.	Montreal, QC	NaCl-P	10	60.0	Ghadiran et al. (1976), Viens (1977)
1976	Public parks	*Toxocara* sp.	Toronto, ON	FEA	12	22.4	Berman (1998)
1994–1995	Parks and playgrounds	*Toxocara* sp.	Toronto, ON	FEA	17	2.9	Berman (1998)
1960–1977	Red foxes (*Vulpes vulpes*)	*Toxocara canis*	New Brunswick, NB; Nova Scotia, NS	Nec	61	70.5	Smith, 1978
1975-1976	Red foxes (*Vulpes vulpes*)	*Toxascaris leonina*	Southwestern MB	Nec	6	100.0	Samuel et al. (1978)
2004–2005	Red foxes (*Vulpes vulpes*)	*Toxocara canis*	PE	SSF-P	271	25.1	Wapenaar et al. (2013)
1983–1986	Red foxes (*Vulpes vulpes*)	*Toxascaris leonina*	Northern QC	Nec	nd	73.0	Curtis et al. (1988)
1978	Arctic foxes (*Vulpes lagopus*)	*Toxascaris leonina*	Banks Island, NT	FEA	50	60.0	Eaton and Secord (1979)
1983–1986	Arctic foxes (*Vulpes lagopus*)	*Toxascaris leonina*	Northern QC	Nec	ns	82.0	Curtis et al. (1988)
2011–2012	Arctic foxes (*Vulpes lagopus*)	*Toxascaris leonina*	Central Nunavut, NU	SSF-DC	95	63.0	Elmore et al. (2013)
1968	Coyotes (*Canis latrans*)	*Toxascaris leonina*	AB	nd	75	52.0	Holmes and Podesta (1968)

1975-1976	Coyotes (*Canis latrans*)	*Toxascaris leonina*	Southwestern MB	Nec	43	65.0	Samuel et al. (1978)
2001–2003	Coyotes (*Canis latrans*)	*Toxocara canis*	Newfoundland, NL	Nec	69	19.0	Bridger et al. (2009)
2001–2003	Coyotes (*Canis latrans*)	*Toxascaris leonina*	Newfoundland, NL	Nec	69	1.0	Bridger et al. (2009)
2004–2005	Coyotes (*Canis latrans*)	*Toxocara canis*	PE	SSF-P	185	2.2	Wapenaar et al. (2013)
2009–2010	Coyote (*Canis latrans*)	*Toxascaris leonina*	Calgary, AB	DM	61	80.3	Liccioli et al., 2012
2009–2010	Coyote (*Canis latrans*)	*Toxascaris leonina*	Calgary, AB	SSF-DC	247	19.0	Liccioli et al. (2012)
1959–1967	Grey wolves (Canis lupus)	*Toxascaris leonina*	AB	nd	98	14.0	Holmes and Podesta (1968)
1975-1976	Gray wolves (*Canis lupus*)	*Toxascaris leonina*	Southwestern MB	Nec	12	9.0	Samuel et al. (1978)
2001–2003	Grey wolves (*Canis lupus*)	*Toxocara* sp.	Riding Mountain National Park, MB	nd	320	0.3	Sallows (2007)
2001–2005	Grey wolves (*Canis lupus*)	*Toxocara* sp.	MB	SSF-DC	601	0.2	Stronen et al. (2011)
2010–2014	Grey wolves (*Canis lupus*)	*Toxascaris*	NT, BC, SK, MB	SSF-DC	191	18.0	Schurer et al. (2016)
2010–2014	Grey wolves (*Canis lupus*)	*Toxascaris leonina*	NT, BC, SK, MB	SSF-DC	151	23.0	Schurer et al. (2016)

Continued

Table 3 Surveys of *Toxocara* and *Toxascaris* spp.in agricultural animals, wild animals and the environment in Canada.—cont'd

Year	Source	Species	Region	Laboratory method/s	Number tested (*n*)	Prevalence of *Toxocara* or *Toxascaris* eggs (%)	References
1961–1963	Lynx (*Felis canadensis*)	*Toxascaris leonina*	Alberta, AB; Mackenzie District	Nec	113	82.0	Van Zyll de Jong (1966)
1961–1964	Lynx (*Felis canadensis*)	*Toxocara cati*	Alberta, AB; Mackenzie District	Nec	113	4.0	Van Zyll de Jong (1966)
1983–1986	Lynx (*Felis canadensis*)	*Toxocara* sp.	Northern QC	Nec	ns	100.0	Curtis et al. (1988)
2001	Lynx (*Felis canadensis*)	*Toxocara cati*	Northern ON	Nec	274	22.0	Smith et al. (1986)
2001	Lynx (*Felis canadensis*)	*Toxascaris leonina*	Northern ON	Nec	274	97.0	Smith et al. (1986)
2011	Bison (*Bison bison*) calves	*Toxocara vitulorum*	MB	SSF-P	15	33.3	Woodbury et al. (2012)
2012	Bison (*Bison bison*) calves	*Toxocara vitulorum*	MB; SK	SSF-DC	54	77.8	Woodbury et al. (2012)
2015	Bison (*Bison bison*)	*Toxocara vitulorum*	Western Canada	$NaNO_3$-Mc	249	0.0	Oostenbrug (2015)

DM, direct microscopy; FEA, formalin-ether/ethyl acetate sedimentation; NaCl-P, saturated salt passive flotation; $NaNO_3$-Mc, sodium nitrate passive flotation McMaster counts; Nec, necropsy; SSF-DC, saturated sucrose double centrifugal flotation; SSF-P, saturated sucrose passive flotation; $ZnSO_4$-C, zinc sulphate centrifugal flotation; nd, no data.

BC, British Columbia; ON, Ontario; MB, Manitoba; NL, Newfoundland and Labrador; NT, Northwest Territories; NU, Nunavut; PE, Prince Edward Island; QC, Quebec; SK, Saskatchewan.

T. leonina, also occurs in Canadian wildlife. Furthermore, bison and cattle may be infected with *Toxocara vitulorum*. Both of these helminth species have been implicated as potential agents of human infection (Sapp et al., 2019; Van Gorp et al., 1987) and exposure to *T. leonina* has been associated with eosinophilia in people from northern Alaska (Rausch and Fay, 2011). Work on cross-reaction of antibodies and antigens from these species and *T. canis* has demonstrated the potential for serologic cross reactions to occur (Page et al., 1991; Smith et al., 1982), including cross reaction of TES antigen with *T. leonina* antibodies (Smith et al., 1982). The degree of interaction of sero-positive rural Canadians with wildlife and *T. vitulorum* infected cattle and *T. leonina* domestic and wild canids should be investigated further in the future.

6. Concluding remarks

The most pressing need in regard to the investigation of toxocariasis and *Toxocara* exposure in Canada is for a broad, large-scale, national study of seroprevalence including all Canadians. Such a study should employ the most recently developed, and most specific, recombinant *T. canis* 32 kDa excretory/secretory C-type lectin-1 antigen, preferably using a multiplex serology assay platform. Such a survey would provide answers to many unknowns about the epidemiology of the disease in Canada. Specific questions about whether Indigenous Canadians or Canadians living in rural areas are at higher risk than others and what regions have the highest rates of *Toxocara* exposure across the nation would be answered by such a study. Evidence of higher rates of overt toxocariasis in poor urban Canadians (Schurer et al., 2016), suggesting increased exposure in this cohort require further investigation by serosurveillance. Without this data, it is difficult to interpret the broad implications of the small cohort serosurveys which have been performed thus far, using less specific TES ELISA or crude antigen ELISA platforms. Surveillance of humans, domestic animals to identify high prevalence foci, followed by public and veterinary health education efforts including, but not limited to, encouraging owners to regularly deworm pet dogs and cats would assist in further reducing exposure to *Toxocara* spp. in the Canadian population. Efforts should also be made to further investigate if *T. leonina* and *T. vitulorum* may also represent a zoonotic disease risk to Canadians in rural and remote communities.

Regardless of the above considerations, it is clear that Canada presents a unique environment for the epidemiology of toxocariasis. A major factor in the varying seroprevalence seen across the nation, and the lower seroprevalences in comparison to the United States, is latitude, particularly in the predominantly Inuit frozen North. In this Arctic Tundra climate, nearly year round frozen temperatures keep the transmission of *Toxocara* spp. to a minimum, despite cultural practices in some groups relating to hunting, raw meat and offal which might otherwise predispose to infection. In the sub-Arctic and, where a short warmer summer occurs, *Toxocara* exposure is more common, but still below that seen in the United States. Once again, the cold winters limit exposure, but also the comparably lower population density of humans, domestic dogs and wildlife reservoir hosts in the region reduces the risk of exposure. In Humid Continental Nova Scotia, on the same latitude as the northern United States, seroprevalence may be quite high and is comparable with similar United States surveys. Much is yet to be learned about the epidemiology of toxocariasis and *Toxocara* seroprevalence in the Arctic and sub-Arctic regions of Canada. Future investigations should include consideration of not only climate, but also local cultural practices and potential exposure to reservoir host wildlife in any research plans.

References

Azam, D., Ukpai, O.M., Said, A., Abd-Allah, G.A., Morgan, E.R., 2012. Temperature and the development and survival of infective *Toxocara canis* larvae. Parasitol. Res. 110, 649–656.

Berman, R.L., 1998. The Prevalence of Parasites Due to Faecal Contamination of Public Parks and Playgrounds in Metropolitan Toronto, Ontario, Canada. Master of Science thesis. University of Toronto, Toronto.

Bridger, K.E., Baggs, E.M., Finney-Crawley, J., 2009. Endoparasites of the coyote (*Canis latrans*), a recent migrant to insular Newfoundland. J. Wildl. Dis. 45, 1221–1226.

Bryan, H.M., Darimont, C.T., Paquet, P.C., Ellis, J.A., Goji, N., Gouix, M., Smits, J.E., 2011. Exposure to infectious agents in dogs in remote coastal British Columbia: possible sentinels of diseases in wildlife and humans. Can. J. Vet. Res. 75, 11–17.

Campagna, S., 2009. Prevalence and Environmental Risk Factors for Ten Zoonoses in Two Cree Communities of James Bay (Canada). Master of Environment thesis. Université de Sherbrooke, Quebec.

Campagna, S., Lévesque, B., Anassour-Laouan-Sidi, E., Côté, S., Serhir, B., Ward, B.J., Libman, M.D., Drebot, M.A., Makowski, K., Adonova, M., Ndao, M., Dewailly, É., 2011. Seroprevalence of 10 zoonotic infections in 2 Canadian Cree communities. Diagn. Microbiol. Infect. Dis. 70, 191–199.

Choquette, L.P.E., Gelinas, L.D.G., 1950. Incidence of intestinal nematodes and protozoa in dogs in the Montreal district. Can. J. Comp. Med. Vet. Sci. 14, 33.

Curtis, M.A., Rau, M.E., Tanner, C.E., Prichard, R.K., Faubert, G.M., Olpinski, S., Trudeau, C., 1988. Parasitic zoonoses in relation to fish and wildlife harvesting by Inuit communities in northern Quebec, Canada. Arctic Med. Res. 47 (Suppl. 1), 693–696.

DesMeules, M., Pong, R.W., Lagacé, C., Heng, D., Manuel, D., Pitblado, R., Bollman, R., Guernsey, J., Kazanjian, A., Koren, I., 2006. How Healthy Are Rural Canadians? An Assessment of Their Health Status and Health Determinants. In: Canadian Institute for Health Information. Public Health Agency of Canada, Ottawa.

Dutra, G.F., Pinto, N.S.F., de Avila, L.F.D.C., de Lima Telmo, P., da Hora, V.P., Martins, L.H.R., Aires Berne, M.E., Scaini, C.J., 2013. Evaluation of the initial and chronic phases of toxocariasis after consumption of liver treated by freezing or cooling. Parasitol. Res. 112, 2171–2175.

Eaton, R.D., Secord, D.C., 1979. Some intestinal parasites of Arctic fox, Banks Island, NWT. Can. J. Comp. Med. 43, 229.

Elmore, S.A., Lalonde, L.F., Samelius, G., Alisauskas, R.T., Gajadhar, A.A., Jenkins, E.J., 2013. Endoparasites in the feces of arctic foxes in a terrestrial ecosystem in Canada. Int. J. Parasitol. Parasites Wildl. 2, 90–96.

Embil, J.A., Tanner, C.E., Pereira, L.H., Staudt, M., Morrison, E.G., Gualazzi, D.A., 1988. Seroepidemiologic survey of *Toxocara canis* infection in urban and rural children. Public Health 102, 129–133.

Fanning, M., Hill, A., Langer, H.M., Keystone, J.S., 1981. Visceral larva migrans (toxocariasis) in Toronto. Can. Med. Assoc. J. 124, 21.

Gaunt, M.C., Carr, A.P., 2011. A survey of intestinal parasites in dogs from Saskatoon, Saskatchewan. Can. Vet. J. 52, 497.

Ghadiran, E., Viens, P., Strykowski, H., Dubreuil, F., 1976. Epidemiology of toxocariasis in the Montreal area: prevalence of *Toxocara* and other helminth ova in dogs and soil. Can. J. Public Health 6, 495–498.

Government of Canada, 2016. https://open.canada.ca/data/en/dataset/09ffaeb5-ec8f-5bb5-bdcb-3436ccf26f58, accessed 10 January 2020.

Goyette, S., Cao, Z., Libman, M.J., Ndao, M., Ward, B.J., 2014. Seroprevalence of parasitic zoonoses and their relationship with social factors among the Canadian Inuit in Arctic regions. Diagn. Microbiol. Infect. Dis. 78, 404–410.

Hamilton, J., 1996. Zoonotic diseases in Canada: an interdisciplinary challenge. Can. Med. Assoc. J. 155, 413.

Herrmann, N., Glickman, L.T., Schantz, P.M., Weston, M.G., Domanski, L.M., 1985. Seroprevalence of zoonotic toxocariasis in the United States: 1971–1973. Am. J. Epidemiol. 122, 890–896.

Holmes, J.C., Podesta, R., 1968. The helminths of wolves and coyotes from the forested regions of Alberta. Can. J. Zool. 46, 1193–1204.

Hoopes, J.H., Polley, L., Wagner, B., Jenkins, E.J., 2013. A retrospective investigation of feline gastrointestinal parasites in western Canada. Can. Vet. J. 54, 359–362.

Hoopes, J., Hill, J.E., Polley, L., Fernando, C., Wagner, B., Schurer, J., Jenkins, E., 2015. Enteric parasites of free-roaming, owned, and rural cats in prairie regions of Canada. Can. Vet. J. 56, 495–501.

Jenkins, E.J., Schurer, J.M., Gesy, K.M., 2011. Old problems on a new playing field: helminth zoonoses transmitted among dogs, wildlife, and people in a changing northern climate. Vet. Parasitol. 182, 54–69.

Jenkins, E.J., Castrodale, L.J., de Rosemond, S.J., Dixon, B.R., Elmore, S.A., Gesy, K.M., Hoberg, E.P., Polley, L., Schurer, J.M., Simard, M., Thompson, R.A., 2013. Tradition and transition: parasitic zoonoses of people and animals in Alaska, northern Canada, and Greenland. In: Rollinson, D. (Ed.), Advances in Parasitology. In: vol. 82. Elsevier Academic Press, London, pp. 33–204.

Joffe, D., Van Niekerk, D., Gagné, F., Gilleard, J., Kutz, S., Lobingier, R., 2011. The prevalence of intestinal parasites in dogs and cats in Calgary, Alberta. Can. Vet. J. 52, 1323.

Khan, R.A., 2001. Zoonoses and new parasites in Canada. In: Proceedings of 1st Congress of Federation of Asian Parasitologists. Federation of Asian Parasitologists, Chiba.

Lévesque, B., Messier, V., Bonnier-Viger, Y., Couillard, M., Côté, S., Ward, B.J., Libman, M.D., Gingras, S., Dewailly, É., 2007. Seroprevalence of zoonoses in a Cree community (Canada). Diagn. Microbiol. Infect. Dis. 59, 283–286.

Li, L., Gao, W., Yang, X., Wu, D., Bi, H., Zhang, S., Hunag, M., Yao, X., 2014. Asthma and toxocariasis. Ann. Allergy Asthma Immunol. 113, 187–192.

Liccioli, S., Catalano, S., Kutz, S.J., Lejeune, M., Verocai, G.G., Duignan, P.J., Fuentealba, M., Hart, E., Ruckstuhl, K.E., Massolo, A., 2012. Gastrointestinal parasites of coyotes (*Canis latrans*) in the metropolitan area of Calgary, Alberta, Canada. Can. J. Zool. 90, 1023–1030.

Liu, E.W., Chastain, H.M., Shin, S.H., Wiegand, R.E., Kruszon-Moran, D., Handali, S., Jones, J.L., 2017. Seroprevalence of antibodies to *Toxocara* species in the United States and associated risk factors, 2011–2014. Clin. Infect. Dis. 66, 206–212.

Ma, G., Holland, C.V., Wang, T., Hofmann, A., Fan, C.K., Maizels, R.M., Gasser, R.B., 2018. Human toxocariasis. Lancet Infect. Dis. 18, e14–e24.

Malloy, W.F., Embil, J.A., 1978. Prevalence of *Toxocara* spp. and other parasites in dogs and cats in Halifax, Nova Scotia. Can. J. Comp. Med. 42, 29.

Mckee, J.A., 1957. Visceral Larva Migrans. 6, The Bulletin of the Hospital for Sick Children (Toronto), pp. 43–46.

Messier, V., Levesque, B., Proulx, J.F., Rochette, L., Serhir, B., Couillard, M., Ward, B.J., Libman, M.D., Dewailly, É., Déry, S., 2012. Seroprevalence of seven zoonotic infections in Nunavik, Quebec (Canada). Zoonoses Public Health 59, 107–117.

Mikhael, N.Z., Montpetit, V.J., Orizaga, M., Rowsell, H.C., Richard, M.T., 1974. *Toxocara canis* infestation with encephalitis. Can. J. Neurol. Sci. 1, 114–120.

Morandi, B., Greenwood, S.J., Conboy, G.A., Galuppi, R., Poglayen, G., VanLeeuwen, J.A., 2020. Endoparasites in dogs and cats diagnosed at the Veterinary Teaching Hospital (VTH) of the University of Prince Edward Island between 2000 and 2017. A large-scale retrospective study. Prev. Vet. Med. 175, 104878.

O'Lorcain, P., 1995. The effects of freezing on the viability of *Toxocara canis* and *T. cati* embryonated eggs. J. Helminthol. 69, 169–171.

Oostenbrug, T.B., 2015. Gastrointestinal Parasites in Farmed Bison: Prevalence in Western Canada. Master of Veterinary Medicine thesis. Utrecht University, Utrecht.

Ota, K.V., Dimaras, H., Héon, E., Babyn, P.S., Yau, Y.C., Read, S., Budning, A., Gallie, B.L., Chan, H.S.L., 2009. Toxocariasis mimicking liver, lung, and spinal cord metastases from retinoblastoma. Pediatr. Infect. Dis. J. 28, 252–254.

Page, A.P., Richards, D.T., Lewis, J.W., Omar, H.M., Maizels, R.M., 1991. Comparison of isolates and species of *Toxocara* and *Toxascaris* by biosynthetic labelling of somatic and ES proteins from infective larvae. Parasitology 103, 451–464.

Pomroy, W.E., 1999. A survey of helminth parasites of cats from Saskatoon. Can. Vet. J. 40, 339–340.

Quattrocchi, G., Nicoletti, A., Marin, B., Bruno, E., Druet-Cabanac, M., Preux, P.M., 2012. Toxocariasis and epilepsy: systematic review and meta-analysis. PLoS Negl. Trop. Dis. 6, e1775.

Rausch, R.L., Fay, F.H., 2011. *Toxascaris leonina* in rodents, and relationship to eosinophilia in a human population. Comp. Parasitol. 78, 236–245.

Rupnik, C., Thompson-James, M., Bollman, R.D., 2001. Measuring Economic Well-Being of Rural Canadians Using Income Indicators. Agriculture and rural working paper no. 45, catalogue no. 21-601-MIE01045. Statistics Canada, Ottawa.

Salb, A.L., Barkema, H.W., Elkin, B.T., Thompson, R.A., Whiteside, D.P., Black, S.R., Dubey, J.P., Kutz, S.J., 2008. Dogs as sources and sentinels of parasites in humans and wildlife, northern Canada. Emerg. Infect. Dis. 14, 60.

Sallows, T.A., 2007. Diet Preference and Parasites of Grey Wolves in Riding Mountain National Park of Canada. Master of Environment thesis. University of Manitoba, Winnipeg.

Sampasa-Kanyinga, H., Lévesque, B., Anassour-Laouan-Sidi, E., Côté, S., Serhir, B., Ward, B.J., Libman, M.J., Drebot, M.A., Ndao, M., Dewailly, É., 2012. Zoonotic infections in native communities of James Bay, Canada. Vector Borne Zoonotic Dis. 12, 473–481.

Samuel, W.M., Ramalingam, S., Carbyn, L.N., 1978. Helminths in coyotes (*Canis latrans* Say), wolves (*Canis lupus* L.), and red foxes (*Vulpes vulpes* L.) of southwestern Manitoba. Can. J. Zool. 56, 2614–2617.

Sapp, S.G.H., Handali, S., Bradbury, R.S., 2019. Larva migrans. In: Wilcke, B.W., Heyman, D.L. (Eds.), Control of Communicable Diseases: Laboratory Practice. American Public Health Association, Washington D.C. pp. 332–343.

Schurer, J.M., Ndao, M., Skinner, S., Irvine, J., Elmore, S.A., Epp, T., Jenkins, E.J., 2013. Parasitic zoonoses: one health surveillance in northern Saskatchewan. PLoS Negl. Trop. Dis. 7, e2141.

Schurer, J.M., Ndao, M., Quewezance, H., Elmore, S.A., Jenkins, E.J., 2014. People, pets, and parasites: one health surveillance in southeastern Saskatchewan. Am. J. Trop. Med. Hyg. 90, 1184–1190.

Schurer, J.M., Rafferty, E., Schwandt, M., Zeng, W., Farag, M., Jenkins, E.J., 2016. Toxoplasmosis and toxocariasis: an assessment of human immunodeficiency virus comorbidity and health-care costs in Canada. Am. J. Trop. Med. Hyg. 95, 168–174.

Seah, S.K., Hucal, G., Law, C., 1975. Dogs and intestinal parasites: a public health problem. Can. Med. Assoc. J. 112, 1191.

Smith, H.J., 1978. Parasites of red foxes in New Brunswick and Nova Scotia. J. Wildl. Dis. 14, 366–370.

Smith, H.V., Quinn, R., Bruce, R.G., Girdwood, R.W., 1982. Development of the serological response in rabbits infected with *Toxocara canis* and *Toxascaris leonina*. Trans. R. Soc. Trop. Med. Hyg. 76, 89–94.

Smith, J.D., Addison, E.M., Joachim, D.G., Smith, L.M., Quinn, N.W.S., 1986. Helminth parasites of Canada lynx (*Felis canadensis*) from northern Ontario. Can. J. Zool. 64, 358–364.

Statistics Canada, 2016. https://www150.statcan.gc.ca/n1/pub/16-201-x/2009000/t071-eng.htm, accessed 8 January 2020.

Statistics Canada, 2019. https://www12.statcan.gc.ca/census-recensement/2016/dp-pd/prof/index.cfm?Lang=E, accessed 8 January 2020.

Statistics Canada, 2020. https://www150.statcan.gc.ca/t1/tbl1/en/tv.action?pid=3610048701, accessed 9 January 2020.

Stojanovic, V., Foley, P., 2011. Infectious disease prevalence in a feral cat population on Prince Edward Island, Canada. Can. Vet. J. 52, 979.

Stronen, A.V., Sallows, T., Forbes, G.J., Wagner, B., Paquet, P.C., 2011. Diseases and parasites in wolves of the Riding Mountain National Park region, Manitoba, Canada. J. Wildl. Dis. 47, 222–227.

Taira, K., Saitoh, Y., Okada, N., Sugiyama, H., Kapel, C.M., 2012. Tolerance to low temperatures of *Toxocara cati* larvae in chicken muscle tissue. Vet. Parasitol. 189, 383–386.

Tanner, C.E., Staudt, M., Adamowski, R., Lussier, M., Bertrand, S., Prichard, R.K., 1987. Seroepidemiological study for five different zoonotic parasites in northern Quebec. Can. J. Public Health 78, 262–266.

Uehlinger, F.D., Greenwood, S.J., McClure, J.T., Conboy, G., O'Handley, R., Barkema, H.W., 2013. Zoonotic potential of *Giardia duodenalis* and *Cryptosporidium* spp. and prevalence of intestinal parasites in young dogs from different populations on Prince Edward Island, Canada. Vet. Parasitol. 196, 509–514.

Unruh, D.H.A., King, J.E., Allen, J.R., Eaton, R.D.P., 1973. Parasites of dogs from Indian settlements in northwestern Canada: a survey with public health implications. Can. J. Comp. Med. 37, 25.

Van Gorp, K., Mangelschots, M., Brandt, J., 1987. *Toxocara vitulorum*: a possible agent of larva migrans in humans? In: Geerts, S., Kumar, V., Brandt, J. (Eds.), Helminth Zoonoses. Springer, Dordrecht, pp. 159–166.

Van Zyll de Jong, C.G., 1966. Parasites of the Canada lynx, *Felis* (*Lynx*) *canadensis* (Kerr). Can. J. Zool. 44, 499–509.

Viens, P., 1977. Visceral larva migrans in Montreal: the tip of the iceberg. Bord. Med. 10, 697–698.

Villeneuve, A., Polley, L., Jenkins, E., Schurer, J., Gilleard, J., Kutz, S., Gagné, F., 2015. Parasite prevalence in fecal samples from shelter dogs and cats across the Canadian provinces. Parasit. Vectors 8, 281.

Wapenaar, W., Barkema, H.W., O'Handley, R., 2013. Fecal shedding of Toxocara canis and other parasites in foxes and coyotes on Prince Edward Island, *Canada*. J. Wildl. Dis. 49, 394–397.

Won, K.Y., Kruszon-Moran, D., Schantz, P.M., Jones, J.L., 2008. National seroprevalence and risk factors for zoonotic *Toxocara* spp. infection. Am. J. Trop. Med. Hyg. 79, 552–557.

Wong, L.C., Laxdal, O.E., 1958. Visceral larva migrans. Can. Med. Assoc. J. 78, 695.

Woodbury, M.R., Copeland, S., Wagner, B., Fernando, C., Hill, J.E., Clemence, C., 2012. *Toxocara vitulorum* in a bison (*Bison bison*) herd from western Canada. Can. Vet. J. 53, 791.

Yang, J., Keystone, J.S., McIntyre, L., Spence, H., 1982. *Toxocara* antibodies in veterinary personnel. Can. Vet. J. 23, 126.

CHAPTER SIXTEEN

Toxocara seroprevalence in the USA and its impact for individuals and society

Richard S. Bradbury[a,*], **Charlotte V. Hobbs**[b]
[a]School of Health and Life Sciences, Federation University Australia, Berwick, VIC, Australia
[b]Children's of Mississippi, University of Mississippi Medical Center, Jackson, MS, United States
*Corresponding author: e-mail address: rbradbury@federation.edu.au

Contents

Abstract

Toxocara species are intestinal helminths of dogs and cats, the larval stages of which may infect humans and cause severe neural, ocular and visceral larva migrans disease. Such cases of severe overt disease represent only a small fraction of the of the US population who have been exposed and infected with *Toxocara*, subsequently developing IgG antibodies to the larvae. The true impact of exposure to *Toxocara* in this large group of Americans remains uncertain. *Toxocara* antibody positivity is associated with poverty, but other specific risk factors have been identified, including sex, age, rural residence, region of residence, race and exposure to pets. This seropositive status has also been associated with several childhood diseases, including asthma and epilepsy, increased serum lead levels, and poor neurocognitive function.

Three large-scale NHANES studies have provided comprehensive datasets, while several smaller studies have explored specific disease associations. Each seroprevalence study must be interpreted in consideration of the sensitivity and specificity of the individual serological methods employed. This chapter summarizes all historical *Toxocara* prevalence data from dogs, cats and soil in the United States. It then carefully examines all previous human *Toxocara* seroprevalence surveys performed in the United States. Data from these surveys is assimilated, compared and discussed to determine the validity of findings and to accurately identify risk factors for *Toxocara* seropositivity. The validity of associations of exposure to *Toxocara* larvae and childhood diseases such as asthma and epilepsy and effects neurocognitive function within the American context are also explored.

Advances in Parasitology, Volume 109
ISSN 0065-308X
https://doi.org/10.1016/bs.apar.2020.01.035

1. Introduction

Paul C. Beaver and colleagues first identified *Toxocara* as a cause of visceral larva migrans in 1952, describing three cases from the United States of America (Beaver et al., 1952). This report also identified an earlier report of eosinophilic granulomas in the liver with associated symptoms in an American child as consistent with *Toxocara* visceral larva migrans disease (Beaver et al., 1952; Perlingiero and György, 1947). Helenor Campbell-Wilder had earlier described a series of nematode endophthalmitis cases from the United States including at least four cases which were later identified being *Toxocara* ocular larva migrans (Wilder, 1950). Since this time, over 200 clinical cases of toxocariasis have been reported from the USA, including at least 9 cases of visceral larva migrans, 184 of ocular larva migrans, 8 of neural larva migrans and 1 of common toxocariasis (Chen et al., 2018; Inagaki et al., 2019). Such cases of overt clinical toxocariasis are relatively rare and represent the "tip of the iceberg" of disease as many cases are undiagnosed or unreported and the many infected persons have subclinical disease or subtle allergic, respiratory or neurocognitive symptoms ("covert" or "common" toxocariasis). These generally go medically unrecognized (Fillaux and Magnaval, 2013; Rostami et al., 2019). Furthermore, a large number of seropositive individuals appear to be asymptomatic (Centers for Disease Control and Prevention, 2019). Indeed, if all cases of exposure and infection with *Toxocara* are considered, toxocariasis represents the most common helminth infection of humans in the United States (Hotez and Wilkins, 2009). Given the relatively ubiquitous presence of *Toxocara canis* and *Toxocara cati* eggs in dogs, cats and urban soils in the USA (Table 1), exposure to infection is difficult to avoid. However, accurate data on the incidence of overt and covert toxocariasis is difficult to find as the disease is not reportable in the USA and no official surveillance program is in place (Woodhall et al., 2014). *Toxocara* larvae cannot reach maturity and cause patent intestinal disease in humans, but rather survive in the organs and tissues for at least 5 years (Nelson et al., 1996), with detection of infection requiring serological methods. These serological IgG titers may remain elevated for an extended period after infection, making interpretation of active infection vs prior exposure (Rostami et al., 2019) a complicated diagnosis, necessitating inclusion of consideration of both clinical symptoms combined with consideration of the serological antibody titers (Fillaux and Magnaval, 2013).

Table 1 Surveys of *Toxocara* spp. from dogs, cats and the environment in the United States of America.

Year/s	Source	Region	Laboratory method/s	Number of samples tested (*n*)	Prevalence of *Toxocara* eggs (%)	Reference
1958	Dogs and cats	New York City, NY	$ZnSO_4$-P	500	1.6	Dorman and Van Ostrand (1958)
1969	Dogs and cats	Philadelphia, PA	$NaNO_3$-C	895	16.6	Dubin et al. (1975)
1970	Dogs and cats	Philadelphia, PA	$NaNO_3$-C	895	18.0	Dubin et al. (1975)
1971	Dogs and cats	Philadelphia, PA	$NaNO_3$-C	1056	20.4	Dubin et al. (1975)
1972	Dogs and cats	Philadelphia, PA	$NaNO_3$-C	1023	19.9	Dubin et al. (1975)
1972	Soil (parks)	Philadelphia, PA	$NaNO_3$-C + Tween	90	11.1	Dubin et al. (1975)
1973	Dogs and cats	Philadelphia, PA	$NaNO_3$-C	922	15.7	Dubin et al. (1975)
1973	Soil (parks)	Philadelphia, PA	$NaNO_3$-C + Tween	46	10.8	Dubin et al. (1975)
1979	Soil (schoolyards)	Manhattan, KS	$ZnSO_4$ + NaOH	11	22.9	Dada and Lindquist (1979)
1979	Soil (parks)	Manhattan, KS	$ZnSO_4$ + NaOH	10	18.4	Dada and Lindquist (1979)
1979	Soil (highway stops)	Manhattan, KS	$ZnSO_4$ + NaOH	15	16.0	Dada and Lindquist (1979)
1979	Soil (sandboxes)	Manhattan, KS	$ZnSO_4$ + NaOH	23	39.1	Dada and Lindquist (1979)
1979	Soil (swings)	Manhattan, KS	$ZnSO_4$ + NaOH	23	17.4	Dada and Lindquist (1979)

Continued

Table 1 Surveys of *Toxocara* spp. from dogs, cats and the environment in the United States of America.—Cont'd

Year/s	Source	Region	Laboratory method/s	Number of samples tested (*n*)	Prevalence of *Toxocara* eggs (%)	Reference
1980	Dogs	Essex County, NJ	$ZnSO_4$-C	246	13.4	Surgan et al. (1980)
1980	Soil (parks)	Essex County, NJ	$ZnSO_4$-C	629	0.3	Surgan et al. (1980)
1985	Soil (backyards)	Baltimore, MD	$ZnSO_4$ + Tween	146	11.0	Childs (1985)
1987	Dogs (puppies)	Atlanta, GA	$ZnSO_4$-C	143	12.0	Stehr-Green et al. (1987)
1988	Dogs and cats	Philadelphia, PA	$ZnSO_4$-C	2294	5.5	Kirkpatrick (1988)
1984–1991	Dogs	Pennsylvania	$ZnSO_4$-C	8077	5.7	Nolan and Smith (1995)
1984–1991	Cats	Pennsylvania	$ZnSO_4$-C	2000	15.0	Nolan and Smith (1995)
1993–1994	Dogs	North East	SSF-C	1480	12.6	Blagburn et al. (1996)
1993–1994	Dogs	South East	SSF-C	1941	17.7	Blagburn et al. (1996)
1993–1994	Dogs	Mid-West	SSF-C	1525	15.8	Blagburn et al. (1996)
1993–1994	Dogs	West	SSF-C	1512	11.0	Blagburn et al. (1996)
2001	Cats (<1 year old)	New York State, NY	SSF-C + $ZnSO_4$-C	263	32.7	Spain et al. (2001)
2003	Cats	National	$ZnSO_4$-C	66,819	2.92	De Santis et al. (2006)
2009	Dogs	Northeastern states	$ZnSO_4$-C	8486	2.2	Little et al. (2009)

2009	Dogs	Midwestern states	$ZnSO_4$-C	5014	2.6	Little et al. (2009)
2009	Dogs	Southern states	$ZnSO_4$-C	4781	1.6	Little et al. (2009)
2009	Dogs	Western states	$ZnSO_4$-C	8514	2.8	Little et al. (2009)
2009	Dogs	National	$ZnSO_4$-C	26,795	2.2	Little et al. (2009)
2009	Dogs	National	$ZnSO_4$-C	2,785,248	5.0	Mohamed et al. (2009)
2010	Dogs	North East	$ZnSO_4$-C	nd*	7.9	Blagburn (2010)
2010	Dogs	South East	$ZnSO_4$-C	nd*	16.4	Blagburn (2010)
2010	Dogs	Mid-West	$ZnSO_4$-C	nd*	12.5	Blagburn (2010)
2010	Dogs	West	$ZnSO_4$-C	nd*	5.9	Blagburn (2010)
2010	Cats	North East	$ZnSO_4$-C	nd*	26.0	Blagburn (2010)
2010	Cats	South East	$ZnSO_4$-C	nd*	21.2	Blagburn (2010)
2010	Cats	Mid-West	$ZnSO_4$-C	nd*	21.2	Blagburn (2010)
2010	Cats	West	$ZnSO_4$-C	nd*	18.1	Blagburn (2010)
2010	Dogs	Huntington, WV	$ZnSO_4$-P	231	6.9	Savilla et al. (2011)
2011	Dogs	National	$ZnSO_4$-C	2,553,250	2.0	Lucio-Forster et al. (2016)
2011	Cats	National	$ZnSO_4$-C	543,961	5.1	Lucio-Forster et al. (2016)

Continued

Table 1 Surveys of *Toxocara* spp. from dogs, cats and the environment in the United States of America.—Cont'd

Year/s	Source	Region	Laboratory method/s	Number of samples tested (*n*)	Prevalence of *Toxocara* eggs (%)	Reference
2012	Dogs	National	$ZnSO_4$-C	2,572,089	2.0	Lucio-Forster et al. (2016)
2012	Cats	National	$ZnSO_4$-C	531,826	5.1	Lucio-Forster et al. (2016)
2013	Dogs	National	$ZnSO_4$-C	2,512,989	1.8	Lucio-Forster et al. (2016)
2013	Cats	National	$ZnSO_4$-C	502,071	4.7	Lucio-Forster et al. (2016)
2014	Dogs	National	$ZnSO_4$-C	2,750,718	1.8	Lucio-Forster et al. (2016)
2014	Cats	National	$ZnSO_4$-C	52,394	4.6	Lucio-Forster et al. (2016)

$NaNO_3$-C: Sodium nitrate centrifugal flotation.
$NaNO_3$-C + Tween: Sodium nitrate centrifugal flotation with Tween 60 pre-treatment.
SSF-C: Saturated sucrose centrifugal flotation.
$ZnSO_4$-C: Zinc sulfate centrifugal flotation.
$ZnSO_4$-P: Zinc sulfate passive flotation.
$ZnSO_4$ + NaOH: Zinc sulfate centrifugal flotation with sodium hydroxide pre-treatment.
$ZnSO_4$ + Tween: Zinc Sulfate centrifugal flotation with Tween 60 pre-treatment.
nd*: no data for number of specimens by region; total number of fecal specimens tested (all regions combined) was 4,278 canine and 1,984 feline samples.

2. *Toxocara* seroprevalance surveys in the USA

Surveys of seroprevalence in the USA have either been localized studies intended to detect specific pathologies associated with sub-clinical toxocariasis (Desowitz et al., 1981; Glickman et al., 1979, 1981; Sharghi et al., 2001), or the production of largescale nationwide seroprevalence data from samples collected during the National Health and Nutrition Examination Surveys (NHANES) conducted since the mid-1970s (Table 2). US surveys have almost exclusively used IgG antibodies to *Toxocara* as the markers of seroprevalence. The results of early seroprevalence surveys must be interpreted with caution given to the sensitivity and specificity of the laboratory methods employed at the time. Some smaller scale studies performed in Hawaii (Jones et al., 1980), Pennsylvania (Desowitz et al., 1981), Connecticut (Sharghi et al., 2001), and others, are of limited utility in extrapolating to the population as a whole, both because of the small sample sizes not reaching statistical significance and the poor specificity of the crude antigen serological methods employed (Table 2). The most reliable and robust data sets and analyses are those generated from the NHANES studies (Berrett et al., 2017; Congdon and Lloyd, 2011; Farmer et al., 2017; Herrmann et al., 1985; Liu et al., 2018; Won et al., 2008) and a largescale study in New York during the early 1980s (Marmor et al., 1987). One moderate size longitudinal study of the effects of *Toxocara* infection on the cognitive development of children in Cleveland has also been undertaken (Nelson et al., 1996). The major demographic and epidemiological data findings are from three of these studies; NHANES I, 1971–1973 (Herrmann et al., 1985); NHANES III, 1988–1994 (Won et al., 2008) and NHANES 2011–2014 (Liu et al., 2018) are summarized in Table 3.

A marked difference in overall *Toxocara* antibody seroprevalence may be observed between the three NHANES datasets (Table 3). When comparing these studies, it should also be noted that each of the NHANES *Toxocara* seroprevalence studies employed differing serological methods, the dataset from NHANES I (1971–1973) samples were analysed using a crude third stage larval antigen ELISA which has a lower sensitivity than the *T. canis* excretory/secretory antigen ELISA used to analyse the NHANES III (1988–1994) dataset (Jacquier et al., 1991; Jin et al., 2013). Both of these methods may cross-react with sera from patients with other helminthiases (Jacquier et al., 1991; Jin et al., 2013). The NHANES 2011–2014 sera were analysed using a recombinant *T. canis* excretory/secretory 32 kDa C-type

Table 2 Seroprevalence surveys of *Toxocara* IgG antibodies in the United States of America.

Year/s of sample collection	Participant group (age range)	Region	Antigen/s employed	Laboratory method	Number of samples tested (*n*)	Sero-prevalence (%)	Reference
1971–1973	Children (1–11 years)	National (NHANES)	TCLA	ELISA	1369	6.4	Herrmann et al. (1985)
1976	Blood donors	New York	TCLA	ELISA	114	7.9	Cypess et al. (1977)
1977	Animal hospital employees	New York	TCLA	ELISA	73	10.9	Glickman and Cypess (1977)
1978	Epileptic children	Pittsburgh	TCLA	ELISA	84	7.1	Glickman et al. (1979)
1978	Nonepileptic children	Pittsburgh	TCLA	ELISA	108	1.9	Glickman et al. (1979)
1980	Rural residents (all ages)	Pennsylvania	TCLA	ELISA	43	23.0	Jones et al. (1980)
1980	Children (1–6 years)	Pennsylvania	TCLA	ELISA	100	8.0	Glickman et al. (1981)
1981	Asthmatic children (1–18 years)	Hawaii	TCLA	CEP	96	2.1	Desowitz et al. (1981)
1981	Nonasthmatic children (1–18 years)	Hawaii	TCLA	CEP	80	4.9	Desowitz et al. (1981)
1980–1981	Children (1–15 years)	New York	TCLA	ELISA	4652	5.4	Marmor et al. (1987)
1984–1990	Children (4–10 years)	Cleveland	TCLA	ELISA	543	12.0	Nelson et al. (1996)

2000	Children (2–15 years)	Connecticut	TCLA	ELISA	324	11.3	Sharghi et al. (2001)
1988–1994	General Public (>6 years)	National (NHANES)	TES	ELISA	20,395	13.9	Won et al. (2008)
2011–2014	General Public (>6 years)	National (NHANES)	rTc-CTL-1	Luminex	13,509	5.1	Farmer et al. (2017)
2011–2014	General Public (>6 years)[a]	National (NHANES)	rTc-CTL-1	Magplex	13,509[a]	5.1[a]	Liu et al. (2018)

[a]Same serum sample set as used by Farmer et al. (2017).
TCLA, *Toxocara canis* crude third stage larval antigen prepared from embryonated eggs;
TES, *Toxocara canis* excretory/secretory antigen;
rTc-CTL-1, recombinant *Toxocara canis* 32 kDa excretory/secretory C-type lectin-1 antigen;
CEP, Counter-immuno-electrophoresis;
ELISA, enzyme-linked immunosorbent assay;
Luminex, Luminex fluorescent multiplex bead assay;
Magplex, Magplex magnetic multiplex bead assay.

Table 3 Summary of selected demographic data from three NHANES *Toxocara* seroprevalence studies.

	NHANES I		**NHANES III**		**NHANES 2011–2014**	
Years	**1971–1973**		**1988–1994**		**2011–2014**	
Antigen and assay employed	**TCL antigen ELISA**		**TES antigen ELISA**		**rTc-CTL-1 antigen Magplex**	
Participant group	**Number of samples tested (*n*)[a]**	**Sero-prevalence (%)**	**Number of samples tested (*n*)**	**Sero-prevalence (%)**	**Number of samples tested (*n*)**	**Sero-prevalence (%)**
Total	1369	6.4	20,395	13.9	13,509	5.0
Sex						
Male	nd	–	9876	15.6	6859	3.8
Female	nd	–	10,519	12.4	6650	6.2
Demographics						
Metropolitan residence[b]	nd	–	9919	12.4	nd	–
Nonmetropolitan residence	nd	–	10,476	15.3	nd	–
At or above poverty line	nd	–	13,439	12.3	9144	3.9
Below poverty line	nd	–	5091	22.9	3374	10.2
United States birthplace	nd	–	16,571	12.7	10,257	3.7
Outside of United States birthplace	nd	–	3769	22.2	3247	11.9

Head of household education						
Some College	nd	–	5668	9.0	7115	3.4
High School Graduate	nd	–	5865	14.1	2863	6.4
Some High School	nd	–	3465	21.8	1872	7.8
<High School	nd	–	5221	21.6	1210	11.1
Region						
North-East	307	6.5	2638	15.6	nd	–
Mid-West	402	3.7	3920	11.4	nd	–
South	339	10.6	8888	17.4	nd	–
West	321	5.3	4949	9.4	nd	–
Ethnicity						
Non-Hispanic White	879	4.3	nd	12.0	4972	3.7
Non-Hispanic Black	142	31.7	nd	21.2	3114	6.6
Non-Hispanic Asian	nd	–	nd	–	1581	7.3
Hispanic	nd	–	nd	10.7	2010	6.1
Reference	Herrmann et al. (1985)		Won et al. (2008)		Liu et al. (2018)	

[a]Adjusted prevalence excluding equivocal serological titre results.
[b]Defined as a city with a population of 1 million or greater.
nd, no data available;
TCL, *Toxocara* crude third stage larval antigen prepared from embryonated eggs;
TES, *Toxocara* excretory/secretory;
rTc-CTL-1, recombinant *Toxocara canis* 32 kDa excretory/secretory C-type lectin-1.

lectin-1 antigen coupled to Magplex beads (Liu et al., 2018), which shows a sensitivity comparable to *T. canis* excretory/secretory antigen ELISA, but very limited cross reactivity with any other parasitic infections (Anderson et al., 2015). Liu et al. suggested that this absence of cross-reactivity for this antigen may extend to not detecting antibodies to the feline *Toxocara* species, *T. cati*, which is thought to play an important role in human toxocariasis. However, this hypothesis is yet to be confirmed by testing against specific serum from *T. cati* exposed/*T. canis* naïve persons (Liu et al., 2018). The decrease in seroprevalence seen between the 1988–1994 and 2011–2014 NHANES studies is more likely due to the far superior specificity of the serological antigen employed than due to a great reduction in cases of past and current infection in the US population. The 1971–1973 total seroprevalence must also be interpreted in consideration of the low specificity of the crude larval antigen serological method employed.

It should also be considered that the NHANES I dataset is limited to US children between 1 and 11 years of age (Herrmann et al., 1985), while the latter two NHANES *Toxocara* seroprevalence datasets (Liu et al., 2018; Won et al., 2008) represent a cohort of US children and adults over 6 years old, making comparison of these demographic datasets difficult. The lower age range of participants in the NHANES I seroprevalence study allowed less opportunity for exposure to infective *Toxocara* larvae over that cohort's lifetime, resulting in lower overall seroprevalence. Comparison of raw seroprevalence results from these three datasets is not informative, but certain distinct risk factors are clear when examining the available NHANES demographic data and these broader epidemiological trends observed are likely to be valid.

3. Associations with age, sex, exposure to pets and place of residence

The 2011–2014 NHANES studies, using the most accurate serological methods found a significantly higher prevalence in males than females; 6.8% vs 4.0% (adjusted odds ratio, aOR of 1.9) in Farmer et al. (2017); and 6.2 vs 3.8% ($P < 0.001$) in Liu et al. (2018). This sex difference was maintained, but did not reach significance, in the cohort sera from 131 children ≤17 years of age with a male seroprevalence of 4.0% and female seroprevalence of 3.2% (Farmer et al., 2017). *Toxocara* seroprevalence increases with age (Farmer et al., 2017), likely to occur with any long-term IgG antibody response, as increasing age allows increased opportunities for exposure and long-term antibody production. Liu and colleagues (Liu et al., 2018) found that the highest odds ratio for possessing *Toxocara* antibodies was in the age groups 50–59 (OR 2.1) and ≥70 years of age (OR 2.6), while the odds for those 12–19 years were much lower (OR 1.1). Another analysis of this 2011–2014 NHANES dataset by Berrett and colleagues demonstrated an incrementally increasing odds ratio of *Toxocara* exposure with each decade of age, from OR 1.00 in the 6–9 age group to OR 2.9 in those older than 80 years of age (Berrett et al., 2017). In the largest childhood cohort study from the USA, carried out by Marmor and colleagues in the 1980s, increasing seroprevalence with increasing age was also reported. The youngest children (0–2 years) had a seroprevalence of 1.3%, which incrementally increased to the oldest age group (12–15 years) at 12.0%. Once again, male seroprevalence (5.8%) was higher than female (5.0%) (Marmor et al., 1987).

In the NHANES III dataset of US residents ≥6 years old, personal dog and cat ownership had no significant influence on the prevalence of *Toxocara* antibodies (Won et al., 2008). This finding was supported by a much smaller and earlier data set of children in Connecticut (Sharghi et al., 2001). However, in the largest dataset from children in the USA, an increased risk ratio was found for those having a dog in the home (RR 2.07), and a marked association between ever having a litter of puppies in the home (RR 4.20) and *Toxocara* antibody positive status, was identified (Marmor et al., 1987). A smaller ($n=543$) longitudinal cohort study of children in Cleveland supported those findings (Nelson et al., 1996). An earlier study (Glickman et al., 1981) of 100 children also found a significant association of dog ownership and the presence of antibodies to *Toxocara*. These associations are consistent with the reservoir and life cycle of the parasite. The relative risks of exposure to dogs or cats outside of the home, having a pet cat in the home or exposure to kittens were less pronounced (RR 1.39, 1.8 and 1.78, respectively) (Marmor et al., 1987).

Although metropolitan residence may expose a person to more *Toxocara* eggs, due to the high number of infected dogs and infective eggs in small, highly frequented geographic areas (Table 1), analysis of the only available data, from the NHANES 1988–1994, showed only a higher overall seroprevalence in those of nonmetropolitan residence (population <1 million or rural), reaching significance in the non-Hispanic white ($P<0.001$) and black ($P<0.01$) population (Won et al., 2008). Risk and prevalence disparities of toxocariasis become more noticeable when one considers the region of residence. Data from NHANES I and NHANES III (Herrmann et al., 1985; Won et al., 2008) both showed the highest seroprevalence in the American South. This is most likely reflective of increased poverty in this region (further discussed in the next section of this chapter), which across all seroprevalence data analyses was a notable risk factor for antibodies to *Toxocara* (Herrmann et al., 1985; Liu et al., 2018; Won et al., 2008).

4. Poverty, race and *Toxocara* seroprevalence

Liu and colleagues' analysis (2018) of the NHANES 2011–2014 dataset found that living below the poverty threshold (as determined by US Department of Health guidelines) was a significant risk factor for *Toxocara* exposure (10.2% seroprevalence vs 3.9%; $P<0.001$) (Liu et al., 2018). Farmer's analysis of the same serum samples employing the poverty level, also finding a greater prevalence and adjusted odds of *Toxocara* antibodies in those below (4.9%) than those above (2.9%) the poverty level (aOR 1.8) (Farmer et al., 2017). The weighted *Toxocara* seroprevalence in this cohort increased markedly with decreased poverty to income ratios (Berrett et al., 2017). Seroprevalence among those with health insurance was 4.3%, while those without was more than double at 9.9%. This level of disparity was also observed in children with and without health insurance (3.2% vs 7.3% seroprevalence; OR 2.4) (Farmer et al., 2017). Analysis of the earlier NHANES III dataset by Congdon and Lloyd showed an almost twofold relative risk for antibodies to *Toxocara* for those in poverty than those not (Congdon and Lloyd, 2011). The greatest disparities in relative risk were seen among nonmetropolitan males in the West (RR 3.38) and females in the Mid-West (RR 2.70). In Southern nonmetropolitan areas, the RR for those in poverty was 1.96 for males and 1.93 for females, higher than the mean average RR for poverty in nonmetropolitan areas overall (1.83 and 1.87, respectively). While metropolitan males in the South had an almost identical RR to the overall mean average, the RR for females in poverty in Southern metropolitan areas (2.21) was notably higher than the overall USA average for those in poverty in metropolitan areas (1.93) (Congdon and Lloyd, 2011). The increased risk of toxocariasis in the poor may be attributable to multiple factors, including access to healthcare, education, poor housing and living conditions and decreased access to veterinary care for pet dogs and cats, including anthelmintic treatment.

Both increased poverty and racial disparities in *Toxocara* seroprevalence may be a reason the increased seroprevalence in Southern states. Poverty is an independent risk factor for toxocariasis (Herrmann et al., 1985; Liu et al., 2018; Won et al., 2008) and the Southern US states have generally higher rates of poverty than the rest of the nation (US Census Bureau, 2018a).

Lower incomes may also feed into the lower percentage of the Southern states' population having health insurance (US Census Bureau, 2012), a further risk factor for infection (Farmer et al., 2017). Surprisingly, Little's (Little et al., 2009) national survey of intestinal parasite in dogs found the lowest prevalence of *T. canis* infection in the South (1.6%, see Table 1). While simplistic interpretation, this data would suggest that overall exposure is lower in this region, Little's samples were exclusively from dogs receiving diagnostic veterinary care. A more accurate picture of prevalence in the South was gained if a survey of dogs from both those who can, and those who cannot, afford veterinary care in the region conducted by Blagburn et al. (1996). In a 1993–1994 survey of shelter dogs, the prevalence of not only *Toxocara canis*, but all common nematodes of dogs were highest in the South East region of the USA (Blagburn et al., 1996). A follow up survey of shelter cats and dogs also found the highest prevalence of *T. canis* in dogs from the South East. Interestingly, this survey found that *T. cati* was the second most common veterinary nematode after hookworm overall, and that the prevalence was slightly higher in cats from the North East (Blagburn, 2010) (Table 1). This unexpected finding raises the question of whether *T. cati* may play a larger role in human toxocariasis in the United States than currently understood.

The impact of environment and climate on the life cycle and transmission of *Toxocara* must be considered as a factor in increased seroprevalence of human *Toxocara* antibodies in the South East region (Blagburn, 2010). The US South East has a sub-tropical climate, high humidity and regions of loamy soil, allowing almost year-round embryonation and infection with *Toxocara* spp. deposited in the soil by cats and dogs. This is a unique situation compared to Northern and Mid-western states, where eggs will not develop over the cold Winters or the Western states, where extremely hot and dry summers will likely also halt the development or kill eggs deposited in the soil.

The increased risk of toxocariasis in the US South may also be affected another significant ($P < 0.001$) independent risk factor, that is to say, race (Liu et al., 2018). The US South East has the highest proportion of African American people as a percentage of overall population (US Census Bureau, 2017). Poverty is higher in this racial group (US Census Bureau, 2018b), and poverty itself is a risk factor for toxocariasis as discussed above. However, even when data is controlled for poverty, non-Hispanic blacks have a higher RR of toxocariasis (Congdon and Lloyd, 2011). Indeed, in the NHANES III data, black non-Hispanic males not in poverty had a higher risk for antibodies to *Toxocara* than Hispanic males in poverty (Congdon and Lloyd, 2011). In the NHANES I dataset, black Americans had more than eight times the seroprevalence of white Americans, while seroprevalence was almost doubled in the NHANES III data (Table 3). Prevalence rates for Hispanic and non-Hispanic black children 6–17 years of age were equivalent in the NHANES 2011–2014 dataset analysed by Farmer (4.5% and 4.7%, respectively), but well above those of non-Hispanic whites (3.1%) and other races/mixed race people (2.7%) (Farmer et al., 2017). Non-Hispanic black Americans have an increased odds ratio (OR 1.4) of exposure to *Toxocara* when compared to the general population (Liu et al., 2018). Herrmann's original NHANES I (1971–1973) study data also found that black American children had significantly higher titers of *Toxocara* antibodies compared to antibody positive white children (Herrmann et al., 1985), suggesting a higher intensity as well as prevalence of exposure to *Toxocara* larvae in the environment.

Liu's analysis of the NHANES 2011–2014 samples found the following seroprevalence rates, non-Hispanic white, 3.7%; non-Hispanic black 6.6%; non-Hispanic Asian, 7.3%; Mexican American, 6.1% and an overall total seroprevalence of 5.0%. Farmer's analysis of the NHANES 2011–2014 adults $\geq$18 years old was roughly concordant with Liu's analysis of all $\geq$6 years old. One marked difference was that Hispanics in Farmer's dataset showed the highest *Toxocara* seroprevalence, at 9.8% (Farmer et al., 2017). The NHANES 2011–2014 participants born outside of the United States had a significantly higher risk for having *Toxocara* antibodies (OR 3.6; $P<0.001$), with an average 11.9% seroprevalence, compared to only 3.9% for American born participants (Liu et al., 2018). This much higher seroprevalence in immigrants is likely due to higher exposure to *Toxocara* in their home countries prior to immigration to the United States.

Regardless of different racial categorizations employed in the NHANES datasets, non-white Americans are always at higher risk of possessing antibodies to *Toxocara* than are white Americans. This racial disparity in past or current infection prevalence has been supported by all NHANES studies and analyses (Berrett et al., 2017; Congdon and Lloyd, 2011; Farmer et al., 2017; Herrmann et al., 1985; Liu et al., 2018; Won et al., 2008).

Education level of the head of household is uniformly related to *Toxocara* seroprevalence in all datasets. Referring to the 2011–2014 NHANES dataset, those with a head of household having less than a high school diploma had a seroprevalence rate of 11.1%, while those with a head of household having attended some college had only a 3.4% seroprevalence rate. Those with a less than college head of household education have almost twice

(OR 1.9) the odds of carrying antibodies to *Toxocara*. These disparities in seroprevalence by head of household education were found to be statistically significant ($P<0.001$) (Liu et al., 2018). Crowding rates in the home also significantly ($P<0.001$) affected seroprevalence, those with ≥1 person per room at home had an overall 10.5% seroprevalence, whereas those <0.5 people per room had only a 3.5% seroprevalence. Lower education level may impact *Toxocara* exposure due to poorer understanding of public health communications and veterinary care requirements for pet animals. Increased household crowding may increase exposure where pets are also present and have smaller areas for defecation outside (*T. canis*) or use cat litter trays inside (*T. cati*), particularly if litter is not regularly changed, as these factors will concentrate exposure to infective *Toxocara* eggs within the home and immediate surrounds. However, the wide effects of lower head of household education level and household crowding are most likely reflective of the independent risk factor for toxocariasis of poverty than any other predisposing factor.

5. Asthma, lead, neurocognitive defects and *Toxocara* seroprevalence

For some time, links have been suggested between exposure to *Toxocara* and asthma. Indeed, some of the earliest seroprevalence studies in the United States, carried out in Hawaii and Connecticut, were initiated to test *Toxocara* seroprevalence in asthmatic and nonasthmatic children (Desowitz et al., 1981; Sharghi et al., 2001). The Hawaii study used a crude third stage larval antigen and counter-immunoelectrophoresis (CEP) to detect IgG. Unlike all other US seroprevalence surveys, this study looked at IgE levels, with a crude larval antigen solid phase radioallergosorbent test (RAST). The results showed that asthmatics had more than double 4.9% vs 2.1% the IgG seroprevalence of nonasthmatics. This was even more marked when IgE antibodies were tested (6.4% vs 28.8%) (Desowitz et al., 1981). Although it is tempting to interpret this data as indicative of a causative correlation, the poor specificity of both tests employed, plus the very high likelihood of nonspecific cross-reactions in the IgE RAST from the asthmatic cohort, make any interpretation of these data fraught. The second and later study in Connecticut which used the relatively nonspecific crude third stage larval antigen ELISA, did not directly compare *Toxocara* seroprevalence in its asthmatic and nonasthmatic cohorts. In addition, this study found no statistically proven association between *Toxocara* risk factors and risk factors for asthma (Sharghi et al., 2001).

More recent work, using the specific rTc-CTL-1 antigen assay provides a clearer summary of the situation, where overall, those with an asthma diagnosis have a slightly lower overall IgG seroprevalence (4.5%) to those without (5.1%). The disparities in seroprevalence were even more marked when divided by racial groups, with the greatest disparity being prevalence in diagnosed asthmatic non-Hispanic black Americans compared to non-asthmatics of the same race (7.1% vs 4.0%). Only Mexican Americans showed a slightly increased *Toxocara* seroprevalence among asthmatics (6.1% vs 4.9%). This data was interpreted as being consistent with the "hygiene hypothesis" of asthma causation (Liu et al., 2018) and refuted the smaller cohort earlier studies suggesting an association between *Toxocara* exposure and asthma which used less specific IgE serology methods (Buijs et al., 1994; Desowitz et al., 1981).

An association of higher *Toxocara* seroprevalence rates in those with elevated serum lead levels found the NHANES III and NHANES 2014–2017 datasets (Farmer et al., 2017; Won et al., 2008) most likely reflects poorer housing, including old lead paint and pipe infrastructure and greater overall exposure to lead in poverty-stricken areas than any direct association. Exposure to soil might represent an independent risk factor for both *Toxocara* and lead exposure (Farmer et al., 2017) and pica in children has been significantly associated with both increased serum lead levels and *Toxocara* antibody titers (Nelson et al., 1996). Glickman and colleagues found a significant association between pica of paint and plaster and elevated lead levels, while pica of faeces, grass and soil (often seen in the same children eating paint and plaster) was significantly associated with the presence of *Toxocara* antibodies in serum (Glickman et al., 1981). The risk ratio of *Toxocara* seropositivity in a large cohort study of children from New York was increased with any history of geophagy (RR 2.65), ingestion of animal faeces (RR 2.40) and ingestion of paint and plaster flakes from housing (RR 1.62) (Marmor et al., 1987). Therefore, although *Toxocara* seropositivity is associated with increased lead levels, this is likely not a direct association, just as increased *Toxocara* antibodies in a case-controlled study of epileptic children was attributed to the propensity of children with epilepsy to engage in pica than due to a direct association of *Toxocara* infection and epileptic disease (Glickman et al., 1979).

An interesting consideration is that two studies in the USA have associated *Toxocara* antibody positivity with neuropsychological deficits in children and poor cognitive outcomes (Erickson et al., 2015; Marmor et al., 1987; Nelson et al., 1996), which will likely lead to poor school performance. It might therefore be considered that early exposure to *Toxocara* may have led to decreased educational achievement in some cases, which in turn entrenches the cycle of poverty and decreased access to suitable housing and healthcare. Although older, studies in children lend some support to the correlation between *Toxocara* positive serology and neurocognitive deficits. Marmor et al had shown associations between *T. canis* infection and poorer performance on a battery of standard neuropsychological tests (including standard neuropsychological tests used in children at the time, such as the Wechsler Preschool and Primary Scales of Intelligence, although these differences were not detected using more behaviourally-oriented tests such as the Goldberg Developmental Progress Chart) even after adjustment for confounders such as socioeconomic status and lead concentrations in children in a case control study (Marmor et al., 1987). In a study following a cohort of children defined as socioeconomically disadvantaged (by Hollingshead social class), children seropositive for *Toxocara* were more likely to have both higher lead levels and seropositivity at ages 4–10, which were assumed to be the results of pica. This was associated with lower IQ as measured by the Weschler Preschool and Primary Scales of Intelligence tests, although after adjustment based on the Bayley Scales of Infant Development test at 1 year old these results were no longer significant (the adjustment was made to attempt to control for preexisting developmental deficits with the Bayley Scales and 1 year being therefore chosen to assess and use in adjusting as this would have presumably predated *Toxocara* exposure) (Nelson et al., 1996). In adults studied in the NHANES III dataset, positive *Toxocara* serology was correlated to performance on various measures of cognitive function in multivariate analysis, controlling for factors such as ethnicity, educational attainment, and poverty-to-income ratio in younger to middle aged adults, although this study also found that there were significant interactions in their analysis indicating decreased cognitive performance is also impacted by demographic factors (Erickson et al., 2015). A study of the children from the same NHANES III cohort found similar associations, with lower scores on both the Wechsler Intelligence Scale for Children-Revised and the Wide Range Achievement Test-Revised tests. These were independent of blood lead levels, socioeconomic status, rural residence, ethnicity, gender and cytomegalovirus infection (Walsh and Haseeb, 2012).

6. Concluding remarks

Specific groups within the US population are at higher risk of *Toxocara* exposure and subsequent IgG antibody response. It is important when interpreting seroprevalence data to consider the sensitivity and specificity of the laboratory diagnostic antigens and methods used and if the size of the cohort examined was sufficient to generate statistically valid results. The most recent (2011–2014) analyses of the nationwide NHANES serum collection (Farmer et al., 2017; Liu et al., 2018) are probably the most reliable results for interpretation of *Toxocara* seroprevalence data. Specifically, these are non-Hispanic black Americans, Hispanic Americans, those in poverty, those with lower head of household education, those in crowded housing and those born outside of the United States of America. American women are more likely to be seropositive than men. Seroprevalence increases with age and is overall higher in the South East of the country, though some Americans living in poverty in other regions have equally high seroprevalences as those in the South. No association between asthma and *Toxocara* exposure has been proven by reliable seroprevalence data from the USA.

Exposure to *Toxocara* larvae is devastating for the few who develop severe overt and debilitating disease such as visceral, ocular or neural larva migrans. The vast majority of seropositive Americans are asymptomatic or do not display overt symptoms of disease. At present, no specific long-term sequelae of covert toxocariasis have been identified, but this does not mean those exposed are unaffected by their infection. *Toxocara* seropositivity has been associated with neurocognitive stunting (Erickson et al., 2015; Marmor et al., 1987; Nelson et al., 1996; Walsh and Haseeb, 2012) and subtle allergic, respiratory and neuropsychiatric symptoms in those affected (Fillaux and Magnaval, 2013; Rostami et al., 2019). While such associations are difficult to separate from other concomitant risk factors, such as poverty likely because of associated poor nutrition and poorer access to high quality education, they must be considered when such a large number of Americans have been exposed to these zoonotic helminths. Further investigation of these associations is warranted, as are public health education programs encouraging hand washing after exposure to soil and dog or cat faeces, regular deworming of household pets and appropriate disposal of dog waste from household and community areas. Development of further serological tests are also indicated, including those with capacity to differentiate active from past infection (Woodhall et al., 2014). The enigma of what the health effects widespread of prior exposure to *Toxocara* larvae are will likely continue for some time. Large cohort studies such as NHANES using highly specific methodologies have provided advances in our understanding of risk factors and may allow detection of any clinical associations, if they exist, in the future.

References

Anderson, J.P., Rascoe, L.N., Levert, K., Chastain, H.M., Reed, M.S., Rivera, H.N., McAuliffe, I., Zan, B., Wiegand, R.E., Hotez, P., Wilkins, P.P., Pohl, J., Handali, S., 2015. Development of a Luminex bead based assay for diagnosis of toxocariasis using recombinant antigens Tc-CTL-1 and Tc-TES-26. PLoS Negl. Trop. Dis. 9, e0004168.

Beaver, P.C., Snyder, C.H., Carrera, G.M., Dent, J.H., Lafferty, J.W., 1952. Chronic eosinophilia due to visceral larva migrans: report of three cases. Pediatrics 9, 7–19.

Berrett, A.N., Erickson, L.D., Gale, S.D., Stone, A., Brown, B.L., Hedges, D.W., 2017. *Toxocara* seroprevalence and associated risk factors in the United States. Am. J. Trop. Med. Hyg. 97, 1846–1850.

Blagburn, B.L., 2010. Where have all the parasites gone? Results of national parasite and vector-borne diseases survey. In: Novartis Parasite Symposium. North American Veterinary Community, Orlando, FL, pp. 1165–1169.

Blagburn, B.L., Lindsay, D.S., Vaughan, J.L., Rippey, N.S., Wright, J.C., Lynn, R.C., Kelch, W.J., Ritchie, G.C., Hepler, D.I., 1996. Prevalence of canine parasites based on fecal flotation. Compend. Contin. Educ. Pract. Vet. 5, 483–509.

Buijs, J., Borsboom, G., van Gemund, J.J., Hazebroek, A., van Dongen, P.A., van Knapen, F., Neijens, H.J., 1994. *Toxocara* seroprevalence in 5-year-old elementary schoolchildren: relation with allergic asthma. Am. J. Epidemiol. 140, 839–847.

Centers for Disease Control and Prevention, 2019. Parasites—Toxocariasis. https://www.cdc.gov/parasites/toxocariasis/disease.html. (accessed 14th October 2019).

Chen, J., Liu, Q., Liu, G.H., Zheng, W.B., Hong, S.J., Sugiyama, H., Zhu, X.Q., Elsheikha, H.M., 2018. Toxocariasis: a silent threat with a progressive public health impact. Infect. Dis. Poverty 7, 59.

Childs, J.E., 1985. The prevalence of *Toxocara* species ova in backyards and gardens of Baltimore, Maryland. Am. J. Public Health 75, 1092–1094.

Congdon, P., Lloyd, P., 2011. *Toxocara* infection in the United States: the relevance of poverty, geography and demography as risk factors, and implications for estimating county prevalence. Int. J. Public Health 56, 15–24.

Cypess, R.H., Karol, M.H., Zidian, J.L., Glickman, L.T., Gitlin, D., 1977. Larva-specific antibodies in patients with visceral larva migrans. J. Infect. Dis. 135, 633–640.

Dada, B.J., Lindquist, W.D., 1979. Studies on flotation techniques for the recovery of helminth eggs from soil and the prevalence of eggs of *Toxocara* spp in some Kansas public places. J. Am. Vet. Med. Assoc. 174, 1208–1210.

De Santis, A.C., Raghavan, M., Caldanaro, R.J., Glickman, N.W., Moore, G.E., Lewis, H.B., Schantz, P.M., Glickman, L.T., 2006. Estimated prevalence of nematode parasitism among pet cats in the United States. J. Am. Vet. Med. Assoc. 228, 885–892.

Desowitz, R.S., Rudoy, R., Barnwell, J.W., 1981. Antibodies to canine helminth parasites in asthmatic and nonasthmatic children. Int. Arch. Allergy Immunol. 65, 361–366.

Dorman, D.W., Van Ostrand, J.R., 1958. A survey of *Toxocara canis* and *Toxocara cati* prevalence in the New York City area. N. Y. State J. Med. 58, 2793–2795.

Dubin, S., Segall, S., Martindale, J., 1975. Contamination of soil in two city parks with canine nematode ova including *Toxocara canis*: a preliminary study. Am. J. Public Health 65, 1242–1245.

Erickson, L.D., Gale, S.D., Berrett, A., Brown, B.L., Hedges, D.W., 2015. Association between toxocariasis and cognitive function in young to middle-aged adults. Folia Parasitol. (Praha) 7, 62.

Farmer, A., Beltran, T., Choi, Y.S., 2017. Prevalence of *Toxocara* species infection in the US: results from the National Health and Nutrition Examination Survey, 2011-2014. PLoS Negl. Trop. Dis. 11, e0005818.

Fillaux, J., Magnaval, J.F., 2013. Laboratory diagnosis of human toxocariasis. Vet. Parasitol. 193, 327–336.
Glickman, L.T., Cypess, R.H., 1977. Toxocara infection in animal hospital employees. Am. J. Public Health. 67, 1193–1195.
Glickman, L.T., Cypess, R.H., Crumrine, P.K., Gitlin, D.A., 1979. *Toxocara* infection and epilepsy in children. J. Pediatr. 94, 75–78.
Glickman, L.T., Chaudry, I.U., Costantino, J., Clack, F.B., Cypess, R.H., Winslow, L., 1981. Pica patterns, toxocariasis, and elevated blood lead in children. Am. J. Trop. Med. Hyg. 30, 77–80.
Herrmann, N., Glickman, L.T., Schantz, P.M., Weston, M.G., Domanski, L.M., 1985. Seroprevalence of zoonotic toxocariasis in the United States: 1971–1973. Am. J. Epidemiol. 122, 890–896.
Hotez, P.J., Wilkins, P.P., 2009. Toxocariasis: America's most common neglected infection of poverty and a helminthiasis of global importance? PLoS Negl. Trop. Dis. 3, e400.
Inagaki, K., Kirmse, B., Bradbury, R.S., Moorthy, R.S., Arguello, I., McGuffey, C.D., Tieu, B., Hobbs, C.V., 2019. Case report: ocular Toxocariasis: a report of three cases from the Mississippi Delta. Am. J. Trop. Med. Hyg. 100, 1223–1226.
Jacquier, P., Gottstein, B., Stingelin, Y., Eckert, J., 1991. Immunodiagnosis of toxocarosis in humans: evaluation of a new enzyme-linked immunosorbent assay kit. J. Clin. Microbiol. 29, 1831–1835.
Jin, Y., Shen, C., Huh, S., Sohn, W.M., Choi, M.H., Hong, S.T., 2013. Serodiagnosis of toxocariasis by ELISA using crude antigen of *Toxocara canis* larvae. Korean J. Parasitol. 51, 433.
Jones, W.E., Schantz, P.M., Foreman, K., Smith, L.K., Witte, E.J., Schooley, D.E., Juranek, D.D., 1980. Human toxocariasis in a rural community. Am. J. Dis. Child. 134, 967–969.
Kirkpatrick, C.E., 1988. Epizootiology of endoparasitic infections in pet dogs and cats presented to a veterinary teaching hospital. Vet. Parasitol. 30, 113–124.
Little, S.E., Johnson, E.M., Lewis, D., Jaklitsch, R.P., Payton, M.E., Blagburn, B.L., Bowman, D.D., Moroff, S., Tams, T., Rich, L., Aucoin, D., 2009. Prevalence of intestinal parasites in pet dogs in the United States. Vet. Parasitol. 166, 144–152.
Liu, E.W., Chastain, H.M., Shin, S.H., Wiegand, R.E., Kruszon-Moran, D., Handali, S., Jones, J.L., 2018. Seroprevalence of antibodies to *Toxocara* species in the United States and associated risk factors, 2011–2014. Clin. Infect. Dis. 66, 206–212.
Lucio-Forster, A., Barbecho, J.S.M., Mohammed, H.O., Kornreich, B.G., Bowman, D.D., 2016. Comparison of the prevalence of *Toxocara* egg shedding by pet cats and dogs in the USA, 2011–2014. Vet. Parasitol. Reg. Stud. Reports 5, 1–13.
Marmor, M., Glickman, L., Shofer, F., Faich, L.A., Rosenberg, C., Cornblatt, B., Friedman, S., 1987. *Toxocara canis* infection of children: epidemiologic and neuropsychologic findings. Am. J. Public Health 77, 554–559.
Mohamed, A.S., Moore, G.E., Glickman, L.T., 2009. Prevalence of intestinal nematode parasitism among pet dogs in the United States (2003–2006). J. Am. Vet. Med. Assoc. 234, 631–637.
Nelson, S., Greene, T., Ernhart, C.B., 1996. *Toxocara canis* infection in preschool age children: risk factors and the cognitive development of preschool children. Neurotoxicol. Teratol. 18, 167–174.
Nolan, T.J., Smith, G., 1995. Time series analysis of the prevalence of endoparasitic infections in cats and dogs presented to a veterinary teaching hospital. Vet. Parasitol. 59, 87–96.
Perlingiero, J.G., György, P., 1947. Chronic eosinophilia: report of a case with necrosis of the liver, pulmonary infiltrations, anemia and ascaris infestation. Am. J. Dis. Child. 73, 34–43.

Rostami, A., Ma, G., Wang, T., Koehler, A.V., Hofmann, A., Chang, B.C., McPherson, C.N., Gasser, R.B., 2019. Human toxocariasis—a look at a neglected disease through an epidemiological 'prism'. Infect. Genet. Evol. 74, 104002.

Savilla, T.M., Joy, J.E., May, J.D., Somerville, C.C., 2011. Prevalence of dog intestinal nematode parasites in south central West Virginia, USA. Vet. Parasitol. 178, 115–120.

Sharghi, N., Schantz, P.M., Caramico, L., Ballas, K., Teague, B.A., Hotez, P.J., 2001. Environmental exposure to *Toxocara* as a possible risk factor for asthma: a clinic-based case-control study. Clin. Infect. Dis. 32, e111–e116.

Spain, C.V., Scarlett, J.M., Wade, S.E., McDonough, P., 2001. Prevalence of enteric zoonotic agents in cats less than 1 year old in central New York State. J. Vet. Intern. Med. 15, 33–38.

Stehr-Green, J.K., Murray, G., Schantz, P.M., Wahlquist, S.P., 1987. Intestinal parasites in pet store puppies in Atlanta. Am. J. Public Health 77, 345–346.

Surgan, M.H., Colgan, K.B., Kennett, S.I., Paffmann, J.V., 1980. A survey of canine toxocariasis and toxocaral soil contamination in Essex County, New Jersey. Am. J. Public Health 70, 1207–1208.

United States Census Bureau, 2012. Health Insurance Coverage in 2012. https://www.census.gov/data/tables/time-series/demo/income-poverty/cps-hi/hi-06.html. (accessed 12th October 2019).

United States Census Bureau, 2017. 2013–2017 American Community Survey 5-Year Estimates. https://factfinder.census.gov.(accessed 12th October 2019).

United States Census Bureau, 2018a. POV-46. Poverty Status by State. https://www.census.gov/data/tables/time-series/demo/income-poverty/cps-pov/pov-46.html. (accessed 12th October 2019).

United States Census Bureau, 2018b. The Black Alone Population in the United States: 2018. https://www.census.gov/data/tables/2018/demo/race/ppl-ba18.html. (accessed 12th October 2019).

Walsh, M.G., Haseeb, M.A., 2012. Reduced cognitive function in children with toxocariasis in a nationally representative sample of the United States. Int. J. Parasitol. 42, 1159–1163.

Wilder, H.C., 1950. Nematode endophthalmitis. Trans. Am. Acad. Opthalmol. Otolaryngol. 55, 99–109.

Won, K.Y., Kruszon-Moran, D., Schantz, P.M., Jones, J.L., 2008. National seroprevalence and risk factors for zoonotic *Toxocara* spp. infection. Am. J. Trop. Med. Hyg. 79, 552–557.

Woodhall, D.M., Eberhard, M.L., Parise, M.E., 2014. Neglected parasitic infections in the United States: toxocariasis. Am. J. Trop. Med. Hyg. 90, 810–813.

Further reading

Lee, R.M., Moore, L.B., Bottazzi, M.E., Hotez, P.J., 2014. Toxocariasis in North America: a systematic review. PLoS Negl. Trop. Dis. 8, e3116.

CHAPTER SEVENTEEN

Toxocara: Seroprevalence in Mexico

Martha Ponce-Macotela, Mario Noé Martínez-Gordillo*
Laboratorio de Parasitología Experimental del Instituto Nacional de Pediatría, Mexico City, Mexico
*Corresponding author: e-mail address: marionmgordillo@yahoo.com

Contents

Abstract

In Mexico, toxocariasis, like some other parasitosis in humans, is not a disease of conventional surveillance or immediate notification. Seroprevalence studies are scarce, six dealing with paediatric populations and eight dealing with adults; the reports were only from four states in Mexico. There were 1596 children, and the seroprevalence was 13.8%. In the case of adults, there were 1827 subjects, and seroprevalence was 4.7%. There is a significant positive association between seroprevalence and the paediatric population $P < 0.0001$ (OR, 3.285; 95% CI, 2.541–4.279). It is advisable to perform competitive ELISAs and add another diagnostic test, such as Western blot or the detection of circulating antigens to reduce diagnostic uncertainty. This neglected parasitosis can be confused with retinoblastoma. Therefore, there is a risk of ocular enucleation. It is necessary to sensitise the authorities of the Ministry of Health and decision-makers, to provide economic support for epidemiological surveillance of this zoonotic parasite.

Advances in Parasitology, Volume 109
ISSN 0065-308X
https://doi.org/10.1016/bs.apar.2020.01.012

1. Background

The most abundant animals on the earth are the roundworms, that is, the nematodes. It has been estimated that there are $4.4 \pm 0.64 \times 10^{20}$ individual worms living in the soil of the planet, a biomass of approximately 0.3 gigatons (300,000 million of kilograms) (Van den Hoogen et al., 2019), not including the animal and plant parasites. The nematodes as parasites of animals are very successful; they have developed all parasitic modalities with the exception of being ectoparasites on animals, i.e., parasites living on the surface of animals rather than inside of the body of the animal. In the human population, it has been estimated that more than 1.6 billion people are infected with adults of the soil-transmitted helminths: *Ascaris lumbricoides, Trichuris trichiura, Necator americanus* and *Ancylostoma duodenale* (Vlaminck et al., 2019). This number does not consider parasites from animals, i.e., those with zoonotic transmission as in the case of the roundworm of dogs and cats *Toxocara canis* and *Toxocara cati*, respectively.

Toxocara spp. is a neglected, zoonotic, soil-transmitted nematode and the canids and felids are the definitive hosts, and in young puppies the rates of infection are often near to 100% (Styles, 1967). The parasite is exquisitely adapted to be successful infecting their hosts. *Toxocara canis* females shed in average 55,000 fertilised eggs daily, as was experimentally demonstrated using a *T. canis* culture method. The eggs are resistant structures that during the maturation process, develop a larva within, and every fertilised egg becomes infective. If the environmental conditions in the soil are favourable, the eggs can live for several years. For this reason, the environment is the primary source of *Toxocara* eggs; they are then infectives to either definitive or paratenic hosts. The life cycle pattern that includes paratenesis connects the trophic gap to allow the larvae to reach definitive hosts. During this unique process of between host transportation, the larval *Toxocara* does not undergo any development. So, here, during the process paratenesis, there is transport from host-to-host that involves an immature parasite that neither undergoes growth or reproduction until it finally reaches its definitive host (Hanelt et al., 2005).

In *Toxocara canis*, vertical transmission is the primary transmission mode, wherein larvae cross the placenta before the puppies' birth, and after delivery, there is potential for the transfer of some worms through maternal milk in a trans-mammary fashion (Burke and Robertson, 1985; Hotez et al., 1993). Vertical transmission is an evolutionary adaptive strategy restricted to pregnancy and lactation events, in which, the larvae in the final host enter a state of hypobiosis and remain arrested in maternal tissues, surviving for years until the next pregnancy. The migrating larvae from eggs or paratenic hosts can somehow sense the hormonal milieu (progesterone, oestradiol and prolactin) of the final host and some larvae develop to adults in dogs, while others, reside as undeveloped larvae in the tissues of both male and female dogs. When the bitch becomes pregnant, then, the larvae that have been present in the tissues will migrate to the uterus or mammary glands to infect the puppies. This evolutionary adaptation allows females to be reservoirs of parasitic stages ready to invade the foetus in such way that the neonate becomes a new definitive host. The cycle closes it when mature parasites shed eggs in the small intestine of the puppies that then enter the environment with the faeces. The eggs mature in the soil, become infective, and if the female reinfects herself again, the larvae hatch, penetrate the intestinal wall and begin the migration. Therefore, the bitch acts as an amphiparatenic host because it can be the definitive host, can be a reservoir, and behave as a paratenic host (Shoop and Corkum, 1987). Finally, the hormonal status of the female dog determines the fate of the larva: arrested in her tissues or migrating to become an adult. On the other hand, if a puppy under 6 months old swallows an infective egg, this reaches the stomach and become subjected to digestion, that involves the acid environment in the stomach, increase of temperature, proteolytic enzymes, and later, arrives at duodenum where the pH becomes neutral or slightly alkaline, allowing the *Toxocara* larva to hatch. After that, the larva penetrates the epithelium of the intestinal wall starting the migration, through mesenteric lymph vessels, travelling via the portal circulation to the liver, passing to the heart, and reaching lungs via pulmonary artery, here the larva perforates alveoli and continues via bronchioles, trachea to the pharynx to be ingested to achieve, again, the digestive system where it develops into an adult (Schnieder et al., 2011).

In dogs older than 6 months, the larvae hatch in the intestine, penetrate the intestinal wall and migrate across the liver, heart and lungs. The infective eggs dose will have effects on how the larvae hatching from eggs behave and develop toxocariasis on naïve dogs (Dubey, 1978). If it ingests only a few eggs, the probability is that the hatching worms will develop to adults. But as higher numbers of eggs are swallowed, there is a significant chance that the larvae will become sequestered in the tissues. When turning arrested in males and non-pregnant female dogs, the larvae enter an hypobiotic state, until the arrival of a stimulus that triggers their migration. In male dogs, the larvae seem to persist in the tissues only; but in female dogs, it has been shown that prolactin and progesterone are inductors of migration (Chávez-Güitrón et al., 2016, 2019) promoting larval concentration in the womb and passing to the foetus, wherein larvae develop to adults after delivery (Strube et al., 2013). Another transmission strategy adapted to the predator-prey relationship is that the parasites infect to the prey, and the victim infects to definitive host; the canids are predators and carnivorous of many paratenic hosts. In this manner, the larvae attain their definitive host when a predator eats the infected paratenic hosts. Many mammals, including the man, birds, and annelids (Cianferoni et al., 2006) act as paratenic hosts, the larvae do not develop but persist in muscle and tissues for a long time (Beaver, 1969). The interaction of humans with a contaminated environment favours the ingestion of embryonated eggs. But, human toxocariasis is an evolutionary mistake; it is a bypass to a dead end because the larva will never develop to the adult stage.

On the other hand, historically, biological research has been developed faster than medical research. For example, the knowledge of the biology of *Toxocara*, life cycle, and hosts have been known since 1782 (Sprent, 1958), while the discovery of humans as paratenic host and the first cases of human toxocariasis dates back to 1952 (Beaver et al., 1952).

2. Mexico on the world

Mexico is a country located in the southern part of North America. Limits to the north with the United States of America. In Central America with Guatemala and Belize. To the west with the Pacific Ocean. The east with the Gulf of Mexico and the Caribbean Sea. It has a very diverse weather system between temperate to tropical. The highest elevation is the Pico de Orizaba at 5700m over sea level. In Mexico, there are approximately 120 million persons, and it is estimated that 41.9% of the population lives in poverty, and that 7.4% live in extreme poverty.

3. *Toxocara* history in Mexico

In Mexico, medical studies on human toxocariasis began in the sixth decade of the 20th century. The first publication of a demonstrated case of visceral larva *migrans* was a histopathological study authored by Martínez-Báez and Alemán (1960), and clinically supported by a description published in the same issue by Molina-Pasquel and Díaz-Muñoz (1960). It was a case of a female patient presenting with eosinophilia, hepatomegaly, and hepatic granulomas. The study of the granulomas showed that they contained nematode larvae that were identified as *Toxocara* larvae. This patient also showed sequelae of perforated keratitis in the left eye, and changes in the fundus of the right eye, but these findings were considered not to be associated with the parasite. Thirty years later, a paediatric case of systemic toxocariasis associated with arthritis, characterised by intermittent fever, anorexia, stiffness, and pain on palpation and limited movement of the metacarpophalangeal and metatarsophalangeal joints was reported. A positive value of the rheumatoid factor, the presence of significant eosinophilia (50%), and a positive *Toxocara* ELISA to a dilution of 1:8192. One year after treatment, the rheumatoid factor became negative, the eosinophilia reduced to 20%, and the IgG response in the ELISA fell to 1:4096 (Richardson-de Corral et al., 1990). This clinical kind of presentation in association with arthritis, eosinophilia, and *Toxocara* has been observed on several occasions (Chiardola et al., 2008; Rayes and Lambertucci, 2001).

4. Seroprevalence in dogs in Mexico

Another approach used in Mexico, as in other places around the world, to probe the impact of the *Toxocara* eggs contamination was to study the rate of infection in dogs.

For an in-depth analysis of *Toxocara* prevalence in dogs in Mexico, see in this issue the chapter entitled: "Prevalence in dogs (and cats), USA, Mexico, Central America".

We found two works on *Toxocara* seroprevalence in dogs. However, it is necessary to put the results in an epidemiological context. The infection frequency on pets under 6 months old, euthanised in a Canine Control Centre was 93% (Styles, 1967). One year later Shantz and Biagi (1968) reported that *T. canis* frequency was of the 75% in the dogs under 6 months and 7.1% in dogs older than 6 months. We (Ponce-Macotela et al., 2005), performed one study in the cold season vs the warm season on samples from adult dogs, found frequencies of 12% and 18%, respectively. Using an indirect hemagglutination assay (IHA), Martínez-Barbabosa et al. (2008a,b) detected a seroprevalence of 66.7% in stray dogs of 6 months old. In the other work using ELISA and WB in samples from puppies under 6-months-old, authors found a seroprevalence of 87.09% (27/31), and they suggest that Western Blot banding patterns showing antigens of low and high molecular weight might be useful for diagnosis in adult dogs (Muñoz-Guzmán and Alba-Hurtado, 2010). The data showed that IHA is less sensitive than ELISA; however, the results with both methods demonstrated high infection rates. The prevalence in puppies is near to 100%; and this is significant because a puppy with a single female of *Toxocara* can shed an average of 55,000 fertile eggs/day (Rodríguez-Caballero et al., 2007)

5. The environment as a *Toxocara* eggs source

In 2008 a study carried out collecting environmental samples in San Cristóbal de las Casas, Chiapas State, a place with many stray dogs, Martínez-Barbabosa et al. (2008a) found 19% (38/200) of samples with *Toxocara* eggs. In Puerto Escondido, Oaxaca close to Chiapas, the prevalence of eggs in faecal samples picked up from streets was 47.78% (Vélez-Hernández et al., 2014). The data support high environmental contamination levels; however, we do not know the seroprevalence in human beings in these areas. It is obligatory to assess the seroprevalence on the population to find a correlation between milieu contamination, and human toxocariasis seroprevalence.

6. *Toxocara* diagnosis problem in humans

Since the last century, a primary goal has been to make a more definitive diagnostic test. The knowledge of fundamental aspects of the biology of the parasite; such as, the migrating larvae ability to survive in a hypobiotic state in the paratenic host, and fundamentally the maintenance of larvae in axenic culture, provided a regular source of antigen that was different from the antigens collected from adult worms (De Savigny, 1975). The *Toxocara* excretory and secretory products from third-stage larvae of *Toxocara canis* (TES) antigens provided an improved means of diagnosis. The characterisation of iodine labelled antigen showed bands of 32, 55, 70, 120, and 400 kDa in TES, and interestingly the presence of antigens of 120 and 32 kDa on the surface of the larvae suggest a protective character against the immune response from the host (Maizels et al., 1984).

In our work, to obtain antigens from larvae, adult worms were collected from the intestines of dogs collected after euthanasia at a local Canine Control Centre. Then, adult *T. canis* females were picked up with forceps and washed with a brush wetted with formalin 1.0% in PBS pH 7.0 to eliminate microbial contamination. Afterwards, the females were cultured in

SGHP medium (PBS pH 7.00, 2% glucose, supplemented with 1% human plasma) at 37 °C. All procedures performed in a vertical laminar flow cabinet. Later the exhausted females were discarded, and the eggs harvested, washed and incubated for 1 month at ambient temperature until the infective stage larvae developed (Rodríguez-Caballero et al., 2007).

To collect larvae, we devised a method very similar to that utilised for the excystation of *Giardia* trophozoites (Ponce-Macotela et al., 2011). The first step was to adjust the pH of the Hank balanced salt solution to a basic pH with sodium bicarbonate, and to then immediately lower it to an acidic pH and incubate the eggs for 30 min at 37 °C. Then, to simulate the passage from the stomach into the duodenum, the pH was returned to normal to allow the larvae to finish hatching. Debris was separated from the larvae using the Lymphoprep™ solution (STEMCELL Technologies Canada) yielding was near 100% of hatched larvae in axenic cultures (Ponce-Macotela et al., 2011). The RPMI-1640 from the cultures was harvested weekly and replaced with fresh RPMI-1640. The antigens were isolated using Amicon filters with a 10 kDa cut off at 12,000*g* at 4 °C, and used in assays to obtain monoclonal antibodies aimed to detect antigens, as a complementary test, owing to cross-reactions.

There are cross-reactions within roundworms of the Order Ascaridida (*Toxocara, Anisakis, Ascaris, Baylisascaris* and others), because they have a common ancestor and therefore their proteins share many antigenic determinants (Park et al., 2011).

7. Seroprevalence of toxocariasis in human

Publications about human toxocariasis seroprevalence, in Mexico, are compilated in Tables 1 and 2. There are only six seroprevalence reports on *Toxocara* in the paediatric population (Table 1). Two from them were carried out in an open community with a low socioeconomic level, in the state of Mexico (near to Mexico City). The authors used a commercial kit, and they found that the risk factors were living with pet dogs under 6 months of age, sleeping with one's pets, or living close to livestock farms (Nava-Cortés et al., 2015; Romero-Núñez et al., 2013).

Another three reports were from Mexico City. One of them was a study of cases with asthma and controls analysed with ELISA (using tools made in-house) and Western Blot; the children were from a hospital of the Ministry of Health that cares for people with low economic resources.

Table 1 Summary of studies of *Toxocara* seroprevalence in Mexican children.

Estate	Method	Population size	Seroprevalence cases (%)	Author (year)
Mexico State (Amecameca and Chalco)	ELISA	183	22 (12.02)	Nava-Cortés et al. (2015)
Mexico State (Ecatepec)	ELISA	108	24 (22.22)	Romero-Núñez et al. (2013)
Mexico City	ELISA and WB	285 with asthma 152 control	88 (31), WB 18 (28) 30 (20), WB 3 (10)	Muñoz-Guzmán et al. (2010)
Baja California (Mexicali)	ELISA	288	25 (10.6)	Tinoco-Gracia et al. (2008)
Mexico City	IHA	207	4 (1.9)	Fernández-Presas et al. (1999)
Mexico City	IHA	373	28 (7.5)	Martínez-Barbabosa et al. (1997)

IHA, indirect haemagglutination assay.

Table 2 Summary of studies of *Toxocara* seroprevalence in Mexican adults.

Estate	Method	Population size	Seroprevalence cases (%)	Author (year)
Durango	ELISA	124 Meat worker 248 Controls	1 (0.8) 5 (2)	Alvarado-Esquivel et al. (2015a)
Durango	ELISA	204 Vision impairment 19 Blindness	5 (2.5) 0 (0)	Alvarado-Esquivel et al. (2015b)
Durango	ELISA	50 Schizophrenic 100 Controls	1 (2) 3 (3)	Alvarado-Esquivel et al. (2014b)
Mexico City	ELISA aa	21 AS with ANGAU 15 AS without ANGAU	8 (38) 1 (7)	Jiménez-Balderas et al. (2014)
Durango	ELISA	168 Gardeners 168 Controls	3 (1.8) 3 (1.8)	Alvarado-Esquivel et al. (2014a)
Durango	ELISA	126 Rural Tepehuanos	33 (26.2)	Alvarado-Esquivel (2014)
Durango	ELISA	128 Psychiatric patients 276 Controls	6 (4.7) 3 (1.1)	Alvarado-Esquivel (2013b)
Durango	ELISA	90 Waste pickers 90 Controls	12 (13) 1 (1)	Alvarado-Esquivel (2013a)

ELISA aa, Elisa with pre-adsorbed sera with *Ascaris*; AS, ankylosing spondylitis; ANGAU, acute non-granulomatous anterior uveitis.

The authors found a high seroprevalence in children with asthma, but they detected a significant number of cross-reactions due to the presence of antigens from *Ascaris*. Therefore, they proposed that to avoid false positives required the absorption of the sera with *Ascaris* antigens (Muñoz-Guzmán et al., 2010). There was a higher prevalence in this work than another reported performed in Baja California State, with a commercial kit, with samples from children from a hospital of the Mexican Institute Social Security (IMSS) (Tinoco-Gracia et al., 2008).

Two other studies were carried out with IHA using tools made in-house. In one study, students were from a primary school (Martínez-Barbabosa et al., 1997). The other study was on sera from 207 children diagnosed with neurologic alterations treated in a neurological rehabilitation centre in Mexico City (Fernández-Presas et al., 1999). In these two paediatric studies using the HIA, the prevalence was lower than those reported with the ELISA method.

There are eight reports utilising sera from adult subjects using a commercial ELISA kit (Table 2). Seven of the studies are from the Durango State, located in the northwest of the country. Six works were comparative studies (cases and controls) to identify possible correlations between some illness or employment being potential risk factors indicating increased contact with larvae or embryonated eggs.

In five of the reports on cases with controls, the seroprevalence was very low in both groups. Neither occupation nor observed human disease was a risk for *Toxocara* infection except in the case of the waste pickers (Alvarado-Esquivel, 2013a). In comparison with the studies of cases and controls, the authors found a high seroprevalence to *T. canis* in an indigenous community (Tepehuanos) in a rural zone with high poverty. In the analysis of sociodemographic and clinical data looking for the association with seropositivity to *Toxocara*, they only found an association with to be unemployed (Alvarado-Esquivel, 2014).

The work from Mexico City was carried out on 36 patients, with ankylosing spondylitis, with or without uveitis, using tools made in-house, and they found nine positives cases (Jiménez-Balderas et al., 2014).

From the reviewed papers, the population of 1596 children had a seroprevalence of 13.8%, and the 1827 adults had an overall seroprevalence of 4.7%. When compared, it shows that there is a significant positive association between increased seroprevalence in the paediatric population $P < 0.0001$ (OR, 3.285; 95% IC, 2.541–4.279).

8. Conclusions relative to human serology in Mexico

The *Toxocara* diagnostic was performed using tools made in-house or with commercial kits based on excretory and secretory antigens. Both methods can be excellent; however, they can produce false-positive results. Only in two of the reports the authors, pre-adsorb the sera with *Ascaris* antigen. Historically to overcome the false-positive diagnosis, it has been proposed to use other methods; for example, finding circulating antigens, detecting specific proteins, competitive immunodiagnostics with antigens from other roundworms or western blot.

The articles are few and regionalised in four from the 32 states. In Baja California and Durango (in the northwest part of Mexico), and in the State of Mexico and Mexico City (central zone of the country).

In Mexico City, live more than 5 million dogs, and 3 million of them are stray dogs producing 625 tons of faeces daily (Acevedo-Ramírez and Peralta-Abarca, 2010), so, why are there so few works on *Toxocara* seroprevalence?

The data support that in Mexico, the neglected diseases, as is the case with toxocariasis in humans, are unimportant for the Ministries of Health. Although, it is known that the parasite produces *visceral larva migrans*, causing weight loss, fever, cough, wheezing, lymphadenopathy, hepatomegaly, Löeffler syndrome; that ocular larva *migrans* can result in irreversible eye damage; and that neuronal toxocariasis can cause meningitis, meningoencephalitis or transverse myelitis (Fillaux and Magnaval, 2013). The fact that the reports showed a high seroprevalence in the paediatric population is of considerable significance, because in Mexico, children make up 30.1% of the nation's total population and represent a need for increased attention of their welfare since they represent the future of Mexico.

It seems that the prevalence in the adult is much lower than in the children. Since the larvae can live several years in the host, it is unclear why there is apparently such a much lower prevalence in the adult population. It may be due to the samples being performed in different geographic locations or that the population is somehow capable of clearing itself of infection over time. Of course, overall, compared with countries that have performed extensive national surveys, it may merely due to those populations chosen and that the sampling was not all performed with the same testing methodologies. With large scale surveys, it might be possible to identify long-term impacts on the health of the infected children, relative to minor deficits caused in overall health or cognitive development.

9. Contributions

Our work on *T. canis* began sampling dogs searching for *Giardia*, and we found that *Toxocara* in adult dogs had a frequency between 12% and 18% in two seasons of the year (Ponce-Macotela et al., 2005), and this was higher than the 7.1% positivity reported by Peter Shantz in 1968.

Later we demonstrated that *T. canis* females, in in vitro cultures, oviposit between 55,000 and 80,000 eggs in the first culture day; but on average, lay 55,000 fertilised eggs (Rodríguez-Caballero et al., 2007). Posteriorly, we made an incursion to improve the efficiency in the *Toxocara* larva hatching.

In *Giardia* excystation, we simulate the digestion process in vitro. First, we place the parasitic structures in an acid environment. When cysts pass to the duodenum, the change from acidic medium to a neutral or alkaline milieu trigger the exit of the trophozoite. The protocol to hatch *Toxocara* larvae was similar and is published elsewhere (Ponce-Macotela et al., 2011), there we demonstrated that two parasites from two different *Phyla* developed convergent strategies to colonise the small intestine of vertebrates.

We also developed a monoclonal antibody, aimed to establish an assay capable of detecting circulating antigens (Rodríguez-Caballero et al., 2015); with this tool we were able to follow in an in vivo model the antigen release, from 50 live larvae, ranging since 267–513 ng/mL through 140 days (Rodríguez-Caballero et al., 2017). Based on this in vivo model, we found antigens at 3 days and IgG after 14 days. The detection of only antigens suggests that infection is recent; antigens and antibodies correlated with active disease; and only antibodies, perhaps indicate chronic infection, immune memory or that larvae are no longer in the host and antibodies are lowering. We, in 2015 also, corroborated that immune complexes are a way to neutralise the TES; therefore, these complexes are circulating throughout the host's body, to make a successful diagnosis, it is necessary to break these immune complexes, freeing both antigens and antibodies (Aguila et al., 1987; Bowman et al., 1987; Rodríguez-Caballero et al., 2015). Besides, to avoid false-positive results that occur with simple detection of IgG is essential absorb sera with antigens from other nematodes, at least with proteins from *Ascaris* spp. (Jiménez-Balderas et al., 2014; Muñoz-Guzmán et al., 2010).

Other exciting findings have been the discovery of a model of ocular toxocariasis performed on gerbils (Alba-Hurtado et al., 2000) and the immunolocalization of prolactin and progesterone receptors in *Toxocara* intestinal cells, with high homology with prolactin (99%) and progesterone (100%) receptors in the dog (Chávez-Güitrón et al., 2016, 2019).

10. Variations on the same theme

It is evident that there are several gaps in the knowledge of *Toxocara* and toxocariasis; surely, from this enormous review in this journal, many propositions shall be made. However, as in many symphonies, some proposals shall be variations of the same theme. For example, to establish a definitive correlation between environmental contamination and infection in paediatric populations; seeking to change the status of *Toxocara* as a neglected parasitic disease, perform national surveys looking for seroprevalence and risk factors, and to investigate the fundamental aspects of the biology and genetics of the parasite. It is necessary for determining diagnostic status, a test must be developed to distinguish the species of the offending nematode and the ability to differentiate between active infections and past exposure. It is vital involves the pet owners in the knowledge of the risk of environmental contamination with faeces, from dogs and cats, as the leading risk factor in the transmission of zoonotic parasites.

11. Conclusions

In Mexico, as in many countries of the world; parasites are not important for the Health Ministries, they belong to the diseases of poverty, catalogued in the box of neglected diseases, and for this reason not subject to epidemiological surveillance or any surveillance, nor subject to notification. It is necessary to sensitise the authorities of the health to provide economic support for epidemiological surveillance for this parasitosis.

Acknowledgement

This work was partially supported to M.P.-M. by the grant 262237 CONACYT.

References

Acevedo-Ramírez, P.M.C., Peralta-Abarca, G.E., 2010. No tiene la culpa el perro, si no quien lo deja en la calle. Rev. Cien. Des. 36, 6–12.

Aguila, C., Cuéllar, C., Fenoy, S., Guillén, J.L., 1987. Comparative study of assays detecting circulating immune complexes and specific antibodies in patients infected with *Toxocara canis*. J. Helminthol. 61, 196–202.

Alba-Hurtado, F., Tórtola, P.J., Tsutsumi, V., Ortega-Pierres, M.G., 2000. Histological investigation of experimental ocular toxocariasis in gerbils. Int. J. Parasitol. 30, 143–147.

Alvarado-Esquivel, C., 2013a. Toxocariasis in waste pickers: a case control seroprevalence study. PLoS One 8, e54897.

Alvarado-Esquivel, C., 2013b. *Toxocara* infection in psychiatric inpatients: a case control seroprevalence study. PLoS One 8, e62606.
Alvarado-Esquivel, C., 2014. Seroepidemiology of toxocariasis in rural Tepehuanos population from Durango, Mexico. J. Helminthol. 88, 173–176.
Alvarado-Esquivel, C., Hernández-Tinoco, J., Sánchez-Anguiano, L.F., 2014a. *Toxocara* infection in gardeners: a case control seroprevalence study. Asian Pac. J. Trop. Med. 7, S79–S81.
Alvarado-Esquivel, C., Hernández-Tinoco, J., Sánchez-Anguiano, L.F., Cisneros-Martínez, J.A., 2014b. Low seroprevalence of *Toxocara* in schizofrenic inpatients in Durango, Mexico: a case control study. Int. J. Biomed. Sci. 10, 269–271.
Alvarado-Esquivel, C., Hernández-Tinoco, J., Sánchez-Anguiano, L.F., Ramos-Nevâres, A., Cerrillo-Soto, S.M., Guido-Arreola, C.A., Saenz-Soto, L., 2015b. Detection of IgG against *Toxocara* in sera of employees of meat industry. Int. J. Biomed. Sci. 11, 152–156.
Alvarado-Esquivel, C., Hernández-Tinoco, J., Sánchez-Anguiano, L.F., 2015a. Seroepidemiology of *Toxocara* infection in patients with vision impairment and blindness in Durango, Mexico. J. Clin. Med. Res. 7, 176–181.
Beaver, P.C., 1969. The nature of visceral larva migrans. J. Parasitol. 55, 3–12.
Beaver, P.C., Snyder, C.H., Carrera, G.M., Dent, J.H., Lafferty, J.W., 1952. Chronic eosinophilia due to visceral larva migrans. Pediatrics 9, 7–19.
Bowman, D.D., Mika-Grieve, M., Grieve, R.B., 1987. Circulating excretory-secretory antigen levels and specific antibody responses in mice infected with *Toxocara canis*. Am. J. Trop. Med. Hyg. 36, 75–82.
Burke, M.T., Robertson, E.L., 1985. Prenatal and lactational transmission of *Toxocara canis* and *Ancylostoma caninum*: experimental infection of the bitch at midpregnancy and parturition. Int. J. Parasitol. 15, 485–490.
Chávez-Güitrón, L.E., Morales-Montor, J., Muñoz-Guzmán, M.A., Nava-Castro, K.E., Ramírez-Álvarez, H., Moreno-Mendoza, N.A., Hernández-Cervantes, R., Alba-Hurtado, F., 2016. The *in vitro* effect of prolactin on the growth, motility and expression of prolactin receptors in larvae of *Toxocara canis*. Vet. Parasitol. 224, 33–38.
Chávez-Güitrón, L.E., Morales-Montor, J., Nava-Castro, K.E., Ramírez-Álvarez, H., Moreno-Mendoza, N.A., Prado-Ochoa, M.G., Muñoz-Guzmán, M.A., Alba-Hurtado, F., 2019. Progesterone *in vitro* increases growth, motility and progesterone receptor expression in third stage of *Toxocara canis*. Exp. Parasitol. 198, 1–6.
Chiardola, F., Schneeberger, E.E., Citera, G., Rosemffet, G.M., Kuo, L., Santillan, G., Maldonado-Cocco, J.A., 2008. Prevalence and clinical significance of eosinophilia in patient with rheumatoid arthritis in Argentina. J. Clin. Rheumatol. 14, 211–213.
Cianferoni, A., Schneider, L., Shantz, P.M., Brown, D., Fox, L.M., 2006. Visceral larva migrans associated with earthworm ingestion: clinical evolution in an adolescent patient. Pediatrics 117, e336–e339.
De Savigny, D.H., 1975. In vitro maintenance of *Toxocara canis* larvae and a simple method for the production of *Toxocara* ES antigen for use in serodiagnostic tests for visceral larva migrans. J. Parasitol. 61, 781–782.
Dubey, J.P., 1978. Patent *Toxocara canis* infection in ascarid-naive dogs. J. Parasitol. 64, 1021–1023.
Fernández-Presas, A.M., Martínez-Barbabosa, I., Gutiérrez-Quiroz, M., Vázquez-Tsuji, O., Pérez-León, M.J., García-Yáñez, Y., 1999. Serología para detección de helmintos extraintestinales en niños con alteración neurológica. Rev. Mex. Patol. Clín. 46, 217–221.
Fillaux, J., Magnaval, J.F., 2013. Laboratory diagnosis of human toxocariasis. Vet. Parasitol. 193, 327–336.
Hanelt, B., Thomas, F., Schmidt-Rhaesa, A., 2005. Biology of the phylum nematomorpha. Adv. Parasitol. 59, 243–305.

Hotez, P., Hawdon, J., Schad, G.A., 1993. Hookworm larval infectivity, arrest and amphiparatenesis: the *Caenorhabditis elegans* Daf-c paradigm. Parasitol. Today 9, 23–26.
Jiménez-Balderas, F.J., García-Jaimes, J., Ríos, R., Zonana-Nacach, A., Tapia-Romero, R., Villanueva, N., Méndez-Samperio, P., delaRosa-Arana, J.L., 2014. Isolation of IgG antibodies to *Toxocara* in ankylosing spondylitis patients with acute anterior uveitis. Korean J. Ophthalmol. 28, 207–212.
Maizels, R.M., De Savigny, D., Ogilvie, B.M., 1984. Characterization of surface and excretory-secretory antigens of *Toxocara canis* infective larvae. Parasite Immunol. 6, 23–37.
Martínez-Báez, M., Alemán, P., 1960. Larva migrans visceral. Primer caso comprobado en México. I estudio histopatológico. Rev. Inst. Salubr. Enferm. Trop. 20, 65–72.
Martínez-Barbabosa, I., Gutiérrez-Quiroz, M., Fernández-Presas, A.M., Pérez-León, M.J., Vázquez-Tsuji, O., García-Yáñez, Y., 1997. Reactividad serológica a antígeno de *Toxocara canis* en una población escolar. Rev. Mex. Patol. Clín. 44, 85–89.
Martínez-Barbabosa, I., Gutiérrez-Cárdenas, E.M., Alpizar-Sosa, E.A., Pimienta-Lastra, R.J., 2008a. Parasitic contamination by dog feces collected from the streets of San Cristóbal de las Casas, Chiapas, Mexico. Vet. Mex. 39, 173–180.
Martínez-Barbabosa, I., Gutiérrez-Quiroz, M., Ruíz-González, L.A., Gutiérrez-Cárdenas, E.M., Alpizar-Sosa, E.A., Valencia-Juárez, J.L., Gaona, E., 2008b. Prevalence of anti-*T. canis* in stray dogs in Mexico City. Vet. Parasitol. 153, 270–276.
Molina-Pasquel, C., Díaz-Muñoz, A., 1960. Larva migrans visceral. Primer caso comprobado en México, II estudio clínico. Rev. Inst. Salubr. Enferm. Trop. 20, 73–80.
Muñoz-Guzmán, M.A., Alba-Hurtado, F., 2010. Secretory-excretory antigens of *Toxocara canis* recognized by puppies of the Mexico City metropolitan area. Vet. Mex. 41, 59–64.
Muñoz-Guzmán, M.A., del Río-Navarro, B.E., Valdivia-Anda, G., Alba-Hurtado, F., 2010. The increase in seroprevalence to *Toxocara canis* in asthmatic children is related to cross-reaction with *Ascaris suum* antigens. Allergol. Immunopathol. 38, 115–121.
Nava-Cortés, N., Romero-Núñez, C., Bautista-Gómez, L.G., Hernández-García, P.A., Heredia-Cárdenas, R., 2015. Presence of anti-*Toxocara canis* antibodies and risk factors in children form the Amecameca and Chalco regions of México. BMC Pediatr. 15, 65. https://doi.org/10.1186/s12887-015-0385-9.
Park, J.K., Sultana, T., Lee, S.H., Kang, S., Kim, H.K., Min, G.S., Eom, K.S., Nadler, S.A., 2011. Monophyly of clade III nematodes is not supported by phylogenetic analysis of complete mitochondrial genome sequences. BMC Genomics 12, 392, 1–16.
Ponce-Macotela, M., Peralta-Abarca, G.E., Martínez-Gordillo, M.N., 2005. *Giardia intestinalis* and other zoonotic parasites: prevalence in adult dogs from the southern part of Mexico City. Vet. Parasitol. 131, 1–4.
Ponce-Macotela, M., Rodríguez-Caballero, A., Peralta-Abarca, G.E., Martínez-Gordillo, M.N., 2011. A simplified method for hatching and isolating *Toxocara canis* larvae to facilitate excretory-secretory antigen collection in vitro. Vet. Parasitol. 175, 382–385.
Rayes, A.A., Lambertucci, J.R., 2001. Human toxocariasis as a possible cause of eosinophilic arthritis. Rheumatology 40, 109.
Richardson-de Corral, V., Lozano-García, J., Ramos-Corona, L.E., 1990. Una presentación poco usual de toxocariasis sistémica. Bol. Med. Hosp. Infant. Mex. 47, 841–844.
Rodríguez-Caballero, A., Luna-Ochoa, R.I., Ponce-Macotela, M., Peralata-Abarca, G.E., Martínez-Gordillo, M.N., 2007. A simple and inexpensive *in vitro* method for retrieving fertilized *Toxocara canis* eggs. Parasitol. Res. 101, 829–832. https://doi.org/10.1007/s00436-007-0539-2.
Rodríguez-Caballero, A., Martínez-Gordillo, M.N., Medina-Flores, Y., Medina-Escutia, M.E., Meza-Lucas, A., Correa, D., Caballero-Salazar, S., Ponce-Macotela, M., 2015. Successful capture of *Toxocara canis* larva antigens from human serum samples. Parasit. Vectors 8, 264.

Rodríguez-Caballero, A., Martínez-Gordillo, M.N., Caballero-Salazar, S., Rufino-González, Y., Ponce-Macotela, M., 2017. *Toxocara canis*: analysis of the kinetics of antigen release and antibody production in an in vivo model for the detection of past or present infection. Vet. Parasitol. 243, 183–187.

Romero-Núñez, C., Mendoza-Martínez, G.D., Yáñez-Arteaga, S., Ponce-Macotela, M., Bustamante-Montes, P., Ramírez-Durán, N., 2013. Prevalence and risk factors associated with *Toxocara canis* infection in children. Sci. World J. 2013, 572089. https://doi.org/10.1155/2013/572089.

Schnieder, T., Laabs, E.M., Wels, C., 2011. Larval development of *Toxocara canis* in dogs. Vet. Parasitol. 175, 193–206.

Shantz, P.M., Biagi, F.F., 1968. Coexistence of *Toxocara* and *Toxascaris* in dogs in Mexico City. J. Parasitol. 54, 185–186.

Shoop, W.L., Corkum, K.C., 1987. Maternal transmission by *Alaria marcianae* (Trematoda) and the concept of amphiparatenesis. J. Parasitol. 73, 110–115.

Sprent, J.F., 1958. Observations on the development of *Toxocara canis* (Werner, 1782) in the dog. Parasitology 48, 184–209.

Strube, C., Heuer, L., Janecek, E., 2013. *Toxocara* spp. infection in paratenic hosts. Vet. Parasitol. 193, 375–389.

Styles, T.J., 1967. Incidence of *Toxocara canis* and other helminth parasites of dogs in Mexico City. J. Parasitol. 53, 822–823.

Tinoco-Gracia, L., Barreras-Serrano, A., López-Valencia, G., Tamayo-Sosa, A.R., Quiroz-Romero, H., Melgarejo, T., 2008. Seroprevalence of larva migrans of *Toxocara canis* and evaluation of associated risk factors among children in a Mexico-United States border region. Int. J. Appl. Res. Vet. Med. 6, 130–136.

Van den Hoogen, J., Geisen, S., Routh, D., Ferris, H., Traunspurger, W., Wardle, D.A., de Goede, R.G.M., Adams, B.J., Ahmad, W., Andriuzzi, W.S., Bardgett, R.D., Bonkowski, M., Campos-Herrera, R., Cares, J.E., Caruso, T., Caixeta, L.B., Chen, X., Costa, S.R., Creamer, R., Castro, J.M.C., Dam, M., Djigal, D., Escuer, M., Griffiths, B.S., Gutiérrez, C., Hohberg, K., Kalinkina, S., Kardol, P., Kergunteuil, A., Korthals, G., Krashevska, V., Kudrin, A.A., Li, Q., Liang, W., Magilton, M., Marais, M., Martín, J.A.R., Matveeva, E., Mayad, E.H., Mulder, C., Mullin, C., Mullin, P., Neilson, R., Nguyen, T.A.D., Nielsen, U.N., Okada, H., Rius, J.E.P., Pan, K., Peneva, V., Pellissier, L., Pereira-daSilva, J.C., Pitteloud, C., Powers, T.O., Powers, K., Quist, C.W., Rasmann, S., Moreno, S.S., Scheu, S., Setälä, H., Sushchuk, A., Tiunov, A.V., Trapa, J., van der Putten, W., Vestargard, M., Villenave, C., Waeyenberge, L., Wall, D.H., Wilschut, R., Wright, D.G., Yang, J.I., Crowther, T.W., 2019. Soil nematode abundance and functional group composition at global scale. Nature 572, 194–198.

Vélez-Hernández, L., Reyes-Barrera, K.L., Rojas-Almaráz, D., Calderón-Oropeza, M.A., Cruz-Vázquez, J.K., Arcos-García, J.L., 2014. Riesgo potencial de parásitos zoonóticos presentes en heces caninas en Puerto Escondido, Oaxaca. Salud Publica Mex. 56, 625–630.

Vlaminck, J., Cools, P., Albonico, M., Ame, S., Ayana, M., Cringoli, G., Dana, D., Keiser, J., Maurelli, M.P., Matoso, L.F., Montresor, A., Mekonnen, Z., Mirams, G., Correa-Oliveira, R., Pinto, S.A., Rinaldi, L., Sayasone, S., Thomas, E., Vercruysse, J., Verweij, J.J., Lovecke, B., 2019. Therapeutic efficacy of albendazole against soil-transmitted helminthiasis in children measured by five diagnostic methods. PLoS Negl. Trop. Dis. 13, e0007471.

CHAPTER EIGHTEEN

Seroprevalence Brazil

Paula Mayara Matos Fialho[a,*,†], **Carlos Roberto Silveira Correa**[b], **Susana Zevallos Lescano**[c]

[a]Institute of Medical Sociology, Centre for Health and Society, Medical Faculty, University of Duesseldorf, Duesseldorf, Germany

[b]Departamento de Saúde Coletiva, Faculdade de Ciências Médicas, São Paulo, Brazil

[c]Universidade de São Paulo, Instituto de Medicina Tropical de São Paulo—FMUSP, Laboratório de Imunopatologia da Esquistossomose, São Paulo, Brazil

*Corresponding author: e-mail address: paulamayara.matosfialho@med.uni-duesseldorf.de

Contents

Abstract

This chapter presents an overview of the seroprevalence of toxocariasis in Brazil and discusses how this zoonosis is studied, diagnosed, and treated in the Brazilian population. Toxocariasis in humans has a high prevalence in several regions of Brazil; however, this disease is neglected because of lack of knowledge, non-specific clinical signs, and difficult diagnosis. Most studies conducted in Brazil have estimated the prevalence of toxocariasis, i.e., the number of people who presented the disease at any given time. However, a few studies have determined disease incidence (number of new cases in a population at risk) and identified risk factors for *Toxocara canis* infection. Despite the high seroprevalence, the Brazilian population is not well aware of toxocariasis. Thus, the need of the hour is to raise awareness about this parasitic infection because of its worldwide distribution and potential health risk.

† Current address: Institute of Medical Sociology, Universitätsstraße 1, 40225 Düsseldorf, Germany.

Advances in Parasitology, Volume 109
ISSN 0065-308X
https://doi.org/10.1016/bs.apar.2020.01.013

1. Introduction

Brazil is located in the Western Hemisphere and has a total area of 8,500,000 km^2; the territory is crossed by the Equator and the Tropic of Capricorn, but most of it is located below the Equator. The large geographical area and diversity explain the variety of soil, flora, and fauna found in Brazil. The country is divided into five regions, and each region contains a predominant biome, including the Amazon rainforest, Cerrado, Atlantic Forest, Caatinga, Pampas, and Pantanal (Brasil, 2012). Eggs of *Toxocara canis* and infected individuals have been found in almost all the biomes (Marchioro et al., 2013).

Toxocariasis is an anthropozoonosis with a high prevalence in Brazil. The prevalence is higher than 20% in several regions, and infection is associated with significant comorbidities (Fialho and Corrêa, 2016).

The prevalence of toxocariasis in Brazil varies from 4.2% to 65.4% (Fialho and Corrêa, 2016). One of the factors that justify this high variability is the age range of the study populations. The prevalence is highest among children because they have the habit of geophagy and onicophagy, along with more contact with dogs (Souza et al., 2011).

This chapter discusses the seroprevalence of toxocariasis in Brazil and how this zoonosis is studied, diagnosed, and treated in the Brazilian population.

2. Epidemiological studies in Brazil

The epidemiology of human infections caused by *T. canis* has been investigated in several cross-sectional and cohort studies. Cross-sectional studies have determined the prevalence of human infections in population segments and identified factors associated with these infections. Some of the factors have been classified as potential risk factors for toxocariasis. Cohort studies have evaluated the incidence of the disease in population segments and identified risk factors for *T. canis* infection.

A few studies have determined the incidence of toxocariasis in Brazil; and to the best of our knowledge, all available studies on this topic have been performed in Brazil. A cohort study in Campinas, state of São Paulo, Brazil, found that the incidence of toxocariasis in children aged 2–12 years was 10.4 cases per 100 children-years (Fialho et al., 2018). Data on the incidence of *Toxocara* sp. in Brazil and other countries are limited because almost all field studies have a cross-sectional design and analysed only one time period in the natural history of infection.

The cross-sectional study by Campos Júnior et al. (2003) indicated a significant difference in the seroprevalence of toxocariasis among children according to their geographical origin. Children from poor neighbourhoods of Brasília had a higher prevalence (21.8%) than those living in wealthy areas (3.0%) (Campos Júnior et al., 2003). Another cross-sectional and population-based study reported that the prevalence of toxocariasis among children aged 2–12 years living in a poor area of Campinas was 16% (Fialho et al., 2017).

2.1 The design effect and intraclass correlation

The epidemiological studies that evaluate the prevalence of positive serology for *T. canis* infections in a particular location, such as a neighbourhood, serological surveillance is not performed in all individuals from the location, and prevalence and confidence intervals are determined in a population segment. The sample size depends on the available resources and study objectives. The study sample is ideally selected from a list of all individuals in the population; however, the list does not exist or may not be available. One strategy to overcome this limitation is randomly selecting households and examining dwellers at the risk of infection. The presence of positive serology for *T. canis* infection may be associated with familial factors, whether genetic or sociocultural. This may be the case when family members have dogs or feed non-domiciled dogs, have contact with dog faeces, or eat vegetables contaminated with parasite eggs. Moreover, the households may be randomly selected to evaluate the presence or absence of these characteristics.

This strategy may involve randomly selecting and screening children from several houses where two children reside. Serological test results can be positive (p) or negative (n). Considering the presence of two children in the same household, the following combination of results is possible: pp. (both are positive), pn (one is positive and the other is negative), or nn (both are negative). The probability of finding the same serological result (pp or nn) in two children from the same household may be higher than that of finding the same result in two children randomly selected from a given neighbourhood. Several statistical software tools can be used to determine these parameters. The association between serological status and environmental factors can be assessed by intraclass correlation. The analysis of this correlation allows the calculation of design effect, which assesses the need to correct a previously calculated sample size (Wejnert et al., 2012). The confidence intervals of the measured prevalence should be corrected after the repeated collection of sample size data (Rowe et al., 2002). The effect design should be taken into consideration in future studies.

The studies performed by our group analysed the design effect and intraclass correlation. There was no intraclass correlation, i.e., the probability of two children in the same household having the same serological result was not higher than that of any other two children who did not live in the same household. The prevalence was 16%, and the obtained confidence interval did not require recalculation of sample size (Fialho et al., 2017).

The cases in which the design effect has not been calculated does not indicate that it cannot be present in other territories. A study has evaluated children who lived in a neighbourhood composed of houses built by a public housing program. These houses had the similar area, physical characteristics, water supply, and sewage systems. Several families owned dogs as pets, and dogs were regularly fed by one or more families (Fialho et al., 2017, 2018).

3. Prevalence and association studies

Previous studies have determined the prevalence of toxocariasis and its association with other diseases in all regions of Brazil. The regions with the highest number of studies did not necessarily have the highest prevalence.

Studies on the seroprevalence of toxocariasis were concentrated in the south-eastern (40%), southern (32%), north-eastern (18%), and northern (9%) regions. Only one study estimated the prevalence of this disease in the centre-west region (Fialho and Corrêa, 2016).

The northeast region had the smallest number of studies but the highest prevalence. A study conducted in Salvador, Bahia, with 1148 children, aged 4–11 years, reported that the prevalence of toxocariasis was 65%. The same study investigated the association of toxocariasis with respiratory factors and atopy (Mendonca et al., 2012).

Another study with 791 children aged 6–13 years reported that the seropositivity of *Toxocara* sp. in São Francisco do Conde, Bahia, Brazil, was 63.6% (Silva et al., 2017).

A study compared the seroprevalence of toxocariasis between low- and middle-income populations in Salvador and found that the prevalence was higher in low-income populations. Moreover, there was a positive and significant correlation between the degree of contact with dogs and cats, and the risk of *T. canis* infection, and a negative and significant correlation between socioeconomic status and the risk of infection (Souza et al., 2011). This may be attributed to the little knowledge of the routes of parasite infection in poorer population, along with increased contact with dogs and cats, while most of these animals have not been dewormed.

In Brazil, the population of stray dogs and cats facilitates *Toxocara* infection because most of these animals are not dewormed. This situation is a public health problem because several diseases are transmitted by stray animals. The lack of knowledge among health authorities about toxocariasis contributes to the neglect of the disease. The high parasite burden in Brazil should stimulate further research on the factors that contribute to this epidemic.

Santarém et al. (2011) evaluated the association between the seroprevalence of toxocariasis and family income in Presidente Prudente, state of São Paulo, and found that high family income was a protective factor for seropositivity for *Toxocara*, both in the total population and subgroups (middle-income and low-income populations) (Santarém et al., 2011).

A population-based study conducted in poor areas of Campinas found that the prevalence of seropositivity for toxocariasis among children aged 2–12 years was 16%. Further, a positive correlation was observed between seropositivity and urticaria (Fialho et al., 2017), which is common in socioeconomically disadvantaged populations.

The prevalence of toxocariasis in children aged 7 months to 12 years was assessed in the public health system (Sistema Único de Saúde—SUS) in nine municipalities in the northwest of Paraná was 32.2% (Marchioro et al., 2011).

Campos Júnior et al. (2003) determined the prevalence of seropositivity for *T. canis* in children from different areas of Brasília and found that there was a significant difference in prevalence between children from poor neighbourhoods (21.8%) and wealthy neighbourhoods (3.0%) (Campos Júnior et al., 2003).

The prevalence of toxocariasis among people aged 5–90 years living in rural Amazonia has been reported to be 26.8%, and the seropositivity rate has been reported to be higher in the age group of 5–14 years (36.6%; 95% CI: 28.1–45.7%) (Rubinsky-Elefant et al., 2008). This result suggests that seroprevalence was higher in preschool/school-age children even among populations with heterogeneous age groups. Moreover, the seropositive groups had a lower socioeconomic status and were less likely to have cats as pets (Rubinsky-Elefant et al., 2008).

The seroprevalence of *Toxocara* sp. among pregnant women in the southeast and centre-west regions of Brazil has been reported to be 6.4% and 22%, respectively (Pereira et al., 2016; Santos et al., 2015). In Brazil, few studies have evaluated disease prevalence in pregnant women.

However, the high prevalence rates suggest that new population groups should be analysed and included in studies on toxocariasis.

The prevalence of toxocariasis is higher than 50% in most regions of Brazil, and the rate is significantly higher in the north-eastern region (Fialho and Corrêa, 2016). The syndromes and diseases caused by *Toxocara* sp. in humans are underdiagnosed, which limits the measurement of disease prevalence and incidence. The lack of knowledge among health professionals and the general population about toxocariasis contributes to underdiagnosis. In Brazil, many health professionals are unaware of *Toxocara* infection and its association with comorbidities. The enhancement of knowledge among health professionals about *Toxocara* infection and its clinical manifestations could help to reduce parasite burden in Brazil.

3.1 Clinical manifestations and association studies

World Health Organisation has recognised toxocariasis as a neglected disease in 2010, among other diseases, including Chagas disease and dengue. The association between *Toxocara* infection and other diseases is unknown because of the lack of knowledge about this roundworm and limited resources for treatment.

The clinical manifestations of toxocariasis, in accordance with the association studies conducted in Brazil, are shown in Fig. 1.

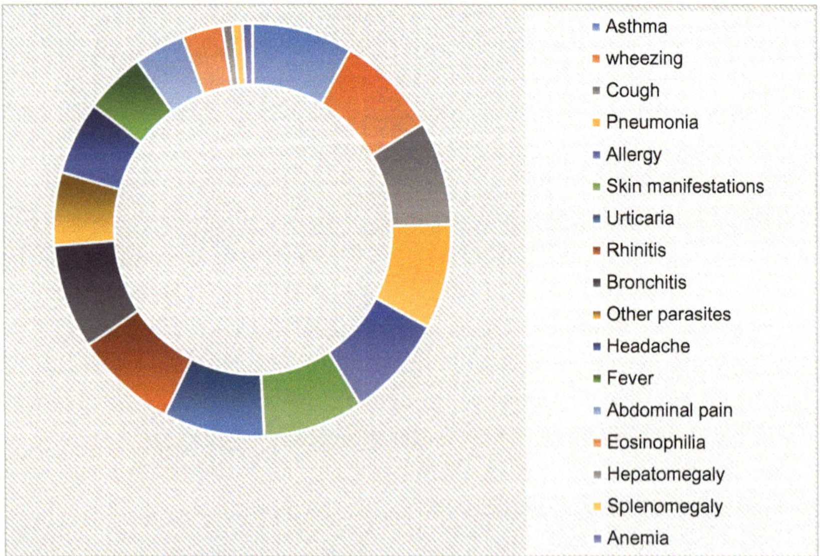

Fig. 1 Main diseases/clinical symptoms of toxocariasis in accordance with the association studies conducted in Brazil.

Most studies have found a correlation between seropositivity and respiratory diseases, including asthma and wheezing (Colli et al., 2010; Fialho and Corrêa, 2014; Fragoso et al., 2011; Guilherme et al., 2013; Manini et al., 2012; Mendonca et al., 2012; Oliart-Guzmán et al., 2014).

Some studies have analysed the association between seropositivity and comorbidities, including skin diseases (urticaria) and atopy (Fialho et al., 2017; Fragoso et al., 2011; Manini et al., 2012; Silva et al., 2017).

These comorbidities affect primarily school-age children, demonstrating the importance of toxocariasis in early childhood.

4. Diagnosis and treatment of toxocariasis in Brazil

The larvae of *Toxocara* sp. do not complete their life cycle to adult worms in humans, who, similar to other hosts such as primates, rodents, chicken, and with pigs or sheep, are considered paratenic hosts, i.e., do not eliminate parasite eggs in the faeces. The definitive diagnosis of infection involves visualising nematode larvae in the granulomatous lesions of infected tissues, morphological and morphometric identification of third-stage larvae (L3), and polymerase chain reaction (PCR) for detecting parasitic DNA. Tissue biopsy is not recommended because the procedure is invasive.

4.1 Visceral toxocariasis

The signs and symptoms of visceral toxocariasis (VT) are caused by the migration of L3 in several organs via the bloodstream. Migration may be asymptomatic or cause different symptoms, depending on the duration and intensity of migration, age, and the immune status of the host. Toxocariasis is rarely fatal, and non-specific symptoms include fever, hepatosplenomegaly, abdominal pain, vomiting, anorexia, diarrhoea, weight loss, fatigue, and in some cases, urticaria. Clinical manifestations are related to repetitive infections and/or parasite load, and may persist for months (Chieffi et al., 2009; Rubinsky-Elefant et al., 2010).

Several serological tests based on the detection of antibodies against the parasite have been developed for diagnosing VT, which are described below.

4.1.1 ELISA

The standard test for diagnosing human toxocariasis is indirect ELISA using *T. canis* larval (L3) excretory-secretory (TES) antigens, which have good specificity and sensitivity. Previous studies have reported several tests based on somatic antigens derived from embryonated eggs, larvae, or adults.

However, these antigens lacked sensitivity and presented a high degree of cross-reactivity with *Ascaris* sp. and other geohelminths common in tropical countries, including hookworms, *Strongyloides stercoralis*, and *Trichuris trichiura*. Although the use of TES antigens has improved the efficiency of this test, it may not have high specificity in countries where parasitic diseases are prevalent. Therefore, serum samples are routinely pre-incubated with the antigenic extract of *A. suum* adults, followed by incubation with TES antigens.

Bach-Rizzatti (1984) standardised an ELISA test for detecting anti-*Toxocara* antibodies in Brazil. The author considered that, after incubating sera with *A. suum* antigen, titres above 1:64 might indicate positivity to toxocariasis in humans (Chieffi et al., 2009). The TES antigen-based test used for detecting IgG antibodies has been reported to have a sensitivity of 78% and a specificity of 92% in the diagnosis of VT (Glickman et al., 1986).

4.1.2 Dot-ELISA

Camargo et al. (1992) standardised a Dot-ELISA test for diagnosing toxocariasis in Brazil and concluded that this test was more effective than ELISA owing to its high stability, low cost, and short processing time. In Dot-ELISA, nitrocellulose membranes are incubated with parasite antigens for screening, and are later incubated with a peroxidase-labelled antibody for reaction and colour development. The advantage of this technique is the possibility of storing blotted membranes at 4 °C for several years; moreover, these membranes remain stable at room temperature and can be shipped to other laboratories (Camargo et al., 1992). The technique is useful in studies in tropical areas where laboratory resources are limited, and parasite infections are common.

De Andrade Lima Coelho et al. (2005) used a dot-blot assay with a *T. canis* recombinant antigen to determine the prevalence of toxocariasis in children in north-eastern Brazil and tested serum samples from individuals infected with *A. lumbricoides* (De Andrade Lima Coelho et al., 2005). This technique was highly specific for diagnosing human toxocariasis as compared to indirect ELISA, especially in tropical regions.

4.1.3 Recombinant proteins

Difficulties in producing sufficient amounts of TES antigens and their cross-reactivity with other helminth antigens led researchers to produce recombinant antigens in *Escherichia coli* and use them in serodiagnosis. This type of antigen has higher sensitivity and specificity in ELISA tests when compared to native TES antigen-based tests. Two recombinant TES proteins are used in the diagnosis of toxocariasis, TES-30, a 30-kDa L3 protein, and TES-120. In immunoblots, rTES-30 reacts specifically with sera from patients with toxocariasis, but not with sera from patients with filariasis or ascariasis. rTES-120 reacts with sera from individuals with toxocariasis, but not with sera from subjects infected with other helminth or protozoan infections (Chieffi et al., 2009).

Coelho et al. (2003) developed an ELISA test using this recombinant antigen immobilised on a solid phase consisting of polysiloxane/polyvinyl alcohol beads. Compared to the conventional test, ELISA showed larger differences in optical density between positive and negative results. Moreover, this test has the advantages of low cost, and ease to obtain the solid phase. This test was used to determine the prevalence of toxocariasis in north-eastern Brazil, with good results.

Santos et al. (2019) evaluated the performance of rTES-30 and rTES-120 in children and adult sera, and found that the sensitivity of rTES-30 was not affected by age (81.8% in children and 87% in adults), whereas the sensitivity of rTES-120 was significantly decreased in children as compared to adults (63.6% vs 95.7%). However, both proteins had high specificity (94%) against other geohelminths, and the authors recommended using rTES-30 with total IgG in indirect ELISA in epidemiological studies (Santos et al., 2019).

4.1.4 Western blotting (WB)

This test is more specific than TES-ELISA, especially in populations with multiple parasitic infections. WB allows identifying *Toxocara* sp. using low molecular weight (24–35 kDa) antigens specific for this roundworm.

Nunes et al. (1997) used WB during a study in Brazil and found that 55–66-kDa antigen complex was responsible for the cross-reactivity between *T. canis* and *A. suum*. Jacob (1995) performed a study in sequential patients with VT, wherein, WB showed the disappearance of standard high molecular weight (97–116 kDa and 200–210 kDa) fractions after treatment, which might be related to the gradual decrease in antibody titres observed in ELISA (Jacob, 1995).

Schoenardie et al. (2013) observed that positivity to anti-*Toxocara* antibodies using ELISA in children aged 1–12 years in southern Brazil was 50.6% ($n=427$). However, WB was used as a confirmatory test in 70 ELISA-positive samples, and these samples were positive for anti-*Toxocara* antibodies, with typical 30 kDa bands, suggesting that this antigen fraction might be useful for the specific diagnosis of toxocariasis (Schoenardie et al., 2013).

Roldan et al. (2017) used WB to identify anti-*Toxocara* IgM antibodies against TES antigens in sera from patients with toxocariasis, patients with other helminth infections, and healthy subjects. Anti-*Toxocara* IgM antibodies were detected in 91.4%, 76%, and 45.3% of sera from patients with toxocariasis, with other helminthic infections, and from healthy individuals, respectively, in ELISA, Whereas, in WB, IgM antibodies were detected in 94.8%, 65.3%, and 41% of sera from patients with toxocariasis, with other helminthiases, and from healthy individuals, respectively. These results demonstrate that the detected IgM antibodies are not specific for the diagnosis of toxocariasis (Roldan et al., 2017).

4.1.5 Immunohistochemistry of granulomatous lesions

The definitive diagnosis of infection is established by visualising nematode larvae in granulomatous lesions in infected tissues, especially from liver, where larvae are present in large numbers. However, a tissue biopsy is not recommended because the procedure is invasive.

Musso et al. (2006) examined 310 paraffin-embedded liver sections from children aged 1–15 years from Vitória, Espírito Santo, Brazil, stained with haematoxylin and eosin to detect *Toxocara* antigens using anti-*Toxocara* rabbit serum. Among the 24 patients with granulomas, 10 patients presented eosinophil-rich lesions that reacted positively to anti-*Toxocara* serum, demonstrating that granulomas in VT are a common cause of granulomatous hepatitis in children. However, only 3.2% of tissue sections presented lesions, whereas, the rate of positive serology was high (30–39%) in this population, possibly because of the low larval burden in infected individuals. Similarly, children with *Toxocara*-induced granulomas had a higher rate of pyogenic infections, thereby, confirming the strong association between *Toxocara* infection and pyogenic liver abscess (Musso et al., 2006).

4.2 Ocular toxocariasis

Clinical findings in ocular toxocariasis (OT) are related to the presence and location of larvae in the eye. The main signs and symptoms include decreased visual acuity, strabismus, unilateral leukocoria, and intermediate or posterior uveitis, potentially leading to visual loss.

Differential diagnosis of ocular toxoplasmosis, intermediate uveitis, diffuse unilateral subacute neuroretinitis, retinoblastoma, and persistent hyperplastic primary vitreous is recommended (Rubinsky-Elefant et al., 2018).

Immunological tests such as ELISA (to determine the level of *T. canis* antibody titres in the serum), blood test, radiography, computed tomography, ocular electrophysiology, and ocular ultrasonography can complement the diagnosis of OT. Ocular ultrasound is essential for differential diagnosis from retinoblastoma in cases where calcium deposits are present. However, the presence of calcification does not exclude the diagnosis of toxocariasis (Morais et al., 2012).

4.2.1 TES-ELISA of the aqueous humour

Aqueous humour samples should be used for detecting anti-*Toxocara* antibodies in cases of OT. Diagnosis can be made by comparing the ELISA results in serum and aqueous humour samples, and applying the Goldmann-Witmer (GW) coefficient: (specific IgG level in aqueous humour/specific IgG level in serum)/(total IgG level in aqueous humour/total IgG in serum). The production of specific antibodies in the intraocular region is defined when the GW coefficient is higher than 3.0 (de Visser et al., 2008). However, ocular fluid examination is not a routine procedure in these cases, and laboratory diagnosis is performed using serum samples in clinical practice.

Few studies have correlated clinical data with serological test results and ophthalmic findings for diagnosing OT. Rubinsky-Elefant et al. (2018) analysed the correlation between the production of serum anti-*Toxocara* antibodies and the diagnosis of OT by evaluating common signs and symptoms in patients from a referral health centre in Brazil. The study has shown that OT affects children predominantly, and is characterised by visual loss, especially in the right eye. In addition, *Toxocara* larvae are located in the peripheral and posterior pole (Rubinsky-Elefant et al., 2018).

4.2.2 Optical coherence tomography

Toxocara larvae migrate through the retina. However, the layers through which larvae migrate, and the effects of larval invasion on the retina are unknown. Lago et al. (2006) analysed optical coherence tomography images in a case of *Toxocara* granuloma and observed that granulomas appeared as hyper-reflective rounded masses above the retinal pigment epithelium and below the neurosensory retina together with two minor satellite lesions. It was concluded that this optical technique might help elucidate the pathophysiology, diagnosis, and treatment of *Toxocara* granuloma (Lago et al., 2006).

4.2.3 *Ultrasound*

Ultrasonography is conducted in cases of OT to determine the type of involvement and perform differential diagnosis from tumour lesions of other aetiologies. However, ultrasonography is useful only in cases involving media opacity, but it does not reveal the pathognomonic findings of OT.

Morais et al. (2012) performed a study in São Paulo, Brazil to evaluate ultrasound findings of the three main forms of presentation of ocular toxocariasis (peripheral granuloma, granulomas in the posterior pole, and chronic endophthalmitis) in patients with confirmed diagnosis of OT (Morais et al., 2012). They reported that the most consistent ultrasound finding in the affected eye was the presence of a highly reflective retinal mass located in the posterior pole or periphery, which might be calcified, and the main characteristic was adherence to vitreous membranes. In conclusion, ultrasound examination combined with clinical history, clinical examination, and serology may help in the diagnosis of OT, especially in cases involving media opacity.

4.3 Neurotoxocariasis (NT)

Infection in the central nervous system (CNS) with *Toxocara* causes non-specific neurological syndromes, and eosinophilia is not detected in many cases. The presence of larvae in the CNS is likely in the cases involving: (a) spinal, brain fluid pleocytosis (CSF with marked eosinophilia); (b) positive serology for anti-*Toxocara* antibodies in serum and CSF, and the absence of antibodies against *Schistosoma mansoni* and *Cysticercus cellulosae* (parasites that invade the CNS); (c) the CSF is sterile, and there is negative serology for other common infections such as toxoplasmosis, syphilis, and cytomegalovirus; and (d) signs and symptoms improve after treatment with albendazole and thiabendazole (Moreira-Silva et al., 2004).

Studies conducted in Brazil suggest that although NT is rare in individuals infected with *Toxocara*, this syndrome should be included in the differential diagnosis of paediatric patients with neurological symptoms associated with high levels of eosinophils in the CSF. Other studies have found that parasitic infection is suspected in cases of meningitis, encephalitis, or myelitis associated with pleocytosis and marked eosinophilia in the humour liquor, and specific serology is necessary for proper diagnosis and treatment. These arguments are justified since eosinophilic meningitis or meningoencephalitis may be idiopathic or caused by larvae of other helminths, including the raccoon roundworm, *Baylisascaris procyonis*, the rodent lungworm,

Angiostrongylus cantonensis, as well as, by *Ascaris lumbricoides*, *Ascaris suum*, *Strongyloides stercoralis*, and *Trichinella spiralis* (Moreira-Silva et al., 2004).

On the contrary, Musso et al. (2006) examined CSF samples from children using anti-*Toxocara* IgG ELISA and found no significant association between *Toxocara* and viral or bacterial infections in the CNS, thereby, demonstrating that infection with this roundworm species was not related to meningitis or meningoencephalitis caused by viruses or bacteria (Musso et al., 2006).

Early diagnosis and treatment can prevent long-term neurological sequelae (Moreira-Silva et al., 2004).

4.4 Treatment

The treatment of human toxocariasis is limited because this infection is often subclinical and self-limiting. However, symptomatic patients should be treated. This infection is chronic (may persist for several years) and may affect the eyes and brain in cases of larval migration (Carvalho and Rocha, 2011). The decision to treat infected individuals depends on the type and severity of clinical signs.

The two main obstacles to treatment are the need for drugs that target larvae in tissues, and the difficulty in assessing drug efficacy in patients. Anthelmintics are recommended for treating acute toxocariasis, especially to prevent larval migration to the brain or eyes. Albendazole and mebendazole are commonly used to treat VT, despite their limited efficacy against larvae in tissues. Albendazole is preferred because of its rapid distribution into tissues after being metabolised, whereas, mebendazole is not absorbed outside the gastrointestinal tract. The recommended duration of treatment is 3–4 weeks. Anti-inflammatory drugs (corticosteroids or non-steroidal anti-inflammatory drugs) are used, together with anthelmintics, to relieve allergic symptoms (Salvador et al., 2010).

OT can be treated with corticosteroids (e.g., prednisolone), and severe cases can be treated with vitreous surgery, depending on the degree of intraocular inflammation and vitreoretinal complications. Surgery may also be necessary in cases of retinal detachment and proliferation of the intravitreal fibrovascular membrane, although albendazole combined with steroids has shown favourable clinical results. Albendazole is recommended for treating neurotoxocariasis because this drug can cross the blood-brain barrier, and the recommended duration of treatment is 3–4 weeks (Rubinsky-Elefant et al., 2010, 2018).

Determination of treatment efficacy in toxocariasis is hampered by the clinical manifestations and unspecific symptoms. Treatment assessment can be improved using eosinophil markers and serology for *T. canis*. However, some studies have shown that *Toxocara* IgG titres are not suitable for monitoring treated patients because titres remain elevated for up to 18 months (Lopez et al., 2005). Bass et al. (1987) evaluated asymptomatic children treated with thiabendazole and observed no significant reduction in eosinophil count after 1 year of therapy (Bass et al., 1987). Souza (1992) found that *Toxocara* IgG levels were normalised 1 year after treatment with thiabendazole; however, there was a significant reduction in the number of leukocytes and eosinophils (Carvalho and Rocha, 2011).

Rubinsky-Elefant et al. (2006) performed a serological follow-up in 27 children aged 1–12 years with VT or OT after treatment with thiabendazole over a period of 22–116 months using ELISA (IgG, IgA, and IgE) with TES antigens and observed that the sensitivity for IgG, IgA, and IgE was 100%, 47.8%, and 78.3%, respectively. There was a significant decrease in specific IgE titres during the first year of treatment, a significant decrease in IgA titres in the second year, and a significant decrease in IgG titres from the fourth year. Patient sera showed a strong affinity to IgG antibodies, indicating that these patients were in the chronic phase of the disease. Further, there was a significant decrease in the number of leukocytes, eosinophils, and anti-A isohaemagglutinin, thereby, suggesting that the measurement of IgE antibody titres together with eosinophil count could improve patient follow-up after therapy (Rubinsky-Elefant et al., 2006).

5. Conclusion

Toxocariasis is a significant public health problem in Brazil. This disease has reached regions that are socioeconomically underdeveloped and inhabited by poorer populations. Toxocariasis is a neglected disease, and the financial resources for diagnosis, control, and treatment are limited.

The increased awareness among health professionals about toxocariasis and parasite burden in Brazil can improve diagnosis and the reliable reports of clinical studies can increase scientific knowledge, and influence decision making by health managers.

Brazilian health authorities should give more attention to this disease, which is highly prevalent in the Brazilian population.

References

Bach-Rizzatti, B.C., 1984. Desenvolvimento de Teste Imuno-enzimático, ELISA, para o Diagnóstico da Toxocaríase Humana. Faculdade de Ciências Farmacêuticas, Universidade de São Paulo, São Paulo.

Bass, J.L., Mehta, K.A., Glickman, L.T., Blocker, R., Eppes, B.M., 1987. Asymptomatic toxocariasis in children. A prospective study and treatment trial. Clin. Pediatr. (Phila) 26, 441–446. https://doi.org/10.1177/000992288702600902.

Brasil, E., 2012. Sistema de Observação e Monitoramento da Agricultura no Brasil (SOMABRASIL).

Camargo, E.D., Nakamura, P.M., Vaz, A.J., da Silva, M.V., Chieffi, P.P., de Melo, E.O., 1992. Standardization of dot-ELISA for the serological diagnosis of toxocariasis and comparison of the assay with ELISA. Rev. Inst. Med. Trop. Sao Paulo 34, 55–60. https://doi.org/10.1590/s0036-46651992000100010.

Campos Júnior, D., Elefant, G.R., Silva, E.O.d.M.e., Gandolfi, L., Jacob, C.M.A., Tofeti, A., Pratesi, R., 2003. Freqüência de soropositividade para antígenos de Toxocara canis em crianças de classes sociais diferentes. Rev. Soc. Bras. Med. Trop. 36, 509–513.

Carvalho, E.A.A., Rocha, R., 2011. Toxocariasis: visceral larva migrans in children. J. Pediatr. 87, 100–110. https://doi.org/10.2223/JPED.2074.

Chieffi, P.P., dos Santos, S.V., de Queiroz, M.L., Lescano, S.A.Z., 2009. Human toxocariasis: contribution by Brazilian researchers. Rev. Inst. Med. Trop. Sao Paulo 51, 301–308.

Coelho, R.A.L., Yamasaki, H., Perez, E., Carvalho Jr., L.B., 2003. The ue of polysiloxane/polyvinyl alcohol beads as solid phase in IgG anti-*Toxocara canis* detection using a recombinant antigen. Mem. Inst. Oswaldo Cruz. 98, 391–393. https://doi.org/10.1590/S0074-02762003000300018.

Colli, C.M., Rubinsky-Elefant, G., Paludo, M.L., Falavigna, D.L.M., Guilherme, E.V., Mattia, S., Araujo, S.M., Ferreira, É., Previdelli, I.T.S., Falavigna-Guilherme, A.L., 2010. Serological, clinical and epidemiological evaluation of toxocariasis in urban areas of south Brazil. Rev. Inst. Med. Trop. Sao Paulo 52, 69–74.

De Andrade Lima Coelho, R., De Carvalho, L.B.J., Perez, E.P., Araki, K., Takeuchi, T., Ito, A., Aoki, T., Yamasaki, H., 2005. Prevalence of toxocariasis in northeastern Brazil based on serology using recombinant Toxocara canis antigen. Am. J. Trop. Med. Hyg. 72, 103–107.

de Visser, L., Rothova, A., de Boer, J.H., van Loon, A.M., Kerkhoff, F.T., Canninga-van Dijk, M.R., Weersink, A.Y.L., de Groot-Mijnes, J.D.F., 2008. Diagnosis of ocular toxocariasis by establishing intraocular antibody production. Am. J. Ophthalmol. 145, 369–374. https://doi.org/10.1016/j.ajo.2007.09.020.

Fialho, P.M.M., Corrêa, C.R.S., 2014. Toxocaríase, asma e índice de massa corporal em crianças e adolescentes em Campinas-SP, 1996 a 1998. Epidemiol. Serv. Saúde 23, 361–368.

Fialho, P.M.M., Corrêa, C.R.S., 2016. A systematic review of toxocariasis: a neglected but high-prevalence disease in Brazil. Am. J. Trop. Med. Hyg. 94, 1193–1199. https://doi.org/10.4269/ajtmh.15-0733.

Fialho, P.M.M., Correa, C.R.S., Lescano, S.Z., 2017. Seroprevalence of toxocariasis in children with urticaria: a population-based study. J. Trop. Pediatr. 63, 352–357. https://doi.org/10.1093/tropej/fmw094.

Fialho, P.M.M., Correa, C.R.S., Lescano, S.Z., 2018. Asthma and seroconversion from Toxocara spp. infection: which comes first? Biomed. Res. Int. 2018, 4280792. https://doi.org/10.1155/2018/4280792.

Fragoso, R.P., Monteiro, M.B.M., Lemos, E.M., Pereira, F.E.L., 2011. Anti-Toxocara antibodies detected in children attending elementary school in Vitoria, state of Espírito Santo, Brazil: prevalence and associated factors. Rev. Soc. Bras. Med. Trop. 44, 461–466.

Glickman, L., Schantz, P., Grieve, R., 1986. Toxocariasis. In: Immunodiagnosis of Parasitic Diseases, first ed. Helminthic Diseases, Academic Press, London.

Guilherme, E.V., Marchioro, A.A., Araujo, S.M., Falavigna, D.L.M., Adami, C., Falavigna-Guilherme, G., Rubinsky-Elefant, G., Falavigna-Guilherme, A.L., 2013. Toxocariasis in children attending a Public Health Service Pneumology Unit in Paraná State, Brazil. Rev. Inst. Med. Trop. Sao Paulo 55, 189–192.

Jacob, C.M.A., 1995. Análise evolutiva dos parâmetros clínico-laboratoriais da toxocaríase visceral na infância. Tese de Doutorado, Faculdade de Medicna da USP, São Paulo.

Lago, A., Andrade, R., Muccioli, C., Belfort, R.J., 2006. Optical coherence tomography in presumed subretinal Toxocara granuloma: case report. Arq. Bras. Oftalmol. 69, 403–405.

Lopez, M.D.L.A., Martin, G., Chamorro, M.D.C., Mario Alonso, J., 2005. Toxocariasis in children from a subtropical region. Medicina (B Aires) 65, 226–230.

Manini, M.P., Marchioro, A.A., Colli, C.M., Nishi, L., Falavigna-Guilherme, A.L., 2012. Association between contamination of public squares and seropositivity for Toxocara spp. in children. Vet. Parasitol. 188, 48–52. https://doi.org/10.1016/j.vetpar.2012.03.011.

Marchioro, A.A., Colli, C.M., Mattia, S., Paludo, M.L., de Melo, G.C., Adami, C.M., Pelloso, S.M., Guilherme, A.L.F., 2011. Avaliação eosinofílica e soropositividade para anticorpos IgG anti-toxocara em crianças atendidas pelo Sistema Único de Saúde. Rev. Paul. Pediatr. 29, 80–84.

Marchioro, A., Colli, C., Ferreira, É., Tiyo, R., Mattia, S., Souza, W., Falavigna-Guilherme, A., 2013. Identification of public areas with potential toxocariasis transmission risk using Geographical Information Systems. Acta Parasitol. 58, 328–333. https://doi.org/10.2478/s11686-013-0142-x.

Mendonca, L.R., Veiga, R.V., Dattoli, V.C.C., Figueiredo, C.A., Fiaccone, R., Santos, J., Cruz, Á.A., Rodrigues, L.C., Cooper, P.J., Pontes-de-Carvalho, L.C., Barreto, M.L., Alcantara-Neves, N.M., 2012. Toxocara seropositivity, atopy and wheezing in children living in poor neighbourhoods in urban Latin American. PLoS Negl. Trop. Dis. 6, e1886 https://doi.org/10.1371/journal.pntd.0001886.

Morais, F.B., Maciel, A.L., Arantes, T.E., Muccioli, C., Allemann, N., 2012. Ultrasonographic findings in ocular toxocariasis. Arq. Bras. Oftalmol. 75, 43–47.

Moreira-Silva, S.F., Rodrigues, M.G., Pimenta, J.L., Gomes, C.P., Freire, L.H., Pereira, F.E.L., 2004. Toxocariasis of the central nervous system: with report of two cases. Rev. Soc. Bras. Med. Trop. 37, 169–174.

Musso, C., Lemos, E.M., Tsanaclis, A.M.C., Pereira, F.E.L., 2006. Toxocara infection is not associated with viral or bacterial central nervous system infection in children. Neuropediatrics 37, 126–129. https://doi.org/10.1055/s-2006-924511.

Nunes, C.M., Tundisi, R.N., Garcia, J.F., Heinemann, M.B., Ogassawara, S., Richtzenhain, L.J., 1997. Cross-reactions between *Toxocara canis* and *Ascaris suum* in the diagnosis of visceral larva migrans by western blotting technique. Rev. Inst. Med. Trop. Sao Paulo 39, 253–256.

Oliart-Guzmán, H., Delfino, B.M., Martins, A.C., Mantovani, S.A.S., Braña, A.M., Pereira, T.M., Branco, F.L.C.C., Ramalho, A.A., Campos, R.G., Fontoura, P.S., de Araujo, T.S., de Oliveira, C.S.M., Muniz, P.T., Rubinsky-Elefant, G., Codeço, C.T., da Silva-Nunes, M., 2014. Epidemiology and control of child toxocariasis in the western Brazilian Amazon—a population-based study. Am. J. Trop. Med. Hyg. 90, 670–681. https://doi.org/10.4269/ajtmh.13-0506.

Pereira, L.C., Elefant, G.R., Nobrega, Y.M., Vital, T., Nitz, N., Gandolfi, L., Pratesi, R., Hecht, M., 2016. Toxocara spp. seroprevalence in pregnant women in Brasilia, Brazil. Rev. Soc. Bras. Med. Trop. 49, 641–643. https://doi.org/10.1590/0037-8682-0106-2016.

Roldan, W.H., Elefant, G.R., Ferreira, A.W., 2017. Immunoglobulin M antibodies are not specific for serodiagnosis of human toxocariasis. Parasite Immunol. 39, e12447. https://doi.org/10.1111/pim.12447.

Rowe, A.K., Lama, M., Onikpo, F., Deming, M.S., 2002. Design effects and intraclass correlation coefficients from a health facility cluster survey in Benin. Int. J. Qual. Health Care 14, 521–523. https://doi.org/10.1093/intqhc/14.6.521.

Rubinsky-Elefant, G., Shimizu, S.H., Sanchez, M.C.A., Jacob, C.M.A., Ferreira, A.W., 2006. A serological follow-up of toxocariasis patients after chemotherapy based on the detection of IgG, IgA, and IgE antibodies by enzyme-linked immunosorbent assay. J. Clin. Lab. Anal. 20, 164–172. https://doi.org/10.1002/jcla.20126.

Rubinsky-Elefant, G., da Silva-Nunes, M., Malafronte, R.S., Muniz, P.T., Ferreira, M.U., 2008. Human toxocariasis in rural Brazilian Amazonia: seroprevalence, risk factors, and spatial distribution. Am. J. Trop. Med. Hyg. 79, 93–98.

Rubinsky-Elefant, G., Hirata, C.E., Yamamoto, J.H., Ferreira, M.U., 2010. Human toxocariasis: diagnosis, worldwide seroprevalences and clinical expression of the systemic and ocular forms. Ann. Trop. Med. Parasitol. 104, 3–23. https://doi.org/10.1179/136485910X12607012373957.

Rubinsky-Elefant, G., Yamamoto, J.H., Hirata, C.E., Prestes-Carneiro, L.E., 2018. Toxocariasis: critical analysis of serology in patients attending a public referral center for ophthalmology in Brazil. Jpn. J. Ophthalmol. 62, 77–83. https://doi.org/10.1007/s10384-017-0543-8.

Salvador, S., Ribeiro, R., Winckler, M.I., Ohlweiler, L., Riesgo, R., 2010. Neurotoxocaríase infantil com acometimento cerebral, cerebelar, e periférico simultâneo: relato de caso e revisão da literatura. J. Pediatr. (Rio J) 86, 531–534.

Santarém, V.A., Leli, F.N.C., Rubinsky-Elefant, G., Giuffrida, R., 2011. Protective and risk factors for toxocariasis in children from two different social classes of Brazil. Rev. Inst. Med. Trop. Sao Paulo 53, 66–72.

Santos, P.C., Lehmann, L.M., Lorenzi, C., Hirsch, C., Telmo, P.L., Mattos, G.T., Cadore, P.S., Klafke, G.B., Berne, M.E.A., Gonçalves, C.V., Scaini, C.J., 2015. The seropositivity of Toxocara spp. antibodies in pregnant women attented at the university hospital in southern Brazil and the factors associated with infection. PLoS One 10, e0131058. https://doi.org/10.1371/journal.pone.0131058.

Santos, L.M.D., Donassolo, R.A., Berne, M.E., Leite, F.P.L., Avila, L.F.d.C., Scaini, C.J., Moreira, Â.N., Conceição, F.R., 2019. The serodiagnostic potential of recombinant proteins TES-30 and TES-120 in an indirect ELISA in the diagnosis of toxocariasis in cattle, horses, and sheep. PLoS One 14, e0213830. https://doi.org/10.1371/journal.pone.0213830.

Schoenardie, E.R., Scaini, C.J., Brod, C.S., Pepe, M.S., Villela, M.M., McBride, A.J.A., Borsuk, S., Berne, M.E.A., 2013. Seroprevalence of Toxocara infection in children from southern Brazil. J. Parasitol. 99, 537–539. https://doi.org/10.1645/GE-3182.

Silva, M.B., Amor, A.L.M., Santos, L.N., Galvao, A.A., Oviedo Vera, A.V., Silva, E.S., Barbosa, C.G., Goncalves, M.S., Cooper, P.J., Figueiredo, C.A., Ribeiro, R.d.C., Alcantara-Neves, N.M., 2017. Risk factors for Toxocara spp. seroprevalence and its association with atopy and asthma phenotypes in school-age children in a small town and semi-rural areas of Northeast Brazil. Acta Trop. 174, 158–164. https://doi.org/10.1016/j.actatropica.2016.04.005.

Souza, F.A., 1992. Parâmetros clínicos laboratoriais na evolução de 104 crianças portadoras de larva migrans visceral por *Toxocara canis* [dissertação]. UFESP, São Paulo.

Souza, R.F., Dattoli, V.C.C., Mendonca, L.R., de Jesus, J.R., Baqueiro, T., Santana, C.d.C., Santos, N.M., Barrouin-Melo, S.M., Alcantara-Neves, N.M., 2011. Prevalência e fatores de risco da infecção humana por Toxocara canis em Salvador, Estado da Bahia. Rev. Soc. Bras. Med. Trop. 44, 516–519.

Wejnert, C., Pham, H., Krishna, N., Le, B., DiNenno, E., 2012. Estimating design effect and calculating sample size for respondent-driven sampling studies of injection drug users in the United States. AIDS Behav. 16, 797–806. https://doi.org/10.1007/s10461-012-0147-8.

CHAPTER NINETEEN

Seroprevalence of human toxocarosis in Europe: A review and meta-analysis

Christina Strube[a,*], Marie-Kristin Raulf[a,b], Andrea Springer[a], Patrick Waindok[a], Herbert Auer[c]

[a]Institute for Parasitology, Centre for Infection Medicine, University of Veterinary Medicine Hannover, Hanover, Germany
[b]Immunology Unit & Research Center for Emerging Infections and Zoonoses, University of Veterinary Medicine Hannover, Hanover, Germany
[c]Department of Medical Parasitology, Center of Pathophysiology, Infectiology and Immunology, Institute of Specific Prophylaxis and Tropical Medicine, Medical University Vienna, Vienna, Austria
*Corresponding author: e-mail address: christina.strube@tiho-hannover.de

Contents

Abstract

Toxocarosis is distributed worldwide and represents the most prevalent zoonotic helminth infection in industrialized countries, thereby posing a substantial risk for public health. Thus, toxocarosis is one of CDC's Neglected Parasitic Infections that has been targeted for public health action. This systematic review and meta-analysis summarizes *Toxocara* seroprevalence in general populations from Europe, populations suspected of *Toxocara* infection and defined risk groups. Random-effects meta-analysis of proportions based on 41 publications resulted in an overall seroprevalence of 6.2% (95% CI: 4.7–8.3%) in the general population of Europe. Subgroup analysis according to decades (1970–2010s) revealed a significant increase in seroprevalence, with the highest value

Advances in Parasitology, Volume 109
ISSN 0065-308X
https://doi.org/10.1016/bs.apar.2020.01.014

(12.4%; 95% CI: 6.5–22.3%) in the 2010s ($\chi^2 = 17.87$, df=4, $P = 0.001$). There were no significant differences between pooled prevalence rates of European sub-regions ($\chi^2 = 3.01$, df=3, $P = 0.389$). Furthermore, meta-analysis of seroprevalence according to age groups, based on data from 22 publications, indicated a significantly higher pooled seroprevalence of 14.9% (95% CI: 8.5–24.8%) in people more than 50 years of age than in younger age cohorts ($\chi^2 = 8.33$, df=2, $P = 0.016$). Occupational groups exposed to contaminated soil and infected animals bear substantial risk for acquiring *Toxocara* infection. Due to the close link between animal infection and human *Toxocara* exposure, a "One Health" approach for the prevention of *Toxocara* infection in both humans and animals is required.

1. Introduction

Toxocara canis and *Toxocara cati*, the roundworms of dogs and cats, are worldwide-distributed zoonotic intestinal helminths and the causative agents of human toxocarosis. More than 60 years ago, Wilder (1950), Beaver et al. (1952), and Nichols (1956) reported the first cases of *Toxocara* infection in humans, thereby discovering that humans act as paratenic hosts for these nematodes. After ingestion of embryonated *Toxocara* eggs, containing infective third-stage larvae, via contaminated soil, water or food, or uptake of larvae via raw or undercooked meat of paratenic hosts, e.g., chicken, the larvae penetrate the intestinal wall and are transported to different tissues with the blood stream (Strube et al., 2013). The persistence of these larvae in the brain, eye, liver and muscle tissue may cause a broad range of clinical symptoms, which most often occur in children (Despommier, 2003). They are classified into four different syndromes, namely, covert toxocarosis, visceral *larva migrans* (VLM), ocular *larva migrans* (OLM) and neural *larva migrans* (NLM), also known as neurotoxocarosis. Covert toxocarosis is characterised by unspecific symptoms, such as headache and behavioural disorders (Taylor et al., 1987). VLM is a multi-systemic disease accompanied by fever, abdominal pain and respiratory symptoms. OLM may lead to retinal granuloma and potentially blindness and NLM may cause myelitis and meningoencephalitis, resulting in various neurological dysfunctions (Strube et al., 2013). In addition, recent studies suggest that *Toxocara* seropositivity may be associated with decreased cognitive function in children and young adults (Erickson et al., 2015; Walsh and Haseeb, 2012). Furthermore, a silent progression to neuropsychiatric disorders, such as schizophrenia and Alzheimer's disease is being discussed (Fan et al., 2015). Thus, even subclinical *Toxocara* infections might lead to long-lasting negative impacts on human health. Due to the potential severity of illness, a high worldwide exposure and the possibility of prevention and treatment, toxocarosis is considered one of the Neglected Parasitic Infections, a group of five parasitic diseases that have been targeted by the Centers for Disease Control and Prevention (CDC) for public health action (CDC, 2019; Woodhall et al., 2014).

Diagnosis of human toxocarosis can be challenging. An acute infection can only be detected by invasive and elaborate methods, e.g., histopathological examination, morphometric identification of larvae or the detection of parasite DNA in tissue samples (Smith and Noordin, 2006). Thus, reports on acute human toxocarosis are scarce with many cases presumably remaining unreported (Chen et al., 2018; Ma et al., 2018). The detection of anti-*Toxocara* antibodies in human body fluids, mainly serum, represents an alternative diagnostic technique. However, the presence of antibodies against *Toxocara* spp. is only an indicator of exposure to the parasite and does not necessarily reflect a current infection. From the end of the 1970s until today, enzyme-linked immunosorbent assays (ELISAs) detecting antibodies directed against excretory-secretory (TES) products of *T. canis* have frequently been used for serodiagnosis (De Savigny et al., 1979). A discrimination between antibodies against *T. canis* and *T. cati* is not possible as TES antigens of both species show a substantial homology at physiochemical and immunological levels (Kennedy et al., 1987). *Toxocara canis* is usually considered more pathogenic to humans; however, *T. cati* has been identified as the causative agent of some VLM, OLM and NLM cases (Fisher, 2003; Fukae et al., 2012) and human exposure due to substantial environmental contamination with *T. cati* eggs is probably high (Otero et al., 2018; Shimizu, 1993). Since the 1990s, ELISA results have additionally been confirmed by immunoblot to exclude false-positive results and cross-reactivity with pathogens other than *Toxocara* spp. (Magnaval et al., 1991). Overall, serodiagnostic data constitute the best indicators of *Toxocara* exposure in human populations.

High seroprevalence rates of more than 50% have been reported in some tropical countries (Baboolal and Rawlins, 2002; Hayashi et al., 2005; Lotsch et al., 2016; Magnaval et al., 1994), whereas lower rates have been observed in industrialized nations (Fan et al., 2013; Jarosz et al., 2010). Environmental contamination with embryonated *Toxocara* eggs constitutes a major risk and the primary route for acquiring infection (Holland, 2017). Estimated pooled contamination rates vary among continents from 13% in North and Central America, 18% in Europe, 21% in South-East Asia, 25% in South America,

27% in Africa up to 35% in Western Pacific regions. The climate in tropical and subtropical regions as well as the presence of a variety of animals in public areas and poor environmental hygiene measures seem to be favourable factors for accumulation and embryonation of eggs, respectively (Fakhri et al., 2018).

This review provides a summary and meta-analysis of *Toxocara* seroprevalence in the general, healthy population of different geographic regions in Europe as well as among different age classes. Furthermore, the development of seroprevalence rates in Europe from the 1970s until today is assessed. Finally, seroprevalence in specific risk groups and suspected cases of toxocarosis is discussed.

2. Selected literature

Pubmed and Google Scholar database literature search was mainly conducted in June and July 2019. Briefly, combinations of the terms "Europe", "*Toxocara*", "seroprevalence", "toxocarosis" and "toxocariasis" together with names of European countries [including the current member states of the European Union, the European Free Trade Association nations Iceland, Norway and Switzerland, the non-EU members Albania, North Macedonia, Montenegro and Serbia (which applied for EU membership) as well as Andorra, Armenia, Azerbaijan, Belarus, Bosnia and Herzegowina, Georgia, Liechtenstein, Moldova, Monaco and Ukraine] were used. Bibliographies of obtained articles were also considered. Original articles in English and different national languages (German, French, Russian, Italian, Spanish, Polish, etc., if available) were included.

3. Conduction of meta-analyses

For the meta-analysis of *Toxocara* seroprevalence in the general, healthy population of Europe, only studies were chosen that were based on a *Toxocara* ELISA and/or Western Blot. Studies based on skin test, microprecipitation, reversed indirect haemagglutination test (RIHA), counterimmunoelectrophoresis (CIE), indirect fluorescent antibody test (IFA) and paper radioimmunosorbent test (PRIST) were excluded to minimize variation due to differences in laboratory tests. Studies that assessed *Toxocara* prevalence among specific risk groups, e.g., patients with symptoms indicative of or associated with toxocarosis, respectively, were excluded, as were studies that only included children, which are often considered as a risk group (cf. Table 1). From case-control studies, only data referring

Table 1 Seroprevalence studies including general, healthy populations in Northern, Eastern, Western and Southern Europe.

Country	Region	Method	Age (years)	Positive/total	Prevalence	Determined risk factors	Reference
Northern Europe							
Denmark	Nationwide	ELISA, conf. WB	20–39	39/2551	1.5%	N/A	Stensvold et al. (2009) *,[a]
Estonia	Nationwide	ELISA, conf. WB	14–18, >18	195/1247	15.6%	N/A	Lassen et al. (2016)*
Iceland	Nationwide	ELISA	Adults	0/307	0.0%	N/A	Woodruff et al. (1982)*
Norway	Nationwide	ELISA	10–63	51/435	11.7%	Age (older), BMI (higher), pet ownership (cat)	Jogi et al. (2018)*
Sweden	Nationwide	ELISA	About 20	23/323	7.1%	Urbanization degree (rural)	Ljungstrom and Van Knapen (1989)*
Eastern Europe							
Azerbaijan	Baku	RIHA	0–60	283/4765	5.9%	N/A	Chobanov et al. (1990)
Bulgaria	Rousse	ELISA, conf. WB	20–59	2/50	4.0%	N/A	Kaneva et al. (2015)*
	N/A	ELISA, conf. WB	20–70	12/350	3.4%	N/A	Rainova (2008)*,[a]
Hungary	Nationwide	ELISA, conf. WB	1–17	273/1605	17.0%	N/A	Bede et al. (2008)

Continued

Table 1 Seroprevalence studies including general, healthy populations in Northern, Eastern, Western and Southern Europe.—cont'd

Country	Region	Method	Age (years)	Positive/total	Prevalence	Determined risk factors	Reference
Poland	Bialystok	ELISA, conf. WB	2–17	8/190	4.2%	N/A	Kroten et al. (2016)[a]
	Kolaczkowo	ELISA	13–17	35/242	14.5%	Pet ownership (dog, cat)	Jarosz et al. (2010)[a]
	North-Eastern	Serological test, not specified	N/A	214/1025	20.9%	N/A	Hermanowska-Szpakowicz et al. (2001)*
	Poznan	ELISA	2–12	5/63	7.9%	Pet ownership (dog), habits (geophagia)	Łużna-Lyskov (2000)
Serbia	Northern, Eastern, South-Eastern	ELISA	2–86	76/338	22.5%	Gender (male), habits (onycophagy, square/park attendance)	Gabrielli et al. (2017)*
Slovakia	Western	ELISA	0–94	1173/7678	15.3%	Gender (male), age (older)	Boldis et al. (2015)*,[a]
	Bratislava, Malacky, Stupava, Pezinok	ELISA	16–44	32/382	8.4%	N/A	Ondriska et al. (2013)*,[a]
	Eastern	ELISA	Adults	12/221	5.5%	N/A	Pavlinová et al. (2011)*
	Nationwide	ELISA	2–15, adults	33/1030	9.6%	Urbanization degree (rural)	Dubinský et al. (1995)*
	Kosice	ELISA	Adults	124/908	13.7%	Gender (female), urbanization degree (rural)	Havasiová et al. (1993)*
Slovenia	Nationwide	ELISA	Children, adults	12/189	6.3%	Age (younger)	Logar et al. (1993)*
Southern Europe							
Greece	Attica	ELISA	<14, 16–56	40/250	16.0%	Age (older)	Papavasilopoulos et al. (2018)*,[a]

Italy	Catania	ELISA	>14	23/287	8.0%	Number of siblings (>3)	Nicoletti et al. (2019)*
	Catania	WB	N/A	13/201	6.6%	N/A	Nicoletti et al. (2008)*
	Marche	ELISA	Adults	7/428	1.6%	N/A	Habluetzel et al. (2003)*
	Ancona	ELISA	0 to >50	1/89	1.1%	Age (younger)	Giacometti et al. (2000)*,[a]
	Rome	ELISA	1–18	26/214	12.1%	Urbanization degree (rural), pet ownership (dog)	Arpino et al. (1990)
	Northern	ELISA	18 to >51	84/2112	4.0%	Age (older), profession (outdoor workers)	Genchi et al. (1990)*
	Sicily	ELISA	Adults	1/79	1.2%	N/A	Di Fiore et al. (1989)
Malta	Valetta	Skin test	<10, >10	2/117	1.7%	N/A	Wiseman and Woodruff (1971)
Spain	A-Estrada	ELISA	Adults	134/463	28.6%	Education (low), urbanization degree (rural), profession (farmers), pet ownership (dog, cat)	Gonzalez-Quintela et al. (2006)*
	Canaries	ELISA	<12, >12	455/14074	3.2%	Climate (humid)	Jimenez et al. (1997)*,[a]
	Madrid, Tenerife	ELISA	Children, adults	156/1413	11.0%, 2.1% in Madrid, 15.4% in Tenerife	N/A	Fenoy et al. (1996)*
	San Sebastián	ELISA	2–16	66/546	12.1%	Age (older), socioeconomic degree (disadvantaged)	Cilla et al. (1996)[a]
	Nationwide	ELISA	1–10	1/100	1.0%	N/A	Guerra et al. (1995)[a]
	Barcelona	ELISA	3–14, adults	2/204	1.0%	N/A	Portus et al. (1989)*
	Salamanca	Dot ELISA	<10, >10	16/650	2.5%	Age (younger)	Conde Garcia et al. (1989) *,[a]

Continued

Table 1 Seroprevalence studies including general, healthy populations in Northern, Eastern, Western and Southern Europe.—cont'd

Country	Region	Method	Age (years)	Positive/total	Prevalence	Determined risk factors	Reference
Western Europe, British Isles							
Austria	Nationwide	ELISA, conf. WB	N/A	1/30	3.3%	N/A	Schneider et al. (2015)
	Nationwide	ELISA	18–60	66/1046	6.3%	Animal contact (occupational)	Poeppl et al. (2013)*
	Styria, Burgenland	ELISA, conf. WB	15–76	1/50	2.0%	N/A	Deutz et al. (2005)
	Western	ELISA, conf. WB	18	281/7656	3.7%	N/A	Auer and Aspöck (1998)*
	North-Eastern	ELISA	Adults	93/6727	1.4%	N/A	Walder and Aspöck (1987)*
Belgium	Nationwide	ELISA	Adults	23/892	2.6%	Age (older)	Cauchie et al. (1990)*
France	Franche-Comté	ELISA, conf. WB	Adults	31/113	27.4%	N/A	Bellanger et al. (2010)*
	Besancon	ELISA	0–97	30/236	12.7%	N/A	Humbert et al. (2000)*
	Toulouse, Midi-Pyrenées	N/A	Adults	21/255	8.2%	N/A	Caucanas et al. (1988)
Germany	Stuttgart	ELISA	Adults	48/1005	4.8%	Pet ownership (dog, cat, livestock), profession (farmer)	Kimmig et al. (1991)*
Ireland	N/A	ELISA	Adults	17/52	32.7%	N/A	Taylor et al. (1996)*,[a]
	Dublin, Kildare, Wicklow	ELISA	4–19	660/2129	31.0%	Gender (male), age, urbanization degree (rural), pet ownership (dog, bird), habits (geophagia)	Holland et al. (1995)
	Dublin	ELISA	<15, >15	8/137	5.8%	N/A	Taylor et al. (1988)*

Netherlands	Nationwide	ELISA	<1 to 79	419/4852	8.6%, 10.7% in 1995/96, 8.0% in 2006/07	Age (older), gender (male), habits (gardening, contact with soil), pet ownership (cat, cattle, pig)	Mughini-Gras et al. (2016)*,[a]
	Utrecht, Brabant	ELISA	4–12	114/1379	8.3%	Gender (male)	Buijs et al. (1997)[a]
	The Hague, Rotterdam	ELISA	4–6	53/694	7.6%	N/A	Buijs et al. (1994) and Buijs and Van Knapen (1994)[a]
	The Hague	ELISA	3–6	26/234	11.0%	N/A	Van Gemund et al. (1989)[a]
	N/A	ELISA	5–6	8/112	7.1%	N/A	Van Knapen et al. (1983)[a]
Switzerland	North-Western	ELISA, conf. WB	Children, 18–77	410/6601	6.3%	Gender (children male), age (older), profession (nature and forest worker)	Jeanneret (1991)*,[a]
	Zürich	ELISA	Children, 20–69	27/1000	2.7%	N/A	Jacquier et al. (1991)*
	Basel, Jura, Zürich	ELISA	Adults	39/765	5.1%	Animal contact (occupational, cattle, sheep)	Stürchler et al. (1986)
	Basel, Entlebuch	ELISA	9–11	4/138	2.9%	N/A	Tönz et al. (1983)[a]
	Nationwide	Multi-antigen ELISA	N/A	34/1998	1.7%	N/A	Speiser (1982)*
	Jura	ELISA	7–16	5/134	3.5%	Pet ownership (cat), paternal profession (father is farmer)	Stürchler and Peter (1981)[a]

Continued

Table 1 Seroprevalence studies including general, healthy populations in Northern, Eastern, Western and Southern Europe.—cont'd

Country	Region	Method	Age (years)	Positive/total	Prevalence	Determined risk factors	Reference
United Kingdom	N/A	ELISA	Adults	5/108	4.6%	N/A	Gillespie et al. (1993)*
	Bredfordshire	ELISA	3–7	19/133	14.3%	N/A	Josephs et al. (1981)[a]
	Nationwide	ELISA	19–65	24/922	2.6%	Gender (male)	Woodruff et al. (1978) and De Savigny et al. (1979)*
	Western Scotland	CIE, IFA, PRIST	Adults	4/200	2.0%	N/A	Girdwood et al. (1978)
	London	Skin test	2–10	7/170	4.1%	N/A	Borg and Woodruff (1973)
	Nationwide	Skin test	N/A	9/485	1.9%	N/A	Woodruff (1970)
	London	Skin test	<10, >10	2/156	1.3%	N/A	Wiseman and Woodruff (1970)
	London	Skin test	>10	7/329	2.1%	N/A	Woodruff et al. (1966) and Wiseman and Woodruff (1971)
	N/A	Skin test	N/A	2/55	3.6%	N/A	Woodruff and Thacker (1964)

[a]Studies included in the random-effects meta-analysis according to age groups. Abbreviations: conf. WB, confirmatory Western Blot; N/A, not available; RIHA, reversed indirect hemagglutination test; CIE, counterimmunoelectrophoresis;, IFA, indirect fluorescent antibody test; PRIST, paper radioimmunosorbent test.

Allocation of countries to geographical regions corresponds to the EuroVoc classification (cf. Fig. 1A). Asterisks indicate studies included in the meta-analysis of the general, healthy population. Literature search was conducted in June and July 2019.

No data is available for Albania, Andorra, Armenia, Belarus, Bosnia and Herzegovina, Croatia, Cyprus, Czech Republic, Finland, Latvia, Liechtenstein, Lithuania, Luxembourg, Moldova, Monaco, Montenegro, North Macedonia, Romania, Ukraine, Portugal, San Marino and Vatican City.

to the healthy control group were extracted. Random-effects meta-analysis of proportions was conducted using the package "meta", version 4.9-5 (Schwarzer, 2007) in R v. 3.5.1 (R Core Team, 2013). The inverse variance method with logit transformation and restricted maximum likelihood estimation of the between-study variance, τ^2, was applied. To assess heterogeneity between studies, Q tests were performed and the I^2 statistic was assessed, with values $\geq$50% considered heterogeneous. To evaluate possible sources of heterogeneity, subgroup analyses were performed according to geographic region of Europe (EuroVoc classification, cf. Fig. 1A; EUROVOC, 2019) and decade of sampling, assuming a common τ^2 across subgroups. Several studies did not report the period of sampling; in these cases, it was assumed that the decade of sampling corresponded to the decade of data publication. If studies reported more than one seroprevalence rate, referring to different geographic regions or data acquisition periods, these were considered separately.

Studies reporting prevalence data in specified age groups were used to assess age-related differences in *Toxocara* seroprevalence. For this purpose, study results were grouped into three categories: Those that reported seroprevalence data from (1) children and young adults up to 20 years of age, (2) persons between 21 and 50 years of age and (3) persons older than 50 years. Seroprevalence data from groups that spanned more than one of these categories (e.g. prevalence among 15- to 25-year-old persons) were excluded. Again, only studies were considered that were based on ELISA and/or Western Blot detection of antibodies, and data referring to specific risk groups were excluded. Subgroup analysis was performed as described above.

Observational prevalence studies are unlikely to suffer from publication bias, as low prevalence rates have a similar probability of being published as higher prevalence rates (Maulik et al., 2011), thus, no assessment of publication bias was performed.

4. *Toxocara* seroprevalence of the general, healthy population in Europe and subgroup analysis of decades and age

Overall, 101 studies originating from 27 countries from a period of 1964 to 2019 were found. Of these, 71 studies originating from 24 countries contained data referring to the general, healthy population (Table 1), including 25 studies from 12 countries reporting data concerning both general and healthy as well as suspected risk populations.

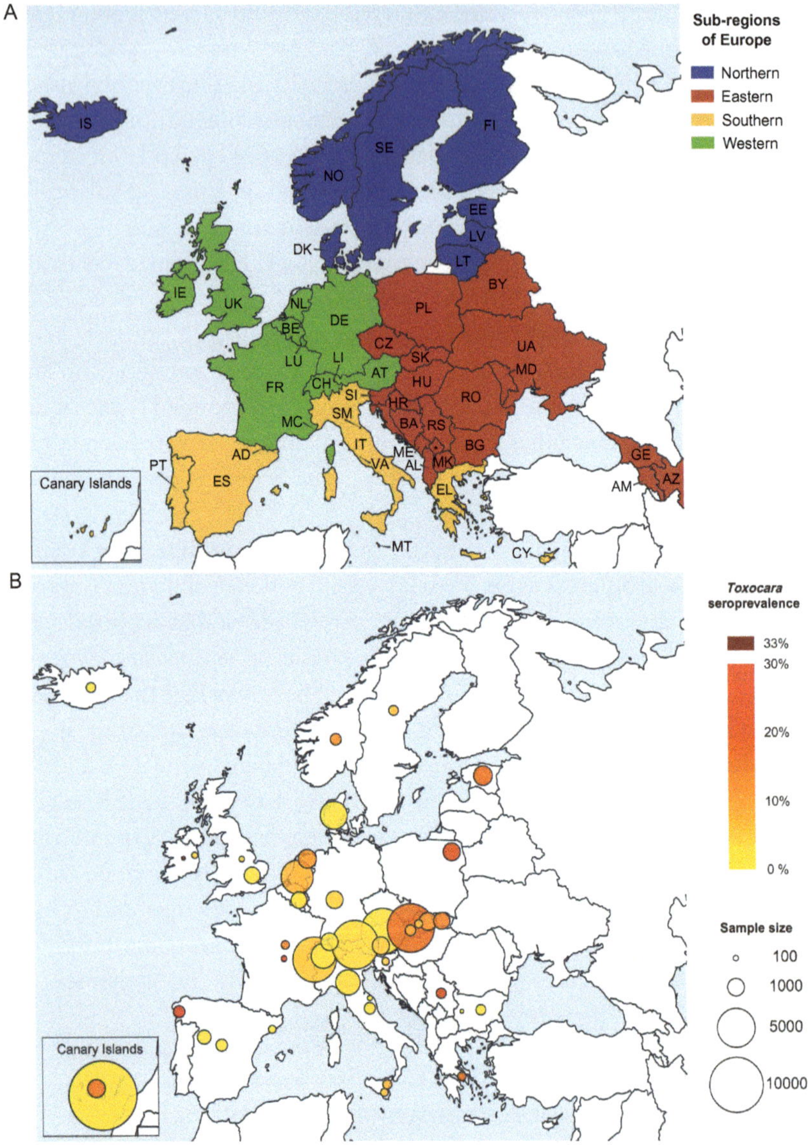

Fig. 1 (A) European sub-regions (Northern, Eastern, Southern and Western Europe) according to EuroVoc. The map of Europe was created using the package "rworldmap" (South, 2011) in R. v. 3.5.1 (R Core Team, 2013). Abbreviations: AD, Andorra; AM, Armenia; AL, Albania; AT, Austria; AZ, Azerbaijan; BA, Bosnia and Herzegovina; BE, Belgium; BG, Bulgaria; BY, Belarus; CH, Switzerland; CY, Cyprus; CZ, Czech Republic; DK, Denmark; DE, Germany; EE, Estonia; EL, Greece; ES, Spain; FI, Finland; FR, France; GE, Georgia; HR, Croatia; HU, Hungary; IE, Ireland; IS, Iceland; IT, Italy; LI, Liechtenstein; LT, Lithuania; LU, Luxembourg; LV, Latvia; MC, Monaco;

(Continued)

In total, 41 publications (marked with asterisks in Table 1) from 22 countries, reporting 43 seroprevalence rates were included in the meta-analysis to assess *Toxocara* seroprevalence in Europe by sub-region and decade. Seroprevalence rates ranged from 0.0% in Iceland (Woodruff et al., 1982) to 32.7% in Ireland (Taylor et al., 1996). Detailed seroprevalence rates in European sub-regions are pictured in Fig. 1B. The overall pooled seroprevalence of these studies was 6.2% (95% CI: 4.7–8.3%), with a significant level of heterogeneity ($I^2=98\%$; 95% CI: 98–99%; $P<0.001$).

Subgroup analysis according to decade indicated a significant increase of pooled *Toxocara* seroprevalence from 1.6% (95% CI: 0.5–4.6%) in the 1970s to 12.4% (95% CI: 6.5–22.3%) in the 2010s (test for subgroup differences: $\chi^2=17.87$, df=4, $P=0.001$; Fig. 2). This apparent increase in *Toxocara* seroprevalence, which is in contrast to several European studies that have found a decrease in environmental contamination with *Toxocara* eggs (Kleine et al., 2017; Mizgajska-Wiktor et al., 2017), may be due to a combination of factors. First, it is probable that the sensitivity of ELISA tests has increased during recent decades, e.g., due to the introduction of fluorescence- and chemiluminescence-based ELISA and Western Blot readers. Furthermore, since 2000, recombinant *Toxocara* antigen is increasingly used for ELISAs and Western Blots (Mohamad et al., 2009; Norhaida et al., 2008; Yamasaki et al., 2000). Second, the different European regions are not equally represented among the different decades, with Eastern European countries being rather underrepresented until 2000, but contributing half of the considered studies from the 2010s. While the estimated pooled seroprevalence in Northern, Southern and Western Europe was approximately equal at 5.0%, the pooled seroprevalence in Eastern Europe was 9.7% (95% CI: 5.4–16.8%; Fig. 3, individual study results shown in Supplementary Fig. 1 in the online version at https://doi.org/10.1016/bs.apar.2020.01.014). Even though this difference was not statistically significant (test for subgroup differences: $\chi^2=3.01$, df=3, $P=0.389$), the unequal

Fig. 1—Cont'd MD, Moldova; ME, Montenegro; MK, North Macedonia; MT, Malta; NL, Netherlands; NO, Norway; PL, Poland; PT, Portugal; RO, Romania; RS, Serbia; SE, Sweden; SI, Slovenia; SK, Slovakia; SM, San Marino; UA, Ukraine; UK, United Kingdom; VA, Vatican City. *States with limited recognition: Kosovo and Northern Cyprus (B) Seroprevalence rates of apparently healthy individuals in different regions of Europe. Forty-one studies from 22 countries based on *Toxocara* ELISA and/or Western Blot are represented. The map of Europe was created using the package "rworldmap" (South, 2011) in R. v. 3.5.1 (R Core Team, 2013). Colour of circles represents prevalence and size of circles represents sample size.

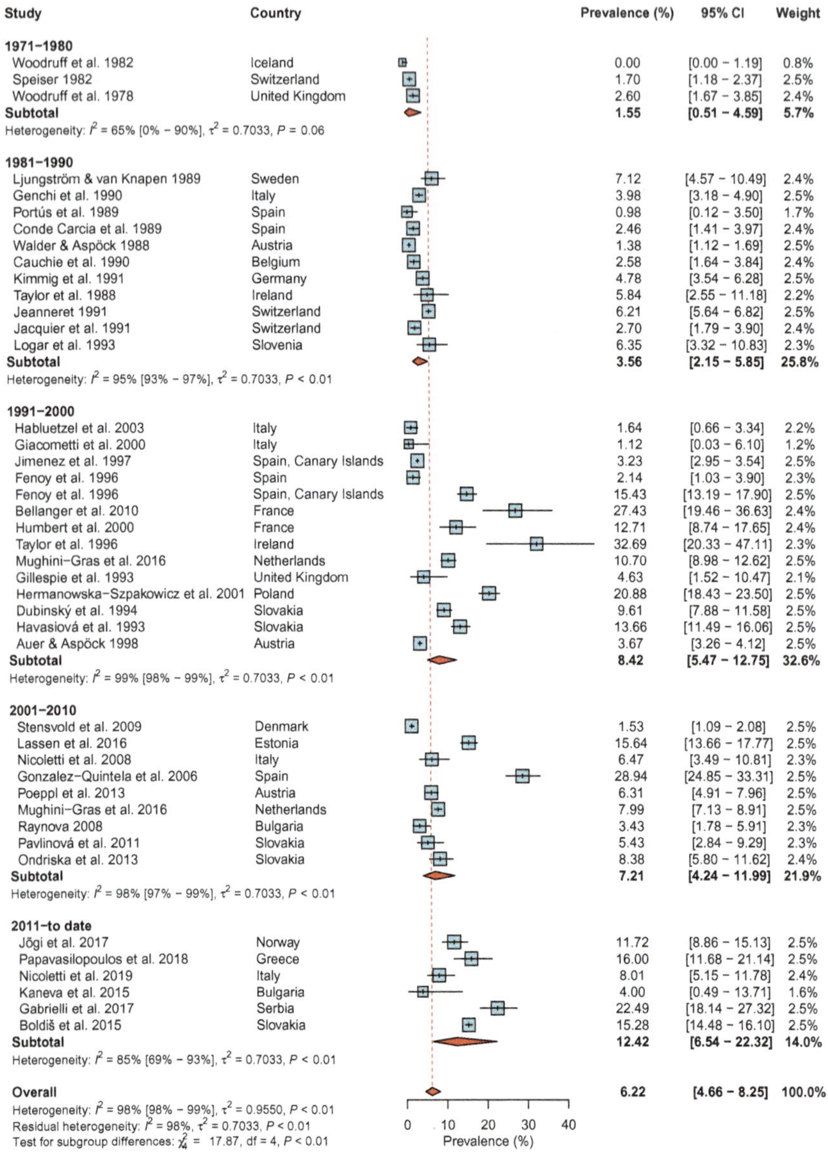

Fig. 2 Forest plot displaying the results of random-effects meta-analysis of *Toxocara* seroprevalence in the general and healthy population of Europe, with subgroup analysis according to decade of sampling. Individual study results are shown as squares, corresponding in size to the weight of the study on the pooled prevalence estimate. Error bars indicate 95% confidence intervals (CI). Pooled prevalences are shown as diamonds and the dotted vertical line indicates the overall pooled prevalence.

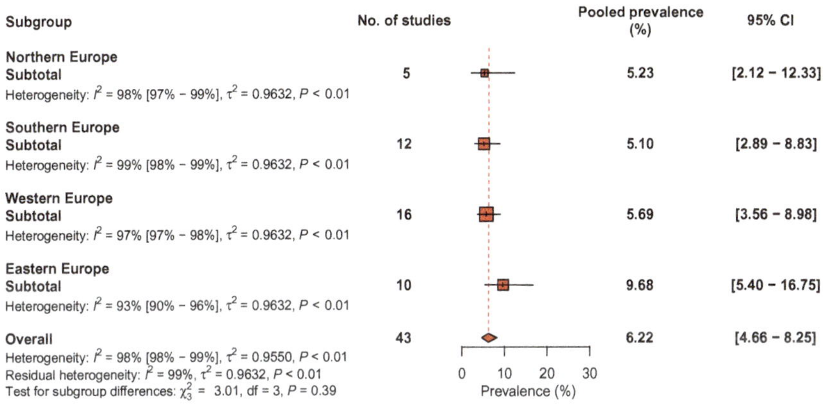

Fig. 3 Forest plot displaying the results of random-effects meta-analysis of *Toxocara* seroprevalence in the general and healthy population of Europe, with subgroup analysis according to geographic region. Squares indicate pooled prevalence estimates for each region, corresponding in size to the weight on the overall pooled prevalence. Error bars indicate 95% confidence intervals (CI). The overall pooled prevalence is indicated by the diamond and the dotted vertical line.

representation may contribute to the apparent increase in seroprevalence. Third, a closer human-animal relationship might be considered as a contributing factor. Several studies have identified pet ownership as a risk factor for *Toxocara* seropositivity (Table 1). However, direct human-pet contact is not considered an important route of infection, as embryonated *Toxocara* eggs may be present in pet fur at low quantities only, and, furthermore, are mostly not viable (Keegan and Holland, 2010; Overgaauw et al., 2009). In contrast, contact with contaminated soil is considered the main route of infection (Holland, 2017). Therefore, changes in recreational activities, especially in cities, with more time spent in public green areas accompanied by an increase of the dog and cat population in the last decades, may have had more impact. For example, according to the European Pet Food Industry Federation (FEDIAF), the European dog population has grown from approximately 75 million in 2012 to approximately 85 million in 2018, while the cat population has increased from 90 million to 104 million during this period (FEDIAF, 2012, 2018).

As small children have a lower hygienic awareness than adults, they are considered especially at risk of infection. Nevertheless, conflicting results with regard to the effect of age have been reported, with some studies identifying a younger age as a risk factor, while others observed an increasing risk of infection with increasing age (Table 1). The meta-analysis of seroprevalence according to age category included data from 22 publications on 42 separate cohorts; however, most reported seroprevalence rates referred to children and young adults (age group 0–20). Meta-analysis indicated a pooled prevalence of 7.8% (95% CI: 5.8–10.5%) among children and young adults up to 20 years of age, while this estimate dropped to 4.6% (95% CI: 2.6–8.1%) in the 21- to 50-year-old population (Fig. 4, individual study results shown in Supplementary Fig. 2 in the online version at

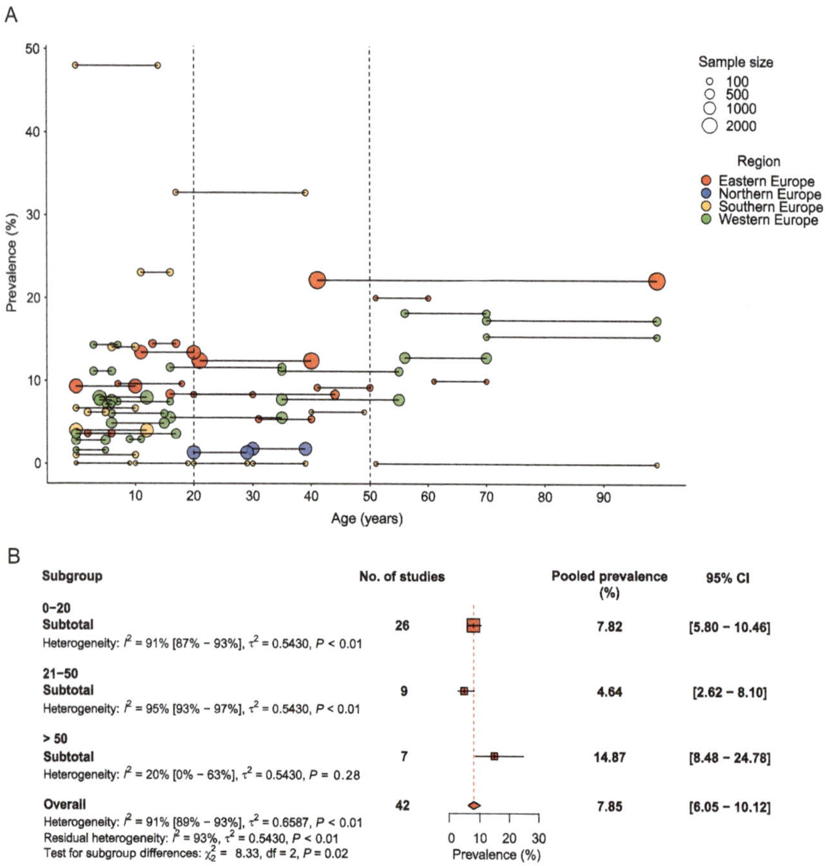

Fig. 4 (A) *Toxocara* seroprevalence in different age groups. Horizontal lines extend from the minimum to the maximum age included in each cohort, while symbol size at each end of the line indicates sample size and symbol colour indicates geographical region. Dotted vertical lines separate the age categories considered in the meta-analysis. (B) Results of random-effects meta-analysis according to age category. Squares indicate pooled prevalence estimates for each age category, corresponding in size to the weight on the overall pooled prevalence. Error bars indicate 95% confidence intervals (CI). The overall pooled prevalence is indicated by the diamond and the dotted vertical line.

https://doi.org/10.1016/bs.apar.2020.01.014). In people more than 50 years of age, a significantly higher pooled seroprevalence of 14.9% (95% CI: 8.5–24.8%) was observed (test for subgroup differences, $\chi^2 = 8.33$, df=2, $P = 0.016$). This increase in the elderly population may be due to a cumulative effect of *Toxocara* exposure over life. Upon *Toxocara* infection, residual antibodies can be detected for at least 2.7 years via ELISA and for more than 5 years via Western Blot (Fillaux and Magnaval, 2013; Jeanneret, 1991; Rubinsky-Elefant et al., 2011). In other studies, VLM-induced IgG antibody titres determined by ELISA declined at the earliest after 4 years subsequent to chemotherapeutic treatment (Cypess et al., 1977; Elefant et al., 2006).

In the following chapters, seroprevalence rates in geographical regions of Europe (Northern, Eastern, Southern and Western Europe, Fig. 1A) according to the EuroVoc classification (EUROVOC, 2019) will be reviewed in detail.

5. Northern Europe

According to the EuroVoc classification (EUROVOC, 2019), Northern Europe is comprised of eight countries, namely Denmark, Finland, Iceland, Norway, Sweden and the Baltic nations Estonia, Latvia and Lithuania (Fig. 1A). Literature search revealed five seroprevalence studies that assessed *Toxocara* exposure in apparently healthy individuals in Denmark, Estonia, Iceland, Norway and Sweden, respectively (Table 1). All of these studies were included in the meta-analysis. Described seroprevalence rates ranged from 0.0% in Iceland (Woodruff et al., 1982) up to 15.6% in Estonia (Lassen et al., 2016). Meta-analysis revealed a pooled seroprevalence of 5.2% (95% CI: 2.1–12.3%) in Northern Europe (Fig. 3).

The absence of *Toxocara*-positive individuals in Iceland is not surprising as dogs were prohibited from 1924 to 1984 in the capital city Reykjavík, harbouring one-third of the country's inhabitants. The main reason for prohibition was the high prevalence of human hydatid disease (Beard, 1973). The seroprevalence study was published in 1982, i.e., during the time of prohibition, indicating that absence of dogs resulted in a lack of *Toxocara* exposure in the human population. Furthermore, in 1986 and 1987 only 2.0% of arctic foxes were infected with *T. canis* (Skírnisson et al., 1993). Until today, strict conditions apply to the ownership of dogs in Iceland and to their import (Skírnisson et al., 2018). Unfortunately, more recent seroprevalence data is not available to see whether the de novo presence of dogs has led to an emergence of *Toxocara* exposure in the Icelandic population. A comparably low exposure to *Toxocara* was reported in Denmark, with a seroprevalence of 1.5% in apparently healthy individuals (Stensvold et al., 2009). A low environmental contamination with infective embryonated eggs due to cold temperatures might be an explanation for this low seroprevalence. Development of eggs to infective stages starts at 4 °C, with accelerated embryonation as ambient temperature increases, while temperatures below 0 °C affect the viability of embryonated eggs (Gamboa, 2005; Kleine et al., 2017; O'lorcain, 1995). Nevertheless, despite the cold climate, the risk for acquiring *Toxocara* infection in Northern European countries should not be underestimated, as seroprevalence rates of 11.7% were found in Norway and 7.1% in Sweden (Jogi et al., 2018; Ljungstrom and Van Knapen, 1989). In Estonia, human exposure to *Toxocara* is estimated as high as 15.6% (Lassen et al., 2016), corresponding to high infection rates in endemic animal hosts. Infection of stray dogs, cats and Eurasian lynx is frequent in this country, with 14.6%, 48.2% and 25.0%, respectively (Talvik et al., 2006; Valdmann et al., 2004). Nevertheless, recent studies indicated a low environmental contamination with *Toxocara* eggs of 4.2% in sandpit samples of the Estonian town Tartu, while 2.7% and 33.3% of collected dog and cat faecal samples, respectively, were positive in this country (Fakhri et al., 2018; Talvik et al., 2006).

Future studies addressing human exposure to *Toxocara* in Northern Europe are needed, as only five studies were published during the last 37 years. Future studies would aid in estimating risk factors that contribute to human *Toxocara* infection and might help to understand the underlying sources for varying seroprevalence rates in Northern European countries.

6. Eastern Europe

Eastern Europe is composed of 19 countries (EUROVOC, 2019; cf. Fig. 1A) and 15 studies originating from the general, healthy population in this region were found, including 5 studies from Slovakia, 4 from Poland, 2 from Bulgaria and one each from Azerbaijan, Hungary, Serbia and Slovenia. Reported seroprevalence rates ranged from 3.4% in Bulgaria (Raynova, 2008) to 22.5% in Serbia (Gabrielli et al., 2017). Ten studies were included in the meta-analysis, resulting in a pooled seroprevalence of 9.7% (95% CI: 5.4–16.8%) in Eastern Europe (Fig. 3).

In western parts of the world, toxocarosis is considered as one of the "neglected infections of poverty", which are mainly endemic in low-income areas. Many Eastern European countries are characterized by a low socioeconomic status, thus, their populations may be at higher risk of *Toxocara* exposure (Hotez and Gurwith, 2011). For instance, in the low-income country Serbia, which endured a long period of wars in the 1990s, 22.5% of the population has been found seropositive for *Toxocara* (Gabrielli et al., 2017). Besides a high level of human *Toxocara* exposure, a high prevalence in dogs (30.5–33.3%) and an abundant soil contamination with infective eggs of 33.5% were reported from this country (Čolović-Čalovski et al., 2014; Kulisic et al., 1998; Nikolić et al., 2008). Stray and pet animals pose a severe risk of contaminating the environment with *Toxocara* eggs, especially in rural areas (Deplazes et al., 2011; Fakhri et al., 2018; Talvik et al., 2006). Awareness regarding zoonotic parasites of pets rises within Serbia and has led to the implementation of preventive methods by the government to improve registration, vaccination and deworming of pets, paving the way for a proper control of toxocarosis (Gabrielli et al., 2017).

No *Toxocara* seroprevalence studies were found concerning other Eastern European countries with a low socioeconomic level, such as North Macedonia, Bosnia and Herzegovina, Albania and Montenegro. In Hungary, a country with a comparably high socioeconomic level, a slightly lower seroprevalence of 17.0% was observed in healthy children aged 1–17 (Bede et al., 2008).

In Poland, seroprevalence rates of 4.2%, 7.9%, 14.5% and 20.9% have been reported (Hermanowska-Szpakowicz et al., 2001; Jarosz et al., 2010; Kroten et al., 2016; Łużna-Lyskov, 2000). Similar observations were made for Slovakia with seroprevalence rates of 5.5%, 8.6%, 9.6%, 13.7% and 15.3%, respectively (Boldis et al., 2015; Dubinský et al., 1995; Havasiová et al., 1993; Ondriska et al., 2013; Pavlinová et al., 2011). A comparably low exposure (seroprevalence of 3.4% and 4.0%, respectively) was reported in healthy adults in Bulgaria (Kaneva et al., 2015; Raynova, 2008) as well as in children in Poland (4.2%, Kroten et al., 2016). In contrast to almost all other data regarding Eastern Europe, the latter studies confirmed ELISA results by Western Blot, which improves specificity. For example, ELISA-based seroprevalence of *Toxocara* was 8.6% in Bulgaria as reported by Raynova (2008), but Western Blot confirmed ELISA results in less than half of the cases. Thus, the high seroprevalence rates determined exclusively by ELISA may be overestimated due to cross-reactivity with other helminth infections, e.g., *Ascaris* spp., which are abundant in Eastern Europe (Avetisian, 2004; Fillaux and Magnaval, 2013; Kroten et al., 2016; Malafiej and Spiewak, 2001; Nikolić et al., 1998; Spinelli et al., 2006).

Overall, the pooled seroprevalence in general and healthy populations of Eastern Europe was not statistically different from those of other European regions. While human *Toxocara* infections seem to be hyperendemic in some Eastern European countries, the seropositivity rates reported from countries with higher socioeconomic status are comparable to other geographical regions of Europe. To gain a more holistic picture of the situation in Eastern Europe, the gap concerning studies from low-income areas needs to be filled by future studies.

7. Southern Europe

According to the EuroVoc classification (EUROVOC, 2019), Cyprus, Greece, Italy, Malta, Portugal, San Marino, Spain and Vatican City are part of Southern Europe. From four of these eight countries, seroprevalence data on the general, healthy population were available. While Italy and Spain contributed seven studies each and were thus well represented, only one study each was available from Greece and Malta. Eleven of these 16 studies were included in the meta-analysis, resulting in an estimated pooled seroprevalence of 5.1% (95% CI: 2.9–8.8%) in Southern Europe (Fig. 3).

In Spanish cities, a low level of human exposure to *Toxocara* was found, with seroprevalence rates of 1.0% in Barcelona, 2.1% in Madrid and 2.5% in Salamanca (Conde Garcia et al., 1989; Fenoy et al., 1996; Portus et al., 1989). In contrast, a seroprevalence of 12.1% was reported in a study from San Sebastián (Cilla et al., 1996). However, this study aimed to elucidate the difference in exposure of severely disadvantaged compared to middle-class children, displaying a seroprevalence of 57.1% and 3.1%, respectively. Furthermore, *Toxocara* seroprevalence in the town A Estrada near Santiago de Compostela was as high as 28.6%, which was attributed to a high frequency of risk factors such as rural environment, farming habitat and pet ownership in this population (Gonzalez-Quintela et al., 2006). High seroprevalence rates were also found on the Canary Islands, a geographically distinct archipelago belonging to Spain. Average exposure to *Toxocara* on the whole archipelago was 3.2%, with highest values of 6.7% in Northern Tenerife and 6.8% on the neighbouring island La Gomera (Jimenez et al., 1997). Even higher values were recorded by Fenoy et al. (1996), who observed a seroprevalence of 15.4% in the city of Santa Cruz located in the Northern area of Tenerife. Overall, seroprevalence rates on the Canary Islands correlated with the De Martonne humidity-aridity index (Jimenez et al., 1997). Moist soil in combination with warm temperatures facilitates the development, long-term survival and infectivity of *T. canis* eggs (Gamboa, 2005; Gaspard et al., 1997). Thus, higher humidity was accompanied by higher *Toxocara* seroprevalence rates (Jimenez et al., 1997).

Geographical differences in seroprevalence rates were also observed in Italy, a country extending from the Alps to the middle of the Mediterranean Sea. From north to south, the Italian climate varies from cold conditions without dry seasons to temperate conditions with dry and hot summers (Beck et al., 2018). In the north and northeast of Italy, human *Toxocara* exposure of 1.1%, 1.6%, and 4.0% was reported (Genchi et al., 1990; Giacometti et al., 2000; Habluetzel et al., 2003), whereas higher seroprevalence rates of 6.6%, 8.0% and 12.1% were observed in southern and southwestern regions (Arpino et al., 1990; Nicoletti et al., 2008, 2019). Only one study from Sicily reported a low seroprevalence of 1.2%. However, this study was conducted in 1989 with a comparably small sample size, whereas more recent studies, which were partly based on the highly sensitive Western Blot technique, reported higher values of 6.6% and 8.0% (Nicoletti et al., 2008, 2019). Overall, these data indicate a gradient in seroprevalence from low values in northern and central Italy to high values in the south, mirroring the gradient in socioeconomic status, which is lower in southern areas (Banca d'Italia, 2018). A similar picture was found regarding environmental contamination with *Toxocara* eggs, which varied from 5.0% and 33.6% in rural and urban soil samples of northern Italy to 54.5% and 63.7% in public playgrounds in central Italy (Genchi et al., 2007; Giacometti et al., 1999, 2000; Habluetzel et al., 2003).

The island nation Malta lies in close proximity to southern Italy. Nevertheless, a comparably low seroprevalence of 1.7% was reported from this country, probably due to the considerably less sensitive detection method of skin testing that was employed at the time (Wiseman and Woodruff, 1971). In addition to the high seroprevalence rates in southern Italy, a study conducted in Greece revealed an even higher *Toxocara* seroprevalence of 16.0% (Papavasilopoulos et al., 2018). In this study, an especially high level of exposure of 48.0% was found in children. The same study reported a soil contamination rate with *Toxocara* eggs of 17.2% of sampled public places in the region of Athens. However, further data, e.g., on northern parts of Greece, are not available.

Overall, human *Toxocara* seroprevalence is well studied in southern parts of Europe, especially in Spain and Italy, leading to a better understanding of relevant risk factors for *Toxocara* exposure.

8. Western Europe

Western Europe is composed of 12 countries as demonstrated in Fig. 1A. In total, 36 seroprevalence studies on the general, healthy population of 8 of these countries were found. Eleven studies were conducted in the United Kingdom (UK), followed by the Netherlands and Switzerland with 6 studies each and Austria with 5 seroprevalence studies. Three studies each were available for France and Ireland and 1 study each was found for Belgium and Germany. Of these 36 seroprevalence studies, 16 were included in the meta-analysis, resulting in an estimated pooled prevalence of 5.7% (95% CI: 3.6–9.0%, Fig. 3) in Western Europe, with a pooled estimate of 7.4% for the British Isles and 5.3% for continental Western Europe (data not shown).

Most of the early seroprevalence studies from the UK should be treated with caution, as they were performed before the introduction of highly sensitive antibody detection methods based on TES antigens (De Savigny et al., 1979) and utilized other, less sensitive techniques. One of the earliest established methods for detection of *Toxocara* exposure was the skin test, introduced by Woodruff and Thacker (1964). This test is based on a local reaction to subcutaneously injected antigens of adult helminths. Within 20 min, swelling of the injection site and erythema can be observed in individuals with previous exposure to *Toxocara*. However, this method is considerably less sensitive compared to serodiagnostic methods. Prevalence rates obtained with the skin test in the UK in the 1960s and 1970s ranged from 1.3% to 4.1% (Borg and Woodruff, 1973; Wiseman and Woodruff, 1970, 1971; Woodruff, 1970; Woodruff and Thacker, 1964; Woodruff et al., 1966), whereas seroprevalence rates assessed via ELISA from the late 1970s until the early 1990s varied from 2.6% to 14.3% (Gillespie et al., 1993; Josephs et al., 1981; Woodruff et al., 1978). Unfortunately, more recent data on *Toxocara* exposure in the UK is not available.

Europe's highest *Toxocara* seroprevalence rates of 32.7% and 31.0% were measured in Ireland (Holland et al., 1995; Taylor et al., 1988, 1996). It is worth noting that the prevalence of 32.7% was based on a small population of women only, while the seroprevalence rate of 31.0% was observed in a population of children, which are often reported to be especially at risk of acquiring *Toxocara* infection (Table 1). Nevertheless, exposure to *Toxocara* seems to vary in Ireland, as Taylor et al. (1988) reported a seroprevalence of only 5.8% in a population composed of children and adults.

One of the factors contributing to high *Toxocara* seroprevalence rates on the British Isles may be a high abundance of pet dogs. Holland et al. (1995) reported that 59.0% of the examined Irish population possessed a dog. In contrast, only 18.2–35.2% of study participants in other Western European seroprevalence studies owned a dog (Buijs et al., 1994; Jogi et al., 2018; Mughini-Gras et al., 2016; Poeppl et al., 2013; Tönz et al., 1983). In the UK, dog ownership was almost as common as in Ireland with 50.4% (Josephs et al., 1981).

France is another Western European country with high seroprevalence rates. Exposure to *Toxocara* ranged from 8.2% in southern and 12.7% to 27.4% in eastern regions (Bellanger et al., 2010; Caucanas et al., 1988; Humbert et al., 2000). In concordance, the level of environmental contamination in public parks of Toulouse amounted to 37.5% (Ferre and Dorchies, 2000), one of the highest contamination rates reported in Europe (Fakhri et al., 2018). In addition, *Toxocara* eggs were detected in up to 48.6% of cat, 11.6% of fox and 33.3% of dog faeces collected from northeastern France (Poulle et al., 2017; Umhang et al., 2017).

Reported human *Toxocara* seroprevalence in the Netherlands was generally lower compared to Ireland and France. Dutch seroprevalence rates showed a high level of consistency, ranging from 7.1% to 11.0% (Buijs and Van Knapen, 1994; Buijs et al., 1994, 1997; Mughini-Gras et al., 2016; Van Gemund et al., 1989; Van Knapen et al., 1983). One study assessed *Toxocara* seroprevalence and associated risk factors during two periods, 1995/96 and 2006/07, reporting a decrease from 10.7% to 8.0% (Mughini-Gras et al., 2016). The authors postulated that this decrease might have been due to improved hygiene and that various factors contribute to seropositivity, such as habits involving contact with soil as well as ownership of a definitive host.

Austria, Switzerland, Germany and Belgium belong to the countries with the lowest *Toxocara* seroprevalence rates in Western Europe. Austria is particularly well studied, as numerous seroprevalence studies with large sample sizes were conducted in this country. Seropositivity was rather low with seroprevalence rates ranging from 1.4% to 6.3% (Auer and Aspöck, 1998; Deutz et al., 2005; Poeppl et al., 2013; Schneider et al., 2015; Walder and Aspöck, 1987). The maximum value of 6.3% may be explained by the fact that the screened population in this study was predominantly composed of males and several studies have identified male gender as a risk factor for *Toxocara* exposure (Table 1). Despite the low seroprevalence rates, environmental contamination and infection of definitive hosts poses a severe risk for acquiring *Toxocara* infection in Austria. Infection rates of 0.6–18.0% for dogs, 9.8–60.0% for cats and 47.0% for red foxes have been reported (Beugnet et al., 2014; Hinaidy, 1971, 1976; Hinney et al., 2017; Kasiecka, 1982; Lassning, 1996; Suchentrunk and Sattmann, 1994; Supperer and Hinaidy, 1986), while up to 14.0% of soil and sand samples in different regions of Austria contained *Toxocara* eggs of different developmental stages (Auer, 2003; Auer and Aspöck, 1995, 2004; Kutzer et al., 1995; Pfeiffer, 1983).

In the neighbouring country of Switzerland, seroprevalence rates in humans were almost the same as in Austria, ranging from 1.7% to 6.3% (Jacquier et al., 1991; Jeanneret, 1991; Speiser, 1982; Stürchler and Peter, 1981; Stürchler et al., 1986; Tönz et al., 1983). Furthermore, similar infection rates of 1.2–17.0% for dogs, 18.5% for cats and 44.0% for red foxes were observed as in Austria (Deplazes et al., 1995; Hauser et al., 2015; Reperant et al., 2007; Sager et al., 2006; Zottler et al., 2019). In both countries, mostly alpine and montane climatic conditions prevail, potentially limiting larval development and survival of *Toxocara* in the environment and thus human exposure.

Only limited data are available regarding Germany and Belgium. In the city of Stuttgart in Southern Germany, human exposure to *Toxocara* was determined at 4.8% (Kimmig et al., 1991). Unfortunately, although Germany constitutes the country with the largest population in Europe (apart from Russia), further seroprevalence studies are not available. Regarding environmental contamination, 23.2% of public playgrounds were contaminated with *Toxocara* eggs in the Northern German city of Hanover in 2010/2011 (Kleine et al., 2017). This represents an almost 50% reduction in environmental contamination as compared to a study conducted in 1985 in the same city (Horn et al., 1990). In Belgium, a similar human seroprevalence of 2.6% and environmental contamination rate of 25.0% have been reported (Cauchie et al., 1990).

In summary, high seroprevalence rates are not only restricted to Eastern and Southern European countries but were also observed in Western European nations. Especially Ireland and France seem to have had a high *Toxocara* exposure of humans in the past, which should be re-examined in future seroprevalence studies. Nevertheless, pooled seroprevalence of continental Western Europe and the British Isles did not differ significantly from other European regions.

9. *Toxocara* seroprevalence in populations suspected of infection and other risk groups

Besides studies that report the seroprevalence of *Toxocara* in apparently healthy general populations, a large number of studies has evaluated seroprevalence rates in populations that are at risk or under suspicion of *Toxocara* infection. For instance, case-control studies often aim to elucidate *Toxocara* seroprevalence in populations suffering from different clinical signs indicative of or associated with toxocarosis, e.g. rash, dermatitis, uveitis, chronic cough, eosinophilia or elevated IgE levels, in comparison to healthy control groups. Literature search resulted in 55 studies from 20 countries yielding data on populations suspected of *Toxocara* infection and/or other risk groups (Table 2). Of these, 25 studies from 12 countries contained data concerning both general and healthy as well as suspected risk populations.

It is not surprising that populations suffering from *Toxocara*-associated symptoms have higher seroprevalence rates (cf. Table 2) compared to the general, healthy population. For example, a seroprevalence of 53.3% has been found in patients displaying eosinophilia (Magnaval et al., 1991). Even lower eosinophilia-related seroprevalence rates, such as 5.3% and 8.1%, were two times or even seven times higher compared to *Toxocara* exposure in the corresponding healthy control groups, respectively (Cauchie et al., 1990; Giacometti et al., 2000). Similar to other helminthoses as well as allergic reactions, eosinophilia seems to be an important indicator of *Toxocara* infection. Another factor associated with *Toxocara* exposure may be asthma, as elevated seroprevalence rates have been found in asthmatic patients compared to healthy populations (Auer and Aspöck, 2004; Fenoy et al., 1997; Girdwood et al., 1978) and the highest seroprevalence of 68.4% was observed in a group of asthmatic children (Cobzaru et al., 2012). A recent meta-analysis stated that *Toxocara* seropositivity is associated with childhood asthma (Aghaei et al., 2018). However, 9 of the 17 studies included in the analysis reported no direct relation between *Toxocara* exposure and asthma, indicating that the role of *Toxocara* infection in asthma and vice versa is still debated. Furthermore, populations suffering from ocular *larva migrans* or other ophthalmic symptoms showed comparably high seroprevalence rates. For instance, seroprevalence of individuals exhibiting ocular lesions was increased almost by the factor 8 compared to healthy individuals within one study (15.3% vs. 2.0%) (Girdwood et al., 1978).

Table 2 Seroprevalence studies including risk groups or symptoms of a potential *Toxocara* infection.

Country	Region	Method	Age (years)	Risk group	Positive/ total	Prevalence	Reference
Austria	Nationwide	ELISA, conf. WB	0–90	Suspected VLM	681/5301	12.9%	Schneider and Auer (2016)
	Nationwide	ELISA, conf. WB	Adults	Farmers	390/1034	37.7%	H. Auer, unpublished results
	Styria, Burgenland	ELISA, conf. WB	15–76	Farmers	67/152	44.1%	Deutz et al. (2005) and Deutz et al. (1996)
				Slaughterhouse workers	37/141	25.2%	
				Hunters	22/149	14.8%	
				Veterinarians	37/137	27.0%	
	Vienna	ELISA, conf. WB	Adults	Employees of the zoological garden	13/60	21.6%	Juncker-Voss et al. (2004)
	Vienna, Burgenland	ELISA, conf. WB	Adults	Canal workers	27/387	7.0%	Auer and Aspöck (2004)
				Dog owners	10/60	16.7%	
				Pregnant women	35/406	8.6%	
				Asthmatics	25/297	8.4%	
				Hunters	70/891	7.9%	
				Patients, not specified	96/525	18.3%	
	Vienna	ELISA, conf. WB	0 to >70	Bronchial hyperreactivity	14/140	10.0%	Zacharasiewicz et al. (2000)
				Atopic patients	6/84	7.1%	
	North-Eastern	ELISA	Adults	Suspected helminthosis	9/736	1.2%	Walder and Aspöck (1987)
				Uveitis	2/150	1.3%	
				Eosinophilia, pica, elevated IgE	16/71	22.5%	

Belgium	Nationwide	ELISA	Adults	International travellers	190/3436	5.5%	Van Den Broucke et al. (2015)
	Nationwide	ELISA	Children, Adults	Paediatrics	1/68	2.6%	Cauchie et al. (1990)
				Neurology	2/99	2.0%	
				Hospital patients	29/789	3.7%	
				Eosinophilia	19/358	5.3%	
Bulgaria	Nationwide	ELISA, conf. WB	N/A	Eosinophilia, allergy	90/466	19.3%	Rainova et al. (2018)
	Rousse	ELISA	0–80	Allergy	4/261	1.5%	Kaneva et al. (2015)
Croatia	Zagreb	ELISA, conf. WB	3–18	Peripheral eosinophilia	44/142	31.0%	Sviben et al. (2009)
Czech Republic	N/A	ELISA	N/A	Multiple sclerosis	1/62	1.6%	Posova et al. (2017)
				Clinically isolated syndrome	0/220	0.0%	
Estonia	Nationwide	ELISA, conf. WB	14–18, >18	Veterinarians	15/158	9.5%	Lassen et al. (2016)
				Animal caretakers	108/375	28.8%	
				Hunters	25/144	17.4%	
France	Franche-Comté	ELISA, conf. WB	Adults	Urticaria, pruritus	52/113	46.0%	Bellanger et al. (2010)
	Besancon	ELISA	N/A	Urticaria	25/128	19.5%	Humbert et al. (2000)
				Pruritus	8/52	15.4%	
				Prurigo	8/21	38.1%	
				Eczema	13/72	18.6%	
				Atopic dermatitis	9/108	8.3%	
	Loire Atlantique, Maine et Loire	ELISA, conf. WB	1–98	Eosinophilia	404/1836	22.0%	Gueglio et al. (1994)
	N/A	ELISA, conf. WB	N/A	Other helminthosis	22/118	18.6%	Magnaval et al. (1991)
				Eosinophilia	66/105	53.3%	

Continued

Table 2 Seroprevalence studies including risk groups or symptoms of a potential *Toxocara* infection.—cont'd

Country	Region	Method	Age (years)	Risk group	Positive/total	Prevalence	Reference
Germany	Stuttgart	ELISA	Adults	Farmers	19/84	22.6%	Kimmig et al. (1991)
	Nationwide	Microprecipitation	N/A	Ophthalmology	111/1511	7.3%	Lamina (1980)
				Internal medicine	152/1632	9.3%	
				Paediatrics	28/281	9.9%	
				Neurology	19/329	5.7%	
				Tropical medicine	57/445	12.8%	
				Laboratory medicine	9/134	6.7%	
				Resident doctors	33/320	10.3%	
Greece	Northern	ELISA	0–15	Different clinical signs	21/511	4.1%	Theodoridis et al. (2001)
Hungary	Nationwide	ELISA, conf. WB	2–17	Chronic cough	136/425	32.0%	Bede et al. (2008)
Ireland	County Dublin	ELISA	N/A	Family members of children with toxocarosis	73/140	52.1%	Holland et al. (1991)
Italy	Catania	ELISA	N/A	Multiple sclerosis	12/132	9.1%	Cicero et al. (2019)
	N/A	ELISA, conf. WB	2–72	Chronic recurrent symptoms	240/753	31.8%	Qualizza et al. (2011)
	Catania	WB	N/A	Epilepsy	38/231	16.4%	Nicoletti et al. (2008)
	Ancona	ELISA	0 to >50	Eosinophilia, elevated IgE, rash	6/74	8.1%	Giacometti et al. (2000)
	Rome	ELISA	1–17	Seizures	20/91	22.0%	Arpino et al. (1990)
	Northern	ELISA	Adults	Strongyloidosis	7/76	9.2%	Genchi et al. (1990)
				Epilepsy	9/207	4.4%	
				Mentally retarded	18/142	12.7%	

Netherlands	Nationwide	ELISA	0 to >70	Suspected toxocarosis	234/2838	8.2%	Pinelli et al. (2011)
Poland	Nationwide	ELISA, conf. WB	<10 to >50	Suspected toxocarosis	366/1681	21.8%	Rudzińska et al. (2017)
	Eastern and Southern	ELISA	Adults	Outdoor forest worker	28/216	13.0%	Żukiewicz-Sobczak et al. (2014)
	North-Eastern	ELISA	0–18	Suspected helminthosis	20/120	16.7%	Żukiewicz et al. (2011)
	Lublin	ELISA	0 to >45	Suspected OLM, eosinophilia	61/151	40.4%	Zwolinski (2000)
Romania	Iasi	ELISA (IgG and IgE)	5–16	Asthma	52/76	68.4%	Cobzaru et al. (2012)
				Rhinitis, dermatitis, rhinosinusitis	12/88	13.6%	
Slovakia	Kosice	ELISA	2–15, adults	Suspected toxocarosis	741/2703	27.4%	Havasiová et al. (1993)
Slovenia	N/A	ELISA, conf. WB	3–82	Suspected OLM	67/239	28.0%	Logar et al. (2004)
	Nationwide	ELISA	3–60	Suspected VLM, suspected OLM	76/319	23.8%	Logar et al. (1993)
Spain	N/A	ELISA	Children, adults	Suspected VLM, eosinophilia, intestinal parasites, asthma	124/407	30.5%	Fenoy et al. (1997)
	Barcelona	ELISA	3–14, adults	Eosinophilia	14/99	14.1%	Portus et al. (1989)
				Ocular complaints	7/116	6.0%	
				Hydatidosis	3/97	3.1%	
				Helminthosis	2/34	5.9%	
				Other symptoms not associated with toxocarosis	9/468	1.9%	

Continued

Table 2 Seroprevalence studies including risk groups or symptoms of a potential *Toxocara* infection.—cont'd

Country	Region	Method	Age (years)	Risk group	Positive/ total	Prevalence	Reference
Sweden	Nationwide	ELISA	>5 to >50	Eosinophilia, ocular disorder	43/175	24.6%	Ljungstrom and Van Knapen (1989)
United Kingdom	N/A	ELISA	N/A	Other helminthosis	2/46	4.3%	Gillespie et al. (1993)
	N/A	ELISA	Adults	Dog exposed personnel in animal husbandry and pharmaceutical research	3/66	4.5%	Slovak (1984)
	Scotland, Ireland, England, Wales	ELISA	<14, >14	Eosinophilia	65/263	24.7%	Ree et al. (1984)
				Endopthalmis	102/497	20.5%	
				Other morbid conditions	104/643	16.2%	
	Bretford, Brentwood, Milton Keynes	ELISA	Adults	Cat breeders and exhibitors	1/67	1.5%	Woodruff et al. (1982)
	N/A	ELISA	Adults	Dog breeders and exhibitors	16/102	15.7%	Woodruff et al. (1978)
	Western Scotland	CIE, IFA, PRIST	N/A	Ocular lesion	22/144	15.3%	Girdwood et al. (1978)
				Eosinophilia	3/19	15.8%	
				Hay fever, asthma, eczema	4/28	14.3%	
				Other helminthosis	0/16	0.0%	
	N/A	Fluorescent antibody test	Adults	Breeding kennel and breeding school	2/34	5.9%	Jacobs et al. (1977)

	Nationwide	Skin test	N/A	Other helminthosis	5/207	2.4%	Woodruff (1970)
				Poliomyelitis	28/191	14.6%	
	London	Skin test	<10, >10	Other helminthosis	3/122	2.5%	Wiseman and Woodruff (1970)
				Suspected toxocarosis	26/237	11.0%	
	Nationwide	Skin test	0 to >31	Toxoplasmosis	2/38	5.3%	Wiseman et al. (1970)
				Patients, not specified	8/67	11.9%	
	N/A	Skin test	N/A	Suspected toxocarosis	24/189	12.9%	Wiseman and Woodruff (1968)
	N/A	Skin test	N/A	Poliomyelitis	26/191	13.6%	Woodruff et al. (1966)
				Epilepsy	26/349	7.5%	
	N/A	Skin test	N/A	Eeosinophilia, choroidoretinitis, allergy	11/35	31.4%	Woodruff and Thacker (1964)
				Other helminthosis	2/85	2.4%	

Literature search was conducted in June and July 2019. Abbreviations: conf. WB, confirmatory Western Blot; N/A, not available; VLM, visceral larva migrans; OLM, ocular larva migrans.
No data is available for Albania, Andorra, Armenia, Azerbaijan, Belarus, Bosnia and Herzegovina, Cyprus, Denmark, Finland, Georgia, Latvia, Liechtenstein, Lithuania, Luxembourg, Malta, Moldova, Monaco, Montenegro, North Macedonia, Norway, Portugal, San Marino, Serbia, Switzerland, Ukraine and Vatican City.

Overall, attributing specific clinical symptoms to *Toxocara* infection is difficult. Seroprevalence data of populations suspected of infection clearly show that *Toxocara* causes a variety of clinical symptoms. However, seroprevalence in patients with these symptoms was mostly less than 50%, indicating that observed symptoms are due to other helminth infections or non-parasitic diseases in the majority of cases.

Apart from studies involving disease manifestations, seroprevalence rates in populations bearing a high risk for *Toxocara* infection have frequently been addressed. Some professions, mostly involving contact to animals and soil, clearly lead to higher *Toxocara* exposure. For instance, farmers display seroprevalence rates ranging from 22.6% to 44.1%, which is up to 22 times higher compared to the general, healthy population (H. Auer, unpublished results; Deutz et al., 2005; Kimmig et al., 1991). These high seroprevalence rates presumably originate from a combination of several risk factors. Farmers reside in rural areas, where seroprevalence rates and environmental contamination are often higher than in urban areas (Table 1), probably due to the overlap of wild animal habitats with those of livestock and companion animals. Furthermore, farm cats may significantly contribute to this contamination as they are often used in farm's pest control as predators for small mammals, thereby acquiring infection via paratenic hosts (Deutz et al., 2005; Kimmig et al., 1991; Nijsse et al., 2016). In addition, specific working procedures such as tilling fields may result in an increased contact of farmers with contaminated soil.

The abundance of infected animals and contact to contaminated faeces or soil is not only a risk factor for farmers but also affects other occupational groups. In Austria, the *Toxocara* seroprevalence in apparently healthy individuals was 2.0%, while 27.0% of veterinarians and 14.8% of hunters were seropositive for *Toxocara* spp. (Deutz et al., 2005). Especially hunters exhibit frequent contact with contaminated forest soil due to infected wild carnivores, which may contribute to an elevated seroprevalence. In addition, slaughterhouse employees seem to be a risk group for *Toxocara* exposure with a seroprevalence of 25.2%. However, it should be mentioned that 25.0% of this group were part time farmers (Deutz et al., 2005).

Juncker-Voss et al. (2004) and Lassen et al. (2016) reported a higher risk for *Toxocara* exposure in populations of animal caretakers in Austria and Estonia. Furthermore, contact to animals and ownership of dogs, cats or both have also been identified as risk factors in general and healthy populations (Table 1). However, the causality of this relationship might rather be based on an increased contamination of pet owners' gardens than direct contact with pets, as the transmission of embryonated eggs from the hairy coat is usually not considered a major route of human infection (Keegan and Holland, 2010; Overgaauw et al., 2009). Thus, gardening may also contribute to *Toxocara* exposure (Mughini-Gras et al., 2016).

Overall, higher *Toxocara* exposure in occupational groups exposed to contaminated soil and faeces of infected animals has frequently been found in Europe. Especially in rural areas, control measures need to be improved to reduce environmental contamination with *Toxocara* eggs. Recent studies have shown that deworming frequencies of dogs and cats in Europe are considerably lower than recommended by the European Scientific Counsel Companion Animal Parasites (ESCCAP) (McNamara et al., 2018; Strube et al., 2019). Based on an individual risk assessment for each pet, ESCCAP recommends faecal examinations or deworming of cats and dogs 2–12 times per year to reduce zoonotic risk (ESCCAP, 2017).

10. Conclusions

With a pooled seroprevalence of 6.2% in the general, healthy population, human *Toxocara* infection is widespread in Europe. Single studies have reported seroprevalence rates as high as 32.7% in general and healthy populations, 68.4% in populations suspected of infection and 44.1% in certain risk groups—values which are comparable to subtropical and tropical regions. Thus, awareness on the zoonotic potential of *Toxocara* should be raised in European countries. Reasons for low deworming frequencies of pets include insufficient knowledge of pet owners, highlighting the importance of counselling by veterinarians and public health institutions. *Toxocara* infections may impact pet health and, furthermore, pose a serious problem for public health as eggs are shed into the environment, where they represent the main source of human infection. The analysed data from the literature suggest an increase in the risk of acquiring *Toxocara* infection in Europe, possibly due to a change in recreational activities over recent decades with more time spent in public green areas and an increasing number of pet animals. Due to the close link between animal infection and human *Toxocara* exposure, a "One Health" approach for the prevention of *Toxocara* infection in both humans and animals is needed. To prevent environmental contamination by companion animals, regular faecal examinations or deworming of dogs and cats according to individual risk group assignment is recommended. In addition, pet owners should be encouraged to remove their animals' faeces. Preventing contamination of children's playgrounds is not only the responsibility of pet owners by preventing access of their animals to these areas, but also of the authorities, e.g., by fencing of playgrounds and/or the periodic change of sand in sand pits or dispensing of sand pits in general. However, environmental contamination by wild carnivores as well as stray dogs and cats is difficult to prevent, but also the elevated *Toxocara* exposure of high-risk groups, such as farmers, remains challenging.

References

Aghaei, S., Riahi, S.M., Rostami, A., Mohammadzadeh, I., Javanian, M., Tohidi, E., Foroutan, M., Esmaeili Dooki, M., 2018. *Toxocara* spp. infection and risk of childhood asthma: a systematic review and meta-analysis. Acta Trop. 182, 298–304.

Arpino, C., Gattinara, G.C., Piergili, D., Curatolo, P., 1990. *Toxocara* infection and epilepsy in children: a case-control study. Epilepsia 31, 33–36.

Auer, H., 2003. *Toxocara*-Infestationen und Toxokarose in Mitteleuropa: Eine Übersicht. In: Infektiologie—Aktuelle Aspekte Jahrbuch 2003/2004. Springer-Verlag, New York, USA, pp. 77–92.

Auer, H., Aspöck, H., 1995. Toxokarose in Österreich-Epidemiologie, Diagnostik und Therapie. Mitt. Österr. Ges. Tropenmed. Parasitol. 17, 61–70.

Auer, H., Aspöck, H., 1998. Toxokarose-Forschung in Österreich—Ergebnisse, Probleme, Herausforderungen. Tropenmed. Parasitol. 20, 17–28.

Auer, H., Aspöck, H., 2004. Nosologie und Epidemiologie der Toxokarose des Menschen-die aktuelle Situation in Österreich. Wien. Klin. Wochenschr. 116, 7–18.

Avetisian, L.M., 2004. Epidemiological surveillance of parasitic diseases in the republic of Armenia. Med. Parazitol. (Mosk) 1, 21–24.

Baboolal, S., Rawlins, S.C., 2002. Seroprevalence of toxocariasis in schoolchildren in Trinidad. Trans. R. Soc. Trop. Med. Hyg. 96, 139–143.

Banca d'Italia, 2018. Survey on Italian Household Income and Wealth, 2016. https://www.bancaditalia.it/pubblicazioni/indagine-famiglie/bil-fam2016/index.html. Accessed 23 August 2019.

Beard, T.C., 1973. The elimination of echinococcosis from Iceland. Bull. World Health Organ. 48, 653–660.

Beaver, P.C., Snyder, C.H., Carrera, G.M., Dent, J.H., Lafferty, J.W., 1952. Chronic eosinophilia due to visceral larva migrans; report of three cases. Pediatrics 9, 7–19.

Beck, H.E., Zimmermann, N.E., Mcvicar, T.R., Vergopolan, N., Berg, A., Wood, E.F.J.S.D., 2018. Present and future Köppen-Geiger climate classification maps at 1-km resolution. Sci. Data 5, 180214.

Bede, O., Szenasi, Z., Danka, J., Gyurkovits, K., Nagy, D., 2008. Toxocariasis associated with chronic cough in childhood: a longitudinal study in Hungary. J. Helminthol. 82, 357–363.

Bellanger, A.P., Humbert, P., Gavignet, B., Deschaseaux, A.D., Barisien, C., Roussel, S., Millon, L., Aubin, F., Piarroux, R., 2010. Comparative assessment of enzyme-linked immunosorbent assay and Western blot for the diagnosis of toxocariasis in patients with skin disorders. Br. J. Dermatol. 162, 80–82.

Beugnet, F., Bourdeau, P., Chalvet-Monfray, K., Cozma, V., Farkas, R., Guillot, J., Halos, L., Joachim, A., Losson, B., Miro, G., Otranto, D., Renaud, M., Rinaldi, L., 2014. Parasites of domestic owned cats in Europe: co-infestations and risk factors. Parasit. Vectors 7, 291.

Boldis, V., Ondriska, F., Spitalska, E., Reiterova, K., 2015. Immunodiagnostic approaches for the detection of human toxocarosis. Exp. Parasitol. 159, 252–258.

Borg, O.A., Woodruff, A.W., 1973. Prevalence of infective ova of *Toxocara* species in public places. Br. Med. J. 4, 470–472.

Buijs, J., Van Knapen, F., 1994. *Toxocara* infection in children and the relation with allergic manifestations. Vet. Q. 16 (Suppl. 1), 13S–14S.

Buijs, J., Borsboom, G., Van Gemund, J.J., Hazebroek, A., Van Dongen, P.A., Van Knapen, F., Neijens, H.J., 1994. *Toxocara* seroprevalence in 5-year-old elementary schoolchildren: relation with allergic asthma. Am. J. Epidemiol. 140, 839–847.

Buijs, J., Borsboom, G., Renting, M., Hilgersom, W.J., Van Wieringen, J.C., Jansen, G., Neijens, J., 1997. Relationship between allergic manifestations and *Toxocara* seropositivity: a cross-sectional study among elementary school children. Eur. Respir. J. 10, 1467–1475.

Caucanas, J.P., Magnaval, J.F., Pascal, J.P., 1988. Prevalence of toxocaral disease. Lancet 1, 1049.

Cauchie, V., Chaillet, P., Bigaignon, G., Tomasi, J.P., Vervoort, T., 1990. Comparative studies of *Toxocara* infections in Belgium and in other countries. Acta Clin. Belg. 45, 227–239.

CDC, 2019. Parasites—Neglected Parasitic Infections (NPIs). https://www.cdc.gov/parasites/npi/index.html. accessed August 23, 2019.

Chen, J., Liu, Q., Liu, G.H., Zheng, W.B., Hong, S.J., Sugiyama, H., Zhu, X.Q., Elsheikha, H.M., 2018. Toxocariasis: a silent threat with a progressive public health impact. Infect. Dis. Poverty 7, 59.

Chobanov, R.E., Gulieva, R.O., Niftullaev, M.Z., 1990. A serological examination for toxocariasis in the population of greater Baku. Med. Parazitol. (Mosk) 3, 35–38.

Cicero, C.E., Patti, F., Lo Fermo, S., Giuliano, L., Rascuna, C., Chisari, C.G., D'amico, E., Paradisi, V., Marin, B., Preux, P.M., Mantella, A., Bartoloni, A., Zappia, M., Nicoletti, A., 2019. Lack of association between *Toxocara canis* and multiple sclerosis: a population-based case-control study. Mult. Scler. https://doi.org/10.1177/1352458518825394.

Cilla, G., Perez-Trallero, E., Gutierrez, C., Part, C., Gomariz, M., 1996. Seroprevalence of *Toxocara* infection in middle-class and disadvantaged children in northern Spain (Gipuzkoa, Basque Country). Eur. J. Epidemiol. 12, 541–543.

Cobzaru, R.G., Rîpă, C., Leon, M.M., Luca, M.C., Ivan, A., Luca, M., 2012. Correlation between asthma and *Toxocara canis* infection. Rev. Med. Chir. Soc. Med. Nat. Iasi. 116, 727–730.

Čolović-Čalovski, I., Jekić, A., Stevanović, O., Dubljanin, E., Kulišić, Z., Dzamić, A., 2014. Anti-*Toxocara* antibodies in patients with suspected visceral larva migrans and evaluation of environmental risk of human infection in Belgrade, Serbia. Arch. Biol. Sci. 66, 545–551.

Conde Garcia, L., Muro Alvarez, A., Simon Martin, F., 1989. Epidemiological studies on toxocariasis and visceral larva migrans in a zone of western Spain. Ann. Trop. Med. Parasitol. 83, 615–620.

Cypess, R.H., Karol, M.H., Zidian, J.L., Glickman, L.T., Gitlin, D., 1977. Larva-specific antibodies in patients with visceral larva migrans. J. Infect. Dis. 135, 633–640.

De Savigny, D.H., Voller, A., Woodruff, A.W., 1979. Toxocariasis: serological diagnosis by enzyme immunoassay. J. Clin. Pathol. 32, 284–288.

Deplazes, P., Guscetti, F., Wunderlin, E., Bucklar, H., Skaggs, J., Wolff, K., 1995. Endoparasite infection in stray and abandoned dogs in southern Switzerland. Schweiz. Arch. Tierheilkd. 137, 172–179.

Deplazes, P., Van Knapen, F., Schweiger, A., Overgaauw, P.A., 2011. Role of pet dogs and cats in the transmission of helminthic zoonoses in Europe, with a focus on echinococcosis and toxocarosis. Vet. Parasitol. 182, 41–53.

Despommier, D., 2003. Toxocariasis: clinical aspects, epidemiology, medical ecology, and molecular aspects. Clin. Microbiol. Rev. 16, 265–272.

Deutz, A., Fuchs, K., Auer, H., Hinterdorfer, F., Schuller, W., Nowotny, N., 1996. Über eine serologische Untersuchung von Tierärzten auf Zoonosen in der Steiermark unter besonderer Berücksichtigung parasitärer Zoonosen. Mitt. Österr. Ges. Tropenmed. Parasitol. 18, 207–214.

Deutz, A., Fuchs, K., Auer, H., Kerbl, U., Aspock, H., Kofer, J., 2005. *Toxocara*-infestations in Austria: a study on the risk of infection of farmers, slaughterhouse staff, hunters and veterinarians. Parasitol. Res. 97, 390–394.

Di Fiore, M., Virga, A., Usticano, V., Di Rosa, S., Rini, G.B., 1989. Antibodies against *Toxocara canis* in human serum from western Sicily. Boll. Ist. Sieroter. Milan. 68, 93–96.

Dubinský, P., Havasiová-Reiterová, K., Petko, B., Hovorka, I., Tomašovičová, O., 1995. Role of small mammals in the epidemiology of toxocariasis. Parasitology 110 (Pt. 2), 187–193.

Elefant, G.R., Shimizu, S.H., Sanchez, M.C., Jacob, C.M., Ferreira, A.W., 2006. A serological follow-up of toxocariasis patients after chemotherapy based on the detection of IgG, IgA, and IgE antibodies by enzyme-linked immunosorbent assay. J. Clin. Lab. Anal. 20, 164–172.

Erickson, L.D., Gale, S.D., Berrett, A., Brown, B.L., Hedges, D.W., 2015. Association between toxocariasis and cognitive function in young to middle-aged adults. Folia Parasitol. 62, 048.

ESCCAP, 2017. Worm Control in Dogs and Cats. ESCCAP Guideline 01, third ed. https://www.esccap.org/page/GL1+Worm+Control+in+Dogs+and+Cats/25/#.XUrpI0FCQuU. accessed August 23, 2019.

EUROVOC, 2019. 7206 Europe. https://publications.europa.eu/en/web/eu-vocabularies/th-concept-scheme/-/resource/eurovoc/100277. accessed August 23, 2019.

Fakhri, Y., Gasser, R.B., Rostami, A., Fan, C.K., Ghasemi, S.M., Javanian, M., Bayani, M., Armoon, B., Moradi, B., 2018. *Toxocara* eggs in public places worldwide—a systematic review and meta-analysis. Environ. Pollut. 242, 1467–1475.

Fan, C.K., Liao, C.W., Cheng, Y.C., 2013. Factors affecting disease manifestation of toxocarosis in humans: genetics and environment. Vet. Parasitol. 193, 342–352.

Fan, C.K., Holland, C.V., Loxton, K., Barghouth, U., 2015. Cerebral toxocariasis: silent progression to neurodegenerative disorders? Clin. Microbiol. Rev. 28, 663–686.

FEDIAF, 2012. Facts and Figures 2012. https://wabbitwiki.com/images/a/ae/Facts_and_figures_2012.pdf. accessed August 26, 2019.

FEDIAF, 2018. Facts and Figures 2018. http://www.fediaf.org/who-we-are/european-statistics.html. accessed August 26, 2019.

Fenoy, S., Cuellar, C., Guillen, J.L., 1996. Seroprevalence of toxocariasis in children and adults in Madrid and Tenerife, Spain. J. Helminthol. 70, 109–113.

Fenoy, S., Cuellar, C., Guillen, J.L., 1997. Serological evidence of toxocariasis in patients from Spain with a clinical suspicion of visceral larva migrans. J. Helminthol. 71, 9–12.

Ferre, P., Dorchies, P., 2000. Recherche des oeufs de *Toxocara* dans le sable des aires de jeux de huit jardins publics de Toulouse. Rev. Med. Vet. (Toulouse) 151, 501–506.

Fillaux, J., Magnaval, J.F., 2013. Laboratory diagnosis of human toxocariasis. Vet. Parasitol. 193, 327–336.

Fisher, M., 2003. *Toxocara cati*: an underestimated zoonotic agent. Trends Parasitol. 19, 167–170.

Fukae, J., Kawanabe, T., Akao, N., Kado, M., Tokoro, M., Yokoyama, K., Hattori, N., 2012. Longitudinal myelitis caused by visceral larva migrans associated with *Toxocara cati* infection: case report. Clin. Neurol. Neurosurg. 114, 1091–1094.

Gabrielli, S., Tasic-Otasevic, S., Ignjatovic, A., Fraulo, M., Trenkic-Bozinovic, M., Momcilovic, S., Cancrini, G., 2017. Seroprevalence and risk factors for *Toxocara canis* infection in Serbia during 2015. Foodborne Pathog. Dis. 14, 43–49.

Gamboa, M.I., 2005. Effects of temperature and humidity on the development of eggs of *Toxocara canis* under laboratory conditions. J. Helminthol. 79, 327–331.

Gaspard, P., Ambolet, Y., Schwartzbrod, J., 1997. Urban sludge reused for agricultural purposes: soils contamination and model development for the parasitological risk assessment. Bull. Acad. Natl. Med. 181, 43–57.

Genchi, C., Di Sacco, B., Gatti, S., Sangalli, G., Scaglia, M., 1990. Epidemiology of human toxocariasis in northern Italy. Parassitologia 32, 313–319.

Genchi, M., Ferroglio, E., Traldi, G., Passera, S., Mezzano, G., Genchi, C., 2007. Fecalizzazione ambientale e rischio parassitario nelle città di Milano e Torino. Professione Veterinaria 41, 15–17.

Giacometti, A., Cerioni, O., Fortuna, M., Caselli, F., D'errico, M., Drenaggi, D., Scalise, G., 1999. Prevalence of *Toxocara* spp. in public playgrounds in a town of Central Italy. Infez. Med. 7, 163–167.

Giacometti, A., Cirioni, O., Fortuna, M., Osimani, P., Antonicelli, L., Del Prete, M.S., Riva, A., D'errico, M.M., Petrelli, E., Scalise, G., 2000. Environmental and serological evidence for the presence of toxocariasis in the urban area of Ancona, Italy. Eur. J. Epidemiol. 16, 1023–1026.

Gillespie, S.H., Bidwell, D., Voller, A., Robertson, B.D., Maizels, R.M., 1993. Diagnosis of human toxocariasis by antigen capture enzyme linked immunosorbent assay. J. Clin. Pathol. 46, 551–554.

Girdwood, R.W., Smith, H.V., Bruce, R.G., Quinn, R., 1978. Human *Toxocara* infection in west of Scotland. Lancet 1, 1318.

Gonzalez-Quintela, A., Gude, F., Campos, J., Garea, M.T., Romero, P.A., Rey, J., Meijide, L.M., Fernandez-Merino, M.C., Vidal, C., 2006. *Toxocara* infection seroprevalence and its relationship with atopic features in a general adult population. Int. Arch. Allergy Immunol. 139, 317–324.

Gueglio, B., De Gentile, L., Nguyen, J.M., Achard, J., Chabasse, D., Marjolet, M., 1994. Epidemiologic approach to human toxocariasis in western France. Parasitol. Res. 80, 531–536.

Guerra, A., Navarro, C., De Guevara, C.L., 1995. Seroprevalence of toxocariasis in children and a case of VLM. Eur. J. Epidemiol. 11, 701–702.

Habluetzel, A., Traldi, G., Ruggieri, S., Attili, A.R., Scuppa, P., Marchetti, R., Menghini, G., Esposito, F., 2003. An estimation of *Toxocara canis* prevalence in dogs, environmental egg contamination and risk of human infection in the Marche region of Italy. Vet. Parasitol. 113, 243–252.

Hauser, M., Basso, W., Deplazes, P., 2015. Kontamination landwirtschaftlicher Nutzflächen durch Hunde-und Fuchskot. Schweiz. Arch. Tierheilkd. 157, 449–455.

Havasiová, K., Dubinský, P., Stefancíková, A., 1993. A seroepidemiological study of human *Toxocara* infection in the Slovak Republic. J. Helminthol. 67, 291–296.

Hayashi, E., Tuda, J., Imada, M., Akao, N., Fujita, K., 2005. The high prevalence of asymptomatic *Toxocara* infection among schoolchildren in Manado, Indonesia. Southeast Asian J. Trop. Med. Public Health 36, 1399–1406.

Hermanowska-Szpakowicz, T., Kondrusik, M., Swierzbinska, R., Zajkowska, J., Pancewicz, S., 2001. Incidence of antibody detection against *Toxocara canis* and clinical symptoms in inhabitants of North-Eastern Poland. Pol. Merkur. Lekarski 10, 168–170.

Hinaidy, H., 1971. Die Parasitenfauna des Rotfuchses, *Vulpes vulpes* (L.), in Österreich. Zentralbl. Veterinarmed. B 18, 21–32.

Hinaidy, H., 1976. Ein weiterer Beitrag zur Parasitenfauna des Rotfuchses, *Vulpes vulpes* (L.), in Österreich. Zentralbl. Veterinarmed. B 23, 66–73.
Hinney, B., Gottwald, M., Moser, J., Reicher, B., Schafer, B.J., Schaper, R., Joachim, A., Kunzel, F., 2017. Examination of anonymous canine faecal samples provides data on endoparasite prevalence rates in dogs for comparative studies. Vet. Parasitol. 245, 106–115.
Holland, C.V., 2017. Knowledge gaps in the epidemiology of *Toxocara*: the enigma remains. Parasitology 144, 81–94.
Holland, C., O'connor, P., Taylor, M.R., Hughes, G., Girdwood, R.W., Smith, H., 1991. Families, parks, gardens and toxocariasis. Scand. J. Infect. Dis. 23, 225–231.
Holland, C.V., O'lorcain, P., Taylor, M.R., Kelly, A., 1995. Sero-epidemiology of toxocariasis in school children. Parasitology 110 (Pt. 5), 535–545.
Horn, K., Schnieder, T., Stoye, M., 1990. Contamination of public children's playgrounds in Hannover with helminth eggs. Dtsch. Tierarztl. Wochenschr. 97 (122), 124–125.
Hotez, P.J., Gurwith, M., 2011. Europe's neglected infections of poverty. Int. J. Infect. Dis. 15, e611–e619.
Humbert, P., Niezborala, M., Salembier, R., Aubin, F., Piarroux, R., Buchet, S., Barale, T., 2000. Skin manifestations associated with toxocariasis: a case-control study. Dermatology 201, 230–234.
Jacobs, D.E., Woodruff, A.W., Shah, A.I., Prole, J.H., 1977. *Toxocara* infections and kennel workers. Br. Med. J. 1, 51.
Jacquier, P., Gottstein, B., Stingelin, Y., Eckert, J., 1991. Immunodiagnosis of toxocarosis in humans: evaluation of a new enzyme-linked immunosorbent assay kit. J. Clin. Microbiol. 29, 1831–1835.
Jarosz, W., Mizgajska-Wiktor, H., Kirwan, P., Konarski, J., Rychlicki, W., Wawrzyniak, G., 2010. Developmental age, physical fitness and *Toxocara* seroprevalence amongst lower-secondary students living in rural areas contaminated with *Toxocara* eggs. Parasitology 137, 53–63.
Jeanneret, J.-P., 1991. Epidémiologie de la toxocarose dans la région jurassienne. Thesis, Université de Neuchâtel.
Jimenez, J.F., Valladares, B., Fernandez-Palacios, J.M., De Armas, F., Del Castillo, A., 1997. A serologic study of human toxocariasis in the Canary Islands (Spain): environmental influences. Am. J. Trop. Med. Hyg. 56, 113–115.
Jogi, N.O., Svanes, C., Siiak, S.P., Logan, E., Holloway, J.W., Igland, J., Johannessen, A., Levin, M., Real, F.G., Schlunssen, V., Horsnell, W.G.C., Bertelsen, R.J., 2018. Zoonotic helminth exposure and risk of allergic diseases: a study of two generations in Norway. Clin. Exp. Allergy 48, 66–77.
Josephs, D.S., Bhinder, P., Thompson, A.R., 1981. The prevalence of *Toxocara* infection in a child population. Public Health 95, 273–275.
Juncker-Voss, M., Prosl, H., Lussy, H., Enzenberg, U., Auer, H., Lassnig, H., Muller, M., Nowotny, N., 2004. Screening for antibodies against zoonotic agents among employees of the Zoological Garden of Vienna, Schonbrunn, Austria. Berl. Munch. Tierarztl. Wochenschr. 117, 404–409.
Kaneva, E., Rainova, I., Harizanov, R., Nikolov, G., Kaftandjiev, I., Mineva, I., 2015. Study of *Toxocara* seroprevalence among patients with allergy and healthy individuals in Bulgaria. Parasite Immunol. 37, 505–509.
Kasiecka, J., 1982. Zur Kontamination öffentlicher Grünflächen und Kinderspielplätze in Wien mit Dauerstadien humanpathogener Endoparasiten von Hund und Katze. Thesis. Veterinärmedizinische Universität Wien.
Keegan, J.D., Holland, C.V., 2010. Contamination of the hair of owned dogs with the eggs of *Toxocara* spp. Vet. Parasitol. 173, 161–164.

Kennedy, M.W., Maizels, R.M., Meghji, M., Young, L., Qureshi, F., Smith, H.V., 1987. Species-specific and common epitopes on the secreted and surface antigens of *Toxocara cati* and *Toxocara canis* infective larvae. Parasite Immunol. 9, 407–420.

Kimmig, P., Naser, K., Frank, W., 1991. Seroepidemiologic studies of human toxocariasis. Zentralbl. Hyg. Umweltmed. 191, 406–422.

Kleine, A., Springer, A., Strube, C., 2017. Seasonal variation in the prevalence of *Toxocara* eggs on children's playgrounds in the city of Hanover, Germany. Parasit. Vectors 10, 248.

Kroten, A., Toczylowski, K., Kiziewicz, B., Oldak, E., Sulik, A., 2016. Environmental contamination with *Toxocara* eggs and seroprevalence of toxocariasis in children of northeastern Poland. Parasitol. Res. 115, 205–209.

Kulisic, Z., Pavlovic, I., Milutinovic, M., Aleksic-Bakrac, N., 1998. Intestinal parasites of dogs and role of dogs in epidemiology of larva migrans in the Belgrade area. Versita Solipska 35, 79–82.

Kutzer, E., Krauthauf, J., Seiler, A., Hejny-Brandl, M., 1995. Öffentliche Grünflächen und Kinderspielplätze als potentielle Infektionsquelle für die Toxokarose des Menschen. Mitt. Österr. Ges. Tropenmed. Parasitol. 17, 71–76.

Lamina, J., 1980. Visceral larva migrans infections caused by *Toxocara* species. Dtsch. Med. Wochenschr. 105, 796–799.

Lassen, B., Janson, M., Viltrop, A., Neare, K., Hutt, P., Golovljova, I., Tummeleht, L., Jokelainen, P., 2016. Serological evidence of exposure to globally relevant zoonotic parasites in the Estonian population. PLoS One 11. e0164142.

Lassning, H., 1996. Beitrag zur Parasitenfauna des Rotfuchses (*Vulpes vulpes*) in der Steiermark. Thesis. Veterinärmedizinische Universität Wien.

Ljungstrom, I., Van Knapen, F., 1989. An epidemiological and serological study of *Toxocara* infection in Sweden. Scand. J. Infect. Dis. 21, 87–93.

Logar, J., Likar, M., Kraut, A., 1993. *Toxocara* antibodies in patients with visceral or ocular disorder in Solvenia. Infection 21, 27–29.

Logar, J., Soba, B., Kraut, A., Stirn-Kranjc, B., 2004. Seroprevalence of *Toxocara* antibodies among patients suspected of ocular toxocariasis in Slovenia. Korean J. Parasitol. 42, 137–140.

Lotsch, F., Obermuller, M., Mischlinger, J., Mombo-Ngoma, G., Groger, M., Adegnika, A.A., Agnandji, S.T., Schneider, R., Auer, H., Ramharter, M., 2016. Seroprevalence of *Toxocara* spp. in a rural population in Central African Gabon. Parasitol. Int. 65, 632–634.

Łużna-Lyskov, A., 2000. Toxocarosis in children living in a highly contaminated area: an epidemiological and clinical study. Acta Parasitol. 45, 40–42.

Ma, G., Holland, C.V., Wang, T., Hofmann, A., Fan, C.K., Maizels, R.M., Hotez, P.J., Gasser, R.B., 2018. Human toxocariasis. Lancet Infect. Dis. 18, e14–e24.

Magnaval, J.F., Fabre, R., Maurieres, P., Charlet, J.P., De Larrard, B., 1991. Application of the western blotting procedure for the immunodiagnosis of human toxocariasis. Parasitol. Res. 77, 697–702.

Magnaval, J.F., Michault, A., Calon, N., Charlet, J.P., 1994. Epidemiology of human toxocariasis in La Reunion. Trans. R. Soc. Trop. Med. Hyg. 88, 531–533.

Malafiej, E., Spiewak, E., 2001. Serological investigation in children infected with *Ascaris lumbricoides*. Wiad. Parazytol. 47, 585–590.

Maulik, P.K., Mascarenhas, M.N., Mathers, C.D., Dua, T., Saxena, S., 2011. Prevalence of intellectual disability: a meta-analysis of population-based studies. Res. Dev. Disabil. 32, 419–436.

McNamara, J., Drake, J., Wiseman, S., Wright, I., 2018. Survey of European pet owners quantifying endoparasitic infection risk and implications for deworming recommendations. Parasit. Vectors 11, 571.

Mizgajska-Wiktor, H., Jarosz, W., Fogt-Wyrwas, R., Drzewiecka, A., 2017. Distribution and dynamics of soil contamination with *Toxocara canis* and *Toxocara cati* eggs in Poland and prevention measures proposed after 20 years of study. Vet. Parasitol. 234, 1–9.

Mohamad, S., Azmi, N.C., Noordin, R., 2009. Development and evaluation of a sensitive and specific assay for diagnosis of human toxocariasis by use of three recombinant antigens (TES-26, TES-30USM, and TES-120). J. Clin. Microbiol. 47, 1712–1717.

Mughini-Gras, L., Harms, M., Van Pelt, W., Pinelli, E., Kortbeek, T., 2016. Seroepidemiology of human *Toxocara* and *Ascaris* infections in the Netherlands. Parasitol. Res. 115, 3779–3794.

Nichols, R.L., 1956. The etiology of visceral larva migrans. I. Diagnostic morphology of infective second-stage *Toxocara* larvae. J. Parasitol. 42, 349–362.

Nicoletti, A., Sofia, V., Mantella, A., Vitale, G., Contrafatto, D., Sorbello, V., Biondi, R., Preux, P.M., Garcia, H.H., Zappia, M., Bartoloni, A., 2008. Epilepsy and toxocariasis: a case-control study in Italy. Epilepsia 49, 594–599.

Nicoletti, A., Cicero, C.E., Mantella, A., Giuliano, L., Rascuna, C., Paradisi, V., Bartoloni, A., Zappia, M., Sofia, V., 2019. Seroprevalence of *Toxocara canis* in the city of Catania, Italy. Mediterr. J. Hematol. Infect. Dis. 11 e2019031.

Nijsse, R., Ploeger, H.W., Wagenaar, J.A., Mughini-Gras, L., 2016. Prevalence and risk factors for patent *Toxocara* infections in cats and cat owners' attitude towards deworming. Parasitol. Res. 115, 4519–4525.

Nikolić, A., Djurković-Djaković, O., Bobić, B., 1998. Intestinal parasitic infections in Serbia. Srp. Arh. Celok. Lek. 126, 1–5.

Nikolić, A., Dimitrijević, S., Katić-Radivojević, S., Klun, I., Bobić, B., Djurković-Djaković, O., 2008. High prevalence of intestinal zoonotic parasites in dogs from Belgrade, Serbia. Acta Vet. Hung. 56, 335–340.

Norhaida, A., Suharni, M., Liza Sharmini, A.T., Tuda, J., Rahmah, N., 2008. rTES-30USM: cloning via assembly PCR, expression, and evaluation of usefulness in the detection of toxocariasis. Ann. Trop. Med. Parasitol. 102, 151–160.

O'lorcain, P., 1995. The effects of freezing on the viability of *Toxocara canis* and *T. cati* embryonated eggs. J. Helminthol. 69, 169–171.

Ondriska, F., Mačuhová, K., Melicherová, J., Reiterová, K., Valentová, D., Beladičová, V., Halgoš, J., 2013. Toxocariasis in urban environment of western Slovakia. Helminthologia 50, 261–268.

Otero, D., Alho, A.M., Nijsse, R., Roelfsema, J., Overgaauw, P., Madeira De Carvalho, L., 2018. Environmental contamination with *Toxocara* spp. eggs in public parks and playground sandpits of Greater Lisbon, Portugal. J. Infect. Public Health 11, 94–98.

Overgaauw, P.A., Van Zutphen, L., Hoek, D., Yaya, F.O., Roelfsema, J., Pinelli, E., Van Knapen, F., Kortbeek, L.M., 2009. Zoonotic parasites in fecal samples and fur from dogs and cats in The Netherlands. Vet. Parasitol. 163, 115–122.

Papavasilopoulos, V., Pitiriga, V., Birbas, K., Elefsiniotis, J., Bonatsos, G., Tsakris, A., 2018. Soil contamination by *Toxocara canis* and human seroprevalence in the Attica region, Greece. Germs 8, 155–161.

Pavlinová, J., Kinčeková, J., Ostró, A., Saksun, L., Vasilková, Z., Königová, A., 2011. Parasitic infections and pregnancy complications. Helminthologia 48, 8–12.

Pfeiffer, H., 1983. Zur Kontamination von öffentlichen Grünanlagen und Kinderspielsand in Wien mit Dauerstadien humanpathogener Parasiten von Hund und Katze. Mitt. Österr. Ges. Tropenmed. Parasitol. 5, 83–87.

Pinelli, E., Herremans, T., Harms, M.G., Hoek, D., Kortbeek, L.M., 2011. *Toxocara* and *Ascaris* seropositivity among patients suspected of visceral and ocular larva migrans in the Netherlands: trends from 1998 to 2009. Eur. J. Clin. Microbiol. Infect. Dis. 30, 873–879.

Poeppl, W., Herkner, H., Tobudic, S., Faas, A., Mooseder, G., Burgmann, H., Auer, H., 2013. Exposure to *Echinococcus multilocularis*, *Toxocara canis*, and *Toxocara cati* in Austria: a nationwide cross-sectional seroprevalence study. Vector Borne Zoonotic Dis. 13, 798–803.

Portus, M., Riera, C., Prats, G., 1989. A serological survey of toxocariasis in patients and healthy donors in Barcelona (Spain). Eur. J. Epidemiol. 5, 224–227.

Posova, H., Hruskova, Z., Havrdova, E., Kolarova, L., 2017. Toxocara spp. seronegativity in Czech patients with early form of multiple sclerosis—clinically isolated syndrome. Epidemiol. Mikrobiol. Imunol. 66, 124–127.

Poulle, M.L., Bastien, M., Richard, Y., Josse-Dupuis, E., Aubert, D., Villena, I., Knapp, J., 2017. Detection of *Echinococcus multilocularis* and other foodborne parasites in fox, cat and dog faeces collected in kitchen gardens in a highly endemic area for alveolar echinococcosis. Parasite 24, 29.

Qualizza, R., Incorvaia, C., Grande, R., Makri, E., Allegra, L., 2011. Seroprevalence of IgG anti-*Toxocara* species antibodies in a population of patients with suspected allergy. Int. J. Gen. Med. 4, 783–787.

R Core Team, 2013. R: A Language and Environment for Statistical Computing. R Foundation for Statistical Computing, Vienna, Austria. http://www.R-project.org/. accessed August 23, 2019.

Rainova, I., Harizanov, R., Kaftandjiev, I., Tsvetkova, N., Mikov, O., Kaneva, E., 2018. Human parasitic diseases in Bulgaria in between 2013-2014. Balkan Med. J. 35, 61–67.

Rainova, I., 2008. Study of *Toxocara* antibody bearing among healthy people in Bulgaria. In: *MEDIMOND International Proceedings X European Multicolloquim of Parasitology (EMOP X) eds. Jean Dupouy-Camet and Eduardo Dei-Cas. Free papers.* Paris (France) 8, pp. 115–118.

Ree, G.H., Voller, A., Rowland, H.A., 1984. Toxocariasis in the British Isles 1982-3. Br. Med. J. (Clin. Res. Ed) 288, 628–629.

Reperant, L.A., Hegglin, D., Fischer, C., Kohler, L., Weber, J.M., Deplazes, P., 2007. Influence of urbanization on the epidemiology of intestinal helminths of the red fox (*Vulpes vulpes*) in Geneva, Switzerland. Parasitol. Res. 101, 605–611.

Rubinsky-Elefant, G., Hoshino-Shimizu, S., Jacob, C.M.A., Sanchez, M.C.A., Ferreira, A.W., 2011. Potential immunological markers for diagnosis and therapeutic assessment of toxocariasis. Rev. Inst. Med. Trop. Sao Paulo 53, 61–65.

Rudzińska, M., Kowalewska, B., Sikorska, K., 2017. Clinical usefulness of Western blotting and ELISA avidity for the diagnosis of human toxocariasis. Parasite Immunol. 39, 1–6.

Sager, H., Moret, C.S., Grimm, F., Deplazes, P., Doherr, M.G., Gottstein, B., 2006. Coprological study on intestinal helminths in Swiss dogs: temporal aspects of anthelminthic treatment. Parasitol. Res. 98, 333–338.

Schneider, R., Auer, H., 2016. Incidence of *Ascaris suum*-specific antibodies in Austrian patients with suspected larva migrans visceralis (VLM) syndrome. Parasitol. Res. 115, 1213–1219.

Schneider, R., Obwaller, A., Auer, H., 2015. Immunoblot for the detection of *Ascaris suum*-specific antibodies in patients with visceral larva migrans (VLM) syndrome. Parasitol. Res. 114, 305–310.

Schwarzer, G., 2007. Meta: an R package for meta-analysis. R News 7, 40–45.

Shimizu, T., 1993. Prevalence of *Toxocara* eggs in sandpits in Tokushima city and its outskirts. J. Vet. Med. Sci. 55, 807–811.

Skírnisson, K., Eydal, M., Gunnarsson, E., Hersteinsson, P., 1993. Parasites of the arctic fox (*Alopex lagopus*) in Iceland. J. Wildl. Dis. 29, 440–446.

Skírnisson, K., Pálsdóttir, G.R., Eydal, M., 2018. Parasites of dogs and cats imported to Iceland during 1989–2017 with remarks on parasites occurring in the native populations. Icel. Agric. Sci. 31, 49–63.

Slovak, A.J., 1984. Toxocaral antibodies in personnel occupationally concerned with dogs. Br. J. Ind. Med. 41, 419.

Smith, H., Noordin, R., 2006. Diagnostic limitations and future trends in the serodiagnosis of human toxocariasis. In: Holland, C.V., Smith, H.V. (Eds.), Toxocara: the enigmatic parasite. CABI Publishing, Cambridge, USA, pp. 89–112.

South, A., 2011. rworldmap: a new R package for mapping global data. R J. 3.

Speiser, F., 1982. Serodiagnosis of tissue dwelling parasites: application of a multi-antigen enzyme-linked immunosorbent assay (ELISA) for screening. Ann. Soc. Belg. Med. Trop. 62, 103–120.

Spinelli, R., Brandonisio, O., Serio, G., Trerotoli, P., Ghezzani, F., Carito, V., Dajci, N., Doci, A., Picaku, F., Dentico, P., 2006. Intestinal parasites in healthy subjects in Albania. Eur. J. Epidemiol. 21, 161–166.

Stensvold, C.R., Skov, J., Moller, L.N., Jensen, P.M., Kapel, C.M., Petersen, E., Nielsen, H.V., 2009. Seroprevalence of human toxocariasis in Denmark. Clin. Vaccine Immunol. 16, 1372–1373.

Strube, C., Heuer, L., Janecek, E., 2013. *Toxocara* spp. infections in paratenic hosts. Vet. Parasitol. 193, 375–389.

Strube, C., Neubert, A., Springer, A., Von Samson-Himmelstjerna, G., 2019. Survey of German pet owners quantifying endoparasitic infection risk and implications for deworming recommendations. Parasit. Vectors 12, 203.

Stürchler, D., Peter, R., 1981. Parasitic disease in schoolchildren in a village in Swiss Jura. Soz. Praventivmed. 26, 317–319.

Stürchler, D., Bruppacher, R., Speiser, F., 1986. Epidemiological aspects of toxocariasis in Switzerland. Schweiz. Med. Wochenschr. 116, 1088–1093.

Suchentrunk, F., Sattmann, H., 1994. Prevalence of intestinal helminths in Austrian red foxes (*Vulpes vulpes* L.) (Cestoda, Nematoda). Ann. Nat. Hist. Mus. Wien Ser. B Bot. Zool. 96B, 29–38.

Supperer, R., Hinaidy, H., 1986. Ein Beitrag zum Parasitenbefall der Hunde und Katzen in Österreich. Dtsch. Tierartztl. Wochenschr. 93, 383–386.

Sviben, M., Čavlek, T.V., Missoni, E.M., Galinović, G.M., 2009. Seroprevalence of *Toxocara canis* infection among asymptomatic children with eosinophilia in Croatia. J. Helminthol. 83, 369–371.

Talvik, H., Moks, E., Mägi, E., Järvis, T., Miller, I., 2006. Distribution of *Toxocara* infection in the environment and in definitive and paratenic hosts in Estonia. Acta Vet. Hung. 54, 399–406.

Taylor, M.R., Keane, C.T., O'connor, P., Girdwood, R.W., Smith, H., 1987. Clinical features of covert toxocariasis. Scand. J. Infect. Dis. 19, 693–696.

Taylor, M.R., Keane, C.T., O'connor, P., Mulvihill, E., Holland, C., 1988. The expanded spectrum of toxocaral disease. Lancet 1, 692–695.

Taylor, M.R., O'connor, P., Hinson, A.R., Smith, H.V., 1996. *Toxocara* titres in maternal and cord blood. J. Infect. 32, 231–233.

Theodoridis, I., Frydas, S., Papazahariadou, M., Hatzistilianou, M., Adamama-Moraitou, K.K., Di Gioacchino, M., Felaco, M., 2001. Toxocarosis as zoonosis. A review of literature and the prevalence of *Toxocara canis* antibodies in 511 serum samples. Int. J. Immunopathol. Pharmacol. 14, 17–23.

Tönz, M., Speiser, F., Tönz, O., 1983. Toxocariasis in Swiss children. Schweiz. Med. Wochenschr. 113, 1500–1507.

Umhang, G., Bastien, M., Renault, C., Faisse, M., Caillot, C., Boucher, J.M., Hormaz, V., Poulle, M.L., Boue, F., 2017. A flotation/sieving method to detect *Echinococcus multilocularis* and *Toxocara* spp. eggs in soil by real-time PCR. Parasite 24, 28.

Valdmann, H., Moks, E., Talvik, H., 2004. Helminth fauna of Eurasian lynx (*Lynx lynx*) in Estonia. J. Wildl. Dis. 40, 356–360.
Van Den Broucke, S., Kanobana, K., Polman, K., Soentjens, P., Vekemans, M., Theunissen, C., Vlieghe, E., Van Esbroeck, M., Jacobs, J., Van Den Enden, E., Van Den Ende, J., Van Gompel, A., Clerinx, J., Bottieau, E., 2015. Toxocariasis diagnosed in international travelers at the Institute of Tropical Medicine, Antwerp, Belgium, from 2000 to 2013. PLoS Negl. Trop. Dis. 9, e0003559.
Van Gemund, J.J., Buijs, J., Van Dongen, P.A., Van Den Bergh, J.P., 1989. Seroprevalence of *Toxocara* infection in young children in the city of the Hague. Trop. Geogr. Med. 41, 294–296.
Van Knapen, F., Van Leusden, J., Polderman, A.M., Franchimont, J.H., 1983. Visceral larva migrans: examinations by means of enzyme-linked immunosorbent assay of human sera for antibodies to excretory-secretory antigens of the second-stage larvae of *Toxocara canis*. Z. Parasitenkd. 69, 113–118.
Walder, M., Aspöck, H., 1987. Untersuchungen über Häufigkeit und Bedeutung von Toxocara-Infektionen des Menschen in Österreich. Mitt. Österr. Ges. Tropenmed. Parasitol. 10, 159–174.
Walsh, M.G., Haseeb, M.A., 2012. Reduced cognitive function in children with toxocariasis in a nationally representative sample of the United States. Int. J. Parasitol. 42, 1159–1163.
Wilder, H.C., 1950. Nematode endophthalmitis. Trans. Am. Acad. Ophthalmol. Otolaryngol. 55, 99–109.
Wiseman, R.A., Woodruff, A.W., 1968. Toxocariasis in Britain as revealed by skin sensitivity tests. Br. Med. J. 1, 677–678.
Wiseman, R.A., Woodruff, A.W., 1970. Evaluation of a skin sensitivity test for the diagnosis of toxocariasis. Trans. R. Soc. Trop. Med. Hyg. 64, 239–245.
Wiseman, R.A., Woodruff, A.W., 1971. Toxocariasis in Africa and Malta. The frequency of infection in host animals and its incidence and distribution in humans as revealed by skin sensitivity tests. Trans. R. Soc. Trop. Med. Hyg. 65, 439–449.
Wiseman, R.A., Fleck, D.G., Woodruff, A.W., 1970. Toxoplasmal and toxocaral infections: a clinical investigation into their relationship. Br. Med. J. 4, 152–153.
Woodhall, D.M., Eberhard, M.L., Parise, M.E., 2014. Neglected parasitic infections in the United States: toxocariasis. Am. J. Trop. Med. Hyg. 90, 810–813.
Woodruff, A.W., 1970. Toxocariasis. Br. Med. J. 3, 663–669.
Woodruff, A.W., Thacker, C.K., 1964. Infection with animal helminths. Br. Med. J. 1, 1001–1005.
Woodruff, A.W., Bisseru, B., Bowe, J.C., 1966. Infection with animal helminths as a factor in causing poliomyelitis and epilepsy. Br. Med. J. 1, 1576–1579.
Woodruff, A.W., De Savigny, D., Jacobs, D.E., 1978. Study of toxocaral infection in dog breeders. Br. Med. J. 2, 1747–1748.
Woodruff, A.W., De Savigny, D.H., Hendy-Ibbs, P.M., 1982. Toxocaral and toxoplasmal antibodies in cat breeders and in Icelanders exposed to cats but not to dogs. Br. Med. J. (Clin. Res. Ed) 284, 309–310.
Yamasaki, H., Araki, K., Lim, P.K., Zasmy, N., Mak, J.W., Taib, R., Aoki, T., 2000. Development of a highly specific recombinant *Toxocara canis* second-stage larva excretory-secretory antigen for immunodiagnosis of human toxocariasis. J. Clin. Microbiol. 38, 1409–1413.
Zacharasiewicz, A., Auer, H., Brath, H., Stohlhofer, B., Frank, W., Aspöck, H., Zwick, H., 2000. *Toxocara* and bronchial hyperreactivity—results of a seroprevalence study. Wien. Klin. Wochenschr. 112, 922–926.
Zottler, E.M., Bieri, M., Basso, W., Schnyder, M., 2019. Intestinal parasites and lungworms in stray, shelter and privately owned cats of Switzerland. Parasitol. Int. 69, 75–81.

Żukiewicz, M., Kaczmarski, M., Topczewska, M., Sidor, K., Tomaszewska, B.M., 2011. Epidemiological and clinical picture of parasitic infections in the group of children and adolescents from north-east region of Poland. Wiad. Parazytol. 57, 179–187.

Żukiewicz-Sobczak, W., Zwoliński, J., Chmielewska-Badora, J., Galińska, E.M., Cholewa, G., Krasowska, E., Zagórski, J., Wojtyła, A., Tomasiewicz, K., Kłapeć, T., 2014. Prevalence of antibodies against selected zoonotic agents in forestry workers from eastern and southern Poland. Ann. Agric. Environ. Med. 21, 767–770.

Zwolinski, J., 2000. The risk factors of *Toxocara canis* infestation in population of patients from the Lublin region. Wiad. Parazytol. 46, 463–473.

CHAPTER TWENTY

Seroprevalence and incidence of human toxocarosis in Russia

Lyudmila V. Akhmadishina[a], Maria N. Ruzina[a], Maria A. Lukasheva[a], Karen K. Kyuregyan[b,c], Mikhail I. Mikhailov[b,c], Alexander N. Lukashev[a,*]

[a]Martsinovsky Institute of Medical Parasitology, Tropical and Vector-Borne Diseases, Sechenov University, Moscow, Russia
[b]Russian Medical Academy of Continuous Professional Education, Moscow, Russia
[c]Mechnikov Research Institute for Vaccines and Sera, Moscow, Russia
*Corresponding author: e-mail address: alexander_lukashev@hotmail.com

Contents

Abstract

Overall incidence of toxocariasis in Russia is low and varies between 1.6 and 2.7 per 100,000, while in several hyper-endemic regions, such as Altay, Kurgan, Perm and Udmurtia, it reaches 43 per 100,000. The seroprevalence of toxocariasis in published references was on average 16% and varied across the regions of Russia from negligible in North Siberia to 40% in southern regions of West Siberia. Seroprevalence in adults in five regions of Russia identified in this study was on average 20%, and varied from 3% in Yakutia (north of East Siberia) to 36% in Rostov-on-Don, South Russia. There was no correlation between seroprevalence and reported incidence of toxocariasis; however, the pattern of seroprevalence variation could be linked to Toxocara prevalence in dogs. Toxocariasis seroprevalence has more than doubled over the last 20 years. Diagnostic antibody titres (1:800 or more) were found in 3.6% of sera, suggesting about five million of acute Toxocara invasions per year.

Advances in Parasitology, Volume 109
ISSN 0065-308X
https://doi.org/10.1016/bs.apar.2020.01.015

1. Toxocariasis incidence in Russia

The registered incidence of parasite infections in Russia has been decreasing over the last few decades, but they remain a significant socio-economic burden and a permanent healthcare concern. All parasitic infections are notifiable, and confirmed human cases have to be submitted to the reporting system and are included within regular incidence reports issued for most of the 85 administrative territories, as well as for the country as a whole; however, the diagnostics quality and the stringency of reporting may vary between diseases and administrative regions. The most common human parasite infections are enterobiasis (215,000 – 240,000 cases per year), ascaridosis (22,000–40,000 cases per year), and opisthorchiasis (20,000–33,000 cases per year) (Rosstat, 2017). Most of these cases are found upon systematic screening, which is mandatory for admission to public kindergartens, schools, swimming pools, permission to work in healthcare, education, food manufacturing, and sales. The screening is done by microscopy of faeces and anal smear/print for enterobiasis screening. As human toxocariasis does not result in the shedding of helminth eggs, it is not detected by this systematic surveillance, and only overt cases, proven by the detection of high anti-Toxocara IgG levels, are registered. Despite this serious limitation, there are around 2000 cases of toxocariasis per year in Russia, or 1.6–2.7 per 100,000 of the population (Yerofeeva, 2017). The registered incidence of toxocariasis was very low in the 1990s, likely due to low awareness and poor diagnostics; the incidence increased several times upon the wide-spread introduction of ELISA, peaking in 2007, and has been slightly decreasing over the last decade (Fig. 1). The incidence is 2–3 times higher than the average in children below 17 years of age, and the highest (about 4–5 times higher than the average, 10–11 per 100,000) in children aged 3–6 years old (Stepanova and Kornachyov, 2013; Yerofeeva, 2017).

The highest incidence of human toxocariasis is registered in West Siberia and the Urals region, followed by Central Russia (Volga region) and the Far East. The incidence in the Altai region (South of West Siberia) is the highest, 43.2 per 100,000, about 20 times higher than the country average, followed by Kurgan, Perm, and Udmurtia (Malkhazova, 2015; Starostina et al., 2015b). A lower incidence is reported in Central and South Russia, even in areas with an extremely high prevalence (up to 100%) of the parasite in dogs and in the environment (Akimova, 2006). The reported regional incidence is patchy, and highly endemic regions may surround regions

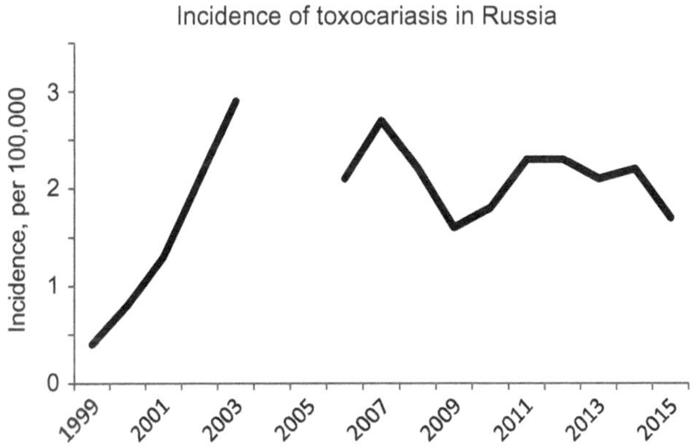

Fig. 1 Incidence of toxocariasis in Russia in 1999–2015 (Guzeeva, 2009; Starostina et al., 2015a; Yerofeeva, 2017).

with more than a ten-fold lower incidence, or vice versa (Malkhazova, 2015; Starostina et al., 2015b). This suggests that the reporting is non-uniform, and the published incidence may reflect the awareness of doctors, the availability of modern diagnostics, and the stringency of the reporting rather than the true incidence. Also, the stringent case definition and laborious reporting (which is rather avoided than overdone by primary care personnel) stress that the higher incidence values are more trustworthy than the lower values.

2. Toxocariasis seroprevalence in Russia

There have been a significant number of toxocariasis seroprevalence studies in Russia beginning from 1990s (Table 1, Fig. 2). Unfortunately, a lack of common guidelines and reference panels seriously complicates comparing the results. This is partially alleviated by the domination of a single ELISA kit on the market in Russia (also used in this study), but even then most studies use a titre cut-off of 1:100, while some may set more stringent titre cut-offs and often do not specify which diagnostic kit was used and which titre was considered positive; so the results of different studies are not directly comparable.

The fraction of the seropositive population in various regions of Russia found in different studies varied between zero and 54% (Table 1). Average seroprevalence among all published reports was 16%. Values below 5% were typically reported before 1990. Values above 20% were found in publications after 2009. This trend was vividly demonstrated in a longitudinal

Table 1 Seroprevalence of Toxocara in Russia.

Region and designation on Fig. 2	Population group	Seroprevalence, %	References
Moscow, 1978 (1)	All age groups	5.4	Yampolskaya and Ignashenkova (1978)
Moscow, 1998 (1)	Adults	21.3	Guzeeva (2009)
	Children	23.5	
Moscow, 2003–2007 (1)	Adults, 50–59 year	29.4	Guzeeva (2009)
	Children, 7–14 year	23.5	
	Children, 4–6 year	11.8	
Moscow region, 2008 (1)	Adults 30–60 year	24	This study
Bryansk, Central Russia, 1983 (2)	Adults	3.5	Avdyukhina (1987)
	Children <14 year	5.4	
St. Petersburgh (3)	Children	4.5	Lebedeva (2006)
Rostov, South Russia (4)	Adults	22.9	Shishkanova (2011)
Rostov, South Russia, 2008 (4)	Adults 30–60 year	36.0	This study
Ekaterinburg, South Urals, 2008 (5)	Adults 30–60 year	13.0	This study
Omsk, south of West Siberia, 2006–2008 (6)	Children <5 year	12.1	Starostina and Romanova (2016)
Omsk, south of West Siberia, 2013–2015 (6)	Children <5 year	32.1	Starostina and Romanova (2016)
Omsk, south of West Siberia (6)	Adults 16–60 year	54.1	Berezina et al. (2011)
	Children <15 year	40.4	
Novosibirsk, south of West Siberia, 1997 (7)	Healthy donors	8.3	Frolova et al. (1997)
Altay, south of West Siberia, <2012 (8)	Endemic districts	15.4–40.6	Pautova et al. (2012)
	Non-endemic districts	2.0–6.0	

Table 1 Seroprevalence of Toxocara in Russia—cont'd

Region and designation on Fig. 2	Population group	Seroprevalence, %	References
Irkutsk, south of East Siberia, 1977–1987 (9)	Healthy donors	2.4	Kupriyanova (1988)
	Healthy adults	4.7	
Yakutia, north-east Siberia, <1994 (10)	Adults	2.6	Avdiukhina and Lysenko (1994)
	Children	0	
Yakutia, north-east Siberia, 2008 (10)	Adults 30–60 year	3.0	This study
Khabarovsk, Far East, 2008 (11)	Adults 30–60 year	24.0	This study
Khabarovsk, Far East, 1999 (11)	All age groups	15.6	Kozyreva (1999)

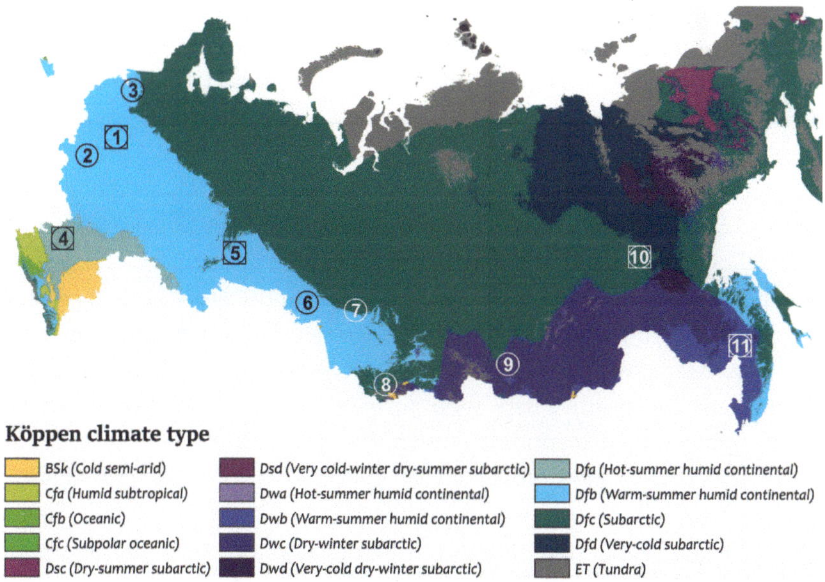

Fig. 2 Map of *Toxocara* seroprevalence study sites in previous publications (circles) and in this study (squares). Numbers correspond to Table 1. Colour indicates Köppen climate zones according to the legend. The original image was taken from https://en.wikipedia.org/wiki/Climate_of_Russia.

study of seroprevalence in Omsk in 1995–2010 (Berezina et al., 2011). That study showed that seroprevalence stayed at around 8% in 1995–2004 and abruptly increased to 18% in 2005 and over 30% in 2006–2008. Another study from Omsk reported that seroprevalence almost tripled between samples collected in 2006–2008 and 2010–2015 (Starostina and Romanova, 2016). It remains unclear if this was an objective increase of seroprevalence, or a hypothetical change in assay sensitivity. Indeed, all studies in Russia use an ELISA kit from a sole manufacturer (see below), and simultaneous rapid increase of seroprevalence in distant areas and in different age groups may be questionable.

There have been no systematic national/multi-region studies in Russia similar to those done in other countries (Poeppl et al., 2013; Won et al., 2008). Moreover, many studies (not discussed in this review) included only risk groups (children, asthma patients, etc.) and are not representative of the general population. To provide a reliable image of toxocariasis seroprevalence in Russia, randomly sampled adult sera from five distant regions of Russia were investigated using a consistent methodology to provide a representative image of toxocariasis seroprevalence.

Serum samples were collected from 2007 to 2008 as a part of a hepatitis B seroprevalence study (Klushkina et al., 2016). Adults aged 30–60 years old were chosen as a target group. The study subjects were randomly selected from an address book, and informed consent was obtained. Anonymous samples were used for this study. Anti-Toxocara antibodies were determined using the Toxocara IgG ELISA kit (Vector-Best, Russia). According to the manufacturer's instructions and state guidelines (2001), antibody titres equal to or above 1:800 (i.e., that give a positive ELISA signal in dilutions of 1:800 or above) are suggested as confirmatory for acute toxocariasis, while titres between 1:100–1:400 may be considered confirmatory in the presence of compatible symptoms. For this seroepidemiological study, a titre of 1:100 was chosen as positive (as was also done in most previously published studies), and the positive sera were further titred to a dilution of 1:800, which was used as a secondary cut-off.

Serum samples were collected in five regions (Fig. 2) representing Central Russia (Moscow region), South Russia (Rostov-on-Don), South Urals (Ekaterinburg), East Siberia (Yakutia) and Far East (Khabarovsk). The seropositivity rates varied from 3% to 36% (Fig. 3). Significantly lower seropositivity (3%) was observed in Yakutia, while in Rostov-on-Don it was higher than in other regions (36%). There was no correlation between seroprevalence and the reported toxocariasis incidence in the study regions

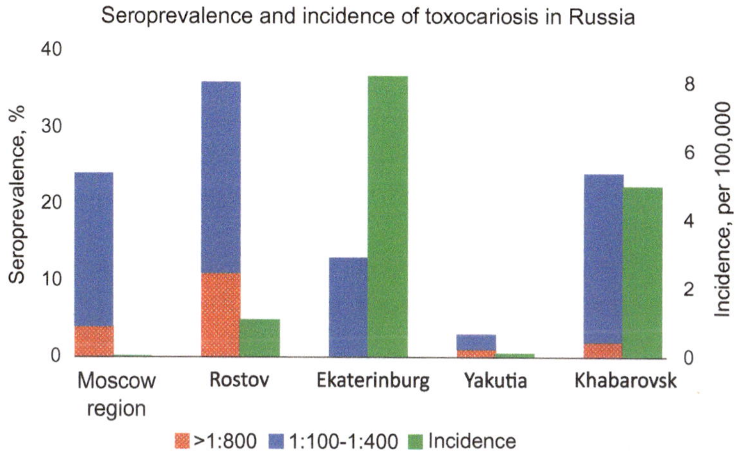

Fig. 3 Seroprevalence and incidence of toxocariasis in five regions of Russia.

(Fig. 3). The Moscow region featured a high seroprevalence (24%), while the incidence was 0.03 per 100,000, almost the lowest in the country. Given the relatively high healthcare level, toxocariasis awareness, and the availability of diagnostics in Moscow, the incidence of overt disease in this case is less likely to be significantly underestimated. On the contrary, the incidence in Ekaterinburg is among the highest in Russia, about four times the country's average, while the seroprevalence (13%) was below average.

The overall fraction of sera with high antibody titres (≥ 1:800) was 3.6%. This titre is recommended as a threshold for acute toxocariasis diagnostics. The fraction of high-titre sera among all positive ones varied from zero to 30%. Similar to general seroprevalence, there was no correlation between high-titre seroprevalence and incidence. The high-titre seroprevalence varied from zero in Ekaterinburg (high registered incidence) to 11% in Rostov (low incidence). In the latter case, an incidence of 1/100,000 was accompanied by 11% high-titre seroprevalence. Therefore, the registered and projected incidence differed about 10,000-fold.

A lack of correlation between incidence and seroprevalence has been also reported in a study done in a hyper-endemic region (Altay, south of West Siberia). While the incidence ranged between 0.7 and 5.1 per 100,000 in the central districts and reached 77.6 in the Northern region, the seroprevalence was 10–20% in moderately endemic districts and 17% in the hyper-endemic ones (Pautova et al., 2012).

Absence of correlation between seroprevalence and incidence can have several explanations. First, it might be due to an absence of typical clinical signs, limited diagnostic capacity and a vague case definition. Second, awareness of medical personnel can have an effect, both negative (lack of knowledge) and positive (over-diagnostics). Antigenic cross-reactivity could also play a role. It is conceivable that all these factors play a role in Russia. However, the gap between seroprevalence and incidence is huge, especially in Moscow. Also, the ratio of high-titre and low-titre sera identified in a single experiment varies across regions.

A lack of correlation between the incidence and the seroprevalence could be also explained by distinct invasion sources or transmission mechanisms. *Toxocara* eggs were found in 4–10% of vegetables and greenery samples in Russia (Sabirova et al., 2012; Suleymanova, 2012). This could lead to common, but low-multiplicity invasion due to a lower number of eggs in these sources, on average 13.8 eggs per kilogram (Bittirov et al., 2018), and explain the significant seroprevalence in the absence of overt disease (as observed in Moscow and Rostov-on-Don) and a low prevalence of infection in pet dogs in the area (Moscow). This hypothetical food-borne route could also explain a high seroprevalence in an area with the highest socioeconomic level (Moscow) because it contradicts the published reports of significantly higher seroprevalence in risk groups or a socially vulnerable population (Alvarado-Esquivel, 2013; Antolova et al., 2015). Higher consumption of vegetables and greenery in this economically privileged region could promote common low-grade invasion. On the contrary, in high-incidence regions, the classical infection directly from contaminated soil may be relatively more common, hypothetically more likely to provide a high infecting dose, and thus a symptomatic disease. Obviously, there is no direct proof for this hypothesis, and further studies are required to test the potential impact of distinct infection routes in Russia.

Although there was no systematic data on *Toxocara* prevalence in primary hosts in all the study regions, it is worth noting that a high seroprevalence was observed in the Moscow region. The previously reported seroprevalence in Moscow was similar to other regions of Russia, but not lower (Avdiukhina and Lysenko, 1994; Guzeeva, 2009). At the same time, the reported incidence of human toxocariasis in Moscow is one of the lowest in Russia and varies between 0.1 and 0.5 per 100,000. This corresponds to a low prevalence of infection in pet dogs, below 5% compared to the 30% average in Russia (Lukashev et al., 2020). In this case, the seroprevalence was not correlated to the hypothetical low exposure risk from infected dogs. This observation further stresses that in the case of toxocariasis, seroprevalence may poorly reflect the overt disease incidence.

Significantly lower seroprevalence was found in Yakutia, which has a cold continental climate with a mean annual temperature of −8.8 °C in the capital (Yakutsk). The mean daytime temperatures go above 20 °C in summer, so the development of *Toxocara* eggs is theoretically possible (Turbabina et al., 2019), but the permissive season is very short, which may explain low seroprevalence compared to other regions of Russia. Unfortunately, there is no data on the prevalence of *Toxocara* infection in dogs in Yakutia, so it is not clear if human infections result from a local circulation, are imported cases, or come from contaminated greenery and vegetables imported from other regions. The latter supposition is favoured by the absence of *Toxocara* seroprevalence in children in Yakutia and low seroprevalence in adults (2.6%) in 1980s (Avdiukhina and Lysenko, 1994).

Toxocariasis seroprevalence in Russia reported in recent studies (about 20%) was higher than in the United States (5.1% (Berrett et al., 2017) or 13.9% (Won et al., 2008)), the Netherlands (10.7–8.0% (Mughini-Gras et al., 2016)), Austria (6.3% (Poeppl et al., 2013)). Among European countries, a comparable seroprevalence (23.5%) was reported in Serbia (Gabrielli et al., 2017). Higher seroprevalence is typical to Asia, for example, 45.2% in Vietnam (Nguyen et al., 2016) and Africa, 57.6% in children in Nigeria (Sowemimo et al., 2017). Seroprevalence in some regions of Russia is very high even compared to many developing countries and generally corresponds to similarly high prevalence of infection in the main hosts.

3. Assay sensitivity

Although dozens of toxocariasis seroepidemiology studies have been published in the world, the data is far from comprehensive, largely due to the limited compatibility of methodology, including sampling and testing approaches. Moreover, some of the popular testing methods may lack both sensitivity and specificity to the degree that would seriously complicate the interpretation of the results (Ma et al., 2018). As antibody titres decrease over time, this may lead to the under-estimation of seroprevalence. This is highlighted by the reports of a seasonal pattern of toxocariasis seroprevalence in Moscow, with the highest values (32–42%) observed in summer and autumn, and the lowest (11–16%) in winter and spring (Guzeeva, 2009). A similar seasonal variation of seroprevalence was observed in Omsk (Berezina et al., 2011). This profile corresponds to seasonal fluctuations in egg shedding by dogs and the contamination of the environment commonly observed in Russia (Lukashev et al., 2020), and suggests that at least some of the seroprevalence studies might predominantly detect recent cases of (re) invasion. Another study reported the absence of a clear cut-off between the titres in the "positive" and "negative" sera (Slobodeniuk et al., 2005), further stressing that the detection of anti-*Toxocara* IgG does not reflect lifetime exposure, but a more or less recent infection.

The concern of low sensitivity of the commonly used ELISA tests is also highlighted by a lower seroprevalence in adults than in children, which was reported in several independent studies (Avdiukhina and Lysenko, 1994; Starostina et al., 2015b). It has also been indicated that a positive ELISA status persists for just a few years after infection (Deplazes et al., 2011). However, in studies done in other countries (Berrett et al., 2017) and some other Russian studies (Avdiukhina and Lysenko, 1994), the seroprevalence increased over age. Unfortunately, this observation does not necessarily indicate that seroprevalence corresponds to cumulative exposure because its increase could have also been attributed to re-infections rather than persisting antibodies (Deplazes et al., 2011). Therefore, it is not clear to what extent toxocariasis seroprevalence studies (especially those done with a stringent titre cut-off) reflect a cumulative life-long exposure (as they do for most other diseases), and the data should be treated as the lower estimate of real toxocariasis exposure.

4. Assay specificity

Specificity is commonly a key limitation of serological tests in helminthology, and in toxocariasis in particular (Ma et al., 2018). Moreover, it may be difficult to distinguish the effect of cross-reactivity from the input of risky behaviour and poor sanitary habits that increase chances of infection with different parasites. In Novosibirsk (Siberia, endemic for *Opisthorchis*), 8.3% of adults had antibodies to *Toxocara*, 7.9% to *Opisthorchis* and 4.6% to both parasites (Frolova et al., 1997). In Khabarovsk (Far East, endemic for Clonorchis) 16.4% adults were positive for Toxocara, 14.8% to *Clonorchis* and 8.6% to both (Kozyreva, 1999). In both studies the fraction of *Toxocara*-positive adults was significantly higher among fluke-seropositive than among fluke-seronegative individuals. Flukes are not universally prevalent in Russia and could not affect the results for all regions. Cross-reactivity with *Ascaris* has been the major concern due to phylogenetic relatedness of the two helminths, relatively high incidence of ascaridosis in Russia, and published reports of cross-reactivity between *Toxocara* and *Ascaris suum* (Munoz-Guzman et al., 2010). To test cross-reactivity

Table 2 Detection of anti-Ascaris IgG in Toxocara-positive sera.

Toxocara IgG titre	Number of Ascaris-positive sera	Percent of Ascaris-positive sera	Geometric mean of anti-Ascaris IgG
1:100–1:200	5/30	17	1:114
1:400–1:800	11/16	69	1:146
Negative	0/30	0	–

between *Toxocara* and *Ascaris*, a panel of randomly selected *Toxocara*-positive and negative sera was tested for presence of antibodies to *Ascaris* using *Ascaris*-IgG-ELISA-Best kit (Vector-Best, Russia). An obvious cross-reactivity was observed. All 30 *Toxocara*-negative sera were also negative for *Ascaris* (Table 2). 16% of sera with a low titre and 67% of sera with a high titre to *Toxocara* were also positive to *Ascaris*. The antibody titres to *Ascaris* were almost always lower than to *Toxocara* in double-positive sera, and most of the low-titre *Toxocara*-positive sera were negative for *Ascaris*. Therefore, it is unlikely that this cross-reactivity has significantly affected the *Toxocara* seroprevalence values, and is rather a concern for the immunodiagnostics of ascaridosis.

5. Conclusion

The results of this and many other studies show that human infection by *Toxocara* is ubiquitous in the human population. The average seroprevalence in adults in Russia was 20%. Based upon a suggestion of rapid antibody clearance in humans (Deplazes et al., 2011), this corresponds to roughly 10 million invasions per year in Russia. A comparable estimate of five million cases can be obtained by extrapolating a ratio of diagnostically relevant high-titre sera (3,6%) on the population of Russia. The reported incidence of toxocariasis (about 2000 cases per year) suggests that significantly less than 1% of infections are diagnosed. The seroprevalence in Russia was roughly double that of Europe and the USA, which corresponds to double the prevalence of *Toxocara* in its primary hosts. However, there was no correlation between the seroprevalence of *Toxocara* in humans and the prevalence in dogs among the regions of Russia.

A lack of correlation between the seroprevalence and incidence suggests that the exposure and egg ingestion are necessary, but not the key factors for the development of the symptomatic human disease. The multiplicity of infection (amount of ingested eggs) may be a critical factor. Immune status, healthcare awareness, and the availability of diagnostics are among other potential explanations.

General improvement of sanitation led to elimination of severe enteric infections, such as cholera and dysentery, in most countries, but apparently did not affect toxocarosis. While the increasing seroprevalence found here may be an artefact, there has been definitely no improvement of the epidemiological situation over the last 30–40 years. It is conceivable that a decreasing awareness to acute enteric infections may even promote an increasing incidence of toxocarosis. So far, toxocariasis remains ubiquitous, yet a neglected disease with poorly understood epidemiology, pathogenesis, and its medical relevance may go beyond our current understanding.

Acknowledgements

This work was supported by the Russian Academic Excellence Project 5-100.

References

Akimova, S.A., 2006. Toxocariasis and Toxascaris of Carnivores in the Lower Volga Region: Epidemiology, Pathogenesis and Treatment. Ph.D. in Veterinary Sciences, Volgograd State Agricultural Academy.

Alvarado-Esquivel, C., 2013. Toxocariasis in waste pickers: a case control seroprevalence study. PLoS One 8, e54897.

Antolova, D., Jarcuska, P., Janicko, M., Madarasova-Geckova, A., Halanova, M., Cislakova, L., Kalinova, Z., Reiterova, K., Skutova, M., Pella, D., Marekova, M., Hepameta, T., 2015. Seroprevalence of human Toxocara infections in the Roma and non-Roma populations of Eastern Slovakia: a cross-sectional study. Epidemiol. Infect. 143, 2249–2258.

Avdiukhina, T.I., Lysenko, A., 1994. How many patients with visceral toxocariasis in Russia? Med. Parazitol. (Mosk) 1, 12–16.

Avdyukhina, T.I., 1987. Comparative Seroepidemiology of Parasitic Zoonoses in Mixed Foci (on Examples of Toxocarosis and Toxoplasmosis). Ph.D. in Medical Sciences, Central Institute of Advanced Medical Education.

Berezina, E.S., Lobkis, D.V., Starostina, O.Y., 2011. Toxocarosis Distribution Peculiarities in the Populations of Small Domestic Carnivoras and the Human Being on the Territory of Russia. vol. 10. Bulletin of Krasnoyarsk State Agrarian University, pp. 168–177.

Berrett, A.N., Erickson, L.D., Gale, S.D., Stone, A., Brown, B.L., Hedges, D.W., 2017. Toxocara Seroprevalence and associated risk factors in the United States. Am. J. Trop. Med. Hyg. 97, 1846–1850.

Bittirov, A.M., Shakhmurzov, M.M., Kagermazov, T.B., Chilayev, A.S., Bittirova, A.A., 2018. Sanitary state of soil and water of the North Caucasus region in relation to contamination by eggs and larvae of parasitic zoonoses. Agrarian Russia 12, 36–39.

Deplazes, P., Van Knapen, F., Schweiger, A., Overgaauw, P.A., 2011. Role of pet dogs and cats in the transmission of helminthic zoonoses in Europe, with a focus on echinococcosis and toxocarosis. Vet. Parasitol. 182, 41–53.

Frolova, S.B., Volkov, G.N., Bormotov, N.I., Zhevachevskii, N.G., Dedkova, L.M., Belanov, E.F., Ofitserov, V.I., 1997. The seroepidemiology of toxocariasis in an opisthorchiasis focus in the western Siberian region. Med. Parazitol. (Mosk) 4, 21–24.

Gabrielli, S., Tasic-Otasevic, S., Ignjatovic, A., Fraulo, M., Trenkic-Bozinovic, M., Momcilovic, S., Cancrini, G., 2017. Seroprevalence and risk factors for Toxocara canis infection in Serbia during 2015. Foodborne Pathog. Dis. 14, 43–49.

Guzeeva, M.V., 2009. The current toxocariasis situation in Moscow. Med. Parazitol. (Mosk) 1, 49–51.

Klushkina, V.V., Kyuregyan, K.K., Kozhanova, T.V., Popova, O.E., Dubrovina, P.G., Isaeva, O.V., Gordeychuk, I.V., Mikhailov, M.I., 2016. Impact of universal hepatitis B vaccination on prevalence, infection-associated morbidity and mortality, and circulation of immune escape variants in Russia. PLoS One 11, e0157161.

Kozyreva, T.G., 1999. Ecologo-Epidemiological Basis for Toxocarosis Prophylactics in the Far-Eastern Region of Russia (on an Example of Khabarovsk Region). Ph.D. in Biology, Far-Eastern State Medical University.

Kupriyanova, N.Y., 1988. Areal of Toxocara Canis in USSR and Epidemiology of Toxocarosis in East Siberia (on an Example of Irkutsk Region). Ph.D. in Medical Sciences, Central Institute of Advanced Medical Education.

Lebedeva, O.V., 2006. Epidemiology of Toxocarosis in St Petersburgh. Ph.D. in Medical Sciences, St Petersburgh State Medical Academy.

Lukashev, A.N., Ruzina, M.N., Akhmadishina, L.V., 2020. *Toxocara* prevalence in dogs, cats and the environment in Russia. Adv. Parasitol. 109, 801–817.

Ma, G., Holland, C.V., Wang, T., Hofmann, A., Fan, C.K., Maizels, R.M., Hotez, P.J., Gasser, R.B., 2018. Human toxocariasis. Lancet Infect. Dis. 18, e14–e24.

Malkhazova, S.M., 2015. Medico-Geographical Atlas of Russia "Natural Focal Diseases". Faculty of Geography, Lomonosov Moscow State University, Moscow.

Mughini-Gras, L., Harms, M., Van Pelt, W., Pinelli, E., Kortbeek, T., 2016. Seroepidemiology of human *Toxocara* and *Ascaris* infections in the Netherlands. Parasitol. Res. 115, 3779–3794.

Munoz-Guzman, M.A., Del Rio-Navarro, B.E., Valdivia-Anda, G., Alba-Hurtado, F., 2010. The increase in seroprevalence to *Toxocara canis* in asthmatic children is related to cross-reaction with *Ascaris suum* antigens. Allergol. Immunopathol. (Madr) 38, 115–121.

Nguyen, T., Cheong, F.W., Liew, J.W., Lau, Y.L., 2016. Seroprevalence of fascioliasis, toxocariasis, strongyloidiasis and cysticercosis in blood samples diagnosed in medic medical center laboratory, Ho Chi Minh City, Vietnam in 2012. Parasit. Vectors 9, 486.

Pautova, E.A., Kurepina, N., Dovgalev, A.S., 2012. Toxocariasis in the republic of Altai. Geoinformation mapping simulation. Med. Parazitol. (Mosk) 4, 11–14.

Poeppl, W., Herkner, H., Tobudic, S., Faas, A., Mooseder, G., Burgmann, H., Auer, H., 2013. Exposure to *Echinococcus multilocularis, Toxocara canis*, and *Toxocara cati* in Austria: a nationwide cross-sectional seroprevalence study. Vector Borne Zoonotic Dis. 13, 798–803.

Rosstat, 2017. Healthcare in Russia 2017. Statistical compendium. Federal State Statistics Service, Moscow.

Sabirova, D.R., Markova, O.P., Belyaeva, M.I., 2012. Incidence of toxocarosis on the territory of Tyumen region. In: 10th VNPOEMP Congress, 2012 Moscow. VNPOEMP.

Shishkanova, L.V., 2011. Toxocariasis in the South of Russia (Epidemiological, Sanitary-Parasitological, Serological Characterization). Ph.D. Rostov Research Institute of Microbiology and Parasitology.

Slobodeniuk, A.V., Kosova, A.A., Rukoleeva, S.I., 2005. Prevalence of toxocariasis in rural and urban areas. Med. Parazitol. (Mosk) 3, 36–38.

Sowemimo, O.A., Lee, Y.L., Asaolu, S.O., Chuang, T.W., Akinwale, O.P., Badejoko, B.O., Gyang, V.P., Nwafor, T., Henry, E., Fan, C.K., 2017. Seroepidemiological study and associated risk factors of *Toxocara canis* infection among preschool children in Osun state, Nigeria. Acta Trop. 173, 85–89.

Starostina, O.Y., Romanova, S.N., 2016. Incidence of toxocariasis and seropositivity to *Toxocara* antigens among children in Omsk region. Public Health Life Environ. 294, 53–56.

Starostina, O.Y., Berezina, E.S., Romanova, S.N., 2015a. Toxocariasis: current state of the Russian Federation. Message 1: risk of Toxocariasis infection of the population on the territory of the Russian Federation. Epidemiol. Vac. Prev. 2 (81), 13–18.

Starostina, O.Y., Romanova, S.N., Panyushkina, I.I., 2015b. Toxocarosis: Current State of Problem in Russian Federation. Omsk Research Institute of Natural Foci Infections of Rospotrebnadzor—Publishing Center "Omsk Scientific Bulletin", Omsk.

Stepanova, T.F., Kornachyov, A.S., 2013. Evaluation of the effectiveness of parasitic diseases prevention in the Russian Federation in 2010–2012. In: Recommendations for Improvement: Monograph in 2 Parts. Tyumen State University, Tyumen.

Suleymanova, G.F., 2012. Epizootological and epidemiological problems of toxocariasis. vol. 210. Scientific Notes of Kazan Bauman State Academy of Veterinary Medicine, pp. 230–234.

Turbabina, N.A., Morozova, L.F., Sergiyev, V.P., Kondrashin, A.V., Stepanova, E.V., Maksimova, M.S., Brazhnikov, A.Y., Morozov, E.N., 2019. Actual situation and area of ascaris in Russia. Med. Parazitol. (Mosk) (1), 41–46.

Won, K.Y., Kruszon-Moran, D., Schantz, P.M., Jones, J.L., 2008. National seroprevalence and risk factors for zoonotic Toxocara spp. infection. Am. J. Trop. Med. Hyg. 79, 552–557.

Yampolskaya, O.V., Ignashenkova, G.V., 1978. Experience of seroepidemiological study of children for toxocariasis using reaction of enzyme labeled antibodies (REMA). In: 2019. Actual Situation and Area of Ascaris in Russia. vol. 4. Meditsinskaya Parazitologiya i Parazitarnye Bolezni, pp. 52–54.

Yerofeeva, V.V., 2017. Ecological and epidemiological problems of toxocarosis in Russia. Int. Res. J. 6 (60), 15–19.

Further reading

MOSCOW: Ministry of Health of Russia, 2001. Toxocarosis Prophylaxis: Methodical Guidelines MU 3.2.1043-01. Ministry of Health.

CHAPTER TWENTY-ONE

Current epidemic situation of human toxocariasis in China

Ling Kong, Hong-Juan Peng*
Department of Pathogen Biology, Guangdong Provincial Key Laboratory of Tropical Disease Research, School of Public Health, Southern Medical University, Guangzhou, China
*Corresponding author: e-mail address: hongjuan@smu.edu.cn

Contents

Abstract

Toxocariasis is a worldwide-distributed helminthic zoonosis, which mainly results from ascarid nematodes *Toxocara canis* and *Toxocara cati*. Humans become infected by accidental ingestion of infective eggs, raw or undercooked meat containing larvae. Keeping and contacting cats and dogs, and bad hygiene situations or habits are the main risk factors for *Toxocara* infection in China. The seroprevalence of *Toxocara* spp. is reported from 12.14% to 44.83%, and the overall seroprevalence in children was 12.14% in 1993 and elevated to 19.3% in 2015. Among the 103 cases reported in China during 1983–2019, ocular larva migrans (OLM), visceral larva migrans (VLM), and neural larva migrans (NLM) occupied 92.23%, 6.80%, and 0.97% of cases, respectively. The diagnosis of toxocariasis is mainly based on the history of exposure to infective eggs or larvae, clinical manifestations, laboratory examinations, and imaging studies. As most individuals who are infected with larval *Toxocara*, are unaware of their infections, patients with mild signs as described under covert toxocariasis (CT) can recover spontaneously, and treatment may not be necessary. Albendazole is the preferred treatment for patients with VLM; steroids, such as prednisolone combined with albendazole, are frequently used in treating patients with OLM, and surgery serves as an alternative treatment; thiabendazole is effective in treating patients with NLM. The true number of cases and prevalence of toxocariasis in China seems to be underestimated and neglected because of the lack of population-based epidemiological studies and insufficient clinical awareness of this disease, which are aspects that need to be improved by the Chinese government.

Advances in Parasitology, Volume 109
ISSN 0065-308X
https://doi.org/10.1016/bs.apar.2020.01.016

1. Introduction

Toxocariasis is a global cosmopolitan and typically neglected helminthic zoonosis. *Toxocara canis* and *Toxocara cati* are the major causative agents (Despommier, 2003). Both *T. canis* and *T. cati* are ascarid nematodes belonging to *Ascaridida*, superfamily *Ascaridoidea*, family *Toxocaridae*, and the genus *Toxocara*, contains a total of some 21 species (Fan et al., 2015; Moreira et al., 2014). Dogs and cats are the most common definitive hosts of *T. canis* and *T. cati*, respectively, while humans can act as one of the many mammalian paratenic hosts (Borecka and Klapec, 2015). After ingestion, the eggs hatch to release larvae in the digestion tract, where they enter the circulation and continue to complete the life cycle (Glickman and Schantz, 1981; Moreira et al., 2014; Schantz, 1989).

Human toxocariasis is a serious contributor to the worldwide disease burden, found in both developing and developed countries (Fialho and Correa, 2016; Hotez and Wilkins, 2009). Human toxocariasis may be severe in regions where basic sanitation conditions are poor and where there is a high occurrence in children (Alderete et al., 2003; Archelli et al., 2014; Fisher, 2003; Paludo et al., 2007). In Western countries, rural areas have a significantly higher prevalence (35–42%) compared with urban areas (2–5%), and children have a seroprevalence ranging from 28.8% to 62.3% (Fillaux and Magnaval, 2013; Magnaval et al., 2001).

Accidental ingestion of embryonated eggs of *T. canis* or *T. cati* is the major route for human infection and later causes larvae migration throughout various organs (Beaver et al., 1952; Magnaval et al., 2001; Morimatsu et al., 2006; Tost et al., 1998). Compared with the histopathological examination (Chieffi et al., 2009), immunological tests are more efficient for diagnosing toxocariasis (Lewis and Maizels, 1993). Using recombinant *Toxocara* excretory-secretory (TES) proteins instead of natural TES proteins has improved the sensitivity and specificity of the immunodiagnostic methods (Despommier, 2003; Moreira et al., 2014; Savigny, 1975), and western blot detection provides a more specific diagnostic result (Smith et al., 2009).

Here, we have reviewed the present situation of human toxocariasis prevalence, as well as the control status in China, to provide suggestions for public health surveillance of this disease.

2. The life cycle of *Toxocara* parasites

After mating in the intestine of a natural (definitive) host, a female adult worm produces approximately 50,000–80,000 unembryonated eggs per day, and those eggs are then excreted with the faeces (Rodríguez-Caballero et al., 2015). Approximately 2 weeks later, the unembryonated eggs will have developed under appropriate temperature and humidity conditions to be infective eggs that will each contain an infective third-stage larva. Ingestion of the infective eggs of *Toxocara* gives rise to infections in both natural hosts, mostly canids and felids, and abnormal hosts such as humans and many other mammals. After ingestion, these eggs hatch to release the third-stage larvae in the small intestine. The larvae then burrow through the intestinal wall, gain access into the circulatory system and migrate through the liver, lung, heart, and brain and are widely distributed in the body via the bloodstream (Wiśniewska-Ligier et al., 2012). In definitive hosts, most of the larvae further migrate from the trachea to oesophagus through the pharynx, reach the stomach and small intestine, and develop to adult worms in the small intestine. Transplacental infection is also common in definitive canine hosts (Parsons, 1987; Smith et al., 2009). The whole life cycle of *Toxocara* spp. from egg to adult in the dog is approximately 60–90 days (Beaver, 1962).

However, humans as paratenic hosts do not provide appropriate settings for larvae to undergo further growth or maturation. After migration throughout the body, the larvae enter various organs and remain viable and alive for several years (Finsterer and Auer, 2013; Rubinsky-Elefant et al., 2010; Woodhall et al., 2014). Humans become infected mainly through accidental ingestion of the embryonated eggs that are abundant in many canine and feline faecal contaminated soils or, less commonly, the ingestion of third-stage larvae through the consumption of raw or undercooked meats and viscera (Woodhall et al., 2014). Human infections are mostly asymptomatic (Macpherson, 2013), whereas in humans, especially children with pica who ingest soil, infections can be symptomatic and, on rare occasions, can be fatal (Beaver, 1956). There are four major clinical presentations for *Toxocara* infection in humans as follows: visceral larva migrans (VLM) or visceral toxocariasis (VT), ocular larva migrans (OLM) or ocular toxocariasis (OT), neural larva migrans (NLM) or neurotoxocariasis (NT), and covert or common toxocariasis (CT) (Borecka and Klapec, 2015).

3. Epidemic distribution of human toxocariasis in China

The epidemiologic studies reported in China are mainly from 1993 to 2019, and the first serological investigation for *Toxocara* infection was conducted in Chengdu, China in 1993 (Zhongjin, 1993). A total of 2 epidemiologic studies involving 7398 samples were reported mainly from Shandong, Jilin, Sichuan, Shanghai and Taiwan (Table 1, Fig. 1). Altogether, 103 recorded cases have been reported from 1983 to 2019, which mainly occurred in the southern provinces of China (Table 2, Fig. 1).

The seroprevalence of *Toxocara* spp. in China ranges from 12.14% to 44.83% (a cross-sectional study and a retrospective study were excluded, see Table 1). The reported serum positivity rates in the subsequent 20 years were higher than those from 1993. As the most common method for human infection, contact with cats and/or dogs was reported in all serological investigations, and *T. canis* was the major pathogeny compared with *T. cati*. Toxocariasis is more prevalent in regions where basic sanitation conditions are poor and with higher occurrence in children. The overall seroprevalence in children was 12.14% in 1993 (Zhongjin, 1993) and increased to 19.3% in 2015 (Cong et al., 2015). The positivity is 17.7% among children living in rural areas and is significantly higher than that of children living in urban areas (2.1%) (Zhongjin, 1993). Asymptomatic infection is common in children with a seroprevalence of 14.4% (Cong et al., 2015). Whether gender is a risk factor is controversial, as the gender components are different in adults and children. In adults, females have a significantly higher incidence of *Toxocara* infection compared with the males (Cong et al., 2014; Yang et al., 2016), while no significant difference was found in children (Zhongjin, 1993). In addition, *Toxocara* infection is different in ethnicity in China, as ethnic minorities have a significantly higher rate of infection than Han (Fan et al., 2004; Yang et al., 2016). Interestingly, compared with healthy individuals, the psychiatric patients show a higher seroprevalence, while pregnant women show a lower seroprevalence (Cong et al., 2014).

Except for epidemiological investigations, cases of human toxocariasis were also reported in China (Fig. 1). Although toxocariasis was first reported in 1950, the first documented case was identified as early as 1924 in Beijing, China, which was resulted by *Toxocara canis* (Qu, 2007). A few decades later, human toxocariasis cases were reported successively. A total of 103 recorded cases have been reported from 1983 to 2019, mainly occurring in southern provinces, and most cases (90.29% of total cases) were concentrated in Shanghai. In China, OLM is the main clinical form, which is the major type in most countries of the world (Chen et al., 2018b). Among the reported 103 cases, 95 cases (92.23%) were OLM, 7 cases (6.80%) were VLM, and only 1 case was NLM (0.97%). However, CT has never been reported in China. More than 90% of reported cases are children under 14 years old, which is

Table 1 Reported epidemiologic study of human *Toxocariasis* in China.

Author	Year	Location	Urban or rural	Species	No. of samples examined	Age range (years)	Seroprevalence (%)	Cats/dogs contact
Zhongjin (1993)	1993	Sichuan	Urban, rural	*T. canis*	519	3–6	Overall 12.14% Urban 2.1% Rural 17.7%	Yes
Fan et al. (2004)	2004	Taiwan	Not defined	*T. canis*	580	20 to ≥60	Overall 44.83% Han 30.2% Aboriginal 46.0%	Yes
Cong et al. (2014)	2014	Shandong	Urban, rural	Not defined	2866	15–93 Clinically healthy individuals 15–93 Pregnant women 18–43 Psychiatric patients 16–91	Overall 12.25% Clinically healthy individuals 13.07% Pregnant women 9.19% Psychiatric patients 16.40%	Yes
Cong et al. (2015)	2015	Shandong and Jilin	Urban, rural	Not defined	1458	1–18	Overall 19.3% Clinically healthy children 14.4% Sick children 26.4%	Yes
Yang et al. (2016)	2016	Shandong and Jilin	Urban, rural	Not defined	1842	≤19 to ≥60	Overall 16.07% Han 14.21% Korean 20.58% Korean 20.58% Mongol 18.89%	Yes
Chen et al. (2018a)	2018	Shanghai	Not defined	*T. canis*	77	4–51	94.81% 92.3% (UBM)	Not defined
Zhang et al. (2019)	2019	Shanghai	Not defined	Not defined	56	3–52	100%	Yes

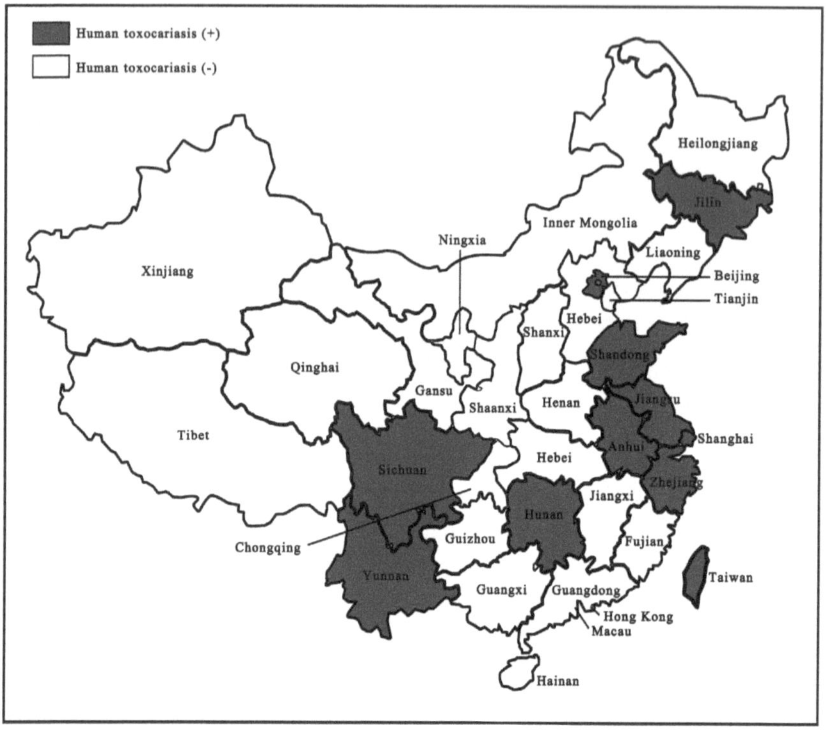

Fig. 1 Geographical distribution of human toxocariasis in China. Human toxocariasis (+): provinces with epidemiologic studies conducted or cases reported. Human toxocariasis (−): provinces with no epidemiologic studies conducted and cases reported. Red dot: the first toxocariasis case reported in Beijing in 1924.

even more prominent than the epidemiological investigations reported above. Consistent with the risk factors reported in epidemiological studies, almost all patients have a history of being in contact with dogs and/or cats.

4. Animal reservoirs of *Toxocara* in China

Animal *Toxocara* infection is distributed in most parts of China (Fig. 2). *T. canis* and *T. cati* are the major culprits of human toxocariasis, and dogs and cats are the most important animal reservoirs of toxocariasis (Ma et al., 2018). In China, *T. canis* serves as the most common parasite species of human *Toxocara* infection (Table 2). Corresponding to this is the widespread prevalence of *T. canis* in dogs, which ranges from 82.0% to 11.5%. Puppies can excrete more *Toxocara* eggs than adult dogs (Saeed et al., 2005) and have a higher prevalence than adult dogs in Sichuan (Table 3). In contrast, *T. cati* infection in humans is rarely reported in China, and a high

Table 2 Reported cases of human *Toxocariasis* in China.

Author	Year	Location	Gender	Species	No. of infections	Age(years)	Cats/dogs contact	Clinical form	Therapeutic
Wang et al. (1983)	1983	Hong Kong	Female	*T. canis*	1	43	Not defined	NLM	Thiabendazole
Liu and Wang (1994)	1994	Sichuan	Male	*T. canis*	1	9	Yes	VLM	Diethylcarbamazine Thiabendazole
Yang et al. (1996)	1996	Sichuan	Male	*T. canis*	3	3–6	Yes	VLM	Albendazole
Xiao (1999)	1999	Sichuan	Male	*T. canis*	1	4	Yes	VLM	Albendazole
Lei et al. (2008)	2008	Hunan	Male	*T. canis*	1	12	Yes	OLM	Prednison Triamcinolone acetonide
Li et al. (2009)	2009	Yunnan	Male	*T. canis*	1	Adults	Yes	VLM	Albendazole
Zhou et al. (2010)	2010	Shanghai	Male 6 female 6	*T. canis*	12	8.4 ± 4.2	Yes	OLM	Not defined
Zhou et al. (2012)	2012	Shanghai	Male 22 female 13	Not defined	35	1.5–33 Children 28, Adults 7	Yes	OLM	Not defined
Zhang et al. (2015)	2015	Jiangsu	Female	*T. canis*	1	6	Yes	OLM	Albendazole Prednisolone
Liu et al. (2016)	2016	Shanghai and surrounding provinces	Male 33 female 13	Not defined	46	≤ 14	Yes	OLM	Prednisolone Surgery
Wang et al. (2019)	2019	Zhejiang	Female	Not defined	1	56	Not defined	VLM	Albendazole

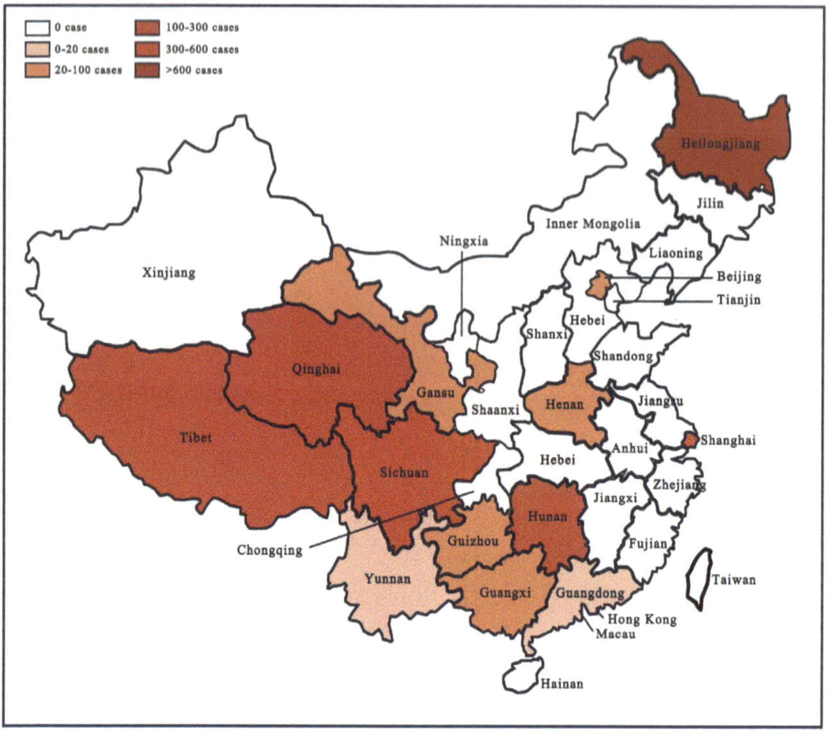

Fig. 2 Geographical distribution of reservoir host infections (animal toxocariasis) in China. Animal *Toxocara* infections have been reported in most parts of China, including the following provinces, municipalities or cities, Heilongjiang, Beijing, Gansu, Qinghai, Tibet, Sichuan, Henan, Shanghai, Hunan, Guizhou, Yunnan, Guangxi, and Guangdong. The colours are labelled based on the number of reported cases.

incidence of *T. cati* in cats exists in Guizhou (Table 3), where cats may serve as potential and important reservoir hosts. Moreover, other species of *Toxocara*, such as *T. leonine*, can infect dogs with a seroprevalence of 1.1%, and cats with a seroprevalence of 7.7% (Fang et al., 2015; Wang et al., 2006). *T. malaysiensis*, which was originally reported in Malaysia, has been reported to infect cats in Guangzhou (Li et al., 2006) and potentially infect humans (Gasser, 2013; Gibbons et al., 2001). Regarding the main source of *Toxocara* infection in China, in addition to dogs and cats, other animals, such as yak calves (Li et al., 2016), sheep (Gao et al., 2017), and even alligators (Zhao et al., 2014), can also serve as reservoirs for parasite dissemination. Therefore, the high prevalence of *Toxocara* infection in these reservoirs continuously exposes humans to infection (Strube et al., 2013). Moreover, the infection of animals also leads to heavy economic losses (Li et al., 2016).

Table 3 Prevalence of *toxocariasis* in definitive hosts and paratenic hosts.

Author	Year	Location	Number examined	Species	Prevalence
Dogs					
Andrews (1937)	1937	Shanghai	590	*T. canis* *T. leonina*	*T. canis/* *T. leonina* 17.63%
Wang et al. (1995)	1995	Guizhou	120	*T. canis*	11.50%
Luo et al. (1999)	1999	Sichuan	255	*T. canis*	1.5–2-mo-old puppies 82% adult dogs 19.5%
Wang et al. (2006)	2006	Heilongjiang	178	*T. leonine* *T. canis*	*T. leonina* 1.1% *T. canis* 36.5%
Dai et al. (2009)	2009	Hunan	438	*T. canis*	45.2%
Li et al. (2009)	2009	Yunnan	10	*T. canis*	70%
Fang et al. (2015)	2015	Guangxi	40	*T. canis*	30%
Cats					
Andrews (1937)	1937	Shanghai	185	*T. mystax*	*T. mystax* 35.14%
Wang et al. (1995)	1995	Guizhou	35	*T. cati*	42.8%
Fang et al. (2015)	2015	Guangxi	39	*T. cati* *T. leonine*	*T. cati* 5.1% *T. leonine* 7.7%
Yang and Liang (2015)	2015	Henan and Beijing	360	*T. cati*	17.78%
Yak calves					
Li et al. (2016)	2016	Qinghai Tibetan Plateau	891	*T. vitulorum*	Qinghai 20.1% Tibet 17.2% Sichuan 40.9% Gansu 7.6%
Sheep					
Gao et al. (2017)	2017	Heilongjiang	7027	*T. cati* *T. canis*	*T. cati* and *T. canis* eggs 74.6%

5. The diagnostic and treatment methods for human toxocariasis

The diagnosis of toxocariasis is mainly based on the history of exposure to infective eggs or larvae and on clinical manifestations, laboratory examinations (histopathological examination and blood tests), imaging studies and immunologic tests (Fan et al., 2015; Fillaux and Magnaval, 2013). Regarding the diagnosis of ocular toxocariasis, due to its complex and nonspecific clinical symptoms, it is also necessary to combine epidemiological investigations and even surgery (Lei et al., 2008). Second-stage larvae identified in biopsy tissue samples by histopathological examination are recognized as the gold standard for the diagnosis of human toxocariasis (Chieffi et al., 2009; Hotez and Wilkins, 2009). However, this method extremely depends on the number and location of larvae present in biopsy materials (Fillaux and Magnaval, 2013). Considering this difficulty, diverse immunological tests become the most common method used for toxocariasis diagnosis (Magnaval et al., 2001). These tests include enzyme-linked immunosorbent assays (ELISA) (Jin et al., 2013; Savigny, 1975), western blot (WB)-based fraction native TES (TES-WB) and indirect TES–IgG–ELISA (Smith et al., 2009; Watthanakulpanich et al., 2008). In China, ELISA using native TES had been in use until approximately 2004 (Fan et al., 2004), and a commercial kit replaced it in recent years (Cong et al., 2014, 2015). A variety of imaging technologies, such as computed tomography, magnetic resonance imaging and high-frequency ultrasonography (Liu et al., 2016; Zhang et al., 2015; Zhou et al., 2012), are also available in China. Among them, ultrasound biomicroscopy (UBM) shows great potential in OLM diagnosis (Chen et al., 2018a). In addition to the diagnosis of human toxocariasis, the use of molecular tools, such as PCR (Chang et al., 2015; He et al., 2017; Li et al., 2006, 2007), assists Chinese researchers in identifying and verifying the species of *Toxocara* spp. from dogs and cats.

An accurate diagnosis of clinical types of human toxocariasis decides whether patients should receive treatment, surgical intervention. Syndromes, such as CT, will recover spontaneously, and treatment may not be necessary, while patients with VLM should be treated at an earlier stage (Magnaval and Glickman, 2006). Benzimidazole derivatives, such as albendazole (ABZ), are a preferred choice for VLM treatment (Despommier, 2003; Hotez and Wilkins, 2009), while mebendazole (MBZ) is a second, optional choice (Chen et al., 2012; Magnaval et al., 2001). The treatment for OLM is more difficult than VLM, and systemic application of corticosteroids combined with albendazole is recommended (Satou et al., 2005). There are not many clinical drug candidates for NLM treatment. Albendazole, corticosteroids, and corticoids used alone or in combination can be considered (Fan et al., 2015). Recent years, novel interventions, such as probiotics, immunomodulators, and DNA vaccines, have shown potential against toxocariasis (Moreira et al., 2014). In China, there is no available vaccine against toxocariasis thus far. Drug treatment is the most important for toxocariasis therapies, which is similar to other countries (Chen et al., 2018b). As shown in Table 2, the use of albendazole is the preferred choice for VLM treatment; the use of steroids, such as prednisolone combined with albendazole, has the highest frequency in OLM treatment. Although the prognosis of the surgical treatment is unfavourable, surgery still can serves as an alternative choice for OLM treatment (Zhang et al., 2019); and the use of thiabendazole for NLM treatment is effective (Table 2).

6. Suggestions for the formulation of control strategies against toxocariasis

Toxocariasis is a typical neglected helminthic zoonosis. *T. canis* and *T. cati* contribute greatly to the prevalence of the disease. An increasing number of dogs and cats have been raised in Chinese families, and this is particularly dangerous for young children and elders (Cong et al., 2014; Wang et al., 2006). Owing to this situation, some suggestions for developing control strategies and measures are offered as follows.

First, human infection with *Toxocara* in China is related to being in contact with dogs and/or cats and hygiene practices. Appropriate preventive measures should be taken to improve the deworming of dogs and cats, to strengthen the management of the pet market and to promote the responsibility of pet ownership in China (Jianjun and Shijia, 2008). Moreover, dogs and cats should be barred from freely entering the fields with surface vegetable crops and parks where children play on the grass and in the dirt (Kozan et al., 2005). In addition, good hygiene practices should be emphasized among the public (Woodhall et al., 2014). For example, washing vegetables harvested from the soil, hands after contacting pets, or having activities on the ground outside.

Second, *Toxocara* eggs released into environments exist alive for a long time (Parsons, 1987), which is a major difficulty in preventing human toxocariasis (Chieffi et al., 2009). Owing to this, surveillance should be strengthened by public health authorities. The prevalence and transmission of toxocariasis, including the transmission of *Toxocara* spp. eggs, the distribution of eggs in public places, and the climate (Liu et al., 2016) should be taken into account in the development of surveillance programs. Only in this way can we develop a more reasonable control strategy to prevent *Toxocara* eggs from contaminating environments. Unexpectedly, we only found one study in the literature concerning the spatial distribution of *T. canis* and *T. cati* eggs in soils in urban areas of China (Gao et al., 2017).

Third, designed and optimized epidemiological investigations and standardized detection methods would help to obtain an accurate prevalence rate of *Toxocara* infection and to identify the role of behavioural habits and environmental factors for human toxocariasis (Smith et al., 2009).

7. Conclusion

Toxocariasis is a worldwide-distributed zoonotic parasitosis, mainly caused by *Toxocara canis* and *Toxocara cati*. Humans are infected through ingesting infective eggs, raw or under cooked meat harbouring larvae. Contact with cats, dogs and poor hygiene habits are the main causes of *Toxocara* infection in China. The serum positivity of *Toxocara* spp. reported in China ranged from 12.14% to 44.83%. The seropositivity rate of children was 12.14% in 1993 and elevated to 19.3% in 2015. During 1983 to 2019, a total of 103 toxocariasis cases were reported in China. The ocular larval migration (OLM), visceral larval migration (VLM) and neurolarval migration (NLM) accounted for 92.23%, 6.80% and 0.97%, respectively. The diagnosis of toxoplasmosis mainly depends on the history of contacting infective eggs or larvae, clinical manifestations, laboratory examinations and imaging diagnosis. In terms of treatment, asymptomatic patients with positive serologic titres will likely recover spontaneously without treatment. Albendazole is the preferred treatment for VLM patients; prednisone and other steroids combined with albendazole are often used to treat OLM patients, and surgery is also an alternative OLM therapy; thiabendazole is effective for treating NLM patients. Due to the lack of population-based epidemiological investigation and insufficient clinical knowledge of this disease, toxocariasis seems to be neglected and underestimated in China. The Chinese government needs to improve its surveillance and pay more attention to toxocariasis.

Acknowledgements

This research was supported by National Key R&D Program of China (2017YFD0500400), National Natural Science Foundation of China (81572012, 81772217, 20180907), Guangdong Provincial Natural Science Foundation Project (2016A030311025, 2017A030313694), Science and Technology Planning Project of Guangdong Province (2018A050506038), and Key Project of Guangzhou Science Research (201904020011) to H.J.P.

References

Alderete, J.M., Jacob, C.M., Pastorino, A.C., Elefant, G.R., Castro, A.P., Fomin, A.B., Chieffi, P.P., 2003. Prevalence of *Toxocara* infection in schoolchildren from the Butanta region, Sao Paulo, Brazil. Mem. Inst. Oswaldo Cruz 98, 593–597.

Andrews, M.N., 1937. The helminth parasites of dogs and cats in Shanghai, China. J. Helminthol. 15 (3), 145–152.

Archelli, S., Santillan, G.I., Fonrouge, R., Cespedes, G., Burgos, L., Radman, N., 2014. Toxocariasis: seroprevalence in abandoned-institutionalized children and infants. Rev. Argent. Microbiol. 46, 3–6.

Beaver, P.C., 1956. Larva migrans. Exp. Parasitol. 5, 587–621.

Beaver, P.C., 1962. Toxocarosis (visceral larva migrans) in relation to tropical eosinophilia. Bull. Soc. Pathol. Exot. Filiales 55, 555–576.

Beaver, P.C., Snyder, C.H., Carrera, G.M., Dent, J.H., Lafferty, J.W., 1952. Chronic eosinophilia due to visceral larva migrans; report of three cases. Pediatrics 9, 7–19.

Borecka, A., Klapec, T., 2015. Epidemiology of human toxocariasis in Poland—a review of cases 1978–2009. Ann. Agric. Environ. Med. 22, 28–31.

Chang, Q.C., Gao, J.F., Sheng, Z.H., Lou, Y., Zheng, X., Wang, C.R., 2015. Sequence variability in three mitochondrial genes among four roundworm species from wild animals in China. Mitochondrial DNA 26, 75–78.

Chen, J., Xu, M.J., Zhou, D.H., Song, H.Q., Wang, C.R., Zhu, X.Q., 2012. Canine and feline parasitic zoonoses in China. Parasit. Vectors 5, 152.

Chen, Q., Gu, J., Jiang, R., Zhou, M., Chang, Q., 2018a. Role of ultrasound biomicroscopy in diagnosis of ocular toxocariasis. Br. J. Ophthalmol. 102, 642–646.

Chen, J., Liu, Q., Liu, G.-H., Zheng, W.-B., Hong, S.-J., Sugiyama, H., Zhu, X.-Q., Elsheikha, H.M., 2018b. Toxocariasis: a silent threat with a progressive public health impact. Infect. Dis. Poverty 7, 59.

Chieffi, P.P., Santos, S.V., Queiroz, M.L., Lescano, S.A., 2009. Human toxocariasis: contribution by Brazilian researchers. Rev. Inst. Med. Trop. Sao Paulo 51, 301–308.

Cong, W., Zhang, X.X., Zhou, N., Yu, C.Z., Chen, J., Wang, X.Y., Li, B., Qian, A.D., Zhu, X.Q., 2014. *Toxocara* seroprevalence among clinically healthy individuals, pregnant women and psychiatric patients and associated risk factors in Shandong Province, Eastern China. PLoS Negl. Trop. Dis. 8, e3082.

Cong, W., Meng, Q.F., You, H.L., Zhou, N., Dong, X.Y., Dong, W., Wang, X.Y., Qian, A.D., Zhu, X.Q., 2015. Seroprevalence and risk factors of *Toxocara* infection among children in Shandong and Jilin provinces, China. Acta Trop. 152, 215–219.

Dai, R.S., Li, Z.Y., Li, F., Liu, D.X., Liu, W., Liu, G.H., He, S.W., Tan, M.Y., Lin, R.Q., Liu, Y., Zhu, X.Q., 2009. Severe infection of adult dogs with helminths in Hunan Province, China poses significant public health concerns. Vet. Parasitol. 160 (3–4), 348–350.

Despommier, D., 2003. Toxocariasis: clinical aspects, epidemiology, medical ecology, and molecular aspects. Clin. Microbiol. Rev. 16, 265–272.

Fan, C.K., Lan, H.S., Hung, C.C., Chung, W.C., Liao, C.W., Du, W.Y., Su, K.E., 2004. Seroepidemiology of *Toxocara canis* infection among mountain aboriginal adults in Taiwan. Am. J. Trop. Med. Hyg. 71, 216–221.

Fan, C.K., Holland, C.V., Loxton, K., Barghouth, U., 2015. Cerebral toxocariasis: silent progression to neurodegenerative disorders? Clin. Microbiol. Rev. 28, 663–686.

Fang, F., Li, J., Huang, T., Guillot, J., Huang, W., 2015. Zoonotic helminths parasites in the digestive tract of feral dogs and cats in Guangxi, China. BMC Vet. Res. 11, 211.

Fialho, P.M., Correa, C.R., 2016. A systematic review of toxocariasis: a neglected but high-prevalence disease in Brazil. Am. J. Trop. Med. Hyg. 94, 1193–1199.

Fillaux, J., Magnaval, J.F., 2013. Laboratory diagnosis of human toxocariasis. Vet. Parasitol. 193, 327–336.

Finsterer, J., Auer, H., 2013. Parasitoses of the human central nervous system. J. Helminthol. 87, 257–270.

Fisher, M., 2003. *Toxocara cati*: an underestimated zoonotic agent. Trends Parasitol. 19, 167–170.

Gao, X., Wang, H., Li, J., Qin, H., Xiao, J., 2017. Influence of land use and meteorological factors on the spatial distribution of *Toxocara canis* and *Toxocara cati* eggs in soil in urban areas. Vet. Parasitol. 233, 80–85.

Gasser, R.B., 2013. A perfect time to harness advanced molecular technologies to explore the fundamental biology of Toxocara species. Vet. Parasitol. 193, 353–364.

Gibbons, L.M., Jacobs, D.E., Sani, R.A., 2001. Toxocara malaysiensis n. sp. (Nematoda: Ascaridoidea) from the domestic cat (*Felis catus* Linnaeus, 1758). J. Parasitol. 87, 660–665.

Glickman, L.T., Schantz, P.M., 1981. Epidemiology and pathogenesis of zoonotic toxocariasis. Epidemiol. Rev. 3, 230–250.

He, X., Lv, M.N., Liu, G.H., Lin, R.Q., 2017. Genetic analysis of *Toxocara cati* (Nematoda: Ascarididae) from Guangdong province, subtropical China. Mitochondrial DNA A DNA Mapp. Seq. Anal. 29, 1–4.

Hotez, P.J., Wilkins, P.P., 2009. Toxocariasis: America's most common neglected infection of poverty and a helminthiasis of global importance? PLoS Negl. Trop. Dis. 3, e400.

Jianjun, W.L.P., Shijia, H., 2008. Problems in pet dog breeding in China and their strategy. Chin. J. Wildl. 6, 013.

Jin, Y., Shen, C., Huh, S., Sohn, W.-M., Choi, M.-H., Hong, S.-T., 2013. Serodiagnosis of toxocariasis by ELISA using crude antigen of *Toxocara canis* larvae. Korean J. Parasitol. 51, 433.

Kozan, E., Gonenc, B., Sarimehmetoglu, O., Aycicek, H., 2005. Prevalence of helminth eggs on raw vegetables used for salads. Food Control 16, 239–242.

Lei, S.B., Guo, X.J., Tang, L.S., 2008. A case of ocular toxocariasis. Chin. J. Ocul. Fundus Dis. 21, 299–300.

Lewis, J., Maizels, R., 1993. *Toxocara* and Toxocariasis: Clinical, Epidemiological and Molecular Perspectives. Institute of Biology.

Li, M.W., Zhu, X.Q., Gasser, R.B., Lin, R.Q., Sani, R.A., Lun, Z.R., Jacobs, D.E., 2006. The occurrence of *Toxocara malaysiensis* in cats in China, confirmed by sequence-based analyses of ribosomal DNA. Parasitol. Res. 99, 554–557.

Li, M.W., Lin, R.Q., Chen, H.H., Sani, R.A., Song, H.Q., Zhu, X.Q., 2007. PCR tools for the verification of the specific identity of ascaridoid nematodes from dogs and cats. Mol. Cell. Probes 21, 349–354.

Li, X.R., Dong, Y.X., Duan, Y.H., Zeng, G.X., Wang, F.Y., Wang, Y.B., 2009. A reported case of *Toxocara canis*. Livestock Poultry Industry 242 (6), 93.

Li, K., Lan, Y., Luo, H., Zhang, H., Liu, D., Zhang, L., Gui, R., Wang, L., Shahzad, M., Sizhu, S., Li, J., Chamba, Y., 2016. Prevalence, associated risk factors, and phylogenetic analysis of *Toxocara vitulorum* infection in yaks on the Qinghai Tibetan Plateau, China. Korean J. Parasitol. 54, 645–652.

Liu, Y.F., Wang, H.Y., 1994. A case with *Toxocara canis* infection. Chin. J. Pediatrics 32 (5), 305.
Liu, Y., Zhang, Q., Li, J., Ji, X., Xu, Y., Zhao, P., 2016. Clinical characteristics of pediatric patients with ocular toxocariasis in China. Ophthalmologica 235, 97–105.
Luo, Z.J., Wang, G.X., Yang, C.I., Luo, C.H., Cheng, S.W., Liao, L., 1999. Detection of circulating antigens and antibodies in *Toxocara canis* infection among children in Chengdu, China. J. Parasitol. 85 (2), 252–256.
Ma, G., Holland, C.V., Wang, T., Hofmann, A., Fan, C.-K., Maizels, R.M., Hotez, P.J., Gasser, R.B., 2018. Human toxocariasis. Lancet Infect. Dis. 18, e14–e24.
Macpherson, C.N., 2013. The epidemiology and public health importance of toxocariasis: a zoonosis of global importance. Int. J. Parasitol. 43, 999–1008.
Magnaval, J.-F., Glickman, L.T., 2006. Management and treatment options for human toxocariasis. *Toxocara*: the enigmatic. Parasite, 113–126.
Magnaval, J.F., Glickman, L.T., Dorchies, P., Morassin, B., 2001. Highlights of human toxocariasis. Korean J. Parasitol. 39, 1–11.
Moreira, G.M., Telmo Pde, L., Mendonca, M., Moreira, A.N., Mcbride, A.J., Scaini, C.J., Conceicao, F.R., 2014. Human toxocariasis: current advances in diagnostics, treatment, and interventions. Trends Parasitol. 30, 456–464.
Morimatsu, Y., Akao, N., Akiyoshi, H., Kawazu, T., Okabe, Y., Aizawa, H., 2006. A familial case of visceral larva migrans after ingestion of raw chicken livers: appearance of specific antibody in bronchoalveolar lavage fluid of the patients. Am. J. Trop. Med. Hyg. 75, 303–306.
Paludo, M.L., Falavigna, D.L., Elefant, G.R., Gomes, M.L., Baggio, M.L., Amadei, L.B., Falavigna-Guilherme, A.L., 2007. Frequency of *Toxocara* infection in children attended by the health public service of Maringa, south Brazil. Rev. Inst. Med. Trop. Sao Paulo 49, 343–348.
Parsons, J.C., 1987. Ascarid infections of cats and dogs. Vet. Clin. North Am. Small Anim. Pract. 17, 1307–1339.
Qu, F.Y., 2007. Historical review on the development of medical parasitology in China during the years of 1871-2006. Zhongguo Ji Sheng Chong Xue Yu Ji Sheng Chong Bing Za Zhi 25, 259–273.
Rodríguez-Caballero, A., Martínez-Gordillo, M.N., Medina-Flores, Y., Medina-Escutia, M.E., Meza-Lucas, A., Correa, D., Caballero-Salazar, S., Ponce-Macotela, M., 2015. Successful capture of *Toxocara canis* larva antigens from human serum samples. Parasit. Vectors 8, 264.
Rubinsky-Elefant, G., Hirata, C.E., Yamamoto, J.H., Ferreira, M.U., 2010. Human toxocariasis: diagnosis, worldwide seroprevalences and clinical expression of the systemic and ocular forms. Ann. Trop. Med. Parasitol. 104, 3–23.
Saeed, I., Taira, K., Kapel, C.M., 2005. *Toxocara canis* in experimentally infected silver and arctic foxes. Parasitol. Res. 97, 160–166.
Satou, T., Horiuchi, A., Akao, N., Koike, K., Fujita, K., Nikaido, T., 2005. *Toxocara canis*: search for a potential drug amongst β-carboline alkaloids—*in vitro* and mouse studies. Exp. Parasitol. 110, 134–139.
Savigny, D.H., 1975. *In vitro* maintenance of *Toxocara canis* larvae and a simple method for the production of *Toxocara* ES antigen for use in serodiagnostic tests for visceral larva migrans. J. Parasitol. 61, 781–782.
Schantz, P.M., 1989. Toxocara larva migrans now. Am. J. Trop. Med. Hyg. 41, 21–34.
Smith, H., Holland, C., Taylor, M., Magnaval, J.F., Schantz, P., Maizels, R., 2009. How common is human toxocariasis? Towards standardizing our knowledge. Trends Parasitol. 25, 182–188.
Strube, C., Heuer, L., Janecek, E., 2013. *Toxocara* spp. infections in paratenic hosts. Vet. Parasitol. 193, 375–389.

Tost, F., Hellmann, A., Ockert, G., 1998. *Toxocara canis* infection. Environmental parasitologic and epidemiologic studies. Ophthalmologe 95, 486–489.
Wang, C., Huang, C., Chan, P., Preston, P., Chau, P., 1983. Transverse myelitis associated with larva migrans: finding of larva in cerebrospinal fluid. The Lancet 321 (8321), 423.
Wang, D.D., Liu, X.M., Han, X., 1995. Investigation of the helminthes infection in dogs and cats in Guizhou Province. Chin. Vet. Sci. Technol. 25 (2), 13–15.
Wang, C.R., Qiu, J.H., Zhao, J.P., Xu, L.M., Yu, W.C., Zhu, X.Q., 2006. Prevalence of helminthes in adult dogs in Heilongjiang Province, the People's Republic of China. Parasitol. Res. 99, 627–630.
Wang, C., Huang, C., Yin, Y., Yang, F., 2019. A case of hepatic visceral larva migrans. Chin. J. Hepatol. 27 (7), 561–562.
Watthanakulpanich, D., Smith, H.V., Hobbs, G., Whalley, A.J., Billington, D., 2008. Application of *Toxocara canis* excretory–secretory antigens and IgG subclass antibodies (IgG1-4) in serodiagnostic assays of human toxocariasis. Acta Trop. 106, 90–95.
Wiśniewska-Ligier, M., Woźniakowska-Gęsicka, T., Sobolewska-Dryjańska, J., Markiewicz-Jóźwiak, A., Wieczorek, M., 2012. Analysis of the course and treatment of toxocariasis in children—a long-term observation. Parasitol. Res. 110, 2363–2371.
Woodhall, D.M., Eberhard, M.L., Parise, M.E., 2014. Neglected parasitic infections in the United States: toxocariasis. Am. J. Trop. Med. Hyg. 90, 810–813.
Xiao, X.M., 1999. Fever and epilepsy induced by *Toxocara canis* infection: a case report. Chin. Pediatr. Emerg. Med. 3, 142.
Yang, Y., Liang, H., 2015. Prevalence and risk factors of intestinal parasites in cats from China. Biomed. Res. Int. 2015, 967238.
Yang, C.L., Luo, C.H., Jia, C.S., Luo, Z.J., Chen, S.W., Wang, G.X., 1996. Asthmatic bronchitis caused by *Toxocara* infection. Chin. J. Appl. Clin. Pediatrics 1, 54–55.
Yang, G.L., Zhang, X.X., Shi, C.W., Yang, W.T., Jiang, Y.L., Wei, Z.T., Wang, C.F., Zhao, Q., 2016. Seroprevalence and associated risk factors of *Toxocara* infection in Korean, Manchu, Mongol, and Han ethnic groups in northern China. Epidemiol. Infect. 144, 3101–3107.
Zhang, H.F., Hua, H.Y., Wang, W., 2015. Pediatric ocular toxocariasis in Jiangsu Province, eastern China. Southeast Asian J. Trop. Med. Public Health 46, 8–14.
Zhang, T., Guo, D., Xu, G., Jiang, R., 2019. Ocular toxocariasis: long-term follow-up and prognosis of patients following vitrectomy. Ocul. Immunol. Inflamm. 1–7. https://doi.org/10.1080/09273948.2019.1597897.
Zhao, J., Zhou, Y., Wang, S., Tu, G., Tang, X., Wu, X., 2014. Preliminary report on the intestinal parasites and their diversity in captive Chinese alligators. Nutr. Hosp. 31, 813–819.
Zhongjin, L., 1993. A survey of serum antibodies against *Toxocara* larvae for preschool children in Chengdu area. Chin. J. Zoonoses 1, 2–4.
Zhou, M., Chang, Q., Xu, G.Z., 2010. Application of intraocular fluid examination in the diagnosis of pediatric uveitis. Chin. J. Ophthalmol. Otorhinolaryngol. 10 (3), 160–162+207.
Zhou, M., Chang, Q., Gonzales, J.A., Chen, Q., Zhang, Y., Huang, X., Xu, G., Wang, W., Jiang, R., 2012. Clinical characteristics of ocular toxocariasis in eastern China. Graefes Arch. Clin. Exp. Ophthalmol. 250, 1373–1378.

CHAPTER TWENTY-TWO

Seroprevalence of *Toxocara* spp. infection in Southeast Asia and Taiwan

Chia-Mei Chou[a], **Chia-Kwung Fan**[a,b,c,*]

[a]Department of Molecular Parasitology and Tropical Diseases, School of Medicine, College of Medicine, Taipei Medical University, Taipei, Taiwan
[b]Research Center of International Tropical Medicine, College of Medicine, Taipei Medical University, Taipei, Taiwan
[c]Tropical Medicine Division, International PhD Program in Medicine, College of Medicine, Taipei Medical University, Taipei, Taiwan
*Corresponding author: e-mail address: tedfan@tmu.edu.tw

Contents

Abstract

Human toxocariasis is a worldwide neglected zoonotic parasitic disease and caused mainly by *Toxocara canis*, and to a lesser event, by *T. cati*. There are only 16 epidemiological studies and 5 clinical toxocariasis case reports in 11 Southeast Asia countries and Taiwan (SEAT) that were found by searching data from PubMed in the period from January 1992 to August 2019. The overall seroprevalence in SEAT varied from 3.9% to 84.6% chiefly detected by using *T. canis* larval excretory-secretory antigen (TcES)-based ELISA. Playing with dogs or contacting *Toxocara* eggs from the contaminated soil or vegetables or eating raw meats/viscera containing encapsulated larvae seem likely the major risk factors leading to human toxocariasis in SEAT. Nevertheless,

Advances in Parasitology, Volume 109
ISSN 0065-308X
https://doi.org/10.1016/bs.apar.2020.01.020

undertaking comprehensive seroepidemiological studies to establish the baseline data and beware of clinical toxocariasis cases by physicians as well as establishing adequate serodiagnostic methods in detection of *Toxocara* infection, e.g., TcES-based immunoblotting method in helminth endemic SEA are strongly required.

1. Introduction

Human toxocariasis is a worldwide zoonotic parasitic disease and caused mainly by *Toxocara canis* and to a lesser extent by *T. cati* (Ma et al., 2018). Humans can get infection by accidental ingestion of *T. canis* and *T. cati* embryonated eggs containing the third-stage larvae through contact with contaminated soil, sandboxes, food and water, as well as, larvae in raw or undercooked viscera and meats of paratenic hosts (Fan et al., 2013; Uga and Kataoka, 1995). Since humans are also a paratenic host of *T. canis* and *T. cati*, the third-stage larvae emerged from the eggs will further penetrate through the small intestine, migrate and invade various internal organs such as the liver or lungs, thus causing visceral larva migrans (VLM), the eyes causing ocular larva migrans (OLM), or the central nervous system (CNS) leading to neurotoxocariasis (NT) (Fan et al., 2015).

The worldwide seroprevalence of toxocariasis varies from 1.6% to 98.8%, indicating the profound impact of *Toxocara* spp. on global human health. Southeast Asia consists of 11 countries that reach from eastern India to China and is generally divided into "mainland" and "island" zones. The mainland (Burma, Thailand, Laos, Cambodia, and Vietnam) is actually an extension of the Asian continent. Island or maritime Southeast Asia includes Malaysia, Singapore, Indonesia, the Philippines, Brunei, and East Timor. Virtually all of Southeast Asia lies between the tropics, and so there are similarities in climate as well as plant and animal life throughout the region. Temperatures are generally warm, although it is cooler in highland areas. Many sea and jungle products are unique to the region (Emmerson, 1984). Even though Taiwan is not one part of SEA, however, there are more than 500 thousands foreign labourers in Taiwan, who mainly come from SEA countries, especially Thailand, Indonesia, Philippines and Vietnam (Cheng, 2016) due to very close geographic location and transportation convenience between Taiwan and SEA. However, the seroprevalence of human toxocariasis among a total of 11 countries of Southeast Asia (SEA) is not well investigated. Herein, we searched for, found, and reviewed epidemiological studies and case reports of toxocariasis in Taiwan and 11 SEA countries from PubMed in the period from January 1992 to August 2019.

The reports included were from Brunei, Cambodia, East Timor (Timor-Leste), Indonesia, Lao People's Democratic Republic (Lao PDR), Malaysia, Myanmar, Philippines, Singapore, Thailand and Vietnam to figure out the prevalence of human toxocariasis and future prospective studies in these countries.

2. Search strategy

To evaluate the overall epidemiological studies and case reports of toxocariasis in Taiwan and 11 SEA countries, we designed a systematic review by searching the literature released online or published in academic journals in English from the PubMed database. For the search was made for papers published from January 1992 to August 2019. The current review was done using medical subject headings (MeSH) terms including: "*Toxocara*", "case", "Southeast Asia" and "individual country name". Using few key-words alone or combined together for searching and eliminating a quantity of unqualified paper by manual assessment, we tried to cover all eligible papers with minimal personal error. In addition, all case reports of toxocariasis among Taiwan and 11 SEA countries published in 1996–2019 were included. To assess the eligibility criteria, all papers were reviewed by two independent reviewers (Chou and Fan). Epidemiological investigations enclosing mass surveys and screening in people living in these countries are also included. The contradictions among selected papers were unravelled by discussion and consensus. In total, 21 papers including 5 case reports (7 clinical cases) and 16 seroepidemiological studies met the criteria for inclusion into this literature review (Tables 1 and 2).

3. Seroprevalence and risk factors of human toxocariasis in SEA and Taiwan

There were a total of 16 seroprevalence studies found from PubMed which were conducted in SEA countries and Taiwan in the period from January 1992 to August 2019 (Table 1). The overall seroprevalence of human toxocariasis varied from 6.0% to 84.6% as conducted by using *T. canis* larval excretory-secretory antigens (TcES)-based ELISA.

3.1 Indonesia

In Indonesia, a high seroprevalence rate (63.2%) was found among children and teenagers from northeast Bali (Chomel et al., 1993) as well as 63.0% of

Table 1 Seroprevalence of *Toxocara* infection in Southeast Asian countries and Taiwan.

Country	Number of studies	Seroprevalence of toxocariasis	Diagnostic method			School children only	Adult only	All aged group/without mention	Risk factors	References
			ELISA	Western blotting	Other methods					
Brunei	0	N/A	N/A	N/A	N/A	N/A	N/A	N/A	N/A	N/A
Cambodia	0	N/A	N/A	N/A	N/A	N/A	N/A	N/A	N/A	N/A
East Timor (Timor-Leste)	0	N/A	N/A	N/A	N/A	N/A	N/A	N/A	N/A	N/A
Indonesia	3	12.2–84.6%	3	0	0	2	0	1	Eating habits and poor hygiene	Chomel et al. (1993), Hayashi et al. (2005), and Uga et al. (1996)
Lao PDR	0	N/A	N/A	N/A	N/A	N/A	N/A	N/A	N/A	N/A
Malaysia	6	3.9–35.5%	6[a]	0	1[a]	2	0	4	Contact with soil	Chan et al. (2001), Hakim et al. (1993), Hakim et al. (1992, 1997), Lim et al. (2015), and Romano et al. (2010)
Myanmar	0	N/A	N/A	N/A	N/A	N/A	N/A	N/A	N/A	N/A

Philippines	1	49.0%	1	0	0	1	0	0	Soil contamination	Fajutag and Paller (2013)
Singapore	0	N/A	N/A	N/A	N/A	N/A	N/A	N/A	N/A	N/A
Taiwan	4	8.4–76.6%	3	1	0	2	2	0	Raise dogs, play in soil and eat raw pig liver	Fan et al. (2004a,b, 2005) and Fu et al. (2015)
Thailand	1	6.0%	1[b]	0	0	1	0	0	Soil contamination	Doi et al. (2017)
Vietnam	1	45.2%	1	0	0	0	0	1	Eating habits and contact with soil	Nguyen et al. (2016)
Overall	16	3.9–84.6%	15	1	1	8	2	6		

[a]One study used both ELISA and rapid diagnostic test to detect the anti-*Toxocara* antibodies.
[b]Using both urine and serum ELISA to determine *Toxocara* antibody.
N/A, not available.

Table 2 Clinical case reports of human toxocariasis in Southeast Asian countries and Taiwan.

Country	Number of clinical cases	Diagnosted method	Type of human toxocariasis	Risk factors	References
Brunei	0	N/A	N/A	N/A	N/A
Cambodia	0	N/A	N/A	N/A	N/A
East Timor (Timor-Leste)	0	N/A	N/A	N/A	N/A
Indonesia	0	N/A	N/A	N/A	N/A
Lao PDR	0	N/A	N/A	N/A	N/A
Malaysia	1	ELISA, indirect ophthalmoscopy[a]	OLM	N/A	Sivaratnam et al. (2008)
	1	ELISA	OLM	Water contamination	Azira and Zeehaida (2011)
	1	Western blot	OLM	Close contact with a cat	Guan-Fook et al. (2012)
Myanmar	0	N/A	N/A	N/A	N/A
Philippines	0	N/A	N/A	N/A	N/A
Singapore	0	N/A	N/A	N/A	N/A
Taiwan	18[c]	Western blot	OLM (7/18) CT suspected (3/18)	Contact with dogs, play in soil, eat raw vegetables	N/A[c]
Thailand	3	ELISA	OLM	N/A	Srimuang et al. (1996)
Vietnam	1	ELISA, PCR[b]	OLM	Contact with dogs	Van De et al. (2013)
Overall	25				

[a]A small larva was seen by indirect ophthalmoscopy.
[b]A larva embedded in the surrounding cyst was collected from patient's left eye by surgery and assessed the *Toxocara* ITS gene by PCR.
[c]Cases unpublished in Fan's lab from 2008 to 2019 August in Taiwan.

224 inhabitants from Sidoarjo of East Java were found as seropositive for *T. canis* infection (Uga et al., 1996). Additionally, a high prevalence of 84.6% of *Toxocara* infection was found in 117 junior high school students from two rural districts near Manado of northern Sulawesi Province of Indonesia, which included 53 subjects (45.3%) with a high sero-titre of specific anti-*Toxocara* antibodies. It is possible that this may have resulted from the local eating habits and poor hygiene in this area compared to the urban districts where there was a comparatively low prevalence of 12.2% among 41 school children in the other urban districts (Hayashi et al., 2005).

3.2 Malaysia

Most epidemiological studies of *Toxocara* infection in SEA were investigated in Malaysia. The seroprevalence of *Toxocara* infection in Malaysia is varied from 3.9% to 35.5% (Table 1). Since Malaysia is a multiracial country, the seroprevalence of human toxocariasis varies from different races and living styles. It has been shown that there was the highest positive rate in Indians (35.5%), followed by Malaysian aborigines, Orang Asli (31.9%), Muslim Malays (14.8%) and Chinese (10.9%) (Hakim et al., 1992, 1993). In the traditional living habits, raising dogs is more common in Chinese society rather than Indians and Muslim Malays; however, eating raw vegetables is more frequent in Indians than traditional Chinese people. Nevertheless, it seems unlikely that contact with dogs is the major risk factors in Malaysia. Several studies have indicated that *Toxocara* ova were the most prevalent zoonotic helminthes contaminating the soil (Azian et al., 2008; Mohd Zain et al., 2015; Ngui et al., 2014), suggesting the contamination of dogs' and cats' faeces in soil might be most important as public health risks. Relative to gender, male Orang Asli indigenous people had a higher level of antibody prevalence than did females as diagnosed by IgG4-ELISA, which were 9.5% and 1%, respectively (Romano et al., 2010). Another study also disclosed a similar seroprevalence difference between males and females (Lim et al., 2015). Moreover, the children in two studies in Malaysia had a higher positive rate than the adults (Hakim et al., 1993; Romano et al., 2010), which differs from studies conducted in Indonesia (Uga et al., 1996). Interestingly, it was found that middle-aged people of Serendah Orang Asli Village conversely have the highest infection rate of *Toxocara* and followed by adolescents, and then children, no matter whether the test that was used was the rTES-30-ELISA or a rapid diagnostic test (Lim et al., 2015). However, it was also found that the overall infection rate of soil-transmitted helminths (STH) was high in subjects diagnosed as seropositive of *Toxocara* infection using TcES-ELISA, suggesting there was a high possibility of antigenic cross-reactivity between *Toxocara* spp. and STH thus resulting in high false-positivity of *Toxocara* infection (Romano et al., 2010). Because *Toxocara* infection might contribute to allergic asthma, children who had asthma or bronchial airway hypersensitivity were subjected to investigation of the relationship between *T. canis* infection and allergic asthma. At the Klang Hospital, Malaysia, children with asthma were found to have significantly more likely to be seropositive (57.8%) than nonasthmatic control (15.4%) (Hakim et al., 1997); another study also showed a similar result among Malaysian children who were *Toxocara* seropositive (Chan et al., 2001).

There were very few studies in Philippines, Thailand and Vietnam.

3.3 Philippines

In Philippines, the seroprevalence of *Toxocara* infection was 49.0% (37/75) among public school children (Fajutag and Paller, 2013). Surprisingly, the soil from participant public schools and participant's backyard were more than 40% positive of *Toxocara* eggs contamination at a concentration of 1 egg/g of soil (Fajutag and Paller, 2013), suggesting that there was a strong correlation between a high seroprevalence of *Toxocara* infection among children due to a high prevalence of soil contamination (Horiuchi et al., 2013).

3.4 Thailand

Even though the seroprevalence of *Toxocara* infection among primary schoolchildren was 6% in Thailand (Doi et al., 2017), which was not as high as Malaysian children (Chan et al., 2001), people in Thailand are still threatened by *Toxocara* infection since the *Toxocara* infection rates are 3.6–37.5% among stray dogs and 2.2–9.7% among stray cats, and oil and raw vegetable were contaminated with *Toxocara* eggs (Doi et al., 2017; Pumidonming et al., 2017; Punsawad et al., 2019; Rojekittikhun et al., 1998, 2014; Wiwanitkit and Waenlor, 2004).

3.5 Vietnam

A seroepidemiological study revealed that 45.2% (34,995/77,356) of blood samples in Medic Medical Center Laboratory, Ho Chi Minh City, Vietnam, was diagnosed as toxocariasis by using ELISA assay (Nguyen et al., 2016). This is much higher than the unpublished data of another study investigated in south (32.5%), middle (30.2%) and northern parts (33.3%) of Vietnam (Van De et al., 2013). The Vietnamese customs and cultures, eating habits and agricultural practices were thought as the risk factors of human toxocariasis in Vietnam (Nguyen et al., 2016; Uga et al., 2009).

3.6 Brunei, Cambodia, East Timor (Timor-Leste), Lao People's Democratic Republic (PDR), Myanmar and Singapore

Unfortunately, there was neither seroepidemiological study nor case reports among Brunei, Cambodia, East Timor (Timor-Leste), Lao People's Democratic Republic (PDR), Myanmar and Singapore from PubMed (Table 1). Nevertheless, a survey for potentially zoonotic parasites in Cambodia revealed that 6.4% of domestic dogs were infected with *T. canis* (Schar et al., 2014). It suggested that contact with *T. canis*-infected domestic dogs might be an important risk factor leading to human toxocariasis in Cambodia; however, the lack of epidemiological investigations might neglect the importance of *Toxocara* infection in this country. Dogs are important sources of several zoonotic diseases including toxocariasis. It had been investigated that dogs living in a rural area of Mekong river basin could walk from 1.4 to 13.3 km per day with a routine of accessing water sources, revealing the critical role of dogs in transmission of *T. canis* ova thus contaminating soil, plants, rivers, and other water sources (Otake Sato et al., 2017). Noteworthy, soil contamination with *Toxocara* eggs is a common problem which threatens people's health in SEA since a recent study indicated that the global prevalence of *Toxocara* eggs in public places from 109 studies investigating 42,797 soil samples in total 40 countries was 21% (13,895/42,797) (Fakhri et al., 2018). Of which, the overall prevalence in studies pooled from India, Malaysia and Thailand was estimated to be 21% (3–49%), indicating people in these three countries are at a potentially high risk in acquisition of *Toxocara* infection (Fakhri et al., 2018).

3.7 Taiwan

There were several seroepidemiological studies describing *T. canis* infection among indigenous schoolchildren and adults living in mountainous areas in Taiwan (Fan et al., 2004a,b, 2005). The overall seroprevalence among Bunun indigenous schoolchildren aged 7 to 12 years in southern eastern Taiwan was high, reaching 76.6% (252/329) and this high infection rate may be related to raising dogs and playing with soil (Fan et al., 2004a). In that study, they found children who washed hands before eating had a lower risk of acquiring *T. canis* infections (Fan et al., 2004a). Indigenous schoolchildren who lived in the mountainous areas of north-eastern Taiwan had a lower seropositive rate (57.5%, 42/73) (Fan et al., 2005) as compared to that in those who lived in Bunun village in southern eastern Taiwan (Fan et al., 2004a). Fan et al. (2004b) in a seroepidemiological study among five indigenous populations resident in mountainous areas, including Ames, Atayal, Bunun, Paiwan and Saisiat, were investigated for the sera anti-*T. canis* antibodies by employing TcES-ELISA, revealing an overall seropositive rate of 46.0% (247/537). Of which, the highest seropositive rate was found in the Saisiat (59.0%, 23/39), following by the Bunun (49.2%, 31/63), the Paiwan (48.2%, 66/137), the Atayal (44.2%, 92/208) then the Ames (38.9%, 35/90). Noteworthy, any of the five indigenous populations showed higher infection rate than that in the Han population (30.2%, 13/43) who also lived in the same districts. Important finding showed that the seropositive participants had a relatively higher percentage eating raw pig liver and raising dogs, indirectly reflecting those persons might acquire such an infection through consumption of the *Toxocara* larvae in swine liver or ingestion of the ova contaminating soil or the dog's fur. The other study by Fan et al. (2015) indicated that the seroprevalence of *T. canis* among college students in Taipei city (8.4%) was much lower than that in indigenous people living in mountain areas; nevertheless, in that study also it was also found that there was a lack of awareness on the knowledge that human toxocariasis was a serious concern that may potentially contribute people to be susceptible to *Toxocara* infection (Fu et al., 2015).

An early study conducted by Fan et al. (1998) indicated that 15% of 83 necropsied stray dogs in Taipei City, northern Taiwan had *T. canis* infections with an average of 5 *T. canis* adult worms per dog. Moreover, a study revealed that 16.8% of quarantined dogs in Taichung city of middle Taiwan were detected as having *T. canis* infections (Ho et al., 2006). However, investigations as to the prevalence of *Toxocara* eggs on soil or contaminating vegetables and further the epidemiological studies of *Toxocara* spp. infection among stray dogs and cats in Taiwan would provide useful epidemiologic information.

On the other hand, the status of *Toxocara* infection among SEA labours and immigrants is not only a challenge in Taiwan but also a gap in other Asia-Pacific countries, such as Australia and Japan (Gordon et al., 2017; Nakayama et al., 2011) since some nonspecific symptoms still happen to *Toxocara*-infected persons such as sleep disturbance or tiredness which may cause a safe issue during the intensive labour-consuming periods.

Recently, raising dogs and cats as accompanying animals, eating raw vegetables to keep better health and resting in the park have become more popular in Taiwan, thus the infection status of animals and human as well as the contamination situation in vegetables, water and soils in the recreation places like parks are serious concerns that need intensive investigation in Taiwan.

4. Immunodiagnostic issues by using TcES-based ELISA in SEA countries

Soil-transmitted helminthes (STH) is endemic in SEA countries (Dunn et al., 2019; Punsawad et al., 2017; Silver et al., 2018). A study has indicated that the overall prevalence of intestinal helminths among village health volunteers in rural communities of southern Thailand was not low, reaching 9.3% (Punsawad et al., 2017). The other study has indicated that *Ascaris* was the most endemic STH with an overall prevalence of 18%, followed by *Trichuris* (14%) and hookworm (12%) (Silver et al., 2018). Thus, it's a big challenge in *Toxocara* serodiagnosis by using TcES-ELISA in SEA countries, e.g., Thailand. The sensitivity and specificity of IgG-TcES-ELISA to detect *Toxocara* specific total IgG antibody in human sera is 97% and 36%, respectively; in contrast, employing IgG-TcES-WB has reliable confidence, 95% sensitivity and 95% specificity, and shows minor antigenic cross-reaction than IgG-TcES-ELISA (Ma et al., 2018; Magnaval et al., 1991). Thus, the seropositive results diagnosed by TcES-ELISA in helminth endemic countries such as SEA are strongly recommended to have a further serological test as confirmed by immunoblotting, i.e., IgG-TcES-WB to avoid possible false-positive results due to antigenic cross-reaction between *Toxocara* and the other helminths (Ma et al., 2018; Moreira et al., 2014).

5. Clinical case reports in SEA and Taiwan

There were five case reports found in the SEA countries and Taiwan, including three human OLM cases reported from Malaysia (Azira and Zeehaida, 2011; Guan-Fook et al., 2012; Sivaratnam et al., 2008), three OLM cases reported from Thailand (Srimuang et al., 1996) and one OLM case from Vietnam (Van De et al., 2013) (Table 2). Contacting contaminated water or soil, playing with dogs and cats as well as eating raw vegetables were considered for these patients as the risk factors contributing to OLM. In Taiwan, 18 unpublished cases were diagnosed as seropositive for *T. canis* infection (Table 2), including 7 OLM cases referred from ophthalmologist and 3 suspected cerebral toxocariasis cases with eosinophilic meningitis referred from Taiwan CDC or neurosurgeon. It was a pity that the type of human toxocariasis and their personal histories have not been further classified in the other 8 seropositive cases. Most of the patients had experienced close contact dogs and eating raw meats which seems likely the possible risk factors.

6. Conclusions and perspectives

The Centers for Disease Control and Prevention announced that human toxocariasis is one of the five major neglected parasitic diseases in the USA that it should be comprehensively monitored and controlled due to nearly 70 blindness cases caused by *Toxocara* infection per year (Woodhall et al., 2014), reflecting this worldwide zoonotic parasitic disease appears a serious public health issue threating human health globally. Substantial epidemiological studies have indicated that the poor hygiene, soil and water contamination, raise or contact with dogs/cats as well as eating raw meats and vegetables that all are the possible risk factors contributing to human toxocariasis in SEA and Taiwan. Moreover, it was found that the infection rate of *Toxocara* spp. infections among stray dogs was significantly higher than that in stray cats ($p < 0.001$) (Tun et al., 2015), thus the prevalence among stray dogs as well as deworming control for stray dogs should need more comprehensive investigations and monitors due to random defecation from these stray dogs in anyplace that may further facilitate contamination of soil, water and vegetables. The knowledge about infection routes for *Toxocara* and the information concerning how to prevent from *Toxocara* infection should be delivered to people properly by public health education and propaganda. Additionally, the consequences of human toxocariasis and the diagnostic methods employing TcES-ELISA for screening and further confirmation by TcES-WB should be also emphasized to clinical physicians in SEA and Taiwan as well.

References

Azian, M.Y., Sakhone, L., Hakim, S.L., Yusri, M.Y., Nurulsyamzawaty, Y., Zuhaizam, A.H., Rodi, I.M., Maslawaty, M.N., 2008. Detection of helminth infections in dogs and soil contamination in rural and urban areas. Southeast Asian J. Trop. Med. Public Health 39, 205–212.

Azira, N.M., Zeehaida, M., 2011. A case report of ocular toxocariasis. Asian Pac. J. Trop. Biomed. 1, 164–165.

Chan, P.W., Anuar, A.K., Fong, M.Y., Debruyne, J.A., Ibrahim, J., 2001. *Toxocara* seroprevalence and childhood asthma among Malaysian children. Pediatr. Int. 43, 350–353.
Cheng, H.I., 2016. On migrant Workers' social status in Taiwan: a critical analysis of mainstream news discourse. Int. J. Commun. 10, 2509–2528.
Chomel, B.B., Kasten, R., Adams, C., Lambillotte, D., Theis, J., Goldsmith, R., Koss, J., Chioino, C., Widjana, D.P., Sutisna, P., 1993. Serosurvey of some major zoonotic infections in children and teenagers in Bali, Indonesia. Southeast Asian J. Trop. Med. Public Health 24, 321–326.
Doi, R., Itoh, M., Chakhatrakan, S., Uga, S., 2017. Epidemiological investigation of parasitic infection of schoolchildren from six elementary schools in Sakon Nakhon Province, Thailand. Kobe J. Med. Sci. 62, E120–E128.
Dunn, J.C., Bettis, A.A., Wyine, N.Y., Lwin, A.M.M., Tun, A., Maung, N.S., Anderson, R.M., 2019. Soil-transmitted helminth reinfection four and six months after mass drug administration: results from the delta region of Myanmar. PLoS Negl. Trop. Dis. 13, e0006591.
Emmerson, D.K., 1984. Southeast Asia: what's in a name? J. Southeast Asian Stud. 15, 1–21.
Fajutag, A.J., Paller, V.G., 2013. Toxocara egg soil contamination and its seroprevalence among public school children in Los Banos, Laguna, Philippines. Southeast Asian J. Trop. Med. Public Health 44, 551–560.
Fakhri, Y., Gasser, R.B., Rostami, A., Fan, C.K., Ghasemi, S.M., Javanian, M., Bayani, M., Armoon, B., Moradi, B., 2018. *Toxocara* eggs in public places worldwide: a systematic review and meta-analysis. Environ. Pollut. 242, 1467–1475.
Fan, C.K., Holland, C.V., Loxton, K., Barghouth, U., 2015. Cerebral toxocariasis: silent progression to neurodegenerative disorders? Clin. Microbiol. Rev. 28, 663–686.
Fan, C.K., Hung, C.C., Du, W.Y., Liao, C.W., Su, K.E., 2004a. Seroepidemiology of *Toxocara canis* infection among mountain aboriginal schoolchildren living in contaminated districts in eastern Taiwan. Trop. Med. Int. Health 9, 1312–1318.
Fan, C.K., Lan, H.S., Hung, C.C., Chung, W.C., Liao, C.W., Du, W.Y., Su, K.E., 2004b. Seroepidemiology of *Toxocara canis* infection among mountain aboriginal adults in Taiwan. Am. J. Trop. Med. Hyg. 71, 216–221.
Fan, C.K., Liao, C.W., Cheng, Y.C., 2013. Factors affecting disease manifestation of toxocarosis in humans: genetics and environment. Vet. Parasitol. 193, 342–352.
Fan, C.K., Liao, C.W., Kao, T.C., Li, M.H., Du, W.Y., Su, K.E., 2005. Sero-epidemiology of *Toxocara canis* infection among aboriginal schoolchildren in the mountainous areas of North-Eastern Taiwan. Ann. Trop. Med. Parasitol. 99, 593–600.
Fan, C.K., Su, K.E., Chung, W.C., Tsai, W.J., Chang, M.H., Lu, J.L., Chao, P.H., 1998. A parasitological survey among stray dogs in Taipei City with Haematological findings. J. Chin. Soc. Vet. Sci. 24, 288–294.
Fu, C.J., Kao, C.Y., Lee, Y.L., Liao, C.W., Chen, P.C., Chuang, T.W., Wang, Y.C., Chou, C.M., Huang, Y.C., Naito, T., Fan, C.K., 2015. Seroprevalence and associated risk factors of Toxocariasis among college students in Taipei City, Taiwan. Iran. J. Parasitol. 10, 482–489.
Gordon, C.A., Kurscheid, J., Jones, M.K., Gray, D.J., McManus, D.P., 2017. Soil-transmitted helminths in tropical Australia and Asia. Trop. Med. Infect. Dis. 2, 56. https://doi.org/10.3390/tropicalmed2040056.
Guan-Fook, N., Hayati, A.A., Raja-Azmi, M.N., Liza-Sharmini, A.T., Wan-Hazabbah, W.H., Zunaina, E., 2012. Diffuse unilateral subacute neuroretinitis in a young boy: a case report. Clin. Ophthalmol. 6, 487–490.
Hakim, S.L., Mak, J.W., Lam, P.L., 1993. ELISA seropositivity for *Toxocara canis* antibodies in Malaysia, 1989-1991. Med. J. Malaysia 48, 303–307.
Hakim, S.L., Mak, J.W., Lam, P.L., Nazma, S., Normaznah, Y., 1992. Seroprevalence of *Toxocara canis* antibodies among orang Asli (aborigines) in Peninsular Malaysia. Southeast Asian J. Trop. Med. Public Health 23, 493–496.

Hakim, S.L., Thadasavanth, M., Shamilah, R.H., Yogeswari, S., 1997. Prevalence of *Toxocara canis* antibody among children with bronchial asthma in Klang Hospital, Malaysia. Trans. R. Soc. Trop. Med. Hyg. 91, 528.

Hayashi, E., Tuda, J., Imada, M., Akao, N., Fujita, K., 2005. The high prevalence of asymptomatic *Toxocara* infection among schoolchildren in Manado, Indonesia. Southeast Asian J. Trop. Med. Public Health 36, 1399–1406.

Ho, S.Y., Watanabe, Y., Lee, Y.C., Shih, T.H., Tu, W.J., Ooi, H.K., 2006. Survey of gastrointestinal parasitic infections in quarantined dogs in Taiwan. J. Vet. Med. Sci. 68, 69–70.

Horiuchi, S., Paller, V.G., Uga, S., 2013. Soil contamination by parasite eggs in rural village in the Philippines. Trop. Biomed. 30, 495–503.

Lim, P.K., Yamasaki, H., Mak, J.W., Wong, S.F., Chong, C.W., Yap, I.K., Ambu, S., Kumarasamy, V., 2015. Field evaluation of a rapid diagnostic test to detect antibodies in human toxocariasis. Acta Trop. 148, 32–37.

Ma, G., Holland, C.V., Wang, T., Hofmann, A., Fan, C.K., Maizels, R.M., Hotez, P.J., Gasser, R.B., 2018. Human toxocariasis. Lancet Infect. Dis. 18, e14–e24.

Magnaval, J.F., Fabre, R., Maurieres, P., Charlet, J.P., de Larrard, B., 1991. Application of the western blotting procedure for the immunodiagnosis of human toxocariasis. Parasitol. Res. 77, 697–702.

Mohd Zain, S.N., Rahman, R., Lewis, J.W., 2015. Stray animal and human defecation as sources of soil-transmitted helminth eggs in playgrounds of peninsular Malaysia. J. Helminthol. 89, 740–747.

Moreira, G.M., Telmo Pde, L., Mendonca, M., Moreira, A.N., McBride, A.J., Scaini, C.J., Conceicao, F.R., 2014. Human toxocariasis: current advances in diagnostics, treatment, and interventions. Trends Parasitol. 30, 456–464.

Nakayama, K., Akao, N., Ohta, N., 2011. Parasitic infections in foreigners living in Japan: estimation of parasitic infection history by serum antibody screening. J. Med. Dent. Sci. 58, 97–102.

Ngui, R., Lee, S.C., Yap, N.J., Tan, T.K., Aidil, R.M., Chua, K.H., Aziz, S., Sulaiman, W.Y., Ahmad, A.F., Mahmud, R., Lian, Y.L., 2014. Gastrointestinal parasites in rural dogs and cats in Selangor and Pahang states in Peninsular Malaysia. Acta Parasitol. 59, 737–744.

Nguyen, T., Cheong, F.W., Liew, J.W., Lau, Y.L., 2016. Seroprevalence of fascioliasis, toxocariasis, strongyloidiasis and cysticercosis in blood samples diagnosed in medic medical center laboratory, Ho Chi Minh City, Vietnam in 2012. Parasit. Vectors 9, 486.

Otake Sato, M., Sato, M., Yoonuan, T., Pongvongsa, T., Sanguankiat, S., Kounnavong, S., Maipanich, W., Chigusa, Y., Moji, K., Waikagul, J., 2017. The role of domestic dogs in the transmission of zoonotic helminthes in a rural area of Mekong river basin. Acta Parasitol. 62, 393–400.

Pumidonming, W., Salman, D., Gronsang, D., Abdelbaset, A.E., Sangkaeo, K., Kawazu, S.I., Igarashi, M., 2017. Prevalence of gastrointestinal helminth parasites of zoonotic significance in dogs and cats in lower Northern Thailand. J. Vet. Med. Sci. 78, 1779–1784.

Punsawad, C., Phasuk, N., Bunratsami, S., Thongtup, K., Siripakonuaong, N., Nongnaul, S., 2017. Prevalence of intestinal parasitic infection and associated risk factors among village health volunteers in rural communities of southern Thailand. BMC Public Health 17, 564.

Punsawad, C., Phasuk, N., Thongtup, K., Nagavirochana, S., Viriyavejakul, P., 2019. Prevalence of parasitic contamination of raw vegetables in Nakhon Si Thammarat province, southern Thailand. BMC Public Health 19, 34.

Rojekittikhun, W., Chaisiri, K., Mahittikorn, A., Pubampen, S., Sa-Nguankiat, S., Kusolsuk, T., Maipanich, W., Udonsom, R., Mori, H., 2014. Gastrointestinal parasites of dogs and cats in a refuge in Nakhon Nayok, Thailand. Southeast Asian J. Trop. Med. Public Health 45, 31–39.

Rojekittikhun, W., Nuamtanong, S., Anantaphruti, M.T., Pubampen, S., Maipanich, W., Visedsuk, K., 1998. *Toxocara* and *Gnathostoma* among stray canines in Bangkok. Southeast Asian J. Trop. Med. Public Health 29, 744–747.

Romano, N., Nor Azah, M.O., Rahmah, N., Lim, Y.A., Rohela, M., 2010. Seroprevalence of toxocariasis among orang Asli (indigenous people) in Malaysia using two immunoassays. Trop. Biomed. 27, 585–594.

Schar, F., Inpankaew, T., Traub, R.J., Khieu, V., Dalsgaard, A., Chimnoi, W., Chhoun, C., Sok, D., Marti, H., Muth, S., Odermatt, P., 2014. The prevalence and diversity of intestinal parasitic infections in humans and domestic animals in a rural Cambodian village. Parasitol. Int. 63, 597–603.

Silver, Z.A., Kaliappan, S.P., Samuel, P., Venugopal, S., Kang, G., Sarkar, R., Ajjampur, S.S.R., 2018. Geographical distribution of soil transmitted helminths and the effects of community type in South Asia and South East Asia—a systematic review. PLoS Negl. Trop. Dis. 12, e0006153.

Sivaratnam, D., Subrayan, V., Ali, N.A., 2008. Transvitreal migration of a *Toxocara* larva resulting in a second chorioretinal granuloma. Jpn. J. Ophthalmol. 52, 416–417.

Srimuang, S., Roongruangchai, K., Lawtiantong, T., Chusattayanond, A.D., Warrasak, S., Sahaphong, S., Tanphaichitra, D., 1996. Immunobiological diagnosis of tropical ocular diseases: *Toxocara*, Pythium insidiosum, *Pseudomonas (Burkholderia) pseudomallei*, *Mycobacterium chelonei* and *Toxoplasma gondii*. Int. J. Tissue React. 18, 23–25.

Tun, S., Ithoi, I., Mahmud, R., Samsudin, N.I., Kek Heng, C., Ling, L.Y., 2015. Detection of helminth eggs and identification of hookworm species in stray cats, dogs and soil from Klang Valley, Malaysia. PLoS One 10, e0142231.

Uga, S., Hoa, N.T., Noda, S., Moji, K., Cong, L., Aoki, Y., Rai, S.K., Fujimaki, Y., 2009. Parasite egg contamination of vegetables from a suburban market in Hanoi, Vietnam. Nepal Med. Coll. J. 11, 75–78.

Uga, S., Kataoka, N., 1995. Measures to control *Toxocara* egg contamination in sandpits of public parks. Am. J. Trop. Med. Hyg. 52, 21–24.

Uga, S., Ono, K., Kataoka, N., Hasan, H., 1996. Seroepidemiology of five major zoonotic parasite infections in inhabitants of Sidoarjo, East Java, Indonesia. Southeast Asian J. Trop. Med. Public Health 27, 556–561.

Van De, N., Trung, N.V., Duyet le, V., Chai, J.Y., 2013. Molecular diagnosis of an ocular toxocariasis patient in Vietnam. Korean J. Parasitol. 51, 563–567.

Wiwanitkit, V., Waenlor, W., 2004. The frequency rate of *Toxocara* species contamination in soil samples from public yards in a urban area "Payathai", Bangkok, Thailand. Rev. Inst. Med. Trop. Sao Paulo 46, 113–114.

Woodhall, D.M., Eberhard, M.L., Parise, M.E., 2014. Neglected parasitic infections in the United States: toxocariasis. Am. J. Trop. Med. Hyg. 90, 810–813.

CHAPTER TWENTY-THREE

Sources and seroprevalence of toxocariasis in Turkey

Aysegul Taylan-Ozkan*
Department of Medical Microbiology, Hitit University School of Medicine, Corum, Turkey
Department of Medical Microbiology and Clinical Microbiology, Near East University School of Medicine, Nicosia, Cyprus
*Corresponding author: e-mail address: aysegultaylanozkan@yahoo.com

Contents

Abstract

Toxocariasis in humans is considered a rare disease in Turkey, and the absence of specific symptoms of this disease is probably the main reason for clinicians to underestimate and underdiagnose the disease. Although there are several seroepidemiological studies on visceral larva migrans in the country, a comparison between them is difficult as the serological tests are not standardised. After the

Advances in Parasitology, Volume 109
ISSN 0065-308X
https://doi.org/10.1016/bs.apar.2020.01.021

introduction of the easily accessible ELISA kit in the market, the number of seroepidemiological studies has increased in which the reported rates ranged between 1% and 56%. Similar to other countries, *Toxocara* seropositivity in Turkey is more common in men, childhood, in those living in rural area, having a low income level, owning dogs, and biting their nails or practicing geophagia. In addition, toxocariasis is a risk factor for veterinarians, farmers, and pet-shop workers. *Toxocara* seroprevalence is significantly higher in respiratory, neuropsychiatric, musculo-skeletal, skin and abdominal disorders. There are also many studies showing the importance of eosinophilia in toxocariasis. In conclusion, although there are many studies on toxocariasis in Turkey, it is still not well understood to what extent the infection is responsible for a plethora ascribed symptoms. Standardisation of the diagnostic methods and the use of molecular techniques could further throw light in the real epidemiology and the role played by the infection to induce signs and symptoms.

1. Introduction

Toxocariasis is considered to be a rare cause of disease in Turkey. The absence of specific and definitive disease findings has caused clinicians to underestimate the number of cases of larval toxocariasis, and thus, the actual prevalence of larva migrans caused by *Toxocara* spp. in Turkey is poorly known. Recently in Turkey; associated signs and symptoms such as fatigue, abdominal pain, cough, headache, liver enlargement, epilepsy, asthma, sleep disorder, increased eosinophil number, and allergic symptoms in different groups of patients have been revealed in different studies that have suggested that the disease perhaps more common than previously expected. Although it is considered rare, practitioners have been aware of its presence as a disease entity in Turkey since 1970, when the syndrome was described in local cases (Merdivenci, 1970). There have also been reports of ocular larva migrans in Turkey associated with strabismus (Berk et al., 2000), retinal detachment (Acar et al., 2007), uveitis (Ozdal et al., 2012), and neuroretinitis (Karaca et al., 2018). The first seroepidemiological study was performed in Izmir in western Turkey (Kuman and Altintas, 1984).

2. Examination of sources of potential infection within Turkey

2.1 Environment

Various studies in different regions of Turkey have examined potential soil sources of infection with samples from children play areas, such as parks and gardens, and the prevalence of *Toxocara* spp. was reported between 4% and 64% (Akdemir, 2010; Avcioglu and Balkaya, 2011; Avcioglu and Burgu, 2008; Ayaz et al., 2003; Aydenizoz Ozkayhan, 2006; Gurel et al., 2005; Oge and Oge, 2000a,b; Simsek et al., 2005). The rate was the lowest (4%) in Konya (Central Anatolia) and in highest (64%) in Erzurum (in Eastern Anatolia) (Ayaz et al., 2003; Guclu and Aydenizoz, 1998). Seasonal variation might play an important role in this discrepancy (Aydenizoz Ozkayhan, 2006). It has been found that the prevalence of *Toxocara* spp., *Toxascaris leonina*, and *Taenia* spp. eggs was the lowest during the summer (4%) but highest during the autumn (13%) (Avcioglu and Burgu, 2008). It is also a possibility that techniques used may be responsible for disparities between studies. Simsek et al. (2005) compared three different techniques using the same soil samples from Elazig, and *Toxocara* spp. eggs were recovered from 7%, 13% and 23% of the samples using flotation by NaCl, $MgSO_4$ and salt/sugar solution, respectively.

Restriction of access of animals to certain areas may also play an important role in that prevalence of *Toxocara* spp. could be as high as 64% in unfenced public parks, while no contamination was observed fenced-off area (Avcioglu and Balkaya, 2011). In Ankara, 170 soil samples from 46 public parks were collected, and 31% of them were found to contain *Toxocara* eggs, most of which were fully embryonated (Oge and Oge, 2000a). Since the human transmission is usually through contact with contaminated soil with embryonated *Toxocara* eggs, this poses a significant risk for children playing in these areas. Children who would be at greatest risk would be those playing in public sand boxes or who practice pica (Gurel et al., 2005).

Usage of contaminated wastewater is another risk for contamination of materials with *Toxocara* eggs. In Afyonkarahisar, helminth eggs were seen in 27% of 240 untreated wastewater samples that were collected at 2-week intervals from 10 different locations, and 6% percent of these helminth eggs observed in the samples were animal derived eggs of *Toxocara* spp. (Kozan et al., 2007).

2.2 Prevalence rates in final hosts

First investigations on animal toxocariasis in Turkey were started at the beginning of the 1960s (Merdivenci, 1962, 1963, 1965, 1970). Doganay (1983) in Ankara found that 24% of 50 stray dogs had toxocariasis. Several investigations in different part of the country revealed the prevalence in dog ranges from 4% to 69% (Atas et al., 1997; Budak et al., 1984; Cicek and Yilmaz, 2012; Doganay, 1983; Doganay and Oge, 1993; Kozan et al., 2007;

Kuru et al., 2013; Oge et al., 2014, 2017a,b, 2019; Orhun and Ayaz, 2006; Sayin İpek and Kochan, 2017; Saygi et al., 1990; Senlik et al., 2006; Yaman et al., 2006). These results can provide an overall impression of the percentage of infected animals, but the studies were performed with different methods (Oge and Oge, 2000b). In Ankara 69% of 182 autopsied stray dogs were found to be infected, whereas the rate was 52% of the faecal samples from these dogs (Doganay and Oge, 1993). When the studies were performed also appeared to have effects on the prevalence rates observed. In Sivas, Saygi et al. (1990) examined 25 stray dogs by microscopy and autopsy and found 28% positive, but 5 years later in 1995 Atas et al. (1997) found a positive rate as high as 50%.

In Turkish military Belgian Malinois dogs, it was found that males had a higher prevalence of infection than females (Senlik et al., 2006). In these dogs, it was found that 22% of the hair samples were found to contain eggs, and of these eggs 20% were found to be embryonated and hence, infective. There was no correlation discovered between the presence of the eggs per gram of hair and age, breed, coat type or hair length; but it was underlined that the age of the dogs was quite important since 82% of the infected dogs were below a year old (Aydenizoz-Ozkayhan et al., 2008). Doganay and Oge (1993) also found *Toxocara* spp. eggs in faecal samples higher in puppies than the adult dogs.

In many studies the species of *Toxocara* have not been mentioned. In Ankara when stray dogs were autopsied, 69.2% of them found to be infected with ascarids; however, 52.2% had *Toxascaris leonina*, while only 21.9% had *T. canis* (Doganay and Oge, 1993). In Diyarbakir, on the other hand, it was found that 15.3% of dogs had *T. canis*, and only 4.8% had *T. leonina* (Sayin İpek and Kochan, 2017). *Toxocara cati* was found 13–82% of cats from different part of the country (Korkmaz et al., 2016; Oge et al., 2014; Yaman et al., 2006). The presence of the *Toxocara* spp. was the highest (82%) in stray cats (Korkmaz et al., 2016). Oge et al. (2014) compared the presence of *Toxocara* eggs in hair and faeces of dogs and cats in Ankara, and the number of cats with contaminated fur was greater than in dogs (22% and 14%, respectively), but the number of the eggs were higher in dogs (136 per dog) than cats (58 per cat). Recently molecular analyses by ITS-2 sequences of *Toxocara* spp. obtained from Van stray cats and dogs showed close resemblance with *T. canis* and *T. cati* collected in other countries of the world (Oguz et al., 2018).

2.3 Food

Although there was no direct evidence, a recent case of neuroretinitis associated with the consumption of raw meat containing *Toxocara* was published (Karaca et al., 2018). In a study from Bursa, 1% of unwashed vegetables such as lettuce and parsley had the eggs of *Toxocara* spp. (Avcioglu et al., 2011). The source of this contamination might be related with the use of untreated wastewater for agricultural purposes (Kozan et al., 2007). Similar results for *Toxocara* egg contamination were found on 1–2% of unwashed vegetables from Ankara (Ozan, 2007), Aydin (Yesilcayir, 2017) and Van (Ketir, 2018).

3. Seroprevalence according to geographical distribution in Turkey

Although there are several seroepidemiological studies on VLM in Turkey, a comparison between them is difficult as the serological tests are not standardised. In addition, most of the studies are based on data from certain defined populations; and therefore, the macro- and micro-epidemiological scales may be different in the level of human exposure to the parasite in the different studies. Also, understanding the relationship between the causative agent and disease formation is difficult and epidemiological data on ocular toxocariasis are missing. All this makes it difficult to evaluate the importance of the disease in terms of public health (Selek and Baylan, 2013). On the other hand, since VLM, imitates many diseases such as rheumatic fever, asthma, and even metastasis of cancer, physicians have difficulty in recognising certain cases of toxocariasis.

The first seroepidemiological study on toxocariasis was conducted in Izmir by Kuman and Altintas (1984). Using adult *Toxocara* antigens in an indirect hemagglutination (IHA) test, 44% of the examined individuals were positive, whereas 25 out of 31 sera showed cross reactivity with *Ascaris* IHA. A few years later in the same region, three different techniques (indirect fluorescent antibody-IFA, IHA and complement fixation tests) were compared, and IHA was found to be the most efficient although also in this study cross reactivity with *Ascaris* was observed (Ozcel and Altintas, 1987). A decade later, Korkmaz (1998) reported similar results (37%) in another study conducted in Izmir using an in-house developed enzyme linked immunosorbent assay (ELISA) coated with the excretion and secretion products of *Toxocara* larvae. After the appearance of a marketed and readily accessible ELISA kit, the number of seroepidemiological studies (Table 1 and Fig. 1), and the reported prevalence rates have ranged between 1% and 56% in the different sero-surveys.

4. Seroprevalence of toxocariasis according to risk factors

4.1 Gender

Toxocara seropositivity has been found to be more common in men than in women (Selek and Baylan, 2013). Yazar et al. (2010) stated that the infection rate is almost twice as high in males than in females (27.8% and 13.7%, respectively). In a study by Kaplan et al. (2008), 51% of men, and 40.4% of women diagnosed with schizophrenia had were seropositive for *Toxocara* antibodies. In some studies, however, no differences between males and females were found (Buyukbaba et al., 1996; Cicek and Yilmaz, 2012; Saglam, 1999).

4.2 Age

Toxocara seropositivity rates are in general higher in the childhood age groups than in other age groups. Oguzturk and Saygi (2002) reported that *Toxocara* seroprevalence was 32.3% in healthy children attending primary school. *Toxocara* seropositivity was significantly higher among subjects less than 10 years-old than in those who were greater than 40 years of age (Demirci et al., 2010). Yazar et al. (2010) found the highest seropositivity in the 11–20-year-old age group (30%), and the lowest in those over 44 years of age (12%). There are, however, studies showing that there is a significant relationship between toxocariasis and increasing age (Cicek and Yilmaz, 2012; Selek et al., 2015). In patients with schizophrenia, the seroprevalence rate increased with the age, and it was highest (80%) in people over 60 years of age (Kaplan et al., 2008). Kaplan et al. (2005) reported that the highest seropositivity rate for toxocariasis (56%) was in those between 35 and 44 years of age, while the lowest seroprevalence (10%) occurred in 45–54-year-old patients with rheumatoid arthritis.

4.3 Socio-economic conditions

It is quite clear that in terms of *Toxocara* seropositivity, those living in rural and more economically deprived regions have a greater risk of being serologically positive than those living in developed regions with middle

Table 1 Seroepidemiological studies conducted on toxocariasis in the regions of Turkey

City	Year	Test(s)	Target population	Seropositivity rate	References
Aegean Region					
Izmir	1984	Inhouse IHA Adult antigen	Adults patients having hepatomegaly	44%, But 81% crossreactivity by ascaris IHA	Kuman and Altintas (1984)
Izmir	1987	Inhouse IHA Adult antigen	Adults	56 Patients	Ozcel and Altintas (1987)
Izmir	1998	In house ELISA E/S *T. cati*	Various	37% in total 39% in suspected patients 29% in healthy children 33% in healthy adults 45% in allergy group	Korkmaz (1998)
Manisa	2004	*T. canis* IgG ELISA	Children with atopia (5–18 ages)	1% in total 1% in control group 0% in atopic children	Hakan (2005)
Aydin	2006	*Toxocara* in house ELISA E/S	Patients with epilepsy	12% in epileptics 5.9% in control	Akyol et al. (2007)
Aydin	2008	*Toxocara* in house ELISA E/S	Various	32.6% in eosinophilic 20.3% in non-eosinophilic	Karadam et al. (2008)
Kutahya	2010	*T. canis* IgG ELISA	Children	7.6% in total	Akdemir (2010)
Mugla	2014	*T. canis* IgG ELISA and WB	Animal husbandry workers and veterinarian	8%	Sozen et al. (2015)

Continued

Table 1 Seroepidemiological studies conducted on toxocariasis in the regions of Turkey—Cont'd

City	Year	Test(s)	Target population	Seropositivity rate	References
Eskisehir[a] Bilecik[b] Kutahya Afyonkarahisar	2007	*T. canis* IgG ELISA	Children	12.95% in total 16.97% in rural 0.71% in urban area	Dogan et al. (2007)
Marmara Region					
Istanbul	1996	ELISA	Children ages between 1 and 10 years	34% in total 12% in urban 42% in rural area There is no difference between male and female	Buyukbaba et al. (1996)
Istanbul	1999	*T. canis* IgG ELISA	Various	10% in people have close contact with dog 6% in veterinarian or veterinary students 5% in hypereosinophilia 0% in control group There is no difference between male and female but higher in contacting of dogs	Saglam (1999)
Istanbul	2005	*T. canis* IgG ELISA and WB	Patients with hypereosinophilia	32.3% by ELISA 48.4% by WB	Artinyan et al. (2014)
Istanbul	2012	*T. canis* IgG ELISA and WB	Patients with chronic urticaria	17.8% in chronic uriticaria 0% in control	Selek et al. (2015)

Mediterranean Region					
Isparta	2002	In house ELISA E/S *T. cati*	Patients with hypereosinophilia	29.1% with eosinophilia 19.4% without eosinophilia 15.5% in control	Demirci et al. (2002)
Isparta	2003	In house ELISA E/S *T. cati*	Patients with chronic urticaria	29.0% in chronic urticarial 16.1% in control	Demirci et al. (2003)
Isparta	2007	In house ELISA E/S IgG and IgE	Adults with allergic rhinitis	*IgG* 28.1% in allergic rhinitis 11.5% in control *Specific IgE* 17.2% in allergic rhinitis 3.3% in control	Yariktas et al. (2007)
Isparta	2010	In house ELISA E/S *T. cati*	Adults	16% in total 14% in urban 28% in rural area There is no difference between male and female	Demirci et al. (2010)
Eastern/Southeastern Anatolia Region					
Elazig	2005	*T. canis* IgG ELISA	Patients with rheumatoid arthritis	35.6% in RA 8.3% in control 42.8% in 25–34 old ages 55.5% in 35–44 old ages 10% in 45–54 old ages 44.4% in 55–64 old ages 30% in 65 and over	Kaplan et al. (2005)

Continued

Table 1 Seroepidemiological studies conducted on toxocariasis in the regions of Turkey—Cont'd

City	Year	Test(s)	Target population	Seropositivity rate	References
Elazig	2006	*T. canis* IgG ELISA	Adult patients with asthma	13.2% in asthma	Kuk et al. (2006a)
Elazig	2006	*Toxocara* IgG and IgM ELISA	Patients with multiple sclerosis and ankylosing spondylitis	10.8% in MS 3.2% in AS No significant difference with control	Kuk et al. (2006b)
Elazig	2008	*T. canis* IgG/IgM ELISA	Patients with schizophrenia	45.9% in patients with schizophrenia 2.0% in control	Kaplan et al. (2008)
Elazig Malatya Diyarbakir[c]	2004	*T. canis* IgG ELISA	Mental retarded children	18.8% in mental retarded 7.1% in control	Kaplan et al. (2004)
Diyarbakir			Patients with chronic urticaria	14.5% in patients	Dal et al. (2013)
Van	2007	*T. canis* IgG ELISA	Various	%15.25 in total 14.65% in male 15.94% in female 18.44% in rural 11.14% in rural 6.54% in children 19.80 in adults	Cicek and Yilmaz (2012)
Van	2016	*T. canis* IgG ELISA	Patients with eosinophilia	15% in eosinophilia 7% in control group	Tileklioglu (2016)

Central Anatolia Region					
Kayseri	2005–2009	*T. canis* IgG ELISA	Various	21.4% 27.8% in male 13.7% in female	Yazar et al. (2010)
Sivas	2002	*T. canis* IgG ELISA	Children from rural area	32% in total	Oguzturk and Saygi (2002)
Ankara	1999	*T. canis* IgG ELISA	Children with unknown abdominal pain	51% in total	Gungor et al. (1999)
Ankara	2007	*T. canis* IgG ELISA	Patients with asthma	9.7% in asthma	Kustimur et al. (2007)

[a]Eskisehir belongs to Central Anatolia Region of Turkey.
[b]Bilecik belongs to Marmara Region of Turkey.
[c]Diyarbakir belongs to Southeastern Region of Turkey.

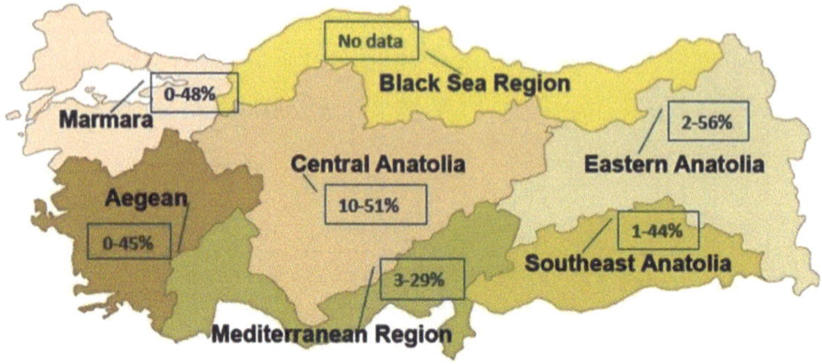

Fig. 1 Seroprevalence of toxocariasis in seven geographical regions of Turkey.

or advanced income levels (Selek and Baylan, 2013). There are many studies in Turkey supporting the finding that the seropositivity rate is higher in rural than urban areas (Buyukbaba et al., 1996; Cicek and Yilmaz, 2012; Demirci et al., 2010; Dogan et al., 2007; Oguzturk and Saygi, 2002). The seropositivity was 35–36% in patients with low or middle income levels, whereas no seropositive subjects in high income patients (Kaplan et al., 2005), while individuals with higher education level showed lower seropositivity for toxocariasis (Demirci et al., 2010; Kaplan et al., 2005).

4.4 Pet ownership

Dog ownership was found as a risk factor for infection with *Toxocara* and seroprevalence among dog owners could be as high as 69% (Saglam, 1999; Selek et al., 2015). Dogan et al. (2007) found that the rate of seropositivity was 12.3% in the group who had pets at home while the average was only 4.6% in those who did not. Kaplan et al. (2005) reported that among 45 patients, *Toxocara* seropositivity was 50% in those feeding their pets, while 30.3% those who were not feeding. On the contrary, owning dogs or cats and hand washing were found as not associated with toxocariasis seropositivity by Hakan (2005) and Demirci et al. (2010).

4.5 Geophagia and nail biting

Seropositivity of *Toxocara* was found to be higher in people with pica than those without this habit (Demirci et al., 2010; Dogan et al., 2007; Ecevit et al., 2013; Kaplan et al., 2005; Selek et al., 2015). It is revealed that insufficient daily hand washing habit increases seropositivity 21 times (Selek et al., 2015). This may explain why nail biting has been associated with high toxocariasis seropositivity (Demirci et al., 2010).

4.6 Occupation

Toxocariasis is a risk factor in veterinarians, farmers, pet-shop workers (Gungor et al., 1999; Selek et al., 2015; Sozen et al., 2015). Kaplan et al. (2008) reported that *Toxocara* seropositivity in farmers were higher than in other occupational groups among schizophrenia patients.

5. Seroprevalence of toxocariasis according to symptoms/diseases

5.1 Respiratory diseases

Toxocara larvae may cause acute bronchiolitis, asthma, or pneumonia-like echocardiography in the lungs (Selek and Baylan, 2013). In our country, the seroprevalence rate of *Toxocara* in asthmatic patients ranged between 9.7% and 13.2% (Kuk et al., 2006a; Kustimur et al., 2007). In another study, 6.11% of 122 patients with asthmatic dyspnea were seropositive for toxocariasis (Cicek and Yilmaz, 2012). Patients with allergic rhinitis had higher (28.1%) toxocariasis seropositivity compared to the control group (11.5%), and specific IgE seropositivity was also higher than in the controls (Yariktas et al., 2007).

5.2 Neuropsychiatric diseases

Kaplan et al. (2004) reported that the rate of *Toxocara* infection was significantly higher in mentally handicapped children, but no correlation was found between age, gender, socio-economic level, owning dogs, and personal hygiene. In another study conducted by Kaplan et al. (2008), the seropositivity of *Toxocara* in 98 patients diagnosed with schizophrenia was 45.9%, while in the control group, it was only 2%.

Toxocara may be a causative agent of idiopathic epilepsy (Kaplan et al., 2002). In a study from Diyarbakir, it was reported that 3.05% of 122 patients with positive toxocariasis had epilepsy (Cicek and Yilmaz, 2012), while none of the patients with epilepsy in Aydin were positive for toxocariasis (Akyol et al., 2007). There was also no correlation between *T. canis* and idiopathic Parkinson's disease in Elazig (Celik et al., 2013).

5.3 Musculoskeletal disorders

In a study conducted in Elazig, *Toxocara* seropositivity was as high as 35.6% in 45 rheumatoid arthritis patients and 8.3% in 48 healthy controls (Kaplan et al., 2005). Cicek and Yilmaz (2012) reported that 9.16% of

122 toxocariasis positive patients had arthralgia. Toxocariasis was detected as 10.8% and 3.2% in multiple sclerosis and ankylosing spondylitis patients, respectively (Kuk et al., 2006b).

5.4 Skin diseases

Demirci et al. (2003), Selek et al. (2015) and Dal et al. (2013) found significantly higher *Toxocara* antibody positivity in patients with chronic urticaria than in healthy individuals. On the other hand, atopic children were negative for toxocariasis when examined by ELISA whereas 1% of the control group showed positive serology, while they did not have a history of feeding or contacting pets at home or in the garden (Hakan, 2005).

5.5 Eosinophilia

There are many studies from around Turkey showing the importance of eosinophilia in toxocariasis. All studies reported a positive correlation between seropositivity to toxocariasis and eosinophilia (Artinyan et al., 2014; Cicek and Yilmaz, 2012; Demirci et al., 2002; Karadam et al., 2008; Tilekliogiu, 2016). It was also found that the Western blot technique was the more sensitive method when compared with the ELISA for diagnosing toxocariasis (Artinyan et al., 2014). Toxocariasis was detected in 42.9% of 163 patients with high total IgE values and in 8.2% of 637 subjects with normal IgE levels, and here it was found that there was a significant correlation both with eosinophilia and IgE elevation and toxocariasis seropositivity (Cicek and Yilmaz, 2012).

5.6 Abdominal disorders

Kaplan et al. (2003) demonstrated that *T. canis* seropositivity was 33% in individuals with non-specific abdominal pain while it was 23% in controls, but the differences were not statistically significant. In a study by Cicek and Yilmaz (2012), 9.8% of patients with abdominal pain, and 4.9% of those with hepatomegaly were positive for toxocariasis. Ecevit et al. (2013) reported cases of hospitalised children with toxocariasis and abdominal pain that imitated tumour or infarction.

6. Concluding remarks

As a conclusion, though there are many studies on toxocariasis in Turkey, it is still not well understood how much the infection with

Toxocara is the reason for a plethora of signs and symptoms. Standardisation of the diagnostic methods and the use of molecular techniques could shed further light on the real epidemiology of this diseases.

Acknowledgement

I would like to thank Prof. Dr. Kosta Y. Mumcuoglu (Department of Microbiology and Molecular Genetics, The Hebrew University-Hadassah Medical School, Jerusalem, Israel) for the critical evaluation of this manuscript.

References

Acar, N., Kapran, Z., Utine, C.A., Buyukbabani, N., 2007. Pars plana vitrectomy revealed *Toxocara canis* organism. Int. Ophthalmol. 27, 277–280. https://doi.org/10.1007/s10792-007-9078-1.

Akdemir, C., 2010. Visceral larva migrans among children in Kutahya (Turkey) and an evaluation of playgrounds for *T. canis* eggs. Turk. J. Pediatr. 52, 158–162.

Akyol, A., Bicerol, B., Ertug, S., Ertabaklar, H., Kiylioglu, N., 2007. Epilepsy and seropositivity rates of *Toxocara canis* and *Toxoplasma gondii*. Seizure 16, 233–237. https://doi.org/10.1016/j.seizure.2006.12.008.

Artinyan, E., Uysal, H.K., Akgul, O., Altiparmak, S., Oner, Y.A., 2014. Research on *Toxocara canis* antibodies obtained from patients with eosinophilia. Indian J. Med. Microbiol. 32, 383–386. https://doi.org/10.4103/0255-0857.142239.

Atas, A.D., Ozcelik, S., Saygi, G., 1997. Helminth species seen in Sivas stray dogs, their spread and importance in terms of public health (in Turkish). Türk. Parazitol. Derg. 21, 305–309.

Avcioglu, H., Balkaya, I., 2011. The relationship of public park accessibility to dogs to the presence of *Toxocara* species ova in the soil. Vector Borne Zoonotic Dis. 11, 177–180. https://doi.org/10.1089/vbz.2009.0244.

Avcioglu, H., Burgu, A., 2008. Seasonal prevalence of *Toxocara* ova in soil samples from public parks in Ankara, Turkey. Vector Borne Zoonotic Dis. 8, 345–350. https://doi.org/10.1089/vbz.2007.0212.

Avcioglu, H., Soykan, E., Tarakci, U., 2011. Control of helminth contamination of raw vegetables by washing. Vector Borne Zoonotic Dis. 11, 189–191. https://doi.org/10.1089/vbz.2009.0243.

Ayaz, E., Yaman, N., Gul, A.N., 2003. Prevalence of *Toxocara* spp. eggs in soil of public parks in Van, Turkey. Indian Vet. J. 80, 574–576.

Aydenizoz Ozkayhan, M., 2006. Soil contamination with ascarid eggs in playgrounds in Kirikkale, Turkey. J. Helminthol. 80, 15–18. https://doi.org/10.1079/joh2005311.

Aydenizoz-Ozkayhan, M., Yagci, B.B., Erat, S., 2008. The investigation of *Toxocara canis* eggs in coats of different dog breeds as a potential transmission route in human toxocariasis. Vet. Parasitol. 25, 94–100. https://doi.org/10.1016/j.vetpar.2007.12.002.

Berk, T.A., Oner, H.F., Saatci, O.A., 2000. Underlying pathologies in secondary strabismus. Strabismus 8, 69–75.

Budak, S., Sermet, İ., Uner, A., 1984. Prevalence of ascaride in stray dogs in and around Izmir (in Turkish). Türk. Parazitol. Derg. 1, 57–65.

Buyukbaba, O., Ozkan, E., Buget, E., 1996. *Toxocara canis* infection and investigation of its seroprevalence in children by ELISA (in Turkish). Infeksiyon Derg. 10, 7–11.

Celik, T., Kaplan, Y., Atas, E., Oztuna, D., Berilgen, S., 2013. *Toxocara* seroprevalence in patients with idiopathic Parkinson's disease: chance association or coincidence? Biomed. Res. Int. 685196. https://doi.org/10.1155/2013/685196.

Cicek, M., Yilmaz, H., 2012. Prevalence of toxocariasis in humans and dogs in Van Province (in Turkish). Kafkas Univ. Vet. Fak. Derg. 18, 531–536. https://doi.org/10.9775/kvfd.2011.5211.

Dal, T., Cicek, M., Ucmak, D., Akkurt, M., Tekin, A., Dal, M.S., Tekin, R., Kalkanli, S.T., 2013. Seroprevalence of IgG anti-*Toxocara canis* antibodies and anti-*Fasciola* sp. antibodies in patients with urticaria. Clin. Ter. 164, 315–317. https://doi.org/10.7417/CT.2013.1579.

Demirci, M., Korkmaz, M., Sakru, N., Kaya, S., Kuman, A., 2002. Diagnostic importance of serological methods and eosinophilia in tissue parasites. J. Health Popul. Nutr. 20, 352–355.

Demirci, M., Yildirim, M., Aridogan, B.C., Baysal, V., Korkmaz, M., 2003. Tissue parasites in patients with chronic urticaria. J. Dermatol. 30, 777–781.

Demirci, M., Kaya, S., Cetin, E., Aridogan, B., Onal, S., Korkmaz, M., 2010. Seroepidemiological investigation of toxocariasis in the Isparta region of Turkey. Iran. J. Parasitol. 5, 52–59.

Dogan, N., Dinleyici, E.C., Bor, O., Toz, S.O., Ozbel, Y., 2007. Seroepidemiological survey for *Toxocara canis* infection in the northwestern part of Turkey. Türk. Parazitol. Derg. 31, 288–291.

Doganay, A., 1983. Helminth species in Ankara stray dogs, their distribution and importance in terms of public health (in Turkish). Ank. Univ. Vet. Fak. Derg. 30, 550–561.

Doganay, A., Oge, S., 1993. The prevalence of ascariasis in stray dogs in Ankara. Ank. Univ. Vet. Fak. Derg. 40, 552–562.

Ecevit, C., Bag, O., Vergin, C., Ozturk, A., 2013. Visceral larva migrans presenting with hypereosinophilia. Türk. Parazitol. Derg. 37, 58–60. https://doi.org/10.5152/tpd.2013.15.

Guclu, F., Aydenizoz, M., 1998. Detection of contamination by dogs and cats helminth eggs in playgrounds (in Turkish). Türk. Parazitol. Derg. 22, 194–198.

Gungor, C., Ciftci, E., Aral Akarsu, G., 1999. Prevalence of *Toxocara* antibody in children with complaints of unknown abdominal pain (in Turkish). Türk. Parazitol. Derg. 23, 24–27.

Gurel, F.S., Ertug, S., Okyay, P., 2005. Prevalence of *Toxocara* spp. eggs in public parks of the city of Aydin, Turkey. Türk. Parazitol. Derg. 29, 177–179.

Hakan, N., 2005. Seroprevalence of *Toxocara canis, Toxoplasma gondii,* and *Echinococcus granulosus* in Atopic Children in Comparison to Healthy Children (in Turkish). Celal Bayar University, Medical Faculty, Department of Child Health and Diseases, Thesis for Residency in Medicine Izmir.

Kaplan, M., Bulut, S., Gokmerdan, A., Kuk, S., Kalkan, A., 2002. Seropositivity of *Toxocara canis* in epileptic patient (in Turkish). Türk. Parazitol. Derg. 26, 415–417.

Kaplan, M., Dogru, O., Kuk, S., Bulbuller, N., Pektas, B., Altas, O., 2003. Can *Toxocara canis* be the cause of non-specific abdominal pain? (in Turkish). Firat Tip Derg. 8, 138–140.

Kaplan, M., Kalkan, A., Hosoglu, S., Kuk, S., Ozden, M., Demirdag, K., Ozdarendeli, A., 2004. The frequency of *Toxocara* infection in mental retarded children. Mem. Inst. Oswaldo Cruz 99, 121–125. https://doi.org/10.1590/s0074-02762004000200001.

Kaplan, M., Kamanli, A., Kalkan, A., Kuk, S., Gulkesen, A., Ardicoglu, O., Demirdag, K., 2005. Toxocariasis seroprevalence in patients with rheumatoid arthritis. Türk. Parazitol. Derg. 29, 251–254.

Kaplan, M., Kalkan, A., Kuk, S., Demirdag, K., Ozden, M., Kilic, S.S., 2008. *Toxocara* seroprevalence in schizophrenic patients in Turkey. Yonsei Med. J. 49, 224–229. https://doi.org/10.3349/ymj.2008.49.2.224.

Karaca, I., Mentes, J., Nalcaci, S., 2018. *Toxocara* neuroretinitis associated with raw meat consumption. Turk. J. Ophthalmol. 48, 258–261. https://doi.org/10.4274/tjo.27085.

Karadam, S.Y., Ertug, S., Ertabaklar, H., Okyay, P., 2008. The comparision of IgG antibodies specific to *Toxocara* spp. among eosinophilic and non-eosinophilic groups. New Microbiol. 31, 113–116.

Ketir, F., 2018. Parasitic Contamination of Raw Vegetables and Salads (in Turkish). Yuzuncu Yil University, Health Sciences Institute, Department of Parasitology, Master Thesis Van.

Korkmaz, M., 1998. Visceral Larva Migrans: Culturing of Second Phase *Toxocara canis* Larvae In-Vitro, Obtaining the Excretory-Secretory Antigens and Diagnosing by the ELISA Method (in Turkish). Ege University, Faculty of Medicine, Department of Parasitology, Thesis for Residency in Medicine Izmir.

Korkmaz, U.F., Gokpinar, S., Yildiz, K., 2016. Prevalence of intestinal parasites in cats and their importance in terms of public health. Türk. Parazitol. Derg. 40, 194–198. https://doi.org/10.5152/tpd.2016.4841.

Kozan, E., Sevimli, F.K., Kose, M., Eser, M., Cicek, H., 2007. Examination of helminth contaminated wastewaters used for agricultural purposes in Afyonkarahisar (in Turkish). Türk. Parazitol. Derg. 31, 197–200.

Kuk, S., Ozgocmen, S., Bulut, S., 2006a. Seroprevalance of *Toxocara* antibodies in multiple sclerosis and ankylosing spondylitis. Indian J. Med. Sci. 60, 297–299.

Kuk, S., Ozel, E., Oguzturk, H., Kirkil, G., Kaplan, M., 2006b. Seroprevalence of *Toxocara* antibodies in patients with adult asthma. South. Med. J. 99, 719–722. https://doi.org/10.1097/01.smj.0000223949.11527.48.

Kuman, H.A., Altintas, N., 1984. Toxocariasis cases diagnosed by serology in Aegean Region (in Turkish). Türk. Parazitol. Derg. 1–2, 113–119.

Kuru, B.B., Aypak, S., Aysul, N., 2013. Prevalence of *Echinococcus granulosus* determined with polymerase chain reaction in dogs in Aydin district (in Turkish). Türk. Parazitol. Derg. 37, 78–83. https://doi.org/10.5152/tpd.2013.20.

Kustimur, S., Dogruman Al, F., Oguzulgen, K., Bakir, H., Maral, I., Turktas, H., Tuzun, H., 2007. *Toxocara* seroprevalence in adults with bronchial asthma. Trans. R. Soc. Trop. Med. Hyg. 101, 270–274. https://doi.org/10.1016/j.trstmh.2006.08.013.

Merdivenci, A., 1962. Research on reservoir of larva migrans in Istanbul (in Turkish). Turk. Vet. Hekim. Dernegi Derg. 32, 382–398.

Merdivenci, A., 1963. Immunologic relations among human, dog and cat ascarids (in Turkish). Mikrobiyol. Derg. 16, 45–69.

Merdivenci, A., 1965. Research on immunity of ascariasis, toxocariasis and toxocariasis (in Turkish). Bornova Vet. Araştirma Enstitüsü Derg. 6, 96–122.

Merdivenci, A., 1970. Visceral larva migrans in man and host-parasite relations in larval toxocariasis (in Turkish). Saglik Derg. 44, 3–24.

Oge, S., Oge, H., 2000a. Prevalence of *Toxocara* spp. eggs in the soil of public parks in Ankara, Turkey. Dtsch. Tierarztl. Wochenschr. 107, 72–75.

Oge, H., Oge, S., 2000b. Quantitative comparison of various methods for detecting eggs of *Toxocara canis* in samples of sand. Vet. Parasitol. 92 (1), 75–79. https://doi.org/10.1016/s0304-4017(00)00276-4.

Oge, H., Oge, S., Ozbakis, G., Gurcan, S., 2014. Comparison of *Toxocara* eggs in hair and faecal samples from owned dogs and cats collected in Ankara, Turkey. Vet. Parasitol. 206, 227–231. https://doi.org/10.1016/j.vetpar.2014.10.005.

Oge, H., Oge, S., Ozbakis, G., Gurcan, I.S., 2017a. Helminth infections by coprological examination in sheep-dogs and their zoonotic importance. Türk. Parazitol. Derg. 41, 22–27. https://doi.org/10.5152/tpd.2017.5123.

Oge, H., Oge, S., Gonenc, B., Sarimehmetoglu, O., Ozbakis, G., 2017b. Coprodiagnosis of *Echinococcus granulosus* infection in dogs from Ankara, Turkey. Vet. Parasitol. 242, 44–46. https://doi.org/10.1016/j.vetpar.2017.05.016.

Oge, H., Oge, S., Ozbakis-Beceriklisoy, G., 2019. Detection and identification of *Toxocara canis* in infected dogs using PCR. Helminthologia 56, 118–123. https://doi.org/10.2478/helm-2019-0008.

Oguz, B., Ozdal, N., Serdar Deger, M., 2018. Genetic analysis of *Toxocara* spp. in stray cats and dogs in Van Province, Eastern Turkey. J. Vet. Res. 62, 291–295. https://doi.org/10.2478/jvetres-2018-0042.

Oguzturk, H., Saygi, G., 2002. Investigation of infection caused by larvae of *Toxocara canis* in elementary school students (in Turkish). Türk. Parazitol. Derg. 26, 409–414.

Orhun, R., Ayaz, E., 2006. Prevalence of helminths in dogs in the Region of Van and their potential public health significance (in Turkish). Türk. Parazitol. Derg. 30, 103–107.

Ozan, Z., 2007. Prevalence of Helminth Eggs for Salads (in Turkish). Afyon Kocatepe University, Health Sciences Institute, Department of (Veterinary) Parasitology, Master Thesis Afyon.

Ozcel, M.A., Altintas, N., 1987. Investigation of visceral larva migrans disease by serological methods (in Turkish). Türk. Parazitol. Derg. 11, 88–95.

Ozdal, P.C., Sen, E., Yazici, A., Ozturk, F., 2012. Patterns of childhood-onset uveitis in a referral center in Turkey. J. Ophthalmic. Inflamm. Infect. 2, 13–19. https://doi.org/10.1007/s12348-011-0044-8.

Saglam, M.G., 1999. Evaluation of *Toxocara canis* Occurrence by the ELISA Method (in Turkish). Istanbul University, Health Sciences Institute, Department of Microbiology and Clinical Microbiology, Master Thesis Istanbul.

Saygi, G., Ozcelik, S., Temizkan, N., 1990. Helminths we found in the small intestine of Sivas Street Dogs (in Turkish). Türk. Parazitol. Derg. 14, 81–93.

Sayin İpek, D.N., Kochan, A., 2017. Gastrointestinal helminths seen in stray dogs in Diyarbakir (in Turkish). Harran Univ. Vet. Fak. Derg. 6, 133–137. https://doi.org/10.31196/huvfd.384244.

Selek, M.B., Baylan, O., 2013. Human toxocariasis (in Turkish). Turk Hij. Deney. Biyol. Derg. 70, 113–134. https://doi.org/10.5505/TurkHijyen.2013.04875.

Selek, M.B., Baylan, O., Kutlu, A., Ozyurt, M., 2015. *Toxocara canis* IgG seropositivity in patients with chronic urticaria. Iran. J. Allergy Asthma Immunol. 14, 450–456.

Senlik, B., Cirak, V.Y., Karabacak, A., 2006. Intestinal nematode infections in Turkish military dogs with special reference to *Toxocara canis*. J. Helminthol. 80, 299–300.

Simsek, S., Utuk, A.E., Koroglu, E., 2005. Prevalence *Toxocara* spp. of eggs in some school gardens in Elazig (in Turkish). Fırat Üniv. Sağlık Bilimleri Derg. 19 (2), 133–136.

Sozen, H., Citil, B.E., Caylak, S., Gokmen, A.A., Kaya, S., Demirci, M., Korkmaz, M., Sahin, C., Kirli, I., 2015. Seroepidemiological study of toxocariasis among volunteers of animal husbandry workers and veterinary in Southern Anatolia region of Turkey in 2014. Iran. J. Parasitol. 10, 473–481.

Tilekliogl u, E., 2016. Fascioliasis, Toxocariasis and Hydatidosis Seroprevalance in Eosinophilic Patients (in Turkish). Yuzuncu Yil University, Health Sciences Institute, Department of Parasitology, Master Thesis Van.

Yaman, M., Ayaz, E., Gul, A., Muz, M.N., 2006. Investigation of helminth infections of cats and dogs in the Hatay Province. Türk. Parazitol. Derg. 30, 200–204.

Yariktas, M., Demirci, M., Aynali, G., Kaya, S., Doner, F., 2007. Relationship between *Toxocara* seropositivity and allergic rhinitis. Am. J. Rhinol. 21, 248–250.

Yazar, S., Yaman, O., Cetinkaya, U., Hamamci, B., Sahin, I., 2010. Investigation of anti-*Toxocara canis* IgG antibodies in patients presenting at the Erciyes University Medical Faculty, Department of Parasitology (in Turkish). Türk. Parazitol. Derg. 34, 24–26.

Yesilcayir, H.E., 2017. Determination of Helminth EGGS on Raw Vegetables used for Salads in Aydin Region (in Turkish). Adnan Menderes University, Health Sciences Institute, Department of (Veterinary) Parasitology, Master Thesis Aydin.

CHAPTER TWENTY-FOUR

Seroprevalence of *Toxocara* spp. antibodies in humans in Africa: A review

Felix Lötsch[a], Martin Peter Grobusch[b,*]

[a]Division of Infectious Diseases and Tropical Medicine, Department of Medicine, Medical University of Vienna, Vienna, Austria

[b]Department of Infectious Diseases, Centre of Tropical Medicine and Travel Medicine, Amsterdam University Medical Centers, location AMC, University of Amsterdam, Amsterdam, The Netherlands

*Corresponding author: e-mail address: m.p.grobusch@amsterdamumc.nl

Contents

Abstract

Background

Human toxocariasis occurs worldwide and is caused by nematodes of the species of the genus *Toxocara*. Infection occurs by the ingestion of eggs and is usually asymptomatic or oligosymptomatic. However, severe manifestations occur. The burden of disease and its public health impact remain ill-defined. The aim of this review was to summarize all available data on the seroprevalence of toxocariasis on the African continent and factors associated with seropositivity.

Methods

Twenty-seven original papers published between 1991 and 2017 were identified that provided data suitable for this review. Case–control studies were included and the seroprevalence in the (healthy) control group was used as a surrogate parameter.

Results

Antibodies against *Toxocara* spp. were found to be frequent in most populations and regions in Africa with the exception of two publications, one from the Democratic

Advances in Parasitology, Volume 109
ISSN 0065-308X
https://doi.org/10.1016/bs.apar.2020.01.022

Republic of the Congo and one from Djibouti, where all participants were seronegative. The highest proportion of participants with antibodies was found on the island of La Réunion with 359 out 387 study participants being positive (92.8%). Factors associated with seropositivity were reported across studies, including—among others—older age, contact with soil via geophagia, agricultural activity or playing with soil, contact with animals, especially dogs, and low socio-economic status, defined as absence of water supply or poor housing. Three Egyptian studies found male gender to be associated with toxocariasis, whereas in La Réunion females were at increased risk.

Conclusions

Exposure to toxocariasis seems to be very frequent and common in large parts of the African continent. However, no data are available for most countries. The public health impact of human toxocariasis and the frequency of severe manifestations remain unclear.

1. Background

Human toxocariasis is a global parasitic zoonosis caused by larvae of *Toxocara* species. *Toxocara* spp. are nematodes belonging to the order of Ascaridida. The most important species relevant for humans are *T. canis*, the dog roundworm, and *T. cati*, the feline roundworm (Ma et al., 2018; Strube et al., 2013). Humans are accidental dead-end hosts of the parasite, which will therefore not develop into adult worms in the human host. It can cause a variety of clinical syndromes mainly depending on the location of its manifestation. These syndromes include covert toxocariasis, larva migrans visceralis, ocular toxocariasis and/or neurotoxocariasis (Macpherson, 2013). Furthermore, associations with asthma (Aghaei et al., 2018; Li et al., 2014), cardiac disease (Kuenzli et al., 2016; Zibaei, 2017) or epilepsy (Luna et al., 2018) have been described. However, most infections are thought to be either asymptomatic or very mild, with unspecific symptoms. Infection occurs through the ingestion of food, fluids or soil contaminated with eggs. After hatching of the eggs, the larvae may migrate through various tissues of the body where they cause respective symptoms, eliciting an immune response.

Although there is an abundance of case reports of severe manifestations of toxocariasis in the literature, there is practically no data on the incidence of such manifestations. To our knowledge, only one publication reports some form of incidence of the condition. In a study with travellers to the African continent, the rate of seroconversion was 4.5/1000 person-months

(Baaten et al., 2011). However, it is not clear what fraction of patients had symptoms attributable to the infection with *Toxocara* larvae. Two other studies aimed to determine the prevalence of ocular toxocariasis in Irish schoolchildren and residents from Alabama, respectively. They estimated the prevalence to be 9.7 cases per 100,000 and 1 per 1000, respectively (Good et al., 2004), Maetz et al., 1987). Additionally, there are no formal studies that have attempted to quantify the impact of toxocariasis both on an individual and societal level by calculating disability-adjusted life years (DALYs), years of life lost (YLLs) or economic losses. Thus, seroprevalence studies currently provide the only data on the epidemiology of human toxocariasis and allow the identification of groups and risk and factors associated with seropositivity. For Africa, some data is available for several countries and several populations, with large gaps in between. The aim of this review was to summarize available data on the seroprevalence of toxocariasis and associated risk factors on the African continent.

2. Methods

A systematic search was performed based on PubMed. The search term combined synonyms for *Toxocara* spp. or toxocariasis with "Africa" or names of all African countries (for details of the search term see Appendix). No time restrictions were applied, and no relevant papers in languages other than English were identified through the respective search term and databases. This resulted in 307 hits. This search strategy was supplemented by a manual search of Google Scholar and findings of a previous systematic review of the authors (Lötsch et al., 2017). Twenty-seven articles provided data on the seroprevalence of *Toxocara* spp. in various African countries and were therefore included. Case–control studies were included, and findings in the respective (healthy) control groups are presented in this review. Case reports, studies in migrants or travellers, animal studies and environmental studies were beyond the scope of this review and excluded. The key outcome was the seroprevalence of anti-*Toxocara* antibodies. Other variables extracted included the study region, population, method of diagnosis and factors associated with toxocariasis. Seroprevalence, the study population and the method of assessment are presented in Table 1. Risk factors for antibodies against *Toxocara* spp. with respective references are listed in Table 2. For a structured arrangement of the results, findings were grouped according to the African subregions (Northern Africa, Central Africa, West Africa, East Africa and Southern Africa).

Table 1 Included studies with region of study, seroprevalence, study population and method of analysis.

Region	Seroprevalence with reference	Population	Method of analysis
North Africa			
Egypt, Alexandria	0/53 (0%) (el Zawawy et al., 1995)	Patients with unexplained eosinophilia	Countercurrent immune-electrophoresis
Egypt, Mansoura	12/200 (3.5%) (Elshazly et al., 2011)	Healthy control children attending Mansoura Children Hospital	ELISA (Bordier Affinity Products)
Egypt, Giza	1/30 (3.3%) (Safar et al., 1995)	Healthcare staff as controls	Immunofluorescence antibody test
Egypt, Sharkia Governorate	18/300 (6.0%) (Hassan et al., 1996)	Children with splenomegaly	Immunofluorescence antibody test
Egypt, Cairo and Zagazig Governorates	1/30 (3.3%) (Mohamed et al., 1991)	Healthy controls in a case–control study	Immunofluorescence antibody test
Egypt, Giza	1/45 (2.2%) (El-Sayed and Ismail, 2012)	Healthy controls in a case–control study	ELISA IgG (R-Biopharma)
Egypt, Mansoura	35/455 (7.7%) (El-Shazly et al., 2009)	Patients attending hospital without allergy, viral hepatitis, malignancy, auto-immune disease, steroid therapy or immunotherapy	ELISA (Bordier Affinity Products)
Egypt, Tanta	8/128 (6.2%) in children 4/22 (18%) in adults (Antonios et al., 2008)	Children and adults with fever of unknown origin or other presumptive symptoms	ELISA (R-Biopharm)
Egypt, Cairo	4/30 (13.3%) (Ismail and Khalafallah, 2005)	Healthy controls in a case–control study on urticaria	In-house ELISA
Egypt, Sharkia Governorate	1/20 (5%) (Nada et al., 1996)	Healthy children as controls in a case control study on renal disease	ELISA

Table 1 Included studies with region of study, seroprevalence, study population and method of analysis.—cont'd

Region	Seroprevalence with reference	Population	Method of analysis
Egypt, Heliopolis	9/30 (30.0%) (Oteifa et al., 1998)	Healthy children as controls in a case control study on allergic diseases	ELISA
Egypt, Benha	2/20 (10%) (Eraky et al., 2016)	Healthy children as controls in a case control study on cryptogenic epilepsy	ELISA (R-Biopharm)
Central Africa			
Gabon, Moyen-Ogooué	199/332 (59.9%) (Lötsch et al., 2016) [53.6% (48.2–59.0%) age-standardized]	Adults from rural region	ELISA (Bordier Affinity Products) and Western Blot IgG (LDBIO Diagnostics)
DR Congo, Titule, Bas-Uélé Province	0/61 (0%) (Colebunders et al., 2016)	Healthy controls from a case–control study on risk factors for epilepsy	ELISA (Bordier Affinity Products)
Cameroon, Tombel Health District	61/168 (36.3%) (Nkouawa et al., 2010)	Volunteers from local villages	ELISA
West Africa			
Nigeria, Jos, Plateau State	31/104 (29.8%) (Ajayi et al., 2000)	Patients and local students	In-house ELISA
Ghana, Central Region	303/566 (53.5%) (Kyei et al., 2015)	Children attending local healthcare institutions	ELISA
Ghana, Kintampo	16/117 (13.7%) in children 36/175 (20.6%) in adults (Ngugi et al., 2013)	Children and adult controls in a case–control study on risk factors for epilepsy	ELISA IgG (Cypress Diagnostics)

Continued

Table 1 Included studies with region of study, seroprevalence, study population and method of analysis.—cont'd

Region	Seroprevalence with reference	Population	Method of analysis
Nigeria, Makoko, Lagos	315/366 (86.1%) (Gyang et al., 2015)	Children in primary school	In-house Western Blot
Nigeria, Osun State	116/308 (37.3%) (Sowemimo et al., 2017)	Preschool children	Western Blot
East Africa			
Tanzania, Haydom	8/20 (40%) Winkler et al., 2008)	Controls without epilepsy from a case control study	In-house ELISA and Western Blot
Tanzania, Ifakara	31/71 (43.7%) in children 48/82 (58.5%) in adults (Ngugi et al., 2013)	Children and adult controls in a case–control study on risk factors for epilepsy	ELISA IgG (Cypress Diagnostics)
Djibouti	0/108 (0%) (Chantal et al., 1996)	Workers in a slaughterhouse	Western Blot (BioMérieux)
Burundi, Kiremba	97/191 (50.8%) (Nicoletti et al., 2007)	Controls of case–control study on epilepsy	Western Blot IgG (LDBIO Diagnostics)
Uganda, Iganga-Mayuge	23/126 (18.3%) in children 26/73 (35.6%) in adults (Ngugi et al., 2013)	Children and adult controls in a case–control study on risk factors for epilepsy	ELISA IgG (Cypress Diagnostics)
Kenya, Kilifi	40/137 (29.2%) in children 38/129 (29.5%) in adults (Ngugi et al., 2013)	Children and adult controls in a case–control study on risk factors for epilepsy	ELISA IgG (Cypress Diagnostics)
Kenya, Turkana district	17/228 (7.5%) (Kenny et al., 1995)	Volunteers from local communities	In-house ELISA

Table 1 Included studies with region of study, seroprevalence, study population and method of analysis.—cont'd

Region	Seroprevalence with reference	Population	Method of analysis
Southern Africa			
Mozambique, Beira	44/601 (7.3%) (Noormahomed et al., 2014)	Adult patients with HIV	Western Blot IgG (LDBIO Diagnostics)
South Africa, Agincourt	13/59 (22.0%) in children 12/152 (7.9%) in adults (Ngugi et al., 2013)	Children and adult controls in a case–control study on risk factors for epilepsy	ELISA IgG (Cypress Diagnostics)
Swaziland, low and middle-veld	41/92 (44.6%) (Liao et al., 2010)	Children from rural slums	Western Blot
Other			
La Réunion	359/387 (92.8%) (Magnaval et al., 1994)	Randomly selected individuals	In-house Western Blot

3. Results

Twenty-seven papers were identified with data that were judged suitable for the purpose of this review. Twelve publications provided data on the seroprevalence in North Africa, all of which were conducted in Egypt. From Central Africa, data was available from Gabon, the Democratic Republic of the Congo (DR Congo) and Cameroon. In West Africa, seroprevalence studies were published from Nigeria (3 publications) and Ghana (2 publications). Regarding East Africa, data was available from Kenya (2 publications), Tanzania (2 publications), Uganda (1 publication), Burundi (1 publication) and Djibouti (1 publication). Studies from Mozambique (1 publication), South Africa (1 publication) and Swaziland (1 publication) were identified in the Southern African region. Additionally, one paper from La Réunion was found. Although politically La Réunion is part of France, it was included on geographical grounds. All data are summarized in Table 1.

Table 2 Risk factors for antibodies against *Toxocara* spp. identified across all included studies.

Associated factors (risk factors)	References
Demographic and socio-economic factors	
Older age	Winkler et al. (2008), Elshazly et al. (2011), Magnaval et al. (1994), Kyei et al. (2015), Gyang et al. (2015), and Antonios et al. (2008)
Male gender	Elshazly et al. (2011), Antonios et al. (2008), and Nada et al. (1996)
Female gender	Magnaval et al. (1994)
Absence of water supply; drinking of unboiled water	Magnaval et al. (1994) and Gyang et al. (2015)
Rural residence	El-Shazly et al. (2009), Antonios et al. (2008), and Nada et al. (1996)
Poor housing	El-Shazly et al. (2009)
Behavioural factors	
Geophagia	Ajayi et al. (2000)
Raw food intake, consumption of raw vegetables	El-Sayed and Ismail, 2012 and Gyang et al. (2015)
Bad personal hygiene; not washing hands	El-Sayed and Ismail, 2012 and Kyei et al. (2015)
Keeping pets	Kyei et al. (2015) and El-Shazly et al. (2009)
Playing with soil, frequent contact with soil	Kyei et al. (2015) and El-Shazly et al. (2009)
Agricultural activity	Lötsch et al. (2016)
Contact with dogs	Gyang et al. (2015) and Sowemimo et al. (2017)
Clinical factors and symptoms	
Active antiretroviral therapy	Noormahomed et al. (2014)
Headache	Noormahomed et al. (2014)
Epilepsy	Nicoletti et al. (2007) and Ngugi et al. (2013)
Visual problems	Kyei et al. (2015)
Mental handicap	Mohamed et al. (1991)
Schizophrenia	El-Sayed and Ismail, 2012
Cough	Kyei et al. (2015)
Eosinophilia	El-Sayed and Ismail, 2012
Other intestinal parasites	El-Sayed and Ismail, 2012

In North Africa, only studies form Egypt were identified. Due to the absence of high-quality, population based seroprevalence surveys, data from (healthy) control groups of case-control studies were included. In summary, the seroprevalence ranged from 0% in patients with eosinophilia in Alexandria to 30% in a control group of children in Heliopolis (el Zawawy et al., 1995; Oteifa et al., 1998).

In Central African rural Gabon, the age-standardized seroprevalence was 53.6% (48.2–59.0%), whereas anti-Toxocara antibodies were found in 36.3% of volunteers from villages in the Tombel Health district in South-West Cameroon. Surprisingly, in a study performed in Bas-Uélé province in the North of the Democratic Republic of the Congo, none of the 61 controls in a case–control study on risk factors of epilepsy had antibodies detected. The reasons for this remain unclear.

In West Africa, five studies report a seroprevalence between 13.7% in children from Kintampo (Ngugi et al., 2013), Ghana, to 86.1% in Makoko, an urban slum in Lagos, Nigeria (Gyang et al., 2015). In Nigeria, high seroprevalences were also found in Jos, Plateau State, with 29.8% (Ajayi et al., 2000) and in pre-school children from Osun state with 37.3% (Sowemimo et al., 2017).

In the East African subregion, the seroprevalence ranged from 0% in slaughterhouse workers in Djibouti (Chantal et al., 1996) to 58.5% in Ifakara, Tanzania, in adults participating as healthy controls in a case control study in risk factors for epilepsy (Ngugi et al., 2013). The same study also provided data from Iganga-Mayuge, Uganda, and Kilifi, Kenya. The seroprevalence in healthy children was 18.3% and 35.6% in adults in Uganda, respectively; and 29.2% in children and 29.5% in Kenyan adults, respectively. Data from two independent studies from Tanzania and Burundi showed comparable results with 40% and 50.8% of participants being positive, respectively.

Only three publications reported data from Southern Africa. In patients with HIV in Beira, Mozambique, only 7.3% were found to have antibodies against *Toxocara* spp. (Noormahomed et al., 2014). The proportion of positive individuals was higher in Agincourt, South Africa; with 22.0% in children 7.9% in adults participating in a case control study on risk factors for epilepsy (Ngugi et al., 2013). The highest seroprevalence, however, was found in Swaziland with 44.6% of children from rural slums being positive (Liao et al., 2010).

The highest seroprevalence of all studies was found on the French island of La Réunion (Magnaval et al., 1994). Among 387 randomly selected individuals, 92.8% had antibodies against *Toxocara* spp.

An abundance of risk factors was reported throughout the included studies and are listed in Table 2. Interestingly, in three Egyptian studies, male gender was reported to be associated with antibodies against *Toxocara* spp. (Antonios et al., 2008; Elshazly et al., 2011; Nada et al., 1996), whereas the only study outside Egypt reporting a significant association between gender and toxocariasis, found females to be at increased risk (Magnaval et al., 1994) with 110/124 (88.7%) male and 249/263 (94.7%) female participants harbouring antibodies. Social and cultural factors including religion may be a possible explanation for this finding. Other reported risk factors such as poor housing, agricultural activity, absence of water supply or drinking of unboiled water may indicate that exposure to *Toxocara* spp. is increased in rural areas and linked to low socio-economic status (Gyang et al., 2015; Lötsch et al., 2016; Magnaval et al., 1994).

Furthermore, also increased contact with soil by various means such as geophagia, playing with soil, or consumption of raw vegetables or food was found to be linked to seropositivity (Ajayi et al., 2000; El-Sayed and Ismail, 2012; El-Shazly et al., 2009; Kyei et al., 2015; Lötsch et al., 2016). This seems comprehensible, considering the mode of transmission of the disease. Although not reported consistently, also pets or contact with dogs and poor personal hygiene were found to be linked to toxocariasis (El-Sayed and Ismail, 2012; El-Shazly et al., 2009; Gyang et al., 2015; Kyei et al., 2015; Sowemimo et al., 2017;). This seems equally comprehensible as dogs are the most important definite hosts for *T. canis*, the species also most relevant for human disease. Last but not least, several symptoms and clinical conditions were linked to the presence of anti-*Toxocara* antibodies. These include visual problems, neuropsychiatric conditions, cough, epilepsy, among others (Colebunders et al., 2016; El-Sayed and Ismail, 2012; Eraky et al., 2016; Hassan et al., 1996; Kenny et al., 1995; Kyei et al., 2015; Ngugi et al., 2013; Nicoletti et al., 2007; Nkouawa et al., 2010; Noormahomed et al., 2014; Safar et al., 1995; Mohamed et al., 1991; Ismail and Khalafallah, 2005; Winkler et al., 2008).

4. Discussion

The aim of this review was to summarize all available data on the seroprevalence of toxocariasis in humans on the African continent. It underlines that exposure to *Toxocara* spp. must be frequent across various geographic, climatic, cultural and political regions in Africa. Only 2 out of 27 publications could not detect any antibodies in their study populations from Bas-Uélé, Democratic Republic of the Congo, and Djibouti (Chantal et al., 1996; Colebunders et al., 2016); whereas seropositivity was frequent in all other publications with the most extreme finding (92.8%) coming from the French island of La Réunion (Magnaval et al., 1994). According to associated factors reported across included studies, human toxocariasis may be seen as a condition linked to low socio-economic status, and contact with soil and animals, especially dogs. This may help to identify regions and populations at risk. Older age was also reported by several studies to be linked to toxocariasis (Antonios et al., 2008; Elshazly et al., 2011; Gyang et al., 2015; Kyei et al., 2015; Magnaval et al., 1994; Winkler et al., 2008). This seems plausible considering that seropositivity may not represent active infection but cumulative previous exposure to the helminth. Although no studies directly have compared different regions in Africa, seroprevalences in dry areas (e.g. Egypt or Djibouti) very roughly seem to be lower than in warm and humid areas. A possible explanation may be the fact that humidity (and warmer temperatures) enhance egg development in the environment (Gamboa, 2005). Socioeconomic and cultural factors, including religion, and their impact on hygiene practices or handling of animals (especially dogs), may also play a role.

Several symptoms or clinical conditions were linked to seropositivity across included studies. These include neuropsychiatric conditions, cough or visual problems (El-Sayed and Ismail, 2012; Hassan et al., 1996; Kyei et al., 2015; Ngugi et al., 2013; Nicoletti et al., 2007). Although it may be intuitive to assume a causative link (i.e. exposure to *Toxocara* spp. leading to these conditions), this can by no means be deflected from the present studies due to their design (i.e. cross-sectional studies and case–control studies). It may also be possible that such conditions (e.g. psychiatric diseases) lead to an increased risk of exposure to toxocariasis.

Unfortunately, to our knowledge, no studies have been published yet aiming to determine the incidence of symptomatic toxocariasis and the frequency of severe manifestations. Thus, the public health impact of the exposure to toxocariasis remains to be elucidated. However, given that exposure seems to be very frequent in many parts of Africa, even mild symptoms may accumulate to a substantial public health burden. For example, children that had antibodies against *Toxocara* spp. performed less well on several neuropsychological tests than those without (Marmor et al., 2011). Thus, its public health impact and its socio-economic impact probably may have been vastly underestimated.

Another issue that has not received much attention in the past is possible interactions between toxocariasis and other infectious diseases mediated by modulations in the immune response. It is known that exposure to toxocariasis is linked to allergic diseases such as asthma (Li et al., 2014). However, possible interactions with vaccines reducing their effectiveness (Cooper et al., 2000; Nookala et al., 2004) or other chronic infectious disease occurring frequently in Africa have so far not been investigated. In the case of tuberculosis, immunomodulatory effects of chronic helminth infections are thought to hamper the effectiveness of BCG vaccination and to impair the cellular immune response to *Mycobacterium tuberculosis*, translating into an increased risk of infection and disease (Chatterjee and Nutman, 2015). Such effects seem especially concerning for Africa, where infectious diseases are still a leading cause of morbidity and mortality in many parts of the continent.

Several studies included in this review report to have used serologic tests (mainly ELISA and WB) to detect antibodies against *T. canis*. However, with current serologic tools differentiation between *T. canis* and *T. cati* is not possible (Poulsen et al., 2015). Thus, the relative importance of each species in humans remains unclear.

In summary, exposure to toxocariasis seems to be very common in most parts of the African continent, with large knowledge gaps remaining, regarding the situation in most countries and regions, the frequency of clinically relevant disease and severe manifestations, and its public health relevance. Future studies need to aim at determining the relative frequency of symptoms and syndromes attributable to *Toxocara* spp. by screening for them using standardized case definitions. When investigating risk factors, environmental and socio-economic factors and practices need to be addressed. Ideally, seroprevalence (or disease) in humans should be linked to infestation in relevant definite hosts in the surroundings and environmental contamination with eggs. We are optimistic that the awareness of toxocariasis as a relevant parasitosis has increased over the last years and that increased efforts in research will lead to a better understanding of the impact of human toxocariasis, with new interventions and strategies ultimately transforming human toxocariasis from a neglected to a negligible condition.

Appendix

Search term #1

("Toxocara"[Mesh] OR "Toxocara canis infection (canine roundworms)" [Supplementary Concept] OR "Toxocariasis"[Mesh] OR "Larva Migrans, Visceral"[Mesh] OR Toxoca*)

Search term #2

(africa* OR "Africa"[Mesh] OR "algeria"[MeSH Terms] OR "algeria"[All Fields] OR "angola"[MeSH Terms] OR "angola"[All Fields] OR "benin"[MeSH Terms] OR "benin"[All Fields] OR "botswana"[MeSH Terms] OR "botswana"[All Fields] OR "burkina faso"[MeSH Terms] OR "burkina faso"[All Fields] OR "burundi"[MeSH Terms] OR "burundi"[All Fields] OR "cameroon"[MeSH Terms] OR "cameroon"[All Fields] OR "cape verde"[MeSH Terms] OR "cape verde"[All Fields] OR "central african republic"[MeSH Terms] OR "central african republic"[All Fields] OR "chad"[MeSH Terms] OR "chad"[All Fields] OR "comoros"[MeSH Terms] OR "comoros"[All Fields] OR "congo"[MeSH Terms] OR "congo"[All Fields] OR "djibouti"[MeSH Terms] OR "djibouti"[All Fields] OR "egypt"[MeSH Terms] OR "egypt"[All Fields] OR "equatorial guinea"[MeSH Terms] OR "equatorial guinea"[All Fields] OR "eritrea"[MeSH Terms] OR "eritrea"[All Fields] OR "ethiopia"[MeSH Terms] OR "ethiopia"[All Fields] OR "gabon"[MeSH Terms] OR "gabon"[All Fields] OR "gambia"[MeSH Terms] OR "gambia"[All Fields] OR "ghana"[MeSH Terms] OR "ghana"[All Fields] OR "guinea"[MeSH Terms] OR "guinea"[All Fields] OR "guinea-bissau"[MeSH Terms] OR "guinea-bissau"[All Fields] OR "guinea bissau"[All Fields] OR "Ivory Coast"[All Fields] OR "Cote d'Ivoire"[Mesh] OR "Cote d'Ivoire"[All Fields] OR "kenya"[MeSH Terms] OR "kenya"[All Fields] OR "lesotho"[MeSH Terms] OR "lesotho"[All Fields] OR "liberia"[MeSH Terms] OR "liberia"[All Fields] OR "libya"[MeSH Terms] OR "libya"[All Fields] OR "madagascar"[MeSH Terms] OR "madagascar"[All Fields] OR "malawi"[MeSH Terms] OR "malawi"[All Fields] OR "mali"[MeSH Terms] OR "mali"[All Fields] OR "mauritania"[MeSH Terms] OR "mauritania"[All Fields] OR "mauritius"[MeSH Terms] OR "mauritius"[All Fields] OR "morocco"[MeSH Terms] OR "morocco"[All Fields] OR "mozambique"[MeSH Terms] OR "mozambique"[All Fields] OR "namibia"[MeSH Terms] OR "namibia"[All Fields] OR "niger"[MeSH Terms] OR "niger"[All Fields] OR "nigeria"[MeSH Terms] OR "nigeria"[All Fields] OR "rwanda"[MeSH Terms] OR "rwanda"[All Fields] OR "senegal"[MeSH Terms] OR "senegal"[All Fields] OR "seychelles"[MeSH Terms] OR "seychelles"[All Fields] OR "Sierra Leone"[All Fields] OR "somalia"[MeSH Terms] OR "somalia"[All Fields] OR "South Africa"[All Fields] OR "Sudan" [MeSH] OR "Sudan" [All Fields] OR "swaziland"[MeSH Terms] OR "swaziland"[All Fields] OR

"Sao Tome"[All Fields] OR "tanzania"[MeSH Terms] OR "tanzania"[All Fields] OR "togo"[MeSH Terms] OR "togo"[All Fields] OR "tunisia"[MeSH Terms] OR "tunisia"[All Fields] OR "uganda"[MeSH Terms] OR "uganda"[All Fields] OR "Western Sahara"[All Fields] OR "zambia"[MeSH Terms] OR "zambia"[All Fields] OR "zimbabwe"[MeSH Terms] OR "zimbabwe"[All Fields] OR "Reunion"[Mesh] OR "La Reunion"[All Fields] OR "Mayotte"[All Fields] OR "Ceuta"[All Fields] OR "Melilla" [All Fields])

References

Safar, E.H., Abd-el Ghaffar, F.M., Saffar, S.A., Makled, K.M., Habib, K.S., el Abiad, R., El-Shabrawy, E., 1995. Incidence of *Toxoplasma* and *Toxocara* antibodies among out-patients in the Ophthalmic Research Institute, Egypt. J. Egypt. Soc. Parasitol. 25, 839–852.

Aghaei, S., Riahi, S.M., Rostami, A., Mohammadzadeh, I., Javanian, M., Tohidi, E., Foroutan, M., Esmaeili Dooki, M., 2018. *Toxocara* spp. infection and risk of childhood asthma: a systematic review and meta-analysis. Acta Trop. 182, 298–304. https://doi.org/10.1016/j.actatropica.2018.03.022.

Ajayi, O.O., Duhlinska, D.D., Agwale, S.M., Njoku, M., 2000. Frequency of human toxocariasis in Jos, Plateau State, Nigeria. Mem. Inst. Oswaldo Cruz 95, 147–149.

Antonios, S.N., Eid, M.M., Khalifa, E.A., Othman, A.A., 2008. Seroprevalence study of *Toxocara canis* in selected Egyptian patients. J. Egypt. Soc. Parasitol. 38, 313–318.

Baaten, G.G., Sonder, G.J., van Gool, T., Kint, J.A., van den Hoek, A., 2011. Travel-related schistosomiasis, strongyloidiasis, filariasis, and toxocariasis: the risk of infection and the diagnostic relevance of blood eosinophilia. BMC Infect. Dis. 11, 84. https://doi.org/10.1186/1471-2334-11-84.

Chantal, J., Bessiere, M., LeGuenno, B., Magnaval, J., Dorchies, P., 1996. A sero-prevalence survey of carriers of the agents of zoonotic diseases on some workers of Djibouti slaughter-house. Bull. Soc. Pathol. Exot. 89, 353–357.

Chatterjee, S., Nutman, T.B., 2015. Helminth-induced immune regulation: implications for immune responses to tuberculosis. PLoS Pathog. 11, e1004582. https://doi.org/10.1371/journal.ppat.1004582.

Colebunders, R., Mandro, M., Mokili, J.L., Mucinya, G., Mambandu, G., Pfarr, K., Reiter-Owona, I., Hoerauf, A., Tepage, F., Levick, B., Begon, M., Laudisoit, A., 2016. Risk factors for epilepsy in Bas-Uélé Province, Democratic Republic of the Congo: a case–control study. Int. J. Infect. Dis. 49, 1–8. https://doi.org/10.1016/j.ijid.2016.05.018.

Cooper, P.J., Chico, M.E., Losonsky, G., Sandoval, C., Espinel, I., Sridhara, R., Aguilar, M., Guevara, R.H., Levine, M.M., Griffin, G.E., Nutman, G.E., 2000. Albendazole treatment of children with ascariasis enhances the vibriocidal antibody response to the live attenuated oral cholera vaccine CVD 103-HgR. J Infect Dis 182, 1199–1206. https://doi.org/10.1086/315837.

el Zawawy, L.A., el Nassery, S.F., al Azzouni, M.Z., Abou el Naga, I.F., el Temsahi, M.M., Awadalla, H.N., 1995. A study on patients with eosinophilia of suspected parasitic origin. J. Egypt. Soc. Parasitol. 25, 245–255.

El-Sayed, N.M., Ismail, K.A., 2012. Relationship between *Toxocara canis* infection and schizophrenia. Rawal Med. J. 37 (02), 155–161.

El-Shazly, A.M., Abdel Baset, S.M., Kamal, A., Mohammed, K.A., Sakrs, T.I., Hammad, S.M., 2009. Seroprevalence of human toxocariasis (visceral larva migrans). J. Egypt. Soc. Parasitol. 39, 731–744.

Elshazly, A.M., Attia, G., El-Ghareeb, A.S.A., Belal, U.S., 2011. Clinical varieties of Toxocariasis canis in Children's hospital, Mansoura University: is it an underestimated problem? J. Egypt. Soc. Parasitol. 41, 263–274.

Eraky, M.A., Abdel-Hady, S., Abdallah, K.F., 2016. Seropositivity of *Toxoplasma gondii* and *Toxocara* spp. in children with cryptogenic epilepsy, Benha, Egypt. Korean J. Parasitol. 54, 335–338. https://doi.org/10.3347/kjp.2016.54.3.335.

Gamboa, M.I., 2005. Effects of temperature and humidity on the development of eggs of *Toxocara canis* under laboratory conditions. J. Helminthol. 79, 327–331. https://doi.org/10.1079/JOH2005287.

Good, B., Holland, C.V., Taylor, M.R.H., Larragy, J., Moriarty, P., O'Regan, M., 2004. Ocular toxocariasis in school children. Clin. Infect. Dis. 39, 173–178. https://doi.org/10.1086/421492.

Gyang, P.V., Akinwale, O.P., Lee, Y.-L., Chuang, T.-W., Orok, A.B., Ajibaye, O., Liao, C.W., Chen, P.C., Chou, C.M., Huang, Y.C., Barghouth, U., Fan, C.K., 2015. Seroprevalence, disease awareness, and risk factors for Toxocara canis infection among primary schoolchildren in Makoko, an urban slum community in Nigeria. Acta Trop. 146, 135–140. https://doi.org/10.1016/j.actatropica.2015.03.018.

Hassan, M.M., Farghaly, A.M., Gaber, N.S., Nageeb, H.F., Hegab, M.H., Galal, N., 1996. Parasitic causes of hepatomegaly in children. J. Egypt. Soc. Parasitol. 26, 177–189.

Ismail, M.A.M., Khalafallah, O., 2005. Toxocara canis and chronic urticaria in Egyptian patients. J. Egypt. Soc. Parasitol. 35, 833–840.

Kenny, J.V., MacCabe, R.J., Smith, H.V., Holland, C., 1995. Serological evidence for the presence of toxocariasis in the Turkana District of Kenya. Trans. R. Soc. Trop. Med. Hyg. 89, 377–378. https://doi.org/10.1016/0035-9203(95)90015-2.

Kuenzli, E., Neumayr, A., Chaney, M., Blum, J., 2016. Toxocariasis-associated cardiac diseases—a systematic review of the literature. Acta Trop. 154, 107–120. https://doi.org/10.1016/j.actatropica.2015.11.003.

Kyei, G., Ayi, I., Boampong, J.N., Turkson, P.K., 2015. Sero-epidemiology of *Toxocara canis* infection in children attending four selected health facilities in the central region of Ghana. Ghana Med. J. 49, 77–83.

Li, L., Gao, W., Yang, X., Wu, D., Bi, H., Zhang, S., Huang, M., Yao, X., 2014. Asthma and toxocariasis. Ann. Allergy Asthma Immunol. 113, 187–192. https://doi.org/10.1016/j.anai.2014.05.016.

Liao, C.-W., Sukati, H., D'Lamini, P., Chou, C.-M., Liu, Y.-H., Huang, Y.-C., Chung, M.-H., Mtsetwa, J.S., Jonato, J., Chiu, W.T., Chang, P.W.S., Du, W.-Y., Chan, H.-C., Chu, T.-B., Cheng, H.-C., Su, W.-W., Tu, C.-C., Cheng, C.-Y., Fan, C.-K., 2010. Seroprevalence of *Toxocara canis* infection among children in Swaziland, southern Africa. Ann. Trop. Med. Parasitol. 104, 73–80. https://doi.org/10.1179/136485910X12607012373795.

Lötsch, F., Obermüller, M., Mischlinger, J., Mombo-Ngoma, G., Groger, M., Adegnika, A.A., Agnandji, S.T., Schneider, R., Auer, H., Ramharter, M., 2016. Seroprevalence of *Toxocara* spp. in a rural population in Central African Gabon. Parasitol. Int. 65, 632–634. https://doi.org/10.1016/j.parint.2016.09.001.

Lötsch, F., Vingerling, R., Spijker, R., Grobusch, M.P., 2017. Toxocariasis in humans in Africa—a systematic review. Travel Med. Infect. Dis. 20, 15–25. https://doi.org/10.1016/j.tmaid.2017.10.009.

Luna, J., Cicero, C.E., Rateau, G., Quattrocchi, G., Marin, B., Bruno, E., Dalmay, F., Druet-Cabanac, F., Nicoletti, A., Preux, P.M., 2018. Updated evidence of the association between toxocariasis and epilepsy: systematic review and meta-analysis. PLoS Negl. Trop. Dis. 12, e0006665. https://doi.org/10.1371/journal.pntd.0006665.

Ma, G., Holland, C.V., Wang, T., Hofmann, A., Fan, C.-K., Maizels, R.M., Hotez, P.J., Gasser, R.B., 2018. Human toxocariasis. Lancet Infect. Dis. 18, e14–e24. https://doi.org/10.1016/S1473-3099(17)30331-6.

Macpherson, C.N.L., 2013. The epidemiology and public health importance of toxocariasis: a zoonosis of global importance. Int. J. Parasitol. 43, 999–1008. https://doi.org/10.1016/j.ijpara.2013.07.004.

Maetz, H.M., Kleinstein, R.N., Federico, D., Wayne, J., 1987. Estimated prevalence of ocular toxoplasmosis and toxocariasis in Alabama. J. Infect. Dis. 156, 414. https://doi.org/10.1093/infdis/156.2.414.

Magnaval, J.F., Michault, A., Calon, N., Charlet, J.P., 1994. Epidemiology of human toxocariasis in La Réunion. Trans. R. Soc. Trop. Med. Hyg. 88, 531–533.

Marmor, M., Glickman, L., Shofer, F., Faich, L.A., Rosenberg, C., Cornblatt, B., Friedman, S., 2011. *Toxocara can*is infection of children: epidemiologic and neuropsychologic findings. Am. J. Public Health 77, 554–559. https://doi.org/10.2105/ajph.77.5.554.

Mohamed, N.H., Salem, S.A., Azab, M.E., Bebars, M.A., Khattab, H.M., Kamal, A.M., Mohamed, M.S., 1991. Parasitic infections associated with mental retardation in Egypt. J. Egypt. Soc. Parasitol. 21 (2), 319–331.

Nada, S.M., Abazza, B.E., Mahmoud, L.A., Habeeb, Y.S., Hussein, H.F., Amer, O.T., 1996. Toxocariasis as a cause of renal disease in children in Sharkia Governorate, Egypt. J. Egypt. Soc. Parasitol. 26, 709–717.

Ngugi, A.K., Bottomley, C., Kleinschmidt, I., Wagner, R.G., Kakooza-Mwesige, A., Ae-Ngibise, K., Osusu-Agyei, S., Masanja, H., Kamuyu, G., Odhiambo, R., Chengo, E., Sander, J., Newton, R.W., for the SEEDS group, 2013. Prevalence of active convulsive epilepsy in sub-Saharan Africa and associated risk factors: cross-sectional and case–control studies. Lancet Neurol. 12, 253–263. https://doi.org/10.1016/S1474-4422(13)70003-6.

Nicoletti, A., Bartoloni, A., Sofia, V., Mantella, A., Nsengiyumva, G., Frescaline, G., Preus, P.-M., 2007. Epilepsy and toxocariasis: a case–control study in Burundi. Epilepsia 48, 894–899. https://doi.org/10.1111/j.1528-1167.2007.01104.x.

Nkouawa, A., Sako, Y., Itoh, S., Kouojip-Mabou, A., Nganou, C.N., Saijo, Y., Knapp, J., Yamsaki, H., Nakao, M., Nakaya, K., Moyou-Somo, R., Ita, A., 2010. Serological studies of neurologic helminthic infections in rural areas of Southwest Cameroon: toxocariasis, cysticercosis and paragonimiasis. PLoS Negl. Trop. Dis. 4, (7), e732. https://doi.org/10.1371/journal.pntd.0000732.

Nookala, S., Srinivasan, S., Kaliraj, P., Narayanan, R.B., Nutman, T.B., 2004. Impairment of tetanus-specific cellular and humoral responses following tetanus vaccination in human lymphatic filariasis. Infect. Immun. 72, 2598–2604. https://doi.org/10.1128/IAI.72.5.2598-2604.2004.

Noormahomed, E.V., Nhacupe, N., Mascaró-Lazcano, C., Mauaie, M.N., Buene, T., Funzamo, C.A., Benson, D.A., 2014. A cross-sectional serological study of cysticercosis, schistosomiasis, toxocariasis and echinococcosis in HIV-1 infected people in Beira, Mozambique. PLoS Negl. Trop. Dis. 8, e3121. https://doi.org/10.1371/journal.pntd.0003121.

Oteifa, N.M., Moustafa, M.A., Elgozamy, B.M., 1998. Toxocariasis as a possible cause of allergic diseases in children. J. Egypt. Soc. Parasitol. 28, 365–372.

Poulsen, C.S., Skov, S., Yoshida, A., Skallerup, P., Maruyama, H., Thamsborg, S.M., Nejsum, P., 2015. Differential serodiagnostics of *Toxocara canis* and *Toxocara cati*—is it possible? Parasite Immunol. 37, 204–207. https://doi.org/10.1111/pim.12181.

Sowemimo, O.A., Lee, Y.-L., Asaolu, S.O., Chuang, T.-W., Akinwale, O.P., Badejoko, B.O., Gyang, V.P., Nwafor, T., Henry, E., Fan, C.K., 2017. Seroepidemiological study and associated risk factors of *Toxocara canis* infection among preschool children in Osun State, Nigeria. Acta Trop. 173, 85–89. https://doi.org/10.1016/j.actatropica.2017.05.030.

Strube, C., Heuer, L., Janecek, E., 2013. *Toxocara* spp. infections in paratenic hosts. Vet. Parasitol. 193, 375–389. https://doi.org/10.1016/j.vetpar.2012.12.033.

Winkler, A.S., Blocher, J., Auer, H., Gotwald, T., Matuja, W., Schmutzhard, E., 2008. Anticysticercal and anti-toxocaral antibodies in people with epilepsy in rural Tanzania. Trans. R. Soc. Trop. Med. Hyg. 102, 1032–1038. https://doi.org/10.1016/j.trstmh.2008.05.004.

Zibaei, M., 2017. Helminth infections and cardiovascular diseases: *Toxocara* species is contributing to the disease. Curr. Cardiol. Rev. 13, 56–62.

CHAPTER TWENTY-FIVE

Seroepidemiology of human toxocariasis in North Africa

Ahmed Awad Adeel*
Independent Consultant, Lawrenceville, GA, United States
*Corresponding author: e-mail address: aaadeel@yahoo.com

Contents

Abstract

Seroprevalence studies on human toxocariasis help to assess the burden and the morbidity associated with this zoonosis. This review searched the seroprevalence studies and case reports in six North African countries: Algeria, Egypt, Libya, Morocco, Sudan and Tunisia, since 1990. The search also included studies on the environmental factors related to the risk of transmission. Most of the published epidemiological studies were done in Egypt. Cross-sectional and case-control studies in Egypt demonstrated that toxocariasis is a significant zoonosis that could be associated with conditions like bronchial asthma allergies and certain neuropsychiatric disorders. The population at risk of this infection includes all ages, both genders, in contact with dogs, resident in rural areas with poor housing conditions. The publications from Tunisia, Morocco and Algeria are limited to case reports and retrospective analyses of cases, but the disease is probably under-diagnosed in these three countries. There are no published reports on human toxocariasis in Libya and Sudan during the period covered by the review. Animal studies confirm high infection rates of dogs with *Toxocara canis* in North Africa. There is also evidence of wide-spread contamination of soil and water with *Toxocara* spp. eggs. Moreover, the use of untreated wastewater for irrigation in parts of North Africa could be a source of contamination of agricultural products with eggs of *Toxocara* spp. Population-based studies on human toxocariasis are recommended, using standardized diagnostic tests. These surveys should also assess risk factors to guide preventive measures.

Advances in Parasitology, Volume 109
ISSN 0065-308X
https://doi.org/10.1016/bs.apar.2020.01.023

1. Introduction

Human toxocariasis is a worldwide zoonosis caused by infection with larvae of *Toxocara canis*, and to a lesser extent by *T. cati* and other ascaridoid species (Hotez and Wilkins, 2009; Macpherson, 2013; Rubinsky-Elefant et al., 2010). Domestic dogs are the main definitive host for *T. canis*, but other canids (including coyotes, dogs, foxes, wolves) could act as definitive hosts (Centre for Disease Control and Prevention, 2019). Eggs of *T. canis* are released in the faeces of the canid host. Under favourable environmental conditions the eggs embryonate to become infective third stage larvae. After ingestion by a canid, the third-stage larvae hatch from the eggs, and penetrate the intestinal wall. In young dogs, larvae migrate through the liver and lungs to the airways and then get swallowed, reaching small intestine, where fourth-stage larvae develop to adult male and female worms, which mate, and reproduce eggs. In some dogs, after oral infection the larvae persist in tissues, where they undergo arrested development. In pregnant female dogs the tissue-dwelling larvae are activated, usually in the last trimester of pregnancy, and undergo trans-placental transmission to pups in utero and trans-mammary transmission to newborn pups. Adult worms become established in the small intestine of pups and become the source of egg contamination. *T. canis* can also be transmitted to accidental (paratenic) hosts (e.g. mice, rats, and rabbits) via the ingestion of infective eggs; in these hosts, larvae hatch from the eggs and penetrate the intestinal wall to then migrate to various organs and tissues, where they persist (Strube et al., 2013). When a canid eats such infected paratenic hosts, adult worms develop in the small intestine and the lifecycle is completed. Human can become infected by ingesting larvae in paratenic hosts or infective eggs from contaminated soil, food, or water. After ingestion, such larvae are released and invade the intestinal wall to then be carried via the blood circulation to various tissues (e.g. liver, lungs, brain, and muscles); although these larvae undergo arrested development in these tissues, they often cause pathogenic effects as a result of inflammatory responses and granuloma formation associated with toxocariasis disease.

Human infections with *T. canis* manifest in a spectrum of clinical syndromes ranging from asymptomatic infection to severe organ injury (Deshayes et al., 2016; Despommier, 2003; Ma et al., 2018). The clinical syndromes of toxocariasis, reviewed by Zinkham (1978), were initially classified as either visceral larva migrans (VLM) and ocular larva migrans (OLM). Cases of neurotoxocariasis (NT) were described at the same time

(Beautyman et al., 1966; Beautyman and Woolf, 1951). More recently, "covert toxocariasis" was described in children with multiple minor symptoms such as abdominal pain, headache and cough (Bass et al., 1983; Taylor et al., 1987). In adults a similar syndrome was described consisting of weakness, pruritis, rash, difficulty in breathing and abdominal named "common toxocariasis" (Glickman et al., 1987). "Covert toxocariasis" and "common toxocariasis" are probably two expressions of same syndrome (CT), one in children and the other in adults (Smith et al., 2009). Thus, the four clinical types of toxocariasis are VLM, OLM, NT and CT. The recommended serodiagnosis of toxocariasis is based on the initial testing by ELISA assays using *T. canis* excretory or secretory (TES) antigen (IgG-TES-ELISA) (de Savigny et al., 1979), after which any positive result should be confirmed by Western blotting (WB) (Fillaux and Magnaval, 2013). In ocular toxocariasis, *Toxocara* spp. antibody levels in serum can be low or absent despite clinical disease. In some cases, *Toxocara* spp. antibody can be detected in the aqueous or vitreous fluid samples from the affected eye and may be due to local antibody production or leakage of antibody from the circulation. The ocular fluid sample may be tested at a lower dilution than serum to improve ELISA sensitivity (Centers for Disease Control and Prevention, 2019).

Human toxocariasis can be prevented and controlled by disrupting the lifecycle at of *Toxocara* spp., first by measures to reduce the transmission by treatment of pet dogs and cats and stray carnivores with an anthelmintic; and second, by preventing human beings from ingesting infective eggs from the environment or larvae in raw or uncooked tissues from infected paratenic hosts (e.g. chicken, duck, and rabbit) (Strube et al., 2013).

The deployment of serodiagnostic tests for toxocariasis enabled a wider recognition of this disease as a global zoonosis, affecting diverse populations and in different geographical areas (Ma et al., 2018). Moreover, increasing human and dog populations, increased population movements and climate change will all serve to change the epidemiology of this zoonosis and call for better understanding of its public health impacts.

Although *T. canis* and *T. cati* were recognized since 1950s as human pathogens, we are still exploring the pathological impacts of *Toxocara* spp. larvae on humans. As a consequence, serological surveys to establish the prevalence of the disease often aim at assessing the clinical impact of infection on infected individuals. After the development of the more sensitive and specific serodiagnostic tests, further clinical epidemiology studies were carried out in different populations to investigate the possible association between *Toxocara* spp. and certain clinical conditions. Such studies contribute to better understanding of the morbidity associated with the high prevalence in any population. The global burden of toxocariasis both in terms of prevalence of infection and morbidity needs to be further explored (Smith et al., 2009). In this context the present review aims at exploring the seroprevalence of toxocariasis in humans in North Africa as shown in epidemiological and clinical reports. We have also assessed the risk of acquiring the disease in this region. We have followed the commonly accepted definition of this subregion of Africa which includes Morocco, Algeria, Tunisia, Libya, Egypt, and Sudan, the six countries that shape the top North of the African continent.

2. Methods

Searches of the databases were completed June 1st, 2019, in PubMed, CAB Abstracts, Web of Science, ScienceDirect, Google Scholar and included English and French articles published since January 1st, 1990.The search terms included "*Toxocara*", "toxocariasis", "visceral larva migrans" and the country names: "Egypt", "Tunisia", "Morocco", "Algeria", "Sudan" and, "Libya". Screening was done by titles and abstracts, and then in full text. Articles were excluded from full-text review if they did not contain original data, were about basic research or a different country. We have identified 53 articles for full-text review and data extraction. The full-texts of six articles, not available in the databases were provided by the WHO Eastern Mediterranean Regional office in Cairo, Egypt. Full-texts of five articles could not be obtained but their abstracts contained the essential data for extraction. In addition, we have included 17 clinical case reports published as meeting abstracts. These abstracts contained the relevant data for clinical case reports.

Publications included in the data extraction tables were classified as containing the following data about Egypt, Sudan, Libya, Tunisia, Morocco or Algeria: (1) original prevalence data for human toxocariasis in cross-sectional or case-control studies (2) original toxocariasis case reports, (3) reports about toxocariasis in domestic animals, (4) reports about environment and food contamination with *Toxocara* spp. eggs.

3. Results

3.1 Evidence of human exposure to *Toxocara* spp. in North Africa

3.1.1 Seroprevalence of Toxocara *spp. in Egypt*

We have identified 22 articles on the seroprevalence of human toxocariasis in Egypt since 1990. Nine articles reported cross-sectional studies (Table 1)

Table 1 Cross-sectional studies on the seroprevalence of toxocariasis in Egypt.

Location	Date	Study population	Age range	Toxocariasis laboratory test	Seroprevalence	References
Zagazig District, Sharkia, Governorate	January to December, 2013	859 schoolchildren aged 6–13 years	6–13 years	(ELISA) technique using the RIDASCREEN *Toxocara* Kit supplied by R-biopharm AG (An der neuen BergstraBe 17, D- 64297 Darmstatdt, Germany)	Urban 1/46 (2.2%), Rural 6/54 = (11.11%)	Farghly et al. (2016)
Research Institute of Ophthalmology, Giza	August 2005 to April 2006	(1) Asymptomatic pregnant women, 28 (2) their infants, 28 (3) other infants 79	(1) Asymptomatic pregnant women:18–32 y (2) infants at least 1 month after delivery	Embryonated Egg Antigen ELISA (ELISA-TEE) and Excretory/secretory or exoantigen ELISA (ELISA-TEX)	(1) Pregnant women: ELISA-TEE: 7/28 (25%), ELISA-TEX: 12/28 (42.2%) (2) Their infants: ELISA-TEE: 3/28 (10.7%), ELISA-TEX: 7/28 (25%) (3) Other infants: ELISA-TEE: 13/79 (16.5%), ELISA-TEX: 20/79 (25%)	Issa (2007)
Different locations in Egypt	June to December 2013	A total of 150 from occupational groups: Military workers (n = 25), Nomads (n = 25), House guards (n = 25), Employees (n = 20), House wives (n = 20), Students (n = 35)	7–45 years	ELISA for detection of anti-*T. canis* antibodies using RIDASCREEN® *Toxocara* IgG Kits	All ages: 36 /150, (24%) 7–15 years: 17/35, (48.57%) 16–25 years: 17.39% (8/46) 26–35 years: 18.18% (8/44) 36–50 years: 12% (3/25)	Awadallah and Salem (2015)

Continued

Table 1 Cross-sectional studies on the seroprevalence of toxocariasis in Egypt.—cont'd

Location	Date	Study population	Age range	Toxocariasis laboratory test	Seroprevalence	References
Cairo University, Cairo	October to December 2007	Five symptomatic dog attendants and 10 other animal house workers	Adults	ELISA (In-house)	3/15 (20%)	Sabry and Lotfy (2009)
Assiut University, Children's Hospital Assiut	May 2014 to May 2015	81 children with suspected VLM	6 months to 13 years	ELISA (Bordier Affinity Products SA, Switzerland)	49/81 (60.5%)	Galal et al. (2016)
Department of Parasitology, Faculty of Medicine, Tanta University, Tanta	NA	150 suspected visceral toxocariasis	(1) 128 children (1–12 years) (2): 22 adults	ELISA (R-Biopharm GmbH, Dramstadt, Germany)	Children: 8/128 (6.2%), Adults: 4/22 (18.2%)	Antonios et al. (2008)
El-Menia University Hospital. El-Menia Sharkia Governorate	NA	300 cases with hepatomegaly	Children (age not specified)	IFAT	18/300 = 6%	Hassan et al. (1996)

Department of Parasitology, Faculty of Medicine, Alexandria University, Alexandria	1993	53 patients with of eosinophilia, suspected of parasitic origin	NA	countercurrent immunoelectrophoresis (CIEP) using crude antigens of *Toxocara canis*	0/53 (0%)	el Zawawy et al. (1995)
Ain Shams University and Research Institute of Ophthalmology. Cairo	NA	(1) 110 IFAT positive toxoplasmosis: One hepatomegaly, 5 asymptomatic, 10 ocular cases, 14 cases with lymphadenopathy and 80 with obstetric implications (2) 12 presumptive cases of toxocariasis.	5–50 years	IFAT	20/110 (18.1%) Toxoplasmosis IFAT +ve in 1/12 presumptive cases to toxocariasis	Azab et al. (1990)

NA, Not available.

and 13 articles reported case-control studies, comparing *Toxocara* spp. seropositivity in cases having certain clinical conditions with matching healthy controls. (Table 2). In all these studies the diagnosis of toxocariasis was confirmed by serologic tests. ELISA was used for diagnosis of toxocariasis in 17/22 (74%) of the studies. Only one of these studies used WB as a confirmatory test after ELISA testing. Four studies published before 2000 used only IFAT and one study used countercurrent immunoelectrophoresis.

Estimates of *Toxocara* spp. seropositivity in asymptomatic, apparently healthy populations were reported in the three cross-sectional studies shown in Table 1, and in healthy controls recruited for 12 case-control studies shown in Table 2. In these apparently healthy populations, 7/15 (46.6%) of the studies reported a prevalence rate of *Toxocara* spp. antibodies of 10% or more. Seropositivity in symptomatic patients was variable, the highest positivity of 60.5% was reported in children with suspected VLM (Galal et al., 2016). Case-control studies confirmed significantly higher *Toxocara* spp. seropositivity in cases with presumptive diagnosis of toxocariasis (El-Shazly et al., 2009a, 2011; Safar et al., 1990). One study reported seropositivity with IFAT significantly lower in ocular cases when compared with non-ocular patients with other conditions and not significantly different from healthy controls (Safar et al., 1995). Case-control studies demonstrated association of *Toxocara* seropositivity with bronchial asthma (Badawey et al., 2018), schizophrenia, (El-Sayed and Ismail, 2012), mental development disorders (Mohamed et al., 1991), and with seropositivity to *Toxoplasma* (Azab et al., 1990). No significant association was found between *Toxocara* spp. seropositivity and epilepsy (El-Tantawy et al., 2013; Eraky et al., 2016; Salama et al., 2019). Also, there was no significant association between seropositivity and renal disease (Nada et al., 1996).

The association of demographic and socioeconomic factors with *Toxocara* spp. seropositivity in Egypt was evaluated in five articles (Awadallah and Salem, 2015; Badawey et al., 2018; El-Shazly et al., 2009a; Galal et al., 2016; Salama et al., 2019). Table 3 summarizes the *P*-values for the statistical tests used to test these associations. In the article by Badawey et al. (2018) the risk analysis was done separately for asthmatic patients and for healthy controls, the results are presented as two separate risk analysis studies. There were no statistically significant differences by gender in all the six studies. Association of seropositivity with age was variable. In the two studies that evaluated all ages, children had higher seropositivity rate in one study (Awadallah and Salem, 2015), but there were no significant differences by age in the other study (El-Shazly et al., 2009a). Three studies found no

Table 2 Case-control studies evaluating the association of seroprevalence of *Toxocara* spp. antibodies with different clinical conditions.

Site	Year	Clinical case group	Control group	Age of participants	Serologic test	Case seroprevalence	Control seroprevalence	*P* value	References
Children's Hospital, Mansoura University	May 2007 to January 2010	480 suspected toxocariasis	200 age and sex matched healthy controls	Children, mean age 7.2 ± 4.22 years	ELISA (Bordier Affinity Products SA, Crissier, Switzerland)	58/480 (12%)	7/200 (3.5%) all controls)	$P < 0.001$ (all patients vs all controls)	El-Shazly et al. (2011)
University' Hospitals of Benha and Mansoura	May 2008 to December 2008	455 Suspected toxocariasis	30 healthy controls	1–67 years	ELISA kit (Bordier Affinity Products SA, Crissier, Switzerland)	35/455 (7.7%)	NA	$P < 0.0001$	El-Shazly et al. (2009a)
Ain Shams University, Cairo	NA	50 suspected OLM, 25 suspected visceral toxocariasis	25 healthy controls	All ages	Precipitin absorption test (PAT), Counter-immunoelectrophoresis (CIEP), indirect and ELISA. Fluorescent antibody test (IFAT)	OLM: PAT: 36% CIEP: 0%, IFAT-EE: 32% IFA-FS: 28% ELISA: 40% VLM: 44%: PAT, 24%: CIEP, 52%: IFAT-EE, 48%: IFAT-S, 52%: ELISA.	PAT (1/25 = 4%) CIEP (0/25 = 0%), ELISA 1/25 = 4%), IFAT 0/25 = (0%)	$P < 0.05$ for PAT, IFAT and ELISA. $P > 0.05$ for CIEP.	Safar et al. (1990)
Department of Parasitology, Research Institute of ophthalmology Giza	NA	70 ocular cases, 30 non ocular cases	30 healthy controls	NA	IFAT	Ocular: 10/70 14.3%), Non-ocular: 13/30 (43.3%)	1/30 (5%)	$P > 0.05$ (ocular vs controls)	Safar et al. (1995)

Continued

Table 2 Case-control studies evaluating the association of seroprevalence of *Toxocara* spp. antibodies with different clinical conditions.—cont'd

Site	Year	Clinical case group	Control group	Age of participants	Serologic test	Case seroprevalence	Control seroprevalence	*P* value	References
Zagazig University Hospital, Zagazig	January to October 2017	118 outpatients with asthmatic bronchitis	Matched controls from other hospital visitors	4–10 years	Rida-Screen Toxocara-IgG ELISA kit (R-Biopharm AG, Germany)	20/118 (17%)	7/100 (7%)	$P = 0.026$	Badawey et al. (2018)
Cairo University	NA	65 patients with chronic urticaria	30 healthy controls	Mean age 32 ± 4.7 years	In house ELISA	18/65 (27.7%)	4/30 (13.3%)	$P < 0.001$	Ismail and Khalafallah (2005)
Paediatric Hospital, Ain Shams University	NA	30 cases of idiopathic bronchial asthma or urticaria	30 healthy controls	4–6 years	ELISA, Behringwerke, Germany	Asthmatic: 8/30 (26.5%) Urticaria: 4/30 (13.3%)	9/30 (30%)	NA	Oteifa et al. (1998)
Neuropsychiatry Department, Ain-Shams University Hospital, Giza, Egypt	NA	90 schizophrenic patients	45 healthy controls	20–60 years	Ridascreen *Toxocara* IgG, R-Biopharm, Germany)	21/90 (23.3%)	1/45 (2.2%)	$P < 0.01$	El-Sayed and Ismail (2012)
Paediatric Neurology Unit of Tanta University Hospital	July 2016 to July 2017	100 cases of epilepsy	50 healthy controls	2–15 years	ELISA kit (Diagnostic Automation/Cortez Diagnostics, Inc., California, USA). Western blotting technique for confirmation (LDBIO Diagnostics, Lyon–France)	7/100 (7%)	0/50 (0%)	$P > 0.05$	Salama et al. (2019)

Benha University Hospital	June 2014 to March 2015	40: cryptogenic epilepsy, 30 non-cryptogenic epilepsy	20 healthy controls	9 months–18 years	Ridascreen *Toxocara* IgG, R-Biopharm, Germany)	Epileptic: 3/40 (7.5%), Non-epileptic: 1/30 (3.3%)	2/20 (10%)	$P = 0.66$	Eraky et al. (2016)
Neurology Unit at Mansoura University Children's Hospital, Mansoura, Egypt	April 2012 to June 2013	132 cryptogenic epilepsy patients	60 age matched volunteers	age range was between 1 and 14 years	RIDASCREEN Toxocara-IgG ELISA (R-Biopharm AG, Germany)	64/132 (48.5%)	28/60 (46.7%)	$P = 0.815$	El-Tantawy et al. (2013)
Abbassiah Psychiatric Hospital Cairo	NA	67 patients with intellectual development disorders	30 healthy controls	10–55 years	IFAT	38/67 (56.7%)	1/30 (5%)	$P < 0.001$	Mohamed et al. (1991)
Zagazig University	1–14 years	84 patients with renal diseases	20 healthy controls	1–14 years	ELISA/microprecipitin in urine	9/84 (10.7%)	1/20 (5%)	$P > 0.05$	Nada et al. (1996)

Table 3 The significance level (*P*-values) of the association of demographic and socio-economic factors with the seropositivity to *Toxocara* spp. in different studies in Egypt.

	References					
	Badawey et al. (2018)[a]		Salama et al. (2019)[a]	El-Shazly et al. (2009a)[b]	Galal et al. (2016)[a]	Awadallah and Salem (2015)[b]
Study population	Asthmatic children, Age 4–10 years ($n=118$)	Control 4–10 years Age 4–10 years ($n=100$)	People with epilepsy Age 2–15 years ($n=100$)	Suspected VLM Age 1–67 years ($n=455$)	Children with presumptive diagnosis of VLM, Age 6 month to 13 years ($n=81$)	Asymptomatic Age 7–45 years ($n=150$)
Age	$P=0.16$ (4–6 years vs 7–10 years)	$P=0.594$ (4–6 years vs 7–10 years)	$P=0.062$ ($2\leq6$ years, $6\leq10$ years, 10—15 years	$P=0.309$ (≤15 vs 15 years +)	$P=0.0001$ (S) more in ≤8 years vs >8 years	$P=0.006$ (S) More in 7–15 years vs 16–45
Sex	$P=0.42$	$P=0.111$	$P=0.458$	$P=0.79$	$P=0.495$	$P=0.35$
Residence: rural/ urban	$P=0.91$	$P=0.02$ (S)	$P=0.918$	$P=0.038$ (S)		
Contact with/ owning dogs	$P=0.001$ (S)	$P=0.078$	$P=0.016$ (S)	$P=0.044$ (S)	$P=0.586$	$P=0.134$
Geophagia/contact with soil	$P=0.000$	$P=0.104$	$P=0.06$	$P=0.004$ (S)	$P=0.475$	$P=0.567$
Not washing hands before eating						$P=0.49$

Family income (High/low)	$P = 0.008$ (S)	$P = 0.126$		$P = 0.068$		
Occupation						
Literacy (Y/N)	$P = 0.000$ (S)	$P = 0.297$		$P = 0.237$		
Education level				$P = 0.884$		
Raw/undercooked meat			$P = 0.61$			
Eating raw vegetables						$P = 0.528$
Body mass index						
Good vs poor housing				$P = 0.036$ (S)		
House floor: paved vs nonpaved					$P = 0.585$	
Water supply underground vs piped water					$P = 0.004$ (S)	
History of parasitic infection					$P = 0.003$ (S)	
Unemployed/employed	$P = 0.927$	$P = 0.921$				

[a] *P*-value based on Chi Square test.
[b] *P*-value based on univariate regression analysis.
S, Statistically significant.

differences in the level of seropositivity by age among children but one study reported higher seropositivity in younger children (Galal et al., 2016). Other significant risk factors identified by at least one of these studies include rural residence, contact with dogs, geophagia, low family income, illiteracy, poor housing, history of parasitic infection, the use of underground water rather than tap water.

3.1.2 *Evidence of human exposure to* Toxocara *spp. in Tunisia, Morocco and Algeria*

The Maghreb countries (Tunisia, Morocco and Algeria) have common borders and share similar environmental and risk factors related to health (Ben Abdelaziz et al., 2018). Also, the data retrieved for these countries demonstrate their similarity with respect to the epidemiology of toxocariasis and warrants that they are analysed together. Published reports on human toxocariasis in Tunisia, Morocco and Algeria were limited to clinical case reports on individual cases or retrospective analyses of cases. We have identified 29 publications reporting toxocariasis cases in Tunisia, Morocco and Algeria. Four publications were duplicates and were therefore excluded in the statistical analysis but still cited as references. Table 4 summarizes the data on human toxocariasis in the three countries. The total number of toxocariasis cases in these reports was 56. According to the reports that indicated the age of cases there were 18/37 (48.6%) children and 19/37 (51.4%) adults. The percentages of the different clinical forms of toxocariasis were as follows: OLM 45/56 (80.3%), VLM 2/56 (3.5%), CT 3/56 (5.3%), NT 3/56 (5.3%), one case with combined NT and OLM and 2 cases of hypereosinophilia. Forty-eight (85.7%) of the cases were reported to have been confirmed by serologic tests. In 21 cases (37.5%) laboratory confirmation was reported as "serology", with no further details. Nine cases (16%) were reported as confirmed by ELISA alone, one case by WB alone. Combination of ELISA and WB was used in 30.4% (17/56) of all cases or 17/27 (62.9%) of the cases in which the type of serologic test used was available. In addition to blood tests, *Toxocara* spp. antibodies were tested in aqueous humour in 8 cases and in CSF in 2 cases. In 8 cases (14.2%) no details were given of the laboratory test done for confirmation.

3.1.3 *Human toxocariasis in Libya and Sudan*

Reports on toxocariasis in Sudan were limited to two articles published before the period covered in this review (Dafalla and Ali Omer, 1977; Woodruff et al., 1981). No human cases of toxocariasis were reported from Libya.

Table 4 Individual cases and case series of toxocariasis reported in Tunisia, Morocco and Algeria

Country	Location	Number of cases	Age	Mode of presentation	Laboratory confirmation	References
Tunisia	Charles-Nicolle Hospital, Tunis, Tunisia	3 out of 10 cases of uveitis	Adults[a]	OLM (uveitis)	Serology[b]	Skouri et al. (2018)
	La Rabta Hospital, Tunis, Tunisia	3/17 eyes (13 cases)	Children[a]	OLM (retinal vasculitis)	NA	Saadouli et al. (2018)
	Tunis Military Hospital, Tunisia	3 cases in 68	Adult[a]	OLM (uveitis)	NA	Ben Achour et al. (2018)
	Tunis Military Hospital, Tunisia	1	24 years	VLM (pancreatitis)	ELISA, WB	Boussetta et al. (2018) Arfaoui et al. (2015a, 2015b)
	Tunis Military Hospital, Tunisia	2	1: 45 years 2: 66 years	1: NT (encephalitis) 2: NT (spastic paraparesis)	ELISA, WB for serum and CSF	Abir et al. (2017), Mrissa et al. (2005), Arfaoui et al. (2015a, 2015b)
	Habib-Thameur Hospital, Tunis, Tunisia	1	52 years	OLM (bilateral granulomatous uveitis)	Blood WB +ve	Fekih et al. (2016) Redissi et al. (2017)

Continued

Table 4 Individual cases and case series of toxocariasis reported in Tunisia, Morocco and Algeria—cont'd

Country	Location	Number of cases	Age	Mode of presentation	Laboratory confirmation	References
	Médecine interne, hôpital militaire principal d'instruction de Tunis, Tunis, Tunisia	2 cases among 100 reviewed	NA	OLM (uveitis)	NA	Alaya et al. (2016)
	Department of Ophthalmology, Fattouma Bourguiba University Hospital, Faculty of Medicine, University of Monastir, Monastir, Tunisia	1 out of 40 cases of optic disc edema with macular star	NA	OLM (neuroretinas)	Serology[b]	Kahloun et al. (2015)
	Médecine interne, hôpital militaire principal d'instruction de Tunis, Tunis, Tunisia.	5	14 years −81 years	1: CT 2 cases, 2: OLM,3 cases	ELISA, WB in all cases	Lajmi et al. (2015)
	Médecine interne, hôpital militaire principal d'instruction de Tunis, Tunis, Tunisia	2	1: 15 years 2: 27 years	1: OLM, 2: OLM	1: Blood WB, 2: Blood WB	Hamrouni et al. (2015)
	Houman Service de médecine interne, CHU La Rabta, Tunis, Tunisia	1 of 22 cases of uveitis	Adult[a]	OLM	Serology	Zoubeidi et al. (2015)
	Department of neurology, Military Hospital, Tunis, Tunisia.	1	62 years	NT	Toxocariasis serologic tests (not specified) for blood and CSF	Riahi et al. (2014a, 2014b)
	Faculté de médecine, université de Sfax, Sfax, Tunisia	1	58 years	OLM	Serum: ELISA, WB	Trabelsi et al. (2014)

Tunisia	Institut Hédi-Rais d'ophtalmologie (service B), Tunis, Tunisia	8 out of 424 cases of uveitis	NA	OLM	Serology[b]	Chebil et al. (2013)
	Institut Hédi-Rais d'ophtalmologie (service B), Tunis, Tunisia	1 in 49 cases of uveitis	Child[a]	OLM (uveitis)	Serology[b]	Chebil et al. (2012)
Tunisia	Rabta Hospital laboratory	9	6 children[a] 3 adults[a]	5 OLM, 1 CT, 1 edema, 2 hypereosinophilia	ELISA	Trabelsi et al. (2004)
	Service de Pédiatrie Générale, Hôpital d'Enfants, Bab-Saadoun, Tunis, Tunisia	1	21 months	OML (global involvement of both eyes with granulomatous inflammation)	Serologic tests[b] negative in blood but positive in aqueous humour	Khaldi et al. (1990)
	Service du Pr Fathi Triki, Institut Hedi Raîs d'Ophtalmologie, Tunis, Tunisia.	1	8 years	OLM	Positive serology[b] of blood and aqueous humour	El-Matri et al. (1990)
Algeria	Laboratoire de parasitologie-mycologie du CHU Mustapha, Algiers, Algria,	1	NA	OLM	serum, aqueous humour: ELISA, WB	Arrache and Hamrioui (2010)
	Oran, Algeria	1	17 years	OLM (retinal detachment)	Negative serology[b], Positive subretinal puncture fluid	Nehili and Boucherit (2009)
	Algiers, Algeria	1 out of 21 cases of uveitis	3 months to 14 years	OLM (uveitis)	NA	Hadoun et al. (2008)

Continued

Table 4 Individual cases and case series of toxocariasis reported in Tunisia, Morocco and Algeria—cont'd

Country	Location	Number of cases	Age	Mode of presentation	Laboratory confirmation	References
Morocco	Service d'ophtalmologie B, hôpital des spécialités, CHU Ibn Sina. Rabat, Maroc	1	40 Years	OLM (granuloma, retinal detachment)	ELISA +ve, WB +ve	Elyadari et al. (2018)
	Service d'Ophtalmologie A de l'Hôpital des Spécialités, Centre Hospitalier Universitaire, Rabat, Maroc	2	1: 12 Years, 2: 4 years	OLM (posterior granuloma in both cases)	1: Serum: ELISA +ve. Aqueous humour: ELISA-ve, and WB +ve. 2: Serum: ELISA -ve. Aqueous humour: ELISA+ve, WB +ve	Daoudi et al. (2014)
	Service d'Ophtalmologie A, Hôpital des Spécialités, Rabat, Maroc	3 out of 20 cases of uveitis	4 years −16 years	OLM (uveitis)	Toxocariasis serology[b] of blood and aqueous humour	Laghmari et al. (2003)
	Service d'Ophtalmologie Pédiatrique, Hôpital 20 Août, CHu Ibn Rochd, université Hassan II, Faculté de Médecine—Casablanca	1	14 years	OLM (papillary granuloma)	Positive blood ELISA, Positive blood WB	Lalami et al. (2017)

[a]Exact age not available.
[b]Exact serologic test not available.
NA, No information available.

3.2 *Toxocara* spp. in domestic animals and the environment in North Africa

Table 5 summarizes studies on the prevalence of *Toxocara* spp. in dogs and cats and contamination of soil, water and raw vegetables in North Africa. Studies on toxocariasis in dogs in Egypt have shown different prevalence rates in different locations (Awadallah and Salem, 2015; El-Tras et al., 2011; Haridy et al., 2009; Khalafalla, 2011; Sabry and Lotfy, 2009). The prevalence rate ranged between 3.3% in dogs housed in high class residential areas in Qalyubia Province to 66.7% in stray dogs in Cairo (Awadallah and Salem, 2015; Sabry and Lotfy, 2009). In Libya the prevalence rates of *T. canis* infection in dogs in the four locations of Tripoli ranged between 20.0% and 31.3% (El Maghrbi et al., 2019). In Tunisia, Oudni-M'rad et al. (2017) reported *T. canis* (27.2%) in a sample of dogs that covered four climatic zones of the country. In Kenitra, Morocco *T. canis* prevalence in rural dogs was reported as 19% (Taboz et al., 2008).

Soil contamination with *Toxocara* eggs has been reported in studies conducted in different locations in North Africa. A study of public parks in Tripoli has found that 62 out of 105 (59.0%) of the soil samples were positive for *T. canis* eggs (Belhage et al., 2016). Variable rates of soil contamination with *T. canis* eggs were reported in soil samples in Egypt (el-Beshbishi et al., 2005; El-Shazly et al., 2009b; Etewa et al., 2016; Farghly et al., 2016; Oteifa and Moustafa, 1997). *T. canis* eggs were also found in drains and canals in Egypt (El Shazly et al., 2003) and in wastewater in Morocco (Hajjami et al., 2012; Zamo et al., 2003). Contamination of fresh vegetables and fruits with *T. canis* has been reported in Egypt (Said, 2012), Libya (Abougrain et al., 2010) and Morocco (Hajjami et al., 2013a, 2013b).

4. Discussion

One notable issue is the lack of standardization of serologic tests used in the studies reviewed. Most of the studies in Egypt are based on TES-ELISA alone although earlier studies used IFAT. TES-ELISA is highly sensitive, but its specificity is reduced in the presence of other parasites, e.g., *Ascaris* and *Strongyloides* (Jacquier et al., 1991; Lynch et al., 1988). The use of fractions of TES in Western blot test gives more specific results (Magnaval et al., 1991). Thus, it has been recommended to use the combination of the two tests, using TES-IgG-ELISA as a screening test followed by TES-WB for confirmation (Fillaux and Magnaval, 2013). In Tunisia, Morocco and

Table 5 Studies on the prevalence of toxocariasis in animals and contamination of the environment and food with *Toxocara* spp. eggs

Date of study	Location	Infection in animals	Soil	Water/Drains	Vegetables/fruits	References
November 2009 and April 2010	Egypt, Kafrelsheikh governorate	Faecal examination, *T. canis* Stray dogs 35.8% (19 out of 53). Domestic dogs 21.3% (10 out of 47).	ND	ND	ND	El-Tras et al. (2011)
June to December 2013	Egypt, Sharkia and Qalyubia provinces	Prevalence of *T. canis* in dogs: High class area: 3.33%, Rural: 6.7% Nomadic:13.3%, Total: 7/130 (5.38%), *T. leonina*: 3.07%	ND	ND	ND	Awadallah and Salem (2015)
2006–2007	Egypt, College of Veterinary Medicine, Cairo University, Cairo	299/3000 (9.83%) of pet dogs passed *T. canis* eggs in stools	ND	ND	ND	Haridy et al. (2009)
October to December 2007	Egypt, College of Veterinary Medicine, Cairo University, Cairo	Stray dogs: 10/15 (66.7%) *T. canis*	ND	ND	ND	Sabry and Lotfy (2009)
January and May 2010	Egypt, Kafrelsheikh province, northern part of the Nile Delta region of Egypt	113 faecal samples from stray cats: *T. cati* (9%), *T. leonina* (5%),	ND	ND	ND	Khalafalla (2011)

January 2014 to June 2015	Libya, Tripoli	The prevalence rates of *T. canis* in dogs ranged between 20.0% and 31.3%.	ND	ND	ND	El Maghrbi et al. (2019)
NA	Four climate zones in Tunisia	The most frequently observed parasites in stray dog samples were *Toxocara spp.* (27.2%)	ND	ND	ND	Oudni-M'rad et al. (2017)
2007/2008	Kenitra, Morocco	*T. canis* were present at 19% and 11% of rural dogs	ND	ND	ND	Taboz et al. (2008)
NA	Tripoli, Libya	ND	Prevalence of *Toxocara* spp. in soil from public parks was 59.0% (62/105 samples).	ND	ND	Belhage et al. (2016)
October 2011 to October 2013	Egypt, Sharkyia Governorate	ND	15/120 of Soil samples contaminated with *T. canis* eggs.	ND	ND	Etewa et al. (2016)
NA	Egypt, Dakahlia Governorate	ND	97/1070 (9.1%) of soil samples contaminated with *T. canis* eggs	ND	ND	el-Beshbishi et al. (2005)

Continued

Table 5 Studies on the prevalence of toxocariasis in animals and contamination of the environment and food with *Toxocara* spp. eggs—cont'd

Date of study	Location	Infection in animals	Soil	Water/Drains	Vegetables/fruits	References
NA	Heliopolis, Egypt	ND	Soil samples contaminated with *T. canis* eggs: 182/600 (30.3%)	ND	ND	Oteifa et al. (1998)
March 2007 to February 2008	Egypt, Dakahlia Governorate, Lower Egypt and Minia Governorate, Upper Egypt.	ND	Soil samples contaminated with *T. canis* eggs: Dakhalia, rural: 18/100 = 18% Dakhalia, rban:10/100 = 10%. El-Minia, rural:22/100 = 22%, El-Minia, rban:22/100 = 22%.	ND	ND	El-Shazly et al. (2009a)
All over the year 2013	Zagazig District	ND	Urban:5/46 (10.9%), Rural: 10/54 (18.6%)	ND	ND	Farghly et al. (2016)
NA	Egypt. Eastern Nile Delta	ND	ND	*Toxocara* spp. In water: 2/2 = 100% of drains, 1/2 = 50% of canals, 0/2 = 0% of river.	ND	El Shazly et al. (2003)

May to November 1999	City of Kenitra (North-East of Morocco)	ND	ND	*Toxocara* spp. In untreated waste water *T. canis* 17 eggs/L.	ND	Zamo et al. (2003)
January 2009 to December 2010	City of Settat, Morocco	ND	ND	*Toxocara* spp. in: Untreated water: 0.96 eggs/L (range: 0–6) Treated water: 0	ND	Hajjami et al. (2012)
January 2009 and December 2010	Settat and Soualem Regions, Morocco	ND	ND	*T. canis* in 4/69 (5.7%) of samples of untreated wastewater	Experimental study confirming *T. canis* contamination in Vegetables irrigated with wastewater.	Hajjami et al. (2013a)
NA	Egypt, Alexandria	ND	ND	ND	*Toxocara* eggs detected in vegetable samples: Total: 57/300 (19%)	Said (2012)
July 2005 and February 2006	Tripoli, Libya	ND	ND	ND	(1) Tomato, (2) cucumber, (3) lettuce, and (4) cress *T. cati* in: (1) 11%, (2) 14%, (3) 48%, (4) 41%. *T. canis* in: (1) 3%, (2) 8%, (3) 37%, (4) 33%	Abougrain et al. (2010)
April 2011 and May 2012	Casablanca, Morocco	ND	ND	ND	*Toxocara spp.* In 11/128 (8.6%) of samples of vegetables	Hajjami et al. (2013b)

ND: Not done; NA: Dates not available.

Algeria the use of combination of ELISA and WB seems to be is the norm. Standardization of *Toxocara* serodiagnosis should take into account the endemicity of other parasites and particular attention should be given to specificity of the immunodiagnostic protocols adopted.

Comparison of prevalence data reported in the different studies is limited by the demographic variability of the study population and diversity of methods for laboratory diagnosis and identification of cases. Available seroprevalence data should be interpreted after taking these variables into account. In general, low seroprevalence rates have been reported from industrialized countries like 0.7% in blood donors in New Zealand whereas much higher rates have been reported in less developed countries in the tropics, e.g., 81.7% in schoolchildren in Indonesia (Hayashi et al., 2005; Zarkovic et al., 2007). The findings in the present review indicate that the seroprevalence of human toxocariasis is high in Egypt, reaching 10% or more in 46.6% of the studies in populations designated as general population or "healthy controls". However, most of these studies used convenience samples, with potential bias in seroprevalence estimates. For more reliable estimates there is need for more community-based studies with representative samples to give more accurate seroprevalence estimates.

The risk analysis studies reviewed show no consistency in the association of seropositivity with age. Reports from other parts of the world also show variable patterns in the association of age with the prevalence of toxocariasis. As examples, studies in Iran and Argentina have found no evidence of correlation with age (Alonso et al., 2000; Sadjjadi et al., 2000). On the other hand, Holland et al. (1995) reported increased seroprevalence in older children, reflecting a cumulative effect of infection. There are no differences in seropositivity by gender in Egypt indicating an almost equal exposure of both sexes to *Toxocara* spp. infection. Rural residence is cited by two studies in Egypt as a risk factor for toxocariasis. Other risk factors cited include ownership of dogs, geophagia/contact with soil, low family income, illiteracy, history of parasitic disease, poor housing, and the use of underground water rather than tap water. Farghly et al. (2016) suggested the increased seroprevalence in rural areas was perhaps due to the low socioeconomic status probably generating some social, cultural and environmental conditions and due to uncleaned and unfenced homes which allow the wandering of stray dogs as well as children. These are generally the conditions that make toxocariasis a disease of poverty even in more affluent societies (Won et al., 2008).

Two studies report association of *Toxocara* seroprevalence with bronchial asthma in Egypt (Badawey et al., 2018; Oteifa et al., 1998). This is consistent with the metanalysis by Li et al. (2014) which found a significantly higher prevalence of *T. canis* infection in patients with asthma than in controls. Intellectual disability (mental retardation) was also reported to be associated with *Toxocara* spp. seropositivity in Egypt (Mohamed et al., 1991). Similar findings were reported by Kaplan et al. (2004) in non-institutionalized individuals with intellectual disabilities in Turkey. In the United States an analysis of data from the Third National Health and Nutrition Examination Survey (NHANES III) concluded that, toxocariasis appears to be associated with decreased cognitive function (Erickson et al., 2015). Association of schizophrenia with *Toxocara* seropositivity reported by El-Sayed and Ismail (2012) has also been reported in Iran (Khademvatan et al., 2014). However, a study in Mexico found no association between *Toxocara* seropositivity and psychiatric diagnosis (Alvarado-Esquivel, 2013). The three studies in Egypt that show no association between seropositivity for toxocariasis and epilepsy are in agreement with similar studies in Turkey and Tanzania that found no such association (Akyol et al., 2007; Winkler et al., 2008). This question has recently been addressed in two meta-analysis studies concluded that there was positive association between toxocariasis and epilepsy (Luna et al., 2018; Quattrocchi et al., 2012). In these cross-sectional studies even if a positive association is statistically established between *Toxocara* spp. seropositivity and conditions like epilepsy, cognitive and psychiatric disorders this would not prove causality. A reverse causality could be true with these disorders acting as a risk factor causing a behaviour favouring infection with *Toxocara* spp. particularly in areas with heavy soil contamination. The fact that toxocariasis is an easily preventable infection makes its etiological association with other serious conditions, all the more important to investigate. Concomitant *Toxocara* seropositivity with *Toxoplasma* seropositivity has been reported in Egypt in two studies (Azab et al., 1990; Safar et al., 1995). This has also been confirmed in data based on the HANES surveys in USA (Jones et al., 2008). Both infections could be acquired through soil contamination, preventable by washing hands before eating.

It is rather surprising that in spite of the large number of publications reporting individual cases with severe clinical complications due to toxocariasis in Tunisia, Morocco and Algeria, there are no published epidemiological studies on this infection in humans in these countries. Moreover, the fact that about 80% of the reported cases are ocular points to possibility that other, milder forms of the disease are under-diagnosed or under-reported or both. Holland et al. (1995) found no cases of toxocaral eye disease among 2129 Irish schoolchildren, 31% of whom were seropositive. The more common visceral forms of toxocariasis are easily missed because they have no pathognomonic clinical features (Smith et al., 2009). An accurate estimate of seroprevalence of *Toxocara* spp. needs to be based on population-based studies with representative samples.

Animal surveys for toxocariasis indicate that infection with *T. canis* is highly prevalent in North Africa. The higher infection rates in stray dogs confirm that pet care could reduce contamination of the environment by *Toxocara* spp. eggs. Contamination of soil, water and vegetables also confirm the high risk of transmission of *Toxocara* spp. in the countries reviewed. Of particular interest is the contamination of untreated wastewater which is frequently used for irrigation in North Africa and could be a source of infection with helminth eggs (Amoah et al., 2018; Ben Ayed et al., 2019; El Kettani et al., 2008; Hajjami et al., 2013a, b). Although no human cases of toxocariasis were published in Libya there is evidence of high rates of infection in dogs and high levels of contamination rates of soil and vegetables with *Toxocara* spp. eggs (Belhage et al., 2016); El Maghrbi et al., 2019; Abougrain et al., 2010). Again, this needs to be further investigated in population-based studies.

Limitations of this study include the inherent inaccuracies of reliance on hospital-based convenience samples and case reports to determine the burden of human toxocariasis. Also, there is lack of standardization of the diagnostic methods and criteria in the different studies. An additional limitation is the difficulty of getting full text articles of local journals, not included in the databases. After scrutinizing the details of case reports in Tunisia, four cases appear to have been presented in multiple publications. For example, cases presented by different departments or at different times. This was taken into consideration in the statistical analysis. Yet, it is still possible that some of the cases presented in individual case reports were also included in retrospective case series.

5. Conclusions

Toxocariasis is a significant public health problem in North Africa but is probably markedly under-diagnosed and under-reported in some countries. The overall purpose of this study was to assess the burden of the disease based on available information. The findings indicate the need for future population-based research with standard methodology to address the knowledge gaps identified in this review. Better awareness of the disease among health workers and the availability of well standardized diagnostic tests could lead to earlier detection and proper management of the milder forms of the disease. Population-based studies are needed to evaluate the true burden of the disease and the role of factors like poor housing, inadequate dog care and wastewater management that lead to contamination of the environment and transmission of infection.

Acknowledgements

The author would like to acknowledge the assistance in obtaining full-text articles kindly provided by the Knowledge Sharing and Production unit (KSP), Department of Information, Evidence and Research (IER), the World Health Organization Regional Office for the Eastern Mediterranean (WHO/EMRO), Cairo, Egypt and Neglected Tropical Diseases unit (NTD), Department of Communicable Diseases Prevention and Control (DCD), the World Health Organization Regional Office for the Eastern Mediterranean (WHO/EMRO) Cairo, Egypt. The database search was made possible by e-access to Cornell University Library.

References

Abir, B., Malek, M., Ridha, M., 2017. Toxocariasis of the central nervous system: with report of two cases. Clin. Neurol. Neurosurg. 154, 94–97. https://doi.org/10.1016/j.clineuro.2017.01.016.

Abougrain, A.K., Nahaisi, M.H., Madi, N.S., Saied, M.M., Ghenghesh, K.S., 2010. Parasitological contamination in salad vegetables in Tripoli-Libya. Food Control 21, 760–762. https://doi.org/10.1016/j.foodcont.2009.11.005.

Akyol, A., Bicerol, B., Ertug, S., Ertabaklar, H., Nn, K., 2007. Epilepsy and seropositivity rates of *Toxocara canis* and *Toxoplasma gondii*. Seizure 16, 233–237. 17239629.

Alaya, N., Boussetta, N., Metoui, L., Ben, A.Y., Louzir, B., Othmani, S., Gharsallah, I., Ajili, F., 2016. CA112 Profil étiologique des uvéites dans un service de médecine interne: à propos de 100 cas. Rev. Med. Interne 37, A141–A267. https://doi.org/10.1016/j.revmed.2016.10.247.

Alonso, J.M., Bojanich, M.V.I., Chamorro, M., Gorodner, J.O., 2000. Toxocara seroprevalence in children from a subtropical city in Argentina. Rev. Inst. Med. Trop. Sao Paulo 42 (4), 235–237. https://dx.doi.org/10.1590/S0036-46652000000400010.

Alvarado-Esquivel, C., 2013. *Toxocara* infection in psychiatric inpatients: a case control seroprevalence study. PLoS One 8, e62606. https://doi.org/10.1371/journal.pone.0062606. 23626838.

Amoah, I.D., Adegoke, A.A., Senström, T.A., 2018. Soil-transmitted helminth infections associated with wastewater and sludge reuse: a review of current evidence. Trop. Med. Int. Health 23, 692–703. doi.org/10.1111/tmi.13076.

Antonios, S.N., Eid, M.M., Khalifa, E.A., Othman, A.A., 2008. Seroprevalence study of *Toxocara canis* in selected Egyptian patients. J. Egypt. Soc. Parasitol. 38, 313–318.

Arfaoui, B., Boussetta, N., Abid, R., Sayhi, S., Batikh, R., Ben, A.N., Salah, O., 2015a. Toxocarose viscérale chez l'adulte, à propos de 2 cas [Visceral visceral toxocariasis in adults, about 2 cases]. Rev. Med. Interne 36 (Suppl. 2), A116–A117.

Arfaoui, B., Boussetta, N., Abid, R., Sayhi, S., Battikh, R., Ben Abdelhafidh, N.N., Othmani, S., 2015b. P23- Toxocarose viscérale chez l'adulte à propos de 2 casP23- Toxocarose viscérale chez l'adulte à propos de 2 cas. Rev. Tunis. Infectiol. 9 (Suppl. 1), S1–S120 p21.

Arrache, D., Hamrioui, B., 2010. Parasitoses oculaires. [Ocular parasitosis]. In: Société Algérienne de Biologie Clinique. Palais de la Culture Moufdi Zakaria 2ème Congrès, 23–r24 Mai 2010, Poster P20. p. 72. Available at: http://www.sante.dz/sabc/congrees2010.pdf.

Awadallah, M.A.I., Salem, L.M.A., 2015. Zoonotic enteric parasites transmitted from dogs in Egypt with special concern to *Toxocara canis* infection. Vet. World 8, 946–957. Available at: www.veterinaryworld.org/Vol.8/August-2015/3.pdf.

Azab, M.E., Safar, E.H., Khattab, H.M., 1990. Concomitant *Toxoplasma* and *Toxocara* infections. J. Egypt. Public Health Assoc. 65, 253–261. 2133900.

Badawey, M.S., Fathy, G.A., Abdel-Rahman, S.A., Abolmaaty, D.A., Abdallah, B.H., 2018. Relation between *Toxocara* infection, atopy and asthmatic bronchitis children in Zagazig University hospitals. J. Egypt. Soc. Parasitol. 48, 93–100.

Bass, J.L., Mehta, K.A., Glickman, L.T., Eppes, B.M., 1983. Clinically inapparent *Toxocara* infection in children. N. Engl. J. Med. 308, 723–724. 6828115.

Beautyman, W., Woolf, A.L., 1951. An ascaris larva in the brain in association with acute anterior poliomyelitis. J. Pathol. Bacteriol. 63, 635–647.

Beautyman, W., Beaver, P.C., Buckley, J.J., Woolf, A.L., 1966. Review of a case previously reported as showing an ascarid larva in the brain. J. Pathol. Bacteriol. 91, 271–273.

Belhage, A.A., Hosni, M.M., El Maghrbi, A.A., 2016. Soil contamination with *Toxocara* spp. eggs in the public parks of Tripoli city, Libya. Libyan J. Vet. Med. Sci. 2, 9–12.

Ben Abdelaziz, A., Melki, S., Ben Abdelaziz, A., Ben Salem, K., Soulimane, A., Serhier, Z., Dahdi, S.A., 2018. Profile and evolution of the Global Burden of Morbidity in the Maghreb (Tunisia, Morocco, Algeria). The Triple burden of morbidity. Tunis. Med. 96, 760–773.

Ben Achour, T., Boussetta, N., Guediche, N.H., Metoui, L., Sayhi, S., Arfaoui, B., Agili, F.B., Louzir, B., 2018. Particularités cliniques, étiologiques et évolutives des uvéites au sein d'un service de médecine interne: étude de 68 cas. [Clinical, etiological and progressive features of uveitis in a department of internal medicine: a study of 68 cases]. Rev. Med. Interne 39 (Suppl. 1), A206.

Ben Ayed, L., Sabbahi, S., Karanis, P., 2019. Waterborne Parasites in North Africa Environment, Reference Module in Earth Systems and Environmental Sciences. Elsevier. ISBN 9780124095489 Available at: https://doi.org/10.1016/B978-0-12-409548-9.11004-8.

Boussetta, N., Arfaoui, B., Metoui, L., Dhahri, R., Louzir, B., Gharsallah, I., Ajili, F., 2018. La toxocarose peut-elle être responsable d'une pancréatite aigue? [Toxocariasis: a possible cause of acute pancreatitis?]. Pan Afr. Med. J. 29, 180. https://doi.org/10.11604/pamj.2018.29.180.9630.

Centers for Disease Control and Prevention, 2019. Parasites -Toxocariasis (also known as Roundworm Infection). Atlanta, GA. Accessed 1st June 2019 at: https://www.cdc.gov/parasites/toxocariasis/health_professionals/index.html#dx.

Chebil, A., Chaabani, L., Kort, F., Ben Youssef, N., Turki, F., El Matri, L., 2012. Étude épidémiologique des uvéites de l'enfant: à propos de 49 cas [Epidemiologic study of pediatric uveitis: A series of 49 cases]. J. Fr. Ophtalmol. 35, 30–34. https://doi.org/10.1016/j.jfo.2011.02.019.

Chebil, A., Baroudi, B., Slim, M., Chaker, N., Lamloum, M., Bouladi, M., Houman, M., El Matri, L., 2013. Profil épidémiologique des uvéites dans la région de Tunis [Epidemiology of uveitis in the Tunis area]. J. Fr. Ophtalmol. 36, 764–768.

Dafalla, A.A., Ali Omer, M.I., 1977. Toxocariasis in a Sudanese boy. Trans. R. Soc. Trop. Med. Hyg. 71, 544–545.

Daoudi, C., Laghmari, M., Naciri, K., Handor, H., Hafidi, Z., Hajji, C., Daoudi, R., 2014. Ocular toxocariasis: report of two cases and review of the literature. [French]. Pan Afr. Med. J. 17, 71. https://doi.org/10.11604/pamj.2014.17.71.3823.

de Savigny, D.H., Voller, A., Woodruff, A.W., 1979. Toxocariasis: serological diagnosis by enzyme immunoassay. J. Clin. Pathol. 32, 284–288. 372253.

Deshayes, S., Bonhomme, J., de La Blanchardière, A., 2016. Neurotoxocariasis: a systematic literature review. Infection 44, 565–574. https://doi.org/10.1007/s15010-016-0889-8. 27084369.

Despommier, D., 2003. Toxocariasis: clinical aspects, epidemiology, medical ecology, and molecular aspects. Clin. Microbiol. Rev. 16, 265–272.

El Kettani, S., Azzouzi, E., Boukachabine, K., El Yamani, M., Maata, A., Rajaoui, M., 2008. Intestinal parasitosis and use of untreated wastewater for agriculture in Settat, Morocco. East. Mediterr. Health J. 14, 1435–1444.

El Maghrbi, A., Hosni, M., Dayhum, A., Belhage, A., 2019. Prevalence and associated risk factors of *Toxocara canis* eggs in dogs in Tripoli, Libya. Adv. Anim. Vet. Sci. 7, 326–334.

El Shazly, A.M., Soliman, M., Nemr, H.I., El Moafyo, N., Abdel Gawad, A.G.E., El Bendary, M., 2003. Nematodes and water pollution in eastern part of Nile Delta. J. Egypt. Soc. Parasitol. 33, 631–636.

el Zawawy, L.A., el Nassery, S.F., al Azzouni, M.Z., Abou el Naga, I.F., el Temsahi, M.M., Awadalla, H.N., 1995. A study on patients with eosinophilia of suspected parasitic origin. J. Egypt. Soc. Parasitol. 25, 245–255. 7602166.

el-Beshbishi, S.N., Abdel-Magied, A.A., el-Nahas, H.A., Azab, M.S., el-Shazly, A.M., Morsy, T.A., Gamal-Edin, M.K., el-Kadi, M.A., 2005. Geoparasites in rural Dakahlia governorate, a preliminary based study for development of the community-based intervention programs. J. Egypt. Soc. Parasitol. 35, 1051–1070.

El-Matri, L., Ghorbal, M., Ayadi, A., Ben-Naceur, B., Triki, M., 1990. Apparently bilateral ocular lesions due to *Toxocara canis*. J. Fr. Ophtalmol. 13, 303–308.

El-Sayed, N.M., Ismail, K.A., 2012. Relationship between *Toxocara canis* infection and schizophrenia. Rawal Med. J. 37, 155–161.

El-Shazly, A.M., Abdel Baset, S.M., Kamal, A., Mohammed, K.A., Sakrs, T.I., Hammad, S.M., 2009a. Seroprevalence of human toxocariasis (visceral larva migrans). J. Egypt. Soc. Parasitol. 39, 731–744.

El-Shazly, A.M., Mohammed, R.M., El-Beshbishi, S.N., Azab, M.S., El-Ghareeb, A.S., Abdeltawab, A.H., Zalook, T.K., 2009b. Soil-parasites particularly *Toxocara* eggs in Egypt. J. Egypt. Soc. Parasitol. 39, 151–162.

El-Shazly, A.M., Attia, G., El-Ghareeb, A.S., Belal, U.S., 2011. Clinical varieties of toxocariasis canis in Children's hospital, Mansoura University: is it an underestimated problem? J. Egypt. Soc. Parasitol. 41, 263–274.

El-Tantawy, N.L., El-Nahas, H.A., Salem, D.A., Salem, N.A., Hasaneen, B.M., 2013. Seroprevalence of *Toxoplasma gondii* and *Toxocara* spp. in children with cryptogenic epilepsy. Am. J. Infect. Dis. Microbiol. 1, 92–95. Available online at: http://pubs.sciepub.com/ajidm/1/5/3.

El-Tras, W.F., Holt, H.R., Ahmed, A., Tayel, A.A., 2011. Risk of *Toxocara canis* eggs in stray and domestic dog hair in Egypt. Vet. Parasitol. 178, 319–323.

Elyadari, M., Zarrouki, M., Elorch, H., Azennoud, S., Harchali, S., Elmerrouni, S., Bouzoubaa, T., Hajji, Z., Abdallah, E., Boulanoir, A., 2018. Toxocarose oculaire [Ocular toxocariasis]. J. Fr. Ophtalmol. 41, 277–279. https://doi.org/10.1016/j.jfo.2017.06.026.

Eraky, M.A., Abdel-Hady, S., Abdallah, K.F., 2016. Seropositivity of *Toxoplasma gondii* and *Toxocara* spp. in children with cryptogenic epilepsy, Benha, Egypt. Korean J. Parasitol. 54, 335–338. https://doi.org/10.3347/kjp.2016.54.3.335.
Erickson, L.D., Gale, S.D., Berrett, A., Brown, B.L., Hedges, D.W., 2015. Association between toxocariasis and cognitive function in young to middle-aged adults. Folia Parasitol. 62, 048. https://doi.org/10.14411/fp.2015.048.
Etewa, S.E., Abdel-Rahman, S.A., Abd El-Aal, N.F., Fathy, G.M., El-Shafey, M.A., Ewis, A.M.G., 2016. Geohelminths distribution as affected by soil properties, physicochemical factors and climate in Sharkyia governorate Egypt. J. Parasit. Dis. 40, 496–504. https://doi.org/10.1007/s12639-014-0532-5.
Farghly, A.M., Mohamed, S.M., Abdel-Rahman, S.A., Mohammed, F.E., El-Bahaie, E.S., El-Shafey, M.A., 2016. The relation between the prevalence of soil transmitted parasites in the soil and among school children in Zagazig district, Sharkyia governorate, Egypt. J. Parasit. Dis. 40, 1021–1029. https://doi.org/10.1007/s12639-014-0627-z.
Fekih, Y., Daoud, F., Kefi, A., Baili, L., Chebbi, A., Bouguila, H., Rachdi, I., Aydi, Z., Ben Dhaou, B., Boussema, F., 2016. CA120: Panuvéite bilatérale granulomatose: pensez à la toxocarose! In: A202 74e *Congrès franc¸ais de médecine interne—Deauville, 8 au 10 décembre 2016/La Revue de médecine interne*. vol. 37, pp. A141–A267. https://doi.org/10.1016/j.revmed.2016.10.255.
Fillaux, J., Magnaval, J.F., 2013. Laboratory diagnosis of human toxocariasis. Vet. Parasitol. 193, 327–336. ISSN 0304017, https://doi.org/10.1016/j.vetpar.2012.12.028.
Galal, L.A., Mahmoud, A.E., Attia, R.A.H., Eltayeb, A., Mahran, D.G., 2016. Sociodemographic, clinical and laboratory predictors for the diagnosis of visceral larva migrans in children—upper Egypt. Int. J. Trop. Dis. Health 19, 1–13.
Glickman, L.T., Magnaval, J.F., Domanski, L.M., Shofer, F.S., Lauria, S.S., Gottstein, B., Brochier, B., 1987. Visceral larva migrans in French adults: a new disease syndrome? Am. J. Epidemiol. 125, 1019–1034. 3578244.
Hadoun, N., Ghemri, S., Yahiaoui, S., Lazreg, S., 2008. Uvéites de l'enfant: à propos de 21 cas [Pediatric uveitis: about 21 cases]. J. Fr. Ophtalmol. 31 (Suppl. 1), 30. Available at: https://doi.org/10.1016/S0181-5512(08)70644-2.
Hajjami, K., Ennaji, M.M., Fouad, S., Oubrim, N., Khallayoune, K., Cohen, N., 2012. Assessment of helminths health risk associated with reuse of raw and treated wastewater of the Settat City (Morocco). Resour. Environ. 2, 193–201. https://doi.org/10.5923/j.re.20120205.03.
Hajjami, K., Ennaji, M.M., Fouad, S., Oubrim, N., Cohen, N., 2013a. Wastewater reuse for irrigation in Morocco: helminth eggs contamination's level of irrigated crops and sanitary risk (A case study of Settat and Soualem regions). J. Bacteriol. Parasitol. 4, 1. https://doi.org/10.4172/2155-9597.1000163.
Hajjami, K., Ennaji, M.M., Amdiouni, H., Fouad, S., Cohen, N., 2013b. Parasistic contamination on fresh vegetable consumed in Casablanca City (Morocco) and risk for consumer. Int. J. Sci. Technol. 2, 543–549.
Hamrouni, S., Boussetta, N., Dhahri, R., Sayhi, S., Gharsallah, I., Metoui, L., 2015. Toxocarose oculaire: à propos de trois cas. [Ocular toxocariasis: about three cases.]. Rev. Med. Interne 36 (Suppl. 2), A116.
Haridy, F.M., Hassan, A.A., Hafez, A.O., El-Sherbini, G.T., Morsy, T.A., 2009. External and intestinal parasites of pet dogs with reference to zoonotic toxocariasis. J. Egypt. Soc. Parasitol. 39, 321–326.
Hassan, M.M., Farghaly, A.M., Gaber, N.S., Nageeb, H.F., Hegab, M.H., Galal, N., 1996. Parasitic causes of hepatomegaly in children. J. Egypt. Soc. Parasitol. 26, 177–189. 8721239.
Hayashi, E., Tuda, J., Imada, M., Akao, N., Fujita, K., 2005. The high prevalence of asymptomatic *Toxocara* infection among schoolchildren in Manado, Indonesia. Southeast Asian J. Trop. Med. Public Health 36, 1399–1406.

Holland, C.V., O'Lorcain, P., Taylor, M.R.H., Kelly, A., 1995. Seroepidemiology of toxocariasis in school children. Parasitology 110, 535–545.

Hotez, P.J., Wilkins, P.P., 2009. Toxocariasis: America's most common neglected infection of poverty and a helminthiasis of global importance? PLoS Negl. Trop. Dis. 3, e400.

Ismail, M.A., Khalafallah, O., 2005. *Toxocara canis* and chronic urticaria in Egyptian patients. J. Egypt. Soc. Parasitol. 35, 833–840. 16333893.

Issa, R.M., 2007. Seroprevalence of *Toxocara* antibodies in asymptomatic pregnant women and children. Middle East Afr. J. Ophthalmol. 14, 16–21.

Jacquier, P., Gottstein, B., Stingelin, Y., Eckert, J., 1991. Immunodiagnosis of toxocariasis in humans: evaluation of a new enzyme-linked immunosorbent assay kit. J. Clin. Microbiol. 29, 1831–1835. PMC270219, 1774303.

Jones, J.L., Kruszon-Moran, D., Won, K., Wilson, M., Schantz, P.M., 2008. *Toxoplasma gondii* and *Toxocara* spp. co-infection. Am. J. Trop. Med. Hyg. 78, 35–39.

Kahloun, R., Khairallah-Ksiaa, I., Abroug, N., Mahmoud, A., Ben Yahia, S., Zaouali, S., Jelliti, B., Khairallah, M., 2015. Final diagnosis in patients referred with a diagnosis of neuroretinitis. Neuro-Ophthalmol. 39, 266–270. https://doi.org/10.3109/01658107.2015.1092561.

Kaplan, M., Kalkan, A., Hosoglu, S., Kuk, S., Ozden, M., Demirdag, K., Ozdarendeli, A., 2004. The frequency of *Toxocara* infection in mental retarded children. Mem. Inst. Oswaldo Cruz 99, 121–125.

Khademvatan, S., Khajeddin, N., Izadi, S., Yousefi, E., 2014. Investigation of Anti-*Toxocara* and Anti-*Toxoplasma* antibodies in patients with schizophrenia disorder. Schizophr. Res. Treat. 2014. 230349. 7 pages, https://doi.org/10.1155/2014/230349.

Khalafalla, R.E., 2011. A survey study on gastrointestinal parasites of stray cats in northern region of Nile Delta, Egypt. PLoS One 6. e20283. https://doi.org/10.1371/journal.pone.0020283.

Khaldi, F., Zaidi, T., Khiari, S., Matri, L., Bennaceur, B., 1990. Ocular toxocariasis Apropos of a case. Ann. Pediatr. 37, 185–188. 2350146.

Laghmari, M., Karim, A., Guedira, K., Ibrahimy, W., Dahreddine, M., Essakalli, N.H., Mohcine, Z., 2003. Uveitis in children: about 20 cases. [French]. J. Fr. Ophtalmol. 26, 609–613. Doi: JFO-06-2003-26-6-0181-5512-101019-ART9, https://www.em-consulte.com/showarticlefile/112619/pdf_51460.pdf.

Lajmi, M., Boussetta, N., Sayhi, S., Dhahri, R., Abid, R., Batikh, R., 2015. Une parasitose rare: la toxocarose (à propos de 5 cas). [Rare parasitosis: toxocariasis (about 5 cases)]. Rev. Med. Interne 36 (Suppl. 2), A118. https://doi.org/10.1016/j.revmed.2015.10.048.

Lalami, S.E., El-Maaloum, L., Allali, B., El kettani, A., Amraoui, A., Zaghloul, K., 2017. Toxocarose oculaire: à propos d'un cas et revue de littérature. Journal de la Société Marocaine d'Ophtalmologie 26, 51–54.

Li, L., Gao, W., Yang, X., Wu, D., Bi, H., Zhang, S., Huang, M., Yao, X., 2014. Asthma and toxocariasis. Ann. Allergy Asthma Immunol. 113, 187–192. https://doi.org/10.1016/j.anai.2014.05.016.

Luna, J., Cicero, C.E., Rateau, G., Quattrocchi, G., Marin, B., Bruno, E., et al., 2018. Updated evidence of the association between toxocariasis and epilepsy: systematic review and meta-analysis. PLoS Negl. Trop. Dis. 12. e0006665. https://doi.org/10.1371/journal.pntd.0006665.

Lynch, N.R., Wilkes, L.K., Hodgen, A.N., Turner, K.J., 1988. Specificity of Toxocara ELISA in tropical populations. Parasite Immunol. 10, 323–337. https://doi.org/10.1111/j.1365-3024.1988.tb00224.x.

Ma, G., Holland, C.V., Wang, T., Hofmann, A., Fan, C.K., Maizels, R.M., Hotez, P.J., Gasser, R.B., 2018. Human toxocariasis. Lancet Infect. Dis. 18, e14–e24. https://doi.org/10.1016/S1473-3099(17)30331-6. 28781085.

Macpherson, C.N.L., 2013. The epidemiology and public health importance of toxocariasis: zoonosis of global importance. Int. J. Parasitol. 43, 999–1008. https://doi.org/10.1016/j.ijpara.2013.07.004 (Epub 2013 Aug 14).

Magnaval, J.F., Fabre, R., Maurières, P., Charlet, J.P., de Larrard, B., 1991. Application of the western blotting procedure for the immunodiagnosis of human toxocariasis. Parasitology research 77, 697–702. 1805214.

Mohamed, N.H., Salem, S.A., Azab, M.E., Bebars, M.A., Khattab, H.M., Kamal, A.M., Mohamed, M.S., 1991. Parasitic infections associated with mental retardation in Egypt. J. Egypt. Soc. Parasitol. 21, 319–331. 1875063.

Mrissa, R., Battikh, R., Abdelhafidh, N.B., Jemli, B., Azzouz, O., Zaouali, J., Louzir, B., Ben Abdallah, N., Gargouri, S., Yedeas, M., Othmani, S., 2005. Méningoencéphalite à *Toxocara canis*: à propos d'un cas. [*Toxocara canis* encephalitis: case report]. Rev. Med. Interne 26, 829–832. https://doi.org/10.1016/j.revmed.2005.04.025.

Nada, S.M., Abazza, B.E., Mahmoud, L.A., Habeeb, Y.S., Hussein, H.F., Amer, O.T., 1996. Toxocariasis as a cause of renal disease in children in Sharkia governorate, Egypt. J. Egypt. Soc. Parasitol. 26, 709–917. 8918044.

Nehili, F.Z., Boucherit, N., 2009. Décollement de rétine révélateur d'une toxocarose oculaire [Retinal detachment indicative of ocular toxocariasis]. J. Fr. Ophtalmol. 32 (Suppl. 1), 1s133. https://doi.org/10.1016/S0181-5512(09)73547-8.

Oteifa, N.M., Moustafa, M.A., 1997. The potential risk of contracting toxocariasis in Heliopolis district, Cairo, Egypt. J. Egypt. Soc. Parasitol. 27, 197–203.

Oteifa, N.M., Moustafa, M.A., Elgozamy, B.M., 1998. Toxocariasis as a possible cause of allergic diseases in children. J. Egypt. Soc. Parasitol. 28, 365–372. 9707665.

Oudni-M'rad, M., Chaâbane-Banaoues, R., M'rad, S., Trifa, F., Mezhoud, H., Babba, H., 2017. Gastrointestinal parasites of canids, a latent risk to human health in Tunisia. Parasit. Vectors 10, 280. https://doi.org/10.1186/s13071-017-2208-3.

Quattrocchi G., Nicoletti A., Marin B., Bruno E., Druet-Cabanac M., Preux P.M. (2012). Toxocariasis and epilepsy: systematic review and meta-analysis. PLoS Negl. Trop. Dis. 6: e1775. [PubMed: 22905274].

Redissi, A., Daoud, F., Aydi, Z., Rachdi, I., Zoubeidi, H., Ben Dhaou, B., Boussema, F., 2017. Uvéo-méningo-encéphalite: quand penser à la toxocarids? [Uveo-meningoencephalitis: when to think of toxocariasis?]. Rev. Med. Interne 38 (Suppl. 2), A246. https://doi.org/10.1016/j.revmed.2017.10.278.

Riahi, A., Messelmani, M., Bedoui, I., Derbali, H., Mansour, M., Zaouali, J., Mrissa, R., 2014a. Acute encephalomyelitis revealing a neurotoxocariasis. Eur. J. Neurol. 21 (Suppl. 1), 388–713.

Riahi, A., Messelmani, M., Bedoui, I., Derbali, H., Mansour, M., Zaouali, J., Mrissa, R., 2014b. Cerbral toxocariasis and rhinocerebral mucormycosis as exceptional etiologies of ischemic strokes, two case report. Cerebrovasc. Dis. 37, 602.

Rubinsky-Elefant, G., Hirata, C.E., Yamamoto, J.H., Ferreira, M.U., 2010. Human toxocariasis: diagnosis, worldwide seroprevalences and clinical expression of the systemic and ocular forms. Ann. Trop. Med. Parasitol. 104, 3–23.

Saadouli, D.S., Yahyaoui, S., Sammoud, A., Afrit, M.A., 2018. Les aspects cliniques et étiologiques des vascularites rétiniennes chez l'enfant [The clinical and etiological aspects of retinal vasculitis in children]. Rev. Med. Interne 39 (Suppl. 1), A205. https://doi.org/10.1016/j.revmed.2018.03.180.

Sabry, M.A., Lotfy, H.S., 2009. Captive dogs as reservoirs of some zoonotic parasites. Res. J. Parasitol. 4, 115–122.

Sadjjadi, S.M., Khosravi, M., Mehrabani, D., Orya, A., 2000. Seroprevalence of *Toxocara* infection in schoolchildren in Shiraz, southern Iran. J. Trop. Pediatr. 46, 327–330.

Safar, E.H., Azab, M.E., Khalil, H.M., Bebars, M.A., el Hady, H., Khattab, H.M., 1990. Immunodiagnostics of *Toxocara canis* in suspected ocular and visceral manifestations. Folia Parasitol. 37, 249–254. https://folia.paru.cas.cz/pdfs/fol/1990/03/09.pdf.

Safar, E.H., Abd-el Ghaffar, F.M., Saffar, S.A., Makled, K.M., Habib, K.S., el Abiad, R., el Shabrawy, E., 1995. Incidence of *Toxoplasma* and *Toxocara* antibodies among out-patients in the ophthalmic research institute, Egypt. J. Egypt. Soc. Parasitol. 25, 839–852. 8586877.

Said, D.E.S., 2012. Detection of parasites in commonly consumed raw vegetables. Alex. J. Med. 48, 345–352.

Salama, A.M., Daoud, A.A., Elshehawy, A.K., Othman, A.A., Eid, M.M., 2019. Toxocariasis and toxoplasmosis in children with idiopathic epilepsy in mid-region of the Nile Delta, Egypt: prevalence and risk factors. Int. J. Curr. Microbiol. App. Sci. 8, 760–767. https://doi.org/10.20546/ijcmas.2019.802.088.

Skouri, W., Boussetta, N., Metoui, L., Arfaoui, B., Ajili, F., Louzir, B., 2018. Uvéites infectieuses dans un service de médecine interne [Infectious Uveitis in a Department of Internal Medicine]. Rev. Med. Interne 39 (Suppl. 1), A206–A207. https://doi.org/10.1016/j.revmed.2018.03.184.

Smith, H., Holland, C., Taylor, M., Magnaval, J.F., Schantz, P., Maizels, R., 2009. How common is human toxocariasis? Towards standardizing our knowledge. Trends Parasitol. 25, 182–188.

Strube, C., Heuer, L., Janecek, E., 2013. *Toxocara* spp. infections in paratenic hosts. Vet. Parasitol. 193, 375–389.

Taboz, Y., El Kharrim, K., Belghyti, D., 2008. Epidemiological survey of dogs gastro-intestinal parasites in the rural zone of the area of Kenitra Morocco. In: Dei-Cas, E., Dupouy-Camet, J. (Eds.), 10th European Multicolloquium of Parasitology, Paris, FRANCE, AUG 24–29. Medimond International Proceedings, Bologna, p. 194. 2008. ISBN:9788875874599 2008.

Taylor, M.R., Keane, C.T., O'Connor, P., Girdwood, R.W., Smith, H., 1987. Clinical features of covert toxocariasis. Scand. J. Infect. Dis. 19, 693–696. https://doi.org/10.3109/00365548709117206. 3441751.

Trabelsi, S., Belhadj, S., Kallel, K., Zouiten, F., Ben, B.S., Ben, A.N., El Matri, L., Hammouda, B., Trabelsi, M., Emna, C., 2004. La toxocarose: Une pathologie sous-estimee. A propos de 9 cas. [Toxocariasis: under-estimated disease. Report of 9 cases]. Tunis. Med. 82, 684–689.

Trabelsi, H., Néji, S., Cheikhrouhou, F., Sellami, H., Guidara, R., Mhiri, W., Makni, F., Ayadi, A., 2014. Toxocarose oculaire: à propos d'un cas [Ocular toxocariasis: a case report]. J. Fr. Ophtalmol. 37, e81. https://doi.org/10.1016/j.jfo.2013.10.005.

Winkler, A.S., Blocher, J., Auer, H., Gotwald, T., Matuja, W., Schmutzhard, E., 2008. Anticysticercal and anti toxocaral antibodies in people with epilepsy in rural Tanzania. Trans. R. Soc. Trop. Med. Hyg. 102, 1032–1038. https://doi.org/10.1016/j.trstmh.2008.05.004. Epub 2008 Jun 20, 18571212.

Won, K.Y., Kruszon-Moran, D., Schantz, P.M., Jones, J.L., 2008. National seroprevalence and risk factors for zoonotic *Toxocara* spp. infection. Am. J. Trop. Med. Hyg. 79, 552–557.

Woodruff, A.W., Salih, S.Y., de Savigny, D., Baya, E.I., Shah, A.I., Dafalla, A.A., 1981. Toxocariasis in the Sudan. Ann. Trop. Med. Parasitol. 75 (5), 559–561. https://doi.org/10.1080/00034983.1981.11687481. 7316582.

Zamo, A.C., Belghyti, D., Lyagoubi, M., Elkharrim, K., 2003. Analyse parasitologique des eaux usées brutes d'un effluent urbain de « la Ville haute » (commune de Mâamora, Kénitra, Maroc). [parasitological analysis of the untreated wastewater of the "Ville haute" urban emissary (Mâamora district, Kenitra, Morocco)]. [article in French]. Sante 13, 269–272.

Zarkovic, A., McMurray, C., Deva, N., Ghosh, S., Whitley, D., Guest, S., 2007. Seropositivity rates for *Bartonella henselae, Toxocara canis* and *Toxoplasma gondii* in New Zealand blood donors. Clin. Experiment. Ophthalmol. 35, 131–134.

Zinkham, W.H., 1978. Visceral larva Migrans: a review and reassessment indicating two forms of clinical expression: visceral and ocular. Am. J. Dis. Child. 132, 627–633. https://doi.org/10.1001/archpedi.1978.02120310091020.

Zoubeidi, H., Abdelkefi, C., Hamzaoui, A., Said, F., Lamloum, M., Ben, G.I., Ben, S.T., Khanfir, M., 2015. Profil étiologique des uvéites infectieuses dans un service de médecine interne [Etiologic Profile of infectious uveitis in an internal medicine department]. Rev. Med. Interne 36 (Suppl. 2), A100–A211. https://doi.org/10.1016/j.revmed.2015.10.021.

Further reading

Arpino, C., Gattinara, G.C., Piergili, D., Curatolo, P., 1990. *Toxocara* infection and epilepsy in children: a case-control study. Epilepsia 31, 33–36.

Worley, G., Green, I.A., Frothingham, T.E., 1984. *Toxocara canis* infection: clinical and epidemiological associations with seropositivity in kindergarten children. J. Infect. Dis. 149, 591–597.

PART IV

Dogs (and cats) disease, diagnosis, prevalence of infection, and treatment

CHAPTER TWENTY-SIX

Pathology of larvae and adults in dogs and cats

Andrew D. Miller*
Department of Biomedical Sciences, Section of Anatomic Pathology, Cornell University, Ithaca, NY, United States
*Corresponding author: e-mail address: adm10@cornell.edu

Contents

Abstract

Endoparasitism remains a significant cause of morbidity and mortality in puppies and kittens. The ascarids of dogs and cats (*Toxocara canis, Toxascaris leonina, Toxocara cati*) cause significant pathology due to either larval migration or adult nematode burden within the gastrointestinal tract. This chapter will review the important pathologic events and lesions that are encountered during ascarid development in dogs and cats with emphasis given to the characteristic gross pathology lesions that are seen in affected animals.

Endoparasitism remains a significant cause of morbidity and mortality in puppies and kittens and environments that promote increased likelihood of transmission (i.e. shelters, hoarding situations) allow for endoparasites to maintain a high prevalence in some of these populations. The ascarids of dogs and cats (*Toxocara canis, Toxascaris leonina, Toxocara cati*) cause a variety of pathologies associated with larval migration through a wide number of tissues in addition to adult nematode burden within the gastrointestinal tract.

Ascarid eggs are able to remain infective in a variety of environmental conditions and in dogs exposure through ingestion, transmammary (in the milk), and transplacental infections will occur (Raza et al., 2018). In cats, the primary route of infection is transmammary (Overgaauw, 1997), although this appears to occur only rarely in natural infection (Coati et al., 2004). In the dog, transmammary and transplacental transmission is often aided by the activation and subsequent migration of tissue-arrested

Advances in Parasitology, Volume 109
ISSN 0065-308X
https://doi.org/10.1016/bs.apar.2020.01.024

larvae in the pregnant or lactating bitch (Buckle et al., 2019; Raza et al., 2018). When ingested, the infective third stage larvae within the ascarid eggs hatch and gain access to the portal circulation through direct intestinal invasion. After invading the portal circulation, the larvae eventually reach the lungs where the parasites migrate through the lung parenchyma to reach the lumen of the trachea. The intratracheal larvae are eventually coughed up and swallowed and subsequently undergo sexual maturity to adult ascarids within the intestine (Raza et al., 2018). A second possibility is that the intravascular larvae migrate through non-pulmonary tissues resulting extra-intestinal lesions in affected organs (somatic migration) (Raza et al., 2018). This book chapter will review the gross and histopathology associated with ascarid infection in dogs and cats.

1. Gross Pathology

In the dog, gross pathology associated with the larval migration stage is often imperceptible; however, miliary pale red to white foci can be seen in the liver and kidney associated with larval migration (Hayden and Kruiningen, 1975; Schnieder et al., 2011). Rarely petechiae can be noted in the lung; however, this is a rare gross finding in natural infections (Hayden and Kruiningen, 1975). In the case of adult ascarid infection, large numbers of parasites are often present in the lumen of the small intestine (Figs 1–3). Extremely heavy intestinal endoparasitism can lead to parasites migrating into the common bile duct and eventually into the liver where

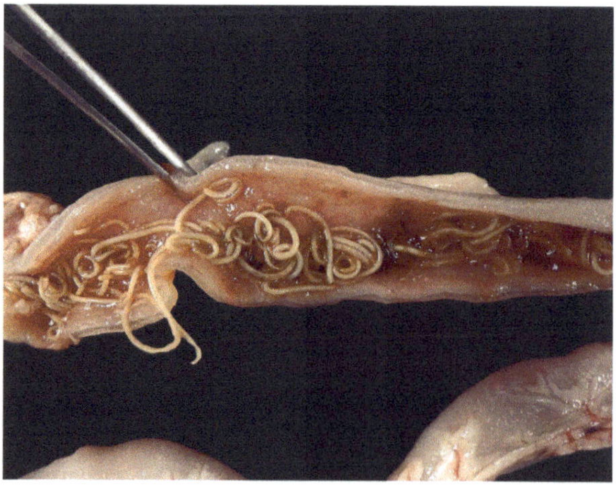

Fig. 1 *Toxocara canis* in the small intestine of a dog. Large numbers of adult ascarids fill the small intestinal lumen.

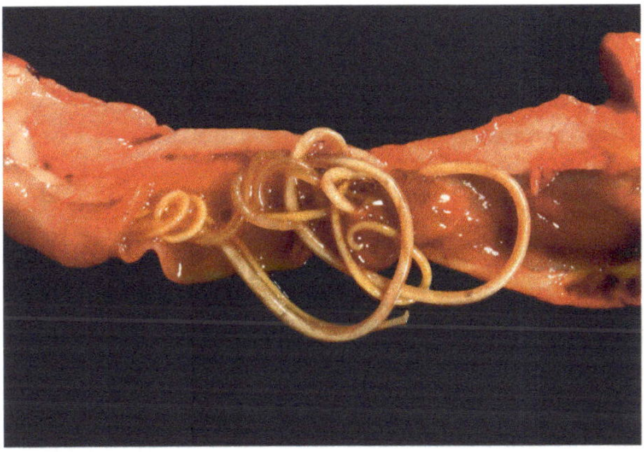

Fig. 2 *Toxocara cati* in the small intestine of a cat. Numerous adult ascarids fill the lumen of the small intestine admixed with mucous. Photo courtesy of Dr. Brian Porter, DVM, Dipl. ACVP, Texas A&M College of Veterinary Medicine.

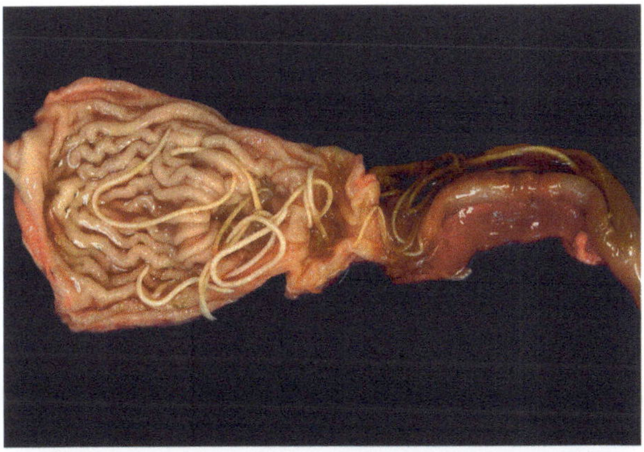

Fig. 3 *Toxocara canis* in the stomach and small intestine of a cat. Photo courtesy of Dr. Taryn Donovan, DVM, Dipl. ACVP, Pathology Department, Animal Medical Center.

severe parenchymal damage ensues (Dade and Williams, 1975; Schnieder et al., 2011). While adult parasites reside in the small intestine, they can be commonly observed in the oesophagus, stomach, or large intestine at necropsy. This non-small intestinal presentation owes itself to the ascarids, still alive after the animal dies, trying to flee a sinking ship. If the parasite load is extremely heavy, animals can present with an impacted small intestine which can lead to intestinal rupture and subsequent septic peritonitis as well as regional haemorrhage, infarction, and possibly intussusception (Schnieder et al., 2011). Diarrhoea is not typically observed in animals infested with adult ascarids, but can be observed, especially when there is co-infection with one or more other pathogens (Duijvestijn et al., 2016). Puppies can often present with a pot-bellied appearance, especially when the parasite load is high and can be a contributing cause of fading puppy syndrome.

Due to the differences in how the infection is transmitted, gross lesions in cats are much less common. Kittens, similar to puppies, will present with a pot-bellied appearance if the parasite load is high enough. As it is in dogs, heavy ascarid loads in cats can be associated with fading kitten syndrome, a nebulous diagnosis that encompasses any number of infectious and non-infectious causes of peri-parturient death in the cat (Duarte et al., 2016). Disseminated granulomatous disease has been reported in a cat infected with *Toxocara canis* in which the animal presented with white to off-white nodules in the kidneys, heart, liver, and other abdominal organs (Parsons et al., 1988).

2. Histopathology

Some of our earliest knowledge regarding ascarid-associated histopathology comes from dogs that were experimentally superinfected with *Toxocara canis* and developed significant transmural eosinophilic gastritis, enteritis, and typhlocolitis (Hayden and Kruiningen, 1975; Lloyd et al., 1991). Atrophic villi, crypt hyperplasia, reduction in goblet cell number and variations in the number of intraepithelial lymphocytes have all been reported in experimental studies of *Toxocarca canis* in puppies (Lloyd et al., 1991). Resultant lymphoid hyperplasia was commonly noted in the draining abdominal lymph nodes where it was accompanied by a significant sinusoidal eosinophilia (Hayden and Kruiningen, 1975). Granulomas were also reported in the stomach, small intestine, and abdominal lymph nodes of these superinfected dogs (Hayden and Kruiningen, 1975). The most severe extra-intestinal lesions were in the liver where severe eosinophilic portal hepatitis predominated, rarely associated with ascarid larvae (Hayden and Kruiningen, 1975) (Figs 4–6). It must be stressed that in a typical necropsy situation, visualizing the larval ascarids in the liver is uncommon as the time passage through the liver is short and transit has likely been completed prior to the death of the puppy. Rarely necrotizing vasculitis has been described in the liver (Buckle et al., 2019). Other histologic lesions of importance in these superinfected dogs included multifocal granulomatous bronchointerstitial pneumonia (Fig. 7), multifocal renal granulomas, myocarditis, pancreatitis,

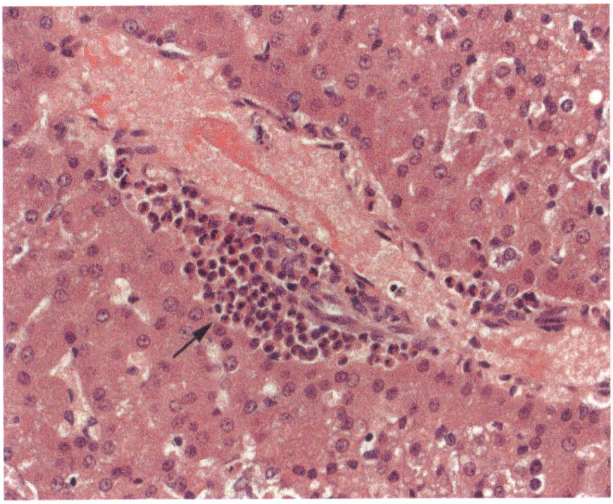

Fig. 4 *Toxocara canis* hepatitis in a puppy. A portal tract is expanded by large numbers of eosinophils (arrow).

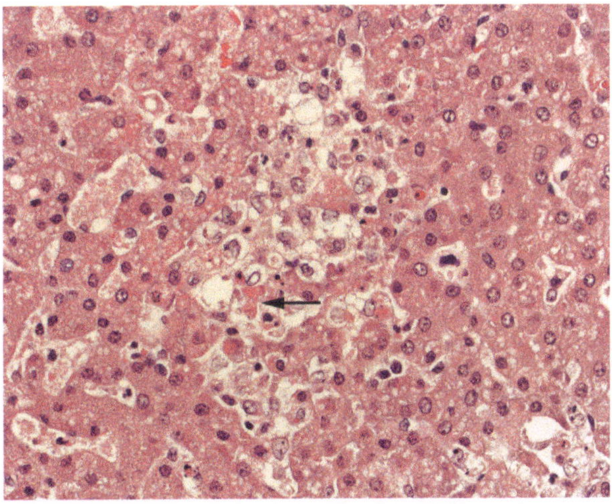

Fig. 5 *Toxocara canis* hepatitis in a puppy. Random areas of necrosis associated (arrow) with a mild inflammatory infiltrate.

and rarely splenitis (Hayden and Kruiningen, 1975; Parsons, 1987). In the lung, lesions often predominate in the interstitium, alveoli, and bronchioles as the larvae migrate towards the trachea (Buckle et al., 2019). As expected, infected animals have a significant increase in eosinophils in the bone marrow (Hayden and Kruiningen, 1975). Rare manifestations associated with larval migration of *Toxocara* sp. are orbital cellulitis in an adult dog and ocular

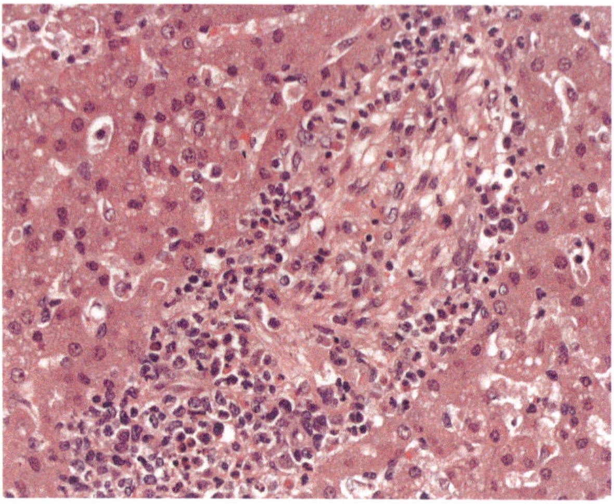

Fig. 6 *Toxocara canis* hepatitis in a puppy. A central vein is shrouded and surrounded by large numbers of eosinophils, lymphocytes, and macrophages.

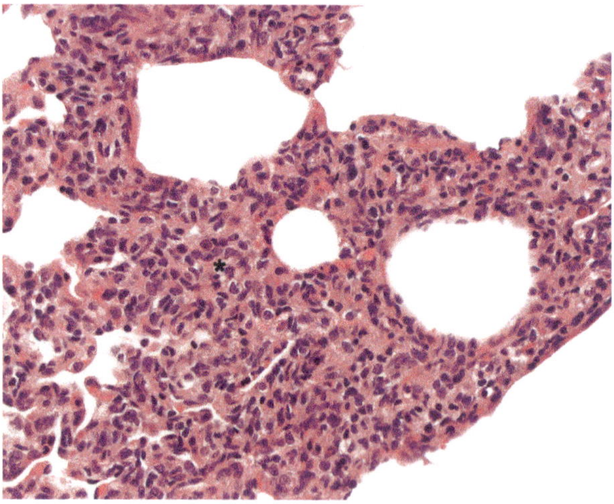

Fig. 7 *Toxocara canis* pneumonia in a puppy. The interstitium is expanded by moderate numbers of infiltrating lymphocytes and macrophages with rare eosinophils (asterisk).

larval migrans presenting predominately as granulomatous retinitis in a population of New Zealand sheep dogs (Hughes et al., 1987; Laus et al., 2003). Adult ascarids are identified histologically by coelomyarian musculature, a uninucleate intestine with a prominent brush border, and thick-shelled eggs (Fig. 8).

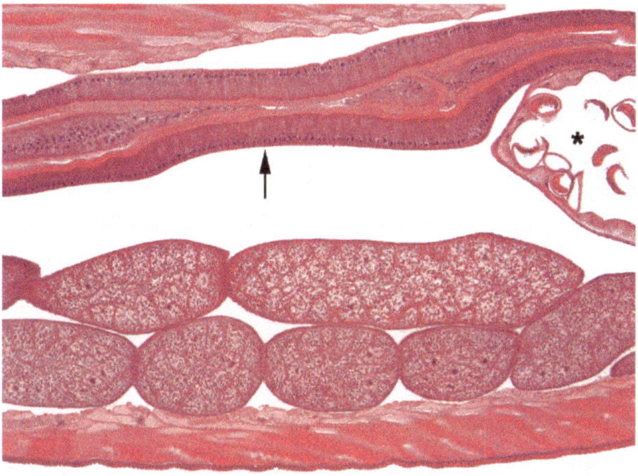

Fig. 8 *Toxocara canis* in a dog. An adult *Toxocara canis* histologic section illustrating the uninucleate intestine with a prominent brush border (asterisk) and uterus with thick shelled eggs (arrow).

In cats, the primary infection is only via transmammary spread and therefore this limits the number of extra-intestinal histologic lesions seen. Additionally, fewer studies have addressed the pathology of ascarid infection in cats compared to dogs; however, cats experimentally infected with *Toxascaris leonina* and *Toxocara cati*, did not develop extraintestinal gross or histologic lesions (Parsons, 1987; Swerczek et al., 1971). Glomerular lesions have been described in cats experimentally infected with *Toxocara cati* in which larvae were lodged in the glomerular capillaries and associated with a variety of thrombotic and degenerative lesions (Hamilton et al., 1982). Additionally, superinfected cats also develop pulmonary arterial disease characterized by intimal proliferation and vasculitis with a correlative role of mastocytosis and elaboration of histamine in the pathogenesis (Weatherley and Hamilton, 1984). The significance of either the glomerular or pulmonary lesions in natural infections is not clear as natural infections of cats with ascarids are limited to the intestinal presentation of adult nematodes.

References

Buckle, K.N., Hardcastle, M.R., Scott, I., Craig, L.E., French, A., Gedye, K., Collett, M.G., 2019. Toxocara canis larval migration causing verminous pneumonia in fading puppies from 2 Scottish terrier litters. Vet. Pathol. 56, 903–906. 300985819852131.

Coati, N., Schnieder, T., Epe, C., 2004. Vertical transmission of Toxocara cati Schrank 1788 (Anisakidae) in the cat. Parasitol. Res. 92, 142–146.

Dade, A.W., Williams, J.F., 1975. Hepatic and peritoneal invasion by adult ascarids (Toxocara Canis) in a dog. Vet. Med. Small Anim. Clin. 70, 947–949.

Duarte, A.M., Jenkins, T.P., Latrofa, M.S., Giannelli, A., Papadopoulos, E., De Carvalho, L.M., Nolan, M.J., Otranto, D., Cantacessi, C., 2016. Helminth infections and gut microbiota—a feline perspective. Parasit. Vectors 9, 625.

Duijvestijn, M., Mughini-Gras, L., Schuurman, N., Schijf, W., Wagenaar, J.A., Egberink, H., 2016. Enteropathogen infections in canine puppies: (co-)occurrence, clinical relevance and risk factors. Vet. Microbiol. 195, 115–122.

Hamilton, J.M., Naylor, J., Weatherley, A., 1982. Glomerular lesions associated with infestation with Toxocara cati. Vet. Rec. 111, 583–584.

Hayden, D.W., Kruiningen, H.J., 1975. Experimentally induced canine toxocariasis: laboratory examinations and pathologic changes, with emphasis on the gastrointestinal tract. Am. J. Vet. Res. 36, 1605–1614.

Hughes, P.L., Dubielzig, R.R., Kazacos, K.R., 1987. Multifocal retinitis in New Zealand sheep dogs. Vet. Pathol. 24, 22–27.

Laus, J.L., Canola, J.C., Mamede, F.V., Almeida, D.E., Godoy, G.S., Oliveira, C.J., Pontin, K., Albuquerque, S., Alessi, A.C., 2003. Orbital cellulitis associated with Toxocara canis in a dog. Vet. Ophthalmol. 6, 333–336.

Lloyd, S., Wijesundera, M.K., Soulsby, E.J., 1991. Intestinal changes in puppies infected with Toxocara canis. J. Comp. Pathol. 105, 93–104.

Overgaauw, P.A., 1997. Aspects of Toxocara epidemiology: toxocarosis in dogs and cats. Crit. Rev. Microbiol. 23, 233–251.

Parsons, J.C., 1987. Ascarid infections of cats and dogs. Vet. Clin. North Am. Small Anim. Pract. 17, 1307–1339.

Parsons, J.C., Bowman, D.D., Gillette, D.M., Grieve, R.B., 1988. Disseminated granulomatous disease in a cat caused by larvae of Toxocara canis. J. Comp. Pathol. 99, 343–346.

Raza, A., Rand, J., Qamar, A.G., Jabbar, A., Kopp, S., 2018. Gastrointestinal parasites in shelter dogs: occurrence, pathology, treatment and risk to shelter workers. Animals (Basel) 8.

Schnieder, T., Laabs, E.M., Welz, C., 2011. Larval development of Toxocara canis in dogs. Vet. Parasitol. 175, 193–206.

Swerczek, T.W., Nielsen, S.W., Helmboldt, C.F., 1971. Transmammary passage of Toxocara cati in the cat. Am. J. Vet. Res. 32, 89–92.

Weatherley, A.J., Hamilton, J.M., 1984. Possible role of histamine in the genesis of pulmonary arterial disease in cats infected with Toxocara cati. Vet. Rec. 114, 347–349.

CHAPTER TWENTY-SEVEN

Antigen detection: Insights into *Toxocara* and other ascarid infections in dogs and cats

David A. Elsemore*
IDEXX Laboratories, Inc., Westbrook, ME, United States
*Corresponding author: e-mail address: david-elsemore@idexx.com

Contents

Abstract

Detection of ascarid excreted or secreted (E/S) molecules is an alternative approach to the identification of infection by egg flotation. E/S molecules serve as direct markers for the ascarid nematode commonly found in cats and dogs (*Toxocara* spp., *Toxascaris leonina* and *Baylisascaris procyonis*). The nematode derived E/S material mixes with the intestinal contents of the host animal and is available for detection as a coproantigen in the host's faeces. Antigen capture immunological techniques allow sensitive coproantigen detection. Different patterns of antigen to egg agreement are demonstrated in an experimental *Toxocara canis* infection throughout the prepatent, patent, and post-treatment phases. Examination of faecal samples from a large field population of dogs and cats tested for both egg shedding and antigen indicates that more infections were identified by antigen. Host age influences the agreement of antigen and *Toxocara* egg results. Older dogs and cats were less likely to have a patent infection (egg positive and antigen positive) result pattern. An egg observation in the absence of antigen detection may indicate a spurious egg. The impact of spurious eggs was further examined by comparisons of cohorts of dogs separated by presence or absence of a pseudoparasite observation or by egg semi-quantification bin. Lastly, the antigen to egg agreement was calculated for other ascarid species.

Advances in Parasitology, Volume 109
ISSN 0065-308X
https://doi.org/10.1016/bs.apar.2020.01.034

1. Introduction

Detection of parasite antigens has been a valuable tool in veterinarian diagnostics since the introduction of *Giardia*, canine parvovirus, and heartworm tests in the 1990s (Church et al., 2005; O'Connor, 2015). These rapid tests are enzyme-linked immunosorbent assays (ELISAs) that rely on a capture antibody and a detection antibody that is commonly conjugated to horseradish peroxidase (Fig. 1).

The capture antibody is immobilized on a solid surface. Antigen produced by the infecting parasite, if present, is bound by the capture antibody. Wash steps eliminate any unbound material from the sample. Addition of the second antibody, the detection phase, completes the ELISA sandwich and another round of wash-steps removes unbound detection molecules and sample material. Finally, addition of substrate allows for product formation often in the form of a chromogenic end point.

Recently, nematode antigen tests, the Fecal Dx® tests, have been introduced to the veterinary market at the IDEXX Reference Laboratories, Inc.

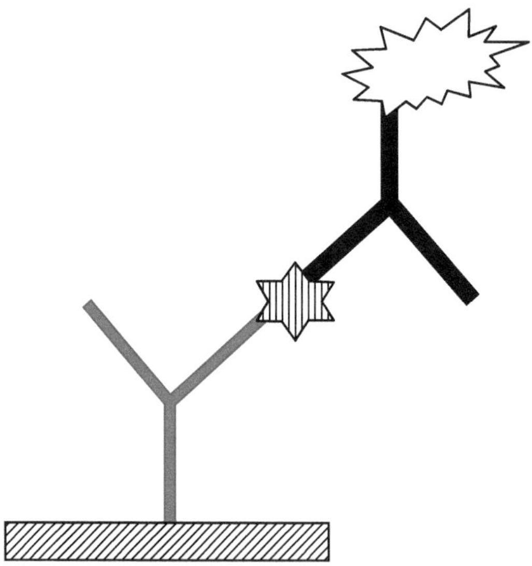

Fig. 1 Antigen capture ELISA schematic. In the presence of a sample containing the specific antigen, capture antibody (grey) immobilized to a surface (hatched rectangle) captures the antigen (hatched star) from the test sample. Binding of the enzyme (HRPO) conjugated detection antibody (black) completes the sandwich ELISA. The HRPO cleaves substrate to provide colorimetric detection. Absence of the antigen in a test sample does not allow the capture and detection antibodies to bridge and results in no signal.

This suite of tests includes assays to detect discrete antigens from ascarid, hookworm, and whipworm infections in dogs and cats. This paper summarizes the field performance for ascarid detection and explores more deeply the relationship between antigen detection and egg detection for *Toxocara canis* and *Toxocara cati*, as well as for the other ascarid species, *Toxascaris leonina* and *Baylisascaris procyonis*.

2. Ascarid antigen detection

Antigen detection requires a biomolecule produced by the nematode to be available in the patient sample. Ideally, this molecule would be abundant and available for detection. Metabolically active nematodes are feeding, avoiding host immune functions, and reproducing within the host. This metabolic activity results in excreted or secreted biomolecules such as carbohydrates, proteins, and/or nucleic acids. E/S proteins are attractive targets because of their molecular size, potential stability, and ability to apply recombinant molecular technology. One such class of E/S proteins has been identified from adult *Ascaris lumbricoides* decades ago (Babin et al., 1984; Fraefel and Acher, 1968; Peanasky et al., 1984). Serine protease inhibitors were one of the first identified proteins from aqueous extracts. This family of inhibitors consists of chymotrypsin/elastase and trypsin inhibitors and is distinct from Kunitz or Kazal domain containing protease inhibitors (Grasberger et al., 1994; Huang et al., 1994). These proteins are interesting because they appear restricted to nematodes. Within *Toxocara*, homologs share high identity (>95% between *T. canis* and *T. cati*) but identity drops off dramatically with homologs from *Ascaris suum* (60–80%) and even further (<50%) with homologs from other non-ascarid nematode species. The conservation in homologs allows for specific detection of *T. canis* and *T. cati* as well as other closely related ascarids of companion animal veterinarian concern.

The biological role of these serine protease inhibitors is most likely maintenance within the host's gastrointestinal system by inhibition of host proteases (Martzen et al., 1985). In *A. suum*, homologs of these proteins line the adult nematode's gut as well as its egg surfaces. It is likely that this class of proteins is produced by the adult nematode throughout its tenure within the host and thus provides a good target molecule for detection. Importantly for diagnostics, expression in a tissue such as gut tissue provides excreted protein in both male and female ascarids.

3. Experimental infections

An experimental infection time course highlights differences between examining infection status by egg observation or by antigen detection (Elsemore et al., 2017). Fig. 2 illustrates an idealized experimental *T. canis* infection time course for dogs infected orally with 150–300 larvated *T. canis* eggs and treated with an anthelmintic at day 89 based on published results.

There are several intervals within the time course that highlight the pattern of antigen detection and egg observation. From study day 0 to 31, both egg and antigen are not detected. At day 31, antigen is detected in the absence of an egg observation. This represents the start of the prepatent period where young adults are present, but egg laying has not commenced. Eggs appear 7 days after antigen detection, i.e., on day 38 post-infection, consistent with the short prepatent period observed for *T. canis*. The patent period is characterized by positive antigen detection results and egg-positive observations. Egg counts are typically in the 100–1000 egg per gram range. The antigen levels are typically 3- to 40-fold above the assay cut-off (0.1 OD). After treatment, both egg observations and antigen return to baseline so that by day 100, results for both tests are negative.

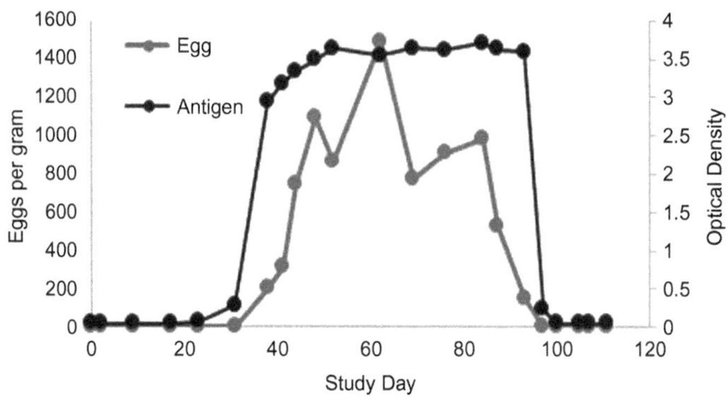

Fig. 2 Idealized experimental *Toxocara canis* infection time course in dog. Antigen signal was first detected between study day 31 and 38 and remained high (OD 4.0 is the maximum value of the plate reader) until treatment. Eggs were observed on study day 38 and fluctuated between 200 and 2000 eggs per gram until treatment. Treatment at study day 89 caused a concurrent drop in both antigen signal and egg enumeration. Both tests were positive on study day 97 (OD = 0.239 and 1 EPG) and then remained negative for the duration of the study.

4. Egg observation and antigen results

The Roundworm Fecal Dx® test detects pan-ascarid secreted or excreted antigen from dog or cat samples. In the following discussion the data groupings are determined by the egg observation. Tables 1 and 2 are pan-ascarid egg-positive results. Subsequent analysis limits the egg-positive groups to *Toxocara* spp. only egg observations (Figs. 3–6). Figs. 7 and 8 group egg-positive samples by the species identified in the flotation assay, *Toxocara* spp., *Toxascaris leonina*, or *Baylisascaris* spp. The figure legends indicate the number of samples in each cohort of dogs or cats.

4.1 Ascarid field data

Since the introduction of the Fecal Dx® test in the IDEXX Reference Laboratories, field data that includes both egg observation by faecal flotation and antigen test results have been collected. Egg flotation was accomplished by zinc sulphate centrifugation, specific gravity equal to 1.24–1.27. A positive egg flotation for ascarid could be an observation recorded as representing eggs of the genera *Toxocara* spp., *Toxascaris*, or *Baylisascaris*. The species is not determined; however, in the case of the eggs

Table 1 Egg flotation results and antigen results for a population of dogs.

		Egg flotation	
		Positive	**Negative**
Antigen	Positive	53,121	22,789
	Negative	15,999	3,889,279

Results where the veterinarian ordered faecal egg flotation and the Roundworm Fecal Dx® tests for dog patients were collected from IDEXX Reference Laboratories, Inc. from January 2017 to 15 June 2019. The table displays positive and negative results for both tests.

Table 2 Egg flotation results and antigen results for a population of cats.

		Egg flotation	
		Positive	**Negative**
Antigen	Positive	25,015	14,854
	Negative	3559	613,411

Results where the veterinarian ordered faecal egg flotation and the Roundworm Fecal Dx® tests for cat patients were collected from IDEXX Reference Laboratories, Inc. from January 2017 to 15 June 2019. The table displays positive and negative results for both tests.

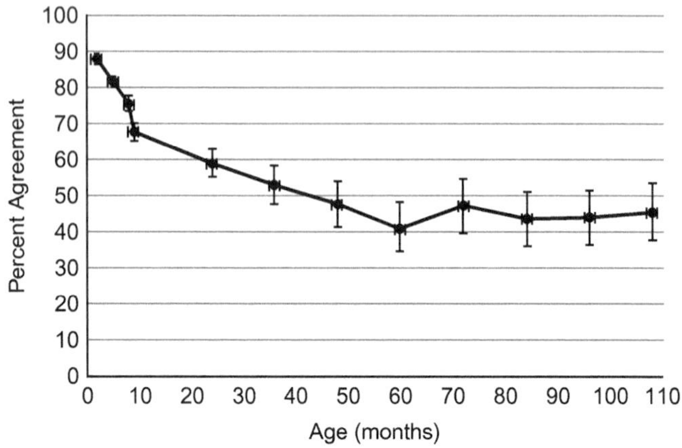

Fig. 3 Antigen to egg agreement by dog age. Proportion of antigen agreement to dogs with a positive *Toxocara* spp. egg observation from a field sample of 37,485 animals. Individual dogs are grouped by 3-month age groups within year one. For 2-year-old and older animals, the 3-month period centred on the anniversary month was pooled (2-year-old dogs were considered 23, 24, and 25-month data). Confidence intervals were calculated using the binomial exact method.

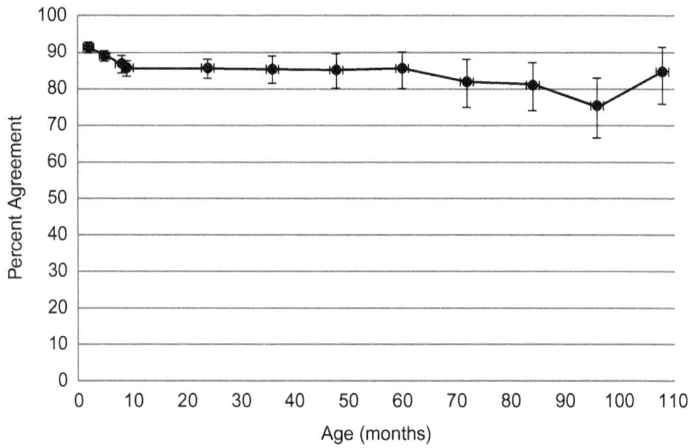

Fig. 4 Antigen to egg agreement by cat age. Proportion of antigen agreement to cats with a positive *Toxocara* spp. egg observation from a field sample of 14,539 animals. Individual cats are grouped by 3-month age groups within year one. For 2-year-old and older animals, the 3-month period centred on the anniversary month was pooled (2-year-old dogs were considered 23, 24, and 25-month data). Confidence intervals were calculated using the binomial exact method.

of the genus *Toxocara*, a *Toxocara* observation is recorded as *T. canis* in a dog sample and *T. cati* when in a cat sample. The antigen test, because of target homology, detects ascarid infections. Data was collected from 1 January 2017 to 15 June 2019.

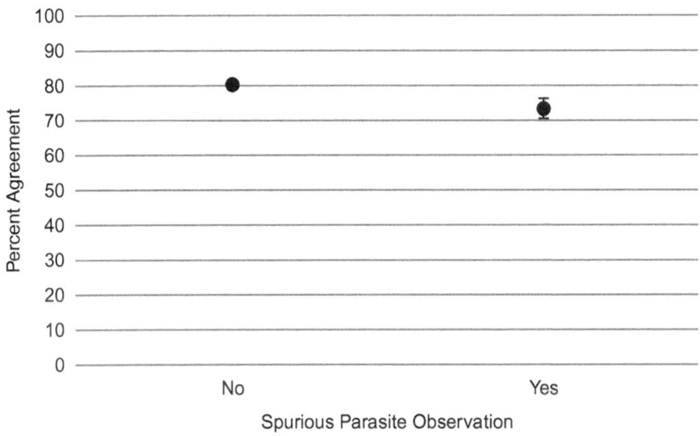

Fig. 5 Impact of pseudoparasite observation on antigen to *Toxocara* egg agreement in dog. *Toxocara* egg positive dogs were divided into two cohorts by the co-observation of the pseudoparasites *Eimeria*, strongyle egg, or *Anoplocephala* egg. There were 41,169 *Toxocara* egg positive samples without a pseudoparasite co observation and 1092 samples where at least one pseudoparasite was noted. Confidence intervals were calculated using the binomial exact method.

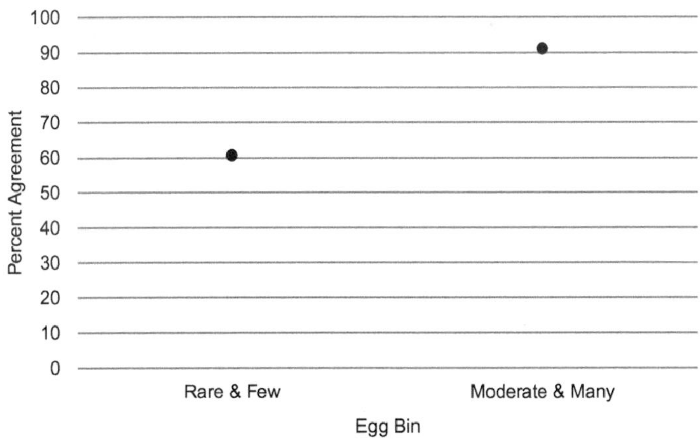

Fig. 6 Percent agreement of antigen to *Toxocara* egg observation by semi-quantitative egg bin. Rare and Few egg bins include samples ($n = 14{,}748$) where 1–10 eggs were observed and moderate and many egg bins include egg counts enumerated to 11–30 and >30 ($n = 27{,}531$). Confidence intervals were calculated using the binomial exact method.

For dogs, Table 1 summarizes the two-by-two relationship between the reference method of ascarid egg detection by flotation and ascarid antigen by the immunologic test.

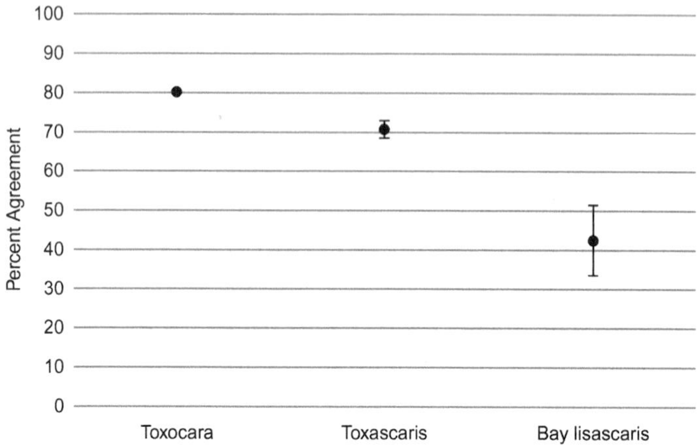

Fig. 7 Antigen to egg agreement for ascarid species in dog. Ascarid egg positive dog samples were identified to the genus level by egg morphology. Agreement of antigen to egg observation was calculated for *Toxocara* spp. (n = 42,261), *Toxascaris* (n = 1602), and *Baylisascaris* (n = 127). Confidence intervals were calculated using the binomial exact method.

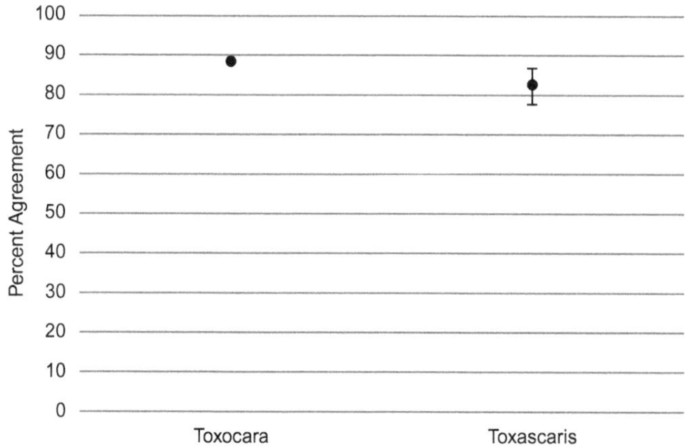

Fig. 8 Antigen to egg agreement for ascarid species in cat. Ascarid egg positive cat samples were identified to the genus level by egg morphology. Agreement of antigen to egg observation was calculated for *Toxocara* spp. (n = 18,072) and *Toxascaris* (n = 289). Confidence intervals were calculated using the binomial exact method.

Of the 3,981,188 total samples, the vast majority (97.7%) were negative on both tests. Overall, 91,909 samples (2.3% of the total samples) had a positive result with eggs being observed, antigen being detected, or being positive on both tests. Of the 91,909 samples positive on one or both tests, there were 53,121 samples (57.8%) positive for both eggs and antigen, 22,789 samples (24.8%) positive only for antigen, and 15,999 samples (17.4%) positive only for eggs. Thus, of the total of 3,981,188 samples tested, of the 91,909 samples positive on any test, there were 1.3% positive on both tests, 0.4% positive only for eggs, and 0.6% positive only for antigen. The egg positive, antigen negative group appears to represent confounding by coprophagia. Studies by Fahrion et al. (2011) and Nijsse et al. (2014) showed that some 23.1% of canine samples contained eggs that represented *Toxocara cati* eggs ingested by coprophagic dogs. The 24.8% of the samples that are antigen positive but without eggs in the sample appears to represent prepatent infections and failure to observe rare eggs due to flotation protocol and/or sampling error (Little et al., 2019). If only a single test is considered to determine infection status, egg-alone observations would indicate 69,120 infections (1.7% of the 3,889,279 samples); whereas, antigen alone would account for 75,910 infections (1.9% of the 3,889,279 samples).

The pattern between egg flotation and antigen test results is slightly different for cats, Table 2.

As in the dog population, most of the 613,411 samples tested negative on both tests (93.4%). The overall prevalence of ascarid detection by egg observation, antigen positive test, or both tests was 6.6% which is 2.9 × higher than observed for dogs. This may reflect poorer compliance in monthly preventative treatment for pet cats than seen for pet dogs and/or an increased risk of infection due to predation of paratenic hosts. The majority of the egg positive samples, 25,015 results (3.8%) were also positive for the antigen test. This proportion is almost 3 × higher than observed for the pet dog population. Interestingly, the proportion (0.5%) of egg positive, antigen negative for the cat population is similar to that observed for the dog population (0.4%) supporting the ubiquitous exposure of environmental eggs in soil, water, and fur. However, the proportion of the egg positive, antigen negative samples was 12.5% of the total egg positive total. This is nearly half the proportion seen for pet dogs (23.1%) and very likely reflects the lack of coprophagic behaviour in cats. An additional 14,854 cat samples were antigen positive in the absence of an egg observation (2.3%). This is 3.8 × higher than was observed for dogs and could reflect challenges in the faecal flotation assay posed by feline samples such as inclusion of kitty litter, dehydration of the faecal sample, and small sample size. If only a single test is considered to determine infection status for cats, egg-alone observations would indicate 28,574 infections (4.4%) whereas antigen alone would account for 39,869 infections (6.1%).

4.2 Antigen agreement to *Toxocara* egg observation by animal age

Morphological identification of *Toxocara* spp. positive dogs and cats allows comparison of the antigen test result, positive or negative, to a cohort of *Toxocara* egg positive samples for both dogs and cats. As seen in the experimental *Toxocara* infection, a patent infection should be positive for antigen. Discrepancy in the antigen result (negative) compared to the egg observation highlights a fundamental difference between egg observation and antigen detection. For example, spurious eggs from coprophagic behaviour or ingestion of eggs from contaminated soil and water would lead to an egg positive, antigen negative pattern. Thus, the agreement of antigen to egg observation may provide a means to access the likelihood of spurious egg and the impact on interpreting infection status. Maximum antigen/egg agreement should be achieved where patent infection is most likely to occur. Conditions that favour spurious eggs should lower antigen/egg agreement. This hypothesis can be directly tested by examining the agreement of antigen and egg result for *Toxocara* egg positive samples from dogs of different age groups. *Toxocara* patency is expected to be at a maximum in young animals as aspects of the life cycle essentially ensure infections of pups and kittens. Fig. 3 shows that the percent antigen/egg agreement rapidly decreases as animal age increases.

There is a precipitous drop within the first 3 years, particularly acute within the first year, followed by a nearly steady agreement of 50% by year four onwards. This pattern of antigen/egg agreement is expected with the *Toxocara* life cycle (Shoop, 1991). More mature dogs inhibit the tracheal migration route preventing ingested, infectious *T. canis* eggs from becoming adult nematodes in the small intestine. Ingestion of eggs from the environment by older dogs would lead to an egg positive, antigen negative result indicative of spurious eggs. In older dogs, *Toxocara* eggs may be more likely to be *T. cati* eggs or non-infective *T. canis* eggs. Presumably, the lower overall rate of patent infections in older dogs reflects a lower rate of infection from egg ingestion plus the rate of predation of paratenic hosts where third-stage larvae would directly infect the gut of the host.

Fig. 4 shows the antigen/egg percent agreement in cats. As in dogs, a decrease in antigen/egg agreement is seen for cats more than a year old. However, the decrease in antigen/egg agreement is not as dramatic as seen for dogs and approaches a steady agreement at a much higher percent agreement than observed for dogs. This may reflect an increased risk in cats to patent *Toxocara* infections by predation of paratenic hosts and/or the lack of outright coprophagy in cats.

4.3 Impact of pseudoparasite observation and semi-quantification of egg count on antigen and *Toxocara* egg agreement

As discussed in the above sections, parasite life cycle parameters, host/parasite biology, and environmental egg contamination are forces that can cloud determination of true infection status of a dog or cat based solely on an egg observation. This can be explored more deeply by dividing the *Toxocara* egg positive dogs ($n = 42{,}261$) into two cohorts based on the co-observation of a pseudoparasite such as *Eimeria*, strongyle egg, and/or *Anoplocephala*. The co-observation of a pseudoparasite is a proxy for animal behaviour and/or environmental exposure that may lead to increased risk of spurious *Toxocara* eggs. This is not to say that behaviours that promote spurious eggs are absent in the cohort of dogs without a pseudoparasite observation. As seen in Fig. 5, the cohort of dogs ($n = 1092$) with a co-observation of a pseudoparasite has lower antigen to egg agreement (80.7% (95% confidence intervals 81.1–80.3%)) than the cohort of dogs ($n = 41{,}169$) without a pseudoparasite observation (73.5% (confidence intervals 76.1–70.8%)). The difference is subtle but significant for *Toxocara* compared to other nematodes like hookworm and whipworm where egg morphology and life cycle parameters influence greater differences (Elsemore, unpublished).

A second means to divide *Toxocara* egg positive dog samples is by semi-quantitative egg count bin. *Toxocara* spp. are prolific egg layers with a single female capable of laying 80,000–100,000 eggs per day. One would expect a patent infection to contain >30 eggs per gram of faecal sample (Nijsse et al., 2015). A patent infection would be predicted to have a relatively high egg count due to *Toxocara* fecundity coupled with the relative ease of flotation and identification of *Toxocara* eggs. Semi-quantification of egg count is described in four egg bins: RARE (1–2 eggs), FEW (3–10 eggs), MODERATE (11–30 eggs), and MANY (>30 eggs). Observation of a low egg count may be more likely caused by spurious egg contamination than a gravid female nematode. Fig. 6 shows that the agreement between antigen and *Toxocara* egg is indeed different for *Toxocara* egg positive samples with a semi-quantification of RARE or FEW ($n = 14{,}748$) compared to samples with higher egg counts ($n = 27{,}531$).

5. Infection of dogs and cats by *Toxocara* and other ascarid species

Two ascarid species, *Toxocara canis* and *Toxascaris leonina* are routinely detected by faecal flotation in dogs, and the raccoon roundworm,

Baylisascaris procyonis does rarely develop patent infections in dogs. Two ascarids, *Toxocara cati* and *Toxascaris leonina*, occur routinely in cats. Fig. 7 demonstrates the overall antigen/egg agreement in dogs for the three ascarid species.

The highest antigen to egg agreement is found for the canonical dog ascarid, *Toxocara*. However, in field samples, this agreement is capped at less than 100% because of the impact of spurious eggs masking the true infection state of all egg positive dogs. *T. leonina* has a lower antigen/egg agreement compared to *Toxocara* but both are much higher than the antigen/egg agreement seen for *Baylisascaris*. The dog has been shown to be a poor host in experimental infections with *B. procyonis* (Dr Michael Yabsley, personal communication). There are several *Baylisascaris* species that infect other hosts such as skunk (*Baylisascaris columnaris*) and bear (*Baylisascaris transfuga*). The low antigen/egg agreement in field dogs could reflect poor host/parasite adaptation for *B. procyonis* and spurious egg contamination with other species of *Baylisascaris*. The intermediate agreement level observed for *T. leonina* may indicate that the dog is not the ideal host for this ascarid species in field settings or that the cat adapted form of this species does not often develop to adulthood in dogs (Okoski and Usui, 1968; Sprent, 1959).

Antigen/egg agreement for both *Toxocara* and *Toxascaris* is higher in cats than observed for dogs, see (Fig. 8).

Cats are less likely to display coprophagic behaviour, but grooming behaviours certainly could be a source of spurious eggs (Overgaauw et al., 2009; Roddie et al., 2008). It is interesting to note that antigen/egg agreement for *Toxascaris leonina* is higher in cats than it is for dogs perhaps reflecting that felids are a better host for this ascarid species or have a higher exposure to infective stages in a field population or again that lack of coprophagia plays a similar role for this parasite as it does for *T. cati*.

6. Concluding remarks

Detection of nematode antigen is a new, non-morphological means to detect ascarid infections in dogs and cats. Protein homology of the marker allows a breadth of detection that is applicable to the veterinary market for both dogs and cats. Experimental infection time courses have demonstrated the ability to detect the prepatent stage in the *T. canis* life cycle. Post anti-helminthic, antigen and eggs both reflected elimination of the *T. canis* nematodes.

Examination of large field populations of pet dogs (>3 million results) and pet cats (>600,000 results) demonstrates the field variation between the reference egg flotation test and the antigen test. Some of the apparent discrepant results can be explained by fundamental differences between the technologies. Egg flotation, by definition, is not able to detect prepatent infections. Antigen, as a marker of the nematode, does identify prepatent infections. Antigen detection may also serve as a "backstop" for situations where eggs from a patent infection are missed in the sample because of sampling error, flotation protocol, and/or failure to visualize an egg during microscopic examination.

The other consideration when evaluating antigen to egg agreement in a large field population is the impact of spurious eggs. A spurious egg passing through the dog or cat may be identified by egg flotation but would be presumed to be antigen negative. Outright coprophagy, in an experimental model, can also lead to spurious antigen although the window of spurious antigen detection is short. This situation would most likely lead to a faecal sample with a false-positive pattern for both egg and antigen (Elsemore, unpublished data). However, it is clear that in large field population, dogs and cats ingest environmental eggs from contaminated water, soil, and fur. Maximum observed agreement of antigen to egg would be capped by the rate of spurious eggs in field populations. Many factors such as preventative treatment, access to the outdoors, and environmental egg contamination levels would influence the agreement. Indeed, drastic difference in antigen to egg agreement have been observed from shelter animals compared to more well-cared for pets. The dog and cat populations described here are mostly comprised of pet animals and most of the testing is routine healthy screening. Even so, there appears to be at least a 10–20% rate of spurious eggs that confound the interpretation of an egg flotation result. Pet dogs and cats serve as egg bio-accumulators as they interact with their environment. This is of import to pet owners as they manage the pet's immediate environs.

Examining *Toxocara* egg positive samples in greater detail revealed a pattern in antigen to egg agreement that correlates with the focus of the *Toxocara* life cycle on young animals. For both dogs and cats, the agreement drops for older animals. This is consistent with abatement of maternal routes of infection in older animals. Interestingly, the antigen to egg agreement is relatively high in cats and may reflect a higher predation rate in pet cats and the lack of coprophagy. Further, the large dog *Toxocara* egg positive population allowed examination of the impact of pseudoparasite co-observation and semi-quantification egg bin on antigen/egg agreement. In both cases, situations that should increase the odds of spurious eggs, pseudoparasite observation or a low egg count, decreased the antigen to egg agreement.

Antigen detection of *Toxocara* and other ascarid species is a new tool for evaluating infection status in dogs and cats. The combination of the two tests provides a comprehensive look into infection status and provides the practitioner with more information to consider for treatment decisions.

References

Babin, D.R., Peanasky, R.J., Goos, S.M., 1984. The isoinhibitors of chymotrypsin/elastase from *Ascaris lumbricoides*: the primary structure. Arch. Biochem. Biophys. 232, 143–161.

Church, D., Miller, K., Lichtenfeld, A., Semeniuk, H., Kirkham, B., Laupland, K., Elsayed, S., 2005. Screening for Giardia/Cryptosporidium infections using an enzyme immunoassay in a centralized regional microbiology laboratory. Arch. Pathol. Lab. Med. 129, 754–759.

Elsemore, D.A., Geng, J., Cote, J., Hanna, R., Lucio-Forster, A., Bowman, D.D., 2017. Enzyme-linked immunosorbent assays for coproantigen detection of *Ancylostoma caninum* and *Toxocara canis* in dogs and *Toxocara cati* in cats. J. Vet. Diagn. Invest. 29, 645–653.

Fahrion, A.S., Schnyder, M., Wichert, B., Deplazes, P., 2011. *Toxocara* eggs shed by dogs and cats and their molecular and morphometric species-specific identification: is the finding of *T. cati* eggs shed by dogs of epidemiological relevance? Vet. Parasitol. 177, 186–189.

Fraefel, W., Acher, R., 1968. The amino acid sequence of a trypsin inhibitor isolated from ascaris (*Ascaris lumbricoides var. suum*). Biochim. Biophys. Acta 154, 615–617.

Grasberger, B.L., Clore, G.M., Gronenborn, A.M., 1994. High-resolution structure of *Ascaris* trypsin inhibitor in solution: direct evidence for a pH-induced conformational transition in the reactive site. Structure 2, 669–678.

Huang, K., Strynadka, N.C., Bernard, V.D., Peanasky, R.J., James, M.N., 1994. The molecular structure of the complex of *Ascaris* chymotrypsin/elastase inhibitor with porcine elastase. Structure 2, 679–689.

Little, S.E., Barrett, A.W., Beall, M.J., Bowman, D.D., Dangoudoubiyam, S., Elsemore, D.A., Liotta, J., Lucio-Forster, A., Mccrann, D.J., Snowden, K.F., Starkey, L.A., Tasse, S., 2019. Coproantigen detection augments diagnosis of common nematode infections in dogs. Top. Companion Anim. Med. 35, 42–46.

Martzen, M.R., Geise, G.L., Hogan, B.J., Peanasky, R.J., 1985. *Ascaris suum*: localization by immunochemical and fluorescent probes of host proteases and parasite proteinase inhibitors in cross-sections. Exp. Parasitol. 60, 139–149.

Nijsse, R., Mughini-Gras, L., Wagenaar, J.A., Ploeger, H.W., 2014. Coprophagy in dogs interferes in the diagnosis of parasitic infections by faecal examination. Vet. Parasitol. 204, 304–309.

Nijsse, R., Mughini-Gras, L., Wagenaar, J.A., Franssen, F., Ploeger, H.W., 2015. Environmental contamination with *Toxocara* eggs: a quantitative approach to estimate the relative contributions of dogs, cats and foxes, and to assess the efficacy of advised interventions in dogs. Parasit. Vectors 8 397.

O'Connor, T.P., 2015. Snap assay technology. Top. Companion Anim. Med. 30, 132–138.

Okoski, S., Usui, M., 1968. Experimental studies on *Toxascaris leonina*, IV. Development of eggs of three ascarids, *T. leonina*, *Toxocara canis* and *Toxocara cati*, in dogs and cats. Jpn. J. Vet. Sci. 30, 29–38.

Overgaauw, P.A., Van Zutphen, L., Hoek, D., Yaya, F.O., Roelfsema, J., Pinelli, E., Van Knapen, F., Kortbeek, L.M., 2009. Zoonotic parasites in fecal samples and fur from dogs and cats in The Netherlands. Vet. Parasitol. 163, 115–122.

Peanasky, R.J., Bentz, Y., Homandberg, G.A., Minor, S.T., Babin, D.R., 1984. The isoinhibitors of chymotrypsin/elastase from *Ascaris lumbricoides*: the reactive site. Arch. Biochem. Biophys. 232, 135–142.

Roddie, G., Stafford, P., Holland, C., Wolfe, A., 2008. Contamination of dog hair with eggs of *Toxocara canis*. Vet. Parasitol. 152, 85–93.

Shoop, W.L., 1991. Vertical transmission of helminths: hypobiosis and amphiparatenesis. Parasitol. Today 7, 51–54.

Sprent, J.F., 1959. The life history and development of *Toxascaris leonina* (von Linstow 1902) in the dog and cat. Parasitology 49, 330–371.

CHAPTER TWENTY-EIGHT

Global prevalence of *Toxocara* infection in dogs

Ali Rostami[a,*], Seyed Mohammad Riahi[b], Andreas Hofmann[c], Guangxu Ma[c], Tao Wang[c], Hamed Behniafar[d], Ali Taghipour[e], Yadolah Fakhri[f], Adel Spotin[g], Bill C.H. Chang[c], Calum N.L. Macpherson[h], Peter J. Hotez[i], Robin B. Gasser[c,*]

[a]Infectious Diseases and Tropical Medicine Research Center, Health Research Institute, Babol University of Medical Sciences, Babol, Iran
[b]Department of Epidemiology and Biostatistics, Faculty of Health, Cardiovascular Diseases Research Center, Birjand University of Medical Sciences, Birjand, Iran
[c]Department of Veterinary Biosciences, Melbourne Veterinary School, Faculty of Veterinary and Agricultural Sciences, The University of Melbourne, Parkville, VIC, Australia
[d]Department of Parasitology and Mycology, School of Medicine, Shahid Beheshti University of Medical Sciences, Tehran, Iran
[e]Department of Parasitology, Faculty of Medical Sciences, Tarbiat Modares University, Tehran, Iran
[f]Department of Environmental Health Engineering, Student Research Committee, School of Public Health, Shahid Beheshti University of Medical Sciences, Tehran, Iran
[g]Immunology Research Center, Tabriz University of Medical Sciences, Tabriz, Iran
[h]School of Graduate Studies, School of Veterinary Medicine, St. George's University, WINDREF, Grenada, West Indies
[i]Texas Children's Hospital Center for Vaccine Development, Departments of Pediatrics and Molecular Virology & Microbiology, National School of Tropical Medicine, Baylor College of Medicine, Houston, TX, United States
*Corresponding authors: e-mail address: a.rostami@mubabol.ac.ir; robinbg@unimelb.edu.au

Contents

Advances in Parasitology, Volume 109
ISSN 0065-308X
https://doi.org/10.1016/bs.apar.2020.01.017

Abstract

Dogs serve as the most important definitive hosts for *Toxocara canis*—a causative agent of human toxocariasis and one of the most widespread zoonotic helminth worldwide. The present study was undertaken to assess the global prevalence of *T. canis* infection in dogs. PubMed, Scopus, Web of Science, EMBASE and SciELO were searched to identify relevant studies. A random-effects model was used to estimate the overall and the subgroup-pooled prevalences across studies, and heterogeneity was assessed via the I^2 test. The data were categorized according to WHO-region, different types of dogs, risk factors and environmental variables. From a total of 4370 peer-reviewed publications, 229 articles that studied 13,010,004 dogs in 60 countries met the final inclusion criteria. The overall prevalence of *Toxocara* infection in dogs was 11.1% (95% CI, 10.6–11.7%). The estimated prevalence in the different WHO-regions ranged from 6.4% to 19.2%: Eastern Mediterranean (19.2%, 13.7–25.5%), Africa (18.5%, 13.7–23.9%), South-East Asia (11.9%, 6.8–18.2%), North America (11.1%, 10.6–11.7%), South America (10.9%, 7.6–14.6%), Europe (10.8%, 8.9–12.9%) and Western Pacific (6.4%, 3.3–10.2%). Young (<1 year of age), stray, rural and male dogs had a significantly ($P < 0.001$) higher prevalence of infection than older, pet, urban or female dogs. The prevalence was higher in low income countries and regions at a low geographical latitude, close to the equator, characterized as having tropical climates. From this review, it is estimated that ≥100 million dogs are infected with *Toxocara* around the world. This highlights the need for an increased focus on implementing affordable, appropriate control programs to reduce the public health threat of toxocariasis as a zoonosis of global importance.

1. Introduction

Dogs (*Canis familiaris*) are ubiquitous and have the widest diversity of roles of any domesticated animal in human societies worldwide. They serve as companion, working or service animals, entertainment or show dogs, working dogs on farms, police or military dogs, shepherds, hunters, guardians, transport, and play an important role in a wide range of comparative animal medicine studies of diseases such as diabetes, narcolepsy and cancer. The dog is widely considered to be 'man's best friend' and has important roles in the psychological and physiological well-being of many people, particularly young children, as well as disabled and elderly people (Serpell and Barrett, 2016). The global dog population is estimated at 900 million (https://www.worldatlas.com), ~500 million of which are stray or feral animals (https://www.carodog.eu). These numbers probably underestimate the true numbers of dogs, as dogs are not registered in many countries. In 2017, the total number of pet dogs in the European Union was estimated at 85 million (https://www.statista.com). According to the 2017–2018 National Pet Owners Survey in the United States, ~60% of households owned a pet, and the number of pet dogs was estimated at 89 million (https://www.iii.org). In addition, according to a previous estimate, 361 million dogs were estimated to live in Asia, 102.2 million in Latin America and the Caribbean, and 87.6 million in Africa (Hughes and Macdonald, 2013).

Although many humans derive great benefits from dogs, these canids can also serve as reservoirs for a wide range of zoonotic pathogens, some of which are of major public health importance (Macpherson et al., 2013; Otranto et al., 2017). In many cases, stray dogs might harbour more infectious agents than pet dogs, such that they represent a significant risk to human populations (Otranto et al., 2017; Paoletti et al., 2015); nevertheless, direct contact of pet dogs with people is a significant risk factor (Dubná et al., 2007; Lucio-Forster et al., 2016; Overgaauw and van Knapen, 2013). Of the important zoonotic pathogens, ascaridoid nematodes of the genus *Toxocara*, including *Toxocara canis* and *T. cati*, are causative agents of human toxocariasis with a worldwide distribution (Aghamolaie et al., 2018; Fisher, 2003; Ma et al., 2018). Toxocariasis can cause four major clinical syndromes in humans, including visceral larva migrans (VLM), ocular larva migrans (OLM), neurotoxocariasis (NT) and common/covert toxocariasis (CT) (Aghaei et al., 2018; Ma et al., 2018; Mohammadzadeh et al., 2018; Rostami et al., 2019). Canids, including dogs, foxes, wolves and jackals serve as definitive hosts of *T. canis*, releasing eggs into the environment, where, under favourable conditions, they can embryonate and eventually become infective. Infective eggs containing third-stage (L_3) larvae can be accidentally ingested by humans and other paratenic hosts via contaminated soil, unwashed raw vegetables, water, or occasionally from the fur of dogs (Ma et al., 2018).

In the past decades, numerous studies have assessed the prevalence of *T. canis* infection in dogs, often in relatively small geographic regions. Consequently, there are significant gaps in the knowledge of the epidemiology of *Toxocara* infection/toxocariasis in many countries. Considering the public health implications of toxocariasis, a more comprehensive understanding of the occurrence and prevalence of *Toxocara* infection would be valuable. This paper provides the first systematic review and meta-analysis of the available data on the global prevalence of *T. canis* in dogs.

2. Methodology

This systematic literature search and meta-analysis study adhered to the protocol recommended by the Preferred Reporting Items for Systematic Reviews and Meta-Analyses (PRISMA) (Moher et al., 2015).

2.1 Search strategy and selection criteria

A comprehensive literature search of the databases PubMed, Scopus, Web of Science, EMBASE and SciELO for peer-reviewed articles published between 1 January 1990 and 1 July 2019 was undertaken, without language or geographical restriction, to identify all studies that reported the prevalence of *Toxocara* infection in dogs. Two authors (A.S. and H.B.) independently searched databases using one or more of the following search terms: '*Toxocara* infection', '*Toxocara*', '*Toxocara* spp.', '*Toxocara canis*', 'gastrointestinal helminth', 'intestinal parasites', 'endoparasites', 'prevalence', 'incidence', 'epidemiology', 'dog', 'puppy' and 'canine'. We also manually appraised all reference lists of all key review articles and of the articles ultimately included in this study. The global prevalence of *Toxocara* infection of dogs was the key topic. *Toxocara* prevalence was defined as the number of dogs that tested positive for *Toxocara* eggs in faecal or hair samples, or harboured adult *Toxocara* at autopsy, divided by the total number of dogs studied.

After the removal of duplicates, the same authors independently screened all abstracts and titles of all retrieved articles to identify all relevant studies. Articles were included in the meta-analysis if they (i) were original, peer-reviewed, cross-sectional studies reporting the prevalence of *Toxocara* in dogs; (ii) represented a sample size of $>$30 dogs; and (iii) used faecal or hair examination to detect *Toxocara* eggs, or postmortem examination to identify *Toxocara* worms. We excluded articles if they did not meet all three of these criteria (i–iii), including case-reports or case-series studies, diagnostic studies, or reviews.

2.2 Data extraction and quality assessment

Two independent authors (A.T. and H.B.) extracted information from eligible studies, in duplicate, using Microsoft Excel (2016 version, Microsoft, Redmond, WA, USA). Any inconsistency was discussed and resolved by an adjudicator (A.R.). All data extracted were assessed for accuracy by the principal investigator/supervisor (A.R.). Data recorded systematically were: the first author's last name; publication year; year(s) of study implementation; country; city; type of diagnostic samples (faecal, hair or carcass) and methods used (faecal examination and/or autopsy); type of dog; sample size and number of dogs that were test-positive. Moreover, we extracted data considering age group ($\leq$12 and $>$12 months), gender (male or female) and geographical location (rural or urban area), if available. Since there were several types of dogs in the studies included, we divided dogs into three groups: (i) *pet (domestic) dogs*: 'pet, household, kennelled, owned or domiciled, sheltered or domestic'; (ii) *working (domestic) dogs*: 'military, hunting, farm, shepherd or guard dogs'; and (iii) *stray (wild) dogs*: 'feral dogs, free-ranging dogs, or semi domestic, refuge, semi stray or stray dogs'.

In each study, we investigated prevalence data in the context of WHO-defined regions (Africa, Eastern Mediterranean, Europe, South-East Asia, the Americas, and Western Pacific) (World Health Organization, 2003), income level in each country (https://datahelpdesk.worldbank.org) as well as geographical latitude and longitude, relative humidity, mean temperature and precipitation rate for each city/area studied. Due to socio-demographic and climate differences among regions, we divided the Americas into North America and South America. We used the following data sources to determine the geographical and climatic status of each city or region studied (https://www.timeanddate.com/, https://en.climate-data.org/, and https://gps-coordinates.org/).

A quality assessment (risk of bias) of studies was performed using the JBI (Joanna Briggs Institute) Prevalence Critical Appraisal Tool (see Supplementary Table S2 in Supplementary material in the online version at https://doi.org/10.1016/bs.apar.2020.01.017). This tool is employed specifically for the quality-appraisal of studies for inclusion into systematic reviews of prevalence datasets (Munn et al., 2014). Two reviewers (A.R. and Y.F.) independently assessed the quality of the methodology employed in each study included here. The level of risk of bias was assessed by combining the percentage of 'yes' responses to each of 10 questions (relating specifically to the collection of a representative sample, recruitment of subjects (dogs) in an appropriate way, sample size, setting description, subject description, outcome measurement, reliable measurements, data analysis, subpopulation analysis, and adjustment for confounders; cf. Munn et al., 2014) for each individual study. A study with 7–10 of 10 questions answered with 'yes' was considered to have a low risk of bias; a study with 4–6 of 10 questions answered with 'yes' was considered to have a moderate risk of bias; and a study with 1–3 of 10 questions answered with 'yes' was considered to have a high risk of bias.

2.3 Meta-analysis

The pooled global prevalence of *Toxocara* infection in dogs was estimated using a random-effects model (DerSimonian and Laird, 1986). Overall summaries of the meta-estimates (95% confidence interval [CI]) were reported separately for the WHO-regions as well as individual countries. Heterogeneity among studies was calculated, and an I^2 statistic with a cut-off of 50% (Higgins et al., 2003), was used to define a statistically significant degree of heterogeneity. To determine the source of heterogeneity, subgroup and meta-regression analyses were implemented. Subgroup analysis was undertaken according to WHO-region, type of dog, type of sample tested, diagnostic method(s) used, dog age, gender, income level in a country, sample size, time period, and geographical (latitude and longitude) and climate (relative humidity, mean temperature and precipitation rate) variables. The χ^2 test was used to compare prevalences among distinct subgroups. Meta-regression analyses were used to examine the effect of over time (1990–2019), income level, geographical and climate parameters on prevalence rates. Since three studies from the United States had a sample size of >12 million (in total), we applied a sensitivity analysis to determine the effect of these three studies on the global prevalence estimate. We did not assess publication bias, as it is not considered relevant in relation to prevalence studies (Hunter et al., 2014). All statistical analyses were conducted using Stata v.13 (Stata Corp., College Station, TX, USA). The results from statistical analyses were significant if the P-value was <0.05.

3. Eligible studies, their characteristics and datasets

Fig. 1 shows a flow diagram for the selection of articles. The search strategy identified 4370 articles, 4064 of which were excluded after the removal of duplicates and the screening of titles and abstracts. A total of 306 articles with full-texts were assessed for eligibility. A total of 229 studies containing 275 datasets were included in this meta-analysis. These studies provided data on 13,010,004 dogs from 60 different countries in six WHO-regions. In total, 93 datasets were available for Europe (117,703 dogs), 42 for Africa (12,056 dogs), 37 for the Eastern Mediterranean region (8482 dogs), 34 for North America (12,845,170 dogs), 29 for the Western Pacific region (10,746 dogs), 25 for South America (11,655 dogs), and 16 for South-East Asia (4192 dogs). Data were from 23 countries in Europe, 8 in Africa, 8 in the Western Pacific region, 6 in North America, 6 in South America, 6 in the Eastern Mediterranean region, and 3 in South-East Asia. Approximately half of the original studies included were from countries with predominantly high income levels (125 datasets; 12,961,852 dogs), 82 datasets (28,304 dogs) were from countries with middle to upper income levels, 48 datasets (14,537 dogs) were from countries with middle to low income levels, and 20 datasets (5311 dogs) represented countries with low income levels. In

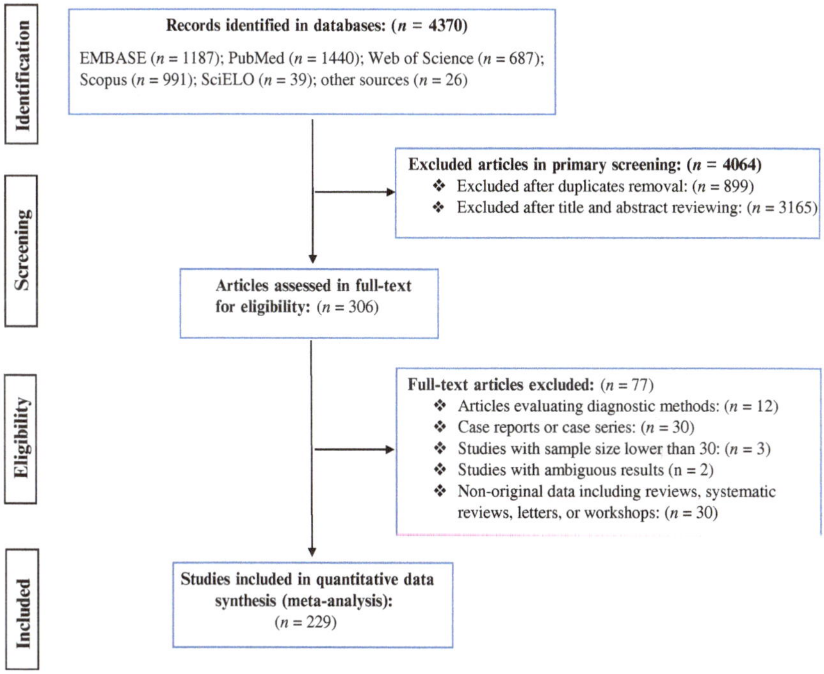

Fig. 1 Flow diagram showing the search and selection methodology used, which follows PRISMA guidelines.

total, 152 datasets were available for pet dogs, 72 for stray dogs, 24 for working dogs and 28 from dogs of an indeterminate type. Most studies (representing 137 datasets) used a faecal flotation technique, combined with microscopy, to detect and identify *Toxocara* eggs; 36 used a sedimentation technique; 67 used a sedimentation or an unspecified flotation technique; 12 used other methods, including Kato–Katz or the McMaster chamber method; and 23 studies used necropsy to detect adult worms in the intestines. Supplementary Table S1 in Supplementary Material in the online version at https://doi.org/10.1016/bs.apar.2020.01.017 summarizes the main characteristics and the geographic distribution of the studies included.

4. Global and regional prevalence rates of *Toxocara* infection in dogs

The random-effects, pooled global prevalence of *Toxocara* infection in dogs was 11.1% (95% CI, 10.6–11.7%; 302,723/13,010,004), with a high heterogeneity among studies ($I^2 = 99.8$). Prevalence was highest in the Eastern Mediterranean region (19.2%, 13.7–25.5%) and lowest in the

Western Pacific region (6.4%, 3.3–10.2%). Pooled prevalences in other WHO-regions were 10.8–18%: Africa (18%, 13.7–23.9%), South-East Asia (11.9%, 6.8–18.2%), North America (11.1%, 10.6–11.7%), South America (10.9%, 7.6–14.6%) and Europe (10.8%, 8.9–12.9%). In a 'sensitivity analysis', we assessed the effect of three studies from the United States (Little et al., 2009; Lucio-Forster et al., 2016; Mohamed et al., 2009) with very large sample sizes (totalling >12 million dogs) on the global prevalence of *Toxocara* infection in dogs. This analysis showed that the global prevalence was not significantly altered by these three studies (i.e., was 11.8%, 10.5–13.1%). For countries with three or more eligible datasets, China (39.1%) in East Asia; Pakistan (37.0%) in the Middle East; Ethiopia (28.3%) in East Africa; Slovakia (18.9%) in East Europe; India (13.0%) in South Asia; Argentina (12.4%) in South America; Mexico (6.9%) in Central America, and Canada (6.9%) in North America exhibited some of the highest prevalences. Additional details pertaining to the prevalence of *Toxocara* infection in dogs in WHO-regions and individual countries are presented in Table 1 and Fig. 2.

Table 1 Global, regional and national prevalences of *Toxocara* infection in dogs, estimated from results extracted from 275 datasets from 60 countries.

WHO-regions / Country	Number of datasets	Total number of samples	Number of test-positive samples	Pooled prevalence (%) established using meta-analysis (95% CI)	Heterogeneity I^2 (%)
Global	***275***	***13,010,004***	***302,723***	***11.1 (10.6–11.7)***	***99.6***
Eastern Mediterranean region	***37***	***8482***	***1284***	***19.2 (13.7–25.5)***	***97.5***
Iran	19	3400	377	15.7 (9.4–23.2)	96.1
Egypt	9	3753	496	14.0 (4.4–27.5)	97.5
Iraq	4	293	160	43.9 (21.6–67.5)	93.6
Pakistan	3	440	159	37.0 (27.1–47.6)	78.4
Jordan	1	340	4	1.2 (0.3–4)	NA
Tunisia	1	256	88	34.4 (28.6–40.5)	NA
African region	***42***	***12,056***	***2269***	***18.5 (13.7–23.9)***	***98.1***
Nigeria	22	6637	1159	16.7 (10.0–24.5)	98.4
Ethiopia	10	2907	773	28.3 (18.8–38.8)	96.9
Tanzania	2	605	42	5.9 (4.2–8)	99.7
Ghana	2	534	51	8.8 (6.5–11.4)	99.7

Table 1 Global, regional and national prevalences of *Toxocara* infection in dogs, estimated from results extracted from 275 datasets from 60 countries.—cont'd

WHO-regions / Country	Number of datasets	Total number of samples	Number of test-positive samples	Pooled prevalence (%) established using meta-analysis (95% CI)	Heterogeneity I^2 (%)
Zambia	2	832	92	10.6 (8.6–12.8)	99.7
South Africa	2	303	31	9.7 (6.6–13.4)	99.7
Malawi	1	40	3	7.5 (1.6–20.4)	NA
Gabon	1	198	118	59.6 (52.4–66.5)	NA
South-East Asian region	***16***	***4192***	***411***	***11.9 (6.8–18.2)***	***96.8***
India	10	3126	328	13.0 (5.8–22.4)	97.9
Thailand	4	976	58	5.4 (3.6–7.6)	35.6
Sri Lanka	2	90	25	27.6 (18.7–37.5)	78.5
North America	***34***	***12,845,170***	***284,925***	***11.1 (10.6–11.7)***	***99.9***
Canada	13	12,966	366	6.9 (3.2–11.8)	97.7
United States	9	12,830,195	284,416	4.5 (3.3–5.9)	100
Mexico	7	1309	115	6.9 (2.8–12.7)	91.2
Cuba	3	195	8	3.2 (0.4–7.8)	44.0
Grenada	1	445	17	3.8 (2.2–6.0)	NA
Costa Rica	1	60	3	5.0 (1.0–13.9)	NA
South America	***25***	***11,655***	***750***	***10.9 (7.6–14.6)***	***96.7***
Brazil	16	8042	316	8.8 (5.5–12.6)	95.7
Argentina	4	2783	323	12.4 (10.1–14.9)	42.2
Venezuela	1	614	70	11.4 (9.0–14.2)	NA
Ecuador	1	97	16	16.5 (9.7–25.4)	NA
Uruguay	1	80	8	10.0 (4.4–18.8)	NA
Colombia	1	39	17	43.6 (27.8–60.4)	NA
Europe region	***93***	***117,703***	***12,349***	***10.8 (8.9–12.9)***	***99.0***
Italy	16	8074	639	8.5 (6.1–11.1)	92.9
Poland	10	5750	388	11.2 (2.8–24.0)	99.0
Greece	6	2396	252	8.9 (5.4–13.3)	89.8
Germany	6	65,454	4765	5.9 (4.5–7.5)	98.2
Spain	6	3595	425	7.7 (3.2–13.8)	96.1

Continued

Table 1 Global, regional and national prevalences of *Toxocara* infection in dogs, estimated from results extracted from 275 datasets from 60 countries.—cont'd

WHO-regions / Country	Number of datasets	Total number of samples	Number of test-positive samples	Pooled prevalence (%) established using meta-analysis (95% CI)	Heterogeneity I^2 (%)
Slovakia	5	1764	312	18.9 (10.2–29.5)	96.3
Portugal	5	1387	104	5.2 (2.7–8.5)	77.4
Serbia	4	695	117	18.1 (6.8–33.0)	93.8
United Kingdom	4	5385	102	4.4 (1.6–8.5)	92.3
Netherlands	4	1373	304	12.5 (0.6–35.4)	99.0
Belgium	4	3483	550	13.0 (5.6–22.9)	97.6
Turkey	3	624	87	12.5 (6.0–20.9)	85.8
Russia	3	8381	3039	9.3 (0.1–43.9)	99.2
Czech Republic	3	4778	383	11.5 (5.3–19.7)	97.0
Romania	2	1314	218	16.6 (14.6–18.7)	98.5
France	2	209	16	7.5 (4.2–11.6)	98.5
Albania	2	713	132	15.5 (12.9–18.3)	98.5
Hungary	2	490	131	26.1 (22.3–30.1)	98.5
Ireland	2	534	305	56.5 (52.3–60.7)	98.5
Denmark	1	178	22	12.4 (7.9–18.1)	NA
Switzerland	1	505	36	7.1 (5.0–9.7)	NA
Bulgaria	1	80	5	6.3 (2.1–14)	NA
Finland	1	541	17	3.1 (1.8–5.0)	NA
Western Pacific region	***29***	***10,746***	***735***	***6.4 (3.3–10.2)***	***98.0***
Japan	10	5027	165	2.0 (0.4–2.8)	96.3
Australia	8	3915	128	3.7 (1.7–6.4)	93.1
China	3	656	275	39.1 (31.1–47.4)	68.6
Cambodia	2	144	10	6.9 (3.1–11.8)	84.2
Malaysia	3	144	23	7.4 (0.1–32.5)	92.7
Philippines	1	200	23	11.5 (7.4–16.8)	NA
Vietnam	1	284	107	37.7 (32.0–43.6)	NA
Taiwan	1	376	4	1.1 (0.3–2.7)	NA

Abbreviations: NA, not applicable; CI, confidence interval.
WHO-regions sorted according to prevalence rates. Countries sorted according to the number of studies included.

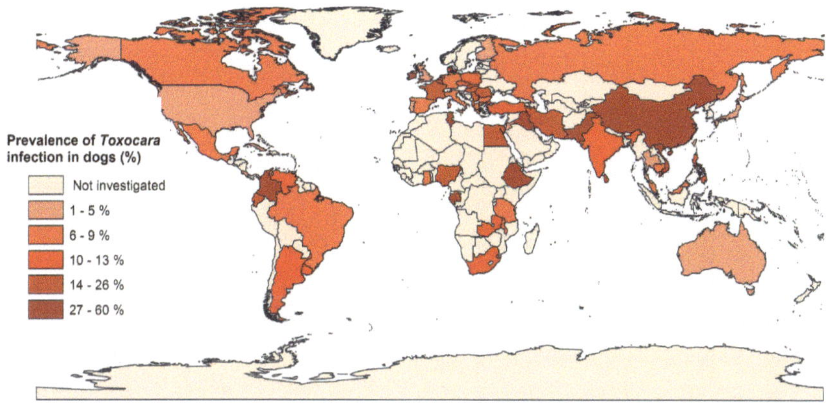

Fig. 2 Prevalence of *Toxocara* infection in dogs in different countries using geographic information system (GIS).

5. Prevalence according to type of dogs, age, gender and area (rural vs urban)

In subgroup analyses, with respect to the type of dogs, the prevalences of *Toxocara* infection worldwide in pet, working and stray dogs were 8.9% (8.3–9.6%), 14.1% (10.1–18.7%) and 18.8% (14.7–23.2%), respectively ($P < 0.001$). In subgroup analyses, according to age and gender, the pooled prevalence of *Toxocara* infection was higher in dogs of ≤12 months of age (28.7%, 23.5–34.2%) and in male dogs (26.8%, 20.2–33.9%) than in dogs of >12 months of age (12.9%, 9.6–16.6%) and female (21.7%, 15.4–28.7%) dogs, respectively ($P < 0.001$). Prevalence in dogs from rural areas (20.1%, 15.0–25.8%) was higher than in dogs from urban areas (14.3%, 11.6–17.2%) ($P < 0.001$). Details of other subgroup analyses are presented in Table 2.

6. Prevalence based on selected study characteristics

With respect to the type of samples, prevalence based on the detection of *Toxocara* eggs in faecal samples (10.9%, 10.3–11.5%) was lower than for the detection of such eggs on hairs (15.8%, 4.0–33.1%) and of *Toxocara* worms (adults) at postmortem (15.6%, 9.8–22.4%). Considering the diagnostic approach used, prevalence rates based on flotation, sedimentation, either flotation or sedimentation (unspecified), necropsy (to detect adult worm),

Table 2 The global prevalences of *Toxocara* infection in dogs estimated according to a priori defined subgroups.

Parameters/subgroups	Number of datasets	Total number of samples	Number of test-positive samples	Pooled prevalence (%) estimated using REM (95% CI)	Heterogeneity I^2 (%)
Type of dogs					
Pet (domestic) dogs	152	12,969,874	297,390	8.9 (8.3–9.6)	99.7
Working (domestic) dogs	24	9659	2813	14.1 (10.1–18.7)	96.8
Stray (wild) dogs	72	16,812	1323	18.8 (14.7–23.2)	97.8
Indeterminate type	27	13,659	1197	8.0 (5.1–11.6)	99.6
Type of sample tested					
Faecal (eggs)	249	13,005,371	302,059	10.9 (10.3–11.5)	99.6
Postmortem (adults or larvae)	23	4345	623	15.6 (9.8–22.4)	96.6
Hair (eggs)	3	288	41	15.8 (4.0–33.1)	89.3
Type of diagnostic method					
Flotation	137	12,915,712	293,572	10.7 (10.0–11.4)	99.7
Sedimentation	36	9237	678	8.7 (5.5–12.4)	96.9
Sedimentation or flotation	67	77,015	6999	11.3 (8.3–14.6)	99.4
Necropsy	23	4345	623	15.6 (9.8–22.4)	96.6
Other (McMaster, Kato-katz, etc.)	12	3695	851	20.8 (12.4–30.6)	97.8
Age (months)					
≤12	44	9718	2092	28.7 (23.5–34.2)	96.4
>12	42	14,374	954	12.9 (9.6–16.6)	96.9

Gender					
Male	34	7657	1292	26.8 (20.2–33.9)	97.6
Female	33	6399	867	21.7 (15.4–28.7)	97.2
Residence					
High standard location (urban)	32	37,860	3758	14.3 (11.6–17.2)	96.5
Low standard location (rural)	13	2491	472	20.1 (15.0–25.8)	89.4
Sample size					
≤500	213	40,222	6241	13.4 (11.4–15.6)	97.2
501–1000	32	20,397	1985	8.3 (6.0–11.1)	97.8
1001–5000	19	43,252	2615	5.6 (3.4–8.2)	99.2
≥5000	11	12,906,133	291,882	5.4 (4.1–6.9)	100
Implementation year					
1990–1995	21	18,752	1916	14.2 (9.0–20.2)	98.9
1996–2000	16	12,088	710	8.7 (4.8–13.7)	98.4
2001–2005	46	1,274,955	64,113	8.3 (6.9–9.7)	98.6
2006–2010	92	1,280,859	33,817	12.9 (11.4–14.8)	99.1
2011–2015	87	10,419,382	201,698	12.4 (9.0–16.3)	99.4
2016–2019	13	3968	469	9.3 (4.1–16.3)	97.6
Risk of bias					
Low risk	213	13,005,254	301,959	10.6 (10.1–11.2)	99.7
Moderate risk	62	4750	764	14.6 (10.6–19.0)	93.9

Abbreviations: REM, random effect meta-analysis; CI, confidence interval.

and other (Kato–Katz or McMaster) techniques were 10.7% (10.0–11.4%), 8.7% (5.5–12.4%), 11.3% (8.3–14.6%), 15.6% (9.8–22.4%) and 20.8% (12.4–30.6%), respectively.

With respect to sample size, the highest prevalence rate was found in studies of <500 dogs (13.4%, 11.4–15.6%), and the lowest prevalence rates were observed in studies of >5000 dogs (5.4%, 4.1–6.9%). Considering risk of bias, subgroup analysis showed that prevalence rates of *Toxocara* infection in studies with low (10.6%, 10.1–11.2%) and moderate (14.6%, 10.6–19.0%) risks of bias were considerable. A slightly lower prevalence was recorded for studies published after 2005 (Table 2). Meta-regression analyses showed a non-statistically significant decreasing trend in prevalence over time (coefficient $[C] = -0.0005$; P-value $= 0.67$) (Fig. 3A).

7. Impact of socio-demographic, geographical and climatic parameters on prevalence

We also performed subgroup analyses with respect to socio-demographic, geographical and climate parameters, to establish the source of heterogeneity and also the effects of these parameters on the prevalence of *Toxocara* infection in dogs. With respect to the income level in a country, the highest and lowest prevalence rates were estimated for countries with low income levels (20.0%, 13.7–27.2%) and high income levels (7.7%, 7.2–8.3%), respectively. Prevalence rates in countries with lower- (16.7%, 12.4–21.4%) and upper-middle (13.7%, 10.1–17.8%) income levels were marked. In subgroup analysis, according to geographical latitude, the highest prevalence rate was found at latitudes of 0–10° (20.7%, 15.0–27.0%), and lowest prevalence rates at latitudes 20–30° (9.3%, 6.5–12.6%) and 40–50° (9.6%, 8.3–11.3%). With respect to geographical longitude, the highest and lowest prevalence rates were estimated at longitudes of 10–20° (14.0%, 10.9–17.4%) and ≥120° (3.6%, 1.9–5.9%), respectively. The highest prevalence rates were estimated at a mean relative environmental humidity of <40% (20%, 3.5–44.8%), a mean environmental temperature of 19–25 °C (15.4%, 11.6–19.6%) and a precipitation range of 0–250 mm (18.2%, 10.8–26.9%). More detail is available in Table 3.

Meta-regression analysis showed a statistically significant, decreasing trend with increasing income ($C = -0.04$, P-value $= 0.001$). Overall, a statistically significant decreasing trend in prevalence was also seen with increasing geographical latitude ($C = 0.0013$, P-value $= 0.02$). However, in a non-linear model (Fig. 3C), we observed a significant decreasing trend

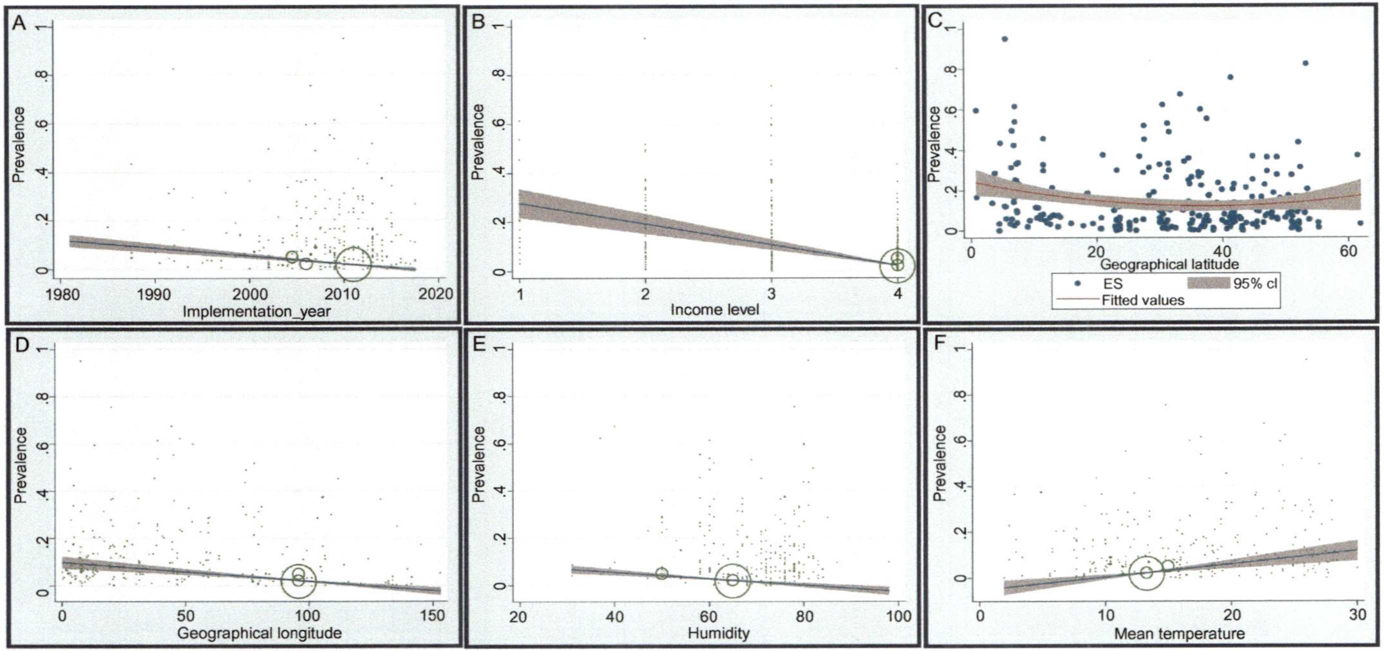

Fig. 3 Results of meta-regression analyses of the prevalence of *Toxocara* infection in dogs according to panel A: implementation years of studies demonstrating a statistically significant downward trend in prevalence in more recent years; panel B: country's income level showing a statistically significant downward trend in prevalence in countries with higher level of income; panel C: ⁂geographical latitude a showing a statistically significant downward trend in prevalence with increasing geographical latitude; panel D: geographical longitude a showing a statistically significant downward trend in prevalence with increasing geographical longitude; panel E: the relative humidity showing a non-statistically significant downward trend in prevalence in areas with higher relative humidity; panel F: the mean temperature showing a statistically significant upward trend in prevalence with increasing mean temperature. "ES" refers to effect size (=prevalence rates). ⁂ All meta-regression analyses, except that for latitude, utilized linear model graphs.

Table 3 The global prevalences of *Toxocara* infection in dogs estimated according to different socio-demographic and geographic parameters.

Parameter/ subgroup	Number of datasets	Total number of samples	Number of test-positive samples	Pooled prevalence (%) established using REM (95% CI)	Heterogeneity I^2 (%)
Income level					
Low	20	5311	1145	20 (13.7–27.2)	97.3
Lower middle	48	14,537	2211	16.7 (12.4–21.4)	98.0
Upper middle	82	28,304	5136	13.7 (10.1–17.8)	98.7
High	125	12,961,852	294,231	7.7 (7.2–8.3)	99.7
Latitude					
0–10°	37	9542	1924	20.7 (15.0–27.0)	98.0
10–20°	27	6139	708	10.1 (7.1–13.6)	94.2
20–30°	42	18,631	1388	9.3 (6.5–12.6)	97.8
30–40°	66	12,819,272	285,687	10.8 (9.8–11.7)	99.8
40–50°	65	121,627	7736	9.8 (8.3–11.3)	98.4
>50°	38	34,793	5280	10.5 (6.0–16)	99.5
Longitude					
0–10°	60	84,624	7698	12.1 (10.0–14.4)	98.7
10–20°	35	22,571	2286	14.0 (10.9–17.4)	97.8
20–30°	25	10,739	939	11.2 (6.6–16.7)	98.3
30–40°	22	7567	1200	17.3 (11.7–23.6)	97.3
40–50°	25	8904	586	14.2 (9.0–20.3)	97.9
50–60°	21	5977	655	15.4 (11.4–19.7)	93.2
60–70°	4	964	54	6.8 (3.2–11.5)	81.9
70–80°	20	41,482	1416	12.6 (9.4–16.0)	98.8
80–90°	11	1038	120	8.2 (3.4–14.8)	89.9
90–100°	8	12,802,855	283,649	5.0 (3.5–6.8)	100.0
100–110°	18	12,289	3515	10.9 (4.7–19.1)	98.9
110–120°	4	1478	223	9.9 (0.1–35.8)	99.3
>120°	22	9516	382	3.6 (1.9–5.9)	96.2

Table 3 The global prevalences of *Toxocara* infection in dogs estimated according to different socio-demographic and geographic parameters.—cont'd

Parameter/ subgroup	Number of datasets	Total number of samples	Number of test-positive samples	Pooled prevalence (%) established using REM (95% CI)	Heterogeneity I^2 (%)
Relative humidity (%)					
<39	7	634	166	20.0 (3.5–44.8)	97.7
40–49	13	1,216,248	61,467	13.1 (9.2–17.6)	95.8
50–59	39	11,441	1748	16.2 (12.2–20.7)	97.1
60–69	67	11,639,928	225,441	6.9 (6.5–7.4)	98.7
70–79	128	13,4301	12,690	10.7 (9.0–12.6)	99.0
≥80	21	7452	1211	18.2 (9.3–29.2)	99.0
Mean temperature (°C)					
≤7.0	17	12,327	3456	10.5 (3.9–19.8)	99.2
7.1–13.0	77	138,021	9031	10.5 (8.9–12.3)	98.9
13.1–19.0	84	12,835,745	286,547	8.7 (8.0–9.4)	99.8
19.1–25.0	53	13,133	2109	15.4 (11.6–19.6)	97.4
25.1–30.0	44	10,778	1580	13.9 (9.7–18.7)	97.7
Precipitation (mm)					
0–250	16	5480	868	18.2 (10.8–26.9)	97.6
251–500	41	15,032	1384	10.9 (8.4–13.8)	95.9
501–1000	118	1,338,901	73,605	11.7 (10.2–13.2)	99.1
1001–2000	87	11,647,433	226,452	9.4 (8.8–9.9)	98.9
>2000	13	3158	414	9.9 (1.8–22.9)	99.0

Abbreviations: REM, random effect meta-analysis; CI, confidence interval.

in latitudes between 0° and 40° ($C = -0.14$, P-value $= 0.01$), and then a non-significant increasing trend for latitudes between 40° and 60° ($C = 0.16$, P-value $= 0.07$). Moreover, a statistically significant decreasing trend was seen with increasing longitude ($C = 0.0005$, P-value $= 0.01$). Furthermore, a statistically significant increasing trend in prevalence was observed for increasing mean environmental temperature ($C = 0.0026$, P-value $= 0.05$); while a non-statistically significant decreasing trend was seen for increasing relative humidity ($C = -0.0003$, P-value $= 0.67$) and increasing annual precipitation ($C = -4.23e-06$, P-value $= 0.81$) (Fig. 3A–F).

8. Discussion and conclusions

This systematic review and meta-analysis of published prevalence studies on *Toxocara* in dogs found a global prevalence of 11.1%, suggesting that at least 100 million dogs are carriers of *Toxocara* worldwide. The results reveal that there are significant differences in prevalence among different regions of the world, which are associated with the type of dog, a country's GDP as well as geographical and climatic parameters. The high global prevalence of *Toxocara* infection is of public health concern, as such a large number of infected dogs pass millions of tons of faeces (Atenstaedt and Jones, 2011; Szwabe and Blaszkowska, 2017) containing billions of *Toxocara* eggs into the environment each year (Fan et al., 2013; Traversa et al., 2014). When deposited in public places, such as playgrounds, parks, public squares and beaches, which serve as recreational areas for people (Fakhri et al., 2018; Otero et al., 2018), places children at increased risk of exposure due to their behaviour (Cong et al., 2015; Kroten et al., 2016). The overall prevalence of *Toxocara* infection in dogs varied among regions, being lowest in the Western Pacific region and highest in Eastern Mediterranean and African countries. Explanations for this variation may include inter alia: differences in the age, ownership (pet or stray), location (rural vs urban), gender and method used to investigate the prevalence of *Toxocara* in the dogs studied. Prevalence also varied depending on the environmental and climatic conditions, regional and national dog control programs, and the level of veterinary care and availability to dogs, which varied according to socio-economic status (Abdel Aziz et al., 2019; Mohamed et al., 2009). Most countries in the Eastern Mediterranean and African regions have a generally lower socio-economic status and lack dog population control and preventive control programs. The more developed countries of the Western pacific, European and American regions were more likely to implement dog control programs. The subgroup and meta-regression analyses indicated a significant decreasing prevalence for countries with higher income levels. This variation might also be due to the types of dogs tested in each specific region. More pet dogs were recruited in Europe (62.3% of datasets) and the Western Pacific region (65.5% of datasets) than in the Eastern Mediterranean region (35% of datasets). Pet dogs (8.9%) had a significantly lower prevalence of *Toxocara* spp. than in working (14.1%) and stray

(18.8%) dogs (Table 2). This variation in prevalence between distinct dog types might relate to animal nutritional, immune and hygiene status, veterinary care and/or anthelmintic treatment availability (Becker et al., 2012; Habluetzel et al., 2003; Nijsse et al., 2015). This finding is similar to that found in a global evaluation of *Toxocara* infection(s) in cats, which found that the prevalence in stray cats (28.6%, 25.1–32.1%) was significantly higher than in pet cats (11.6%, 10.6–12.5%).

The types of samples used and the techniques employed to test them can have a bearing on prevalence estimates. Prevalence was higher for postmortem examination for adult *T. canis* (15%) compared with those studies that used coproscopic examination(s) to detect eggs (10.9%). A higher prevalence (15.6%) was estimated for surveys using postmortem examination than faecal flotation (10.7%) or sedimentation (8.7%) methods. The variability in diagnostic sensitivity and specificity of these different methods is a likely source of heterogeneity, resulting in an over- or under-estimation of the true prevalence.

Young dogs (<1 year of age) have a higher prevalence of *Toxocara* infection than older dogs (>1 year of age)—a finding consistent in most previous studies of both domestic (e.g., Abdel Aziz et al., 2019; Mohamed et al., 2009; Moro and Abah, 2019) and wild definitive hosts (Kapel and Nansen, 1996). This is due to the efficiency of vertical (transplacental and/or lactogenic/transmammary) transmission to puppies, which avoids the vagaries of survival and accidental transmission through the environmental/paratenic host transmission route (Blagburn et al., 1996; Glickman and Schantz, 1981). The acquired age-associated immunity in dogs of >12 weeks of age typically decreases the establishment and intensity of *Toxocara* infection (Abdel Aziz et al., 2019; Greve, 1971). Male dogs had a significantly ($P < 0.001$) higher prevalence than female dogs, which has also been reported previously (Overgaauw, 1997). This could be explained by female dogs spreading *T. canis* infection via reactivated (somatic) larvae to their offspring (predominantly via transplacental transmission), whereas males can only transmit via patent intestinal infection (Overgaauw, 1997; Schnieder et al., 2011). Another explanation could be the immunosuppressive effect of testosterone in male dogs (Abdel Aziz et al., 2019; Curi et al., 2017).

A higher prevalence of *Toxocara* infection in dogs was found in regions at lower latitudes, and with higher average temperatures. These variables coincided and relate to the survival rate of *Toxocara* eggs in the environment that is higher in areas with moderate temperatures (20–30 °C) and damp soil, whereas survival and embryonation rates are lower in areas where temperatures are <10 °C or >37 °C (cf. Despommier, 2003; Overgaauw, 1997).

In agreement with the present results, previous studies of *Toxocara* eggs in the environment and of the prevalence of anti-*Toxocara* serum antibodies in people in areas with high mean temperatures and relative humidity indicate a higher risk of *Toxocara* infection in humans than in regions with moderate or cold climates (Fakhri et al., 2018; Foroutan et al., 2019; Rostami et al., 2017). Comparisons of prevalence rates among areas with different climatic conditions should be made with caution, because confounding factors such as differences in preventive measures, veterinary care, deworming programs and environmental hygiene among countries, might have an impact (Foroutan et al., 2019). *Toxocara* prevalence was significantly lower in developed countries, which are located at higher latitudes, and are characterized by colder climates. Prevalence was found to be higher in regions at lower latitudes, where many countries are of lower socio-economic status, and have lower access rates to veterinary care (Aiello and Larson, 2002; McMichael, 2000; Montgomery and Elimelech, 2007).

The findings of this review must be interpreted cautiously, considering a number of possible limitations. First, although this worldwide meta-analysis of the prevalence of *Toxocara* infection in dogs is the largest thus far, only eligible published studies were included, and it is possible that useful data were missed from the 'grey' literature. Second, prevalence data for *Toxocara* infection in dogs were not available for a number of countries, including several countries in Central and West Africa, East Europe and Central Asia; also, for some selected countries, data were available for only one location or region. Therefore, our estimates may not be representative of all countries that were included, and results for comprehensive future studies might significantly alter the national prevalence rate for some countries. Third, a common limitation of meta-analyses is heterogeneity among prevalence studies (Rossi et al., 2012; Singh et al., 2018; Stockdale et al., 2017); the source of this heterogeneity could not be identified based on subgroup analyses of data/information available for sample size, study year, WHO-region, income level or methods. Despite these limitations, and to the best of our knowledge, this is the first systematic review and meta-analysis to provide a global estimate of the prevalence of *Toxocara* infection in dogs. Data were compiled for >13 million dogs from 60 countries using major electronic databases, utilizing rigorous methodological and statistical procedures to estimate prevalence. Sensitivity analysis—conducted by removing studies with large sample sizes, and by including studies with a low risk of bias—estimated prevalences similar to the 'crude' prevalences, which gives us confidence about the findings.

Toxocariasis is a neglected parasitic disease of major human health importance (Ma et al., 2018; Rostami et al., 2019). The findings of the present review demonstrate that more needs to be done to prevent and control this zoonosis. The estimated 11.1% prevalence of *Toxocara* infection in dogs represents ≥100 million infected dogs and should serve as a reminder to public health experts and policy makers of the need to implement effective intervention programs (Ma et al., 2018).

Acknowledgements

This research was supported by Health Research Institute at the Babol University of Medical Sciences (IR.MUBABOL.HRI.REC.1398.129), Babol, Iran (A.R.). RBG's research program is presently supported through funds from the National Health and Medical Research Council (NHMRC) of Australia, the Australian Research Council (ARC), Yourgene Health, Melbourne Water Corporation and The University of Melbourne.

References

Abdel Aziz, A.R., Hassan, A.A., Elmahallawy, E.K., Elshahawy, I.S., Almuzaini, A.M., 2019. Prevalence and associated risk factors of *Toxocara* infection in dogs in northern and southern Egypt. Vet. Parasitol. 17, 100305.

Aghaei, S., Riahi, S.M., Rostami, A., Mohammadzadeh, I., Javanian, M., Tohidi, E., Foroutan, M., Esmaeili Dooki, M., 2018. *Toxocara* spp. infection and risk of childhood asthma: a systematic review and meta-analysis. Acta Trop. 182, 298–304.

Aghamolaie, S., Seyyedtabaei, S.J., Behniafar, H., Foroutan, M., Saber, V., Hanifehpur, H., Mehravar, S., Rostami, A., 2018. Seroepidemiology, modifiable risk factors and clinical symptoms of *Toxocara* spp. infection in northern Iran. Trans. R. Soc. Trop. Med. Hyg. 113, 116–122.

Aiello, A.E., Larson, E.L., 2002. What is the evidence for a causal link between hygiene and infections? Lancet Infect. Dis. 2, 103–110.

Atenstaedt, R.L., Jones, S., 2011. Interventions to prevent dog fouling: a systematic review of the evidence. Public Health 125, 90–92.

Becker, A.C., Rohen, M., Epe, C., Schnieder, T., 2012. Prevalence of endoparasites in stray and fostered dogs and cats in Northern Germany. Parasitol. Res. 111, 849–857.

Blagburn, B.L., Lindsay, D.S., Vaughan, J.L., Rippey, N.S., Wright, J.C., Lynn, R.C., Kelch, W.J., Ritchie, G., Hepler, D.I., 1996. Prevalence of canine parasites based on fecal flotation. Compend. Contin. Educ. Pract. Vet. 18, 483–509.

Cong, W., Meng, Q.F., You, H.L., Zhou, N., Dong, X.Y., Dong, W., Wang, X.Y., Qian, A.D., Zhu, X.Q., 2015. Seroprevalence and risk factors of *Toxocara* infection among children in Shandong and Jilin provinces, China. Acta Trop. 152, 215–219.

Curi, N.H.A., Paschoal, A.M.O., Massara, R.L., Santos, H.A., Guimarães, M.P., Passamani, M., Chiarello, A.G., 2017. Risk factors for gastrointestinal parasite infections of dogs living around protected areas of the Atlantic Forest: implications for human and wildlife health. Braz. J. Biol. 77, 388–395.

DerSimonian, R., Laird, N., 1986. Meta-analysis in clinical trials. Control. Clin. Trials 7, 177–188.

Despommier, D., 2003. Toxocariasis: clinical aspects, epidemiology, medical ecology, and molecular aspects. Clin. Microbiol. Rev. 16, 265–272.

Dubná, S., Langrová, I., Nápravník, J., Jankovská, I., Vadlejch, J., Pekár, S., Fechtner, J., 2007. The prevalence of intestinal parasites in dogs from Prague, rural areas, and shelters of the Czech Republic. Vet. Parasitol. 145, 120–128.

Fakhri, Y., Gasser, R.B., Rostami, A., Fan, C.K., Ghasemi, S.M., Javanian, M., Bayani, M., Armoon, B., Moradi, B., 2018. *Toxocara* eggs in public places worldwide—a systematic review and meta-analysis. Environ. Pollut. 242, 1467–1475.
Fan, C.K., Liao, C.W., Cheng, Y.C., 2013. Factors affecting disease manifestation of toxocarosis in humans: genetics and environment. Vet. Parasitol. 193, 342–352.
Fisher, M., 2003. *Toxocara cati*: an underestimated zoonotic agent. Trends Parasitol. 19, 167–170.
Foroutan, M., Fakhri, Y., Riahi, S.M., Ebrahimpour, S., Namroodi, S., Taghipour, A., Spotin, A., Gamble, H.R., Rostami, A., 2019. The global seroprevalence of *Toxoplasma gondii* in pigs: a systematic review and meta-analysis. Vet. Parasitol. 269, 42–52.
Glickman, L.T., Schantz, P.M., 1981. Epidemiology and pathogenesis of zoonotic toxocariasis. Epidemiol. Rev. 3, 230–250.
Greve, J.H., 1971. Age resistance to *Toxocara canis* in ascarid-free dogs. Am. J. Vet. Res. 32, 1185–1192.
Habluetzel, A., Traldi, G., Ruggieri, S., Attili, A.R., Scuppa, P., Marchetti, R., Menghini, G., Esposito, F., 2003. An estimation of *Toxocara canis* prevalence in dogs, environmental egg contamination and risk of human infection in the Marche region of Italy. Vet. Parasitol. 113, 243–252.
Higgins, J.P., Thompson, S.G., Deeks, J.J., Altman, D.G., 2003. Measuring inconsistency in meta-analyses. Br. Med. J. 327, 557–560.
Hughes, J., Macdonald, D.W., 2013. A review of the interactions between free-roaming domestic dogs and wildlife. Biol. Conserv. 157, 341–351.
Hunter, J.P., Saratzis, A., Sutton, A.J., Boucher, R.H., Sayers, R.D., Brown, M.J., 2014. In meta-analyses of proportion studies, funnel plots were found to be an inaccurate method of assessing publication bias. J. Clin. Epidemiol. 67, 897–903.
Kapel, C.M.O., Nansen, P., 1996. Gastrointestinal helminths of arctic foxes (*Alopex lagopus*) from different bioclimatological regions in Greenland. J. Parasitol. 82, 17–24.
Kroten, A., Toczylowski, K., Kiziewicz, B., Oldak, E., Sulik, A., 2016. Environmental contamination with *Toxocara* eggs and seroprevalence of toxocariasis in children of northeastern Poland. Parasitol. Res. 115, 205–209.
Little, S.E., Johnson, E.M., Lewis, D., Jaklitsch, R.P., Payton, M.E., Blagburn, B.L., Bowman, D.D., Moroff, S., Tams, T., Rich, L., Aucoin, D., 2009. Prevalence of intestinal parasites in pet dogs in the United States. Vet. Parasitol. 166, 144–152.
Lucio-Forster, A., Barbecho, J.S., Mohammed, H.O., Kornreich, B.G., Bowman, D.D., 2016. Comparison of the prevalence of *Toxocara* egg shedding by pet cats and dogs in the USA, 2011–2014. Vet. Parasitol. Reg. Stud. Reports 5, 1–13.
Ma, G., Holland, C.V., Wang, T., Hofmann, A., Fan, C.K., Maizels, R.M., Hotez, P.J., Gasser, R.B., 2018. Human toxocariasis. Lancet Infect. Dis. 18, e14–e24.
Macpherson, C.N.L., Meslin, F.-X., Wandeler, A. (Eds.), 2013. Dogs, Zoonoses and Public Health, second ed. CAB International Publishing, Wallingford, UK, p. 277.
McMichael, A.J., 2000. The urban environment and health in a world of increasing globalization: issues for developing countries. Bull. World Health Organ. 78, 1117–1126.
Mohamed, A.S., Moore, G.E., Glickman, L.T., 2009. Prevalence of intestinal nematode parasitism among pet dogs in the United States (2003–2006). J. Am. Vet. Med. Assoc. 234, 631–637.
Mohammadzadeh, I., Riahi, S.M., Saber, V., Darvish, S., Amrovani, M., Arefkhah, N., Rostami, A., 2018. The relationship between *Toxocara* species seropositivity and allergic skin disorders: a systematic review and meta-analysis. Trans. R. Soc. Trop. Med. Hyg. 112, 529–537.
Moher, D., Shamseer, L., Clarke, M., Ghersi, D., Liberati, A., Petticrew, M., Shekelle, P., Stewart, L.A., PRISMA-P Group, 2015. Preferred reporting items for systematic review and meta-analysis protocols (PRISMA-P) 2015 statement. Syst. Rev. 4, 1.

Montgomery, M.A., Elimelech, M., 2007. Water and sanitation in developing countries: including health in the equation. Environ. Sci. Technol. 41, 17–24.

Moro, K.K., Abah, A.E., 2019. Epizootiology of zoonotic parasites of dogs in Abua Area of Rivers State, Nigeria. Vet. Anim. Sci. 7, 100045.

Munn, Z., Moola, S., Riitano, D., Lisy, K., 2014. The development of a critical appraisal tool for use in systematic reviews addressing questions of prevalence. Int. J. Health Policy Manag. 3, 123–128.

Nijsse, R., Ploeger, H.W., Wagenaar, J.A., Mughini-Gras, L., 2015. *Toxocara canis* in household dogs: prevalence, risk factors and owners' attitude towards deworming. Parasitol. Res. 114, 561–569.

Otero, D., Alho, A.M., Nijsse, R., Roelfsema, J., Overgaauw, P., Madeira de Carvalho, L., 2018. Environmental contamination with *Toxocara* spp. eggs in public parks and playground sandpits of Greater Lisbon, Portugal. J. Infect. Public Health 11, 94–98.

Otranto, D., Dantas-Torres, F., Mihalca, A.D., Traub, R.J., Lappin, M., Baneth, G., 2017. Zoonotic parasites of sheltered and stray dogs in the era of the global economic and political crisis. Trends Parasitol. 33, 813–825.

Overgaauw, P.A., 1997. Aspects of *Toxocara* epidemiology: toxocarosis in dogs and cats. Crit. Rev. Microbiol. 23, 233–251.

Overgaauw, P.A., van Knapen, F., 2013. Veterinary and public health aspects of *Toxocara* spp. Vet. Parasitol. 193, 398–403.

Paoletti, B., Traversa, D., Iorio, R., De Berardinis, A., Bartolini, R., Salini, R., Di Cesare, A., 2015. Zoonotic parasites in feces and fur of stray and private dogs from Italy. Parasitol. Res. 114, 2135–2141.

Rossi, C., Shrier, I., Marshall, L., Cnossen, S., Schwartzman, K., Klein, M.B., Schwarzer, G., Greenaway, C., 2012. Seroprevalence of chronic hepatitis B virus infection and prior immunity in immigrants and refugees: a systematic review and meta-analysis. PLoS One 7, e44611.

Rostami, A., Riahi, S.M., Fakhri, Y., Saber, V., Hanifehpour, H., Valizadeh, S., Gholizadeh, M., Pouya, R.H., Gamble, H.R., 2017. The global seroprevalence of *Toxoplasma gondii* among wild boars: a systematic review and meta-analysis. Vet. Parasitol. 244, 12–20.

Rostami, A., Ma, G., Wang, T., Koehler, A.V., Hofmann, A., Chang, B.C., Macpherson, C.N., Gasser, R.B., 2019. Human toxocariasis—a look at a neglected disease through an epidemiological 'prism'. Infect. Genet. Evol. 74, 104002.

Schnieder, T., Laabs, E.M., Welz, C., 2011. Larval development of *Toxocara canis* in dogs. Vet. Parasitol. 175, 193–206.

Serpell, J., Barrett, P., 2016. The Domestic Dog: Its Evolution, Behaviour and Interactions With People. Cambridge University Press, UK, ISBN: 0521425379, pp. 182–210.

Singh, P., Arora, A., Strand, T.A., Leffler, D.A., Catassi, C., Green, P.H., Kelly, C.P., Ahuja, V., Makharia, G.K., 2018. Global prevalence of celiac disease: systematic review and meta-analysis. Clin. Gastroenterol. Hepatol. 16, 823–836.

Stockdale, A.J., Chaponda, M., Beloukas, A., Phillips, R.O., Matthews, P.C., Papadimitropoulos, A., King, S., Bonnett, L., Geretti, A.M., 2017. Prevalence of hepatitis D virus infection in sub-Saharan Africa: a systematic review and meta-analysis. Lancet Glob. Health 5, e992–e1003.

Szwabe, K., Blaszkowska, J., 2017. Stray dogs and cats as potential sources of soil contamination with zoonotic parasites. Ann. Agric. Environ. Med. 24, 39–43.

Traversa, D., Frangipane di Regalbono, A., Di Cesare, A., La Torre, F., Drake, J., Pietrobelli, M., 2014. Environmental contamination by canine geohelminths. Parasit. Vectors 7, 67.

World Health Organization, 2003. List of Member States by WHO region and mortality stratum. In: World Health Report. 2003, p. 182.

CHAPTER TWENTY-NINE

Sources of environmental contamination with *Toxocara* spp.: An omnipresent parasite

Rolf Nijsse[a,*], Paul Overgaauw[b], Harm Ploeger[a], Lapo Mughini-Gras[b,c]
[a]Department of Infectious Diseases and Immunology, Faculty of Veterinary Medicine, Utrecht University, Utrecht, The Netherlands
[b]Division of Veterinary Public Health, Faculty of Veterinary Medicine, Institute for Risk Assessment Sciences, Utrecht University, Utrecht, The Netherlands
[c]National Institute for Public Health and the Environment, Centre for Infectious Disease Control (CIb), Bilthoven, The Netherlands
*Corresponding author: e-mail address: e.r.nijsse@uu.nl

Contents

Abstract

Embryonated *Toxocara* eggs in the environment are considered to be the most important source of human toxocariasis. These eggs, however, are also a source of infection for the definitive and paratenic hosts. Most available literature focuses on *Toxocara canis* in dogs, or other canids. There are, however, other *Toxocara* species with their accompanying definitive hosts. Results from studies that modelled patent infections in dogs, cats and foxes show that although dogs are a very important source for environmental contamination with *Toxocara* eggs, other sources cannot be ignored. For a good

Advances in Parasitology, Volume 109
ISSN 0065-308X
https://doi.org/10.1016/bs.apar.2020.01.010

understanding of the relative contributions of different definitive hosts to environmental contamination with *Toxocara* eggs, computational models should be built and fed with data from different fields of expertise as is discussed in this paper.

1. Background

The presence of parasitic nematodes of the genus *Toxocara* is documented in every continent. Reports often communicate information on the prevalence of faecal shedding of *Toxocara* spp. eggs in definitive hosts (DHs) (Brochier et al., 2007; Bruzinskaite-Schmidhalter et al., 2012; Daryani et al., 2009; Le et al., 2016; Lucio-Forster et al., 2016; Millan and Casanova, 2009; Mohamed et al., 2009; Rodríguez Gallegos et al., 2016; Sowemimo, 2012), the presence of *Toxocara* spp. eggs in the environment (Amoah et al., 2017; Bojanich et al., 2015; Ghadirian et al., 1976; Gurel et al., 2005; Otero et al., 2018; Uga et al., 1995; Wiwanitkit and Waenlor, 2004), the infection of paratenic hosts (PHs) containing larval stages in arrested development (Davidson et al., 2012; Helwigh et al., 1999; Santarem et al., 2011; Talvik et al., 2006; Zibaei et al., 2017), or seroprevalence studies (Araujo et al., 2015; Cong et al., 2014; Giacometti et al., 2000; Jarosz et al., 2010; Kanafani et al., 2006; Kanobana et al., 2013; Mughini-Gras et al., 2016; Sharif et al., 2010; Won et al., 2008) and clinical case reports of *Toxocara* infections in humans (Agarwal et al., 2019; Coskun and Akinci, 2013; Ghoroobi et al., 2017; Hatzipantelis et al., 2017; Inagaki et al., 2019; Noh et al., 2012; Pinelli et al., 2011; Ranasuriya et al., 2014). In many human cases suspected of larva migrans interna, *Toxocara canis* is presumed to be involved. Most of the time, diagnosis is based on serology using techniques that cannot discriminate between different *Toxocara* species. In such a scenario, questions about the patient's history usually focus on the presence of canids in the direct living environment as the source of infection. However, other genera of DHs cannot be excluded as a source of environmental contamination. Various groups of mammals can be DHs for certain species of the genus *Toxocara* (Table 1) (Borecka, 2010; Delgado and Rodríguez-Morales, 2009; Gallas and da Silveira, 2013; Gibbons et al., 2001; Mozgovoĭ, 1953; Vega et al., 2018). Patent infections of *T. canis* and *T. cati* occur worldwide in populations of dogs and cats, respectively. These patent infections are of public health relevance because hundreds of thousands of eggs can be shed daily by a single DH, and these eggs can survive

Table 1 *Toxocara* species displayed as combined from information and tables of Mozgovoĭ (1953), Gibbons et al. (2001), Delgado and Rodríguez-Morales (2009), Borecka (2010), and Gallas and da Silveira (2013).

Species	Definitive host	Locality	Reference
Toxocara alienata (Rudolphi, 1819)	*Nasua rufus*	Brazil	Warren (1970)
Toxocara anakumae (Noda, 1966)	*Meles anakuma*	Japan	Noda (1966)
Toxocara apodemi (Olsen, 1957)	*Apodemus peninsulae*, *Apodemus agrarius*	Korea	Warren (1970)
		China	Asakawa et al. (1994)
Toxocara canarisi (Puylaert, 1967)[a]	*Felis serval*	Kenya	Puylaert (1967b)
Toxocara canis (Werner, 1782) (=*T. vulpis* (Froelich, 1789), type species) (=*Lumbricus canis* (Stiles in Stiles and Hassal, 1905))	*Alopex lagopus*, *Alopex beringensis*, *Canis mexicanus*, *Canis lupus*, *Canis occidentalis*, *Canis dingo*, *Canis aureus*, *Canis familiaris*, *Canis pallipes*, *Crocuta crocuta*, *Fennecus zerda*, *Lycaon pictus*, *Meles anakuma*, *Nyctereutes procyonoides ussuriensis*, *Procyon lotor*, *Urocyon cinereoargentatus scotti*, *Vulpes bengalensis*, *Vulpes fulva pennyslvanicus*, *Vulpes fulva regalis*, *Vulpes vulpes*, *Vulpes vulpes japonicus*	Cosmopolitan	Sprent (1958)
	Fennucus zerda, *Ichneumia albicauda*, *Panthero leo*		Round (1968)
	Herpestes sanguineus		Warren (1972)
Toxocara canis (Werner, 1782) (=*Toxocara canis* (Werner, 1782)) (=*Toxocara cati* (Schrank, 1788)) (=*Toxocara mystax* (Zeder, 1800)), *Toxocara crenulata* (Bremser, 1824)	*Acinonyx jubilatus*, *Felis* spp., *Lynx baileyi*, *Lynx canadensis*, *Lynx lynx*, *Lynx rufus*, *Lynx rufus texensis*	Cosmopolitan	Sprent (1956)
	Genetta sp., *Panthera leo*, *Panthera pardus*		Round (1968)
	Helogale parvula, *Civettictis civetta*		Warren (1972)

Continued

Table 1 *Toxocara* species displayed as combined from information and tables of Mozgovoĭ (1953), Gibbons et al. (2001), Delgado and Rodríguez-Morales (2009), Borecka (2010), and Gallas and da Silveira (2013).—Cont'd

Species	Definitive host	Locality	Reference
	Leopardus colocolo *Leopardus geoffroyi* *Puma yagouaroundi* *Leopardus tigrinus*	Brazil	Gallas and da Silveira (2013)
Toxocara cynonycteridis (Parona, 1889)[b]	*Cynonycteris amplexicaudata*	Myanmar (Burma)	Warren (1970)
Toxocara elephantis (Rudolphi, 1819)[b]	*Elephas maximus*	Switzerland, United States	Warren (1970)
Toxocara genettae (Warren, 1972)	*Genetta felina*	South Africa	Warren (1972)
	Genetta genetta	Spain	Alvarez et al. (1990)
Toxocara herpestum (Vuylsteke, 1956)	*Herpestes ichneunon*	Asia	Vuylsteke (1956)
Toxocara hippopotami (Canavan, 1931)	*Hippopotamus amphibius*	Uganda	Round (1968)
Toxocara indica (Naidu, 1981)	*Bandicota indica*	India	Naidu (1981)
Toxocara lyncis (Macchioni, 1999)	*Lynx caracal*	Asia, Africa	Macchioni (1999)
Toxocara mackerrasae (Sprent, 1957)	*Rattus fuscipes*, *Hydromys chrysogaster*	Australia	Warren (1970)
Toxocara malaysiensis (Zhu, 1998)	*Felis catus*	Malaysia, China, Vietnam	Zhu et al. (1998)
Toxocara manzadiensis (Vuylsteke, 1956)[b]	*Syncerus caffer*	The Congo	Round (1968)
Toxocara marginata (=*Belascaris marginata*) (Rudolphi, 1802)	*Canis familiaris*	Africa	Ortlepp (1924)
Toxocara masculior (Railliet & Henry, 1911)	*Vulpes zerda*	North Africa	Round (1968)
(*Toxocara melis* (Gedoelst, 1920))[c] =*Baylisascaris melis* (Gedoelst, 1920)	*Meles* sp.		Hartwich (1958)

Toxocara mystax (Zeder, 1800) = *Toxocara cati*			
Toxocara paradoxura (Kou, 1958)	*Paradoxurus minor exitus*	China	Warren (1970)
Toxocara pearsei (Chitwood, 1935)[b]	*Synalpheus brooksi*	United States	Warren (1970)
Toxocara pteropodis (Baylis, 1936)	*Pteropus geddiei*	Vanuatu	Warren (1970)
	Pteropus hypomelanus	United States	Heard et al. (1995)
	Pteropus conspicullatus, *Pteropus poliocephalus*	Australia	Prociv (1990)
Toxocara sprenti (Warren, 1972)	*Viverricula indica*	Thailand	Warren (1972)
Toxocara suricattae (Ortlepp, 1940)	*Suricata suricatta*	South Africa	Mozgovoĭ (1953) and Warren (1970)
	Mungos mungos		Warren (1972)
Toxocara tanuki (Yamaguti, 1941)	*Nyctereutes procyonoides viverrinus*	Japan	Warren (1970)
Toxocara vajrasthirae (Sprent, 1972)	*Arctonyx collaris*	Thailand	Sprent (1972)
Toxocara vincenti (Puylaert, 1967)	*Civettictis civetta*	Democratic Republic of Congo	Puylaert (1967a) and Warren (1970)
Toxocara vitulorum (Goeze, 1782)	*Bos taurus*, *Bos indicus*, *Bubalus bubalis*	Tropical, subtropical regions	Mozgovoĭ (1953)
	Bos spp., *Capra* spp., *Ovis* spp.		Warren (1970)
Toxocara vulpis (Froelich, 1789) = *Toxocara canis*			
Toxocara warreni (Durette-Desset and Chabaud, 1974)	*Hyemoschus aquaticus*	Gabon	Durette-Desset and Chabaud (1974)

[a]Species inquirendae in Warren (1972).
[b]Species inquirendae in Warren (1970).
[c]Species inquirendae in Hartwich (1958).

for years in the environment depending on climatic conditions (Azam et al., 2012; Pautova et al., 2015). Several weeks after being shed, eggs will contain an infective larva (embryonated eggs) and then become a risk for infection of DHs and PHs, including humans, upon ingestion.

For carnivorous DHs, next to the ingestion of embryonated eggs, an additional route of infection in the lifecycle of *Toxocara* spp. (Fig. 1) is known. This route concerns PHs, including vertebrates such as rodents and birds (Krucken et al., 2017; Schnieder et al., 2011; Strube et al., 2013; Talvik et al., 2006; Warren, 1969; Zibaei et al., 2017), which acquire infection by ingesting embryonated eggs. After ingestion of these eggs, larvae will begin their migration, but they are unable to pass the lungs and will remain as dormant or migrating larvae in the tissues. When a PH is eaten by a DH, the larvae are set free during the process of digestion and can directly mature in the intestines without having to complete the hepato-tracheal migration, leading to patent infections even in the presence of a functional age resistance. The larvae develop directly into adult worms in the intestine because they already migrated in the preceding PH, and thereby presumably reached an appropriate stage of biological development to continue maturation in the intestine without further migration (Overgaauw, 1997a; Sprent, 1958). This extra route of infection has been investigated and confirmed for *T. canis* and *T. cati* (Sprent, 1956, 1958). This does not necessarily mean that larvae of other *Toxocara* species lack this additional route of infection. However, the evolutionary advantages of an infection route involving PHs in a predator–prey relationship will be less obvious for *Toxocara* spp. of non-carnivores.

Embryonated eggs can accidentally be ingested by humans. In the human intestines, the larvae hatch from the eggs, penetrate the intestinal mucosa, migrate through the body via blood and lymphatic vessels, and can invade various tissues. Humans can therefore be considered as incidental PHs. The number and location of the larvae in the human body and the intensity of the individual immune response against them determine the outcome of such an infection, which varies from asymptomatic to severe disease in various described syndromes (Fan et al., 2015; Overgaauw, 1997b; Pawlowski, 2001; Smith et al., 2009).

From the parasite perspective, *Toxocara* spp. in carnivores are very successful nematodes. Their lifecycle is continued even in populations with relatively high hygiene standards (Akao and Ohta, 2007; Davidson et al., 2012). Infection levels can be high, both in PHs (up to 87% seropositive schoolchildren) and DHs (51–100% egg shedding in puppies)

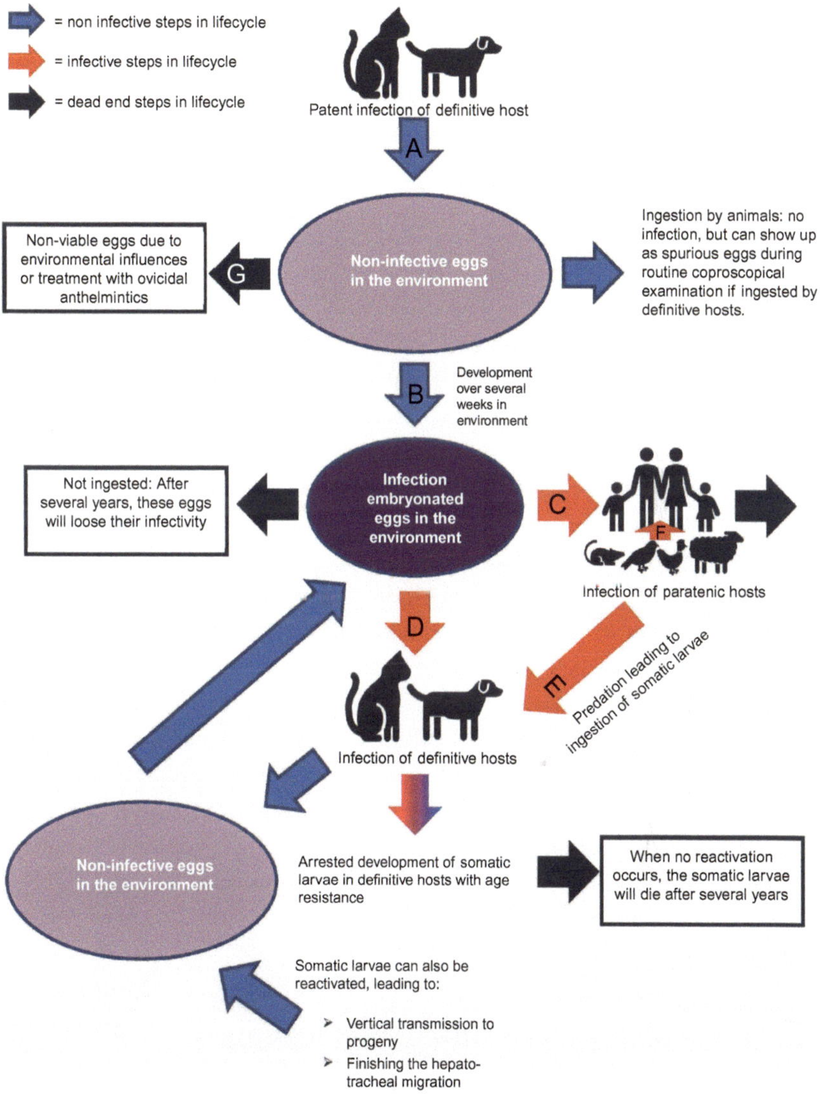

Fig. 1 Key elements of environmental contamination with eggs of *Toxocara canis* and *Toxocara cati*. (A) Patent infections in definitive host contaminate the environment with not yet infective eggs (unembryonated). (B) Eggs need to mature for several weeks in the environment to become infective (embryonated) depending on soil type and climatic conditions such as temperature and humidity. (C) Embryonated eggs can infect paratenic hosts leading to a pool of infective larvae in potential prey animals. (D) Embryonated eggs can infect definitive hosts leading to patent infections when age resistance is absent or to somatic larvae when age resistance is present. (E) Paratenic hosts (containing viable somatic larvae) eaten by definitive hosts are a source of infection that will lead to patent infection in definitive hosts without a migration outside the intestines. (F) Non-definitive hosts eating paratenic hosts (containing viable somatic larvae) can become infected leading to somatic larvae in this new, from that moment on 'paratenic host'. (G) The effect of directly cleaning up faeces after dogs or cats. This will lead to a less contaminated environment.

(Fu et al., 2014; Ma et al., 2018). Seroprevalence data in humans show that exposure to *Toxocara* spp. is common (Mughini-Gras et al., 2016; Strube et al., 2013). This success can be explained by the fact that several reservoirs of different stages of these nematodes are present in the environment (i) as extremely resistant eggs, (ii) as somatic larvae within infected paratenic hosts, but also (iii) as an internal reservoir in the somatic tissues of infected DHs. For some *Toxocara* spp., arrested larvae in somatic tissues of DHs can be reactivated in pregnant DHs and subsequently infect the next generation of DHs, either via the intrauterine (canids) or lactogenic route (canids, felids, bovids). It also can be hypothesized that somatic larvae in the lung tissues of nonpregnant DHs get reactivated when the immune system of the animal is compromised. Dormant somatic larvae in or nearby the lung tissues might be able to complete their hepato-tracheal migration and return to the intestinal lumen to become reproductive adults in, e.g., animals treated with corticosteroids (Lloyd et al., 1981; Nijsse et al., 2016).

Besides PHs, other animals including invertebrates may function as mechanical transport hosts. These animals simply transport eggs from one place to another without becoming actually infected themselves. These so-called transport hosts can transport *Toxocara* eggs from DHs' defecation areas to areas that are not directly polluted by DHs' faeces.

Clearly, there is a focus in published literature on *Toxocara* infections in dogs as a source for human toxocariasis. However, it is also clear that other DH species and *Toxocara* spp. can contribute to infections in humans as PHs and in pets as DHs. Therefore, this paper will discuss different sources of eggs and larvae of *Toxocara* and their contribution to environmental contamination.

2. Definitive hosts with patent infections

2.1 Ingesting embryonated eggs

A *Toxocara* infection in a DH cannot be considered to be synonymous to a patent infection. Due to environmental exposure to embryonated *Toxocara* eggs, it can be assumed that, e.g., most household dogs and cats with an active outdoor life do become infected, but this does not mean that they will start shedding eggs. The absence or presence of age resistance defines the outcome of ingesting embryonated eggs as becoming a patent infection or not. As in dogs, infections with embryonated eggs in animals without age resistance (which mostly affect dogs younger than 6 months) will lead to hepato-tracheal migration of the hatched larvae and, after being coughed up and swallowed, to maturation to adult reproductive worms in the intestines. This latter scenario will therefore lead to patent infections. Age resistance in dogs older than 6 months, a known feature in the epidemiology of *Toxocara* infections, will prevent the development of patent infections after ingestion of infective eggs in most dogs (Greve, 1971). In dogs with age resistance, the migration route differs. Here, after hatching in the intestines, the larvae that penetrate the intestinal mucosa and start their hepato-tracheal migration, are not able to pass the alveoli (Schnieder et al., 2011). These larvae will then return in the systemic circulation to end up in the somatic tissues of the DH as arrested larvae. These arrested larvae can be reactivated in some dogs due to different known and unknown factors. Known factors are, for example, pregnancy (Burke and Roberson, 1985; Overgaauw, 1997a; Overgaauw et al., 1998) and use of corticosteroids (Lloyd et al., 1981; Nijsse et al., 2016). Reactivation is expected in female DHs due to pregnancy leading to infection of their progeny. In some cases, reactivation may lead to patent infections in the DH individual itself, however, this is, as far as known by the authors, neither supported nor invalidated in literature.

2.2 Ingesting paratenic hosts

When dogs, even with a functional age resistance, are not infected with embryonated eggs but by ingesting larvae from somatic tissues of a PH, these larvae will mature directly in the intestines, in spite of that age resistance. This will lead to patent infections (Sprent, 1956, 1958). This can partly explain the difference in prevalence of patent infections between household animals on commercial food and predating stray or wild animals. Therefore, PHs are another important source in the epidemiology of patent *Toxocara* infections in carnivores. The outcomes of infections in different categories of animals infected with different infective stages are displayed in Table 2.

Table 2 Different infection routes of, e.g., *Toxocara canis* and their outcomes.

	Embryonated eggs	Paratenic hosts
Definitive hosts without age resistance	**PI**/sl	**PI**/sl
Definitive hosts with age resistance	**SL**/pi	**PI**/sl
Paratenic hosts (including humans)	**SL**	**SL**

In bold capitals the most likely outcome is mentioned with PI; pi, patent infection; SL, sl = somatic larvae. The most likely outcome is capitalized.

2.3 Required information to estimate environmental contamination

Patent infections in DHs are responsible for the contamination of the environment with *Toxocara* spp. eggs, and therefore infections in PHs (including humans) and DHs. Data on prevalence of patent infections and the intensity of these infections (i.e. eggs per gram of faeces or EPG) in DHs are necessary to estimate the relative importance of the different sources for environmental contamination with eggs leading to human and animal exposure to these infective stages.

Studies on the prevalence of patent infections are more elaborately discussed in other chapters of this thematic issue. For optimal use of data from previous and future prevalence studies these should preferably be standardized. Organizations like the 'World Association for the Advancement of Veterinary Parasitology' (WAAVP), but also the 'Companion Animal Parasite Council' (CAPC), the 'European Scientific Counsel Companion Animal Parasites' ESCCAP and the 'Tropical Council for Companion Animal Parasites' (TroCCAP) can play an important role in promoting standardization within new research projects. One important aspect of standardization concerns the methods used, which will contribute to improved comparability between different studies (i.e. comparable detection limits and specificity) without compromising method feasibility in countries with limited research facilities. Further, a seasonal pattern in both the prevalence of egg shedding (Barutzki and Schaper, 2011; Kirkpatrick, 1988; Nijsse et al., 2016; Nolan and Smith, 1995) and the presence of worms in the intestines (Radwan et al., 2009) are reported for *Toxocara* spp., which should be considered when prevalence studies are compared with each other. It is, however, unclear how and why these seasonal differences occur in different climatic zones.

A source of bias in prevalence studies concerns coprophagy and predation leading to the so-called 'spurious eggs' in the faeces of animals (Fahrion et al., 2011; Nijsse et al., 2014). Prevalence studies based on faecal egg shedding need confirmation of actual patent infection of the *Toxocara* species in question. Spurious eggs, in this case unembryonated *Toxocara* eggs, which are present in the faeces of an animal or in the intestines of a prey animal, are ingested by another animal, will pass the gastrointestinal tract and end up in the faeces of this latter animal while it does not have a patent infection (see Fig. 1). The issue of spurious eggs in faecal samples of pet animals can be avoided by letting the owner/caretaker prevent the dog or cat from displaying coprophagy or predatory behaviour 3–4 days prior to sampling.

However, in wild or stray animals, this is not feasible and therefore there is a need for confirmation of patent infections and proper identification of the recovered eggs. Confirmation of patent infections can be done, for example, by detecting the presence of adult worms in the intestine of DHs (Radwan et al., 2009), and determine the species of these worms. The number of adult worms present in the intestines combined with the intensity of shedding will provide additional useful information about the fecundity of the adult worms. The specific identification of viable spurious eggs may provide relevant information on the egg distribution of different *Toxocara* spp. If it is not possible to obtain adult worms, the identification of the species can be performed based on egg morphology. However, this can be problematic for both *T. canis* and *T. cati*, as 'intermediate types' of eggs in terms of size and pitting are reported (Uga et al., 2000). These two species can also be differentiated using molecular techniques (Durant et al., 2012; Fogt-Wyrwas et al., 2007; Khademvatan et al., 2013; Macuhova et al., 2010). Coproantigens, instead of eggs, can also be detected using ELISA techniques specific for ascarids, but this technique does not discriminate between *Toxocara* spp. and *Toxascaris leonina* or other ascarids (Elsemore et al., 2017).

Several studies report abundance of infection and intensity of shedding (Mikaeili et al., 2013; Radwan et al., 2009; Saeed and Kapel, 2006; Sowemimo, 2007, 2012). For better understanding of the relative importance of the contribution of different DHs to environmental contamination, these parameters are essential. Especially the intensity of shedding (EPG) should be feasible to report, provided that faecal samples are available. Information on population density and distribution of DHs, their faecal output, the prevalence of patent infections, confirmation of the nematode species and intensities of patent infections are key elements for quantifying the different sources of environmental contamination with eggs of *Toxocara* spp.

2.4 Quantifying relative contributions to environmental contamination

Morgan et al. (2013) proposed a stochastic model based on the levels of patent infections in different DHs in Bristol, United Kingdom, to determine the relative contributions of different DH populations and groups therein to the environmental contamination with *Toxocara* spp. eggs (Morgan et al., 2013). The model also calculates these relative contributions in different regions with different compositions of DH populations. The outcome of the model suggested that dogs younger than 12 weeks of age dominate the total egg output. However, they may be less important to the contamination of public areas because access to public parks by puppies is limited. They are often dewormed every 14 days, and their faeces are usually disposed of. Therefore, foxes, due to their high prevalence of patent infections, with their faeces not removed from public areas, and a total absence of any anthelmintic treatment, could take over as the primary source of *Toxocara* spp. eggs in the environment. Building on this model by adding further layers of complexity from the known epidemiology of *Toxocara* spp., Nijsse et al. (2015) estimated the relative contributions of different non-juvenile (i.e. >6 months old) DHs to the environmental contamination with *Toxocara* eggs in the Netherlands. This latter model took into account host density, faecal output, prevalence and intensity of *Toxocara* infection, but also frequency of coprophagic behaviour, faeces disposal by owners, cats' outdoor access and practiced anthelmintic treatment regimens of the participating pet owners. It is important to mention that there is no stray dog population in the Netherlands (Sternheim, 2012). The outcomes of the relative contributions of different hosts to the environmental contamination are shown in Fig. 2. From these results, it can be concluded that (stray) cats

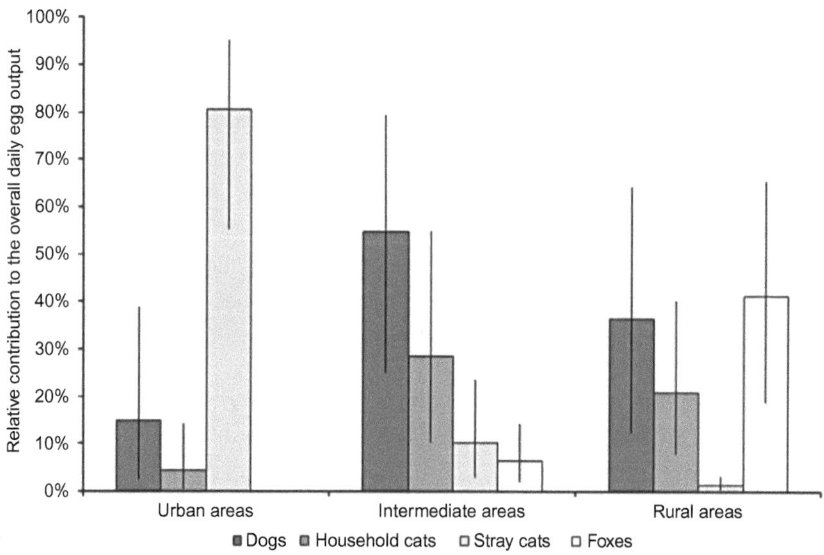

Fig. 2 Relative contributions to environmental contamination with *Toxocara* eggs in urban, intermediate and rural areas. Estimated relative contributions (%) of non-juvenile (≥6 month old) dogs, household cats, stray cats, and foxes to the environmental contamination with *Toxocara* eggs in urban, intermediate and rural areas in the Netherlands. Error bars represent 95% confidence intervals (Nijsse et al., 2015).

are the most important contributors in urban areas. Household cats in urban areas however, due to the use of litterboxes, limited access to the outdoors and periodical use of anthelmintic treatments appear to contribute relatively less than dogs. However, they often bury their faeces in private gardens or sandboxes, possibly leading to a greater chance of exposure of humans to cat faeces than to dog faeces (Jansen et al., 1993; Kleine et al., 2016; Shimizu, 1993; Uga, 1993). Both studies stress the importance of incorporating information on the above-mentioned parameters when planning control strategies. In Islamic countries, where keeping dogs as pets is very uncommon for religious reasons and cats are favored pets, the seroprevalence of *Toxocara* infections is considerable as well (Romano et al., 2010; Zibaei and Sadjjadi, 2017). In other countries the underestimated role of cats in the epidemiology of human toxocariasis is also recognized by other authors (Deplazes et al., 2011; Fisher, 2003; Overgaauw and van Knapen, 2013; Talvik et al., 2006).

3. *Toxocara* eggs in the environment

Embryonated eggs in the environment are depicted in the centre point of Fig. 1. No matter what source of infection for humans or animals is considered, the actual presence of embryonated, viable *Toxocara* eggs in soil and sand samples is the key factor in the continuation of the lifecycle of *Toxocara* spp. The topic of environmental contamination will be discussed more elaborately in another chapter of this thematic issue about *Toxocara* spp., in this paragraph some highlights of recent literature will be addressed.

A selected number of articles ($n = 109$) on the topic of the presence of eggs in soil samples from public parks and sand samples from sandboxes, from all over the world was recently systematically analysed (Fakhri et al., 2018). Simplified data from that study are summarized in Table 3 to present the range in positive samples in different regions of the world. The pooled global prevalence of samples with *Toxocara* eggs in soils of public places was 21%. The authors discuss the problems comparing the outcomes of different studies due to the lack of uniformity in the methods used and materials. Mizgajska-Wiktor (2005), Nikolay et al. (2014), Kleine et al. (2016), Fakhri et al. (2018), and Rostami et al. (2019) all recently stressed the need for a more standardized approach in the methods of studying soil samples for the presence of soil-transmitted helminths. Standardization of the methods used involves distribution of sample points over an area (Collender et al., 2015), the depth in which the soil sample is taken (Jansen et al., 1993; Mizgajska, 2001)

Table 3 Estimated pooled prevalences of *Toxocara* eggs positive soil/sand samples per WHO region, and countries in that region with lowest and highest reported prevalence (Fakhri et al., 2018).

WHO regions	Pooled prevalence (%)	Country in region with lowest prevalence (%)		Country in region with highest prevalence (%)	
South America	25	Argentina	8	Uruguay	53
North and Central America	13	Costa Rica	3	Canada	33
Europe	18	Estonia	4	Portugal	53
Middle East and North Africa	18	Iraq/Egypt	13	Iran	20
Africa	27	Zimbabwe	4	Sudan	75
Southeast Asia	21	Thailand	8	Malaysia	38
Western Pacific Region	35	Australia	0	China	75

and the method used to recover the eggs from the samples, including use of detergents, passive flotation or centrifugal flotation, type of flotation solution, materials used (e.g. glass vs plastic) and viability check of the recovered eggs (Kleine et al., 2016).

Some publications also mention a seasonal pattern in contamination rates of the environment (Avcioglu and Burgu, 2008; Gao et al., 2017; Kleine et al., 2017). Therefore, knowledge about the seasonal patterns of sampled areas is needed to facilitate comparison between different studies. The underlying mechanism to explain these differences needs to be looked into. This might be related to the above-mentioned seasonal patterns in shedding of *Toxocara* spp. eggs in dogs that have been evidenced in longitudinal studies (Barutzki and Schaper, 2011; Kirkpatrick, 1988; Nijsse et al., 2016; Nolan and Smith, 1995). However, results differ according to the climate of the countries in question, indicating that the season can also influence the defecation behaviour of DHs. The more hostile a season for a DH is, probably the closer to their home base the animal will defecate.

Rostami et al. (2019) reported on the scarcity of published studies that report the recovered *Toxocara* eggs from soil samples on a species level. The studies that do, mostly use molecular techniques (Durant et al., 2012; Macuhova et al., 2010; Ozlati et al., 2016). Though the advantage and need of species identification is clear, these techniques are not available in every area and are sometimes preceded with flotation methods that, again, need to be standardized. Soil is a substance that can vary a lot in composition. Inhibiting factors present in the soil samples, can influence the outcomes of these molecular techniques. Some of these molecular techniques (e.g. PCR) are more susceptible to these factors than others (e.g. LAMP) (Collender et al., 2015). Advanced digital automated image identification software, based on specific algorithms, could also facilitate the identification of *Toxocara* eggs to species level (Jimenez et al., 2016). As described earlier, for constructing and validating of models that estimate the relative contributions of different DHs, quantification and specific identification of recovered eggs from soil is essential. The actual exposure of different hosts to the contaminated environment depends on the use of the affected area by humans or other animals.

4. Paratenic hosts

Reservoir parasitism for Ascarididae was described in 1963 by Mozgovoi and the term reservoir host was proposed by Skryabin and Shul'ts in 1940 defined as: 'animals in which parasites up to the infective stage simply collect and do not develop' (cf. Mozgovoĭ and Shakhmatova, 1986). Today these animals are called paratenic hosts. PHs play a very important role in the life cycle of *Toxocara* spp. of carnivores. The larvae in the somatic tissues from the PH will bypass age resistance because they will mature in the intestines of the DH without further migration (Overgaauw, 1997a; Sprent, 1956, 1958). The availability of PHs is a major reason why sylvatic predating DHs show higher patent infections rates than household animals (Brochier et al., 2007; Bruzinskaite-Schmidhalter et al., 2012; Franssen et al., 2014; Saeed et al., 2006). For different animal species, including humans, larval migration to somatic tissues is reported (Borecka et al., 2008; Cardillo et al., 2009; Davidson et al., 2012; Helwigh et al., 1999; Krucken et al., 2017; Merdivenci and Sezen, 1965; Santarem et al., 2011; Strube et al., 2013; Talvik et al., 2006; Zibaei et al., 2017). Humans as PHs, however, can be considered as a dead end in the life cycle of *Toxocara* spp., as we humans are hardly a meal for DHs anymore. There are many publications about humans as PHs. Exposure to the larval stages of *Toxocara* spp. evokes the production of antibodies. Seroprevalence studies in both the general population and groups of people suspected of suffering from migrating *Toxocara* third-stage larvae show comparable and considerably high prevalence estimates (Mughini-Gras et al., 2016; Pinelli et al., 2011). Seroprevalence in humans from different parts of the world will be discussed in more detail in other chapters of this thematic issue. Most serodiagnostics, although highly specific for detecting antibodies against the genus *Toxocara*, do not discriminate to the species level (Chen et al., 2018; Poulsen et al., 2015). Many case studies report on direct evidence of migrating larvae or larvae in arrested development (Agarwal et al., 2019; Coskun and Akinci, 2013; Ghoroobi et al., 2017; Hatzipantelis et al., 2017; Inagaki et al., 2019; Noh et al., 2012; Ranasuriya et al., 2014), e.g., based on visual or molecular confirmation of the larva present in the eye (OLM) (Choi et al., 2018; Hare and Franco-Paredes, 2014; Lim et al., 2014; Van De et al., 2013) or central nervous system (NT) (Caldera et al., 2013), or indirect evidence based on serology and eosinophilia (VLM, NT, CT), being the cause of symptoms, in patients. The question about which *Toxocara* species are involved in human infections remains mostly unanswered. The answer to this question will shed some light on the relative contribution of each *Toxocara* sp. on the human burden of illness. This burden of illness is mostly defined by the level of exposure, because a specific diagnosis in patients suspected of disease due to migrating larvae is difficult to make.

Compared to the seroprevalence studies or case reports in humans, there are far fewer publications about non-human PHs (Borecka et al., 2008; Cardillo et al., 2009; Correa et al., 2014; Dutra et al., 2013; Flecher et al., 2016; Helwigh et al., 1999; Janecek et al., 2014; Klockiewicz et al., 2019; Kusnoto et al., 2017; Maruyama et al., 1994; Mata-Santos et al., 2016; Moura et al., 2018; Özbakış and Doğanay, 2019; Springer et al., 2019; Strube et al., 2013; Taira et al., 2012). Available articles mostly concern experimental infections of PHs as a model for human toxocariasis. Even fewer studies focus on the sylvatic PH populations from an epidemiological point of view (Dubinsky et al., 1995; Krucken et al., 2017; Reiterová et al., 2013; Webster and MacDonald, 1995). One study from Estonia studied somatic larvae in stray dogs, cats and brown rats. No somatic larvae could be recovered from cats and rats and about 12% of the dogs tested positive for larval infection of kidney and liver (Talvik et al., 2006). However, in this study no serology was used to assess exposure to *Toxocara* spp. Limited amounts of tissue samples (hindlimb muscle, kidney, liver, and lung tissue) were digested for larval recovery. The migrating behaviour and pattern of larvae in PHs can differ with different roundworm species, the duration of the infection, but also different species of PHs (Janecek et al., 2014; Strube et al., 2013). This could have led to an underestimation of the infection rate of the studied animals. This is also apparent from data from a study from the Slovak Republic (Dubinsky et al., 1995). It showed a seroprevalence among different species of small mammals ($n=582$) of 15%, whereas *Toxocara* larvae could only be recovered from minced brain tissue and hindleg muscle digestion in 6.3% of 476 small mammals. The highest prevalence rates were found in synanthropic rodent species caught in urban areas. This again emphasizes that to achieve comparable information from studies focusing on prevalence data from PHs, standardization of methods is important. Knowledge about normal territorial behaviour and biotopes of the species of PHs, can provide useful information about exposure to contaminated areas. Seroprevalence data, larval recovery and identification, including viability testing, are all missing pieces of the epidemiological puzzle that is *Toxocara*.

5. Transport hosts

Next to PHs that are actually infected for longer periods of time, some publications also describe hosts that serve as so-called transport hosts (THs) (Atiokeng Tatang et al., 2017; Caldera et al., 2013; Cardillo et al., 2016; Gonzalez-Garcia et al., 2017; Romeu et al., 1991; Sasmal et al., 2008; Umeche and Mandah, 1989; Yu et al., 2012). These animals serve as a way of mechanically transporting eggs or larvae, without acquiring long-lasting infection. In some publications on the possible transport hosts for *Toxocara*, these, mostly invertebrate, animals are also referred to as PHs. Though THs can be consumed at a moment when eggs or larvae are present, it can be questioned whether long-lasting tissue invasion of the somatic tissues in THs occurs. In a study using earthworms (*Pheretima posthuma*), no larvae could be detected in these annelids 20 days after experimental infection (Pahari and Sasmal, 1991). Examples of acknowledged THs are slugs, snails, earthworms, cockroaches and houseflies. These animals can contribute to the dissemination of *Toxocara* eggs in the environment. Their role in the aetiology of *Toxocara* infections in humans is very circumstantial. People who eat insects, earthworms, and/or gastropods probably live in, and will probably also indirectly consume, sand and soil from a contaminated environment (Fellrath and Magnaval, 2014). From this perspective, these THs are just one of the transport media available for infective organisms. When modelling the epidemiology of *Toxocara* spp. these factors should be considered but are difficult to incorporate and quantify. The same applies for 'inanimate' objects, e.g., fur, vegetables and shoes, for which a transport role, as fomites, for *Toxocara* is described

(Klapec and Borecka, 2012; Merigueti et al., 2017; Overgaauw et al., 2009; Panova and Khrustalev, 2018; Paoletti et al., 2015; Uga et al., 2009).

6. Discussion

Toxocara spp. eggs are very resilient in the environment and can retain their infectivity for years. Reducing the environmental contamination with these eggs should be the main aim of control strategies to reduce animal and human exposure to infective stages of *Toxocara* spp. Control strategies should consist of (i) removal of faeces of DHs from the environment and (ii) control of patent infections in DHs, which includes preventing consumption of raw PHs by DHs.

6.1 Removal of faeces of DHs from the environment

Removal of faeces will, if feasible for all DHs, lead to a decline in infection rates of PHs, including humans, and also to a loss of function for THs as they will have nothing to transport. Reducing the contribution to the contamination of the environment with *Toxocara* eggs from household animals can be achieved very effectively by the proper disposal of their faeces with the regular garbage rather than in organic waste, thus preventing the eventual survival of eggs during the process of composting (Morgan et al., 2013; Nijsse et al., 2015). For sylvatic or stray DHs this is unfeasible. Therefore, it can be assumed that parks in urban areas, especially those that are accessible to stray cats and stray dogs, are contaminated (Becker et al., 2012; Ferreira et al., 2017; Giacometti et al., 2000; Millan and Casanova, 2009; O'Lorcain, 1994). This is confirmed in the many publications on the presence of helminth eggs in soil and sand samples. So, it can be assumed that exposure to infective eggs will occur in areas not exclusively accessible to household animals of which the faeces are disposed of immediately after defecation.

6.2 Controlling patent infections in DHs

Control strategies of patent infections almost exclusively concern owned (companion) animals. Control of patent infections is attempted by the use of anthelmintics for treating animals blindly in different schemes. The efficacy of blind treatments is currently under debate. For the control of patent infections of *Toxocara* spp. in companion animals, the logical frequency for blind treatment should be based on the prepatent period leading to a frequency of treatment of 10–12 times a year. In countries where the prevalence of patent infections in dogs in cross-sectional studies is about 5%, it is questionable whether the use of anthelmintics is justified mainly related to the responsible use of medicines and possible environmental issues. Besides, in countries where monthly treatment is advised and practiced to control infections of other parasites, like *Dirofilaria immitis*, prevalence of patent *Toxocara* infections still is 2–5% (Little et al., 2009; Lucio-Forster et al., 2016; Mohamed et al., 2009), which is comparable to some other countries where *D. immitis* is not endemic and monthly treatment is practiced less often. So, just propagating monthly treatments and leaving this up to the dog owners is not likely to significantly decrease the prevalence of patent *Toxocara* infections, at least not in household dogs. Identifying and differentiating low- from high-frequent shedders based on both risk factors and frequent use of diagnostics may be a good alternative or complementary strategy to control companion animals as a source of environmental contamination with *Toxocara* eggs (Nijsse et al., 2016).

Feasibility of preventing ingestion of PHs is low in unowned (stray) DHs. For companion animals, predation of and feeding raw meat from animals that are possible PHs should be prevented. For owners that do not want to stop feeding raw meat to their pets, this means that meat should only be fed from slaughter animals originating from a high biosecurity setting or they should practice high frequency anthelmintic treatments.

6.3 Concluding remarks

It is clear that most parks and unprotected sandboxes in urban areas can be assumed to be contaminated with *Toxocara* eggs. The contribution of companion animals with outdoor access can, and should be, controlled. This, however, will not lead to the absence of *Toxocara* eggs in these environments because other sources do contribute to environmental contamination. For more effective strategies in reducing environmental contamination, it may help to investigate the actual sources of that contamination and their relative contributions. This can be facilitated using models. These models should be fed with data (Table 4) generated from periodically repeated studies using standardized methods. Available data will also help to validate already existing models in which intervention scenarios can be tested. Simulated intervention scenarios dealing with, e.g., different compliance rates of owners properly disposing the faeces of their DHs, practiced deworming regimes, faeces clean-up regimes in the environment, and population control of DHs, can provide information on the effects of the individual and combined interventions. This way the feasibility and necessity of these measures can be weighed against each other.

Table 4 Elements to include in models to quantify the different sources of environmental contamination.

Elements concerning	DHs[a]	PHs[a]	Environment
Animal itself	Species	Species	Which DHs have access
	Numbers (population size)	Numbers (population size)	
	Biotopes	Biotopes	
	Defecation behavior	Behavior related to ingestion of eggs	
	Faecal output	Behavior related to being eaten by DH or other PH	
	Age category	Age category	
	Coprophagy		
	Predation		
'Pet related'	Practiced deworming regime		Clean-up management, e.g., park or sandbox
	Clean up behaviour owner		
Worms/larvae	Abundance	Abundance	n.a.
	Specific identification	Specific identification Localization somatic tissues	
Eggs	Egg shedding prevalence		Intensity (EPG)
	Intensity (EPG)		Specific identification
	Specific identification		Localization
	Seasonality		Seasonality
Serology	Prevalence exposure	Prevalence exposure	n.a.
	Specific identification	Specific identification	

[a]DH, definitive host; PH, paratenic host.

Additionally, because *Toxocara* eggs are still ingested by humans, stressing the importance to the general public of standard hygiene measures and risks of infection are equally important as measures to control contamination of the environment. In some countries where the prevalence of patent infections in dogs and cats is stable, a decline in seroprevalence can be observed (Mughini-Gras et al., 2016; Pinelli et al., 2011). This can be explained by higher hygiene measures, including covering sandboxes, stimulating cleaning up after their dogs, etc. Finally, to attribute different sources to infections in humans, serodiagnostic techniques that can differentiate between the different *Toxocara* species are highly desirable.

Acknowledgements

The authors like to thank the journal Parasites and Vectors (BMC publishers, Springer Nature) for making Fig. 2 available for the use in this chapter.

References

Agarwal, A., Das, P., Kumar, A., Sharma, S., Aggarwal, K., Sehgal, S., Gupta, V., 2019. Multiple granulomas of ocular toxocariasis in an immunocompetent male. Ocul. Immunol. Inflamm. 3, 1–5.

Akao, N., Ohta, N., 2007. Toxocariasis in Japan. Parasitol. Int. 56 (2), 87–93.

Alvarez, F., Iglesias, R., Bos, J., Tojo, J., Sanmartin, M.L., 1990. New findings on the helminth fauna of the common European genet (*Genetta genetta* L.): first record of *Toxocara genettae* Warren, 1972 (Ascarididae) in Europe. Ann. Parasitol. Hum. Comp. 65 (5–6), 244–248.

Amoah, I.D., Singh, G., Stenstrom, T.A., Reddy, P., 2017. Detection and quantification of soil-transmitted helminths in environmental samples: a review of current state-of-the-art and future perspectives. Acta Trop. 169, 187–201.

Araujo, Z., Brandes, S., Pinelli, E., Bochichio, M.A., Palacios, A., Wide, A., Rivas-Santiago, B., Jimenez, J.C., 2015. Seropositivity for ascariosis and toxocariosis and cytokine expression among the indigenous people in the Venezuelan Delta region. Rev. Inst. Med. Trop. Sao Paulo 57 (1), 47–55.

Asakawa, M., Li, J.F., Guo, A.H., Yang, X.Y., Huhebateer, Liu, Z.L., Liu, Y., Cao, X.M., Chen, K.Y., 1994. A new host and locality for Toxocara apodemi (Olsen, 1957) (Nematoda: Ascarididae) from striped field mice, Apodemus agrarius (Pallas). J. Rakuno Gakuen Univ. Nat. Sci. 19 (1), 193–196.

Atiokeng Tatang, R.J., Tsila, H.G., Wabo Pone, J., 2017. Medically important parasites carried by cockroaches in Melong subdivision, Littoral, Cameroon. J. Parasitol. Res. 2017, 7967325.

Avcioglu, H., Burgu, A., 2008. Seasonal prevalence of *Toxocara* ova in soil samples from public parks in Ankara, Turkey. Vector Borne Zoonotic Dis. 8 (3), 345–350.

Azam, D., Ukpai, O.M., Said, A., Abd-Allah, G.A., Morgan, E.R., 2012. Temperature and the development and survival of infective *Toxocara canis* larvae. Parasitol. Res. 110 (2), 649–656.

Barutzki, D., Schaper, R., 2011. Results of parasitological examinations of faecal samples from cats and dogs in Germany between 2003 and 2010. Parasitol. Res. 109 (Suppl. 1), 45.

Becker, A.C., Rohen, M., Epe, C., Schnieder, T., 2012. Prevalence of endoparasites in stray and fostered dogs and cats in Northern Germany. Parasitol. Res. 111 (2), 849–857.

Bojanich, M.V., Alonso, J.M., Caraballo, N.A., Itati Scholler, M., Lopez, M.L., Garcia, L.M., Basualdo, J.A., 2015. Assessment of the presence of Toxocara eggs in soils of an arid area in central-western Argentina. Rev. Inst. Med. Trop. Sao Paulo 57 (1), 73–76.

Borecka, A., 2010. The spread of nematodes from *Toxocara* genus in the world. Wiad. Parazytol. 56 (2), 117–124.

Borecka, A., Gawor, J., Niedworok, M., Sordyl, B., 2008. Detection of *Toxocara canis* larvae by PCR in the liver of experimentally infected Mongolian gerbils (*Meriones unguiculatus*). Helminthologia 45 (3), 147–149.

Brochier, B., De Blander, H., Hanosset, R., Berkvens, D., Losson, B., Saegerman, C., 2007. *Echinococcus multilocularis* and *Toxocara canis* in urban red foxes (*Vulpes vulpes*) in Brussels, Belgium. Prev. Vet. Med. 80 (1), 65–73.

Bruzinskaite-Schmidhalter, R., Sarkunas, M., Malakauskas, A., Mathis, A., Torgerson, P.R., Deplazes, P., 2012. Helminths of red foxes (*Vulpes vulpes*) and raccoon dogs (*Nyctereutes procyonoides*) in Lithuania. Parasitology 139 (1), 120–127.

Burke, T.M., Roberson, E.L., 1985. Prenatal and lactational transmission of *Toxocara canis* and *Ancylostoma caninum*: experimental infection of the bitch before pregnancy. Int. J. Parasitol. 15 (1), 71–75.

Caldera, F., Burlone, M.E., Genchi, C., Pirisi, M., Bartoli, E., 2013. *Toxocara* encephalitis presenting with autonomous nervous system involvement. Infection 41 (3), 691–694.

Cardillo, N., Rosa, A., Ribicich, M., López, C., Sommerfelt, I., 2009. Experimental infection with *Toxocara cati* in BALB/c mice, migratory behaviour and pathological changes. Zoonoses Public Health 56 (4), 198–205.

Cardillo, N., Prous, C.G., Krivokapich, S., Pittaro, M., Ercole, M., Perez, M., Pasqualetti, M., Farina, F., Rosa, A., Gatti, G., Ribicich, M., 2016. First report of *Toxocara cati* in the domestic land snail *Rumina decollata*. Rev. Argent. Microbiol. 48 (3), 206–209.

Chen, J., Liu, Q., Liu, G.H., Zheng, W.B., Hong, S.J., Sugiyama, H., Zhu, X.Q., Elsheikha, H.M., 2018. Toxocariasis: a silent threat with a progressive public health impact. Infect. Dis. Poverty 7 (1), 59.

Choi, K., Choi, J., Choi, S., Jung, J.H., 2018. *Toxocara* optic neuropathy: clinical features and ocular findings. Int. J. Ophthalmol. 11 (3), 520–523.

Collender, P.A., Kirby, A.E., Addiss, D.G., Freeman, M.C., Remais, J.V., 2015. Methods for quantification of soil-transmitted helminths in environmental media: current techniques and recent advances. Trends Parasitol. 31 (12), 625–639.

Cong, W., Zhang, X.X., Zhou, N., Yu, C.Z., Chen, J., Wang, X.Y., Li, B., Qian, A.D., Zhu, X.Q., 2014. *Toxocara* seroprevalence among clinically healthy individuals, pregnant women and psychiatric patients and associated risk factors in Shandong Province, Eastern China. PLoS Negl. Trop. Dis. 8 (8), e3082.

Correa, F.M., Chieffi, P.P., Lescano, S.A., Santos, S.V., 2014. Behavioral and memory changes in *Mus musculus* coinfected by *Toxocara canis* and *Toxoplasma gondii*. Rev. Inst. Med. Trop. Sao Paulo 56 (4), 353–356.

Coskun, F., Akinci, E., 2013. Hepatic toxocariasis: a rare cause of right upper abdominal pain in the emergency department. Turkiye Parazitol. Derg. 37 (2), 151–153.

Daryani, A., Sharif, M., Amouei, A., Gholami, S., 2009. Prevalence of *Toxocara canis* in stray dogs, northern Iran. Pak. J. Biol. Sci. 12 (14), 1031–1035.

Davidson, R.K., Mermer, A., Oines, O., 2012. *Toxocara cati* larva migrans in domestic pigs—detected at slaughterhouse control in Norway. Acta Vet. Scand. 54, 6–66.

Delgado, O., Rodríguez-Morales, A.J., 2009. Aspectos clínico-epidemiológicos de la toxocariasis: una enfermedad desatendida en Venezuela y América Latina. Bol. Mal. Salud Amb. 49 (1), 1–33.

Deplazes, P., van Knapen, F., Schweiger, A., Overgaauw, P.A., 2011. Role of pet dogs and cats in the transmission of helminthic zoonoses in Europe, with a focus on echinococcosis and toxocarosis. Vet. Parasitol. 182 (1), 41–53.

Dubinsky, P., Havasiova-Reiterova, K., Petko, B., Hovorka, I., Tomasovicova, O., 1995. Role of small mammals in the epidemiology of toxocariasis. Parasitology 110 (2), 187–193.

Durant, J.F., Irenge, L.M., Fogt-Wyrwas, R., Dumont, C., Doucet, J.P., Mignon, B., Losson, B., Gala, J.L., 2012. Duplex quantitative real-time PCR assay for the detection and discrimination of the eggs of *Toxocara canis* and *Toxocara cati* (Nematoda, Ascaridoidea) in soil and fecal samples. Parasit. Vectors 5, 288.

Durette-Desset, M.C., Chabaud, A.G., 1974. Three new nematodes parasites of the water-chevrotain *Hyemoschus aquaticus* in Gabon (collected by G. Dubost). In: Bulletin du Muséum National d'Histoire Naturelle, Third Series (205, Zoology 135), pp. 75–87.

Dutra, G.F., Pinto, N.S., da Costa de Avila, L.F., de Lima Telmo, P., da Hora, V.P., Martins, L.H., Berne, M.E., Scaini, C.J., 2013. Evaluation of the initial and chronic phases of toxocariasis after consumption of liver treated by freezing or cooling. Parasitol. Res. 112 (6), 2171–2175.

Elsemore, D.A., Geng, J., Cote, J., Hanna, R., Lucio-Forster, A., Bowman, D.D., 2017. Enzyme-linked immunosorbent assays for coproantigen detection of *Ancylostoma caninum* and *Toxocara canis* in dogs and *Toxocara cati* in cats. J. Vet. Diagn. Invest. 29 (5), 645–653.

Fahrion, A.S., Schnyder, M., Wichert, B., Deplazes, P., 2011. *Toxocara* eggs shed by dogs and cats and their molecular and morphometric species-specific identification: is the finding of *T. cati* eggs shed by dogs of epidemiological relevance? Vet. Parasitol. 177 (1–2), 186–189.

Fakhri, Y., Gasser, R.B., Rostami, A., Fan, C.K., Ghasemi, S.M., Javanian, M., Bayani, M., Armoon, B., Moradi, B., 2018. *Toxocara* eggs in public places worldwide—a systematic review and meta-analysis. Environ. Pollut. 242 (Pt. B), 1467–1475.

Fan, C.K., Holland, C.V., Loxton, K., Barghouth, U., 2015. Cerebral toxocariasis: silent progression to neurodegenerative disorders? Clin. Microbiol. Rev. 28 (3), 663–686.

Fellrath, J.M., Magnaval, J.F., 2014. Toxocariasis after slug ingestion characterized by severe neurologic, ocular, and pulmonary involvement. Open Forum Infect. Dis. 1 (2), ofu063.

Ferreira, A., Alho, A.M., Otero, D., Gomes, L., Nijsse, R., Overgaauw, P.A.M., Madeira de Carvalho, L., 2017. Urban dog parks as sources of canine parasites: contamination rates and pet owner behaviours in Lisbon, Portugal. J. Environ. Public Health 2017, 5984e086.

Fisher, M., 2003. *Toxocara cati*: an underestimated zoonotic agent. Trends Parasitol. 19 (4), 167–170.

Flecher, M.C., Musso, C., Martins, I.V., Pereira, F.E., 2016. Larval migration of the ascarid nematode *Toxocara canis* following infection and re-infection in the gerbil *Meriones unguiculatus*. J. Helminthol. 90 (5), 569–576.

Fogt-Wyrwas, R., Jarosz, W., Mizgajska-Wiktor, H., 2007. Utilizing a polymerase chain reaction method for the detection of *Toxocara canis* and *T. cati* eggs in soil. J. Helminthol. 81 (1), 75–78.

Franssen, F., Nijsse, R., Mulder, J., Cremers, H., Dam, C., Takumi, K., van der Giessen, J., 2014. Increase in number of helminth species from Dutch red foxes over a 35-year period. Parasit. Vectors 7, 166.

Fu, C.J., Chuang, T.W., Lin, H.S., Wu, C.H., Liu, Y.C., Langinlur, M.K., Lu, M.Y., Hsiao, W.W., Fan, C.K., 2014. Seroepidemiology of *Toxocara canis* infection among primary schoolchildren in the capital area of the Republic of the Marshall Islands. BMC Infect. Dis. 15 (14). https://doi.org/10.1186/1471-2334-14-261.

Gallas, M., Da Silveira, E.F., 2013. *Toxocara cati* (Schrank, 1788) (Nematoda, Ascarididae) in different wild feline species in Brazil: new host records. Biotemas 26 (3), 117–125.

Gao, X., Wang, H., Li, J., Qin, H., Xiao, J., 2017. Influence of land use and meteorological factors on the spatial distribution of *Toxocara canis* and *Toxocara cati* eggs in soil in urban areas. Vet. Parasitol. 233, 80–85.

Ghadirian, E., Viens, P., Strykowski, H., Dubreuil, F., 1976. Epidemiology of Toxocariasis in the Montreal area. Prevalence of *Toxocara* and other helminth ova in dogs and soil. Can. J. Public Health 67 (6), 495–498.

Ghoroobi, J., Mohajerzadeh, L., Khoddami, M., Mirshemirani, A., Sadeghian, N., Mahdavi, A., Hatefi, S., 2017. Abdominal mass secondary to human toxocariasis. APSP J. Case. Rep. 8 (1), 4.

Giacometti, A., Cirioni, O., Fortuna, M., Osimani, P., Antonicelli, L., Del Prete, M.S., Riva, A., D'Errico, M.M., Petrelli, E., Scalise, G., 2000. Environmental and serological evidence for the presence of toxocariasis in the urban area of Ancona, Italy. Eur. J. Epidemiol. 16 (11), 1023–1026.

Gibbons, L.M., Jacobs, D.E., Sani, R.A., 2001. *Toxocara malaysiensis* n. sp. (Nematoda: Ascaridoidea) from the domestic cat (*Felis catus* Linnaeus, 1758). J. Parasitol. 87 (3), 660–665.

Gonzalez-Garcia, T., Munoz-Guzman, M.A., Sanchez-Arroyo, H., Prado-Ochoa, M.G., Cuellar-Ordaz, J.A., Alba-Hurtado, F., 2017. Experimental transmission of *Toxocara canis* from *Blattella germanica* and *Periplaneta americana* cockroaches to a paratenic host. Vet. Parasitol. 246, 5–10.

Greve, J.H., 1971. Age resistance to *Toxocara canis* in ascarid-free dogs. Am. J. Vet. Res. 32 (8), 1185–1192.

Gurel, F.S., Ertug, S., Okyay, P., 2005. Prevalence of *Toxocara* spp. eggs in public parks of the city of Aydin, Turkey. Türk. Parazitol. Derg. 29 (3), 177–179.

Hare, A., Franco-Paredes, C., 2014. Ocular larva migrans: a severe manifestation of an unseen epidemic. Curr. Trop. Med. Rep. 1 (1), 69–73.

Hartwich, G., 1958. Der Dachsspulwurm "*Belascaris meli*" Gedoelst, 1920, (Nematoda, Ascaridoidea) und seine systematische Stellung. Mitt. Zool. Mus. Berl. 34 (1), 57–61.

Hatzipantelis, E., Pana, Z., Tsotoulidou, V., Kalogera, A., Diakou, A., Pantoleon, A., Papageorgiou, T., 2017. Visceral larva migrans due to *Toxocara canis* in a 9-year-old boy mimicking hepatic hemangiomas. J. Paediatr. Child Health 53 (5), 517–519.

Heard, D.J., Garner, M., Greiner, E., 1995. Toxocariasis and intestinal volvulus in an island flying fox (*Pteropus hypomelanus*). J. Zoo Wildl. Med. 26 (4), 550–552.

Helwigh, A.B., Lind, P., Nansen, P., 1999. Visceral larva migrans: migratory pattern of *Toxocara canis* in pigs. Int. J. Parasitol. 29 (4), 559–565.

Inagaki, K., Kirmse, B., Bradbury, R.S., Moorthy, R.S., Arguello, I., McGuffey, C.D., Tieu, B., Hobbs, C.V., 2019. Case report: ocular toxocariasis: a report of three cases from the Mississippi delta. Am. J. Trop. Med. Hyg. 100 (5), 1223–1226.

Janecek, E., Beineke, A., Schnieder, T., Strube, C., 2014. Neurotoxocarosis: marked preference of *Toxocara canis* for the cerebrum and *T. cati* for the cerebellum in the paratenic model host mouse. Parasit. Vectors 7, 194.

Jansen, J., van Knapen, F., Schreurs, M., van Wijngaarden, T., 1993. *Toxocara* ova in parks and sandboxes in the city of Utrecht. Tijdschr. Diergeneeskd. 118 (19), 611–614.

Jarosz, W., Mizgajska-Wiktor, H., Kirwan, P., Konarski, J., Rychlicki, W., Wawrzyniak, G., 2010. Developmental age, physical fitness and *Toxocara* seroprevalence amongst lower-secondary students living in rural areas contaminated with *Toxocara* eggs. Parasitology 137 (1), 53–63.

Jimenez, B., Maya, C., Velasquez, G., Torner, F., Arambula, F., Barrios, J.A., Velasco, M., 2016. Identification and quantification of pathogenic helminth eggs using a digital image system. Exp. Parasitol. 166, 164–172.

Kanafani, Z.A., Skoury, A., Araj, G.F., El-Khoury, M., Sawaya, R.A., Atweh, S.F., Kanj, S.S., 2006. Seroprevalence of toxocariasis in Lebanon: a pilot study. Parasitology 132 (5), 635–639.

Kanobana, K., Devleesschauwer, B., Polman, K., Speybroeck, N., 2013. An agent-based model of exposure to human toxocariasis: a multi-country validation. Parasitology 140 (8), 986–998.

Khademvatan, S., Rahim, F., Tavalla, M., Abdizadeh, R., Hashemitabar, M., 2013. PCR-based molecular characterization of *Toxocara* spp. using feces of stray cats: a study from Southwest Iran. PLoS One 8 (6), e65293.

Kirkpatrick, C.E., 1988. Epizootiology of endoparasitic infections in pet dogs and cats presented to a veterinary teaching hospital. Vet. Parasitol. 30 (2), 113–124.

Klapec, T., Borecka, A., 2012. Contamination of vegetables, fruits and soil with geohelmints eggs on organic farms in Poland. Ann. Agric. Environ. Med. 19 (3), 421–425.

Kleine, A., Janecek, E., Waindok, P., Strube, C., 2016. Flotation and adherence characteristics of *Toxocara canis* and *T. cati* and a reliable method for recovering *Toxocara* eggs from soil. Vet. Parasitol. 227, 35–41.

Kleine, A., Springer, A., Strube, C., 2017. Seasonal variation in the prevalence of *Toxocara* eggs on children's playgrounds in the city of Hanover, Germany. Parasit. Vectors 10 (1), 248.

Klockiewicz, M., Sobczak-Filipiak, M., Jakubowski, T., Dlugosz, E., 2019. Histopathological lesions caused by experimental Toxocara canis and Toxascaris leonina infections in farm mink (Neovison vison). J. Vet. Res. 63 (2), 205–214.

Krucken, J., Blumke, J., Maaz, D., Demeler, J., Ramunke, S., Antolova, D., Schaper, R., von Samson-Himmelstjerna, G., 2017. Small rodents as paratenic or intermediate hosts of carnivore parasites in Berlin, Germany. PLoS One 12 (3), e0172829.

Kusnoto, Koesdarto, S., Mumpuni, S., Prasetyo, R.H., 2017. Immunoglobulin subclass in experimental murine *Toxocara cati* infection. Vet. World 10 (11), 1333–1336.

Le, T.H., Anh, N.T., Nguyen, K.T., Nguyen, N.T., Thuy do, T.T., Gasser, R.B., 2016. *Toxocara malaysiensis* infection in domestic cats in Vietnam—an emerging zoonotic issue? Infect. Genet. Evol. 37, 94–98.

Lim, S.J., Lee, S.E., Kim, S.H., Hong, S.H., You, Y.S., Kwon, O.W., Kim, H.S., 2014. Prevalence of *Toxoplasma gondii* and *Toxocara canis* among patients with uveitis. Ocul. Immunol. Inflamm. 22 (5), 360–366.

Little, S.E., Johnson, E.M., Lewis, D., Jaklitsch, R.P., Payton, M.E., Blagburn, B.L., Bowman, D.D., Moroff, S., Tams, T., Rich, L., Aucoin, D., 2009. Prevalence of intestinal parasites in pet dogs in the United States. Vet. Parasitol. 166 (1–2), 144–152.

Lloyd, S., Kristensen, S., Soulsby, E.J.L., 1981. The effect of corticosteroid therapy on infection with *Toxocara canis* in dogs. Z. Parasitenkd. 66 (1), 57–61.

Lucio-Forster, A., Mizhquiri Barbecho, J.S., Mohammed, H.O., Kornreich, B.G., Bowman, D.D., 2016. Comparison of the prevalence of *Toxocara* egg shedding by pet cats and dogs in the U.S.A., 2011–2014. Vet. Parasitol. Reg. Stud. Rep. 5, 1–13.

Ma, G., Holland, C.V., Wang, T., Hofmann, A., Fan, C.K., Maizels, R.M., Hotez, P.J., Gasser, R.B., 2018. Human toxocariasis. Lancet Infect. Dis. 18 (1), e14–e24.

Macchioni, G., 1999. A new species, *Toxocara lyncis*, in the caracal (*Lynx caracal*). Parassitologia 41 (4), 529–532.

Macuhova, K., Kumagai, T., Akao, N., Ohta, N., 2010. Loop-mediated isothermal amplification assay for detection and discrimination of *Toxocara canis* and *Toxocara cati* eggs directly from sand samples. J. Parasitol. 96 (6), 1224–1227.

Maruyama, S., Yamamoto, K., Katsube, Y., 1994. Infectivity of *Toxocara canis* larvae from Japanese quails in mice. J. Vet. Med. Sci. 56 (2), 399–401.

Mata-Santos, T., Mata-Santos, H.A., Carneiro, P.F., De Moura, K.C., Fenalti, J.M., Klafke, G.B., Cruz, L.A., Martins, L.H., Pinto, N.F., Pinto, M.C., Berne, M.E., Da Silva, P.E., Scaini, C.J., 2016. *Toxocara canis*: anthelmintic activity of quinone derivatives in murine toxocarosis. Parasitology 143 (4), 507–517.

Merdivenci, A., Sezen, Y., 1965. The resistance of tortoises, *Testudo graeca* L., against *Toxocara canis* infection. Z. Parasitenkd. 25, 387–392.

Merigueti, Y.F.F.B., Santarem, V.A., Ramires, L.M., da Silveira Batista, A., da Costa Beserra, L.V., Nuci, A.L., de Paula Esposte, T.M., 2017. Protective and risk factors associated with the presence of *Toxocara* spp. eggs in dog hair. Vet. Parasitol. 244, 39–43.

Mikaeili, F., Mirhendi, H., Hosseini, M., Asgari, Q., Kia, E.B., 2013. *Toxocara* nematodes in stray cats from Shiraz, southern Iran: intensity of infection and molecular identification of the isolates. Iran. J. Parasitol. 8 (4), 593–600.

Millan, J., Casanova, J.C., 2009. High prevalence of helminth parasites in feral cats in Majorca Island (Spain). Parasitol. Res. 106 (1), 183–188.

Mizgajska, H., 2001. Eggs of *Toxocara* spp. in the environment and their public health implications. J. Helminthol. 75 (2), 147–151.

Mizgajska-Wiktor, H., 2005. Recommended method for recovery of *Toxocara* and other geohelminth eggs from soil. Wiad. Parazytol. 51 (1), 21–22.

Mohamed, A.S., Moore, G.E., Glickman, L.T., 2009. Prevalence of intestinal nematode parasitism among pet dogs in the United States (2003–2006). J. Am. Vet. Med. Assoc. 234 (5), 631–637.

Morgan, E.R., Azam, D., Pegler, K., 2013. Quantifying sources of environmental contamination with *Toxocara* spp. eggs. Vet. Parasitol. 193 (4), 390–397.

Moura, M.Q., Macedo, M.R.P., Terto, W.D.D.S., Avila, L.F.D.C., Leivas Leite, F.P., Scaini, C.J., Pinto, N.B., Capella, G.A., Strothmann, A.L., Villela, M.M., Berne, M.E.A., 2018. Detection of *Toxocara canis* DNA in tissues of experimentally infected mice. Acta Trop. 187, 51–56.

Mozgovoĭ, A.A., 1953. Principles of nematodology, edited by K. I. Skryabin. Vol. II. Ascaridata of animals and man and diseases caused by them. Part II. (Askaridaty Zhivotnykh i Cheloveka i Vyzyvaemye Imi Zabolevaniya). Izdatelstvo Akademii Nauk, Moscow.

Mozgovoĭ, A.A., Shakhmatova, V.I., 1986. Ascaridata of animals and man and the diseases caused by them. In: Fundamentals of Nematodology, 3. vol. 23. Oxonian Press.

Mughini-Gras, L., Harms, M., van Pelt, W., Pinelli, E., Kortbeek, T., 2016. Seroepidemiology of human *Toxocara* and *Ascaris* infections in the Netherlands. Parasitol. Res. 115 (10), 3779–3794.

Naidu, T.S.V., 1981. Two new ascarid nematodes from vertebrate hosts from India. Folia Parasitol. 28 (4), 327–334.

Nijsse, R., Mughini-Gras, L., Wagenaar, J.A., Ploeger, H.W., 2014. Coprophagy in dogs interferes in the diagnosis of parasitic infections by faecal examination. Vet. Parasitol. 204 (3–4), 304–309.

Nijsse, R., Mughini-Gras, L., Wagenaar, J.A., Franssen, F., Ploeger, H.W., 2015. Environmental contamination with *Toxocara* eggs: a quantitative approach to estimate the relative contributions of dogs, cats and foxes, and to assess the efficacy of advised interventions in dogs. Parasit. Vectors 8, 397.

Nijsse, R., Mughini-Gras, L., Wagenaar, J.A., Ploeger, H.W., 2016. Recurrent patent infections with *Toxocara canis* in household dogs older than six months: a prospective study. Parasit. Vectors 9 (1), 531.

Nikolay, B., Brooker, S.J., Pullan, R.L., 2014. Sensitivity of diagnostic tests for human soil-transmitted helminth infections: a meta-analysis in the absence of a true gold standard. Int. J. Parasitol. 44 (11), 765–774.

Noda, R., 1966. A new species of *Neoascaris* (Nematoda) from a Japanese badger. Bull. Univ. Osaka Pref., Ser. B Agric. Life Sci. 18, 11–16.

Noh, Y., Hong, S.T., Yun, J.Y., Park, H.K., Oh, J.H., Kim, Y.E., Jeon, B.S., 2012. Meningitis by *Toxocara canis* after ingestion of raw ostrich liver. J. Korean Med. Sci. 27 (9), 1105–1108.

Nolan, T.J., Smith, G., 1995. Time series analysis of the prevalence of endoparasitic infections in cats and dogs presented to a veterinary teaching hospital. Vet. Parasitol. 59 (2), 87–96.
O'Lorcain, P., 1994. Epidemiology of *Toxocara* spp. in stray dogs and cats in Dublin, Ireland. J. Helminthol. 68 (4), 331–336.
Ortlepp, R.J., 1924. On a collection of helminths from Dutch Guiana. J. Helminthol. 2 (1), 15–40.
Otero, D., Alho, A.M., Nijsse, R., Roelfsema, J., Overgaauw, P., Madeira de Carvalho, L., 2018. Environmental contamination with *Toxocara* spp. eggs in public parks and playground sandpits of Greater Lisbon, Portugal. J. Infect. Public Health 11 (1), 94–98.
Overgaauw, P.A.M., 1997a. Aspects of *Toxocara* epidemiology: toxocarosis in dogs and cats. Crit. Rev. Microbiol. 23 (3), 233–251.
Overgaauw, P.A.M., 1997b. Aspects of *Toxocara* epidemiology: human toxocarosis. Crit. Rev. Microbiol. 23 (3), 215–231.
Overgaauw, P.A.M., van Knapen, F., 2013. Veterinary and public health aspects of *Toxocara* spp. Vet. Parasitol. 193 (4), 398–403.
Overgaauw, P.A.M., Okkens, A.C., Bevers, M.M., Kortbeek, L.M., 1998. Incidence of patent *Toxocara canis* infection in bitches during the oestrous cycle. Vet. Q. 20 (3), 104–107.
Overgaauw, P.A.M., van Zutphen, L., Hoek, D., Yaya, F.O., Roelfsema, J., Pinelli, E., van Knapen, F., Kortbeek, L.M., 2009. Zoonotic parasites in fecal samples and fur from dogs and cats in The Netherlands. Vet. Parasitol. 163 (1–2), 115–122.
Özbakış, G., Doğanay, A., 2019. Visceral larva migrans detection using PCR-RFLP in BALB/c mice infected with *Toxocara canis*. J. Helminthol. 94, 1–8.
Ozlati, M., Spotin, A., Shahbazi, A., Mahami-Oskouei, M., Hazratian, T., Adibpor, M., Ahmadpour, E., Dolatkhah, A., Khoshakhlagh, P., 2016. Genetic variability and discrimination of low doses of *Toxocara* spp. from public areas soil inferred by loop-mediated isothermal amplification assay as a field-friendly molecular tool. Vet. World 9 (12), 1471–1477.
Pahari, T.K., Sasmal, N.K., 1991. Experimental infection of Japanese quail with *Toxocara canis* larvae through earthworms. Vet. Parasitol. 39 (3–4), 337–340.
Panova, O.A., Khrustalev, A.V., 2018. Dog walking brings *Toxocara* eggs to people's homes. Vet. Parasitol. 262, 16–19.
Paoletti, B., Traversa, D., Iorio, R., De Berardinis, A., Bartolini, R., Salini, R., Di Cesare, A., 2015. Zoonotic parasites in feces and fur of stray and private dogs from Italy. Parasitol. Res. 114 (6), 2135–2141.
Pautova, E.A., Shchuchinova, L.D., Dovgalev, A.S., 2015. The development and survival of *Toxocara canis* eggs in the natural climatic conditions of Gorno-Altaisk. Med. Parazitol. (Mosk) 2, 42–44.
Pawlowski, Z., 2001. Toxocariasis in humans: clinical expression and treatment dilemma. J. Helminthol. 75 (4), 299–305.
Pinelli, E., Herremans, T., Harms, M.G., Hoek, D., Kortbeek, L.M., 2011. *Toxocara* and *Ascaris* seropositivity among patients suspected of visceral and ocular larva migrans in the Netherlands: trends from 1998 to 2009. Eur. J. Clin. Microbiol. Infect. Dis. 30 (7), 873–879.
Poulsen, C.S., Skov, S., Yoshida, A., Skallerup, P., Maruyama, H., Thamsborg, S.M., Nejsum, P., 2015. Differential serodiagnostics of *Toxocara canis* and *Toxocara cati*—is it possible? Parasite Immunol. 37 (4), 204–207.
Prociv, P., 1990. Aberrent migration by *Toxocara pteropodis* in flying foxes. J. Wildl. Dis. 26 (4), 532–534.
Puylaert, F.A., 1967a. Un nouvel ascardide Toxocara vincenti sp.n. parasite de Civettictis civetta Schreber. Bulletin du Muséum national d'histoire naturelle 39, 736.

Puylaert, F.A., 1967b. Un nouvel ascaride, *Toxocara canarisi* sp. n. parasite de *Felis (Leptailurus) serval* Schreber (Vermes-Nematoda). Rev. Zool. Bot. Africaines 76, 77–82.

Radwan, N.A., Khalil, A.I., El Mahi, R.A., 2009. Morphology and occurrence of species of *Toxocara* in wild mammal populations from Egypt. Comp. Parasitol. 76 (2), 273–282.

Ranasuriya, G., Mian, A., Boujaoude, Z., Tsigrelis, C., 2014. Pulmonary toxocariasis: a case report and literature review. Infection 42 (3), 575–578.

Reiterová, K., Antolová, D., Zalesny, G., Stanko, M., Špilovská, S., Mošanský, L., 2013. Small rodents—permanent reservoirs of toxocarosis in different habitats of Slovakia. Helminthologia 50 (1), 20–26.

Rodríguez Gallegos, L.M., Romero Núñez, C., Bautista Gómez, L., Martínez Castañeda, J., Heredia Cardenas, R., 2016. Presence of Toxocara spp. in domestic cats in the state of Mexico. Acta Sci. Vet. 44, 1351.

Romano, N., Nor Azah, M.O., Rahmah, N., Lim, Y.A.L., Rohela, M., 2010. Seroprevalence of toxocariasis among Orang Asli (Indigenous people) in Malaysia using two immunoassays. Trop. Biomed. 27 (3), 585–594.

Romeu, J., Roig, J., Bada, J.L., Riera, C., Munoz, C., 1991. Adult human toxocariasis acquired by eating raw snails. J. Infect. Dis. 164 (2), 438.

Rostami, A., Ma, G., Wang, T., Koehler, A.V., Hofmann, A., Chang, B.C.H., Macpherson, C.N., Gasser, R.B., 2019. Human toxocariasis—a look at a neglected disease through an epidemiological 'prism'. Infect. Genet. Evol. 74, 104002.

Round, M.C., 1968. Check list of the helminth parasites of African mammals of the orders carnivora, tubulidentata, proboscidea, hyracoidea, artiodactyla and perissodactyla. In: Commonwealth Agricultural Bureaux, Farnham Royal. Commonwealth Agricultural Bureaux, United Kingdom, Technical Communication No. 38.

Saeed, I.S., Kapel, C.M., 2006. Population dynamics and epidemiology of *Toxocara canis* in Danish red foxes. J. Parasitol. 92 (6), 1196–1201.

Saeed, I., Maddox-Hyttel, C., Monrad, J., Kapel, C.M., 2006. Helminths of red foxes (*Vulpes vulpes*) in Denmark. Vet. Parasitol. 139 (1–3), 168–179.

Santarem, V.A., Chesine, P.A., Lamers, B.E., Rubinsky-Elefant, G., Giuffrida, R., 2011. Anti-*Toxocara* spp. antibodies in sheep from southeastern Brazil. Vet. Parasitol. 179 (1–3), 283–286.

Sasmal, N.K., Pahari, T.K., Laha, R., 2008. Experimental infection of the cockroach *Periplaneta americana* with *Toxocara canis* and the establishment of patent infections in pups. J. Helminthol. 82 (2), 97–100.

Schnieder, T., Laabs, E.M., Welz, C., 2011. Larval development of *Toxocara canis* in dogs. Vet. Parasitol. 175 (3–4), 193–206.

Sharif, M., Daryani, A., Barzegar, G., Nasrolahei, M., Khalilian, A., 2010. Seroprevalence of toxocariasis in schoolchildren in Northern Iran. Pak. J. Biol. Sci. 13 (4), 180–184.

Shimizu, T., 1993. Prevalence of *Toxocara* eggs in sandpits in Tokushima city and its outskirts. J. Vet. Med. Sci. 55 (5), 807–811.

Smith, H., Holland, C., Taylor, M., Magnaval, J., Schantz, P., Maizels, R., 2009. How common is human toxocariasis? Towards standardizing our knowledge. Trends Parasitol. 25 (4), 182–188.

Sowemimo, O.A., 2007. Prevalence and intensity of *Toxocara canis* (Werner, 1782) in dogs and its potential public health significance in Ile-Ife, Nigeria. J. Helminthol. 81 (4), 433–438.

Sowemimo, O.A., 2012. Prevalence and intensity of gastrointestinal parasites of domestic cats in Ode—Irele and Oyo communities, Southwest Nigeria. J. Parasitol. Vector Biol. 4 (1), 7–13.

Sprent, J.F.A., 1956. The life history and development of *Toxocara cati* (Schrank 1788) in the domestic cat. Parasitology 46 (1–2), 54–78.
Sprent, J.F.A., 1958. Observations on the development of *Toxocara canis* (Werner, 1782) in the dog. Parasitology 48 (1–2), 184–209.
Sprent, J.F.A., 1972. *Toxocara vajrasthirae* sp. nov. from the hog-badger (*Arctonyx collaris*) of Thailand. Parasitology 65 (3), 491–498.
Springer, A., Heuer, L., Janecek-Erfurth, E., Beineke, A., Strube, C., 2019. Histopathological characterization of *Toxocara canis* and *T. cati* induced neurotoxocarosis in the mouse model. Parasitol. Res. 118 (9), 2591–2600.
Sternheim, I., 2012. Hoe Nederland zwerfhondenarm is geworden. Report of Dog Research Initiative, pp. 1–9. https://www.stray-afp.org/nl/wp-content/uploads/sites/2/2015/11/DR_Dutch_Straydogs1.pdf.
Strube, C., Heuer, L., Janecek, E., 2013. *Toxocara* spp. infections in paratenic hosts. Vet. Parasitol. 193 (4), 375–389.
Taira, K., Saitoh, Y., Okada, N., Sugiyama, H., Kapel, C.M., 2012. Tolerance to low temperatures of *Toxocara cati* larvae in chicken muscle tissue. Vet. Parasitol. 189 (2–4), 383–386.
Talvik, H., Moks, E., Magi, E., Jarvis, T., Miller, I., 2006. Distribution of *Toxocara* infection in the environment and in definitive and paratenic hosts in Estonia. Acta Vet. Hung. 54 (3), 399–406.
Uga, S., 1993. Prevalence of Toxocara eggs and number of faecal deposits from dogs and cats in sandpits of public parks in Japan. J. Helminthol. 67 (1), 78–82.
Uga, S., Ono, K., Kataoka, N., Safriah, A., Tantular, I.S., Dachlan, Y.P., Ranuh, I.G., 1995. Contamination of soil with parasite eggs in Surabaya, Indonesia. Southeast Asian J. Trop. Med. Public Health 26 (4), 730–734.
Uga, S., Matsuo, J., Kimura, D., Rai, S.K., Koshino, Y., Igarashi, K., 2000. Differentiation of *Toxocara canis* and *T. cati* eggs by light and scanning electron microscopy. Vet. Parasitol. 92 (4), 287–294.
Uga, S., Hoa, N.T., Noda, S., Moji, K., Cong, L., Aoki, Y., Rai, S.K., Fujimaki, Y., 2009. Parasite egg contamination of vegetables from a suburban market in Hanoi, Vietnam. Nepal Med. Coll. J. 11 (2), 75–78.
Umeche, N., Mandah, L.E., 1989. *Musca domestica* as a carrier of intestinal helminths in Calabar, Nigeria. East Afr. Med. J. 66 (5), 349–352.
Van De, N., Trung, N.V., Duyet le, V., Chai, J.Y., 2013. Molecular diagnosis of an ocular toxocariasis patient in Vietnam. Korean J. Parasitol. 51 (5), 563–567.
Vega, R.M., Gonzalez Prous, C., Krivokapich, S., Gatti, G., Brugni, N.L., Semenas, L., 2018. Toxocariasis in carnivora from Argentinean Patagonia: species molecular identification, hosts, and geographical distribution. Int. J. Parasitol. Parasites Wildl. 7 (1), 106–110.
Vuylsteke, C., 1956. Note sur quelques nematodes parasites avec description de neuf espèces nouvelles. Revue zool. bot. Africaines 53, 441–477.
Warren, E.G., 1969. Infections of *Toxocara canis* in dogs fed infected mouse tissues. Parasitology 59 (4), 837–841.
Warren, E.G., 1970. Studies on the morphology and taxonomy of the genera *Toxocara* Stiles, 1905 and *Neoascaris* Travassos 1927. Zool. Anz. 185 (5/6), 393–442.
Warren, E.G., 1972. Two new species of *Toxocara* from viverrid hosts. Parasitology 65 (2), 179–187.
Webster, J.P., MacDonald, D.W., 1995. Parasites of wild brown rats (*Rattus norvegicus*) on UK farms. Parasitology 111, 247–255.
Wiwanitkit, V., Waenlor, W., 2004. The frequency rate of *Toxocara* species contamination in soil samples from public yards in a urban area "Payathai", Bangkok, Thailand. Rev. Inst. Med. Trop. Sao Paulo 46 (2), 113–114.

Won, K.Y., Kruszon-Moran, D., Schantz, P.M., Jones, J.L., 2008. National seroprevalence and risk factors for zoonotic *Toxocara* spp. infection. Am. J. Trop. Med. Hyg. 79 (4), 552–557.

Yu, T., Zhao, L.N., Fan, M.J., Wu, H., Chen, Q.K., 2012. Visceral larva migrans associated with earthworm and gecko ingestion: a case report. J. Med Case Reports 6, 21–210.

Zhu, X.Q., Jacobs, D.E., Chilton, N.B., Sani, R.A., Cheng, N.A.B.Y., Gasser, R.B., 1998. Molecular characterization of a *Toxocara* variant from cats in Kuala Lumpur, Malaysia. Parasitology 117 (2), 155–164.

Zibaei, M., Sadjjadi, S.M., 2017. Trend of toxocariasis in Iran: a review on human and animal dimensions. Iran. J. Vet. Res. 18 (4), 233–242.

Zibaei, M., Sadjjadi, S.M., Maraghi, S., 2017. The occurrence of *Toxocara* species in naturally infected broiler chickens revealed by molecular approaches. J. Helminthol. 91 (5), 633–636.

CHAPTER THIRTY

Global prevalence of *Toxocara* infection in cats

Ali Rostami[a,*], Mahdi Sepidarkish[b], Guangxu Ma[c], Tao Wang[c], Maryam Ebrahimi[d], Yadolah Fakhri[e], Hamed Mirjalali[f], Andreas Hofmann[c], Calum N.L. Macpherson[g], Peter J. Hotez[h], Robin B. Gasser[c,*]

[a]Infectious Diseases and Tropical Medicine Research Center, Health Research Institute, Babol University of Medical Sciences, Babol, Iran
[b]Department of Epidemiology and Biostatistics, School of Medicine, Babol University of Medical Sciences, Babol, Iran
[c]Department of Veterinary Biosciences, Melbourne Veterinary School, Faculty of Veterinary and Agricultural Sciences, The University of Melbourne, Parkville, VIC, Australia
[d]Department of Parasitology and Mycology, School of Medicine, Shahid Beheshti University of Medical Sciences, Tehran, Iran
[e]Department of Environmental Health Engineering, Student Research Committee, School of Public Health, Shahid Beheshti University of Medical Sciences, Tehran, Iran
[f]Foodborne and Waterborne Diseases Research Center, Research Institute for Gastroenterology and Liver Diseases, Shahid Beheshti University of Medical Sciences, Tehran, Iran
[g]School of Graduate Studies, School of Veterinary Medicine, St. George's University, WINDREF, Grenada, West Indies
[h]Texas Children's Hospital Center for Vaccine Development, Departments of Pediatrics and Molecular Virology & Microbiology, National School of Tropical Medicine, Baylor College of Medicine, Houston, TX, United States
*Corresponding authors: e-mail address: alirostami1984@gmail.com; robinbg@unimelb.edu.au

Contents

Advances in Parasitology, Volume 109
ISSN 0065-308X
https://doi.org/10.1016/bs.apar.2020.01.025

Abstract

Zoonotic parasites, including *Toxocara* species, of pet and stray cats are of public health importance. Justification for, and the design and implementation of prevention and control of human toxocariasis may benefit from an understanding of the zoonotic potential and prevalence of parasites in this definitive host species. This is the first systematic review and meta-analysis of cross-sectional studies, conducted to estimate the prevalence of *Toxocara* infection(s) in cats by geographical location, type (rural vs urban and stray vs pet), gender and age. Pooled data were assessed using a random effects-model as well as several meta-regression and stratified analyses conducted. Of 1733 peer-reviewed articles, 143 were included in this review and represented 2,158,069 cats from 51 countries. The global pooled (95% CI) prevalence of *Toxocara* infection in cats was 17.0% (16.1–17.8%), being highest in African (43.3%, 28.3–58.4%) and lowest in South American (12.6%, 8.2–17.0%) countries. In other WHO regions, prevalence rates of *Toxocara* were as follows: Eastern Mediterranean (21.6%, 15.1–28.1%), North America (18.3%, 15.4–21.2%), Europe (17.8%, 15.9–19.7%), Western Pacific (17.3%, 14.7–19.9%), and South-East Asia (14.9%, 9.8–20.1%). Prevalence of *Toxocara* was higher in low-income tropical countries and also in stray (28.6%, 25.1–32.1%) and young ($\leq$12 months of age) (27.7%, 23.4–32.0%) cats than in pet (11.6%, 10.7–12.5%) and older cats (>12 months of age) (23.8%, 14.8–32.7%). This review indicates that ~118–150 million cats worldwide serve as definitive hosts of *Toxocara*, shedding eggs and thus contributing to the public health risk of human infection. Prevention and control of this zoonosis in cats should receive greater attention by health officials and cat owners, particularly in countries where risk factors and prevalence are highest.

1. Introduction

There is a long history of domestic cats (*Felis catus*) having a close relationship with humans. Cats are important human companions and can play a significant role in enhancing mental health and well-being of people (Beck and Meyers, 1996; Paul et al., 2010). The global cat population is estimated at 700 million (https://www.carocat.eu). Depending on "life-style", cats can be classified as pets (owned and kept indoors) and stray/feral cats (unowned domestic animals that live outdoors and avoid human contact) (Greene, 2006). It is estimated that there are 220 million pet cats and 480 million stray cats worldwide (https://www.carocat.eu). These numbers are likely to under-estimate the global cat population, as a pet owner survey conducted in the USA revealed that there were ~95.6 million pet cats in the USA alone in 2017 (http://statista.com).

Some taxa of *Toxocara* (order Ascaridida) are zoonotic, with *T. canis* likely being the most important and geographically widespread species, with canids as the main definitive hosts (Holland and Smith, 2006; Overgaauw and van Knapen, 2013; Rostami et al., 2019a). In humans, there are four main syndromes resulting from zoonotic *Toxocara* infection, including visceral larva migrans (VLM), ocular larva migrans (OLM), neurotoxocariasis (NT) (e.g. eosinophilic meningoencephalitis) and common/covert toxocariasis (CT) (Ma et al., 2018; Macpherson, 2013; Rostami et al., 2019a). Associations with neurological and allergic disorders have been described (Aghaei et al., 2018; Aghamolaie et al., 2018; Luna et al., 2018; Mohammadzadeh et al., 2018). An additional finding that human co-infections with *Toxocara* and *Toxoplasma* are common in North America and possibly elsewhere (Jones et al., 2008; Liu et al., 2019) suggests that cats may contribute a higher percentage of *Toxocara* eggs into the environment (relative to dogs) than previously realised.

To date, only a few clinical cases in humans have been attributed to infection with *T. cati* (syn. *T. mystax*) (Fisher, 2003; Shimokawa et al., 1982). The syndrome most commonly associated with *T. cati* infection in human cases has been OLM, diagnosed using the Ouchterlony test (Fillau and Magnaval, 2013), and a single case by ELISA (Sakai et al., 1998). A case of *T. cati* causing VLM in a patient has also been reported (Shimokawa et al., 1982). A number of cases of children vomiting adult worms, identified as *T. cati*, have also been reported, but whether they represent a zoonotic infection remains controversial (Eberhard and Alfano, 1998; Fisher, 2003). The *Toxocara* species causing human infection are rarely characterised molecularly. Without such information, the true zoonotic potential of *T. cati* remains unclear. Thus, additional study of *T. cati* is required. The same applies to *T. malaysiensis*, which has also been recorded in cats in Malaysia, China and Vietnam (cf. Gasser, 2013; Gibbons et al., 2001; Holland and Smith, 2006; Le et al., 2016; Oguz et al., 2018).

Cats are infected with *T. cati* via the ingestion of embryonated eggs from soil or larvae within paratenic hosts (e.g. rodents) or milk (transmammary or lactogenic transmission in kittens) from the queen cat (Coati et al., 2004; Overgaauw and van Knapen, 2013). Following ingestion by the cat, infective larvae in milk or from *T. cati* eggs, penetrate the intestinal wall and then migrate through liver and lungs to the airways, and make their way to the small intestine, where fourth-stage larvae (L4s) develop to the adult stage (within 2–3 months) (Despommier, 2003). Fertilised female worms may release thousands of unembryonated eggs in faeces per day, contributing to often substantial environmental contamination (Fakhri et al., 2018; Fan et al., 2013). In suitable environments (depending on the temperature and humidity), embryonation occurs within 2–5 weeks, and the eggs can remain viable in soil for up to several years under favourable conditions (Despommier, 2003; Fan et al., 2013). Both stray and, to a lesser extent, pet cats can play a role in contaminating the environment with *Toxocara* eggs by defaecating in public places, after which *Toxocara* eggs embryonate and then become infective to a range of mammals including humans; such infective eggs represent a risk to people, as it was indicated that about one fifth (21%, 16–27%) of public places around the world are contaminated with *Toxocara* eggs (Fakhri et al., 2018). Moreover, some recent studies reported that direct contact with contaminated fur of an infected cat might be a source of *Toxocara* eggs (Bakhshani et al., 2019; Öge et al., 2014; Overgaauw et al., 2009).

T. cati may also cause significant disease in cats, with heavy worm burdens in kittens resulting in the feline host failing to thrive and, in some instances, infection being fatal (Overgaauw and van Knapen, 2013). Some food animals, including pigs, sheep and chickens, can served as paratenic hosts for *Toxocara* species including *T. cati* (see Strube et al., 2013; Ziegler and Macpherson, 2019). In these hosts, larvae undergo migration into various tissues and would appear to survive there for years (Sommerfelt et al., 2014; Strube et al., 2013; Taira et al., 2011). If raw or undercooked meat or viscera, including liver, from such animals are consumed by humans, this may result in infection or disease (e.g. Choi et al., 2008; Morimatsu et al., 2006; Strube et al., 2013; Yoshikawa et al., 2008). Clearly, studies of the prevalence of *T. cati* and its infection intensity in cats are important from both the veterinary and public health perspectives. In the past decades, many epidemiological studies have been carried out in different parts of the world to estimate the prevalence of *Toxocara* infection in cats (Fisher, 2003), but most studies were focused on limited geographical areas, and knowledge gaps remains for many countries and territories.

Considering the public health issues relating to cats as a source of *Toxocara* infection, a summary of data on the global prevalence of *Toxocara* infection in cats is important for public health officials, medical practitioners and veterinarians alike. There had not been a comprehensive analysis of prevalence data for *T. cati* or *T. malaysiensis* infection in cats. This review provides the first systematic overview and meta-analysis to assess the global and regional prevalence rates of *T. cati* infection in cats, and also evaluates specific risk factors, and the impact of geographical and climate features on prevalence.

2. Methodology

This meta-analysis study was conducted according to recommendations from the Preferred Reporting Items for Systematic Reviews and Meta-Analyses (PRISMA) statement (Moher et al., 2015).

2.1 Search strategy and selection criteria

We extensively searched the electronic databases EMBASE, PubMed, Scopus, SciELO and Web of Science for records in the time period from 1 January 1990 to 1 July 2019, using the following search terms: "*Toxocara* infection", "*Toxocara* spp.", "*Toxocara cati*", "gastrointestinal helminth", "intestinal parasites", "endoparasites", "prevalence", "epidemiology", "cat", "kitten" and "feline". The literature search was enhanced via searches using the Google Scholar search engine as well as manual appraisals of the bibliographies of key reviews and studies. No language or geographical restrictions were applied. For the present meta-analysis, a cat was considered infected if *Toxocara* eggs were detected by faecal flotation or hair examination, or adult worms of *Toxocara* were identified at postmortem examination.

All search results were imported into the Endnote (v.X8) reference management software and any duplicates were removed. Two independent investigators (M.E. and H.M.) screened all publications by title and abstract and eliminated irrelevant studies. The full texts of the remaining studies were reviewed in depth against the eligibility criteria. Where discrepancies arose, studies were discussed with a third investigator (A.R.) to resolve any issues.

Inclusion criteria were: (i) cross-sectional studies reporting the prevalence of *Toxocara* (in at least 30 cats), (ii) published in a peer-reviewed journal; and (iii) a faecal or hair examination to detect and identify *Toxocara* eggs, or an autopsy to identify adult worms of *Toxocara*. We excluded: articles without the abovementioned criteria or studies that focused only on the comparative evaluation of diagnostic methods; case-reports; case-series studies; and review articles.

2.2 Data extraction and quality assessment

Two of the authors (H.M. and M.E.) worked independently, in a blinded manner, on data extraction. They used a comprehensive form and extracted the following information from each study: first author's last name; year of publication; time period during which the study was conducted; country;

city; types of samples tested (faecal, hair and/or carcass); diagnostic test used (faecal flotation, smear or other); type of cat (pet or stray); number of cats studied; and number of cats with a positive test result. In addition, if possible, prevalence was stratified by age ($\leq$12 vs >12 months of age), gender and geographical origin. Since various types of cats were studied in previous publications, for convenience, we divided cats into: (i) *pet (domestic) cats*: "pet, household, sheltered or domestic"; (ii), *stray cats*: "stray, free-roaming or feral". We excluded studies performed on "jungle" cats. Any discrepancy was resolved by a third reviewer (A.R.). All extracted data were assessed for accuracy by the principal author/supervisor (A.R.).

All geographical areas (i.e. countries and cities) studied were classified according to WHO-region (Africa, Eastern Mediterranean, Europe, Southeast Asia, the Americas or Western Pacific) (World Health Organization, 2003); World Bank's income category (https://datahelpdesk.worldbank.org); geographical latitude and longitude; mean relative environmental humidity; and mean environmental temperature. The Americas were further divided into North America and South America, because there is significant variance in socio-demographic and climatic status between these two areas. The following data sources were used to define the geographical and climatic status of cities, regions or areas studied: https://www.timeanddate.com/, https://en.climate-data.org/ and https://gps-coordinates.org/.

To critically assess quality and the risk of bias in each study included in this meta-analysis, we used a well-defined method (Supplementary Table S2 in Supplementary material in the online version at https://doi.org/10.1016/bs.apar.2020.01.025) that is usually applied to systematic reviews exploring prevalence (Munn et al., 2014). Y.F. and A.R. independently appraised the quality of each study, and any disagreement was reconciled in a team discussion. Each individual study (article) was ranked according to 10 criteria (collection of a representative sample, recruitment of participants in an appropriate way, sample size, setting description, subject description, outcome measurement, reliable measurements, data analysis, subpopulations analysis and adjustment for confounders) (Munn et al., 2014). Publications that met 7–10, 4–6 and 1–3 criteria were ranked as "low risk", "moderate risk", and "high risk", respectively.

2.3 Meta-analysis

As high heterogeneity was expected among studies, all analyses were performed using the random effect model (REM) as described by

DerSimonian and Laird (1986). The global and regional prevalences established for all studies were combined to generate a "pooled estimate" with a 95% confidence interval (CI). Heterogeneity was assessed using the I^2 statistic; I^2 values of >50% indicate high heterogeneity (cf. Higgins et al., 2003). We applied several meta-regression and subgroup analyses to identify the source of heterogeneity. Subgroup analyses were undertaken according to geographic region, income level in a country, sample size, type of cat, type of diagnostic method, age, gender, geographical and climate variables (including latitude, longitude, mean relative humidity, mean temperature and precipitation) and risk of bias. The χ^2 test was used to compare prevalences among distinct subgroups. Meta-regression analyses were used to examine the effects of time, income level, geographical and climate parameters on prevalence. Publication bias was not assessed in this study, as it is not considered relevant for prevalence studies (Hunter et al., 2014). All statistical analyses were conducted using STATA v.13 (STATA Corp., College Station, Texas, USA). The results from statistical analyses were regarded as significant if the *P*-value was <0.05.

3. Eligible studies, their characteristics and data sets

Our literature search returned 1733 publications. In total, 143 unique studies containing 180 data sets were scored as eligible and were thus selected for data extraction (Fig. 1). All 180 data sets represented 2,158,069 cats from 51 countries in all WHO regions. The highest number of studies (74 data sets) were conducted in the European region, while most cats (2,109,397) were studied in the USA. Data were from 23 countries in the European region, 10 in the Western Pacific region, 6 in the Eastern Mediterranean region, 5 in North America, 3 in South America, two in the African region, and 2 in the Southeast Asian region. Most data sets were from countries with high-level of income (166 data sets; 2,145,256 cats), while 52 data sets (11,521 cats) were from countries with a middle to upper level of income, and only 12 data sets (1340 cats) were from countries with a middle to low-income level. There was no study from countries with a low level of income. Ninety-five data sets were available for pet cats, 72 for stray cats; in 13 studies, the type of cats was not described. One hundred and three data sets used faecal flotation for the detection of *Toxocara* infection. Supplementary Table S1 in Supplementary material in the online version at https://doi.org/10.1016/bs.apar.2020.01.025 (appendix) details the main characteristics of all studies included in this investigation.

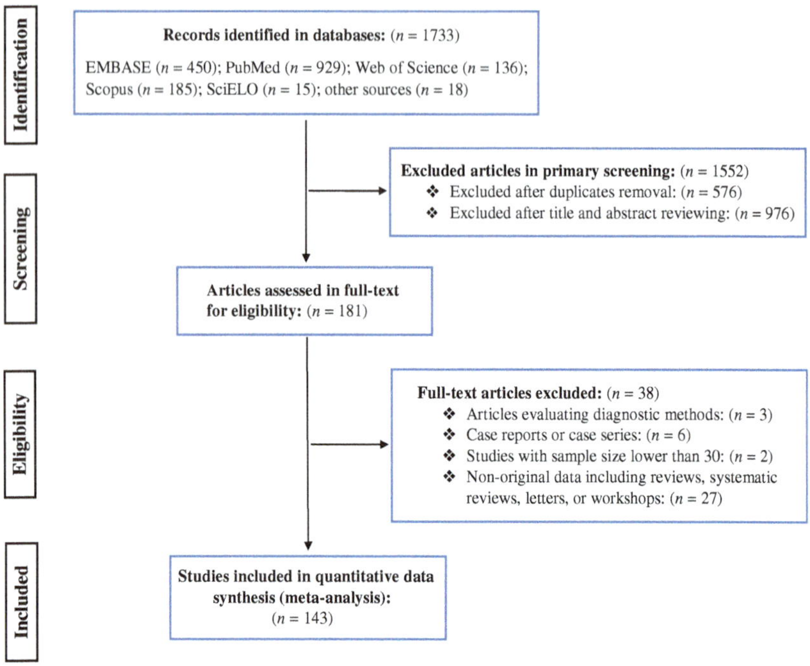

Fig. 1 Flow diagram showing the search and selection methodology used, which follows PRISMA guidelines.

4. Global and regional prevalences of *Toxocara* infection in cats

The pooled global prevalence of *Toxocara* infection in cats was 17.0% (95% CI, 16.1–17.8%; Table 1). The heterogeneity among studies was significant ($I^2 = 98.3\%$, $P < .001$). In relation to WHO-regions, prevalences were: 43.3% (28.3–58.4%) in the African region; 21.6% (15.1–28.1%) in the Eastern Mediterranean region; 18.3% (15.4–21.2%) in North American countries; 17.8% (15.9–19.7%) in the European region; 17.3% (14.7–19.9%) in the Western Pacific region; 14.9% (9.8–20.1%) in the South-East Asia region; and 12.6% (8.2–17.0%) in South America. In sensitivity analysis, we assessed the effect of one study with a very large sample size (>2 million cats) from the USA (Lucio-Forster et al., 2016) on the global prevalence rate. This analysis showed that the global prevalence rate altered to 22.6% (21.4–23.8%) following the removal of data reported in this study (Lucio-Forster et al., 2016) from the present investigation. For

Table 1 Global, regional and national prevalence of *Toxocara* infection in cats (results from 180 data sets performed in 51 countries).

WHO regions / Country	Number of data sets	Total number of samples	Number of test-positive samples	Pooled prevalence (%) established using meta-analysis (95% CI)	Heterogeneity I^2 (%)
Global	**180**	**2,158,069**	**110,148**	**17.0 (16.1–17.8)[a]**	**98.35**
African region	**4**	**422**	**183**	**43.3 (28.3–58.4)**	**89.78**
Nigeria	3	319	159	50.0 (44.0–55.0)	NA
Kenya	1	103	24	23.0 (16.0–33.0)	NA
Eastern Mediterranean region	**24**	**3542**	**621**	**21.6 (15.1–28.1)**	**98.35**
Iran	17	2055	520	26.0 (15.1–36.9)	97.80
Egypt	2	283	24	8.47 (5.2–11.7)	NA
Iraq	2	206	60	28.12 (3.5–52.7)	NA
Pakistan	1	100	5	5.0 (1.6–11.3)	NA
United Arab Emirates	1	658	5	2.9 (1.2–5.9)	NA
Qatar	1	240	7	0.1 (0.002–1.8)	NA
North America	**34**	**2,113,108**	**104,670**	**18.3 (15.4–21.2)**	**98.70**
USA	15	2,109,397	103,909	20.3 (15.7–24.9)	99.09
Canada	12	2032	267	14.5 (8.8–20.3)	96.90
Mexico	5	1538	172	24.5 (7.4–41.6)	99.34
West Indies	2	141	5	3.4 (0.1–6.3)	NA
Colombia	1	121	45	37.2 (28.5–46.4)	NA
European region	**74**	**26,075**	**3035**	**17.8 (15.9–19.7)**	**97.81**
Spain	9	1555	254	19.8 (13.5–26.1)	91.56
Greece	8	1779	375	18.2 (11.4–25.1)	89.67
Italy	7	1507	297	20.4 (14.2–26.7)	90.17
Netherlands	6	1380	78	5.4 (1.9–8.9)	87.42
Germany	6	14,674	898	7.7 (4.3–11.1)	99.25
Poland	5	322	81	27.6 (8.6–46.6)	94.73
Turkey	4	372	74	19.5 (15.5–23.5)	0

Continued

Table 1 Global, regional and national prevalence of *Toxocara* infection in cats (results from 180 data sets performed in 51 countries).—cont'd

WHO regions / Country	Number of data sets	Total number of samples	Number of test-positive samples	Pooled prevalence (%) established using meta-analysis (95% CI)	Heterogeneity I^2 (%)
Switzerland	3	664	123	22.3 (1.3–43.4)	NA
Russia	3	334	10	2.8 (1.0–4.6)	NA
United Kingdom	3	199	44	18.8 (9.4–28.1)	NA
France	3	234	98	40.3 (14.7–65.8)	97.85
Portugal	3	146	16	10.8 (5.8–15.9)	NA
Belgium	2	85	22	14.2 (7.9–20.6)	NA
Romania	2	535	91	22.8 (19.7–25.8)	NA
Hungary	2	714	165	17.0 (13.8–20.2)	NA
Finland	1	411	22	5.3 (3.3–7.9)	NA
Czech Republic	1	135	24	17.7 (11.7–25.3)	NA
Ireland	1	181	76	42.0 (34.7–49.5)	NA
Sweden	1	205	43	20.9 (15.6–27.2)	NA
Serbia	1	107	17	15.9 (9.5–24.2)	NA
Denmark	1	99	84	84.8 (76.2–91.2)	NA
Albania	1	252	121	48.0 (41.7–54.3)	NA
Cyprus	1	185	22	11.9 (7.6–17.4)	NA
Western Pacific region	**24**	**8370**	**1086**	**17.3 (14.7–19.9)**	**98.63**
Japan	6	3595	429	10.6 (6.6–14.7)	99.03
Australia	7	2809	112	8.0 (4.5–11.5)	97.56
China	2	399	66	14.6 (11.2–18.1)	NA
Malaysia	2	571	68	10.9 (8.4–13.4)	NA
Kerguelen	2	91	81	63.8 (53.8–72.9)	NA
Laos	1	55	6	10.9 (4.1–22.2)	NA
Vietnam	1	253	121	47.8 (41.5–54.1)	NA
Taiwan (China)	1	94	4	4.1 (1.1–10.3)	NA
New Zealand	1	63	42	66.6 (53.–78.0)	NA
South Korea	1	438	157	35.8 (31.3–40.5)	NA

Table 1 Global, regional and national prevalence of *Toxocara* infection in cats (results from 180 data sets performed in 51 countries).—cont'd

WHO regions / Country	Number of data sets	Total number of samples	Number of test-positive samples	Pooled prevalence (%) established using meta-analysis (95% CI)	Heterogeneity I^2 (%)
South-East Asian region	**8**	**2342**	**174**	**14.9 (9.8–20.1)**	**95.51**
Thailand	5	2115	126	11.7 (5.9–17.4)	94.79
India	3	227	48	29.6 (1.0–60.2)	NA
South America	**12**	**4210**	**379**	**12.6 (8.2–17.0)**	**97.66**
Brazil	9	3394	145	8.9 (5.6–12.2)	94.86
Argentina	1	230	23	35.7 (31.3–40.2)	NA
Chile	1	465	166	10.0 (6.4–14.6)	NA

[a]In sensitive analysis the global prevalence rate was changed to 22.6% (21.4–23.8) after removing the study by Lucio-Forster et al. (2016) in USA that tested 2,101,792 of cats.
Abbreviations: NA, not applicable; CI, confidence intervals.
WHO regions sorted according to prevalence rates.
Countries sorted according to number of studies included.
Bold represents region details and unbold represents country details.

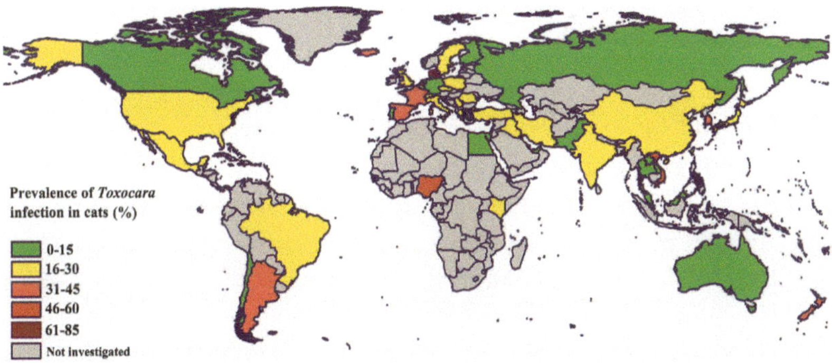

Fig. 2 Prevalence of *Toxocara* infection(s) in cats in different countries using geographic information system (GIS).

countries with three or more eligible data sets, Nigeria (50.0%) in West Africa; France (40.0%) in West Europe; Poland (27.6%) in Central Europe; India (29.6%) in South Asia; Iran (26.0%) in Middle East; and Mexico (24.5%) exhibited some of the highest prevalences. Other details pertaining to the prevalence of *Toxocara* infection in cats in WHO-regions and individual countries are presented in Table 1 and Fig. 2.

5. Prevalence according to type of cats, age, gender and area (rural vs urban)

In a subgroup analysis, according to type of studied cats, the global prevalence of *Toxocara* infection was 11.6% (10.7–12.5%) in pet cats, and 28.6% (25.1–32.2%) in stray cats, indicating a significant difference between the two groups (P-value$=$0.001). Considering age, meta-analysis results showed that the prevalence rate in cats of $\leq$12 months of age (27.7%, 23.4–32.0%) was significantly higher (P-value $<$ 0.001) than in cats of $>$12 months of age (23.8%, 14.8–32.7%). Considering gender, the pooled prevalences of *Toxocara* infection in female and male cats were 25.6% (20.0–31.1%) and 24.3% (19.0–29.6%), respectively, indicating no significant difference. Moreover, the prevalence was significantly higher (P-value$<$0.001) in rural cats (28.6%, 13.2–44.0%) than in urban cats (24.3%, 12.8–35.9%). Additional details are given in Table 2.

6. Prevalence according to selected study characteristics

Considering sample size, results of a subgroup analysis revealed that the highest and lowest prevalences of *Toxocara* infection were observed in studies with sample sizes of $<$500 cats (20.9%, 19.0–22.8%) and $>$5000 cats (4.8%, 4.8–4.9%). In addition, meta-regression analysis showed a significant decreasing trend in prevalence with increasing sample size (coefficient [C]$=-$0.00034, P-value$=$0.035) (Table 2 and Supplementary Fig. S1 in Supplementary material in the online version at https://doi.org/10.1016/bs.apar.2020.01.025). Other results showed that the prevalence of *Toxocara* infection in studies with a low risk of bias (14.9%, 14.1–15.8%) was significantly lower than in studies with a moderate risk of bias (26.9%, 21.3–32.5%). In addition, a lower prevalence was recorded for studies published after 2005 (Table 2). However, meta-regression analysis for the years of study-implementation showed a non-significant decreasing trend in prevalence over time ($C=-0.0033$, P-value$=$0.1) (Fig. 3A).

Table 2 The global prevalence of *Toxocara* infection in cats according to *a priori* defined subgroups.

Parameters/ subgroups	Number of data sets	Total number of samples	Number of test-positive samples	Pooled prevalence (%) established by REM (95% CI)	Heterogeneity I^2 (%)
Type of cats					
Pet (domestic) cats	95	2,140,199	106,273	11.6 (10.7–12.5)	98.46
Stray (wild) cats	72	12,272	2809	28.6 (25.1–32.1)	98.53
Indeterminate (not specified type)	13	5646	1024	15.4 (10.0–20.7)	97.05
Type of sample tested					
Faecal	149	2,153,014	109,205	16.2 (15.3–17.1)	98.56
Post mortem	28	4093	796	25.5 (20.2–30.8)	98.26
Hair	3	326	42	11.5 (2.4–20.6)	97.41
Type of diagnosis method					
Flotation	103	2,139,925	107,558	18.1 (16.9–19.2)	98.54
Sedimentation	22	5608	528	13.1 (10.8–15.5)	96.75
Sedimentation and Flotation	18	5918	655	8.4 (5.5–11.2)	97.77
Necropsy	27	3993	764	25.3 (19.9–30.6)	98.35
Other (McMaster, Kato-katz, etc.)	10	2625	643	23.8 (14.8–32.7)	98.51
Age					
≤12 months	40	9385	1459	27.7 (23.4–32.0)	98.39
>12 months	40	11,177	1028	23.8 (14.8–32.7)	98.51
Gender					
Male	38	4663	703	24.3 (19.0–29.6)	97.79
Female	38	4910	600	25.6 (20.1–31.1)	97.91
Residence					
High standard location (Urban)	8	1851	419	24.3 (12.8–35.9)	98.69
Low standard location (Rural)	9	536	189	28.6 (13.2–44.0)	94.89

Continued

Table 2 The global prevalence of *Toxocara* infection in cats according to *a priori* defined subgroups.—cont'd

Parameters/ subgroups	Number of data sets	Total number of samples	Number of test-positive samples	Pooled prevalence (%) established by REM (95% CI)	Heterogeneity I^2 (%)
Sample size					
<500	156	23,762	4836	20.9 (19.0–22.8)	97.84
501–1000	12	8299	930	9.6 (7.0–12.2)	99.12
1001–5000	9	12,537	1428	11.8 (6.9–16.7)	99.45
>5000	3	2,113,519	102,912	4.8 (4.8–4.9)	94.23
Implementation year					
1990–1995	7	3652	593	27.5 (19.3–35.7)	97.27
1996–2000	12	2110	482	25.1 (16.5–33.7)	98.56
2001–2005	17	6546	1114	28.6 (23.0–34.1)	98.87
2006–2010	33	10,349	1072	12.7 (10.4–15.1)	96.63
2011–2015	64	21,702	2535	16.1 (14.2–17.9)	97.94
2016–2019	47	2,113,758	104,310	18.0 (16.4–19.6)	99.06
Risk of bias					
Low Risk	124	2,154,617	109,161	14.9(14.1–15.9)	98.68
Moderate Risk	56	3500	945	26.9 (21.3–32.5)	97.52

Abbreviations: NA, not applicable; CI, confidence intervals.

7. Impact of socio-demographic, geographical and climatic parameters on prevalence

A subgroup analysis, according to income level in a country, revealed lowest prevalences (15.7%, 14.7–16.7%) in countries with a high-income level, and highest prevalence (28.1%, 17.2–38.9%) in countries with low- to middle-income levels (Table 3). Based on geographical latitude, the highest and lowest prevalence rates were observed at latitudes of 0–10° (32.7%, 19–46.4%) and 20–30° (6.0%, 4.3–7.8%), respectively. Considering relative humidity, the highest and lowest prevalence rates were observed in climes with mean relative humidities of ≥80%

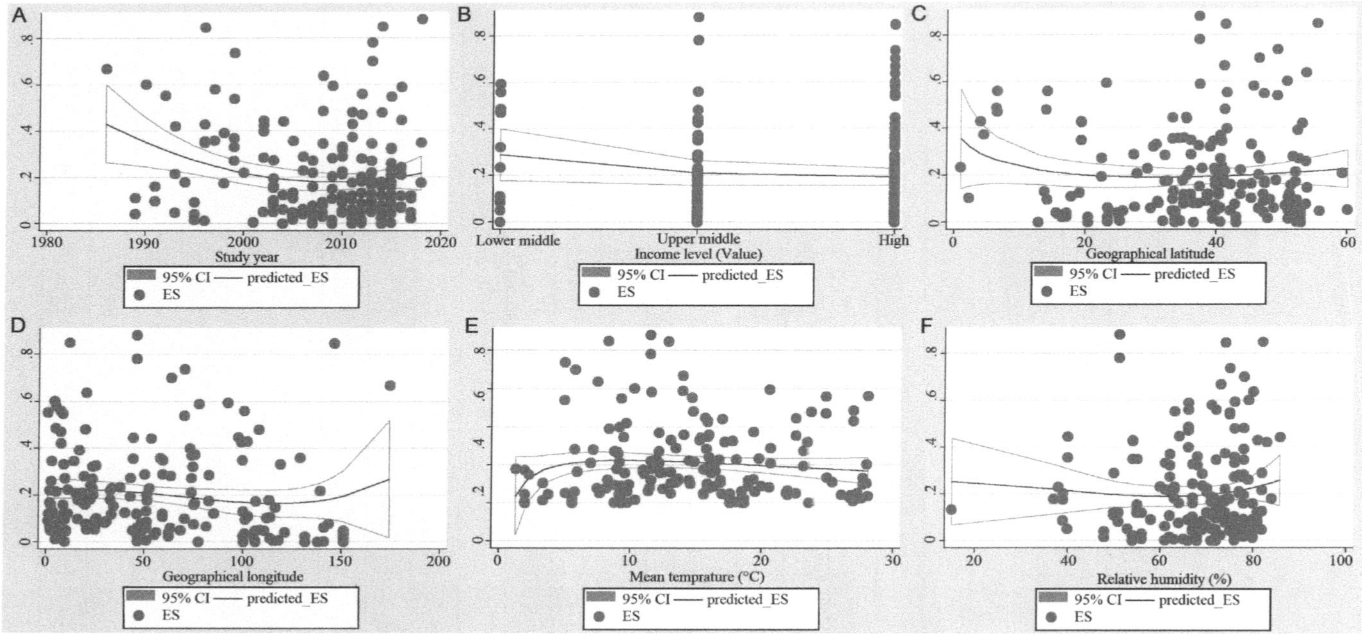

Fig. 3 Results of meta-regression analyses of the prevalence of *Toxocara* infection in cats according to: (A) demonstrating a statistically non-significant decreasing trend in prevalence over time in more recent years; (B) country's income level, showing a statistically non-significant downward trend in prevalence in countries with a higher level of income; (C and D) geographical latitude and longitude, showing statistically non-significant downward trend in prevalence with increasing geographical latitude and longitude; and (E and F) mean environmental temperature and relative humidity, showing non-statistically significant upward trend in prevalence in areas with a higher mean temperature and relative humidity. "ES" refers to effect size (= prevalence rates).

Table 3 The global prevalence of *Toxocara* infection in cats based on subgroups according to different socio-demographic and geographic parameters.

Parameters/ subgroups	Number of data sets	Total number of samples	Number of test-positive samples	Pooled prevalence (%) established by REM (95% CI)	Heterogeneity I^2 (%)
Income					
Lower middle	12	1340	388	28.1 (17.2–38.9)	97.78
Upper middle	52	11,521	1826	20.1 (17.1–23.0)	98.38
High	116	2,145,256	107,892	15.7 (14.7–16.7)	98.47
Latitude					
0–10°	8	1155	297	32.7 (19.0–46.4)	96.99
10–20°	14	4109	767	19.6 (12.7–26.5)	98.56
20–30°	17	4556	189	6.0 (4.3–7.8)	92.70
30–40°	59	2,117,197	105,003	17.9 (16.1–19.7)	98.43
40–50°	48	12,356	2436	23.8 (20.0–27.6)	98.57
>50°	34	18,744	1414	13.5 (11.3–15.7)	97.98
Longitude					
0–10°	40	8549	1355	19.4 (16.2–22.7)	97.87
10–20°	15	13,920	1108	23.6 (19.0–28.2)	98.45
20–30°	16	3330	614	17.3 (12.2–22.4)	93.71
30–40°	7	773	130	16.8 (12.3–21.3)	66.71
40–50°	15	3857	398	22.5 (16.0–29.1)	98.88
50–60°	17	3309	512	17.1 (11.8–22.3)	97.28
60–70°	6	537	113	18.7 (4.9–32.5)	97.65
70–80°	14	7085	1366	29.5 (22.9–36.1)	98.41
80–90°	4	399	79	16.2 (5.8–26.6)	88.16
90–100°	5	2053	876	42.3 (38.2–46.3)	65.15
100–110°	17	4062	325	9.4 (6.5–12.3)	95.27
110–120°	9	2,103,892	102,599	8.9 (6.1–11.7)	98.09
>120°	15	6351	631	11.2 (8.4–13.9)	98.54

Table 3 The global prevalence of *Toxocara* infection in cats based on subgroups according to different socio-demographic and geographic parameters.—cont'd

Parameters/ subgroups	Number of data sets	Total number of samples	Number of test-positive samples	Pooled prevalence (%) established by REM (95% CI)	Heterogeneity I^2 (%)
Humidity (%)					
<40	7	2,102,407	102,451	13.9 (7.7–20.0)	98.54
40–49	9	1348	233	16.3 (8.9–23.7)	98.54
50–59	18	3825	819	22.5 (15.3–29.6)	98.54
60–69	50	29,048	3450	16.2 (14.2–18.3)	98.54
70–79	81	18,549	2578	17.7 (16.1–19.2)	98.54
≥ 80	14	2740	478	23.9 (15.5–32.4)	98.54
Mean temperature (°C)					
<7.0	19	3406	470	16.6 (12.1–21.2)	98.5
7.1–13.0	58	2,118,092	104,842	18.3 (16.8–19.9)	98.8
13.1–19.0	64	29,347	3771	18.4 (16.5–20.3)	98.6
19.1–25.0	23	2632	614	22.9 (16.8–28.9)	96.38
25.1–30.0	16	4640	409	11.3 (8.1–14.5)	96.4
Precipitation (mm)					
0–250	18	3341	571	17.3 (11.6–23.0)	97.4
251–500	36	4915	660	16.9 (13.2–20.5)	97.22
501–1000	65	2,116,847	105,322	19.2 (17.5–20.8)	98.65
1001–2000	56	32,542	3379	16.5 (14.9–18.1)	98.60
≥2001	4	272	77	34.9 (8.9–60.9)	96.3

Abbreviations: REM, random effect meta-analysis; CI, confidence intervals.

(23.9%, 15.5–32.4%) and <40 (13.9%, 7.7–20.0%), respectively. More details and also additional subgroup analyses with respect to geographic longitude, mean temperature and precipitation are given in Table 3.

In meta-regression analyses, there was a statistically non-significant decreasing trend with increasing income in a country ($C = -0.03$, P-value $= 0.10$). With respect geographical parameters, meta-regression analyses showed a non-significant decreasing trend in prevalence with increasing geographical latitudes ($C=-0.00047$, P-value$=0.67$) and geographical longitudes ($C=-0.00041$, P-value$=0.17$). Considering climatic parameters, a non-significant decreasing prevalence was observed with increasing mean environmental temperature ($C=-0.00074$, P-value$=0.72$), while non-significant increasing prevalence rates were seen with increasing mean relative humidity ($C=-0.00002$, P-value$=0.46$) (Fig. 3B–F).

8. Discussion and conclusions

This review demonstrates that globally, cats have a prevalence of *Toxocara* of ~17%. This represents an estimated number of 118–150 million cats infected with *T. cati* (and/or one or more other species) and can release (initially unembryonated) *Toxocara* eggs via defaecation inside the household in sandboxes and externally in playgrounds, garden soil and other outdoor recreational areas. When embryonated, such eggs likely represent a considerable public health problem. Substantial variation in the prevalence of *T. cati* occurs depending on location, type (rural vs urban; pet vs stray) and age of cats, socio-demographic status of cat owners and climate. The findings indicated that the prevalence of *Toxocara* infection in cats was highest in African and Eastern Mediterranean regions and lowest in South-East Asia and South America, which is relatively consistent with results from our recent study of dogs (Rostami et al., 2020). These results should be interpreted with some caution due to the limited number of studies reported from Africa, South-East Asia and South America. In addition, it should be noted that the type of cats recruited varied among studies—the majority of studies being in the Eastern Mediterranean region examined stray cats, while most studies in South America investigated pet cats (Supplementary Table S1 in Supplementary material in the online version at https://doi.org/10.1016/bs.apar.2020.01.025).

Subgroup analysis revealed that the prevalence in stray cats (28.6%) was significantly higher than in pet cats (11.6%). This finding confirms our knowledge that stray cats, unlike pets, live outdoors, are often neglected and are not under routine veterinary preventative care and are not treated for parasites. They harbour more infectious agents and, thus, pose a greater risk of contaminating the environment with *Toxocara* eggs and represent a potential health threat to wildlife, domestic animals and humans (cf. Gerhold and Jessup, 2013; Taetzsch et al., 2018). Our results also indicated a significantly higher prevalence in young cats and rural cats, whereas there was no significant difference in prevalence in relation to gender. These findings confirm those from earlier studies (Barutzki and Schaper, 2003; Barutzki and Schaper, 2013; Buehl et al., 2006; Daugschies et al., 2000), demonstrating that young animals are more likely to be infected with helminths and protozoa than older cats. The higher prevalence in younger cats might be explained, for example, by a lesser-developed immune system in younger than in older cats, and transmammary transmission of *T. cati* to kittens (Blagburn et al., 1996; Glickman and Schantz, 1981; Swerczek et al., 1971). Male cats had a similar prevalence (24.3%) to females (25.6%), which contrasts with results seen for *T. canis* infection in dogs (Rostami et al., 2020), where the prevalence in male dogs was higher than in females. The higher prevalence found in rural cats may be as a result of a poor health status, reduced immunity and/or access to infected rodents or other small mammals that serve as paratenic hosts (Goldstein and Abrahamian, 2016; Ngui et al., 2014; Overgaauw and van Knapen, 2013).

In this review, *Toxocara* prevalence decreased with increasing latitude. This result is in accordance with findings of other recent meta-analyses (Fakhri et al., 2018; Rostami et al., 2019b, 2020), which demonstrated a similar trend in dogs and humans as well as the environmental contamination of public places with *Toxocara* eggs. It can be suggested that this decreasing trend in prevalence of infection with increasing geographical latitude may be due to the fact that countries in higher latitudes are more developed, and veterinary care for pets, preventive measures for stray animals and environmental hygiene practices are relatively common, regular and accessible (Beck and Meyers, 1996; Einav et al., 2017). In such countries, people are perhaps more aware of zoonotic diseases and their accessibility to a health care centre is better (Pittet et al., 2008). In agreement with these statements, our findings in the present and previous studies (Fakhri et al., 2018; Rostami et al., 2019b, 2020) have shown that the prevalence rates of *Toxocara* infection in dogs, humans and cats and the contamination of soil with *Toxocara* eggs are significantly lower in countries with high mean income levels compared with those with low or low to moderate incomes. Another explanation would be that low environmental temperatures at higher latitudes affect the rate of embryonation and the survival of *Toxocara* eggs (Azam et al., 2012; Gamboa, 2005). Conditions that favour the embryonation and survival of *Toxocara* eggs are shade, suitable environmental temperature (15–30 °C), high mean relative humidity (>60%) and high oxygen content in soil (Azam et al., 2012; Fakhri et al., 2018;

Gamboa, 2005). The prevalence of *Toxocara* in dogs and humans and environmental contamination with *Toxocara* eggs are high in areas with mean annual environmental temperatures of 20–30 °C, with high relative humidities of 70–80% (Fakhri et al., 2018; Rostami et al., 2019b, 2020). In addition, the decreasing prevalence of *Toxocara* infection in cats with increasing geographical longitude is similar to findings for *T. canis* in dogs (Rostami et al., 2020). Results for human infection and environmental contamination were somewhat conflicting, and high prevalence rates of *Toxocara* infection/exposure in humans (24.2% and 34.1%) and *Toxocara* eggs in public places (35% and 21%) were recorded for the Western Pacific and South-East Asia regions, respectively (Fakhri et al., 2018; Rostami et al., 2019b). Therefore, it might be concluded that a lower rate of *Toxocara* infection is seen in animals in Far East and East Asian countries, while the seropositivity rate for human toxocariasis and environmental contamination with *Toxocara* eggs in these regions were relatively high (Fakhri et al., 2018; Rostami et al., 2019b). These findings suggest that environmental and personal hygiene and/or eating habits in these countries should be improved to reduce the risk of infection in humans.

The strengths of this review include a comprehensive literature search using robust methods, the number of cats investigated and the subgroup analyses, according to geographical location, gender, age and diagnostic approaches. However, our systematic review and meta-analysis might have some limitations. First, although we undertook a comprehensive search of the available peer-reviewed literature and included a large number of studies that had assessed the prevalence of *Toxocara* infection in cats, we cannot exclude the possibility that some studies may have been missed in the "grey literature". Second, the studies included were not proportionately distributed across all WHO-regions, and only small numbers of studies were available for the African, South-East Asian, and South American regions, emphasizing the paucity of epidemiological data for countries in these regions. Moreover, in some countries, only one study was available from a particular region, such that our results may not be representative for all parts of a country. Third, there was significant heterogeneity across studies, although this is a common finding for meta-analyses of prevalence studies (e.g. Ahmed et al., 2014; Hill et al., 2016; Hooi et al., 2017; Rostami et al., 2017). While subgroup analyses were conducted, we were not able to identify precisely the reason(s) for this heterogeneity.

In conclusion, our comprehensive analysis of prevalence studies confirms that *Toxocara* infection is prevalent (~17%) in cats around the world. Given that cats represent reservoirs for *Toxocara*, in particular *T. cati*, and are the source of eggs that disseminate and become infective in the environment to then infect humans and other animals, there is a need to establish the contributions of *T. cati* as well as *T. malaysiensis*, *Toxascaris leonina* and/or other ascaridoids to human disease in both developed and underprivileged regions of the world using advanced molecular and/or immunological/serological tools. The findings of this review suggest that both stray and pet cat populations in all parts of the world need to be monitored, and that pet cats be regularly dewormed for *Toxocara*.

Acknowledgements

This research was supported by Health Research Institute at the Babol University of Medical Sciences (IR.MUBABOL.HRI.REC.1398.129), Babol, Iran (A.R.). Research in R.B.G.'s group is supported through funds from the National Health and Medical Research Council (NHMRC) of Australia, the Australian Research Council (ARC), Yourgene Health, Melbourne Water Corporation and The University of Melbourne.

References

Aghaei, S., Riahi, S.M., Rostami, A., Mohammadzadeh, I., Javanian, M., Tohidi, E., Foroutan, M., Esmaeili Dooki, M., 2018. *Toxocara* spp. infection and risk of childhood asthma: a systematic review and meta-analysis. Acta Trop. 182, 298–304.

Aghamolaie, S., Seyyedtabaei, S.J., Behniafar, H., Foroutan, M., Saber, V., Hanifehpur, H., Mehravar, S., Rostami, A., 2018. Seroepidemiology, modifiable risk factors and clinical symptoms of *Toxocara* spp. infection in northern Iran. Trans. R. Soc. Trop. Med. Hyg. 113, 116–122.

Ahmed, S.M., Hall, A.J., Robinson, A.E., Verhoef, L., Premkumar, P., Parashar, U.D., Koopmans, M., Lopman, B.A., 2014. Global prevalence of norovirus in cases of gastroenteritis: a systematic review and meta-analysis. Lancet Infect. Dis. 14, 725–730.

Azam, D., Ukpai, O.M., Said, A., Abd-Allah, G.A., Morgan, E.R., 2012. Temperature and the development and survival of infective *Toxocara canis* larvae. Parasitol. Res. 110, 649–656.

Bakhshani, A., Maleki, M., Haghparast, A., Parande Shirvan, S., Borji, H., 2019. A survey on *Toxocara cati* eggs on the hair of stray cats: a potential risk factor for human toxocariasis in Northeastern Iran. Comp. Immunol. Microbiol. Infect. Dis. 64, 10–13.

Barutzki, D., Schaper, R., 2003. Endoparasites in dogs and cats in Germany 1999–2002. Parasitol. Res. 90, S148–S150.

Barutzki, D., Schaper, R., 2013. Age-dependant prevalence of endoparasites in young dogs and cats up to one year of age. Parasitol. Res. 112, 119–131.

Beck, A.M., Meyers, N.M., 1996. Health enhancement and companion animal ownership. Ann. Rev. Public Health 17, 247–257.

Blagburn, B.L., Lindsay, D.S., Vaughan, J.L., Rippey, N.S., Wright, J.C., Lynn, R.C., Kelch, W.J., Ritchie, G., Hepler, D.I., 1996. Prevalence of canine parasites based on fecal flotation. Comp. Cont. Ed. Pract. Vet. 18, 483–509.

Buehl, I.E., Prosl, H., Mundt, H.C., Tichy, A., Joachim, A., 2006. Canine isosporosis–epidemiology of field and experimental infections. J. Vet. Med. Series B. 53, 482–487.

Paul, M., King, L., Carlin, E.P., 2010. Zoonoses of people and their pets: a US perspective on significant pet-associated parasitic diseases. Trends Parasitol. 26, 153–154.

Pittet, D., Allegranzi, B., Storr, J., Bagheri Nejad, S., Dziekan, G., Leotsakos, A., Donaldson, L., 2008. Infection control as a major World Health Organization priority for developing countries. J. Hosp. Infect. 68, 285–292.

Rostami, A., Ma, G., Wang, T., Koehler, A.V., Hofmann, A., Chang, B.C.H., Macpherson, C.N., Gasser, R.B., 2019a. Human toxocariasis—a look at a neglected disease through an epidemiological 'prism'. Infect. Genet. Evol. 74, 104002.

Rostami, A., Riahi, S.M., Fakhri, Y., Saber, V., Hanifehpour, H., Valizadeh, S., Gholizadeh, M., Pouya, R.H., Gamble, H.R., 2017. The global seroprevalence of *Toxoplasma gondii* among wild boars: a systematic review and meta-analysis. Vet. Parasitol. 244, 12–20.

Rostami, A., Riahi, S.M., Holland, C.V., Taghipour, A., Khalili Fomeshi, M., Fakhri, Y., Omrani, V.F., Hotez, P.J., Gasser, R.B., 2019b. Seroprevalence estimates for toxocariasis in people worldwide: a systematic review and meta-analysis. PLoS Negl. Trop. Dis. 13 (12), e0007809.

Rostami, A., Riahi, S.M., Hofmann, A., Ma, G., Wang, T., Behniafar, H., Taghipour, A., Fakhri, Y., Spotin, A., Chang, B.C.H., Macpherson, C.N.L., Hotez, P.J., Gasser, R.B., 2020. Global prevalence of *Toxocara* infection in dogs. Adv. Parasitol. 108, 561–583. (Chapter 28–This Special Issue).

Sommerfelt, I.E., Duchene, A., Daprato, B., Lopez, C.M., Cardillo, N., Franco, A.J., 2014. Experimental infection with *Toxocara cati* in pigs: migratory pattern and pathological response in early phase. Rev. Inst. Med. Trop. Sao Paulo 56, 347–352.

Strube, C., Heuer, L., Janecek, E., 2013. *Toxocara* spp. infections in paratenic hosts. Vet. Parasitol. 193, 375–389.

Swerczek, T.W., Nielsen, S.W., Helmboldt, C.F., 1971. Transmammary passage of *Toxocara cati* in the cat. Ain. J. Vet. Res. 32, 89–92.

Taetzsch, S.J., Bertke, A.S., Gruszynski, K.R., 2018. Zoonotic disease transmission associated with feral cats in a metropolitan area: a geospatial analysis. Zoonoses Public Health 65, 412–419.

Taira, K., Saitoh, Y., Kapel, C.M., 2011. *Toxocara cati* larvae persist and retain high infectivity in muscles of experimentally infected chickens. Vet. Parasitol. 180, 287–291.

Sakai, R., Kawashima, H., Shibui, H., Kamata, K., Kambara, C., Matsuoka, H., 1998. *Toxocara cati*-induced ocular toxocariasis. Arch. Ophthalmol. 116 (12), 1686–1687.

Shimokawa, H., Nakashima, T., Akagi, K., Omae, T., Tsuji, M., 1982. Visceral larva migrans by *Toxocara cati*. Fukuoka. Igaku. Zasshi. 73, 64–69.

World Health Organization, 2003. List of Member States by WHO Region and Mortality Stratum. 2003 World Health Report, p. 182.

Yoshikawa, M., Nishiofuku, M., Moriya, K., Ouji, Y., Ishizaka, S., Kasahara, K., Mikasa, K., Hirai, T., Mizuno, Y., Ogawa, S., Nakamura, T., Maruyama, H., Akao, N., 2008. A familial case of visceral toxocariasis due to consumption of raw bovine liver. Parasitol. Int. 57, 525–529.

Ziegler, M.A., Macpherson, C.N., 2019. *Toxocara* and its species. CAB Rev. 1749-8848. 2019, 14, No. 053. Online.

Further reading

Arbabi, M., Hooshyar, H., 2009. Gastrointestinal parasites of stray cats in Kashan. Iran. Trop. Biomed. 26, 16–22.

Baneth, G., Thamsborg, S.M., Otranto, D., Guillot, J., Blaga, R., Deplazes, P., Solano-Gallego, L., 2016. Major parasitic zoonoses associated with dogs and cats in Europe. J. Comp. Pathol. 155, S54–S74.

Paul, M., King, L., Carlin, E.P., 2010. Zoonoses of people and their pets: a US perspective on significant pet-associated parasitic diseases. Trends Parasitol. 26, 153–154.

Pittet, D., Allegranzi, B., Storr, J., Bagheri Nejad, S., Dziekan, G., Leotsakos, A., Donaldson, L., 2008. Infection control as a major World Health Organization priority for developing countries. J. Hosp. Infect. 68, 285–292.

Rostami, A., Ma, G., Wang, T., Koehler, A.V., Hofmann, A., Chang, B.C.H., Macpherson, C.N., Gasser, R.B., 2019a. Human toxocariasis—a look at a neglected disease through an epidemiological 'prism'. Infect. Genet. Evol. 74, 104002.

Rostami, A., Riahi, S.M., Fakhri, Y., Saber, V., Hanifehpour, H., Valizadeh, S., Gholizadeh, M., Pouya, R.H., Gamble, H.R., 2017. The global seroprevalence of *Toxoplasma gondii* among wild boars: a systematic review and meta-analysis. Vet. Parasitol. 244, 12–20.

Rostami, A., Riahi, S.M., Holland, C.V., Taghipour, A., Khalili Fomeshi, M., Fakhri, Y., Omrani, V.F., Hotez, P.J., Gasser, R.B., 2019b. Seroprevalence estimates for toxocariasis in people worldwide: a systematic review and meta-analysis. PLoS Negl. Trop. Dis. 13 (12), e0007809.

Rostami, A., Riahi, S.M., Hofmann, A., Ma, G., Wang, T., Behniafar, H., Taghipour, A., Fakhri, Y., Spotin, A., Chang, B.C.H., Macpherson, C.N.L., Hotez, P.J., Gasser, R.B., 2020. Global prevalence of *Toxocara* infection in dogs. Adv. Parasitol. 108, 561–583. (Chapter 28–This Special Issue).

Sommerfelt, I.E., Duchene, A., Daprato, B., Lopez, C.M., Cardillo, N., Franco, A.J., 2014. Experimental infection with *Toxocara cati* in pigs: migratory pattern and pathological response in early phase. Rev. Inst. Med. Trop. Sao Paulo 56, 347–352.

Strube, C., Heuer, L., Janecek, E., 2013. *Toxocara* spp. infections in paratenic hosts. Vet. Parasitol. 193, 375–389.

Swerczek, T.W., Nielsen, S.W., Helmboldt, C.F., 1971. Transmammary passage of *Toxocara cati* in the cat. Ain. J. Vet. Res. 32, 89–92.

Taetzsch, S.J., Bertke, A.S., Gruszynski, K.R., 2018. Zoonotic disease transmission associated with feral cats in a metropolitan area: a geospatial analysis. Zoonoses Public Health 65, 412–419.

Taira, K., Saitoh, Y., Kapel, C.M., 2011. *Toxocara cati* larvae persist and retain high infectivity in muscles of experimentally infected chickens. Vet. Parasitol. 180, 287–291.

Sakai, R., Kawashima, H., Shibui, H., Kamata, K., Kambara, C., Matsuoka, H., 1998. *Toxocara cati*-induced ocular toxocariasis. Arch. Ophthalmol. 116 (12), 1686–1687.

Shimokawa, H., Nakashima, T., Akagi, K., Omae, T., Tsuji, M., 1982. Visceral larva migrans by *Toxocara cati*. Fukuoka. Igaku. Zasshi. 73, 64–69.

World Health Organization, 2003. List of Member States by WHO Region and Mortality Stratum. 2003 World Health Report, p. 182.

Yoshikawa, M., Nishiofuku, M., Moriya, K., Ouji, Y., Ishizaka, S., Kasahara, K., Mikasa, K., Hirai, T., Mizuno, Y., Ogawa, S., Nakamura, T., Maruyama, H., Akao, N., 2008. A familial case of visceral toxocariasis due to consumption of raw bovine liver. Parasitol. Int. 57, 525–529.

Ziegler, M.A., Macpherson, C.N., 2019. *Toxocara* and its species. CAB Rev. 1749-8848. 2019, 14, No. 053. Online.

Further reading

Arbabi, M., Hooshyar, H., 2009. Gastrointestinal parasites of stray cats in Kashan. Iran. Trop. Biomed. 26, 16–22.

Baneth, G., Thamsborg, S.M., Otranto, D., Guillot, J., Blaga, R., Deplazes, P., Solano-Gallego, L., 2016. Major parasitic zoonoses associated with dogs and cats in Europe. J. Comp. Pathol. 155, S54–S74.

Hunter, J.P., Saratzis, A., Sutton, A.J., Boucher, R.H., Sayers, R.D., Bown, M.J., 2014. In meta-analyses of proportion studies, funnel plots were found to be an inaccurate method of assessing publication bias. J. Clin. Epidemiol. 67, 897–903.

Jones, J.L., Kruszon-Moran, D., Won, K., Wilson, M., Schantz, P.M., 2008. *Toxoplasma gondii* and *Toxocara* spp. co-infection. Am. J. Trop. Med. Hyg. 8, 35–39.

Le, T.H., Anh, N.T., Nguyen, K.T., Nguyen, N.T., Gasser, R.B., 2016. *Toxocara malaysiensis* infection in domestic cats in Vietnam—an emerging zoonotic issue? Infect. Genet. Evol. 37, 94–98.

Liu, E.W., Elder, E.S., Rivera, H.N., Kruszon-Moran, D., Handali, S., Jones, J.L., 2019. Concurrent seroprevalence of antibodies to *Toxoplasma gondii* and *Toxocara* species in the United States, 2011-2014. Clin. Infect. Dis. 68, 712–713.

Lucio-Forster, A., Mizhquiri Barbecho, J.S., Mohammed, H.O., Kornreich, B.G., Bowman, D.D., 2016. Comparison of the prevalence of *Toxocara* egg shedding by pet cats and dogs in the U.S.A., 2011-2014. Vet. Parasitol. Reg. Stud. Rep. 5, 1–13.

Luna, J., Cicero, C.E., Rateau, G., Quattrocchi, G., Marin, B., Bruno, E., Dalmay, F., Druet-Cabanac, M., Nicoletti, A., Preux, P.M., 2018. Updated evidence of the association between toxocariasis and epilepsy: systematic review and meta-analysis. PLoS Negl. Trop. Dis. 12, e0006665.

Ma, G., Holland, C.V., Wang, T., Hofmann, A., Fan, C.K., Maizels, R.M., Hotez, P.J., Gasser, R.B., 2018. Human toxocariasis. Lancet. Infect. Dis. 18, e14–e24.

Macpherson, C.N., 2013. The epidemiology and public health importance of toxocariasis: a zoonosis of global importance. Int. J. Parasitol. 43, 999–1008.

Mohammadzadeh, I., Riahi, S.M., Saber, V., Darvish, S., Amrovani, M., Arefkhah, N., Rostami, A., 2018. The relationship between *Toxocara* species seropositivity and allergic skin disorders: a systematic review and meta-analysis. Trans. R. Soc. Trop. Med. Hyg. 112, 529–537.

Moher, D., Shamseer, L., Clarke, M., Ghersi, D., Liberati, A., Petticrew, M., Shekelle, P., Stewart, L.A., PRISMA-P Group, 2015. Preferred reporting items for systematic review and meta-analysis protocols (PRISMA-P) 2015 statement. Syst. Rev. 4, 1.

Morimatsu, Y., Akao, N., Akiyoshi, H., Kawazu, T., Okabe, Y., Aizawa, H., 2006. A familial case of visceral larva migrans after ingestion of raw chicken livers: appearance of specific antibody in bronchoalveolar lavage fluid of the patients. Am. J. Trop. Med. Hyg. 75, 303–306.

Munn, Z., Moola, S., Riitano, D., Lisy, K., 2014. The development of a critical appraisal tool for use in systematic reviews addressing questions of prevalence. Int. J. Health Policy. Manag. 3, 123–128.

Ngui, R., Lee, S.C., Yap, N.J., Tan, T.K., Aidil, R.M., Chua, K.H., Aziz, S., Sulaiman, W.Y., Ahmad, A.F., Mahmud, R., Lian, Y.L., 2014. Gastrointestinal parasites in rural dogs and cats in Selangor and Pahang states in Peninsular Malaysia. Acta Parasitol. 59, 737–744.

Öge, H., Öge, S., Özbakış, G., Gürcan, S., 2014. Comparison of *Toxocara* eggs in hair and faecal samples from owned dogs and cats collected in Ankara. Turkey. Vet. Parasitol. 206, 227–231.

Oguz, B., Ozdal, N., Deger, M., 2018. Genetic analysis of *Toxocara* spp. in stray cats and dogs in Van province, Eastern Turkey. J. Vet. Res. 62, 291–295.

Overgaauw, P.A., van Knapen, F., 2013. Veterinary and public health aspects of *Toxocara* spp. Vet. Parasitol. 193, 398–403.

Overgaauw, P.A., van Zutphen, L., Hoek, D., Yaya, F.O., Roelfsema, J., Pinelli, E., van Knapen, F., Kortbeek, L.M., 2009. Zoonotic parasites in fecal samples and fur from dogs and cats in The Netherlands. Vet. Parasitol. 163, 115–122.

Choi, D., Lim, J.H., Choi, D.C., Paik, S.W., Kim, S.H., Huh, S., 2008. Toxocariasis and ingestion of raw cow liver in patients with eosinophilia. Korean J. Parasitol. 46, 139–143.

Coati, N., Schnieder, T., Epe, C., 2004. Vertical transmission of *Toxocara cati* Schrank 1788 (Anisakidae) in the cat. Parasitol. Res. 92, 142–146.

Daugschies, A., Mundt, H.C., Letkova, V., 2000. Toltrazuril treatment of cystoisosporosis in dogs under experimental and field conditions. Parasitol. Res. 86, 797–799.

DerSimonian, R., Laird, N., 1986. Meta-analysis in clinical trials. Control Clin. Trials 7, 177–188.

Despommier, D., 2003. Toxocariasis: clinical aspects, epidemiology, medical ecology, and molecular aspects. Clin. Microbiol. Rev. 16, 265–272.

Eberhard, M.L., Alfano, E., 1998. Adult *Toxocara cati* infections in US children: report of four cases. Am. J. Trop. Med. Hyg. 59 (3), 404–406.

Einav, L., Finkelstein, A., Gupta, A., 2017. Is American pet health care (also) uniquely inefficient? Am. Economic. Rev. 107, 491–495.

Fakhri, Y., Gasser, R.B., Rostami, A., Fan, C.K., Ghasemi, S.M., Javanian, M., Bayani, M., Armoon, B., Moradi, B., 2018. *Toxocara* eggs in public places worldwide—a systematic review and meta-analysis. Environ. Pollut. 242, 1467–1475.

Fan, C.K., Liao, C.W., Cheng, Y.C., 2013. Factors affecting disease manifestation of toxocarosis in humans: genetics and environment. Vet. Parasitol. 193, 342–352.

Fillaux, J., Magnaval, J.-F., 2013. Laboratory diagnosis of human toxocariasis. Vet. Parasitol. 193, 327–336.

Fisher, M., 2003. *Toxocara cati*: an underestimated zoonotic agent. Trends Parasitol. 19, 167–170.

Gamboa, M.I., 2005. Effects of temperature and humidity on the development of eggs of *Toxocara canis* under laboratory conditions. J. Helminthol. 79, 327–331.

Gasser, R.B., 2013. A perfect time to harness advanced molecular technologies to explore the fundamental biology of *Toxocara* species. Vet. Parasitol. 193, 353–364.

Gerhold, R.W., Jessup, D.A., 2013. Zoonotic diseases associated with free-roaming cats. Zoonoses Public Health 60, 189–195.

Gibbons, L.M., Jacobs, D.E., Sani, R.A., 2001. *Toxocara malaysiensis* n. sp. (Nematoda: Ascaridoidea) from the domestic cat (Felis catus Linnaeus, 1758). J. Parasitol. 87, 660–665.

Glickman, L.T., Schantz, P.M., 1981. Epidemiology and pathogenesis of zoonotic toxocariasis. Epidemiol. Rev. 3, 230–250.

Goldstein, E.J.C., Abrahamian, F.M., 2016. Diseases transmitted by cats. In: Schlossberg, D. (Ed.), Infections of Leisure, fifth ed. The American Society for Microbiology, pp. 133–150.

Greene, C.E., 2006. Infectious Diseases of the Dog and Cat. W.B. Saunders\Elsevier Science, United Kingdom. ISBN: 072160062X.

Higgins, J.P., Thompson, S.G., Deeks, J.J., Altman, D.G., 2003. Measuring inconsistency in meta-analyses. BMJ 327, 557–560.

Hill, N.R., Fatoba, S.T., Oke, J.L., Hirst, J.A., O'Callaghan, C.A., Lasserson, D.S., Hobbs, F.D., 2016. Global prevalence of chronic kidney disease—a systematic review and meta-analysis. PLoS One 11, e0158765.

Holland, C., Smith, H.V., 2006. *Toxocara*: the Enigmatic Parasite. CABI, United Kingdom, ISBN: 1-84593-026-6.

Hooi, J.K.Y., Lai, W.Y., Ng, W.K., Suen, M.M.Y., Underwood, F.E., Tanyingoh, D., Malfertheiner, P., Graham, D.Y., Wong, V.W.S., Wu, J.C.Y., Chan, F.K.L., Sung, J.J.Y., Kaplan, G.G., Ng, S.C., 2017. Global prevalence of *Helicobacter pylori* infection: systematic review and meta-analysis. Gastroenterology 153, 420–429.

that cats represent reservoirs for *Toxocara*, in particular *T. cati*, and are the source of eggs that disseminate and become infective in the environment to then infect humans and other animals, there is a need to establish the contributions of *T. cati* as well as *T. malaysiensis*, *Toxascaris leonina* and/or other ascaridoids to human disease in both developed and underprivileged regions of the world using advanced molecular and/or immunological/serological tools. The findings of this review suggest that both stray and pet cat populations in all parts of the world need to be monitored, and that pet cats be regularly dewormed for *Toxocara*.

Acknowledgements

This research was supported by Health Research Institute at the Babol University of Medical Sciences (IR.MUBABOL.HRI.REC.1398.129), Babol, Iran (A.R.). Research in R.B.G.'s group is supported through funds from the National Health and Medical Research Council (NHMRC) of Australia, the Australian Research Council (ARC), Yourgene Health, Melbourne Water Corporation and The University of Melbourne.

References

Aghaei, S., Riahi, S.M., Rostami, A., Mohammadzadeh, I., Javanian, M., Tohidi, E., Foroutan, M., Esmaeili Dooki, M., 2018. *Toxocara* spp. infection and risk of childhood asthma: a systematic review and meta-analysis. Acta Trop. 182, 298–304.

Aghamolaie, S., Seyyedtabaei, S.J., Behniafar, H., Foroutan, M., Saber, V., Hanifehpur, H., Mehravar, S., Rostami, A., 2018. Seroepidemiology, modifiable risk factors and clinical symptoms of *Toxocara* spp. infection in northern Iran. Trans. R. Soc. Trop. Med. Hyg. 113, 116–122.

Ahmed, S.M., Hall, A.J., Robinson, A.E., Verhoef, L., Premkumar, P., Parashar, U.D., Koopmans, M., Lopman, B.A., 2014. Global prevalence of norovirus in cases of gastroenteritis: a systematic review and meta-analysis. Lancet Infect. Dis. 14, 725–730.

Azam, D., Ukpai, O.M., Said, A., Abd-Allah, G.A., Morgan, E.R., 2012. Temperature and the development and survival of infective *Toxocara canis* larvae. Parasitol. Res. 110, 649–656.

Bakhshani, A., Maleki, M., Haghparast, A., Parande Shirvan, S., Borji, H., 2019. A survey on *Toxocara cati* eggs on the hair of stray cats: a potential risk factor for human toxocariasis in Northeastern Iran. Comp. Immunol. Microbiol. Infect. Dis. 64, 10–13.

Barutzki, D., Schaper, R., 2003. Endoparasites in dogs and cats in Germany 1999–2002. Parasitol. Res. 90, S148–S150.

Barutzki, D., Schaper, R., 2013. Age-dependant prevalence of endoparasites in young dogs and cats up to one year of age. Parasitol. Res. 112, 119–131.

Beck, A.M., Meyers, N.M., 1996. Health enhancement and companion animal ownership. Ann. Rev. Public Health 17, 247–257.

Blagburn, B.L., Lindsay, D.S., Vaughan, J.L., Rippey, N.S., Wright, J.C., Lynn, R.C., Kelch, W.J., Ritchie, G., Hepler, D.I., 1996. Prevalence of canine parasites based on fecal flotation. Comp. Cont. Ed. Pract. Vet. 18, 483–509.

Buehl, I.E., Prosl, H., Mundt, H.C., Tichy, A., Joachim, A., 2006. Canine isosporosis–epidemiology of field and experimental infections. J. Vet. Med. Series B. 53, 482–487.

Chen, J., Xu, M.J., Zhou, D.H., Song, H.Q., Wang, C.R., Zhu, X.Q., 2012. Canine and feline parasitic zoonoses in China. Parasit. Vectors 5, 152.
Duarte, A., Castro, I., Pereira da Fonseca, I.M., Almeida, V., Madeira de Carvalho, L.M., Meireles, J., Fazendeiro, M.I., Tavares, L., Vaz, Y., 2010. Survey of infectious and parasitic diseases in stray cats at the Lisbon Metropolitan Area. Portugal. J. Feline Med. Surg. 12, 441–446.
Robertson, I.D., Thompson, R.C., 2002. Enteric parasitic zoonoses of domesticated dogs and cats. Microb. Infect. 4, 867–873.
Sweatman, G.K., Henshall, T.C., Manktelow, B.W., 1962. Experimental observations on parasitic liver white spot in New Zealand sheep. N. Z. Vet. J. 10, 99–107.
Tan, J.S., 1997. Human zoonotic infections transmitted by dogs and cats. Arch. Intern. Med. 157, 1933–1943.

CHAPTER THIRTY-ONE

Toxocara spp. in dogs and cats in Canada

Emily J. Jenkins*
Zoonotic Parasite Research Unit, Department of Veterinary Microbiology, Western College of Veterinary Medicine, University of Saskatchewan, Saskatoon, SK, Canada
*Corresponding author: e-mail address: emily.jenkins@usask.ca

Contents

Abstract

Toxocara spp. (*T. canis* and *T. cati*) are the dominant ascarids of domestic dogs and cats, respectively, in populated regions of southern Canada, where they pose animal and public health concerns. A review of the published literature indicated that prevalence of both parasites is declining in more recent studies (post 2000), likely due to changes in animal husbandry as well as use of anthelmintics. Geographically, prevalence was higher in the east (Atlantic), and in more southerly locations, possibly due to more favourable climate conditions for egg survival and development. At northern latitudes and in wild felids and canids in general, the non-zoonotic ascarid *Toxascaris leonina* appears to outcompete *Toxocara* spp.; however, *T. leonina* is rare in domestic cats in Canada. Prevalence of *Toxocara* spp. was higher in cats than dogs, shelter/rural/remote/feral/stray vs owned animals, and young vs adult animals, as has been observed in many other studies and regions of the world. While the regional prevalences in this review should be interpreted carefully in light of variation in diagnostic methods and study populations, they generally follow the same trends observed in a recent national study of shelter animals. This review is a timely summary of the state of the published knowledge on prevalence of *Toxocara* spp. in Canada, and highlights knowledge gaps to be addressed, including the northern

Advances in Parasitology, Volume 109
ISSN 0065-308X
https://doi.org/10.1016/bs.apar.2020.01.026

distributional limits of these species in Canada, the potential for transmission to and from wildlife hosts, and the public health significance of the parasite in the mainstream Canadian population.

1. Introduction

Toxocara spp. are the dominant ascarids of domestic dogs (*T. canis*) and cats (*T. cati*) in populated regions of southern Canada, where they pose a public health concern and may have clinical effects in pups and kittens. The non-zoonotic *Toxascaris leonina* is the dominant ascarid in dogs in northern Canada, as well as wild canids and felids in Canada generally (Holmes and Podesta, 1968; Smith et al., 1986; Van Zyll de Jong, 1966). While *T. leonina* can be present in domestic cats, it was not detected in faecal samples from 636 cats in shelters across the country in a recent national study (Villeneuve et al., 2015) and has only rarely been reported in domestic cats (Hoopes et al., 2015; Threlfall, 1969). It is important (and easy) to distinguish these two ascarid species on faecal diagnostic tests, since the eggs are morphologically distinct and the public health significance is quite different (Fig. 1). In light of the importance of *Toxocara* spp. from both animal and human health perspectives, and the timeliness of the recent national study, the published literature on distribution, prevalence, and risk factors for *Toxocara* spp. in dogs and cats in Canada was reviewed.

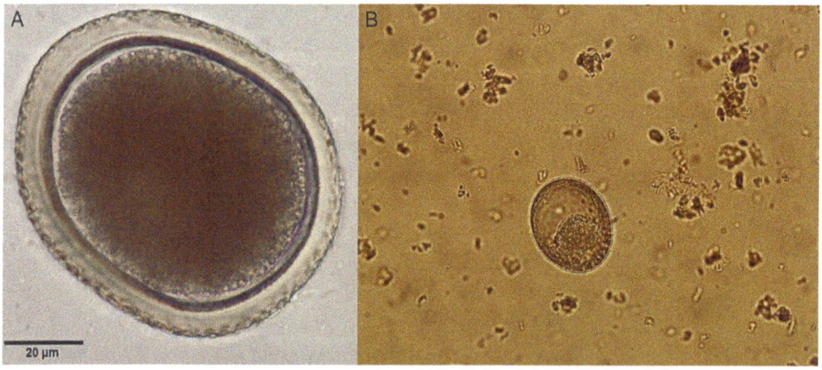

Fig. 1 Eggs of (a) *Toxocara canis* and (b) *Toxascaris leonina* at 400 × magnification. Eggs are easily distinguished by the pebbled vs smooth appearance of the outer wall and the greater space between the ovum and the eggshell in *T. leonina*. As *T. canis* is zoonotic and *T. leonina* is not, it is important to distinguish the eggs of these two ascarid species. *Photo credits: Pratap Kafle and Rajnish Sharma.*

2. Methods

Search terms "*Toxocara*", "Canada", "dog", and "cat" were used to search the published literature in Google Scholar. As well, the works cited in recent synoptic reviews were mined (Hoopes et al., 2013; Jenkins et al., 2013; Villeneuve et al., 2015). For each study, Table 1 captures the sample size, nature of the study population (low risk: owned and/or diagnostic laboratory specimens vs high risk: shelter, feral, rural, remote, and/or stray), and study prevalence (proportion of samples positive in each population). Results were reported by region: Atlantic—Newfoundland Labrador, New Brunswick, Nova Scotia, and Prince Edward Island; Central—Ontario and Québec; and West—British Columbia, Alberta, Saskatchewan, and Manitoba. Overall regional and risk group prevalences were calculated by taking the sum of the number of positive samples/sum of the total number of samples in studies from 2000 and onwards, to best reflect the current situation in Canada. Confidence intervals were calculated using the binomial, or Clopper-Pearson Exact method at http://epitools.ausvet.com.au/content.php?page=CIProportion. There are obvious limitations to this approach, including variation in the diagnostic methods (generally some kind of faecal flotation) used among the different studies and differences in age, season of collection, and other risk factors among the different study populations; however, the goal was to provide the big picture of regional differences in prevalence of these parasites, using the best available data in the peer reviewed literature. Finally, some mention is made of the host and geographic distribution in wildlife, since this more accurately reflects the ability of the parasite to establish under regional climate conditions, without interference from treatment, which is a confounding factor in domestic dogs and cats.

3. Geographic distribution

Toxocara spp. are present in domestic dogs and cats across southern Canada, the most densely populated regions of the country (Fig. 2). In a recent national study of shelter animals, the majority of which were in major urban centres, eggs of *Toxocara* spp. were present in faecal samples from dogs and cats in all 10 provinces (NL, NS, NB, PEI, QC, ON, MB, SK, AB, and BC) (Villeneuve et al., 2015), with the exception of *T. canis* in dogs in NL; however, this parasite has previously been reported

Table 1 Published reports of *Toxocara canis* in dogs in Canada, ordered chronologically within three regions (Atlantic, Central, and West, province abbreviations as for Fig. 1).

Location	Population	Prevalence % (n)	References
Atlantic (NL, NB, NS, PEI)			
NL	Euthanized	26% (35)[a]	Threlfall (1969)
NS	Stray	27% (474)	Malloy and Embil (1978)
St Pierre and Miquelon	Owned Shelter	24% (42) 20% (15)	Bridger and Whitney (2009)
PEI	Shelter	10% (555)	CPEP, 2009
NL, NB, NS, PEI	Shelter	10% (101)	Villeneuve et al. (2015)
Atlantic region (95% CI)		*11% (9–14%)*	Since 2000
Central (ON and QC)			
ON	Owned, Dx	10% (5069)	Slocombe (1973)
QC	Owned	34% (332)	Ghadirian et al. (1976)
ON	Owned	2% (102)	Lefebvre et al. (2006)
ON	High risk	14% (70)	Shukla et al. (2006)
ON	Shelter	10% (49)	Blagburn et al. (2008)
ON	Owned, Dx	4% (1110)	CPEP (2009)
QC	Owned, Dx	4% (1108)	CPEP (2009)
ON and QC	Shelter	12% (622)	Villeneuve et al. (2015)
Central region (95% CI)		*6% (5–7%)*	Since 2000
West (BC, AB, SK, MB)			
SK	Not specified	30% (3370)	Allen and Mills (1971)
SK	Remote	48% (160)	Unruh et al. (1973)
SK	Shelter	2% (623)	Anvik et al. (1974)
AB	Remote	3% (59)	Salb et al. (2008)
SK	Rural	17% (155)	Himsworth et al. (2010)
BC	Remote	4% (75)	Bryan et al. (2011)
SK	Owned	0.2% (457)	Gaunt and Carr (2011)
AB	Owned Shelter	1% (477) 9% (142)	Joffe et al. (2011)

Table 1 Published reports of *Toxocara canis* in dogs in Canada, ordered chronologically within three regions (Atlantic, Central, and West, province abbreviations as for Fig. 1).—cont'd

Location	Population	Prevalence % (n)	References
SK	Rural/ remote	12% (254)	Schurer et al. (2012)
SK	Shelter	8% (231)	Schurer et al. (2014a)
AB	Owned	0.3% (355)	Smith et al. (2014)
BC, AB, SK, MB	Shelter	14% (363)	Villeneuve et al. (2015)
Western region (95% CI)		*6% (5–7%)*	Since 2000
Canada overall (95% CI)		*6% (6–7%)*	Since 2000
Low risk (95% CI)		*3% (2–4%)*	Since 2000
High risk (95% CI)		*11% (10–12%)*	Since 2000

[a]Detection of adult nematodes on necropsy (vs detection of eggs in faecal flotation).
Two populations of dogs were considered: (1) low risk (owned dogs and samples submitted to a veterinary diagnostic laboratory—Dx) and (2) high risk (rural, remote, stray, and shelter).

in both dogs and coyotes in NL (Bridger et al., 2009; Threlfall, 1969). Reports of *T. canis* north of 60°N (in the three northern territories) are rare; the most northerly reports of *T. canis* are 63°N and for *T. cati*, 54°N (Cameron et al., 1940; Unruh et al., 1973; Van Zyll de Jong, 1966). While there have not been extensive surveys of dogs, and none of cats, at northern latitudes, various necropsy and faecal surveys in both wild and domestic canids have found *Toxascaris leonina*, but not *Toxocara* spp. (Choquette et al., 1973; Desrochers and Curtis, 1987; Eaton and Secord, 1979; Schurer et al., 2016). The lack of success of *T. canis* at northern latitudes in Canada is further supported by low human seroprevalence in these regions (reviewed in Jenkins et al., 2013). Eggs of *T. cati* are more freeze tolerant and therefore may have a higher northern distributional limit (O'Lorcain, 1995); however, cats are not commonly kept as pets in northern Canada, and lynx are distributed only as far north as the northern limit of the boreal forest.

Potential wildlife hosts for *T. cati* in Canada include the following: bobcat (*Lynx rufus*), present in the southern regions of all provinces except NL and PEI; cougar (*Puma concolor*), primarily present in mountainous

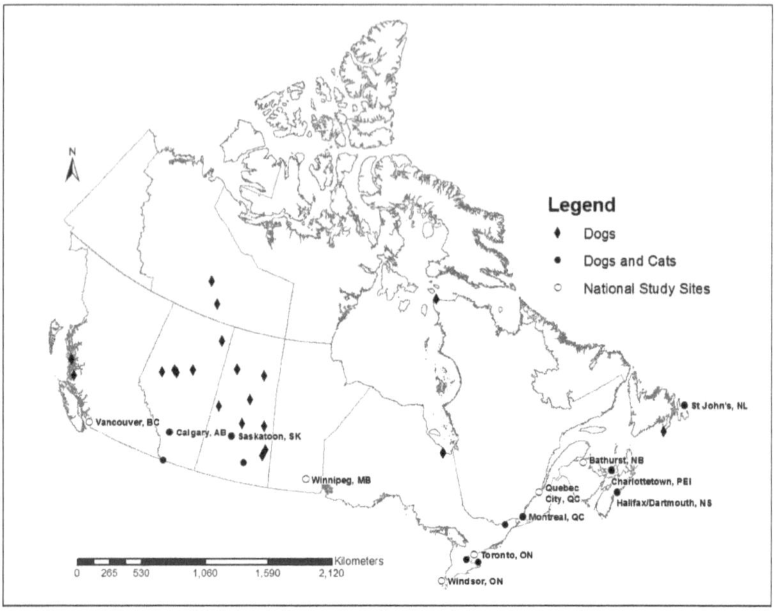

Fig. 2 *Toxocara* spp. have been reported in dogs (diamond) and dogs and cats (filled circle) in all 10 Canadian provinces (British Columbia—BC, Alberta—AB, Saskatchewan—SK, Manitoba—MB, Ontario—ON, Québec—QC, Newfoundland—NL, New Brunswick—NB, Nova Scotia—NS, and Prince Edward Island = PEI) and the southernmost Northwest Territories. *Toxocara* spp. have not been reported in the Yukon Territory, Nunavut, or Labrador (the mainland portion of NL). Named cities/open circles are sites for the national survey in shelter dogs and cats (Villeneuve et al., 2015). *Map credit Lianne McLeod.*

regions of BC and AB; and lynx (*Lynx canadensis*), present in boreal regions of all provinces and the southern regions of the northern territories (Dare and Watkins, 2013; Hiestand et al., 2014; Naughton, 2012; Smith et al., 1986; Van Zyll de Jong, 1966). Potential wildlife hosts for *T. canis* in Canada include coyote (*Canis latrans*), present everywhere except the Arctic coast and islands; grey fox (*Urocyon cinereoargenteus*), present in southern MB and ON; red fox (*Vulpes vulpes*), present everywhere except some Arctic islands and the northern BC coast; swift fox (*Vulpes velox*), present only vestigially in southern AB and SK; and wolves (*Canis lupus*), present everywhere except the prairies, southernmost ON and QC, the Maritime provinces, and the island of Newfoundland (Bridger et al., 2009; Bryan et al., 2012; Davidson et al., 1992; Holmes and Podesta, 1968; Miller et al., 1998; Naughton, 2012; Stronen et al., 2011; Wapenaar et al., 2013). *Toxocara canis* has not been reported in Arctic fox (*Vulpes lagopus*), despite necropsy and faecal surveys (Eaton and Secord, 1979; Elmore et al., 2013); this may well reflect absence of the parasite at high latitudes rather than lack of host suitability.

4. Temporal and geographic trends in prevalence in pets in Canada

Prevalences of both *T. canis* and *T. cati* were lower in more recent studies (since 2000) as compared to older studies (Tables 1 and 2). This declining prevalence has also been observed in the United States (Little et al., 2009), and likely reflects use of anthelmintics, as well as decreased exposure due to more stringent faecal hygiene practices and increased feeding of commercial pet foods (thus reducing transmission via consumption of paratenic hosts) within the pet population in North America. As well, several older studies were based on finding of adult nematodes on necropsy, which generally has higher sensitivity than faecal based methods. Prevalence of *Toxocara* spp. was higher in cats (11%) vs dogs (6%) in Canada, similar to findings in the United States (Lucio-Forster et al., 2016). This is likely due to the fact that cats (many of which have at least some access to the outdoors) have more exposure through hunting paratenic hosts, and cats are less likely to receive anthelmintic treatment for financial and logistical reasons.

Overall, Canadian prevalence (11% in cats, 6% in dogs) based on studies since 2000 was higher than in recent studies of veterinary diagnostic laboratory submissions in the United States (5% in cats, 2% in dogs) (Little et al., 2009; Lucio-Forster et al., 2016); this likely reflects that many of the Canadian studies were in higher risk populations, including feral, shelter, rural, remote, and stray animals. In low risk (owned) pets in Canada, prevalence of 5% in cats and 3% in dogs was almost identical to United States findings. It is also important to note that samples submitted to veterinary diagnostic laboratories (although they are from owned, well-maintained pets) are not representative of the general healthy pet population, since faecal samples are rarely submitted unless some clinical illness (such as diarrhoea) is present. Therefore, true prevalence in healthy, owned pets (especially adult animals) is likely much lower.

The finding of higher prevalence in recent Canadian vs United States studies is counter-intuitive, as one would expect to see higher levels of transmission of *Toxocara* spp. in the United States, where the climate is more favourable for egg survival and development. However, it is also likely that many United States pet owners (especially dog owners) are following the national guidelines for monthly deworming, largely to protect against

Table 2 Study prevalence of *Toxocara cati* in cats in Canada, ordered chronologically within three regions (Atlantic, Central, and West, province abbreviations as for Fig. 1).

Location	Method	Prevalence % (n)	References
Atlantic (NL, NB, NS, PEI)			
NL	Euthanized	46% (35)[a]	Threlfall (1969)
NS	Stray	25% (299)	Malloy and Embil (1978)
PEI	Shelter	10% (145)	CPEP (2009)
PEI	Feral	35% (78)	Stojanovic and Foley (2011)
PEI	Feral &shelter	38% (200)	Raab et al. (2016)
NL, NB, NS, PEI	Shelter	24% (81)	Villeneuve et al. (2015)
Atlantic region (95% CI)		*27% (23–31%)*	Since 2000
Central (ON and QC)			
ON	Owned, Dx	30% (458)	Slocombe (1973)
ON	High Risk	12% (41)	Shukla et al. (2006)
ON	Shelter	11% (47)	Blagburn et al. (2008)
ON	Owned, Dx	5% (360)	CPEP (2009)
QC	Owned, Dx	5% (442)	CPEP (2009)
QC and ON	Shelter	19% (285)	Villeneuve et al. (2015)
Central region (95% CI)		*9% (7–11%)*	Since 2000
West (BC, AB, SK, MB)			
SK	Shelter	17% (52)[a]	Pomroy (1999)
AB	Owned, Shelter	1% (68) 11% (85)	Joffe et al. (2011)
SK	Owned, Dx	5% (635)	Hoopes et al. (2013)
AB	Rural	15% (27)	Hoopes et al. (2015)
SK	Owned Other	0% (31) 1% (161)	Hoopes et al. (2015)
West (BC, AB, SK, MB)	Shelter	12% (270)	Villeneuve et al. (2015)

Table 2 Study prevalence of *Toxocara cati* in cats in Canada, ordered chronologically within three regions (Atlantic, Central, and West, province abbreviations as for Fig. 1).—cont'd

Location	Method	Prevalence % (n)	References
Western region (95% CI)		*6% (5–8%)*	Since 2000
Canada overall (95% CI)		*11% (10–12%)*	Since 2000
Low risk (95% CI)		*5% (4–6%)*	Since 2000
High risk (95% CI)		*18% (16–20%)*	Since 2000

[a]Detection of adult nematodes on necropsy (vs detection of eggs in faecal flotation).
Two populations of cats were considered: (1) low risk (owned cats and samples submitted to a veterinary diagnostic laboratory—Dx) and (2) high risk (feral, rural, stray, and shelter)

heartworm (*Dirofilaria immitis*). In contrast, heartworm has a low prevalence and patchy distribution in southern Canada and seasonally limited transmission (May–October); therefore, year-round monthly prophylaxis, even in heartworm endemic regions, is not recommended (CPEP, 2019). This may also contribute to the higher prevalence of *Toxocara* spp. observed in companion animals in Canada vs the United States.

Within Canada, there appears to be an East-West trend, with highest prevalence of both species of *Toxocara* in the Atlantic provinces, which may reflect a more temperate climate (Tables 1 and 2). In the recent national study of shelter animals, the prevalence of *T. cati* was highest in the Atlantic region (East coast) and the prevalence of *T. canis* highest in British Columbia (West coast), suggesting that coastal environments may be more conducive to transmission (Villeneuve et al., 2015); there may also be higher pet densities, although this is difficult to capture since there are no formal estimates in Canada. As well, there appears to be higher prevalence of *T. canis* in more southern populations of dogs—for example, prevalence was three times higher in a population of dogs in southern vs northern Saskatchewan (Schurer et al., 2013, 2014b); likewise, prevalence of *T. cati* was much higher in cats in southern Alberta than central Saskatchewan (Hoopes et al., 2015). Older studies also report that *T. canis* becomes increasingly rare in dogs as one moves north (Cameron et al., 1940; Unruh et al., 1973).

5. Other risk factors

Several studies demonstrated higher prevalence in younger animals (generally less than 1 year) vs adult animals (Joffe et al., 2011;

Malloy and Embil, 1978; Villeneuve et al., 2015). This is not surprising in light of the ability of these parasites to transmit via transplacental (primarily *T. canis*) and transmammary routes (primarily *T. cati*), and the immature immune systems of young animals. It should, however, be taken into consideration when comparing among different study populations; for example, shelter animals and animals brought to remote spay and neuter clinics are frequently younger than the general pet population, biasing the results towards higher prevalence. For purposes of this study, feral/shelter/stray/remote and rural animals were grouped together as "high risk"; however, there are differences in prevalence even within these groups—for example, prevalence of *T. cati* was 70% in feral cats vs 6% in shelter cats (Raab et al., 2016). As well, prevalence of *T. canis* was significantly higher in shelter dogs from rural vs urban origins (Schurer et al., 2014a). On the positive side, control efforts targeting these known high risk groups (young, rural, feral, etc.) will have greater effects on decreasing parasite transmission than prophylactic deworming of healthy, owned, adult pets, which may also contribute to growing anthelmintic resistance in canine parasites, such as hookworm (*Ancylostoma caninum*) and heartworm.

6. Conclusions and the way forward

These findings reinforce current best practice guidelines for companion animal parasite management in Canada (CPEP, 2019), which recommend routine deworming of pups and kittens under 6 months, and deworming adult pets only when they have clear risk factors (hunting and scavenging, for example) or have a positive faecal test (ideally a combination of flotation and coproantigen/coproPCR). If temporal trends continue, the prevalence of these important helminth parasites may continue to decline in Canada. However, increasingly pet owners are seeking to decrease "unnecessary" treatments, and are indulging in high risk behaviours including raw food diets, free roaming access to the outdoors, and pet daycares and classes. Therefore, this review is a timely opportunity to remind practitioners and pet owners to remain vigilant about these zoonoses, especially in young and high risk animals. As these parasites have wildlife reservoirs, eradication will never be possible, and preventing pets from sharing environments (such as periurban dog parks) with wildlife is important to protect pets (and people) from exposure to important zoonoses such as *Toxocara* and *Echinococcus* spp. Finally, this review highlights knowledge gaps to be addressed, including the northern distributional limits of

Toxocara spp. in Canada, the potential for transmission to and from wildlife hosts, and the public health significance of the parasite in the mainstream Canadian population; there is a great need for national human seroprevalence data on these and other important parasitic zoonoses.

Acknowledgements

Many thanks to Pratap Kafle and Rajnish Sharma for sharing egg images, Sarah Parker for guidance in analysis, Lianne McLeod for mapping, Janna Schurer and Jessica Hoopes for previous reviews of the subject, and the Canadian Parasitology Expert Panel.

References

Allen, J.R., Mills, J.H., 1971. *Alaria arisaemoides* in Saskatchewan dogs. Can. Vet. J. 12, 24–28.

Anvik, J.O., Hague, A.E., Rahaman, A., 1974. A method of estimating urban dog populations and its application to the assessment of canine fecal pollution and endoparasitism in Saskatchewan. Can. Vet. J. 15, 219–223.

Blagburn, B.L., Schenker, R., Gagne, F., Drake, J., 2008. Prevalence of intestinal parasites in companion animals in Ontario and Quebec, Canada, during the winter months. Vet. Ther. 9, 169–175.

Bridger, K.E., Whitney, H., 2009. Gastrointestinal parasites in dogs from the island of St. Pierre off the south coast of Newfoundland. Vet. Parasitol. 162, 167–170.

Bridger, K.E., Baggs, E.M., Finney-Crawley, J., 2009. Endoparasites of the coyote (*Canis latrans*), a recent migrant to insular Newfoundland. J. Wildl. Dis. 45, 1221–1226.

Bryan, H.M., Darimont, C.T., Paquet, P.C., Ellis, J.A., Goji, N., Gouix, M., Smits, J.E., 2011. Exposure to infectious agents in dogs in remote coastal British Columbia: possible sentinels of diseases in wildlife and humans. Can. J. Vet. Res. 75, 11–17.

Bryan, H.M., Darimont, C.T., Hill, J.E., Paquet, P.C., Thompson, R.C.A., Wagner, B., Smits, J.E.G., 2012. Seasonal and biogeographical patterns of gastrointestinal parasites in large carnivores: wolves in a coastal archipelago. Parasitology 139, 781–790.

Cameron, T.W.M., Parnell, I.W., Lyster, L.L., 1940. The helminth parasites of sledge-dogs in northern Canada and Newfoundland. Can. J. Res. 18, 325–332.

Choquette, L.P.E., Gibson, G.G., Kuyt, E., Pearson, A.M., 1973. Helminths of wolves, *Canis lupus* L., in the Yukon and Northwest Territories. Can. J. Zool. 51, 1087–1091.

CPEP, 2009. Canadian Parasitology Expert Panel (CPEP) Guidelines for the Treatment of Parasites in Dogs and Cats. University of Saskatchewan, Saskatoon, SK, p. 32.

CPEP, 2019. Canadian Parasitology Expert Panel (CPEP) Guidelines for the Management of Parasites in Dogs and Cats. University of Saskatchewan, Saskatoon, SK, p. 71.

Dare, O.K., Watkins, W.G., 2013. First record of parasites from cougars (*Puma concolor*) in Manitoba, Canada. Can. Field-Nat. 126, 324–327.

Davidson, W.R., Appel, M.J., Doster, G.L., Baker, O.E., Brown, J.F., 1992. Diseases and parasites of red foxes, gray foxes, and coyotes from commercial sources selling to fox-chasing enclosures. J. Wildl. Dis. 28, 581–589.

Desrochers, F., Curtis, M.A., 1987. The occurrence of gastrointestinal helminths in dogs from Kuujjuaq (fort Chimo), Quebec, Canada. Can. J. Public Health 78, 403–406.

Eaton, R.D., Secord, D.C., 1979. Some intestinal parasites of Arctic fox, Banks Island, NWT. Can. J. Comp. Med. 43, 229–230.

Elmore, S.A., Lalonde, L.F., Samelius, G., Alisauskas, R.T., Gajadhar, A.A., Jenkins, E.J., 2013. Endoparasites in the feces of arctic foxes in a terrestrial ecosystem in Canada. Int. J. Parasitol. Parasites Wildl. 2, 90–96.

Gaunt, M.C., Carr, A.P., 2011. A survey of intestinal parasites in dogs from Saskatoon, Saskatchewan. Can. Vet. J. 52, 497–500.

Ghadirian, E., Viens, P., Strykowski, H., Dubreuil, F., 1976. Epidemiology of toxocariasis in the Montreal area: prevalence of *Toxocara* and other helminth ova in dogs and soil. Can. J. Public Health 67, 495–498.

Hiestand, S.J., Nielsen, C.K., Jiménez, F.A., 2014. Epizootic and zoonotic helminths of the bobcat (*Lynx rufus*) in Illinois and a comparison of its helminth component communities across the American Midwest. Parasite 21, 4.

Himsworth, C.G., Skinner, S., Chaban, B., Jenkins, E., Wagner, B.A., Harms, N.J., Leighton, F.A., Thompson, R.C., Hill, J.E., 2010. Multiple zoonotic pathogens identified in canine feces collected from a remote Canadian indigenous community. Am. J. Trop. Med. Hyg. 83, 338–341.

Holmes, J.C., Podesta, R., 1968. The helminths of wolves and coyotes from the forested regions of Alberta. Can. J. Zool. 46, 1193–1204.

Hoopes, J.H., Polley, L., Wagner, B., Jenkins, E.J., 2013. A retrospective investigation of feline gastrointestinal parasites in western Canada. Can. Vet. J. 54, 359–362.

Hoopes, J., Hill, J.E., Polley, L., Fernando, C., Wagner, B., Schurer, J.M., Jenkins, E.J., 2015. Enteric parasites of free-roaming, owned, and rural cats in prairie regions of Canada. Can. Vet. J. 56, 495–501.

Jenkins, E.J., Castrodale, L.J., de Rosemond, S.J., Dixon, B.R., Elmore, S.A., Gesy, K.M., Hoberg, E.P., Polley, L., Schurer, J.M., Simard, M., Thompson, R.C.A., 2013. Tradition and transition: parasitic zoonoses of people and animals in Alaska, northern Canada, and Greenland. Adv. Parasitol. 82, 33–204.

Joffe, D., Van Niekerk, D., Gagné, F., Gilleard, J., Kutz, S., Lobingier, R., 2011. The prevalence of intestinal parasites in dogs and cats in Calgary, Alberta. Can. Vet. J. 52, 1323–1328.

Lefebvre, S.L., Waltner-Toews, D., Peregrine, A.S., Reid-Smith, R., Hodge, L., Arroyo, L.G., Weese, J.S., 2006. Prevalence of zoonotic agents in dogs visiting hospitalized people in Ontario: implications for infection control. J. Hosp. Infect. 62, 458–466.

Little, S.E., Johnson, E.M., Lewis, D., Jaklitsch, R.P., Payton, M.E., Blagburn, B.L., Bowman, D.D., Moroff, S., Tams, T., Rich, L., Aucoin, D., 2009. Prevalence of intestinal parasites in pet dogs in the United States. Vet. Parasitol. 166, 144–152.

Lucio-Forster, A., Mizhquiri Barbecho, J.S., Mohammed, H.O., Kornreich, B.G., Bowman, D.D., 2016. Comparison of the prevalence of *Toxocara* egg shedding by pet cats and dogs in the U.S.A., 2011–2014. Vet. Parasitol. Reg. Stud. Reports 5, 1–13.

Malloy, W.F., Embil, J.A., 1978. Prevalence of *Toxocara* spp. and other parasites in dogs and cats in Halifax, Nova Scotia. Can. J. Comp. Med. 42, 29–31.

Miller, D.S., Campbell, B.G., McLean, R.G., Campos, E., Covell, D.F., 1998. Parasites of swift fox (*Vulpes velox*) from Southeastern Colorado. Southwest. Nat. 43, 476–479.

Naughton, D., 2012. The Natural History of Canadian Mammals. Canadian Museum of Nature and University of Toronto Press, Toronto.

O'Lorcain, P., 1995. The effects of freezing on the viability of *Toxocara canis* and *T. cati* embryonated eggs. J. Helminthol. 69, 169–171.

Pomroy, W.E., 1999. A survey of helminth parasites of cats from Saskatoon. Can. Vet. J. 40, 339–340.

Raab, O., Greenwood, S., Vanderstichel, R., Gelens, H., 2016. A cross-sectional study of *Tritrichomonas foetus* infection in feral and shelter cats in Prince Edward Island, Canada. Can. Vet. J. 57, 265–270.

Salb, A.L., Barkema, H.W., Elkin, B.T., Thompson, R.C.A., Whiteside, D.P., Black, S.R., Dubey, J.P., Kutz, S.J., 2008. Dogs as sources and sentinels of parasites in humans and wildlife, northern Canada. Emerg. Infect. Dis. 14, 60–63.

Schurer, J.M., Hill, J.E., Fernando, C., Jenkins, E.J., 2012. Sentinel surveillance for zoonotic parasites in companion animals in indigenous communities of Saskatchewan. Am. J. Trop. Med. Hyg. 87, 495–498.

Schurer, J.M., Ndao, M., Skinner, S., Irvine, J., Elmore, S.A., Epp, T., Jenkins, E.J., 2013. Parasitic zoonoses: one health surveillance in northern Saskatchewan. PLoS Negl. Trop. Dis. 7, e2141.

Schurer, J.M., Hamblin, B., Davenport, L., Wagner, B., Jenkins, E.J., 2014a. Rural origin, age, and endoparasite fecal prevalence in dogs surrendered to the Regina Humane Society, 2013. Can. Vet. J. 55, 1192–1195.

Schurer, J.M., Ndao, M., Quewezance, H., Elmore, S.A., Jenkins, E.J., 2014b. People, pets, and parasites: one health surveillance in southeastern Saskatchewan. Am. J. Trop. Med. Hyg. 90, 1184–1190.

Schurer, J.M., Pawlik, M., Huber, A., Elkin, B., Cluff, D., Pongracz, J., Gesy, K., Wagner, B., Dixon, B., Merks, H., Bal, M., Jenkins, E., 2016. Intestinal parasites of wolves (*Canis lupus*) in northern and western Canada. Can. J. Zool. 94, 643–650.

Shukla, R., Giraldo, P., Kraliz, A., Finnigan, M., Sanchez, A.L., 2006. *Cryptosporidium* spp. and other zoonotic enteric parasites in a sample of domestic dogs and cats in the Niagara region of Ontario. Can. Vet. J. 47, 1179–1184.

Slocombe, J.O., 1973. Parasitisms in domesticated animals in Ontario. I. Ontario Veterinary College Records 1965-70. Can. Vet. J. 14, 36–42.

Smith, J.D., Addison, E.M., Joachim, D.G., Smith, L.M., Quinn, N.W.S., 1986. Helminth parasites of Canada lynx (*Felis canadensis*) from northern Ontario. Can. J. Zool. 64, 358–364.

Smith, A.F., Semeniuk, C.A., Kutz, S.J., Massolo, A., 2014. Dog-walking behaviours affect gastrointestinal parasitism in park-attending dogs. Parasit. Vectors 7, article 429.

Stojanovic, V., Foley, P., 2011. Infectious disease prevalence in a feral cat population on Prince Edward Island, Canada. Can. Vet. J. 52, 979–982.

Stronen, A.V., Sallows, T., Forbes, G.J., Wagner, B., Paquet, P.C., 2011. Diseases and parasites in wolves of the Riding Mountain National Park region, Manitoba, Canada. J. Wildl. Dis. 47, 222–227.

Threlfall, W., 1969. Further records of helminths from Newfoundland mammals. Can. J. Zool. 47, 197–201.

Unruh, D.H.A., King, J.E., Eaton, R.D.P., Allen, J.R., 1973. Parasites of dogs from Indian settlements in northwestern Canada: a survey with public health implications. Can. J. Comp. Med. 37, 25–32.

Van Zyll de Jong, C.G., 1966. Parasites of the Canada lynx, *Felis (lynx) canadensis* (Kerr). Can. J. Zool. 44, 499–509.

Villeneuve, A., Polley, L., Jenkins, E., Schurer, J., Gilleard, J., Kutz, S., Conboy, G., Benoit, D., Seewald, W., Gagné, F., 2015. Parasite prevalence in fecal samples from shelter dogs and cats across the Canadian provinces. Parasit. Vectors 8, e281.

Wapenaar, W., Barkema, H.W., O'Handley, R., 2013. Fecal shedding of *Toxocara canis* and other parasites in foxes and coyotes on Prince Edward Island, Canada. J. Wildl. Dis. 49, 394–397.

CHAPTER THIRTY-TWO

Toxocara canis and *Toxocara cati* in domestic dogs and cats in the United States, Mexico, Central America and the Caribbean: A review

Jennifer K. Ketzis[a,]*, Araceli Lucio-Forster[b]

[a]Department of Biomedical Sciences, Ross University School of Veterinary Medicine, Basseterre, St. Kitts and Nevis, West Indies

[b]Department of Microbiology and Immunology, Cornell University College of Veterinary Medicine, Ithaca, NY, United States

*Corresponding author: e-mail address: jketzis@rossvet.edu.kn

Contents

Abstract

Toxocara prevalence ranges from 0 to >87% and 0 to >60% in dogs and cats, respectively, within the United States, Mexico, Central America and the Caribbean. Higher prevalence occurs in animals less than 1 year of age. Overall, prevalence is higher in cats compared to dogs. The lowest prevalence occurs in the US owned dog population. Specific populations in this industrialized nation, in animal shelters or resource-limited locations, have prevalences similar to those seen in populations from other regions reviewed here. Conversely, subpopulations in Central America and the Caribbean have very low prevalence. Apparent contributors to prevalence, excluding animal age and climate, are socio-economic factors, attitudes towards pet management and animal population density. The lack of data from some regions pose a challenge in assessing trends; however, with the exception of the US owned dog population, there is no strong indication of any decrease in prevalence from historical levels.

Advances in Parasitology, Volume 109
ISSN 0065-308X
https://doi.org/10.1016/bs.apar.2020.01.027

1. Introduction

Assessing the prevalence of *Toxocara canis* and *Toxocara cati* in dogs and cats, respectively, in the United States, Mexico, Central America and the Caribbean Islands is a daunting task, although critical to understanding the risk these parasites pose to dog, cat and human health. Many interrelated factors influence their prevalence in animals and their surroundings, including human interventions, attitudes and behaviours, host (dog, cat, and wild felid and canid) behaviours, and host and parasite biology. More specifically, some of these factors include: attitudes towards pet ownership, socio-economic factors, access to veterinary care, frequency of use of anthelmintics (particularly in puppies), spaying and neutering of dogs and cats, level of free-roaming allowed for pets, removal of faeces from the environment, age distribution of dog and cat populations, presence and density of wild and domestic animals serving as final or paratenic hosts (including presence of community and feral dog and cat populations), soil composition, and climatic conditions. Additionally, the method used to diagnose infection can influence the apparent prevalence within the population tested. As there is inter-play between all these factors, and none are consistent within or across the countries or studies included in this review, it is difficult to extrapolate with any certainty the prevalence determined in one study to a wider population. With that said, there may be identifiable themes that can be used to better understand the risk posed by these parasites to animal and human health in given regions, as well as to identify areas in which targeted education, anthelmintic treatment, and perhaps other interventions could be of most benefit.

To obtain an understanding of the current situation of *Toxocara* in dogs and cats in these regions, and to identify similarities and areas where further studies are required, data from peer reviewed and grey literature (e.g., theses) have been compiled. In this review, for simplicity, the term 'prevalence' is used to indicate the proportion of positive animals within the total population tested.

2. United States

The available national and regional data for dogs and cats since the 1960s are summarized in Tables 1 and 2, respectively. With few exceptions, all studies for the United States have been geographically limited, with only four national studies in dogs (two each in owned and animal shelters) and

Table 1 Summary of *Toxocara canis* in dogs for the United States.

Location	Year[a]	Per cent positive for *Toxocara*		Description	Analysis method	Reference
National						
	1993–1994	14.5	Overall	6458 dogs in animal shelters Dogs not known to be treated with an anthelmintic 1224 dogs: <6 mo of age 2014 dogs: 6–12 mo of age 1983 dogs: 1–3 y of age 77 dogs: 3–7 y of age 230 dogs: > 7 y of age	CF; sucrose	Blagburn et al. (1996)
		30.2	<6 mo			
		12.1	6–12 mo			
		10.1	1–3 y			
		10.6	3–7 y			
		6.1	> 7 y			
	2003–2006	5.0		1,213,061 dogs at 547 Banfield veterinary clinics in 44 states Data excludes repeat testing of the same dog Including additional testing of the same dog, prevalence decreases Higher in younger dogs (<6 mo) and in intact dogs	Flotation (Fecalyzer®); $ZnSO_4$ Direct smear with saline 0.9% NaCl when insufficient quantity for flotation	Mohamed et al. (2009)
	2006	2.2[b]	Overall	1,199,293 samples submitted to Antech Diagnostic Laboratories 141,970 samples: dog <6 mo of age 21,410 samples: dog 6 mo to 1 y of age 103,165 samples: dogs 1–2 y of age 162,124 samples: dogs 3–7 y of age 123,179 samples: dogs >7 y of age Some specific locations had much higher prevalence (e.g., 10.6% Roanike Rapids, NC; 11% Montgomery, AL; 13.5% Victoria TX; 21% Greensboro NC)	CF; $ZnSO_4$ spg 1.18	Little et al. (2009)
		6.5	<6 mo			
		3.3	6–12 mo			
		1.1	1–2 y			
		0.5	3–7 y			
		0.5	>7 y			

Continued

Table 1 Summary of *Toxocara canis* in dogs for the United States.—cont'd

Location	Year[a]	Per cent positive for *Toxocara*		Description	Analysis method	Reference
	2008–2009	14.2		2603 dogs in animal shelters	CF; sucrose spg 1.2	Blagburn (2009)
			Number of samples	Prevalence based on data from the Companion Animal Parasite Council (capcvet.org) website analysed using a general linear model Prevalence estimates corrected based on the model Faecal data on the CAPC site are from results from commercial laboratories	CF	Lucio-Forster et al. (2016)
	2011	2.0	2,553,250			
	2012	2.0	2,572,089			
	2013	1.8	2,512,989			
	2014	1.8	2,750,718			
South						
Regional data			Number of samples			
	1993–1994	17.7	ND	Dogs in animal shelters	CF; sucrose	Blagburn et al. (1996)
	2006	1.6[b]	307,076	Samples submitted to Antech Diagnostic Laboratories	CF; $ZnSO_4$ spg 1.18	Little et al. (2009)
	2008–2009	17.4	ND	Dogs in animal shelters	CF; sucrose spg 1.2	Blagburn (2009)
	2011	1.7	632,635	Based on CAPC data; see national data	CF	Lucio-Forster et al. (2016)
	2012	1.7	644,122			
	2013	1.8	651,788			
	2014	1.6	714,428			

Louisiana	1956	8.2	170 faecal samples from ground/sidewalk in areas with limited homeless dogs Largely well-cared dogs in area New Orleans	Direct smear CF; $ZnSO_4$	Vaughn and Jordan (1960)
	1957	6.5	325 dogs at four veterinary clinics Considered 'well cared' for dogs 14.6% of dogs <9 mo of age were positive 2.7% of dogs >9 mo of age were positive New Orleans	Direct smear CF; $ZnSO_4$ Formalin-ether sedimentation	Vaughn and Jordan (1960)
	1977–1980	8.5[b]	4058 dogs at the Louisiana State University Veterinary Teaching Hospital and Clinics	SF; sodium nitrate	Hoskins et al. (1982)
Oklahoma	1981–1990	5–8%	12,515 faecals (mean 1250/y) Lower prevalence in 1990; higher in 1981 Oklahoma State University Veterinary Medical Teaching Hospital	Direct smear with 0.9% NaCl SF; saturated sodium nitrate	Jordan et al. (1993)
Texas	1968–1969	27.3	44 dogs from a shelter Brazos County	Necropsy	Costa et al. (1971)
	1974–1975	6.6	105 dog faeces from the ground Suburban, upper middle-class neighbourhood with no stray dogs Houston	Brine flotation	Arambulo and Steele (1976)
	1976*	13	50 stray dogs and 50 surrendered dogs Houston	Necropsy	Arambulo and Steele (1976)

Continued

Table 1 Summary of *Toxocara canis* in dogs for the United States.—cont'd

Location	Year[a]	Per cent positive for *Toxocara*		Description	Analysis method	Reference
	1977–1978	21		100 stray dogs >50% of the dogs were 0–6 mo of age Tarrant County	Necropsy	Stewart et al. (1979)
	1978	30		60 dogs from animal shelters 50% of 2–6 mo dogs were positive; none of the dogs >2 y of age (8 dogs) were positive Results not different from 10 y previously	Necropsy	Smith and Seaton (1981)
West Virginia	2009	6.9	Overall	231 dogs at a veterinary clinic 86 dogs: ≤12 mo of age 64 dogs: 13–83 mo of age 81 dogs: >83 mo of age Charleston	SF (FecaTect®); $ZnSO_4$	Savilla et al. (2011)
		17.4	≤12 mo			
		0	13–83 mo			
		1.2	>83 mo			
Northeast						
Regional data			Number of samples			
	1993–1994	12.6	ND	Dogs in animal shelters	CF; sucrose	Blagburn et al. (1996)
	2006	2.2[b]	390,429	Samples submitted to Antech Diagnostic Laboratories	CF; $ZnSO_4$ spg 1.18	Little et al. (2009)
	2008–2009	9.1	ND	Dogs in animal shelters	CF; sucrose spg 1.2	Blagburn (2009)

	2011	3.4	950,490	Based on CAPC data; see national data	CF	Lucio-Forster et al. (2016)
	2012	4.4	968,974			
	2013	3.0	942,271			
	2014	2.2	1,007,473			
New Jersey	1960–1966	8.4		2737 stray dogs 685 of the dogs were necropsied with flotation results indicating 11.4% and necropsy and flotation indicating 22.5%	CF; $ZnSO_4$ spg 1.2 Necropsy	Lillis (1967)
	1971–1974	18.9[3]		387 dogs entering a research facility	CF; $ZnSO_4$ spg 1.2	Loebenberg and Waitz (1977)
New Jersey and New York	1957	1.6		500 faecal samples from the ground New York City and suburbs in NY and New Jersey	Flotation; $ZnSO_4$ spg 1.18	Dorman and Van Ostrand (1958)
Pennsylvania	1983–1986[c]	5.5[3]		2294 owned dogs Mean age 1.9 y; median age 0.5 *Toxocara* more common than *Toxascaris* Dogs presented at the School of Veterinary Medicine Teaching Hospital, University of Pennsylvania	CF; $ZnSO_4$ If high lipids, reanalysed with formalin-ethyl acetate sedimentation	Kirkpatrick (1988)
	1984–1991[c]	5.7[3]		8077 faecal samples from owned dogs Due to repeat years, potentially the same dogs was tested more than once Dogs presented at the School of Veterinary Medicine Teaching Hospital, University of Pennsylvania	CF; $ZnSO_4$ Samples with high lipids reanalysed using formalin-ethyl acetate sedimentation followed by CF with $ZnSO_4$ on the sediment	Nolan and Smith (1995)

Continued

Table 1 Summary of *Toxocara canis* in dogs for the United States.—cont'd

Location	Year[a]	Per cent positive for *Toxocara*		Description	Analysis method	Reference
	1997–2007[d]	2.0		6555 dog samples from owned dogs Due to repeat years, potentially the same dogs was tested more than once Dogs presented at the School of Veterinary Medicine Teaching Hospital, University of PA	CF; $ZnSO_4$ Samples with high lipids reanalysed using formalin-ethyl acetate sedimentation followed by CF with $ZnSO_4$ on the sediment	Gates and Nolan (2009)
	2000–2007[d]	2.0[3]		12,914 owned dogs (calculated based on Nolan and Smith, 1995) Due to repeat years, potentially the same dogs was tested more than once 89.1% *Toxocara* and 10.9% *Toxascaris* Approximately 79.8% on monthly heartworm prevention Dogs presented at the School of Veterinary Medicine Teaching Hospital, University of PA	CF; $ZnSO_4$ Samples with high lipids reanalysed using formalin-ethyl acetate sedimentation followed by CF with $ZnSO_4$ on the sediment	Gates and Nolan (2014)
Midwest						
Regional data			Number of samples			
	1993–1994	15.8	ND	Dogs in animal shelters	CF; sucrose	Blagburn et al. (1996)
	2006	2.6[b]	191,840	Samples submitted to Antech Diagnostic Laboratories	CF; $ZnSO_4$ spg 1.18	Little et al. (2009)

	2008–2009	14.9	ND	Dogs in animal shelters	CF; sucrose spg 1.2	Blagburn (2009)
	2011	3.5	377,662	Based on CAPC data; see national data	CF	Lucio-Forster et al. (2016)
	2012	3.9	377,203			
	2013	3.4	368,612			
	2014	3.8	395,940			
Illinois	1966–1968	2.0		846 faecal samples from the ground Neighbourhood consisted of well cared for dogs Residential area of Chicago (Edgewater and Rogers Park)	CF; Sheather's sugar	Jaskoski (1971)
	1979–1980	4.3		806 samples from the ground Compared to 1970 study, changes in demographics and more stray dogs in the city Residential area of Chicago (Edgewater and Rogers Park)	CF; Sheather's sugar	Jaskoski et al. (1982)
	1980	24.5		110 samples from the Chicago Animal Control Center	CF; Sheather's sugar	Jaskoski et al. (1982)
Indiana	1974–1976	18.3		104 dogs from a humane shelter All >1 y of age Tippecanoe County	Necropsy	Kazacos (1978)

Continued

Table 1 Summary of *Toxocara canis* in dogs for the United States.—cont'd

Location	Year[a]	Per cent positive for *Toxocara*		Description	Analysis method	Reference
Iowa	1958, 1960, 1961	14[b]		224 random-source dogs >6 mo of age State University of Iowa	CF; sugar Flotation; $ZnSO_4$	Braun and Thayer (1962)
	1966–1974	2.0[b]		33,594 owned dogs visiting the Iowa State University Veterinary Clinic Higher per cent positive in puppies and intact dogs All data from dogs from urban areas of Ames	Not indicated	Lightner et al. (1978)
	1965–1968	18.5[3]	Overall	2049 faecal samples from owned dogs Iowa State University Vet Teaching Hospital 530 dogs: 0–6 mo of age 1200 dogs: ≥12 mo of age Iowa State University Veterinary Teaching Hospital	CF; sucrose	Greve and O'Brien (1989)
		44.3	0–6 mo			
		6.9	≥12 mo			
	1988	4.5[3]	Overall	935 faecal samples from owned dogs 176 samples: 0–6 mo of age 673 samples: ≥12 mo of age Iowa State University Veterinary Teaching Hospital	CF; sucrose	Greve and O'Brien (1989)
		18.2	0–6 mo			
		1.2	≥12 mo			
Kansas	1991	5.0	Overall	218 Greyhounds submitted to Kansas State University for necropsy 25 dogs: <12 mo of age 149 dogs: 12–47 mo of age 44 dogs: ≥48 mo of age	Necropsy and quantitative faecal examination in duplicate	Ridley et al. (1994)
		24	<12 mo			
		3.4	12–47 mo			
		0	≥48 mo			

Michigan	1964*	35.8	123 stray adult dogs Detroit	Flotation; NaCl or $ZnSO_4$ Necropsy	Worley (1964)
Missouri	1975	17.9[3]	1468 owned dogs Higher per cent positive in intact dogs compared to castrated and spayed dogs Higher per cent in dogs 0–6 mo of age than older dogs University of Missouri Veterinary Teaching Hospital	Flotation; $MgSO_4$ spg 1.25	Visco et al. (1977)
Ohio	1974–1975	19.2	500 dogs in an animal shelter Franklin County	SF; sucrose spg 1.15; drops from flotation examined	Streitel and Dubey (1976)
South Dakota	2017*	7.1	84 dogs spay/neuter clinic Pine Ridge Indian Reservation	CF; Sheather's sugar	Scorza and Lappin (2017)
Wisconsin	1994–1995	21.4	309 dogs in one animal shelter Higher per cent positive in warmer months Higher per cent positive in stray dogs compared to previously owned dogs Higher per cent positive in intact dogs compared to spay/neutered dogs Milwaukee County	CF; $ZnSO_4$ spg 1.18 (most samples) or Sheather's sugar	Coggins (1998)

Continued

Table 1 Summary of *Toxocara canis* in dogs for the United States.—cont'd

Location	Year[a]	Per cent positive for *Toxocara*		Description	Analysis method	Reference
West						
Regional data			Number of samples			
	1993–1994	11.0	ND	Dogs in animal shelters	CF; sucrose	Blagburn et al. (1996)
	2006	2.8[b]	309,948	Samples submitted to Antech Diagnostic Laboratories	CF; $ZnSO_4$ spg 1.18	Little et al. (2009)
	2008–2009	6.6	ND	Dogs in animal shelters	CF; sucrose spg 1.2	Blagburn (2009)
	2011	1.3	592,463	Based on CAPC data; see national data	CF	Lucio-Forster et al. (2016)
	2012	1.5	588,810			
	2013	0.6	550,318			
	2014	1.5	605,877			
California	1976	49.5		182 dogs from five animal shelters Estimated to be 2–6 mo of age Los Angeles County	Flotation; saturated sodium nitrate	Marron and Schroeder (1978)

Colorado	1997–1998	3.1	Overall	130 owned dogs	CF; $ZnSO_4$ with lugol's iodine	Hackett and Lappin (2003)
		5.6	Diarrhoea	71 with diarrhoea and 59 age matched healthy dogs		
		0	Healthy	Veterinary Teaching Hospital at Colorado State University		
Hawaii	1962*	24	Overall	96 stray dogs	Necropsy	Ash (1962)
		57	<6 mo	35 dogs: <6 mo of age 61 dogs: >6 mo of age		
		7	>6 mo	Honolulu and rural Oahu		
Utah	1976*	26		50 dogs from animal control facilities Provo and Orem	Necropsy	Sawyer et al. (1976)
	1978*	49		100 dogs from an animal shelter Designated positive if worms or eggs seen Most infected dogs were estimated to be 3–12 mo of age 13 communities in Utah County	Necropsy CF; Sheather's sugar	Palmieri et al. (1978)

[a]Year of study; if study year not specified, year of publication which is denoted by an asterisk *.
[b]Per cent positive is for ascarids, *Toxocara canis* and *Toxascaris leonina*.
[c]Data overlap in these studies.
[d]Data overlap in these studies.
CF, centrifugation flotation; SF simple flotation, flotation method not further described; Spg, specific gravity; ND, number of samples per region could not be determined from the data presented; TNR, trap-neuter/spay-release program.
Notes: Many studies compare per cent positive between male and female cats; these data are not included since consistently no difference was found.

Table 2 Summary of *Toxocara cati* for the United States.

Location	Year[a]	Per cent positive for *Toxocara*		Description	Analysis method	Reference
National						
	2003	3.5^{b} (2.9)	Overall	66,819 owned cats from 359 Banfield clinics in 40 states 18.4% of cats had more than one faecal exam resulting in 80,278 faecals; data for total faecals is in parentheses 17,780 (20831) cats: <6 mo of age 8141 (8758) cats: 6 to <12 mo of age 22,453 (25776) cats: 1 to <4 y of age 15,815 (18335) cats: 4 to <10 y of age 5619 (6567) ≥ 10 y of age More positive in summer > fall > winter > spring More positive in intact then spayed/castrated cats Regional differences with highest in northeast and lowest in California	SF (Fecalyzer®); $ZnSO_4$ Direct smear with saline 0.9% NaCl when insufficient quantity for flotation	De Santis et al. (2006)
		9.8 (8.5)	<6 mo			
		2.6 (2.4)	6–12 mo			
		1.1 (1.0)	1 to <4 y			
		0.6 (0.5)	4 to <10 y			
		0.5 (0.4)	≥10 y			
	2008–2009	22.2		1179 cats in animal shelters	CF; sugar spg 1.2	Blagburn (2009)
			Number of samples	Prevalence based on data from the Companion Animal Parasite Council (capcvet.org) website analysed using a general linear model Prevalence estimates corrected based on the model Faecal data on the CAPC site are from results from commercial laboratories	CF	Lucio-Forster et al. (2016)
	2011	5.1	543,961			
	2012	5.1	531,826			
	2013	4.7	502,071			
	2014	4.6	523,934			

South						
Regional data			Number of samples			
	2008–2009	19.8	ND	Portion of 1179 cats in animal shelters	CF; sugar spg 1.2	Blagburn (2009)
	2011	4.9	103,338	CAPC data; see national data	CF	Lucio-Forster et al. (2016)
	2012	4.3	103,777			
	2013	4.5	102,496			
	2014	4.6	111,330			
Alabama	2004*	23.3		120 random-source cats >1 y of age 1/3 previously owned; 2/3 free-roaming[c] East-central Alabama	CF; Sheather's sugar Necropsy	Eiland et al. (2004)
Florida	2009	11		100 cats in an animal shelter for ≤24 h Approximately ¾ were <6 mo of age 50 with and 50 without diarrhoea; not different in per cent positive Alachua County	SF (Fecalyzer®); sodium nitrate	Sabshin et al. (2012)
Florida	2012–2018[d]	12.6[b]		127 free-roaming cats in five TNR programs Cats were selected such that approximately half had diarrhoea 18% ≤ 6 mo of age; 60% adults; 22% age unknown	CF; $ZnSO_4$ spg >1.2	Andersen et al. (2018)

Continued

Table 2 Summary of *Toxocara cati* for the United States.—cont'd

Location	Year[a]	Per cent positive for *Toxocara*	Description	Analysis method	Reference
Florida	2012–2018[d]	26.4[b]	121 cats resident in five long-term sanctuaries; group housed with outdoor access Cats were selected such that approximately half had diarrhoea Age and treatment history not assessed; most cats present in facility for several months or years	CF; $ZnSO_4$ spg >1.2	Andersen et al. (2018)
Florida and Georgia	2012–2018[d]	5.4[b]	112 cats in 13 short-term shelters for ≤1 mo Cats were selected such that approximately half had diarrhoea 63% ≤ 6 mo of age; 38% adults 96% reported to have been treated for roundworms	CF; $ZnSO_4$ spg >1.2	Andersen et al. (2018)
Florida and Georgia	2012–2018[d]	6.6[b]	122 cats in 24 foster care programs for ≤6 mo Cats were selected such that approximately half had diarrhoea 74% ≤ 6 mo of age; 25% adults; 1% age unknown 80% reported to have been treated for roundworms	CF; $ZnSO_4$ spg >1.2	Andersen et al. (2018)

Florida	2014	10.9[b]		64 free-roaming cats in a TNR program Miami-Dade County	IDEXX Faecal DxTM coproantigen ELISA	Geng et al. (2018)
Florida	2016	6.6		76 cats in an animal shelter Citrus County	CF; Sheather's sugar spg 1.275	Wyrosdick et al. (2017)
North Carolina	2004*	21	Feral	87 free-roaming cats 66 owned cats Randolph County	Formalin–ethyl acetate sedimentation	Nutter et al. (2004)
		18	Pet			
Oklahoma	2009–2010	41.4	Necropsy	116 cats ≥1 y of age in an animal shelter Necropsy and both faecal methods used for each cat; flotation detected 68.8% and CF detected 77.1% of the cats that were positive on necropsy Northeastern OK	SF (Fecasol®); sodium nitrate CF; Sheather's sugar Necropsy	Little et al. (2015)
Oklahoma	2015–2016	44.6	Overall	846 free-roaming cats 161 cats: 3–5 mo of age 297 cats: 6–12 mo of age 388 cats: >12 mo of age TNR from 14 counties Analysed at the Boren Veterinary Medical Hospital, Oklahoma State University	CF; $ZnSO_4$ spg 1.18	Nagamori et al. (2018)
		63.4	3–5 mo			
		40.1	6–12 mo			
		40.7	>12 mo			

Continued

Table 2 Summary of *Toxocara cati* for the United States.—cont'd

Location	Year[a]	Per cent positive for *Toxocara*		Description	Analysis method	Reference
Virginia	2016	58.9		275 free-roaming cats in a TNR program Per cent positive higher in younger cats Richmond	CF; $ZnSO_4$ spg 1.18	Taetzsch et al. (2018)
Northeast						
Regional data			Number of samples			
	2008–2009	28.1	ND	Portion of 1179 cats in animal shelters	CF; sugar spg 1.2	Blagburn (2009)
	2011	6.6	250,845	CAPC data; see national data	CF	Lucio-Forster et al. (2016)
	2012	6.9	248,016			
	2013	5.7	233,881			
	2014	6.1	239,838			
Connecticut	2003*	39.8	Overall	450 cats Owned 336 cats; shelter 114 cats Urban 255 cats; suburb 195 cats 127 cats: <1 y of age 323 cats: adult	SF (Ovassay® Plus); $ZnSO_4$ spg 1.18	Rembiesa and Richardson (2003)
		30.4	Owned			
		67.5	Shelter			
		36.5	Urban			
		44.1	Suburb			
		41.7	<1 y			
		39.0	Adult			

New Jersey	1960–1966	36.2	Overall	1480 free-roaming cats 318 were necropsied	CF; $ZnSO_4$ spg 1.2 Necropsy	Lillis (1967)
		45.3	Faecal only			
		55.7	Faecal + necropsy			
New York	1957	10		100 cats from 'well-patient' boarding section of an animal hospital New York City	Flotation; $ZnSO_4$ spg 1.18	Dorman and Van Ostrand (1958)
New York	1998–1999	32.7	Overall	263 cats 114 owned cats seen at a clinic; 149 in three animal shelters All 1–12 mo of age Central New York (including Tompkins County)	CF; sugar spg 1.33 CF; $ZnSO_4$ spg 1.18	Spain et al. (2001)
New York	2006–2010	21.0		1322 cats from two animal shelters; 50 of the cats were in foster homes Cortland and Tompkins County	CF; sugar spg 1.3 CF; $ZnSO_4$ spg 1.18	Lucio-Forster and Bowman (2011)

Continued

Table 2 Summary of *Toxocara cati* for the United States.—cont'd

Location	Year[a]	Per cent positive for *Toxocara*	Description	Analysis method	Reference
Pennsylvania[e]	1983–1986	16.4[b]	454 owned cats Mean age 1.5 y; median age 0.5 y (*Toxocara* more common than *Toxascaris*) Cats presented at the School of Veterinary Medicine Teaching Hospital, University of PA	CF; $ZnSO_4$ Samples with high lipids reanalysed using formalin-ethyl acetate sedimentation	Kirkpatrick (1988)
Pennsylvania[e]	1984–1991	16[b]	2000 cat samples Due to repeat years, some samples could be from the same cat Cats presented at the School of Veterinary Medicine Teaching Hospital, University of PA	CF; $ZnSO_4$ Samples with high lipids reanalysed using formalin-ethyl acetate sedimentation followed by CF with $ZnSO_4$ on the sediment	Nolan and Smith (1995)
Pennsylvania	1997–2007	7.5	1566 cat samples Due to repeat years, some samples could be from the same cat Cats presented at the School of Veterinary Medicine Teaching Hospital, University of PA	CF; $ZnSO_4$ Samples with high lipids reanalysed using formalin-ethyl acetate sedimentation followed by CF with $ZnSO_4$ on the sediment	Gates and Nolan (2009)

Midwest						
Regional data			Number of samples			
	2008–2009	24.4	ND	Portion of 1179 cats in animal shelters	CF; sugar spg 1.2	Blagburn (2009)
	2011	6.7	72,692	CAPC data; see national data	CF	Lucio-Forster et al. (2016)
	2012	6.5	69,604			
	2013	6.1	66,128			
	2014	6.8	70,161			
Illinois and Kentucky	1968–1969	26		100 cats from a dealer 78 from Illinois and 22 from Kentucky	Necropsy	Power (1971)
Iowa	1966–1974	2.8 [b]		11,995 owned cats visiting the Iowa State University Veterinary Clinic Higher per cent positive in kittens and intact cats All data from cats from urban areas of Ames	Not indicated	Lightner et al. (1978)
Missouri	1974–1976	24.4[b]		1294 owned cats Per cent positive higher in cats <6 mo and in intact cats University of Missouri Teaching Hospital	Flotation; $MgSO_4$ spg 1.25	Visco et al. (1978)

Continued

Table 2 Summary of *Toxocara cati* for the United States.—cont'd

Location	Year[a]	Per cent positive for *Toxocara*		Description	Analysis method	Reference
South Dakota	2017*	0		9 cats attending a spay/neuter clinic Pine Ridge Indian Reservation	CF; Sheather's sugar	Scorza and Lappin (2017)
West						
Regional data			Number of samples			
	2008–2009	17.9	ND	Portion of 1179 cats in animal shelters	CF; sugar spg 1.2	Blagburn (2009)
	2011	4.5	117,086	CAPC data; see national data	CF	Lucio-Forster et al. (2016)
	2012	4.0	110,429			
	2013	3.3	99,566			
	2014	4.4	102,605			
Colorado	1993–1995	1.6		129 owned cats (76 with diarrhoea; 53 healthy) 27 cats <1 y of age Excluded if known cause of diarrhoea or treated with anthelmintic in the previous 7 days Per cent positive similar in diarrhoea and non-diarrhoea cats	CF; $ZnSO_4$	Hill et al. (2000)

Colorado	1993–1995	7.8	77 cats in a humane society animal shelter 12 with diarrhoea; 53 healthy; 12 unknown 8 cats <1 y of age All positive cats were healthy Larimer County, Fort Collins	CF; $ZnSO_4$	Hill et al. (2000)
Hawaii	1962*	8	107 free-roaming cats Honolulu and rural Oahu	Necropsy	Ash (1962)
Utah	1976*	43	100 free-roaming cats Provo and American Fork	Necropsy Flotation; sugar	Sawyer et al. (1976)

[a]Year of study; if study year not specified, year of publication which is denoted by an asterisk *.
[b]Per cent positive is for ascarids, *Toxocara cati* and *Toxascaris leonina*.
[c]Free-roaming is used to denote unowned, stray, friendly or feral cats.
[d]Institutional Animal Care and Use Committee approval was in 2012; publication in 2018.
[e]Data overlap in these studies.
CF, centrifugation flotation; SF simple flotation, flotation method not further described; Spg, specific gravity; TNR, trap-neuter/spay-release program; ND, not able to determine based on the data presented.
Notes: Many studies compare per cent positive between male and female cats; these data are not included since consistently no difference was found.

two studies in cats (one each in owned and animal shelters). National studies were conducted between 1996 and 2009 and, except for one local study within a Native American Reservation, there have been no studies that include *T. canis* prevalence since 2010. In contrast, there have been five studies with cats since 2010, all in free-roaming or shelter populations. Prevalence maps generated by the Companion Animal Parasite Council™ (CAPC) using data from two commercial laboratories (ANTECH Diagnostics and IDEXX Laboratories), provide more recent information and were recently reviewed by Lucio-Forster et al. (2016). It is expected that samples submitted to these laboratories represent animals receiving some degree of veterinary care and are less likely to be from stray, free-roaming or shelter populations.

There are several limitations in interpreting changes in prevalence and estimating current prevalence in dogs and cats in the United States on a national and regional level. First, there is no national data prior to 1996. Second, while centrifugation methods are used in the commercial laboratories and were used in the studies by Blagburn et al. (1996), Blagburn (2009), and Little et al. (2009), the studies by Mohamed et al. (2009) and De Santis et al. (2006) used simple flotation methods, which are considered less sensitive than centrifugation. Third, while *Toxascaris* typically makes up only a small portion of ascarid infections in dogs and cats (Blagburn et al., 1996; Gates and Nolan, 2014), lack of differentiation in most national studies could influence interpretation of changes in prevalence. Lastly, given that the most up-to-date data are from the CAPC maps, their limitations need special consideration. These data only capture an estimated third of the total number of positive tests in any area. Additionally, some animals may have been tested more than once, and there may be influences cast by the motivation behind the requested tests (wellness versus diagnosis of disease testing). Hence, these data might underestimate prevalence if the number of wellness tests is high. Also, the 2015 addition of the IDEXX coproantigen test, which in combination with centrifugal flotation, has been shown to increase overall detection of ascarids, could indicate an increase in prevalence based solely on improved diagnostics (Little et al., 2019). With recognized limitations, these national studies provide the most comprehensive regional data and, combined with the numerous geographically focused studies, provide the best overview regarding changes in prevalence.

On a national level prevalence in stray dogs and those in animal shelters has not appeared to change; however, prevalence in owned dogs appears to be decreasing. Most focal studies in owned dogs prior to the 1990s indicate a prevalence >5%. The 2% found by Lightner et al. (1978) might reflect the diagnostic method used or the population tested (one visiting a referral clinic) and not be applicable to a wider population. Based on studies since 2006, prevalence in owned dogs has decreased and is ≤5% with several studies suggesting an even lower prevalence of <2%. Reasons for this decrease include, but are not exclusive of, better control in puppies and young dogs, overall increased use of anthelmintics, and potentially a change in the population with fewer puppies (Gates and Nolan, 2014; Jordan et al., 1993; Little et al., 2009).

Owned dogs in focal areas can have much higher levels that the national average (Savilla et al., 2011; Scorza and Lappin, 2017). Differences may be attributable to climate or soil conditions impacting egg development and longevity of viability, dog demographics (e.g., proportion of urban and rural dogs) and the presence of wild canids and paratenic hosts (Blagburn, 2009; Gates and Nolan, 2014; Little et al., 2009). Socio-economic factors also could play a role by limiting access to veterinary care. Additionally, prevalence in pets might be related to differences in veterinary recommendations (Brophy and Peregrine, 2009; Little et al., 2009; Overgaauw and Nederland, 1997). Given the increasing concern regarding *Toxocara* infection in people (Holland, 2017; Hotez, 2014; Lee et al., 2014; Woodhall et al., 2014), a better understanding of the factors leading to these hot spots is needed.

Publications on *Toxocara* in cats nationally consistently report higher overall prevalence in shelter versus owned cats receiving veterinary care (Blagburn, 2009; De Santis et al., 2006; Lucio-Forster and Bowman, 2011). In regional studies prevalence in shelter and free-roaming cats are 5.45–67.5%, while in owned populations they are 1.6–30.4% (excluding the Scorza and Lappin (2017) study with only nine cats) (Table 2). Taken as a whole, prevalence results for cats in regional studies range from 1.6% to 67.5% (excluding the study with nine cats), with the lowest prevalence in cats visiting a veterinary hospital and the highest in a population of shelter cats (Hill et al., 2000; Rembiesa and Richardson, 2003). Additionally, a study in Colorado (Hill et al., 2000) comparing owned and shelter cats in the same area found an almost fivefold increase in prevalence in the shelter population when compared to the owned population. These findings are likely explained by the increased likelihood of deworming, routine veterinary care, and prevention of access to prey and faecal contaminated environments for pets versus stray cat populations. Overall, regional studies support the findings of national studies, and no significant changes in prevalence are evident when compared to studies reported prior to the 1990s.

As previously noted, there are too few reports per region, too much variability in populations sampled, sample sizes and methods of analysis to draw meaningful conclusions on regional trends in prevalence. An exception may be in Pennsylvania, where three studies were published reporting prevalence for cats presented to the University of Pennsylvania's School of Veterinary Medicine Teaching Hospital (Gates and Nolan, 2009; Kirkpatrick, 1988; Nolan and Smith, 1995). The first two publications report prevalence of 16.4% in 1983–1986 and 16% from 1984 to 1991. However, by 1997–2007 infection rates had dropped practically by half (7.5%), likely as a result of the increased routine use of anthelmintics (Gates and Nolan, 2009).

Age has also been found to consistently have a significant impact on prevalence, with young animals, especially those less than 6 months old, having a higher likelihood of infection than those older than a year (De Santis et al., 2006; Lightner et al., 1978; Nagamori et al., 2018; Taetzsch et al., 2018; Visco et al., 1978). The national data from De Santis et al. (2006) exemplifies this beautifully: prevalence in kittens less than 6 months of age was 3.8 times higher than that seen in kittens 6–12 months of age, and 8.9–16.3 times higher than for cat populations older than 1 year of age. A few earlier studies also found that intact cats had a higher likelihood of infection (Lightner et al., 1978; Visco et al., 1978). Thus, it appears that in the United States cat population, age, deworming status with access to veterinary care, and free-roaming capacity remain more highly predictive of infection than national region or year of study.

3. Mexico

Fifty-two studies on *Toxocara* prevalence in Mexico were accessible as published reports or graduate level theses. These works span from 1955 to 2018 and report data from 12 of Mexico's 32 states. The majority of these studies were conducted in central and southern states of Mexico [mainly the state of Mexico and adjoining Federal District (a.k.a. Mexico City)]. Baja California is the only northern state from which studies were available. Of these studies, eight examined dog faecal samples collected from the ground with some also including direct sampling of dogs in the same area, 35 report *Toxocara* prevalence in dogs, and 10 studies are available on prevalence in cats.

In the studies investigating presence of *Toxocara* eggs in faecal samples collected from the environment (Table 3), all sampling locations (parks, sidewalks, traffic-refuges, public and private gardens, etc.) were contaminated with faeces

Table 3 Summary of *Toxocara* reports from environmental (faeces collected from the ground) samples in Mexico.

State	Year[a]	Per cent positive for *Toxocara*	Description	Analysis method	Reference
Campeche	2018	14.3	Pooled dog faecal samples ($n=5$ per park) from strays in 14 parks	McMaster's	Cortez-Aguirre et al. (2018)
Chiapas	2005	19.0	200 dog faecal samples from 31 streets ($n=176$), 1 traffic-refuge ($n=14$) and 1 public garden ($n=10$)	Direct smear CF; $ZnSO_4$ spg 1.18	Martínez-Barbabosa et al. (2008a)
Mexico	2010	20.3 overall (range 18–23)	171 dog faecal samples from streets near 4 municipal parks	Flotation McMaster's; $MgSO_4$	Romero et al. (2010)
	2011	28.3 overall (range 18.7–39)	346 faecal samples from streets, traffic-refuges and sidewalks near 5 municipal parks	CF; $ZnSO_4$ spg 1.18	Romero-Núñez et al. (2011)
	2013	31.7 overall (range 12.1–45)	199 faecal samples from streets, traffic-refuges and sidewalks near 7 recreational areas	Flotation McMaster's; $MgSO_4$	Romero-Núñez et al. (2013)
Mexico City	2004–2005	overall 67.5 (range 62.5–80)	200 dog faecal samples from 5 municipal parks ($n=40$ per park)	Flotation	Romero-Núñez et al. (2009)
Oaxaca	2012	47.8	180 dog faecal samples from natural, urban and suburban areas	Direct smear SF	Vélez-Hernández et al. (2014)
Yucatán	2015	1.0	100 dog faecal samples from 20 municipal parks ($n=5$ per park)	CF McMaster's; sucrose spg 1.28	Medina-Pinto et al. (2018)

[a]Year of publication if year of study not specified.
CF, centrifugation flotation; SF simple flotation, flotation method not further described; Spg, specific gravity.

from infected dogs. The proportions of *Toxocara*-positive faecal samples collected from different areas ranged from 1% to 80%, with the lowest per cent positive reported in a study from Yucatan (Medina-Pinto et al., 2018) and the highest from a study area in Mexico City (Romero-Núñez et al., 2009). Some of these studies report 40–100% viability of eggs recovered, generally trending towards the higher ranges (Romero et al., 2010; Romero-Núñez et al., 2011, 2013). Although *Toxocara* eggs may not persist or develop as efficiently under suboptimal environmental conditions, or in certain types of soils, the potential for high rates of viable eggs contaminating public and private areas is concerning. These eggs penetrate soil slowly and are thus most likely to be found in the top few centimetres of soil (Mizgajska, 2001), increasing the risk of host exposure to infection through subsequent ingestion.

In dogs, the reported prevalence of *Toxocara* nationwide ranged broadly between 0% and 93% (Table 4) in the 10 states where studies have been conducted. The complete absence of *Toxocara* detection in a population of 101 stray dogs where centrifugal flotation methods were employed is noteworthy (Alvarado-Esquivel et al., 2015); these dogs were housed in a shelter environment and would expectedly have some level of infection and, therefore, faecal shedding. However, the dogs had been treated with mebendazole a couple of months prior to sampling. This finding highlights the known capacity to interrupt faecal shedding by the use of appropriate anthelmintics, and to prevent reinfection through depriving dogs of free access to prey and contaminated environments. On the opposite end of the reported range, the 93% prevalence is not unexpected when considering the population sampled (by necropsy) was 120 stray puppies all less than 6 months of age (Styles, 1967). In light of the parasite's ability to cross the placenta, all puppies born to infected females are expected to be born infected, thus age is routinely found to be an important risk factor for infection in dogs (e.g., Encalada-Mena et al., 2011; Martínez-Barbabosa et al., 1998; Quiñones-Ávila et al., 1998; Romero-Núñez et al., 2009, 2011; Schantz and Biagi, 1968).

In addition to faecal examination and necropsy studies, three studies investigated antibody levels to *Toxocara* in dogs (Martínez-Barbabosa et al., 2008b; Muñoz-Guzmán and Alba-Hurtado, 2010; Tinoco-Gracia et al., 2007). Seropositivity levels in these studies are high (57.8–87.1%) likely due to the successful life history of the parasite, whereby use of multiple modes of transmission ensure high likelihood of infection and reinfection in canine populations (eggs and prey ensuring reinfection of mature populations, and guaranteeing the infection of new generations (puppies) though vertical transmission).

Table 4 Summary of *Toxocara* reports from dogs in Mexico.

State	Year[a]	Per cent positive for *Toxocara*	Description	Analysis method	Reference
Baja California	2001–2002	57.8	344 owned dogs attending 33 clinics (10–11 per clinic)	ELISA	Tinoco-Gracia et al. (2007)
	2014	7.1	380 stray dogs	Necropsy CF; $ZnSO_4$ spg 1.25	Trasviña-Muñoza et al. (2017)
Campeche	2008	14.4	270 owned dogs	McMasters NaCl	Encalada-Mena et al. (2011)
Jalisco	2006–2007	1.3	75 stray dogs (1–36 mo)	CF; $ZnSO_4$ spg 1.18	Jiménez-Cardoso et al. (2010)
Mexico	2005	6.0	441 owned dogs	CF; $ZnSO_4$ spg 1.18	Rodríguez-Prado et al. (2014)
	2010	64.6	31 stray puppies (1–3 mo)	Necropsy	Muñoz-Guzmán and Alba-Hurtado (2010)
	2010	87.1		ELISA	
	2010	34.2	221 owned dogs	Flotation	Romero et al. (2010)
	2010	39.3 overall	346 owned dogs	CF; $ZnSO_4$ spg 1.18 n	Romero-Núñez et al. (2011)
	2010	38	199 owned dogs	Flotation $MgSO_4$ McMasters	Romero-Núñez et al. (2013)

Continued

Table 4 Summary of *Toxocara* reports from dogs in Mexico.—cont'd

State	Year[a]	Per cent positive for *Toxocara*	Description	Analysis method	Reference
Mexico City	1955	25	100 stray and surrendered	Direct smear CF; $ZnSO_4$ spg 1.18	Flores-Barroeta (1955)
		30.0		Necropsy	
	1965–66	53.1 overall 75.6 53.1	128 stray dogs <6 mo ($n=86$) >6mo ($n=42$)	Necropsy	Schantz and Biagi (1968)
	1967	93.0	120 stray dogs (<6 mo)	Necropsy	Styles (1967)
	1972	9.5	105 stray, bought, surrendered dogs	Necropsy	Cruz-Reyes (1971)
	1997–1998	13.3	120 stray dogs	Necropsy	Eguía-Aguilar et al. (2005)
	1997–1998	27[b]	200 stray and surrendered dogs	Necropsy; small intestine exam only	Ponce-Macotela et al. (2005)
	1996	21.2 owned	500 owned dogs	CF; $ZnSO_4$ spg 1.18	Martínez-Barbabosa et al. (1998)
		12.4 stray	210 stray dogs		
	2004–2005	60.5	100 owned dogs presenting to a veterinary clinic	Flotation	Romero-Núñez et al. (2009)
	2005	66.7	141 stray dogs aged 45–120 mo	Hemagglutination (IHA) technique	Martínez-Barbabosa et al. (2008b)
	2006–2007	25.0	72 stray dogs (1–36 mo)	CF; $ZnSO_4$ spg 1.18	Jiménez-Cardoso et al. (2010)
	2008	14	200 owned dogs	Stoll method	Martínez-Barbabosa et al. (2011)

	2013	41 overall 0 12.2 10 18.9	180 stray puppies (3–5 mo) Urban zone ($n=90$) Rural, stray ($n=30$) Rural, owned ($n=30$) Rural, canine control centre ($n=30$)	Formalin-ether sedimentation	De la Rosa-Arana and Tapia-Romero (2018)
	2013	6	183 pets (3 mo-12 y)	Direct smear CF; $ZnSO_4$ spg 1.18	Martínez-Barbabosa et al. (2015)
	2015	3.6	1603 pets	CF; $ZnSO_4$ spg 1.18	Romero et al. (2015)
Queretaro	2000	17.9	201 stray dogs	Necropsy	Campos and Alarcon (2002)
	2008	15.1	378 stray dogs	Necropsy	Cantó et al. (2011)
Tabasco	2013	2.3	302 owned dog presenting to a veterinary clinic	Gross examination CF; Sheather's sugar	Torres-Chable et al. (2015)
Veracruz	2013	0.0	101 stray dogs	CF; Sheather's sugar CF; $ZnSO_4$ spg 1.18	Alvarado-Esquivel et al. (2015)
	2016	12.4	89 owned dogs	McMaster's Flotation; saturated $NaCl_2$ CF; $ZnSO_4$ spg 1.18	Mata-Ramos and Castañeda Ortega (2018)

Continued

Table 4 Summary of *Toxocara* reports from dogs in Mexico.—cont'd

State	Year[a]	Per cent positive for *Toxocara*	Description	Analysis method	Reference
Yucatán	1984–1999	7.8	993 owned dogs visiting veterinary clinic(s)	CF; unspecified	Rodríguez-Vivas et al. (2001)
	2011	6.2	130 owned dogs	CF; McMaster's; sucrose spg 1.3 spg	Rodríguez-Vivas et al., 2011
	1998	34.2	38 stray dogs	Necropsy	Quiñones-Ávila et al. (1998)
	2015	12.5	52 owned dogs	CF; unspecified McMaster's	Ortega-Pacheco et al. (2015)
Zacatecas	2012	59.6 *T. canis*; 4.9 *T. cati*	163 owned dogs	Direct smear Flotation; zinc solution Flotation; sugar solution Flotation; saturated $NaCl_2$ Kato Katz technique	Chávez-Ruvalcaba et al. (2012)

[a]Year of publication if year of study not specified.
[b]Given in figure only. *Toxocara* and *Toxascaris* reported together.
CF, centrifugation flotation; SF simple flotation, flotation method not further described; Spg, specific gravity.

There were 10 reports investigating the prevalence of *Toxocara* in cats from 5 Mexican states (Table 5). Two of these had sample sizes smaller than 50 animals, and all but 2 of the studies examined owned populations. Prevalence in these studies ranged from 2.4% to 50.3%, with the lowest detection found in owner-surrendered cats. Although two studies report prevalence less than 4.5% (Cantó et al., 2013; Rodríguez-Vivas et al., 2001), the majority report rates above 20%, with some of the highest observed in owned cats (Cantó et al., 2013; Flores-Barroeta, 1955; Romero-Callejas et al., 2014) included stray cat populations in their studies. Unfortunately, the 1955 study

Table 5 Summary of *Toxocara* reports from cats in Mexico.

State	Year[a]	Per cent positive for *Toxocara*	Description	Analysis method	Reference
Mexico	1996	34.7	259 urban and rural cats aged 3–120 months	Direct smear CF; $ZnSO_4$ spg 1.18spg	Martínez-Barbabosa et al. (1997)
		36.4	231 urban areas owned cats (in houses)		
		21.4	28 rural areas owned cats (in houses)		
	2016	42.0	229 owned cats	CF; $NaNO_3$ spg 1.3	Rodriguez Gallegos et al. (2016)
Mexico City	1955	40 *T. cati* 2 *T. canis*	100 cats stray and surrendered	Direct smear CF; $ZnSO_4$ spg 1.18spg	Flores-Barroeta (1955)
		50 *T. cati* 2 *T. canis*		Necropsy	
	1986	13[b]	200 owned cats visiting veterinary clinics (50 per clinic)	Flotation; saturated sugar	Guevara Collazo et al. (1990)
	1996	42.9	401 owned cats (in houses and apartments) aged 3–120 months	Direct smear CF; $ZnSO_4$ spg 1.18spg	Martínez-Barbabosa et al. (1997)
		50.3	308 owned cats (in houses)		
		18.3	93 owned cats (in apartments)		

Continued

Table 5 Summary of *Toxocara* reports from cats in Mexico.—cont'd

State	Year[a]	Per cent positive for *Toxocara*	Description	Analysis method	Reference
	2003	42.5	520 owned cats (in houses and apartments) (aged 3–120 months, avg. 19 mo)	CF; $ZnSO_4$ spg 1.18spg	Martínez-Barbabosa et al. (2003)
		49.1	399 owned (in houses)		
		20.7	121 owned (in apartments)		
	2017	33.1	121 owned cats in apartments; 2–96 mo	Direct smear CF; $ZnSO_4$ spg 1.18spg	Martínez-Barbabosa et al. (2018)
Queretaro	2010–2011	3.4 overall; 3.7 stray; 2.4 surrendered	358 stray and surrendered cats (273 stray, 85 owner surrendered)	Necropsy	Cantó et al. (2013)
Tabasco	2009–2013	31.8	22 stray cats (17 feral, 5 roadkill)	Necropsy	Romero-Callejas et al. (2014)
Yucatán	1984–1999	4.3	46 owned cats visiting veterinary clinic(s)	CF	Rodríguez-Vivas et al. (2001)

[a]Year of publication if year of study not specified.
[b]*Toxocara* and *Toxascaris* reported together.
CF, centrifugation flotation; SF simple flotation, flotation method not further described; Spg, specific gravity.

included both stray and owner-surrendered cats and gives insufficient detail to determine the infection rate in each population. Prevalence in this study of 100 cats from Mexico City was high (40–50%) depending on the examination method [Notably, this study also detected *T. canis* (worms and eggs) in two of these cats.]. The second study, from Queretaro had low prevalence (2.4%) in necropsied stray cats. Finally, the study in Tabasco included only 22 cats, and found approximately a third to be infected. It is interesting to note, that in this small group of nationwide studies, some of the lowest prevalence levels were found in stray cats, while the highest levels were reported from owned cats living in houses (Martínez-Barbabosa et al., 1997). It has been noted that there is a significant difference in infection rates among owned cats living in apartments and those living in houses (Martínez-Barbabosa et al., 1997, 2003), the latter having more access to outdoor environments and thus at higher risk for infection. In addition to outdoor access, age is routinely found to be a significant risk factor. Although infection is reported from all age groups, animals less than a year old are regularly found to have a higher prevalence of infection (Martínez-Barbabosa et al., 1997, 2003, 2018; Rodriguez Gallegos et al., 2016).

It is estimated that there are 23 million dogs in Mexico, 70% of which are classified as street or stray (Cortez-Aguirre et al., 2018); estimates of stray cats in Mexico are not available. In 2011 the estimated pet population was 19 million (12 million dogs, and 7 million cats), 10–17% of which defecate outdoors (Martínez-Barbabosa et al., 2011; Martinez-Barrios, 2014). Faecal contamination of private and public outdoor environments is therefore high. Without municipal faecal collection there is an elevated risk of infection for animals and humans, especially in light of the fact that out of the 35 million homes reported in the 2010 census, 1.7 million have soil floors (where *Toxocara* eggs tracked in from outside may persist) and 3.1 million lack piped water (Martinez-Barrios, 2014).

Although studies in Mexico are overall limited, especially in the northern states, it is evident that unlike the situation seen in the United States, where 'ownership status' (i.e., pet versus unowned) impacts the likelihood of infection, in Mexico it has little bearing; pets are commonly allowed to roam free, may not be routinely dewormed, and may be fed fresh viscera (Rodríguez-Prado et al., 2014). Thus, access to the environment and age are the more likely contributors to risk of infection for animals and people alike.

Overall the information available on prevalence of infection in Mexico reflects the knowledge we have amassed globally: prevalence is highly variable dependent on host population sampled (final or paratenic), age, use of anthelmintics (and frequency of use), method of assessment (e.g., faecal shedding, necropsy, antibody detection), and access to the outdoors. In Mexico, important factors associated with the risk of infection of host populations include the large number of final hosts, their uncontrolled access to the outdoors, the lack of responsible pet ownership education programs, lack of programs to control stray populations, no practice of faecal removal from the environment by owners or municipalities, and socio-economic factors (Chávez-Ruvalcaba et al., 2012; Cortez-Aguirre et al., 2018; Tinoco-Gracia et al., 2007; Vélez-Hernández et al., 2014).

4. Central America

More information is available on *Toxocara* in dogs than in cats within Central America and the information is skewed towards some countries with no data available for Belize, El Salvador and Panama (Table 6). One drawback to much of the information available for the region is that it is in grey literature, not readily accessible, with small sample sizes, very local datasets, insufficient information about the social and cultural setting for someone unfamiliar with the study location, and often the use of diagnostic methods of low sensitivity. Despite this, the information on *Toxocara* in Central America is consistent with what is known about the parasite, with higher number of puppies infected than adult dogs, regardless if owned, contained or free-roaming, or stray.

Studies from Costa Rica consistently use the more sensitive centrifugation with Sheather's flotation solution diagnostic method and provide good background information on the study sites. The prevalence of *T. canis* ranged from 5% to 25.3% in the overall population with the lowest seen in adult owned dogs (1.2%) and the highest in <1-year-old dogs in animal shelters (39.5%) (Alemán Laporte, 2011; Valverde Alvarado, 2010). The oldest study located, from 2002 to 2004, was conducted with dogs visiting a veterinary clinic and identified the highest prevalence (17.7%) in adult dogs (ZeLedón et al., 2006). A later study with adult dogs from a limited resource region showed a lower prevalence, suggesting that prevalence might be decreasing (Valverde Alvarado, 2010). To confirm this, studies from similar settings (urban and rural and representing the different climatic zones) need to be performed.

All studies from Guatemala are in grey literature and most use less sensitive diagnostic methods or examine only a small portion of material from sedimentation. The studies represent several areas of the country with large differences in the findings ranging from no *Toxocara* eggs seen in a study with free-roaming dogs to, in another region, >20% in adult dogs and 100% in <1-year-old dogs. All the studies were conducted over a 4-year-time period; hence, changes over time cannot be determined. Data from Nicaragua are similar to that from Guatemala with the three studies located all from grey literature and the diagnostic methods being of low sensitivity for *Toxocara*. The lowest prevalence (5.1%) was seen in the most recent study but no inferences regarding change over time can be made due to the differences in the populations.

Both studies with cats had very small sample sizes, making their reliability limited. While 26.64% of the 15 cats from Guatemala were infected, the study had the requirement that they were not dewormed in the previous 6 months, biasing the results. While more historical, Schantz and Glickman (1983) reference a 50.2% infection rate in a study with 237 cats from Costa Rica.

Table 6 Summary of *Toxocara canis* and *Toxocara cati* in dogs and cats, respectively, for Central American Countries.

Country	Year[a]	Per cent positive for *Toxocara*		Description	Analysis method	Reference
Dogs						
Costa Rica	2002–2004	25.3 32 17.7	Overall <1 y >1 y	1136 dogs visiting a veterinary clinic 610 dogs: <1 y of age 526 dogs: >1 y of age San Jose	Direct smear with Lugol's iodine CF; Sheather's sugar spg 1.3	ZeLedón et al. (2006)
	2008	18.5		184 dogs at pet shops All <6 mo of age	CF; Sheather's sugar spg 1.3	Calderón et al. (2012)
	2008–2009	5.1 9.7 1.2	Overall <1 y >1 y	158 owned dogs 72 dogs: <1 y of age 86 dogs: >1 y of age Communities with limited access to resources	CF; Sheather's sugar spg 1.3 When sufficient faecal material, also direct smear with Lugol's iodine	Valverde Alvarado (2010)
	2009	5		60 dogs presented at a spay/neuter clinic San Isidro de El General	CF; Sheather's sugar	Scorza et al. (2011)
	2011*	6.7 39.5 3.7	Overall <1 y >1 y	465 dogs in animal shelters 38 dogs: <1 y of age 427 dogs: >1 y of age Valle Central	Direct smear with Lugol's iodine CF; Sheather's sugar spg 1.3	Alemán Laporte (2011)

Continued

Table 6 Summary of *Toxocara canis* and *Toxocara cati* in dogs and cats, respectively, for Central American Countries.—cont'd

Country	Year[a]	Per cent positive for *Toxocara*		Description	Analysis method	Reference
Guatemala	2011	53	Overall	62 owned dogs 22 dogs: <1 y of age 40 dogs: >1 y of age Quetzal city in San Juan Sacatepéquez	McMaster; sugar	Mena Pérez (2014)
		100	<1 y			
		23	>1 y			
	2011*	8		100 free-roaming dogs Aldea Monterrico, Taxisco, Santa Rosa	SF; sugar	Choc Martínez (2011)
	2013*	65		49 owned dogs Zone 7 of the capital of Guatemala	Sedimentation	Arevalo Garcia (2013)
	2014*	20		70 free-roaming[b] dogs San Marcos La Laguna, Sololá	Direct smear with Kato solution	Cornejo Arriola (2014)
	2014	8.4		71 owned dogs Santo Domingo El Tuerto zona 1, Departamento de Guatemala	Sedimentation	Guerra Ruíz et al. (2017)
	2014*	2.5		81 owned dogs Not dewormed in previous 6 mo Four neighbourhoods in the municipality of Amatitlán	Sedimentation	Fuentes Soto and Salas Lémus (2014)
	2016	0		40 free-roaming adult dogs at a food market municipality of Palín, Escuintla	McMaster; sugar	Matute Argueta (2017)

Honduras	2012–2013	3.8	Overall	207 dogs 82 owned; 69 commercial kennel; 56 stray or free-roaming dogs Age for owned and kennel only: 38 dogs: <1 y of age 13 dogs: >1 y of age Tegucigalpa, Tatumbla, Zambrano and Danlí	Direct smear with Lugol's iodine SF; saturated salt	Kaminsky et al. (2014)
		2.4	Owned			
		1.4	Kennel			
		8.9	Stray			
		5.3	<1 y			
		0.9	>1 y			
Nicaragua	2006–2007	33		100 owned dogs <3 mo of age and not dewormed in the previous week Zaragoza and la Providencia, León	Direct smear with Lugol's iodine	Moreira Chévez and Velásquez García (2007)
	2008	11.5		78 owned dogs <1 y of age South-east León	Ritchie formol-ether SF; $ZnSO_4$ spg 1.18	Barcenas Barcenas and Solis Rodriguez (2009)
	2016–2017	5.1		196 owned dogs visiting a veterinary clinic Managua	Direct smear	Navarrete Úbeda and Gómez Guevara (2017)
Cats						
Guatemala	2014*	26.6		15 owned cats Not dewormed in previous 6 mo Four neighbourhoods of the Amatitlán municipality	Sedimentation	Fuentes Soto and Salas Lémus (2014)
Costa Rica	2009	11.1		9 cats at a spay/neuter clinic San Isidro de El General	CF; Sheather's sugar	Scorza et al. (2011)

[a]Year of study; if study year not specified, year of publication which is denoted by an asterisk *.
[b]Free-roaming is used to denote owned free-roaming, community and unowned dogs. The term 'stray' is only used when it is clear that the dog is not owned.
CF, centrifugation flotation; SF, simple flotation; Spg, specific gravity.

In Costa Rica, with the increase in veterinary access, this infection rate is unlikely to still be accurate but highlights the need for comprehensive studies in the region.

As a region, little can be said about prevalence in cats due to the lack of studies. However, for dogs, there are large differences in prevalence within and between countries with location appearing to be more of an influencing factor than ownership of the dog, even when accounting for differences in the diagnostic sensitivity of the methods used in different regions. Reasons for this potentially include the level of free-roaming owned and stray dogs, access to veterinary care and veterinary recommendations regarding deworming protocols. For example, within Costa Rica where veterinary care is available, there is an estimated population of 1.3 million owned dogs with over 25% being free-roaming and an estimated one million stray dogs (Rojas et al., 2017; World Animal Protection, 2016). In El Salvador the dog population in 2013 was estimated to be almost 724,000 with over 100,000 of these being street dogs (Fuentes Vásquez and Luna Martínez, 2015). Even if all owned dogs received regular anthelmintic treatments, the population of stray dogs would drive *T. canis* prevalence and increase the risk of human toxocarosis. Access to veterinary care for owned dogs can be limited in rural areas and, given, the low incomes within much of the region, care and regular use of anthelmintics might not be affordable for many households. In areas with more access to veterinary care, a variety of parasite control programs are recommended by the veterinarians with few recommending monthly deworming and many recommending only annual deworming in adult dogs and cats (Fernández et al., 2012).

From the data available, *Toxocara* is an important infection in dogs and cats in Central America with many of the issues highlighted in the discussion on *Toxocara* in Mexico being the same. More and better designed studies are required to make comparisons within the region and to understand the impact of veterinary services. Efforts to decrease stray populations would likely be needed to impact human exposure and prevalence in owned dogs.

5. Caribbean

In general, there is a lack of accessible data on *Toxocara* for the region with much of what is available being reported in grey literature (theses, conference abstracts) or local publications. Data for 10 and 5 islands for dogs and cats, respectively, were accessible and are presented in Table 7. While for five islands, studies have been conducted since the 2000s, the remainder

Table 7 Summary of *Toxocara canis* and *Toxocara cati* in dogs and cats, respectively, for the Caribbean Islands and Countries.

Country/Island	Year[a]	Per cent positive for *Toxocara*		Description	Analysis method	Reference
Dogs						
Aruba	1974	37.0		27 dogs[b]	Necropsy	Rep (1975)
Bahamas	1957–1958	63.9		36 dogs New Providence	Necropsy	Clarkson and Owen (1959)
Bonaire	1974	20.0		10 dogs	Necropsy	Rep (1975)
Cuba	1992	17.9		330 owned dogs Havana	Willis brine flotation	Duménigo et al. (1994) as referenced in Sariego et al. (2012)
	2003	27.1	Overall	321 owned dogs 116 dogs: <1 y of age 205 dogs: >1 y of age Villa Clara Province	Faecal flotation	de la Fe Rodríguez (2004) as referenced in Sariego et al. (2012)
		62.1	<1 y			
		7.3	>1 y			
	2005–2006	19.7	Overall	461 stray dogs 248 dogs: <1 y of age 213 dogs: >1 y of age No difference in the dry and rainy seasons seen Havana	Necropsy	Merlo et al. (2007)
		29.6	<1 y			
		11.3	>1 y			

Continued

Table 7 Summary of *Toxocara canis* and *Toxocara cati* in dogs and cats, respectively, for the Caribbean Islands and Countries.—cont'd

Country/Island	Year[a]	Per cent positive for *Toxocara*		Description	Analysis method	Reference
	2015	9	Urban	49 urban owned dogs 59 rural owned dogs No age difference seen Municipality Santa Clara	Preserved 10% phenol Sheather's sugar flotation	Castillo-Cuenca et al. (2016)
		40	Rural			
	2015	27.6		547 samples from the ground Municipality Camagüey	Flotation in duplicate	Iván Peña et al. (2016)
Curaçao	1974	5.6		54 dogs	Necropsy	Rep (1975)
	1986	7.5	Overall	133 dogs 74 pets (with 'no history of medical treatment') 59 stray	Faecal examination by formalin-ethyl acetate sedimentation	Saleh et al. (1988)
		10.8	Pets			
		3.4	Stray			
	2011	0		157 dogs 6 mo to 17 y of age 26 from a shelter, remainder owned and examined at a veterinary clinic	Centrifugation with sugar flotation solution	El Amrani (2011)
Dominican Republic	2018*	4		113 dogs Primarily free-roaming[c] adult dogs San Cristobal	McMaster; saturated salt solution	Joubert Canelo and Mallén Moré (2018)

Grenada	2006–2007	5		20 dogs Free roaming	CF; zinc sulphate spg 1.18–1.2	Neill (2009)
	2006–2007	4		170 dogs Free roaming	CF; zinc sulphate spg 1.18–1.2	Coomansingh et al. (2007)
	2007*	7		100 dogs All seen at a veterinary clinic	Method could not be determined	Erskine (2007) as referenced in Neill (2009)
	2008–2012	3.8	Overall	445 stray dogs Age estimated 8 dogs: <12 wk of age 32 dogs: 12–24 wk of age 405 dogs: adult	Stored 10% formalin Flotation; saturated NaCl	Tiwari et al. (2016)
		50	<12 wk			
		0	12–24 wk			
		0.7	adult			
	2017	48		306 owned dogs All <1 y of age	CF; zinc sulphate spg 1.18–1.2	Schwartz et al. (2018, 2019)
Guadeloupe	1982–1983	17		44 dogs Ownership not specified	Necropsy Faecal examination; method not described	Esterre and Maitre (1985)
Jamaica	1986	7.8		122 dogs Primarily adult and owned	Ritchie formol-ether in duplicate	Robinson et al. (1989)

Continued

Table 7 Summary of *Toxocara canis* and *Toxocara cati* in dogs and cats, respectively, for the Caribbean Islands and Countries.—cont'd

Country/Island	Year[a]	Per cent positive for *Toxocara*		Description	Analysis method	Reference
St. Kitts	2014	19	Overall	97 owned dogs 6 dogs: ≤6 mo of age 91 dogs: >6 mo of age Primarily confined, not free-roaming	CF; Sheather's sugar spg 1.27–1.28	Ketzis et al. (2015b)
		33	≤6 mo			
		18	>6 mo			
St. Lucia	1983	32		22 samples from the ground Samples from free-roaming and non-free-roaming dogs	Modified Ritchie formol-ether	Thompson et al. (1986)
Cats						
Aruba	1974	0.0		18 cats	Necropsy	Rep (1975)
Bahamas	1957–1958	19		21 cats	Necropsy	Clarkson and Owen (1959)
Bonaire	1974	0.0		12 cats	Necropsy	Rep (1975)
Curaçao	1974	3.8		53 cats	Necropsy	Rep (1975)
Grenada	2018	8.8		57 free-roaming[d] and domestic cats	CF	Paterson et al. (2019)

Guadeloupe	1982–1983	60	31 cats	Necropsy Faecal examination; method not described	Esterre and Maitre (1985)
Puerto Rico	1964	75	70 cats La Perla and Santurce San Juan	Necropsy	de León and Kolodziej (1969)
St. Kitts	2005–2006	4	100 free-roaming cats	CF; Sheather's sugar spg 1.27–1.28	Krecek et al. (2010)
	2013–2014	7	41 owned indoor and indoor/ outdoor cats All >10 mo of age	CF; Sheather's sugar spg 1.27–1.28	Ketzis et al. (2015a)
	2014–2015	8.6	35 free-roaming cats All >6 mo of age	Necropsy	Geng et al. (2018)
	2017	16	50 free-roaming All >6 mo of age	CF; Sheather's sugar spg 1.27–1.28	Eisenbraun et al. (2019)

[a]Year of study; if study year not specified, year of publication which is denoted by an asterisk *.
[b]When only 'cats' or 'dogs' is used to describe the population, data on ownership was not provided; however, based on the study design these are likely unowned.
[c]Free-roaming dogs is used to denote owned free-roaming, community and unowned dogs. The term 'stray' is only used when it is clear that the dog is not owned.
[d]Free-roaming cats are used to denote unowned, stray, friendly or feral cats.
CF, centrifugation flotation; SF, simple flotation; spg, specific gravity.

is more historical. No accessible data could be located for Anguilla, Antigua and Barbuda, Barbados, British Virgin Islands, Cayman Islands, Dominica, Haiti, Martinique, Montserrat, Saba, Saint Barthelemy, Saint Martin and Sint Maarten, Saint Vincent and the Grenadines, Trinidad and Tobago, Turks and Caicos Islands, and the US Virgin Islands. Bundy and Steele (1984) noted that with four languages in the region (Dutch, English, French and Spanish), few regional journals, and obscure local journals, obtaining scientific data for the region can be challenging and this appears to still be the case today.

The most information on *Toxocara* in dogs comes from Cuba, Curaçao, and Grenada. Prevalence in dogs ranged from 63.9%, historical data from the Bahamas (Clarkson and Owen, 1959), to 0% in Curaçao in 2011. However, the per cent of positive dogs appears to be less related to the year of the study than the population sampled, as with studies from Central America. For example, data from 2006 to 2012 from Grenada found 3.8–7% of adult dogs to be infected while a study from 2017 with dogs <1 year of age found 48% to be infected. Data from Cuba also indicate that occurrence is driven more by age of the dogs examined as well as differences in urban and rural areas with rural being higher, than the year of the study (Castillo-Cuenca et al., 2016). Within urban areas, population density also impacted the number of positive dogs, with more dogs found to be infected in higher density areas (Iván Peña et al., 2016).

The majority of the studies in the region were with owned but free-roaming dogs. While one might expect more of these dogs to be infected with *Toxocara*, most free-roaming dogs are adults (Neill, 2009; Tiwari et al., 2016). At the same time, puppies are brought to veterinary clinics for vaccination at which time deworming with or without faecal sampling could occur. Within this context, the higher number of infected dogs seen in the study conducted with dogs at a veterinary clinic in Grenada compared to that seen in a free-roaming population in Grenada (7% versus 3.8–5%) is likely reflective of the age of the animals.

Only on Curaçao is there an indication that infections might be decreasing. In 2011, *Toxocara* was not identified in any dogs at a veterinary clinic nor at any animal shelter (El Amrani, 2011). This is in contrast to a study from 1986 in which 10.3% domestic and 3.4% feral dogs were positive (Saleh et al., 1988). El Amrani (2011) interviewed dog owners and found that 36.2% of the dogs were never dewormed, 33.1% were administered a monthly broad-spectrum heartworm preventative, and the remainder were dewormed less frequently. As a result of these practices, 86.2% had been dewormed within the 6 months prior to the faecal sampling. This level of deworming in Curaçao is in agreement with what Meijer (2012) found in interviews with veterinarians and dog owners. One can contrast this to the dogs on St. Kitts where approximately 47% were dewormed 4 months prior to the study and <13% were on a monthly heartworm preventative with 19% being positive for *Toxocara*.

Most of the data on *Toxocara* in cats is from St. Kitts and from feral cats. Studies from the 1950s–1980s from the Bahamas, Puerto Rico and Guadalupe showed high numbers to be infected (19–75%), and data from the last 12 years from St. Kitts shows no decrease. In addition, no difference in feral versus owned cats was seen on St. Kitts, even with over half of the cats being indoor only.

While data are limited for the region, some generalities can be made. While there are some exceptions, most of the islands have high free-roaming dog populations despite laws attempting to prevent this (Alie et al., 2007; Cleaton et al., 2019; Fielding, 2008; Fielding et al., 2012; Iván Peña et al., 2016; Perilhou, 2003). In the case of cats, feral populations also can be high, and, with both cats and dogs, spaying and neutering is infrequent (Alie et al., 2007; Castro-Prieto and Andrade-Núñez, 2018; Fielding, 2009; Moura et al., 2007). While free-roaming populations can have a large impact on environmental contamination and host exposure, the free-roaming populations often consist of older dogs, which could limit environmental contamination (Joubert Canelo and Mallén Moré, 2018; Neill, 2009). In addition, from the studies in Curaçao and unpublished data from St. Kitts, even when adult dogs are not treated, owners tend to treat the puppies, again limiting environmental contamination and subsequent host exposure. However, the lack of treatment of adult female dogs could contribute to higher infections and negatively impact the overall health of puppies.

Despite the lack of data for many islands, given the similarities in management attitudes and climate, it is likely that for islands without data, prevalence is similar to those for which there are data with free-roaming populations, generally high populations, lack of treatment of adult animals and lack of spaying and neutering all contributing to the prevalence.

6. Summary

Within these regions, the quantity and quality of data are highest from the United States and Mexico with no data available for many of the Caribbean islands and Central American countries. This is consistent with data availability for human *Toxocara* and vector-borne diseases in pet animals in these regions (Delgado and Rodríguez-Morales, 2009; Fakhri et al., 2018; Maggi and Krämer, 2019). Even in areas with extensive data, such as the United States, some regions and animal populations may be under-represented. Most of the data have the limitation that it is reliant on the presence of eggs in faeces as an indicator of infection, which may underestimate the true prevalence. Conversely, analysis of single samples could overestimate prevalence in some canine populations if coprophagia is high (Nijsse et al., 2014).

Regardless of the issues with the data available, with the exception of owned dogs in the United States, prevalence in owned dogs in Mexico, Latin America, the Caribbean, and economically constrained areas of the United States and cats in all regions is high and not much different in pets than what is seen in shelter and feral populations. This high prevalence of *Toxocara* is not only a health issue for dogs and cats, but a potential risk for visceral, neural, and ocular larval migrans in people, particularly children. Toxocarosis is considered a neglected disease with associations to poverty and areas with limited resources (Hotez and Wilkins, 2009). Serum antibody prevalence and cases of larval migrans in human populations within regions covered in this review are a concern (Bolivar-Mejia et al., 2014; Guerra Ruíz et al., 2017; Heredia et al., 2014; Sariego et al., 2012; Tinoco-Gracia et al., 2008), with human exposure occurring not only from soil contamination, but also potentially through contaminated poultry and livestock (Romero et al., 2016; Taira et al., 2004).

Decreasing prevalence is not as simple as increasing anthelmintic use in these populations of dogs and cats. Increasing spaying and neutering of dogs and cats and control of free-roaming owned and stray dog and feral cat populations is essential. The impact of treating puppies and young dogs on prevalence can be greater than that achieved with treatment of adult dogs (Gates and Nolan, 2014). Targeting treatment to this population combined with promoting spaying and neutering might have a greater impact than promoting monthly control in dogs of all ages. In areas where stray dog populations can be almost 50% of the total population, owned dogs, even if treated regularly, will be constantly exposed to reinfection. Given the interaction of these factors, cost-benefit analyses are needed to determine how best to allocate resources regarding education, treatment and population control, especially in resource-limited areas.

Feral cat populations can be as large of an issue as stray and free-roaming dogs with some populations in focal areas estimated to be almost equivalent to the owned cat population (Ireland and Neilan, 2016; Kilgour et al., 2017). The impact of trap-neuter-release programs on these populations, and ultimately the environmental levels of *T. cati*, are beyond the scope of this review but do need consideration. Also, of importance is the attitude of cat owners towards the need of anthelmintic treatments for cats and the frequency of veterinary visits, with cats typically attending a veterinary clinic less frequently than dogs and normally not on monthly preventatives (AVMA, 2018; Levy et al., 2017). Given that prevalence of *T. cati* in adult cats, including owned and indoor cats, can be high and much higher than dogs, this is an area that requires attention if prevalence is to be decreased.

In some locations, wild canids and felids can add to the environmental levels and host exposure. In a study in Bristol, UK, the primary source of *Toxocara* in soil was determined to be from puppies and dogs; however better control of dog faeces would result in fox and cat populations becoming the primary source (Morgan et al., 2013). This situation also could occur in places in the United States and Central America where wild animal populations overlap with urban and rural pet populations. When considering means of decreasing the occurrence of infection and considering the impact of deworming programs, these sources could become critical.

Despite the development of highly effective anthelmintics, the review of the data from these regions shows that there has been limited impact on prevalence in cats and dogs. More studies on *Toxocara* in dogs and cats, including owner socio-economic data, are needed to develop educational and intervention programs and to have baseline data to evaluate the impact of such programs. A multi-systems approach will be needed if prevalence is to be decreased and dog, cat and human health improved.

References

Alemán Laporte, J.M., 2011. Prevalencia de parásitos gastrointestinales en siete refugios de perros abandonados del Valle Central. Escuela de Medicina Veterinaria, Facultad de Ciencias de la Salud, Universidad Nacional, Costa Rica, Costa Ricad. Thesis.

Alie, K., Witkind Davis, B., Fielding, W.J., Maldonado, F.G., 2007. Attitudes towards dogs and other "pets" in Roseau, Dominica. Anthrozoös 20, 143–154.

Alvarado-Esquivel, C., Romero-Salas, D., Aguilar-Domínguez, M., Cruz-Romero, A., Ibarra-Priego, N., Pérez-de-León, A.A., 2015. Epidemiological assessment of intestinal parasitic infections in dogs at animal shelter in Veracruz, Mexico. Asian Pac. J. Trop. Biomed. 5, 34–39. https://doi.org/10.1016/S2221-1691(15)30167-2.

Andersen, L.A., Levy, J.K., McManus, C.M., McGorray, S.P., Leutenegger, C.M., Piccione, J., Blackwelder, L.K., Tucker, S.J., 2018. Prevalence of enteropathogens in cats with and without diarrhea in four different management models for unowned cats in the southeast United States. Vet. J. 236, 49–55.

Arambulo, P.V., Steele, J.H., 1976. Urban dogs in Houston, Texas—parasitic infection and environmental health impact. Int. J. Zoonoses 3, 114–144.

Arevalo Garcia, C.J., 2013. Determinación de helmintos gastrointestinales zoonóticos en perros y sus dueños (niños), en la Colonia Santa Elena 1 zona 7 de la Ciudad de Guatemala. Thesis, Facultad de Medicina Veterinaria Y Zootecnia, Escuela de Medicina Veterinaria, Universidad de San Carlos de Guatemala.

Ash, L.R., 1962. Helminth parasites of clogs and cats of Hawaii. J. Parasitol. 48, 65–68.

AVMA, 2018. Pet Ownership and Demographics Sourcebook, 2017-2018 edition. American Veterinary Medical Association.

Barcenas Barcenas, L.A., Solis Rodriguez, C.A., 2009. Prevalencia de *Giardia canis* en los barrios del Sur-Este de León (Alfonso Cortes, Rubén Darío y Salomón de la Selva) en el period Septiembre-Noviembre 2008. Thesis submitted to the Escuela de Medicina Veterinaria, Universidad Nacional Autónoma de Nicaragua.

Blagburn, B.L. (2009) National parasite prevalence survey: an interim report. NAVC Conference. 233. Proceeding, pp. 1168-1171.

Blagburn, B.L., Lindsay, D.S., Vaughan, J.L., Rippey, N.S., Wright, J.C., Lynn, R.C., Kelch, W.J., Ritchie, G.C., Hepler, D.I., 1996. Prevalence of canine parasites based on fecal flotation. Compend. Contin. Educ. Pract. Vet. 18, 483–509.

Bolivar-Mejia, A., Alarcón-Olave, C., Calvo-Betancourt, L.S., Paniz-Mondolfi, A., Delgado, O., Rodriguez-Morales, A.J., 2014. Toxocariasis in the Americas: burden and disease control. Curr. Trop. Med. Rep. 1, 62–68.

Braun, J.L., Thayer, C.B., 1962. A survey for intestinal parasites in Iowa dogs. J. Am. Vet. Med. Assoc. 141, 1049–1050.

Brophy, J., and Peregrine, A.S. (2009) .Parasitic zoonoses of dogs and cats: a medical and veterinary perspective in Canada. Conference Proceedings, Ontario Veterinary Medical Association (OVMA), 29–31 January, unpaginated.

Bundy, D.A.P., Steele, J.H., 1984. Parasitic zoonoses in the Caribbean region—a review. Int. J. Zoonoses 11, 1–38.

Calderón, S., de Oliveira, J., Hernández, J., Jiménez, M., Muñoz, P., 2012. Parásitos gastrointestinales en caninos menores de seis meses comercializados en tiendas de mascotas de la Gran Área Metropolitana de Costa Rica [Gastrointestinal parasites in dogs 6 months old or younger sold in 18 pet stores in the great metropolitan area of Costa Rica]. Cienc. Vet. 26, 21–35.

Campos, F.F., Alarcon, G.J.C., 2002. Intestinal helminth frequency in stray dogs sacrificed in the City of Queretaro, in the State of Queretaro, in Mexico. Vet. Mex. 33, 247–253.

Cantó, G.J., Garcia, M.P., Garcia, A., Guerrero, M.J., Mosqueda, J., 2011. The prevalence and abundance of helminth parasites in stray dogs from the city of Queretaro in central Mexico. J. Helminthol. 85, 263–269.

Cantó, G.J., Guerrero, R.I., Olvera-Ramirez, A.M., Milian, F., Mosqueda, J., Aguilar-Tipacamu, G., 2013. Prevalence of fleas and gastrointestinal parasites in free-roaming cats in central Mexico. PLoS One 8, e60744.

Castillo-Cuenca, J.C., Iannacone-Oliver, J., Fimia-Duarte, R., Cepero-Rodríguez, O., Morales-Morales, A., 2016. Prevalencia y factores de riesgo asociados con la infección de *Toxocara canis* y *Ancylostoma caninum* en canes de compañía. [Prevalence and risk factors associate with *Toxocara canis* and *Ancylostoma caninum* infection in companion dogs]. Biologist 14, 103–108.

Castro-Prieto, J., Andrade-Núñez, M.J., 2018. Health and ecological aspects of stray cats in old San Juan, Puerto Rico: baseline information to develop an effective control program. P. R. Health Sci. J. 37, 110–114.

Chávez-Ruvalcaba, F., Moreno Garcia, M.A., de Muñoz Escobedo, J.J., Chavez Ruvalcaba, M.I., 2012. Detection of gastroenteric parasites in dogs in the suburbs of Guadalupe Zacatecas, Mexico. [Deteccion de parasitosis gastroentericas en canideos en la zona conurbada Zacatecas-Guadalupe, Mexico.]. REDVET 13, 101213.

Choc Martínez, L.F., 2011. Determinación de la presencia de parásitos gastrointestinales en heces de perros deambulantes, en la Aldea Monterrico, Taxisco, Santa Rosa. Thesis, Facultad de Medicina Veterinaria Y Zootecnia, Escuela de Medicina Veterinaria, Universidad de San Carlos de Guatemala.

Clarkson, M.J., Owen, L.N., 1959. The parasites of domestic animals in the Bahama islands. Ann. Trop. Med. Parasitol. 53, 341–346.

Cleaton, J.M., Blanton, J.D., Dilius, P., Ludder, F., Crowdis, K., Medley, A., Chipman, R., Estime, F., Maciel, E., Wallace, R.M., 2019. Use of photography to identify free-roaming dogs during sight-resight surveys: impacts on estimates of population size and vaccination coverage, Haiti 2016. Vaccine: X 2, 100025.

Coggins, J.R., 1998. Effect of season, sex, and age on prevalence of parasitism in dogs from southeastern Wisconsin. J. Helminthol. Soc. Wash. 65, 219–224.

Coomansingh, C.-M., Pinckney, R.D., Macpherson, C.N.L., Stone, D.I., 2007. Helminth parasites in dogs in Grenada, West Indies. In: American Association of Veterinary Parasitologists 52nd Annual Meeting, July 14-17, 2007, Washington D.C., USA.

Cornejo Arriola, P.A., 2014. Determinación de la carga parasitaria en perros de la región de San Marcos La Laguna, Sololá. Thesis, Facultad de Medicina Veterinaria Y Zootecnia, Escuela de Medicina Veterinaria, Universidad de San Carlos de Guatemala.

Cortez-Aguirre, G.R., Jimenez-Coello, M., Gutierrez-Blanco, E., Ortega-Pacheco, A., 2018. Stray dog population in a city of southern Mexico and its impact on the contamination of public areas. Vet. Med. Int. 2018, 2381583.

Costa, J.O., Galvin, T.J., Bell, R.R., Smith, J.P., 1971. Survey of helminth parasites of dogs from Brazos County, Texas. Southwest. Vet. 24, 305–306.

Cruz-Reyes, A., 1971. Frequency of some helminth parasites of dogs (*Canis familiaris* Linnaeus, 1758) in the Federal District (Mexico). [Frecuencia de algunos helmintos parasitos de perros (*Canis familiaris* Linnaeus, 1758) del Distrito Federal. (Mexico)]. Thesis, Universidad Nacional Autonoma de Mexico, p. 133.

de la Fe Rodríguez, P.Y., 2004. Prevalencia de Toxocara canis en perros caseros de la provincia Villa Clara. Thesis, Institute of Tropical Medicine "Pedro Kourí", Havana, Cuba. As summarized in Sariego, I., Kanobana, K., Rojas, L., Speybroeck, N., Polman, K., and Núñez, F.A. (2012) Toxocariasis in Cuba: a literature review. PLoS Negl. Trop. Dis. 6, e1382. https://doi.org/10.1371/journal.pntd.0001382.

De la Rosa-Arana, J.L., Tapia-Romero, R., 2018. Frequency of helminth eggs in faeces of puppies living in urban or rural environments of Mexico City. Iran. J. Parasitol. 13, 632–636.

de León, D.D., Kolodziej, F., 1969. Helminth parasites of cats. J. Agric. Univ. Puerto Rico 53, 77–78.

De Santis, A.C., Raghavan, M., Caldanaro, R.J., Glickman, N.W., Moore, G.E., Lewis, H.B., Schantz, P.M., Glickman, L.T., 2006. Estimated prevalence of nematode parasitism among pet cats in the United States. J. Am. Vet. Med. Assoc. 228, 885–892.

Delgado, O., Rodríguez-Morales, A., 2009. Aspectos clínico-epidemiológicos de la toxocariasis: una enfermedad desatendida en Venezuela y América Latina. B. Malariol. Salud. Amb. 49, 1–33.

Dorman, D.W., Van Ostrand, J.R., 1958. A survey of *Toxocara canis* and *Toxocara cati* prevalence in the New York City area. N. Y. State J. Med. 58, 2793–2795.

Duménigo, B., Lau, N., Bravo, J.R., 1994. Prevalencia de *Toxocara canis* en perros caseros de Ciudad de La Habana. Rev. Cubana Med. Trop. 46, 99–102. As summarized in Sariego, I., Kanobana, K., Rojas, L., Speybroeck, N., Polman, K., and Núñez, F.A. (2012) Toxocariasis in Cuba: a literature review. PLoS Negl. Trop. Dis. 6, e1382. https://doi.org/10.1371/journal.pntd.0001382.

Eguía-Aguilar, P., Cruz-Reyes, A., Martinez-Maya, J.J., 2005. Ecological analysis and description of the intestinal helminths present in dogs in Mexico City. Vet. Parasitol. 127, 139–146.

Eiland, C.B., Tamblyn, K., Rynders, P., Dillon, A.R., Newton, J.C., Spencer, J.A., Blagburn, B.L., 2004. Prevalence of *Dirofilaria immitis, Toxocara cati, Ancylostoma tubaeforme*, and other endo- and ectoparasites of random-source cats from east central Alabama. In: Proc. Annual Mtg A Assoc. Vet. Parasitol., Philadelphia, PA July 2004 Abstract 116.

Eisenbraun, H., Alluwie, A., Connolly, S., Nair, R., Verocai, G.G., Ketzis, J.K., 2019. Comparison of fecal analysis methods for the detection of *Platynosomum fastosum* in naturally infected cats. J. Feline Med. Surg. 1–4. https://doi.org/10.1177/1098612X19848173.

El Amrani, F., 2011. *Spirocerca lupi* Infections in Dogs on the Island of Curaçao. Thesis, Faculty of Veterinary Medicine, Utrecht University, the Netherlands.

Encalada-Mena, L.A., Duarte-Ubaldo, E.I., Vargaz-Magaña, J.J., García-Ramírez, M.J., Medina-Hernández, R.E., 2011. Prevalence of gastroenteric parasites of dogs in the city of Escárcega, Campeche, México. [Prevalencia de parásitos gastroentéricos de cánidos en la ciudad de Escárcega, Campeche, México.]. Universidad y Ciencia 27, 209–217.

Erskine, A., 2007. A comparative study into the prevalence of intestinal parasites in owned dogs in Grenada. Senior Project. St. George's University, Grenada as referenced in Neill, K.G. (2009) The public health importance of dogs, Grand Anse, Grenada. Thesis, School of Medicine, St George's University, Grenada.

Esterre, P., Maitre, M.J., 1985. Les affections parasitaires des monogastriques en Guadeloupe. Rev. Elev. Med. Vet. Pays Trop. 38, 43–48.

Fakhri, Y., Gasser, R.B., Rostami, A., Fan, C.K., Ghasemi, S.M., Javanian, M., Bayani, M., Armoon, B., Moradi, B., 2018. Toxocara eggs in public places worldwide—a systematic review and meta-analysis. Environ. Pollut. 242 (Pt .B), 1467–1475. https://doi.org/10.1016/j.envpol.2018.07.087.

Fernández, D., de Oliveira, J.B., Calderón, S., Romero, J.J., 2012. Prácticas de diagnóstico y control de parásitos de caninos y felinos en 50 clínicas veterinarias del área metropolitana de Costa Rica [Diagnosis and control procedures of the parasites of canines and felines in 50 clinics in the metropolitan area of Costa Rica]. Cienc. Vet. 26, 51–71.

Fielding, W.J., 2008. Dogs: a continuing and common neighborhood nuisance of New Providence, The Bahamas. Soc. Anim. 16, 61–73.

Fielding, W.J., 2009. A comparison of Bahamian cat and dog caregivers on New Providence. J. Appl. Anim. Welf. Sci. 12, 30–43. https://doi.org/10.1080/10888700802536616.

Fielding, W.J., Gall, M., Green, D., Eller, W.S., 2012. Care of dogs and attitudes of dog owners in Port-au-Prince, the Republic of Haiti. J. Appl. Anim. Welf. Sci. 153, 236–253. https://doi.org/10.1080/10888705.2012.683760.

Flores-Barroeta, L., 1955. Helminths of dogs (*Canis familiaris*) and cats (*Felis catus*) in Mexico City. English title not available, 8, Anales de la Escuela Nacional de Ciencias Biologicas, pp. 159–202.

Fuentes Soto, E.A., Salas Lémus, J.E.G., 2014. Prevalencia de parásitos intestinales en los habitantes y sus mascotas en los barrios Hospital, San Lorenzo, Amanecer Y San Antonio Del Municipio De Amatitlán. Thesis, Facultad de Ciencias Químicas Y Farmacia, Universidad de San Carlos De Guatemala.

Fuentes Vásquez, C.G., Luna Martínez, D.E., 2015. Desarrollo de campaña social sobre la tenencia responsible de perros, dirigida a la asociación para la rehabilitación de animales "El Santuario". Thesis, Facultad de Ciencias Y Artes Francisco Gavidia, Escuela de Ciencias de la Comunicación, Universidad Dr. José Matías Delgado, El Salvador.

Gates, M.C., Nolan, T.J., 2009. Endoparasite prevalence and recurrence across different age groups of dogs and cats. Vet. Parasitol. 166, 153–158.

Gates, M.C., Nolan, T.J., 2014. Declines in canine endoparasite prevalence associated with the introduction of commercial heartworm and flea preventatives from 1984 to 2007. Vet. Parasitol. 204, 265–268.

Geng, J., Elsemore, D.A., Oudin, N., Ketzis, J.K., 2018. Diagnosis of feline whipworm infection using a coproantigen ELISA and the prevalence in feral cats in southern Florida. Vet. Parasitol. Reg. Study. Rep. 14, 181–186.
Greve, J.H., O'Brien, S.E., 1989. Prevalence of intestinal parasites in Iowa dogs: a comparison between 1965-68 and 1988. Iowa State Univ. Vet. 51, 24–25.
Guerra Ruíz, M.A., Pereira Castillo, R.A., Pérez Ardón, S.A., 2017. Prevalencia de anticuerpos anti-Toxocara IGg en personas que conviven con perros como mascotas. Thesis, Facultad de Ciencias Químicas Y Farmacia, Universidad de San Carlos de Guatemala.
Guevara Collazo, D., Torres Montoya, J.T., Chernitzky Waissman, J., 1990. Examination of cats' faeces for *Toxoplasma gondii* oocysts in Mexico City. [Situacion de los ooquistes de *Toxoplasma gondii* en heces de gatos del Distrito Federal, Mexico.]. Vet. Mex. 21, 45–48.
Hackett, T., Lappin, M.R., 2003. Prevalence of enteric pathogens in dogs of north-central Colorado. J. Am. Anim. Hosp. Assoc. 39, 52–56.
Heredia, R., Romero, C., Mendoza, G.E., Ponce, M., Portal, A., Gonzalez, L., Bautista, L.G., 2014. Occurrence of *Toxocara canis* in students of veterinary and graphic design in a Mexican university. Acta Sci. Vet. 42, 1219.
Hill, S.L., Cheney, J.M., Taton-Allen, G.F., Reif, J.S., Bruns, C., Lappin, M.R., 2000. Prevalence of enteric zoonotic organisms in cats. J. Am. Vet. Med. Assoc. 216, 687–692.
Holland, C.V., 2017. Knowledge gaps in the epidemiology of *Toxocara*: the enigma remains. Parasitology 144, 81–94. https://doi.org/10.1017/S0031182015001407. Epub 2015 Dec 16.
Hoskins, J.D., Malone, J.B., Smith, P.H., Uhl, S.A., 1982. Prevalence of parasitism diagnosed by fecal examination in Louisiana dogs. Am. J. Vet. Res. 43, 1106–1109.
Hotez, P.J., 2014. Neglected parasitic infections and poverty in the United States. PLoS Negl. Trop. Dis. 8, e3012. https://doi.org/10.1371/journal.pntd.0003012.
Hotez, P.J., Wilkins, P.P., 2009. Toxocariasis: America's most common neglected infection of poverty and a helminthiasis of global importance? PLoS Negl. Trop. Dis. 3, e400.
Ireland, T., Neilan, R.M., 2016. A spatial agent-based model of feral cats and analysis of population and nuisance controls. Ecol. Model. 337, 123–136.
Iván Peña, G., Florangel Vidal, F., Aliesky Hernández, R., 2016. Población de perros callejeros del municipio Camagüey, Cuba. Rev. Inv. Vet. Perú 27, 840–844. https://doi.org/10.15381/rivep.v27i4.12570.
Jaskoski, B.J., 1971. Intestinal parasites of well cared for dogs. Am. J. Trop. Med. Hyg. 20, 441–444.
Jaskoski, B.J., Barr, V., Borges, M., 1982. Intestinal parasites of well-cared-for dogs: an area revisited. Am. J. Trop. Med. Hyg. 31, 1107–1110.
Jiménez-Cardoso, E., Eligio-Garcia, L., Cortes-Campos, A., Estrada, A.C., Pinto-Sagahon, M., Noguera-Estrada, C., 2010. The frequency of intestinal parasites in puppies from Mexican kennels. Health 2, 1316–1319.
Jordan, H.E., Mullins, S.T., Stebbins, M.E., 1993. Endoparasitism in dogs: 21,583 cases (1981-1990). J. Am. Vet. Med. Assoc. 203, 547–549.
Joubert Canelo, M.F., Mallén Moré, L.L., 2018. Presencia del parásito *Linguatula serrata* en perros callejeros alrededor de los mataderos informales de ovicaprinos en la provincia de San Cristóbal, República Dominicana. Thesis, Facultad de Ciencias Agropecuarias y Recursos Naturales, Escuela de Medicina Veterinaria, Universidad Nacional Pedro Henríquez Ureña.
Kaminsky, R., Groothousen, C.M., Zúniga, A.M., Contreras, M., Ferrera, A.M., Henríquez, K.C., 2014. Infección por *Toxocara canis* en perros y riesgo de toxocariasis humana, Honduras [*Toxocara canis* infection in dogs and risk of human toxocariasis, Honduras]. Rev. Med. Hondur. 82, 50–57.

Kazacos, K.R., 1978. Gastrointestinal helminths in dogs from a humane shelter in Indiana. J. Am. Vet. Med. Assoc. 173, 995–997.
Ketzis, J.K., Shell, L., Chinault, S., Pemberton, C., Mauldin Pereira, M., 2015a. The prevalence of *Trichuris* spp. infection in indoor and outdoor cats on St. Kitts. J. Infect. Dev. Ctries. 9, 111–113. https://doi.org/10.3855/jidc.5778.
Ketzis, J.K., Shell, L., Scorpio, D., 2015b. A survey of ectoparasites and vector-borne diseases of dogs on St. Kitts. In: American Association of Veterinary Parasitologists 60th Annual Meeting, 59th Livestock Insect Workers' Conference, 13th International Symposium on Ectoparasites of Pets, July 11-14, 2015, Boston, USA.
Kilgour, R.J., Magle, S.B., Slater, M., Christian, A., Weiss, E., DiTullio, M., 2017. Estimating free-roaming cat populations and the effects of one year Trap-Neuter-Return management effort in a highly urban area. Urban Ecosyst. 20, 207–216. https://doi.org/10.1007/s11252-016-0583-8.
Kirkpatrick, C.E., 1988. Epizootiology of endoparasitic infections in pet dogs and cats presented to a veterinary teaching hospital. Vet. Parasitol. 30, 113–124.
Krecek, R.C., Moura, L., Lucas, H., Kelly, P., 2010. Parasites of stray cats (*Felis domesticus* L., 1758) on St. Kitts, West Indies. Vet. Parasitol. 172, 147–149.
Lee, R.M., Moore, L.B., Bottazzi, M.E., Hotez, P.J., 2014. Toxocariasis in North America: a systematic review. PLoS Negl. Trop. Dis. 8, e3116.
Levy, J.K., Burling, A.N., Crandall, M.M., Tucker, S.J., Wood, E.G., Foster, J.D., 2017. Seroprevalence of heartworm infection, risk factors for seropositivity, and frequency of prescribing heartworm preventives for cats in the United States and Canada. J. Am. Vet. Med. Assoc. 250, 873–880. https://doi.org/10.2460/javma.250.8.873.
Lightner, L., Christensen, B.M., Beran, G.W., 1978. Epidemiologic findings on canine and feline intestinal nematode infections from records of the Iowa State University Veterinary Clinic. J. Am. Vet. Med. Assoc. 172, 564–567.
Lillis, W.G., 1967. Helminth survey of dogs and cats in New Jersey. J. Parasitol. 53, 1082–1084.
Little, S.E., Johnson, E.M., Lewis, D., Jaklitsch, R.P., Payton, M.E., Blagburn, B.L., Bowman, D.D., Moroff, S., Tams, T., Rich, L., Aucoin, D., 2009. Prevalence of intestinal parasites in pet dogs in the United States. Vet. Parasitol. 166, 144–152.
Little, S., Adolph, C., Downie, K., Snider, T., Reichard, M., 2015. High prevalence of covert infection with gastrointestinal helminths in cats. J. Am. Anim. Hosp. Assoc. 51, 359–364.
Little, S.E., Barrett, A.W., Beall, M.J., Bowman, D.D., Dangoudoubiyam, S., Elsemore, D.A., Liotta, J., Lucio-Forster, A., McCrann, D.J., Snowden, K.F., Starkey, L.A., Tasse, S., 2019. Coproantigen detection augments diagnosis of common nematode infections in dogs. Top. Companion Anim. Med. 35, 42–46. https://doi.org/10.1053/j.tcam.2019.04.001. Epub 2019 Apr 6.
Loebenberg, D., Waitz, J.A., 1977. Intestinal helminths and protozoa of New Jersey dogs. J. Parasitol. 63, 1139–1140.
Lucio-Forster, A., Bowman, D.D., 2011. Prevalence of fecal-borne parasites detected by centrifugal flotation in feline samples from two shelters in upstate New York. J. Feline Med. Surg. 13, 300–303. https://doi.org/10.1016/j.jfms.2010.12.013.
Lucio-Forster, A., Mizhquiri Barbecho, J.S., Mohammed, H.O., Kornreich, B.G., Bowman, D.D., 2016. Comparison of the prevalence of *Toxocara* egg shedding by pet cats and dogs in the U.S.A., 2011-2014. Vet. Parasitol. Reg. Study Rep. 5, 1–13. https://doi.org/10.1016/j.vprsr.2016.08.002. Epub 2016 Aug 16.
Maggi, R.G., Krämer, F., 2019. A review on the occurrence of companion vector-borne diseases in pet animals in Latin America. Parasit. Vectors 12, 145.

Marron, J.A., Schroeder, R.J., 1978. Survey of *Toxocara canis* infection in Los Angeles county. J. Am. Vet. Med. Assoc. 172, 713.

Martínez-Barbabosa, I., Ruiz Gonzalez, L.A., Gutierrez Quiroz, M., Fernandez Presas, A.M., Vasquez Tsuji, O., 1997. Frequency of *Toxocara cati* eggs in domestic cats in Mexico city and the state of Mexico. [Frecuencia de hallazgo de huevos de *Toxocara cati* en gatos domesticos de la Ciudad de Mexico y el Estado de Mexico.]. Bol. Chil. Parasitol. 52, 12–17.

Martínez-Barbabosa, I., Fernandez, P.A.M., Vazquez, T.O., Ruiz, H.A., 1998. Prevalence of *Toxocara canis* in dogs and in green areas of the south of Mexico City. [Frecuencia de *Toxocara canis* en perros y areas verdes del sur de la ciudad de Mexico, Distrito Federal.]. Vet. Mex. 29, 239–244.

Martínez-Barbabosa, I., Vazquez Tsuji, O., Romero Cabello, R., Gutierrez Cardenas, E.M., Amancio Chasin, O., 2003. The prevalence of *Toxocara cati* in domestic cats in Mexico City. Vet. Parasitol. 114, 43–49.

Martínez-Barbabosa, I., Gutierrez Cardenas, E.M., Alpizar Sosa, E.A., de Pimienta Lastra, R.J., 2008a. Parasitic contamination by dog feces collected from the streets of San Cristobal de Las Casas, Chiapas, Mexico. Vet. Mex. 39, 173–180.

Martínez-Barbabosa, I., Gutierrez Quiroz, M., Ruiz Gonzalez, L.A., Gutierrez Cardenas, E.M., Sosa Edubiel, A.A., Valencia Juarez, J.L., Gaona, E., 2008b. Prevalence of anti-*T. canis* antibodies in stray dogs in Mexico City. Vet. Parasitol. 153, 270–276.

Martínez-Barbabosa, I., Gutierrez-Cardenas, E.M., Aguilar Venegas, J., Lastra, P., R.deJ., and Shea, M., 2011. Frequency of geohelminths in pet dogs from seven municipalities of Mexico City. Vet. Mex. 42, 83–91.

Martínez-Barbabosa, I., Gutierrez, M., Ruiz, L.A., Fernandez, A.M., Gutierrez, E.M., Aguilar, J.M., Shea, M., Gaona, E., 2015. Detection of *Cryptosporidium* spp. and other enteric zoonotic parasites in pet dogs of Mexico City. [Deteccion de *Cryptosporidium* spp. y otros parasitos zoonoticos entericos en perros domiciliados de la Ciudad de Mexico.]. Arch. Med. Vet. 47, 347–353.

Martínez-Barbabosa, I., Pimienta Lastra, R., Ortiz Pérez, H., Marcos, J.R., Venegas, A., Fernández Presas, A.M., 2018. Presence of zoonotichelminths in cats (*Felis catus*) of condominiums in City of Mexico with special concern to *Toxocara cati* infection. Bioffin Access 1.1, 102. Manuscript ID: MMMB-1-102.

Martinez-Barrios, A.B., 2014. Seroprevalencia de *Toxocara* spp en niños de Chalco Estado de México. Thesis, Centro Universitario Uaem-Amecameca, Licenciatura En Medicina Veterinaria Y Zootecnia, Universidad Autónoma Del Estado De México.

Mata-Ramos, M., Castañeda Ortega, J., 2018. Identification of gastrointestinal parasites in domestic dogs from a housing complex in San José de Abajo de Córdoba, Veracruz. [Identificación de parásitos gastrointestinales en perros domésticos en la unidad habitacional San José de Abajo de Córdoba, Veracruz.]. Actual. Medicina Veterinaria Zootec. Méx. 22, 42–47.

Matute Argueta, P.M.R., 2017. Determinación de la presencia de *Ancylostoma caninum* Y *Toxocara canis* en heces de perros (*Canis Lupus Familiaris*) que deambulan en el mercado municipal del Municipio De Palín, Escuintla. Thesis submitted to the Facultad de Medicina Veterinaria Y Zootecnia, Escuela de Veterinaria, Universidad de San Carlos de Guatemala.

Medina-Pinto, R.A., Rodriguez-Vivas, R.I., Bolio-Gonzalez, M.E., 2018. Zoonotic intestinal nematodes in dogs from public parks in Yucatan, Mexico. [Nematodos intestinales de perros en parques publicos de Yucatan, Mexico.]. Biomedica 38, 105–110.

Meijer, C., 2012. Prevalence and awareness of zoonotic parasites of dogs on Curaçao. Thesis, Faculty of Veterinary Medicine, Utrecht University, Netherlands.

Mena Pérez, M.J., 2014. Determinación de la prevalencia de *Ancylostoma caninum* y *Toxocara canis* por medio del método de McMaster en heces de perros, de la comunidad Las Estrellas, Ciudad Quetzal, en San Juan Sacatepéquez, en el primer semestre del año 2011. Thesis, Facultad de Medicina Veterinaria Y Zootecnia, Escuela de Medicina Veterinaria, Universidad de San Carlos de Guatemala.

Merlo, R.H., Núñez, F.A., Durán, L.P., 2007. Potencial zoonótico de las infecciones por helmintos intestinales en perros callejeros de Ciudad de La Habana. Rev. Cubana Med. Trop. 59, 234–240.

Mizgajska, H., 2001. Eggs of *Toxocara* spp. in the environment and their public health implications. J. Helminthol. 75, 147–151.

Mohamed, A.S., Moore, G.E., Glickman, L.T., 2009. Prevalence of intestinal nematode parasitism among pet dogs in the United States (2003-2006). J. Am. Vet. Med. Assoc. 234, 631–637. https://doi.org/10.2460/javma.234.5.631.

Moreira Chévez, K.P., Velásquez García, J.L., 2007. Prevalencia de *Toxocara canis* en cachorros de canidos domésticos en los repartos Héroes y Mártires de Zaragoza y la Providencia en el período de Noviembre 2006 a Marzo del 2007. Thesis submitted to the Facultad de Ciencias Médicas, Universidad Nacional Autónoma de Nicaragua.

Morgan, E.R., Azam, D., Pegler, K., 2013. Quantifying sources of environmental contamination with *Toxocara* spp. eggs. Vet. Parasitol. 193, 390–397. https://doi.org/10.1016/j.vetpar.2012.12.034.

Moura, L., Miller, T., Thurk, J., Kelly, P., Krecek, T., 2007. Animal ownership and attitudes to feral cats on St. Kitts, West Indies. West Indian Vet. J. 7, 72–77.

Muñoz-Guzmán, M.A., Alba-Hurtado, F., 2010. Secretory-excretory antigens of *Toxocara canis* recognized by puppies of the Mexico City metropolitan area. Vet. Mex. 41, 59–64.

Nagamori, Y., Payton, M.E., Duncan-Decocq, R., Johnson, E.M., 2018. Fecal survey of parasites in free-roaming cats in northcentral Oklahoma, United States. Vet. Parasitol. Reg. Stud. Reports 14, 50–53. https://doi.org/10.1016/j.vprsr.2018.08.008. Epub 2018 Sep 2.

Navarrete Úbeda, G.J., Gómez Guevara, J.G., 2017. Parásitos gastrointestinales de caninos (*Canis lupus familiaris*), atendidos en la Clínica Veterinaria Valverde, colonia Villa libertad, Managua, Noviembre 2016 – Marzo 2017. Thesis submitted to the Facultad de Ciencia Animal, Departamento de Veterinaria, Universidad Nacional Agraria, Nicaragua.

Neill, K.G., 2009. The public health importance of dogs, Grand Anse, Grenada. Thesis, School of Medicine, St George's University, Grenada.

Nijsse, R., Mughini-Gras, L., Wagenaar, J.A., Ploeger, H.W., 2014. Coprophagy in dogs interferes in the diagnosis of parasitic infections by faecal examination. Vet. Parasitol. 204, 304–309.

Nolan, T.J., Smith, G., 1995. Time series analysis of the prevalence of endoparasitic infections in cats and dogs presented to a veterinary teaching hospital. Vet. Parasitol. 59, 87–96.

Nutter, F.B., Dubey, J.P., Levine, J.F., Breitschwerdt, E.B., Ford, R.B., Stoskopf, M.K., 2004. Seroprevalences of antibodies against *Bartonella henselae* and *Toxoplasma gondii* and fecal shedding of *Cryptosporidium* spp, *Giardia* spp, and *Toxocara cati* in feral and pet domestic cats. J. Am. Vet. Med. Assoc. 225, 1394–1398.

Ortega-Pacheco, A., Torres-Acosta, J.F.J., Alzina-Lopez, A., Gutierrez-Blanco, E., Bolio-Gonzalez, M.E., Aguilar-Caballero, A.J., Rodriguez-Vivas, R.I., Gutierrez-Ruiz, E., Acosta-Viana, K.Y., Guzman-Marin, E., Rosado-Aguilar, A., Jimenez-Coello, M., 2015. Parasitic zoonoses in humans and their dogs from a rural community of tropical Mexico. J. Trop. Med. 2015, 481086.

Overgaauw, P.A., Nederland, V., 1997. Aspects of *Toxocara* epidemiology: toxocarosis in dogs and cats. Crit. Rev. Microbiol. 23, 233e251.

Palmieri, J.R., Thurman, J.B., Andersen, F.L., 1978. Helminth parasites of dogs in Utah. J. Parasitol. 64, 1149–1150.

Paterson, T., Hockley, T., Elsemore, D., Hanscom, J., Tyrrell, P., Leutenegger, C., Chandrashekar, R., 2019. Comprehensive survey of parasitic and infectious diseases in feral & domesticated cats in Grenada, West Indies. In: 27th Conference of the World Association for the Advancement of Veterinary Parasitology, July 7-11, Madison WI, USA.

Perilhou, M., 2003. Le chien errant en Guadeloupe. Thesis, Ecole Nationale Vétérinaire de Toulouse, France.

Ponce-Macotela, M., Peralta-Abarca, G.E., Martinez-Gordillo, M.N., 2005. *Giardia intestinalis* and other zoonotic parasites: prevalence in adult dogs from the southern part of Mexico City. Vet. Parasitol. 131, 1–4.

Power, L.A., 1971. Helminths of cats from the midwest with a report of *Ancylostoma caninum* in this host. J. Parasitol. 57, 610.

Quiñones-Ávila, F., Espaine-Aliet, L.E., Rodríguez-Vivas, R.I., Domínguez-Alpízar, J.L., 1998. Contribution to the study of helminths of the digestive tract of dogs in the city of Merida, Yucatan, Mexico. [Contribución al estudio de los helmintos del tracto digestivo en perros de la ciudad de Mérida, Yucatán, México.]. Revista AMMVEPE 9, 191–193.

Rembiesa, C., Richardson, D.J., 2003. Helminth parasites of the house cat, *Felis catus*, in Connecticut, U.S.A. Comp. Parasitol. 70, 115–119.

Rep, B.H., 1975. Intestinal helminths of dogs and cats in the Antillean islands of Aruba, Bonaire and Curaçao. Trop. Geogr. Med. 27, 317–323.

Ridley, R.K., Dryden, M.W., Gabbert, N.H., Schoning, P., 1994. Epidemiology and control of helminth parasites in Greyhound breeding farms. Compend. Contin. Educ. Pract. Vet. 16, 585–599.

Robinson, R.D., Thompson, D.L., Lindo, J.F., 1989. A survey of intestinal helminths of well-cared-for dogs in Jamaica, and their potential public health significance. J. Helminthol. 63, 32–38.

Rodriguez Gallegos, L.M., Romero Nunez, C., Bautista Gomez, L.G., Martinez Castaneda, J.S., Heredia Cardenas, R., 2016. Presence of *Toxocara* spp. in domestic cats in the state of Mexico. Acta Sci. Vet. 44, 1351.

Rodríguez-Prado, U., Gutierrez-Marin, A., Martinez-Ocana, J., Romero-Valdovinos, M., Olivo-Diaz, A., Hernandez-Castro, R., Flisser, A., Maravilla, P., Martinez-Maya, J.J., 2014. Coprological and ultrasonographic study in dogs and sheep of a suburban community in the Estado de Mexico in search of *Echinococcus* spp. Vet. Mex. 45 (Special Issue), 53–58.

Rodríguez-Vivas, R.I., Cob-Galera, L., Domínguez-Alpizar, J., 2001. Frecuencia de parásitos gastrointestinales en animales domésticos diagnosticados en Yucatán, México. Rev. Biomed. 12, 19–25.

Rodríguez-Vivas, R.I., Gutierrez-Ruiz, E., Bolio-Gonzalez, M.E., Ruiz-Pina, H., Ortega-Pacheco, A., Reyes-Novelo, E., Manrique-Saide, P., Aranda-Cirerol, F., Lugo-Perez, J.A., 2011. An epidemiological study of intestinal parasites of dogs from Yucatan, Mexico, and their risk to public health. Vector Borne Zoonotic Dis. 11, 1141–1144.

Rojas, N., Rojas, J.J., Herrera, S., Valerio, E., 2017. 1. Percepciones de la influencia de los perros callejeros en la salud pública. In: Encuesta Actualidades 2017. Universidad De Costa Rica Escuela De Estadística Curso Diseño Y Ejecución De Encuestas.

Romero, C., Mendoza, G.D., Bustamante, L.P., Yanez, S., Ramirez, N., 2010. Contamination and viability of *Toxocara* sp. in feces collected from public parks, streets and dogs in Tejupilco at the subhumid tropic of Mexico. J. Anim. Vet. Adv. 9, 2996–2999.

Romero, C., Mendoza, G.E., Pineda, M.A., Nava, N., Bautista, L.G., Heredia, R., 2015. Prevalence of intestinal parasites with zoonotic potential in canids in Mexico City. Acta Sci. Vet. 43, 1307.

Romero, C., Heredia, R., Aguilar, S., Nava, N., Pineda, J., 2016. Presence of anti-*Toxocara* antibodies in sheep from the state of Mexico. Acta Vet. Brno 85, 223–226.

Romero-Callejas, E., Rendón-Franco, E., Villanueva-García, C., Osorio-Sarabia, D., Muñoz-García, C., 2014. Risk of cutaneous larva migrans and other zoonotic parasites infections due to feral cats from a touristic tropical park. Travel Med. Infect. Dis. 12, 684–686.

Romero-Núñez, C., del Garcia Contreras, A.C., Mendoza Martinez, G.D., Torres Corona, N.C., Ramirez Duran, N., 2009. Contamination for *Toxocara* spp. in Tulyehualco parks, Mexico. [Contaminacion por *Toxocara* spp. en parques de Tulyehualco, Mexico.]. Revista Cientifica, Facultad de Ciencias Veterinarias, Universidad del Zulia 19, 253–256.

Romero-Núñez, C., Mendoza Martiñez, G.D., Bustamante, L.P., Crosby Galvan, M.M., Ramirez Duran, N., 2011. Presence and viability of Toxocara spp. in soils of public parks, gardens of houses and feces from dogs in Nezahualcoyotl, Mexico. [Presencia y viabilidad de Toxocara spp. en suelos de parques publicos, jardines de casas y heces de perros en Nezahualcoyotl, Mexico]. Revista Cientifica, Facultad de Ciencias Veterinarias, Universidad del Zulia 21, 195–201.

Romero-Núñez, C., Yanez-Arteaga, S., Mendoza-Martinez, G.D., Bustamante-Montes, L.P., Ramirez-Duran, N., 2013. Contamination and viability of eggs of *Toxocara* spp. in soil and feces collected from public parks, streets and dogs in Toluca, Mexico. [Contaminacion y viabilidad de huevos de Toxocara spp. en suelo y heces colectadas en parques publicos, calles y perros en Toluca, Mexico]. Revista Cientifica, Facultad de Ciencias Veterinarias, Universidad del Zulia 23, 475–479.

Sabshin, S.J., Levy, J.K., Tupler, T., Tucker, S.J., Greiner, E.C., Leutenegger, C.M., 2012. Enteropathogens identified in cats entering a Florida animal shelter with normal feces or diarrhea. J. Am. Vet. Med. Assoc. 241, 331–337. https://doi.org/10.2460/javma.241.3.331.

Saleh, F.C., Kirkpatrick, C.E., De Haseth, O., Lok, J.B., 1988. Occurrence of some blood and intestinal parasites in dogs in Curaçao, Netherlands Antilles. Trop. Geogr. Med. 40, 318–321.

Sariego, I., Kanobana, K., Rojas, L., Speybroeck, N., Polman, K., Núñez, F.A., 2012. Toxocariasis in Cuba: a literature review. PLoS Negl. Trop. Dis. 6, e1382. https://doi.org/10.1371/journal.pntd.0001382.

Savilla, T.M., Joy, J.E., May, J.D., Somerville, C.C., 2011. Prevalence of dog intestinal nematode parasites in south central West Virginia, USA. Vet. Parasitol. 178, 115–120.

Sawyer, T.W., Cowgill, L.M., Andersen, F.L., 1976. Helminth parasites of cats and dogs from central Utah. Great Basin Nat. 36, 471–474.

Schantz, P.M., Biagi, F.F., 1968. Coexistence of *Toxocara* and *Toxascaris* in dogs in Mexico City. J. Parasitol. 54, 185–186.

Schantz, P.M., Glickman, L.T., 1983. Ascaridos de perros y gatos: un problema de salud publica, y de medicina veterinaria. Bol. Oficina Sanit. Panam. 94, 571–585.

Schwartz, R., Macpherson, C., Bidaisee, S., 2018. Public health significance of pets: case of dogs. Acta Sci. Microbiol. 1, 13–16.

Schwartz, R., Bidaisee, S., Macpherson, C., 2019. *Toxocara canis* in puppies and their public health importance in Grenada. Caribb. Med. J. 81, 7–12.

Scorza, A.V., Lappin, M.R., 2017. Prevalence of selected zoonotic and vector-borne agents in dogs and cats on the Pine Ridge Reservation. Vet. Sci. 4, 43. https://doi.org/10.3390/vetsci4030043.

Scorza, A.V., Duncan, C., Miles, L., Lappin, M.R., 2011. Prevalence of selected zoonotic and vector-borne agents in dogs and cats in Costa Rica. Vet. Parasitol. 183, 178–183.

Smith, J.P., Seaton, A., 1981. Helminth infections of dogs in central Texas. Vet. Med. Small Anim. Clin. 76, 1627–1629.

Spain, C.V., Scarlett, J.M., Wade, S.E., McDonough, P., 2001. Prevalence of enteric zoonotic agents in cats less than 1 year old in central New York State. J. Vet. Intern. Med. 15, 33–38.

Stewart, G.L., Reddington, J.J., Smyth, W.G., 1979. Intestinal helminth parasites of dogs from Tarrant County, Texas. Southwest. Vet. 32, 29–32.

Streitel, R.H., Dubey, J.P., 1976. Prevalence of Sarcocystis infection and other intestinal parasitisms in dogs from a humane shelter in Ohio. J. Am. Vet. Med. Assoc. 168, 423–424.

Styles, T.J., 1967. Incidence of *Toxocara canis* and other helminth parasites of dogs in Mexico City. J. Parasitol. 53, 822–823.

Taetzsch, S.J., Gruszynski, K.R., Bertke, A.S., Duey, J.P., Monti, K.A., Zajac, A.M., Lindsay, D.S., 2018. Prevalence of zoonotic parasites in feral cats of Central Virginia, USA. Zoonoses Public Health 65, 728–735. https://doi.org/10.1111/zph.12488.

Taira, K., Saeed, I., Permin, A., Kapel, C.M.O., 2004. Zoonotic risk of *Toxocara canis* infection through consumption of pig or poultry viscera. Vet. Parasitol. 121, 115–124.

Thompson, D.E., Bundy, D.A.P., Cooper, E.S., Schantz, P.M., 1986. Epidemiological characteristics of *Toxocara canis* zoonotic infection of children in a Caribbean community. Bull. World Health Organ. 64, 283–290.

Tinoco-Gracia, L., Barreras-Serrano, A., Lopez-Valenci, G., Tamayo-Sosa, A.R., 2007. Seroprevalence and risk factors associated with larva migrans of *Toxocara canis* in dogs from Mexicali Baja California, Mexico. J. Anim. Vet. Adv. 6, 198–202.

Tinoco-Gracia, L., Barreras-Serrano, A., Lopez-Valencia, G., Tamayo-Sosa, A.R., Quiroz-Romero, H., Melgarejo, T., 2008. Seroprevalence of larva migrans of *Toxocara canis* and evaluation of associated risk factors among children in a Mexico-United States border region. Int. J. Appl. Res. Vet. Med. 6, 130–136.

Tiwari, K., Thomas, J.C.D., de Allie, C., Chikweto, A., Hegamin-Younger, C., Sharma, R.N., 2016. Prevalence of gastrointestinal parasites in stray dogs (*Canis familiaris*) from Grenada, West Indies. J. Anim. Res. 6, 1–5.

Torres-Chable, O.M., Garcia-Herrera, R.A., Hernandez-Hernandez, M., Peralta-Torres, J.A., Ojeda-Robertos, N.F., Blitvich, B.J., Baak-Baak, C.M., Garcia-Rejon, J.E., Machain-Wiliams, C., 2015. Prevalence of gastrointestinal parasites in domestic dogs in Tabasco, southeastern Mexico. Braz. J. Vet. Parasitol. 24, 432–437.

Trasviña-Muñoza, E., López-Valencia, G., Álvarez Centeno, P., Cueto-Gonzáleza, S.A., Monge-Navarro, F.J., Tinoco-Gracia, L., Núñez-Castro, K., Pérez-Ortiza, P., Medina-Basulto, G.E., Tamayo-Sosa, A.R., Gómez-Gómez, D., 2017. Prevalence and distribution of intestinal parasites in stray dogs in the northwest area of Mexico. Aust. J. Vet. Sci. 49, 105–111.

Valverde Alvarado, M., 2010. Diagnóstico de parásitos gastrointestinales de caninos de áreas de riesgo social: impacto en la salud pública y salud animal. Thesis submitted to the Facultad de Ciencias de la Salud, Escuela de Medicina Veterinaria, Universidad Nacional, Costa Rica.

Vaughn, J., Jordan, R., 1960. Intestinal nematodes in well-cared-for dogs. Am. J. Trop. Med. Hyg. 9, 29–31. https://doi.org/10.4269/ajtmh.1960.9.29.

Vélez-Hernández, L., Reyes-Barrera, K.L., Rojas-Almaraz, D., Calderon-Oropeza, M.A., Cruz-Vazquez, J.K., Arcos-Garcia, J.L., 2014. Potential hazard of zoonotic parasites present in canine feces in Puerto Escondido, Oaxaca. [Riesgo potencial de parasitos zoonoticos presentes en heces caninas en Puerto Escondido, Oaxaca.]. Salud Publica Mex. 56, 625–630.

Visco, R.J., Corwin, R.M., Selby, L.A., 1977. Effect of age and sex on the prevalence of intestinal parasitism in dogs. J. Am. Vet. Med. Assoc. 170, 835–837.

Visco, R.J., Corwin, R.M., Selby, L.A., 1978. Effect of age and sex on the prevalence of intestinal parasitism in cats. J. Am. Vet. Med. Assoc. 172, 797–800.

Woodhall, D.M., Eberhard, M.L., Parise, M.E., 2014. Neglected parasitic infections in the United States: Toxocariasis. Am. J. Trop. Med. Hyg. 90, 810–813.

World Animal Protection, 2016. Estudio nacional sobre tenecia de perros en Costa Rica. 2016. https://issuu.com/wspalatam/docs/estudioperros-web-singles.
Worley, D.E., 1964. Helminth parasites of dogs in southeastern Michigan. J. Am. Vet. Med. Assoc. 144, 42–46.
Wyrosdick, H.M., Chapman, A., Martinez, J., Schaefer, J.J., 2017. Parasite prevalence survey in shelter cats in Citrus County, Florida. Vet. Parasitol. Reg. Stud. Reports 10, 20–24. https://doi.org/10.1016/j.vprsr.2017.07.002. Epub 2017 Jul 11.
ZeLedón, D.A., Bitter, E., de Oliveira, J., Romero, J.J., 2006. Prevalencia de *Toxocara canis* y otros parásitos gastrointestinales en perros atendidos en un clínica veterinaria en San José, Costa Rica. Cienc. Vet. 24, 137–150.

CHAPTER THIRTY-THREE

Toxocara prevalence in dogs and cats in Brazil

Filipe Dantas-Torres*
Department of Immunology, Aggeu Magalhães Institute, Oswaldo Cruz Foundation (Fiocruz), Recife, Pernambuco, Brazil
*Corresponding author: e-mail address: filipe.dantas@cpqam.fiocruz.br

Contents

Abstract

I herein review published studies reporting the prevalence of *Toxocara* infection in dogs and cats in Brazil. Based on data gathered from faecal examinations of approximately 38,940 dogs and 5600 cats from different Brazilian studies, the mean prevalence of *Toxocara* infection is 11.4% (range: 0.7–48.9%) in dogs and 16.7% (0.3–43.1%) in cats. These mean values based on faecal examinations should be interpreted with cautious, considering the obvious differences in terms of sample size, diagnostic tests and animal populations. Accordingly, necropsy investigations reveal higher mean prevalence values (21.9% for *Toxocara canis* and 27.6% *Toxocara cati* in dogs and cats, respectively). The contamination with *Toxocara* eggs in different environments and the significance of these parasites from a public health perspective in Brazil are briefly discussed.

1. Introduction

Brazil is a South American country with continental dimensions, being thus extremely diverse in terms of landscape. Contrary to common sense, the climate of this country is not always tropical, spanning from tropical (north of the Equator) to temperate zones (south of the Tropic of

Advances in Parasitology, Volume 109
ISSN 0065-308X
https://doi.org/10.1016/bs.apar.2020.01.028

Capricorn). As such, this land provides a splendid opportunity for a multitude of parasites affecting both animal and human populations (Dantas-Torres and Otranto, 2014). It is not by chance that Brazil leads the Americas in terms of number of cases of several neglected parasitic diseases, including Chagas disease, both cutaneous and visceral leishmaniasis, vivax malaria, schistosomiasis, and intestinal helminth infections (e.g., ascariasis, trichuriasis, and hookworm infection) (Hotez and Fujiwara, 2014; Martins-Melo et al., 2018). For instance, almost 12 million children (both preschool-aged and school-aged children) require preventive chemotherapy, accounting for approximately one-quarter of the children in the Latin American and Caribbean region with intestinal helminths (Hotez and Fujiwara, 2014). Nonetheless, according to the World Health Organization, only about 15% of children at risk in Brazil actually receive regular chemotherapy (Hotez and Fujiwara, 2014).

Intestinal helminth infections are also among the most prevalent parasites of dogs and cats worldwide, including in Brazil (Beugnet et al., 2014; Dantas-Torres and Otranto, 2014; Deplazes et al., 2011; Wright et al., 2016). Along with hookworms (Rhabditida: Ancylostomatidae), whipworms (Trichocephalida: Trichuridae), and flea tapeworms (Cyclophyllidea: Dipylidiidae), ascarids (Ascaridida: Ascarididae, Toxocaridae) are among the most prevalent intestinal helminths of dogs and cats in Brazil. Different species, including *Toxocara canis* (in dogs), *Toxocara cati* (in cats), *Toxascaris leonina* (in both dogs and cats), and *Lagochilascaris minor* (in both dogs and cats), may be found in dogs, cats, or both, in Brazil (Dantas-Torres and Otranto, 2014). Nonetheless, *T. canis* and *T. cati* are by far the most widespread and prevalent ascarids infecting dogs and cats, respectively, in this country (Heukelbach et al., 2012; Labarthe et al., 2004). These parasites have also been reported in a range of wild canids and felids in Brazil (Gallas and Silveira, 2013; Holsback et al., 2013; Santos et al., 2012; Vieira et al., 2008).

Toxocara canis and *T. cati* are significant parasites for dogs and cats, not only causing clinical disease in their primary hosts, but also in humans, especially children (Deplazes et al., 2011). The level of environmental contamination by *Toxocara* eggs in public squares, parks, and beaches is very high in some Brazilian regions (Fontes et al., 2017; Marques et al., 2012), probably also due to the large stray dog and cat populations existing in this country. As a consequence, the level of exposure to *Toxocara* spp. in humans, as determined by serological tests, is incredibly high in most Brazilian regions, eventually reaching over 70%, as recently reported among patients

(18 years or older) referred to a basic healthcare unit in a rural area in Pelotas city (Rio Grande do Sul state, southern Brazil) (Araújo et al., 2018).

I herein review published studies reporting the prevalence of *T. canis* and *T. cati* infections in dogs and cats in Brazil. The contamination with *Toxocara* eggs in different environments and the significance of these parasites from a public health perspective in this country are also briefly discussed.

2. Prevalence in dogs

Both privately-owned and stray dogs in Brazil are highly exposed to *T. canis*. Based on data gathered from coprological examinations of 38,939 dogs from different Brazilian studies, the prevalence of *T. canis* in dogs ranged from 0.7% to 48.9% (mean $\pm$ standard deviation $=$ 11.4% $\pm$ 9.6%) (Table 1). This mean value should, for several reasons, be interpreted with caution. The sample size, diagnostic methods and the dog populations (e.g., level of restriction and dependence on humans, and age class) varied widely

Table 1 Prevalence of *Toxocara canis* infection in dogs ($n = 38{,}939$) in different Brazilian regions, based on faecal examinations.

State	Region	Sample size	Prevalence (%)	References
São Paulo	South-east	903	10.1	Fenerich et al. (1972)
Paraná	South	135	48.9	Chieffi and Müller (1976)
Rio de Janeiro	South-east	286	24.9	Ferreira et al. (1976)
Minas Gerais	South-east	437	9.2	Araújo et al. (1986)
São Paulo	South-east	9150	11.7	Côrtes et al. (1988)
Bahia	North-east	277	18.4	Alcântara et al. (1989)
Rio Grande do Sul	South	316	8.2	Hoffmann et al. (1990)
Minas Gerais	South-east	11,563	6.8	Oliveira et al. (1990)
São Paulo	South-east	314	16.6	Farias et al. (1995)
Paraná	South	889	13.7	Guimarães Junior et al. (1996)
São Paulo	South-east	353	8.5	Gennari et al. (1999)

Continued

Table 1 Prevalence of *Toxocara canis* infection in dogs ($n = 38{,}939$) in different Brazilian regions, based on faecal examinations.—cont'd

State	Region	Sample size	Prevalence (%)	References
São Paulo	South-east	65	4.6	Hoffmann et al. (2000)
São Paulo	South-east	871	5.5	Gennari et al. (2001)
São Paulo	South-east	271	5.5	Oliveira-Sequeira et al. (2002)
Goiás	Centre-west	434	2.5	Alves et al. (2005)
Santa Catarina	South	158	14.5	Blazius et al. (2005)
São Paulo	South-east	257	1.2	Castro et al. (2005)
São Paulo	South-east	41	39.0	Muradian et al. (2005)
Paraná	South	280	1.8	Tesserolli et al. (2005)
Minas Gerais	South-east	734	14.4	Araújo (2006)
Rio Grande do Sul	South	120	5.0	Ginar et al. (2006)
Roraima	North	95	18.9	Labruna et al. (2006)
Rio de Janeiro	South-east	204	8.8	Vasconcellos et al. (2006)
Mato Grosso	Centre-west	121	5.8	Almeida et al. (2007)
São Paulo	South-east	1755	2.6	Funada et al. (2007)
Paraná	South	387	3.4	Leite et al. (2007)
Rio Grande do Sul	South	1473	4.1	Lorenzini et al. (2007)
Bahia	North-east	119	4.2	Campos Filho et al. (2008)
São Paulo	South-east	254	8.7	Katagiri and Oliveira-Sequeira (2008)
Distrito Federal	Centre-west	193	12.4	Santos et al. (2008)
Sergipe	North-east	150	5.3	Ferreira et al. (2009)
Goiás	Centre-west	201	8.0	Oliveira et al. (2009)
Paraná	South	81	2.5	Prates et al. (2009)
Rio Grande do Norte	North-east	60	13.3	Ferreira et al. (2010)

Table 1 Prevalence of *Toxocara canis* infection in dogs ($n = 38{,}939$) in different Brazilian regions, based on faecal examinations.—cont'd

State	Region	Sample size	Prevalence (%)	References
Pernambuco	North-east	96	28.1	Ostermann et al. (2011)
Paraná	South	171	10.5	Martins et al. (2012)
Minas Gerais	South-east	141	22.7	Ribeiro et al. (2013)
São Paulo	South-east	640	8.1	Alves et al. (2014)
Sergipe	North-east	93	10.8	Lima et al. (2014)
Acre	North	230	17.4	Monteiro et al. (2014)
Espírito Santo	South-east	345	6.1	Campos et al. (2016)
São Paulo	South-east	3099	0.7	Ferreira et al. (2016)
Santa Catarina	South	50	16.0	Frizzo et al. (2016)
Minas Gerais	South-east	129	18.6	Curi et al. (2017)
São Paulo	South-east	278	11.9	Oliveira-Arbex et al. (2017)
Maranhão	North-east	720	4.6	Silva et al. (2017a)

in these studies. For instance, the sensitivity of different methods for detecting *T. canis* eggs in faecal samples of dogs may vary significantly (Katagiri and Oliveira-Sequeira, 2010; Mandarino-Pereira et al., 2010; Ostermann et al., 2011). The sample size and age class of sampled animals may directly affect prevalence data. A study carried out with 41 young dogs (up to 10 months old) in São Paulo (São Paulo state, south-eastern Brazil) reported a positivity of 39% (Muradian et al., 2005). On the other hand, different studies conducted in the same city but using larger sample sizes (from 353 up to 9159 dogs), with no age restriction, have reported prevalence values ranging from 0.7% to 11.7% (Côrtes et al., 1988; Fenerich et al., 1972; Ferreira et al., 2016; Funada et al., 2007; Gennari et al., 1999, 2001). Finally, one should consider that some dogs found with "ascarid eggs" in their faeces may also be (co)infected with *T. leonina*, as demonstrated in a study combining coprological examinations and necropsies (Ostermann et al., 2011).

Information from necropsies is relatively limited, but studies indicate *T. canis* prevalence values ranging from 3.2% to 71.4% (mean ± standard

Table 2 Prevalence of *Toxocara canis* infection in dogs ($n = 973$) in different Brazilian regions, based on necropsies.

State	Region	Sample size	Prevalence (%)	References
Amazonas	North	50	14.0	Gordon and Young (1922)
Bahia	North-east	10	10.0	Menezes (1954)
São Paulo	South-east	81	42.0	Zago Filho and Barreto (1957)
Minas Gerais	South-east	100	14.0	Costa et al. (1962)
Goiás	Centre-west	40	17.7	Carneiro et al. (1973)
Bahia	North-east	100	9.0	Brust et al. (1976)
Paraná	South	23	17.4	Chieffi and Müller (1976)
Rio Grande do Sul	South	118	26.7	Lara et al. (1981)
Espírito Santo	South-east	61	3.2	Costa et al. (1990)
São Paulo	South-east	28	71.4	Silva et al. (2001)
São Paulo	South-east	65	24.6	Bresciani et al. (2008)
Ceará	North-east	46	8.7	Klimpel et al. (2010)
Pernambuco	North-east	96	32.3	Ostermann et al. (2011)
Minas Gerais	South-east	155	15.5	Heukelbach et al. (2012)

deviation = 21.9% ± 17.6%) (Table 2). According to these studies, the mean intensity of *T. canis* infection (i.e., adult worms per infected dog) may vary widely. In two more recent studies, it varied from 3.0 in Fortaleza (Ceará state, north-eastern Brazil) (Klimpel et al., 2010) to 7.54 in Uberlândia (Minas Gerais state, south-eastern Brazil) (Heukelbach et al., 2012). Furthermore, in these necropsy investigations, the three most prevalent intestinal helminths of dogs in Brazil were generally, in descending order, *Ancylostoma caninum*, *Dipylidium caninum*, and *T. canis* (Bresciani et al., 2008; Brust et al., 1976; Carneiro et al., 1973; Chieffi and Müller, 1976; Costa et al., 1962, 1990; Gordon and Young, 1922; Heukelbach et al., 2012; Klimpel et al., 2010; Lara et al., 1981; Menezes, 1954; Ostermann et al., 2011; Silva et al., 2001; Zago Filho and Barreto, 1957).

Limited information on the prevalence of *T. canis* infection in dogs from different Brazilian regions is available, but data suggest that it may be higher

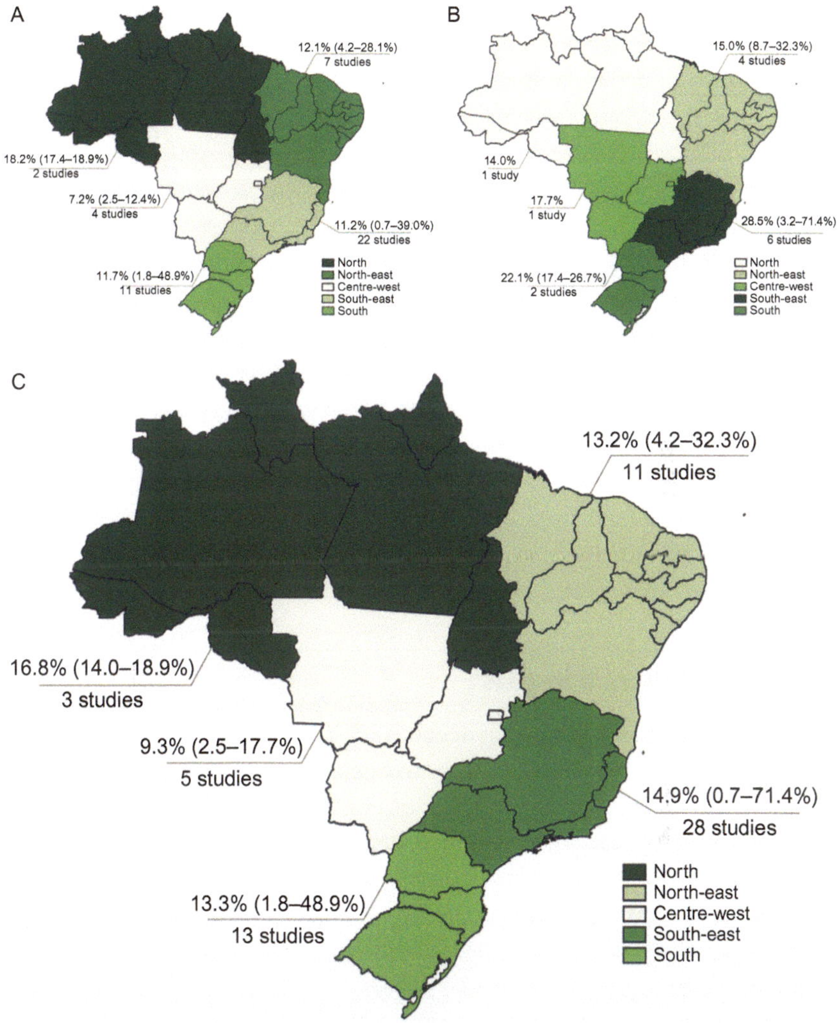

Fig. 1 Prevalence of *Toxocara canis* infection in dogs in different Brazilian regions, based on faecal examinations (A), necropsies (B), or both datasets combined (C).

in northern Brazil as compared to other regions (Fig. 1). However, it is important to underline that many Brazilian studies analysed a limited number of dogs and that prevalence may vary widely from city to city or from state to state, within a given geographic region. It is also worth mentioning that very limited information, mostly from local journals (some cited herein) and abstract books (not considered herein), is available for some Brazilian regions. As such, comparative figures from different Brazilian region should, once again, be interpreted with caution.

Studies evaluating the risk factors associated to *T. canis* infection in dogs in Brazil are also relatively restricted (Balassiano et al., 2009; Curi et al., 2017; Heukelbach et al., 2012; Katagiri and Oliveira-Sequeira, 2008; Martins et al., 2012; Regis et al., 2011). Nonetheless, studies are generally congruent in indicating little or no sex influence, but a higher risk of infection among young dogs as compared to adults, and among dogs receiving infrequent or no anti-helminthic treatment (Balassiano et al., 2009; Curi et al., 2017; Katagiri and Oliveira-Sequeira, 2008; Regis et al., 2011). However, data are not always congruent. A seroprevalence study conducted in Salvador (Bahia state, north-eastern Brazil) reported a higher risk among males as compared to females (odds ratio = 2.19, 95% confidence interval = 1.19–4.05, *P*-value = 0.02) (Regis et al., 2011). In the same way, a necropsy investigation conducted in Uberlândia reported a higher risk among males (odds ratio = 3.60, 95% confidence interval = 1.24–10.40, *P*-value = 0.02) as compared to females (Heukelbach et al., 2012). These findings may suggest that, in some areas, males are more exposed to *T. canis* than females, probably due to sex-related features of local dog populations.

3. Prevalence in cats

In a similar fashion to what occurs with *T. canis* in dogs in Brazil, *T. cati* is widespread and prevalent in both privately-owned and stray cats in this country. However, a limited number of prevalence studies have been conducted in different Brazilian regions, particularly studies with an adequate sample size. The relatively low number of studies with cats as compared to dogs may be partly attributed to the inherent difficulties to work with cats, which generally translates into a relatively lower number of parasitological studies with this animal species. As for dogs, some studies with cats have been published in local journals (some cited herein) or in abstract books (not considered herein).

Based on data from coprological examinations of 5598 cats from different Brazilian studies, the prevalence of *T. cati* in cats ranges from 0.3% to 43.1% (mean ± standard deviation = 16.7% ± 12.8%) (Table 3). It is important to underline that these studies have used different faecal examination methods, which may lead to different results. For instance, a study conducted in Andradina (São Paulo state) reported the finding of *Toxocara* eggs in 43.1% and 9.8% of the cats ($n = 51$) using sodium chloride floatation and zinc-sulphate centrifugation floatation, respectively (Coelho et al., 2009).

Necropsy studies for recovering intestinal helminths from cats in Brazil are even more scarce. In these studies, the prevalence of *T. cati* infection

Table 3 Prevalence of *Toxocara cati* infection in cats ($n = 5598$) in different Brazilian regions, based on faecal examinations.

State	Region	Sample size	Prevalence (%)	Reference
São Paulo	South-east	215	21.9	Ogassawara et al. (1986a)
São Paulo	South-east	674	17.6	Côrtes et al. (1988)
São Paulo	South-east	32	6.3	Farias et al. (1995)
São Paulo	South-east	187	34.2	Gennari et al. (1999)
São Paulo	South-east	303	10.2	Gennari et al. (2001)
São Paulo	South-east	138	31.2	Ragozo et al. (2002)
Rio de Janeiro	South-east	131	19.1	Serra et al. (2003)
Paraná	South	30	10.0	Tesserolli et al. (2005)
São Paulo	South-east	327	6.1	Funada et al. (2007)
Rio Grande do Sul	South	288	5.9	Lorenzini et al. (2007)
São Paulo	South-east	51	43.1	Coelho et al. (2009)
Santa Catarina	South	111	32.4	Stalliviere et al. (2009)
Rio Grande do Sul	South	191	30.4	Pivoto et al. (2013)
Espírito Santo	South-east	160	12.5	Campos et al. (2016)
São Paulo	South-east	502	2.2	Gennari et al. (2016)
Pernambuco	North-east	173	26.6	Monteiro et al. (2016)
Pernambuco	North-east	37	19.0	Lima et al. (2017)
Rio de Janeiro	South-east	263	1.5	Pereira et al. (2017)
Maranhão	North-east	60	3.3	Silva et al. (2017a)
São Paulo	South-east	1725	0.3	Souza et al. (2017)

ranged from 4.1% to 53.7% (mean ± standard deviation = 27.6% ± 19.0%) (Table 4). The three most prevalent intestinal helminths of cats in these studies were generally, in descending order, *A. braziliense*, *D. caninum*, and *T. cati* (Campos et al., 1974; Costa et al., 1966; Federman et al., 1973; Gordon and Young, 1922; Labarthe et al., 2004; Mudim et al., 2004; Ogassawara et al., 1986b; Ramos et al., 2013; Zago Filho and Barreto, 1957).

Table 4 Prevalence of *Toxocara cati* infection in cats ($n = 701$) in different Brazilian regions, based on necropsies.

State	Region	Sample size	Prevalence (%)	References
Amazonas	North	9	44.4	Gordon and Young (1922)
São Paulo	South-east	196	49.0	Zago Filho and Barreto (1957)
Minas Gerais	South-east	63	36.5	Costa et al. (1966)
Minas Gerais	South-east	11	6.7	Federman et al. (1973)
Goiás	Centre-west	37	19.0	Campos et al. (1974)
São Paulo	South-east	54	53.7	Ogassawara et al. (1986b)
Rio de Janeiro	South-east	135	25.2	Labarthe et al. (2004)
Minas Gerais	South-east	50	10.0	Mudim et al. (2004)
Mato Grosso	Centre-west	146	4.1	Ramos et al. (2013)

A study conducted with 135 cats in Rio de Janeiro (Rio de Janeiro state, south-eastern Brazil) revealed that 25.2% of the cats subjected to necropsy were infected by *T. cati*, with a mean intensity of 2.9 adult worms per cat (Labarthe et al., 2004). The prevalence and intensity of *T. cati* infection was higher in stray cats as compared to shelter cats, although differences were not statistically significant (Labarthe et al., 2004). In another study carried out in Cuiabá (Mato Grosso state, central-western Brazil), out of 146 cats subjected to necropsy, 4.1% were infected by *T. cati*, with a mean intensity of 28.3 adult worms per cat (Ramos et al., 2013). These studies suggest a lower prevalence and a higher intensity of *T. cati* in cats in Cuiabá as compared to Rio de Janeiro, but data are limited to draw any conclusion in this sense. In this respect, as for dogs, data suggest that the prevalence of *T. cati* in cats is higher in northern Brazil as compared to other regions (Fig. 2).

4. Environmental contamination

A number of investigations have been carried out in different Brazilian regions to assess the contamination of soil with *Toxocara* eggs in a range of environments, including in public squares, parks, and beaches (Alcântara et al., 1989; Araújo et al., 1999; Capuano and Rocha, 2005;

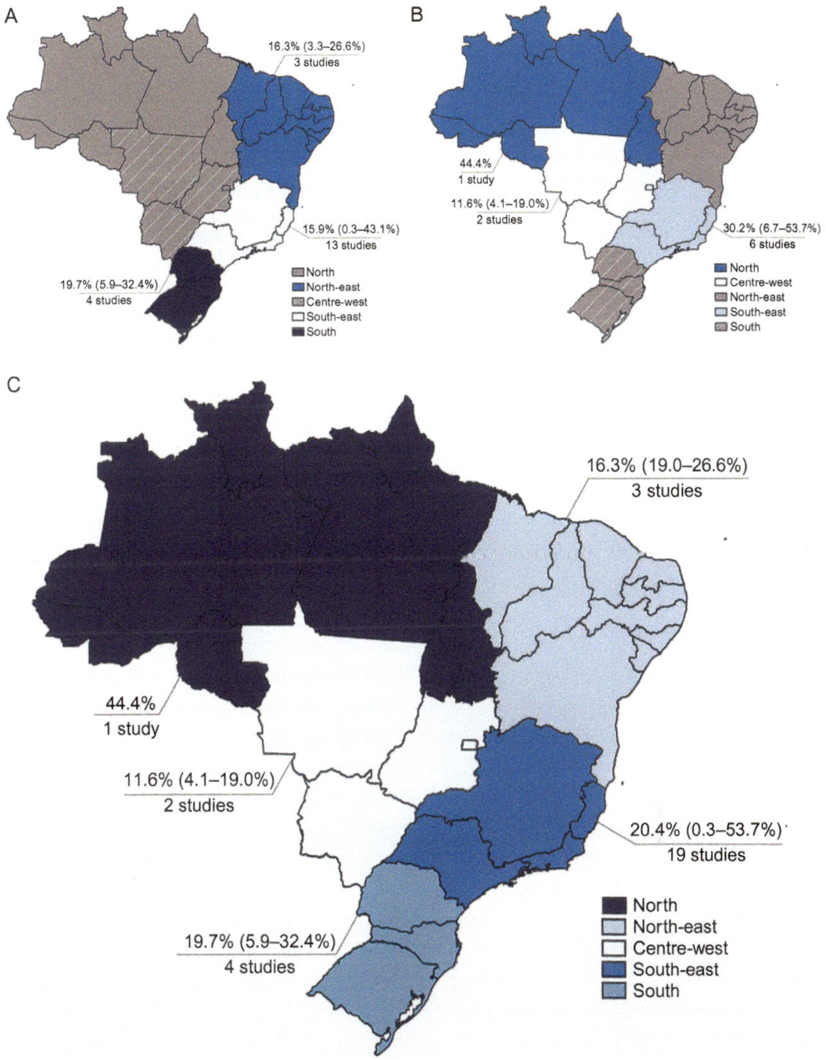

Fig. 2 Prevalence of *Toxocara cati* infection in cats in different Brazilian regions, based on faecal examinations (A), necropsies (B), or both datasets combined (C).

Cassenote et al., 2011; Castro et al., 2005; Coelho et al., 2001; Corrêa et al., 1995; Costa-Cruz et al., 1994; Fontes et al., 2017; Gallina et al., 2011; Guimarães et al., 2005; Lima et al., 2005; Manini et al., 2012; Marchioro et al., 2013; Marques et al., 2012; Mattia et al., 2012; Moura et al., 2010, 2013; Nunes et al., 2000; Rocha et al., 2011; Santarém et al., 1998, 2008, 2012; Scaini et al., 2003; Sprenger et al., 2014;

Tiyo et al., 2008). The frequency of soil contamination with *Toxocara* eggs is very high, reaching as high as 91.7% in a study conducted in 24 - public squares in Santa Maria (Rio Grande do Sul state, southern Brazil) (Corrêa et al., 1995).

Sandboxes in recreational areas constitute an important source of *Toxocara* spp. infection for children. In fact, the level of soil contamination with *Toxocara* eggs in these areas is impressive. For instance, a study conducted in São Mateus (Espírito Santo state, south-eastern Brazil) reported that six (75%) out of eight public schools investigated presented *Toxocara* eggs in soil samples collected from recreational areas (Fontes et al., 2017).

Free-roaming dogs and cats are frequently seen in areas contaminated with *Toxocara* eggs (Araújo et al., 1999; Guimarães et al., 2005). As a matter of fact, free-roaming dogs and cats are abundant in all Brazilian regions and have free-access to public squares, parks, beaches, and gardens (Figs. 3 and 4). For instance, it is acknowledged that not only feral dogs (independent on human care and unrestricted), but also family dogs (fully dependent and semi-restricted), neighbourhood dogs (semi-dependent and semi-restricted), and unrestricted dogs (semi-dependent and unrestricted) may play a role in

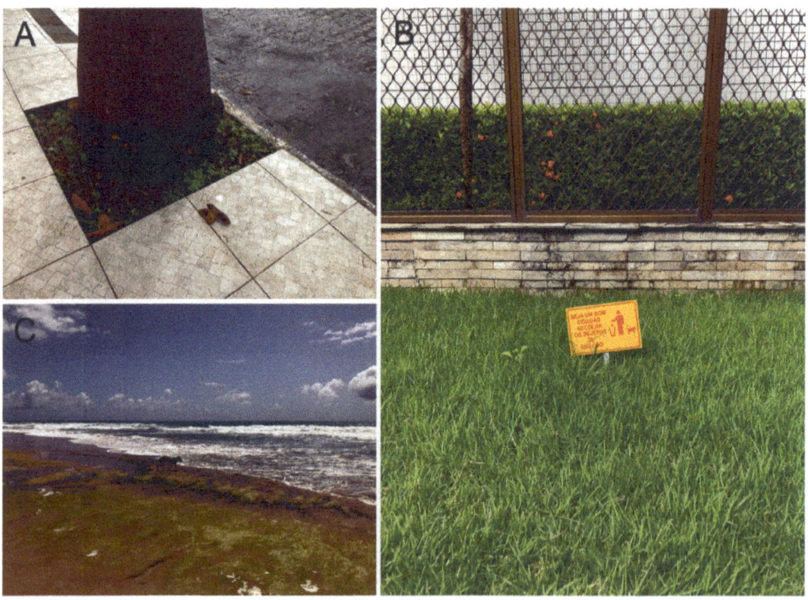

Fig. 3 Fresh faeces in a high-income neighbourhood (A) and a sign advising the owners to collect their dog waste (from Portuguese, "Be a good citizen, collect your dog's waste") (B). A free-roaming dog on a famous beach in north-eastern Brazil (C).

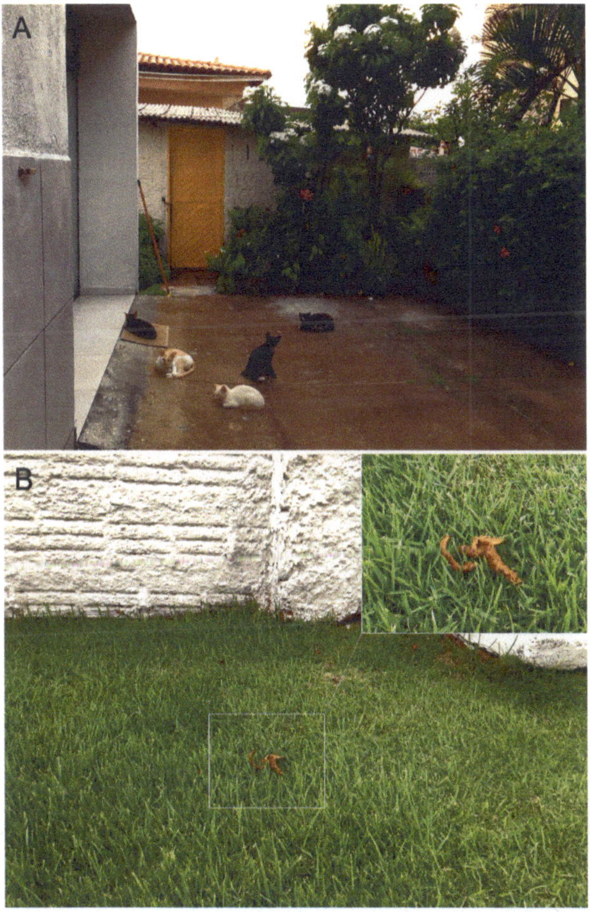

Fig. 4 Free-roaming cats in the backyard of an apartment complex (A), where daily contamination with cat faeces (closeup image) is common (B).

the dissemination of zoonotic parasites, including *T. canis* (Otranto et al., 2017). Many (if not most) dogs and cats seen wandering in the streets in Brazil have some level of dependence on humans. In fact, family dogs are often allowed to go out alone to urinate or defecate.

The environmental contamination with *Toxocara* eggs appears to vary seasonally, with higher frequencies during certain periods of the year (Chieffi and Müller, 1978; Queiroz et al., 2006; Tiyo et al., 2008). This may be related to local dog population dynamics (e.g., mating season), but also to meteorological variables, considering that rain may also favour the dispersion of *Toxocara* eggs in the environment.

5. Public health significance

Toxocara canis and *T. cati* are recognised agents of human toxocariasis, an important zoonotic parasitic disease of worldwide distribution (Ma et al., 2018; Macpherson, 2013; Rubinsky-Elefant et al., 2010). Numerous studies have been conducted in Brazil to assess the frequency of anti-*Toxocara* antibodies in humans, particularly children (Chieffi et al., 2009; Ma et al., 2018). According to these studies, the seroprevalence in Brazil generally ranges from less than 5% up to 52% (Bolivar-Mejia et al., 2014; Ma et al., 2018), but may reach as high as 71.8% as reported in a recent study conducted in Cerrito Alegre (Rio Grande do Sul state) (Araújo et al., 2018).

From a clinical perspective, studies have reported significant associations between exposure to *Toxocara* spp. and atopy, asthma, urticaria, or wheezing in humans in Brazil (Alcântara-Neves et al., 2014; Cadore et al., 2016; Chieffi et al., 2009; Grama et al., 2014; Matos Fialho et al., 2017; Mendonça et al., 2012; Silva et al., 2016, 2017b). Rare cases of neurotoxocariasis with central nervous system involvement have also been reported in this country (Marx et al., 2007; Moreira-Silva et al., 2004; Salvador et al., 2010). In spite of the widespread distribution, high prevalence, and clinical significance of *Toxocara* spp. infection in humans in Brazil, the burden of toxocariasis in this country is largely underestimated.

Risk factors for *Toxocara* spp. infection in humans identified in studies conducted in Brazil include contact with contaminated soil, dogs and cats, poor personal hygiene habits, and socioeconomic conditions (Alderete et al., 2003; Anaruma Filho et al., 2002; Campos Júnior et al., 2003; Coelho et al., 2004; Coêlho et al., 2005; Fragoso et al., 2011; Marchioro et al., 2015; Negri et al., 2013; Rubinsky-Elefant et al., 2010; Santarém et al., 2011; Souza et al., 2011; Teixeira et al., 2006). A study conducted in São Paulo state identified dog ownership as a risk factor for *Toxocara* spp. exposure in women, whereas men with occupational contact with dogs were not at a significantly higher risk (Chieffi et al., 1988).

Contact with dog hair contaminated with *T. canis* eggs has also been suggested as a potential risk factor (Amaral et al., 2010). However, eggs present in dog hair are usually not embryonated (thus, non-infective) (Merigueti et al., 2017). Moreover, even considering that a small proportion of these eggs may be embryonated, *Toxocara* eggs are very adhesive and difficult to remove from the hair of animals, thus rendering the ingestion of sufficient infective eggs very unlikely (Deplazes et al., 2011).

Children are at a higher risk of *Toxocara* spp. infection due to their increased level of exposure to contaminated environments (e.g., sandboxes in recreational areas) and due to some of their habits (e.g., geophagy) that may increase the probability of ingesting embryonated eggs (Cassenote et al., 2014).

Humans may become infected by ingesting infective *Toxocara* eggs from contaminated soil, water, raw vegetables, or fruits (Ma et al., 2018). A study conducted in a large public food market located in the metropolitan region of São Paulo reported that 2.5% of vegetables examined were contaminated with *Toxocara* eggs (Oliveira and Germano, 1992). The aforementioned study, which was conducted in the largest public food market in Brazil at that time, underlines that the consumption of unwashed vegetables could be a potential route of *Toxocara* spp. infection in humans in this country. A more recent study reported that, among several other potential risk factors, 72.2% of the parents/guardians of children testing positive for anti-*Toxocara* antibodies reported using only water for sanitising raw vegetables and fruits (Araújo et al., n.d.).

Another possible infection route is the ingestion of tissue dwelling third-stage larvae in raw or undercooked or raw meat or organs from paratenic hosts, such as rabbits, sheep, cattle, and chickens (Ma et al., 2018; Strube et al., 2013). For instance, the ingestion of raw chicken livers has been implicated as the route of *T. canis* infection in a familial outbreak of visceral larva migrans in Japan (Morimatsu et al., 2006). In this perspective, recent studies have reported high levels of exposure to *Toxocara* spp. in broiler chickens in Brazil (Campos-da-Silva et al., 2015; Oliveira et al., 2018). An experimental study conducted in Brazil concluded that the consumption of raw chicken liver could pose a risk of infection, even when chickens are inoculated with low doses of *T. canis* infective eggs (Dutra et al., 2014). Another study concluded that chickens have the potential of dispersing *T. canis* eggs into the environment and that eggs passed through the intestine are infective after being incubated under experimental conditions (Merigueti et al., 2018). Furthermore, it has been demonstrated that *T. cati* larvae retain infective in the muscles of chickens for half a year (Taira et al., 2011). While these studies suggest that chickens may play a role in the epidemiology of *Toxocara* spp. infection in humans in Brazil, further studies are needed to confirm this hypothesis.

6. Future directions

Considering the continental size of Brazil, a relatively restricted number of field studies assessing the prevalence of *Toxocara* spp. infection in dogs and cats have been conducted in this country. Studies are disproportionally concentrated in south-eastern and southern regions, which makes the current picture of *Toxocara* spp. infection in dogs and cats in this country geographically-biased. Furthermore, there is an even more limited number of studies using a properly randomised sampling strategy and including a representative number of animals. For instance, hospital-based studies may not necessarily reflect the reality of an animal population in a city, state or region. Therefore, further randomised, population-based studies, using a representative sample of animals, should be conducted in Brazil, particularly in the northern, north-eastern, and central-western regions.

Toxocara cati eggs have been reported in coprolites from small and large wild felids retrieved in archaeological sites in Piauí state (north-eastern Brazil), dating from 9150 (±60) to 410 (±40) years before present (Sianto et al., 2014). This finding indicates an ancient parasite-host association between wild felids and *T. cati* in Brazil, but there is virtually no genetic data regarding *Toxocara* spp. circulating in this country, which preclude us from making any inference in this way. Considering that wild canids and felids can play a role in the spreading of parasites to dogs and cats and vice versa (Otranto et al., 2015; Sevá et al., 2018), further studies are needed to better understand the epidemiological picture and transmission patterns of *Toxocara* spp. infecting domestic and wild canids and felids in Brazil.

There is a wide clinical spectrum of *Toxocara* spp. in humans in Brazil (Alcântara-Neves et al., 2014; Cadore et al., 2016; Colli et al., 2010; Dattoli et al., 2011; Grama et al., 2014; Matos Fialho et al., 2017; Mendonça et al., 2012; Recuero et al., 2019; Salvador et al., 2010; Silva et al., 2017b; Vasconcelos-Santos et al., 2010; Viola et al., 2016) and genetic studies could also help in understating if there any species/genotype difference in terms of clinical presentation in these accidental hosts.

Animal population control is far from being achieved in Brazil and in Latin America in general. The number of free-roaming dogs and cats is huge, yet underestimated. Governmental and non-governmental initiatives (e.g., spay/neuter programmes, adoption, veterinary trainings, and capacity-building workshops) to reduce stray animal overpopulation and abandonment of animals should be encouraged. Responsible ownership should be continuously promoted among pet owners. Increased awareness on the importance of prompt removal and discharge of animal faeces (Fig. 3B) is also imperative to reduce overall environmental contamination.

Regular and frequent anthelmintic treatment of dogs and cats, starting at an early age, constitute an important control strategy for *Toxocara* spp.

(Macpherson, 2013; Rehbein et al., 2017). In this perspective, continuous education of veterinary practitioners is also pivotal. Current guidelines for the control of *Toxocara* spp. infection in dogs and cats are available and should be promoted. For instance, the Tropical Council for Companion Animal Parasites (TroCCAP) have elaborated guidelines for the diagnosis, treatment and control of canine and feline endoparasites (including *Toxocara* spp.) in the tropics. These guidelines are open access and available in several languages, including Portuguese and Spanish (see https://www.troccap.com), making then fully accessible for the continuous education of veterinary practitioners, medical physicians and any other health professionals dealing directly or indirectly with these parasites in Brazil and other Latin American countries.

Acknowledgements

I would like to thank Prof. Dwight Bowman for inviting me to contribute to this book series. I am grateful also to Kamila Gaudêncio da Silva Sales, Luciana Aguiar Figueredo and Lucas Christian de Sousa-Paula (who also kindly elaborated Figs 1 and 2) for their help with the preparation of Tables 1–4. Finally, thanks to the National Council for Scientific and Technological Development (CNPq) for a research fellowship (Bolsa de Produtividade; grant number: 313118/2018-3).

References

Alcântara, N., Bavia, E., Silvão, R.M., Carvalho, E., 1989. Environmental contamination by *Toxocara* sp. eggs in public areas of Salvador, Bahia state, Brazil. Rev. Soc. Bras. Med. Trop. 22, 187–190.

Alcântara-Neves, N.M., Britto, G.S.G., Veiga, R.V., Figueiredo, C.A., Fiaccone, R.L., Conceição, J.S., Cruz, Á.A., Rodrigues, L.C., Cooper, P.J., Pontes-de-Carvalho, L.C., Barreto, M.L., 2014. Effects of helminth co-infections on atopy, asthma and cytokine production in children living in a poor urban area in Latin America. BMC. Res. Notes 7, 817.

Alderete, J.M., Jacob, C.M., Pastorino, A.C., Elefant, G.R., Castro, A.P., Fomin, A.B., Chieffi, P.P., 2003. Prevalence of *Toxocara* infection in schoolchildren from the Butantã region, São Paulo, Brazil. Mem. Inst. Oswaldo Cruz 98, 593–597.

Almeida, A.B.P.F., Sousa, V.R.F., Dalcin, L., Justino, C.H.S., 2007. Contaminação por fezes canina das praças públicas de Cuiabá, Mato Grosso. Braz. J. Vet. Res. Anim. Sci. 44, 132–136 [Article in Portuguese].

Alves, O.F., Gomes, A.G., Silva, A.C., 2005. Ocorrência de Enteroparasitos em cães do município de Goiânia, Goiás: comparação de técnicas de diagnóstico. Cienc. Anim. Bras. 6, 127–133 [Article in Portuguese].

Alves, A.P.S.M., Coelho, F.A.S., Coelho, M.D.G., 2014. Frequency of enteroparasites collected in feces of dogs in public squares in the city of Pindamonhangaba, SP. Brazil. Rev. Patol. Trop. 43, 341–350.

Amaral, H.L., Rassier, G.L., Pepe, M.S., Gallina, T., Villela, M.M., Nobre, M.O., Scaini, C.J., Berne, M.E., 2010. Presence of *Toxocara canis* eggs on the hair of dogs: a risk factor for visceral larva migrans. Vet. Parasitol. 174, 115–118.

Anaruma Filho, F., Chieffi, P.P., Correa, C.R., Camargo, E.D., Silveira, E.P., Aranha, J.J., Ribeiro, M.C., 2002. Human toxocariasis: a seroepidemiological survey in the municipality of Campinas (SP), Brazil. Rev. Inst. Med. Trop. Sao Paulo 44, 303–307.

Araújo, J.V., 2006. Helmintoses intestinais em cães da microrregião de Viçosa, Minas Gerais. Rev. Ceres 53, 363–365 [Article in Portuguese].

Araújo, R.B., Assis, C.B., Del Carlo, R.J., 1986. Helmintoses intestinais em cães da microregião de Viçosa, Minas Gerais. Arq. Bras. Med. Vet. Zootec. 38, 197–203 [Article in Portuguese].

Araújo, F.R., Crocci, A.J., Rodrigues, R.G., Avalhaes, J.S., Miyoshi, M.I., Salgado, F.P., da Silva, M.A., Pereira, M.L., 1999. Contaminação de praças públicas de Campo Grande, Mato Grosso do Sul, Brasil, por ovos de *Toxocara* e *Ancylostoma* em fezes de cães. Rev. Soc. Bras. Med. Trop. 32, 581–583 [Article in Portuguese].

Araújo, A.C., Villela, M.M., Sena-Lopes, Â., Farias, N.A.D.R., Faria, L.M.J., Avila, L.F.C., Berne, M.E.A., Borsuk, S., 2018. Seroprevalence of *Toxoplasma gondii* and *Toxocara canis* in a human rural population of southern Rio Grande do Sul. Rev. Inst. Med. Trop. Sao Paulo 60, e28.

Araújo, G.M.S., Walcher, D.L., Previtali, I.F., Lehman, L.M., Costa, M.P., Susin, L.O., Avila, L.F.C., Scaini, C.J., n.d. Frequency of enteroparasitic infections and serum positivity for *Toxocara* spp. in children from a public day care center in southern Brazil. Braz. J. Biol., in press.

Balassiano, B.C., Campos, M.R., Menezes, R.C., Pereira, M.J., 2009. Factors associated with gastrointestinal parasite infection in dogs in Rio de Janeiro, Brazil. Prev. Vet. Med. 91, 234–440.

Beugnet, F., Bourdeau, P., Chalvet-Monfray, K., Cozma, V., Farkas, R., Guillot, J., Halos, L., Joachim, A., Losson, B., Miró, G., Otranto, D., Renaud, M., Rinaldi, L., 2014. Parasites of domestic owned cats in Europe: co-infestations and risk factors. Parasit. Vectors 7, 291.

Blazius, R.D., Emerick, S., Prophiro, J.S., Romão, P.R., Silva, O.S., 2005. Ocorrência de protozoários e helmintos em amostras de fezes de cães errantes da Cidade de Itapema, Santa Catarina. Rev. Soc. Bras. Med. Trop. 38, 73–74 [Article in Portuguese].

Bolivar-Mejia, A., Alarcón-Olave, C., Calvo-Betancourt, L.S., Paniz-Mondolfi, A., Delgado, O., Rodriguez-Morales, A.J., 2014. Toxocariasis in the Americas: burden and disease control. Curr. Trop. Med. Rep. 1, 62–68.

Bresciani, K.D.S., Ishizaki, M.N., Kaneto, C.N., Montano, T.R.P., Perri, S.H.V., Vasconcelos, R.O., Nascimento, A.A., 2008. Frequência e intensidade parasitária de helmintos gastrintestinais em cães na área urbana do município de Araçatuba, SP. Ars Vet. 24, 181–185 [Article in Portuguese].

Brust, M.B., Motta, J.G., Caldas, E.M., Jacques, S.A., 1976. Localização de helmintos nos diversos segmentos do intestino delgado de cães (*Canis familiaris*) na cidade de Salvador, Bahia. Arq. EMV 1, 115–122 [Article in Portuguese].

Cadore, P.S., Zhang, L., Lemos, L.L., Lorenzi, C., Telmo, P.L., Santos, P.C., Mattos, G.T., Vignol, F.S., Prietsch, S.O., Berne, M.E., Scaini, C.J., 2016. Toxocariasis and childhood asthma: a case-control study. J. Asthma 53, 601–606.

Campos Filho, P.C., Barros, L.M., Campos, J.O., Braga, V.B., Cazorla, I.M., Albuquerque, G.R., Carvalho, S.M., 2008. Parasitas zoonóticos em fezes de cães em praças públicas do município de Itabuna, Bahia, Brasil. Rev. Bras. Parasitol. Vet. 17, 206–209 [Article in Portuguese].

Campos Júnior, D., Elefant, G.R., de Melo e Silva, E.O., Gandolfi, L., Jacob, C.M., Tofeti, A., Pratesi, R., 2003. Freqüência de soropositividade para antígenos de *Toxocara canis* em crianças de classes sociais diferentes. Rev. Soc. Bras. Med. Trop. 36, 509–513 [Article in Portuguese].

Campos, D.M.B., Garibaldi, I.M., Carneiro, J.R., 1974. Prevalência de helmintos em gatos (*Felis catus domesticus*) de Goiânia. Rev. Pat. Trop. 3, 355–359 [Article in Portuguese].

Campos, D.R., Oliveira, L.C., Siqueira, D.F., Perin, L.R., Campos, N.C., Aptekmann, K.P., Martins, I.V., 2016. Prevalence and risk factors associated with endoparasitosis of dogs and cats in Espírito Santo, Brazil. Acta Parasitol. 61, 544–548.

Campos-da-Silva, D.R., Paz, J.S., Fortunato, V.R., Beltrame, M.A., Valli, L.C., Pereira, F.E., 2015. Natural infection of free-range chickens with the ascarid nematode *Toxocara* sp. Parasitol. Res. 114, 4289–4293.

Capuano, D.M., Rocha, G.M., 2005. Environmental contamination by *Toxocara* sp. eggs in Ribeirão Preto, São Paulo state, Brazil. Rev. Inst. Med. Trop. Sao Paulo 47, 223–226.

Carneiro, J.R., Freitas, J.S., Pereira, E., Campos, D.M.B., Jardim, S.V., 1973. Prevalência de helmintos em "*Canis familiaris*" no município de Goiânia. Rev. Patol. Trop. 2, 401–404 [Article in Portuguese].

Cassenote, A.J., Pinto Neto, J.M., Lima-Catelani, A.R., Ferreira, A.W., 2011. Contaminação do solo por ovos de geo-helmintos com potencial zoonótico na municipalidade de Fernandópolis, Estado de São Paulo, entre 2007 e 2008. Rev. Soc. Bras. Med. Trop. 44, 371–374 [Article in Portuguese].

Cassenote, A.J., Lima, A.R., Pinto Neto, J.M., Rubinsky-Elefant, G., 2014. Seroprevalence and modifiable risk factors for *Toxocara* spp. in Brazilian schoolchildren. PLoS Negl. Trop. Dis. 8, e2830.

Castro, J.M., Santos, S.V., Monteiro, N.A., 2005. Contaminação de canteiros da orla marítima do município de Praia Grande, São Paulo, por ovos de *Ancylostoma* e *Toxocara* em fezes de cães. Rev. Soc. Bras. Med. Trop. 38, 199–201 [Article in Portuguese].

Chieffi, P.P., Müller, E.E., 1976. Prevalência de parasitismo por *Toxocara canis* em cães e presença de ovos de *Toxocara* sp. no solo de localidades públicas da zona urbana do município de Londrina, estado do Paraná, Brasil. Rev. Saude Publica 10, 367–372 [Article in Portuguese].

Chieffi, P.P., Müller, E.E., 1978. Estudo da variação mensal na contaminação do solo por ovos de *Toxocara* sp. (Nematoda, Ascaroidea), na zona urbana do município de Londrina, estado do Paraná, Brasil. Rev. Inst. Adolfo Lutz 38, 13–16 [Article in Portuguese].

Chieffi, P.P., Ueda, M., Camargo, E.D., Souza, A.M.C., Silva, C.L., Nova, A.V., Guedes, M.L.S., 1988. Contacto domiciliar e profissional com cães como fatores de risco para infecção humana por larvas de *Toxocara*. Rev. Inst. Med. Trop. Sao Paulo 30, 379–382 [Article in Portuguese].

Chieffi, P.P., Santos, S.V., Queiroz, M.L., Lescano, S.A., 2009. Human toxocariasis: contribution by Brazilian researchers. Rev. Inst. Med. Trop. Sao Paulo 51, 301–308.

Coelho, L.M., Dini, C.Y., Milman, M.H., Oliveira, S.M., 2001. *Toxocara* spp. eggs in public squares of Sorocaba, São Paulo state, Brazil. Rev. Inst. Med. Trop. Sao Paulo 43, 189–191.

Coelho, L.M., Silva, M.V., Dini, C.Y., Giacon Neto, A.A., Novo, N.F., Silveira, E.P., 2004. Human toxocariasis: a seroepidemiological survey in schoolchildren of Sorocaba, Brazil. Mem. Inst. Oswaldo Cruz 99, 553–557.

Coêlho, R.A.L., Carvalho Jr., L.B., Perez, E.P., Araki, K., Takeuchi, T., Ito, A., Aoki, T., Yamasaki, H., 2005. Prevalence of toxocariasis in northeastern Brazil based on serology using recombinant *Toxocara canis* antigen. Am. J. Trop. Med. Hyg. 72, 103–107.

Coelho, W.M., Amarante, A.F., Soutello, R.V., Meireles, M.V., Bresciani, K.D., 2009. Ocorrência de parasitos gastrintestinais em amostras fecais de felinos no município de Andradina, São Paulo. Rev. Bras. Parasitol. Vet. 18, 46–49 [Article in Portuguese].

Colli, C.M., Rubinsky-Elefant, G., Paludo, M.L., Falavigna, D.L., Guilherme, E.V., Mattia, S., Araújo, S.M., Ferreira, E.C., Previdelli, I.T., Falavigna-Guilherme, A.L., 2010. Serological, clinical and epidemiological evaluation of toxocariasis in urban areas of south Brazil. Rev. Inst. Med. Trop. Sao Paulo 52, 69–74.

Corrêa, G.L.B., Michelon, E., Lagaggio, V.R.A., Moreira, W.S., Moraes, R.Q., Leite, C.R., Ribas, H.O., Adamy, M., Pit, G.L., Colombo, F.H., 1995. Contaminação do solo por ovos, larvas de helmintos e oocistos de protozoários, em praças públicas de Santa Maria e sua importância em saúde pública. Rev. Bras. Parasitol. Vet. 4, 137–141 [Article in Portuguese].

Côrtes, V.A., Paim, G.V., Alencar Filho, R.A., 1988. Infestação por ancilostomídeos e toxocarídeos em cães e gatos apreendidos em vias públicas, São Paulo (Brasil). Rev. Saude Publica 22, 341–343 [Article in Portuguese].

Costa, H.M.A., Batista Jr., J.A., Freitas, M.G., 1962. Endo e ecto parasitos de *Canis familiares* em Belo Horizonte. Arq. Esc. Vet. UFMG 14, 103–112 [Article in Portuguese].

Costa, H.M.A., Costa, J.O., Freitas, M.G., 1966. Parasitos de *Felis domestica* em Belo Horizonte, Minas Gerais. Arq. Esc. Vet. UFMG 18, 65–69 [Article in Portuguese].

Costa, J.O., Guimarães, M.P., Lima, W.S., Lima, E.A.M., 1990. Freqüência de endo e ecto parasitos de cães capturados nas ruas de Vitória—ES—Brasil. Arq. Bras. Med. Vet. Zootec. 42, 451–452 [Article in Portuguese].

Costa-Cruz, J.M., Nunes, R.S., Buso, A.G., 1994. Presença de ovos de *Toxocara* spp em praças públicas da cidade de Uberlândia, Minas Gerais, Brasil. Rev. Inst. Med. Trop. Sao Paulo 36, 39–42 [Article in Portuguese].

Curi, N.H.A., Paschoal, A.M.O., Massara, R.L., Santos, H.A., Guimarães, M.P., Passamani, M., Chiarello, A.G., 2017. Risk factors for gastrointestinal parasite infections of dogs living around protected areas of the Atlantic Forest: implications for human and wildlife health. Braz. J. Biol. 77, 388–395.

Dantas-Torres, F., Otranto, D., 2014. Dogs, cats, parasites, and humans in Brazil: opening the black box. Parasit. Vectors 7, 22.

Dattoli, V.C., Freire, S.M., Mendonça, L.R., Santos, P.C., Meyer, R., Alcantara-Neves, N.M., 2011. *Toxocara canis* infection is associated with eosinophilia and total IgE in blood donors from a large Brazilian centre. Trop. Med. Int. Health 16, 514–517.

Deplazes, P., van Knapen, F., Schweiger, A., Overgaauw, P.A., 2011. Role of pet dogs and cats in the transmission of helminthic zoonoses in Europe, with a focus on echinococcosis and toxocarosis. Vet. Parasitol. 182, 41–53.

Dutra, G.F., Pinto, N.S., Avila, L.F., Dutra, P.C., Telmo, P.L., Rodrigues, L.H., Silva, A.M., Scaini, C.J., 2014. Risk of infection by the consumption of liver of chickens inoculated with low doses of *Toxocara canis* eggs. Vet. Parasitol. 203, 87–90.

Farias, N.A., Christovão, M.L., Stobbe, N.S., 1995. Freqüência de parasitas intestinais em cães (*Canis familiaris*) e gatos (*Felis catus domestica*) em Araçatuba, São Paulo. Rev. Bras. Parasitol. Vet. 4, 57–60 [Article in Portuguese].

Federman, H.B., Holanda, J.C., Evangelista, A., 1973. Ocorrência de parasitos em gatos (*Felis catus domesticus*) e pombos (*Columba livia*) procedentes de algumas localidades de Minas Gerais. Rev. Patol. Trop. 2, 207–215 [Article in Portuguese].

Fenerich, F.L., Santos, S.M., Amaral, V., 1972. Análise dos resultados obtidos em 903 amostras de fezes oriundas da espécie canina. Biológico 38, 175–177 [Article in Portuguese].

Ferreira, L.F., Silva, M.L., Camillo-Coura, L., 1976. *Toxocara* e outros helmintos, em cães, na cidade do Rio de Janeiro. Rev. Soc. Bras. Med. Trop. 10, 361–365 [Article in Portuguese].

Ferreira, M.A.S., Rodrigues, J.S., Andrade, R.L.F.S., Jesus, H.A., Barros, S.L.B., 2009. Avaliação de endoparasitos em cães domiciliados, de abrigo e errantes na cidade de Aracaju—Sergipe. Med. Vet. 3, 20–25 [Article in Portuguese].

Ferreira, C.G.T., Bezerra, A.C.D.S., Ahid, S.M.M., 2010. Endoparasitas em cães (*Canis familiaris* L.) em Apodi, Rio Grande do Norte, Brasil. PUBVET 4, 844–849 [Article in Portuguese].

Ferreira, J.I., Pena, H.F., Azevedo, S.S., Labruna, M.B., Gennari, S.M., 2016. Occurrences of gastrointestinal parasites in fecal samples from domestic dogs in São Paulo, SP, Brazil. Rev. Bras. Parasitol. Vet. 25, 435–440.

Fontes, A.M., Gusson, V.P., Souza, A.A., Souza, M.A., 2017. Identification of enteroparasites in recreation areas of elementary schools in Northern Espírito Santo, Brazil. Rev. Salud Publica. (Bogota) 19, 795–799.

Fragoso, R.P., Monteiro, M.B., Lemos, E.M., Pereira, F.E., 2011. Anti-*Toxocara* antibodies detected in children attending elementary school in Vitoria, state of Espírito Santo, Brazil: prevalence and associated factors. Rev. Soc. Bras. Med. Trop. 44, 461–466.

Frizzo, C., Schimidt, A.P., Wagner, G., Muller, G.A., 2016. Intestinal parasites present in canine fecal samples collected in rural areas of municipalities in the Midwest of Santa Catarina, Brazil. Rev. Patol. Trop. 45, 227–232.

Funada, M.R., Pena, H.F.J., Soares, R.M., Amaku, M., Gennari, S.M., 2007. Freqüência de parasitos gastrintestinais em cães e gatos atendidos em hospital-escola veterinário da cidade de São Paulo. Arq. Bras. Med. Vet. Zootec. 59, 1338–1340 [Article in Portuguese].

Gallas, M., Silveira, E.F., 2013. *Toxocara cati* (Schrank, 1788) (Nematoda, Ascarididae) in different wild feline species in Brazil: new host records. Biotemas 26, 117–125.

Gallina, T., Silva, M.A., Castro, L.L., Wendt, E.W., Villela, M.M., Berne, M.E., 2011. Presence of eggs of *Toxocara* spp. and hookworms in a student environment in Rio Grande do Sul, Brazil. Rev. Bras. Parasitol. Vet. 20, 176–177.

Gennari, S.M., Kasai, N., Pena, H.F.J., Cortez, A., 1999. Ocorrência de protozoários e helmintos em amostras de fezes de cães e gatos da cidade de São Paulo. Braz. J. Vet. Res. Anim. Sci. 36, 87–91 [Article in Portuguese].

Gennari, S.M., Pena, H.F.J., Blasques, L.S., 2001. Frequência de ocorrência de parasitos gastrintestinais em amostras de fezes de cães e gatos da cidade de São Paulo. Vet News 8, 10–12 [Article in Portuguese].

Gennari, S.M., Ferreira, J.I., Pena, H.F., Labruna, M.B., Azevedo, S.D., 2016. Frequency of gastrointestinal parasites in cats seen at the University of São Paulo Veterinary Hospital, Brazil. Rev. Bras. Parasitol. Vet. 25, 423–428.

Ginar, R.M.B., Galarça, R.C.G., Picavêa, J.P., Petry, H., 2006. Índice de contaminação do solo por ovos dos principais nematoides de caninos nas praças públicas da cidade de Uruguaiana-RS, Brasil. Rev. FZVA 13, 103–111 [Article in Portuguese].

Gordon, R.M., Young, C.J., 1922. Parasites in dogs and cats in Amazonas. Ann. Trop. Med. Parasitol. 16, 297–300.

Grama, D.F., Lescano, S.Z., Mota, K.C.P., Pultz, B.A., Miranda, J.S., Silva Segundo, G.R., Taketomi, E.A., Fernandes, K.P., Limongi, J.E., de Paula, F.M., Chieffi, P.P., Cury, M.C., 2014. Seroprevalence of *Toxocara* spp. in children with atopy. Trans. R. Soc. Trop. Med. Hyg. 108, 797–803.

Guimarães Junior, J.S., Vidotto, O., Yamamura, M.H., Ross, G.M., Fonseca, N.A.N., Pereira, A.B.L., 1996. Helmintos gastrointestinais em cães (*Canis familiaris*) na região de Londrina, PR. Semina Cienc. Agrar. 17, 29–32 [Article in Portuguese].

Guimarães, A.M., Alves, E.G., de Rezende, G.F., Rodrigues, M.C., 2005. Ovos de *Toxocara* sp. e larvas de *Ancylostoma* sp. em praça pública de Lavras, MG. Rev. Saude Publica 39, 293–295 [Article in Portuguese].

Heukelbach, J., Frank, R., Ariza, L., Sousa Lopes, I., Assis e Silva, A., Borges, A.C., Limongi, J.E., Alencar, C.H., Klimpel, S., 2012. High prevalence of intestinal infections and ectoparasites in dogs, Minas Gerais state (southeast Brazil). Parasitol. Res. 111, 1913–1921.

Hoffmann, R.P., Fortes, E., Pandolfo, R.A., Kaiser, J.C., Belló, A.R.R., Motta-Neto, A.A., 1990. Prevalência de helmintos gastrointestinais do cão errante do município de Porto Alegre, Rio Grande do Sul. Arq. Fac. Vet. UFRGS 18, 61–68 [Article in Portuguese].

Hoffmann, A.N., Beltrão, N., Botton, S.A., Caminha, B.X., Rue, M.L., 2000. Intestinal nematodes of stray dogs as zoonoses agents in D. Pedrito city RS-Brazil. Bol. Chil. Parasitol. 55, 92–93.

Holsback, L., Cardoso, M.J., Fagnani, R., Patelli, T.H., 2013. Natural infection by endoparasites among free-living wild animals. Rev. Bras. Parasitol. Vet. 22, 302–306.

Hotez, P.J., Fujiwara, R.T., 2014. Brazil's neglected tropical diseases: an overview and a report card. Microbes Infect. 16, 601–606.

Katagiri, S., Oliveira-Sequeira, T.C., 2008. Prevalence of dog intestinal parasites and risk perception of zoonotic infection by dog owners in São Paulo state, Brazil. Zoonoses Public Health 55, 406–413.

Katagiri, S., Oliveira-Sequeira, T.C., 2010. Comparison of three concentration methods for the recovery of canine intestinal parasites from stool samples. Exp. Parasitol. 126, 214–216.

Klimpel, S., Heukelbach, J., Pothmann, D., Rückert, S., 2010. Gastrointestinal and ectoparasites from urban stray dogs in Fortaleza (Brazil): high infection risk for humans? Parasitol. Res. 107, 713–719.

Labarthe, N., Serrão, M.L., Ferreira, A.M., Almeida, N.K., Guerrero, J., 2004. A survey of gastrointestinal helminths in cats of the metropolitan region of Rio de Janeiro, Brazil. Vet. Parasitol. 123, 133–139.

Labruna, M.B., Pena, H.F.J., Souza, S.L.P., Pinter, A., Silva, J.C.R., Ragozo, A.M.A., Camargo, L.M.A., Gennari, S.M., 2006. Prevalência de endoparasitas em cães da área urbana do município de Monte Negro, Rondônia. Arq. Inst. Biol. 3, 183–193 [Article in Portuguese].

Lara, S.I.M., Tarouco, M.R.R., Ribeiro, P.B., 1981. Helmintos parasitos de *Canis familiaris* de Pelotas, Rio Grande do Sul. Arq. Esc. Vet. UFMG 33, 293–297 [Article in Portuguese].

Leite, L.C., Círio, S.M., Navarro-Silva, M.A., Zadorosnei, A.C.B., Luz, E., Marinoni, L.P., Leite, S.C., Lunelli, D., 2007. Ocorrência de endoparasitas em amostras de fezes de cães (*Canis familiaris*) da região metropolitana de Curitiba, Paraná—Brasil. Rev. Estud. Biol. 29, 319–326 [Article in Portuguese].

Lima, J.L., Andrade, L.D., Aguiar-Santos, A.M., Alves, L.C., Medeiros, Z., 2005. Contaminação por ovos de Toxocara sp. em solo no município de Moreno, Estado de Pernambuco, Brasil. Braz. J. Vet. Res. Anim. Sci. 42, 339–346 [Article in Portuguese].

Lima, V.F.S., Santos, T.J., Bezerra, T.L., Silva-Santos, M., Meira-Santos, P.O., 2014. Helmintozoonoses e protozoonoses caninas no bairro Rosa Elze, São Cristóvão/ Sergipe—Brasil. Enciclopédia Biosfera 10, 1133–1145.

Lima, V.F.S., Ramos, R.A.N., Lepold, R., Borges, J.C.G., Ferreira, C.D., Rinaldi, L., Cringoli, G., Alves, L.C., 2017. Gastrointestinal parasites in feral cats and rodents from the Fernando de Noronha Archipelago, Brazil. Rev. Bras. Parasitol. Vet. 26, 521–524.

Lorenzini, G., Tasca, T., Carli, G.A., 2007. Prevalence of intestinal parasites in dogs and cats under veterinary care in Porto Alegre, Rio Grande do Sul, Brazil. Braz. J. Vet. Res. Anim. Sci. 44, 137–145.

Ma, G., Holland, C.V., Wang, T., Hofmann, A., Fan, C.K., Maizels, R.M., Hotez, P.J., Gasser, R.B., 2018. Human toxocariasis. Lancet Infect. Dis. 18, e14–e24.

Macpherson, C.N., 2013. The epidemiology and public health importance of toxocariasis: a zoonosis of global importance. Int. J. Parasitol. 43, 999–1008.

Mandarino-Pereira, A., Souza, F.S., Lopes, C.W., Pereira, M.J., 2010. Prevalence of parasites in soil and dog feces according to diagnostic tests. Vet. Parasitol. 170, 176–181.

Manini, M.P., Marchioro, A.A., Colli, C.M., Nishi, L., Falavigna-Guilherme, A.L., 2012. Association between contamination of public squares and seropositivity for *Toxocara* spp. in children. Vet. Parasitol. 188, 48–52.

Marchioro, A.A., Colli, C.M., Ferreira, É.C., Tiyo, R., Mattia, S., Souza, W.F., Falavigna-Guilherme, A.L., 2013. Identification of public areas with potential toxocariasis transmission risk using geographical information systems. Acta Parasitol. 58, 328–333.

Marchioro, A.A., Colli, C.M., Ferreira, É.C., Viol, B.M., Araújo, S.M., Falavigna-Guilherme, A.L., 2015. Risk factors associated with toxoplasmosis and toxocariasis in populations of children from nine cities in southern Brazil. J. Helminthol. 89, 428–432.
Marques, J.P., Guimarães, C.R., Boas, A.V., Carnaúba, P.U., Moraes, J., 2012. Contamination of public parks and squares from Guarulhos (São Paulo state, Brazil) by *Toxocara* spp. and *Ancylostoma* spp. Rev. Inst. Med. Trop. Sao Paulo 54, 267–271.
Martins, C.M., Barros, C.C., Bier, D., Marinho, A.P., Figueiredo, J.M.G., Hoffmann, J.L., Molento, M.B., Biondo, A.W., 2012. Dog parasite incidence and risk factors, from sampling after one-year interval, in Pinhais, Brazil. Rev. Bras. Parasitol. Vet. 21, 101–106.
Martins-Melo, F.R., Carneiro, M., Ramos Jr., A.N., Heukelbach, J., Ribeiro, A.L.P., Werneck, G.L., 2018. The burden of neglected tropical diseases in Brazil, 1990–2016: a subnational analysis from the Global Burden of Disease Study 2016. PLoS Negl. Trop. Dis. 12, e0006559.
Marx, C., Lin, J., Masruha, M.R., Rodrigues, M.G., Rocha, A.J., Vilanova, L.C., Gabbai, A.A., 2007. Toxocariasis of the CNS simulating acute disseminated encephalomyelitis. Neurology 69, 806–807.
Matos Fialho, P.M., Correa, C.R.S., Lescano, S.Z., 2017. Seroprevalence of toxocariasis in children with urticaria: a population-based study. J. Trop. Pediatr. 63, 352–357.
Mattia, S., Colli, C.M., Adami, C.M., Guilherme, G.F., Nishi, L., Rubinsky-Elefant, G., Marchioro, A.A., Gomes, M.L., Falavigna-Guilherme, A.L., 2012. Seroprevalence of *Toxocara* infection in children and environmental contamination of urban areas in Paraná state, Brazil. J. Helminthol. 86, 440–445.
Mendonça, L.R., Veiga, R.V., Dattoli, V.C., Figueiredo, C.A., Fiaccone, R., Santos, J., Cruz, Á.A., Rodrigues, L.C., Cooper, P.J., Pontes-de-Carvalho, L.C., Barreto, M.L., Alcantara-Neves, N.M., 2012. *Toxocara* seropositivity, atopy and wheezing in children living in poor neighbourhoods in urban Latin American. PLoS Negl. Trop. Dis. 6, e1886.
Menezes, O.B., 1954. Parasitos de *Canis familiaris* em Salvador. Bol. Inst. Biol. Bahia 1, 75–78 [Article in Portuguese].
Merigueti, Y.F.F.B., Santarém, V.A., Ramires, L.M., Batista, A.S., Beserra, L.V.C., Nuci, A.L., Esposte, T.M.P., 2017. Protective and risk factors associated with the presence of *Toxocara* spp. eggs in dog hair. Vet. Parasitol. 244, 39–43.
Merigueti, Y.F.F.B., Raposo, R.S., Zampieri, B.P., Cerazo, L.M.L., Pereira, L., Santarém, V.A., 2018. Dispersion and infectivity of *Toxocara canis* eggs after passage through chicken intestine. Parasitol. Res. 117, 3481–3486.
Monteiro, M.B., Medeiros, L.S., Ribeiro, V.M.F., Carvalho, Y.K., Souza, S.F., 2014. Endoparasitas em cães domiciliados no município de Rio Branco, Acre. Enciclopédia Biosfera 10, 982–989 [Article in Portuguese].
Monteiro, M.F., Ramos, R.A., Calado, A.M., Lima, V.F., Ramos, I.C., Tenório, R.F., Faustino, M.A., Alves, L.C., 2016. Gastrointestinal parasites of cats in Brazil: frequency and zoonotic risk. Rev. Bras. Parasitol. Vet. 25, 254–257.
Moreira-Silva, S.F., Rodrigues, M.G., Pimenta, J.L., Gomes, C.P., Freire, L.H., Pereira, F.E., 2004. Toxocariasis of the central nervous system: with report of two cases. Rev. Soc. Bras. Med. Trop. 37, 169–174.
Morimatsu, Y., Akao, N., Akiyoshi, H., Kawazu, T., Okabe, Y., Aizawa, H., 2006. A familial case of visceral larva migrans after ingestion of raw chicken livers: appearance of specific antibody in bronchoalveolar lavage fluid of the patients. Am. J. Trop. Med. Hyg. 75, 303–306.
Moura, F.T., Falavigna, D.L., Mota, L.T., Toledo, M.J., 2010. Enteroparasite contamination in peridomiciliar soils of two indigenous territories, state of Paraná, southern Brazil. Rev. Panam. Salud Publica 27, 414–422.

Moura, M.Q., Jeske, S., Vieira, J.N., Corrêa, T.G., Berne, M.E., Villela, M.M., 2013. Frequency of geohelminths in public squares in Pelotas, RS, Brazil. Rev. Bras. Parasitol. Vet. 22, 175–178.

Mudim, T.C.D., Oliveira Júnior, S.D., Rodrigues, D.C., Cury, M.C., 2004. Freqüência de helmintos em gatos de Uberlândia, Minas Gerais. Arq. Bras. Med. Vet. Zootec. 56, 562–563 [Article in Portuguese].

Muradian, V., Gennari, S.M., Glickman, L.T., Pinheiro, S.R., 2005. Epidemiological aspects of visceral larva migrans in children living at São Remo community, São Paulo (SP), Brazil. Vet. Parasitol. 134, 93–97.

Negri, E.C., Santarém, V.A., Rubinsky-Elefant, G., Giuffrida, R., 2013. Anti-*Toxocara* spp. antibodies in an adult healthy population: serosurvey and risk factors in southeast Brazil. Asian Pac. J. Trop. Biomed. 3, 211–216.

Nunes, C.M., Pena, F.C., Negrelli, G.B., Anjo, C.G., Nakano, M.M., Stobbe, N.S., 2000. Ocorrência de larva migrans na areia de áreas de lazer das escolas municipais de ensino infantil, Araçatuba, SP, Brasil. Rev. Saude Publica 34, 656–658 [Article in Portuguese].

Ogassawara, S., Benassi, S., Larsson, C.E., Hagiwara, M.K., 1986a. Prevalência de endoparasitas em gatos na cidade de São Paulo. Rev. Fac. Med. Vet. Zootec. Univ. Sao Paulo 23, 39–46 [Article in Portuguese].

Ogassawara, S., Benassi, S., Larsson, C.E., Leme, P.T.Z., Hagiwara, M.K., 1986b. Prevalência de infecções helmínticas em gatos na cidade de São Paulo. Rev. Fac. Med. Vet. Zootec. Univ. Sao Paulo 23, b, 145–149, 1986. [Article in Portuguese].

Oliveira, C.A., Germano, P.M., 1992. Estudo da ocorrência de enteroparasitas em hortaliças comercializadas na região metropolitana de São Paulo, SP, Brasil. I—Pesquisa de helmintos. Rev. Saude Publica 26, 283–289 [Article in Portuguese].

Oliveira, P.R., Silva, P.L., Parreira, V.F., Ribeiro, S.C.A., Gomes, J.B., 1990. Prevalencia de endoparasitos em cães da região de Uberlândia, Minas Gerais. Braz. J. Vet. Res. Anim. Sci. 27, 193–197 [Article in Portuguese].

Oliveira, V.S.F., Melo, D.P.G., Fernandes, P.R., Schulze, C.M.B., Guimarães, M.S., Silva, A.C., 2009. Ocorrência de helmintos gastrintestinais em cães errantes na cidade de Goiânia—Goiás. Rev. Patol. Trop. 38, 279–283 [Article in Portuguese].

Oliveira, A.C., Rubinsky-Elefant, G., Merigueti, Y.F.F.B., Batista, A.D.S., Santarém, V.A., 2018. Frequency of anti-*Toxocara* antibodies in broiler chickens in southern Brazil. Rev. Bras. Parasitol. Vet. 27, 141–145.

Oliveira-Arbex, A.P., David, E.B., Oliveira-Sequeira, T.C., Katagiri, S., Coradi, S.T., Guimarães, S., 2017. Molecular identification of *Ancylostoma* species from dogs and an assessment of zoonotic risk in low-income households, São Paulo state, Brazil. J. Helminthol. 91, 14–19.

Oliveira-Sequeira, T.C., Amarante, A.F., Ferrari, T.B., Nunes, L.C., 2002. Prevalence of intestinal parasites in dogs from São Paulo state, Brazil. Vet. Parasitol. 103, 19–27.

Ostermann, A.M., Lima, M.M., Farias, M.P.O., d'Alencar, A.S., Galindo, M.K.F., Silva, C.T., Alves, L.C., Faustino, M.A.G., 2011. Comparação entre exames coproparasitológicos e necroscópicos para diagnóstico da infecção por helmintos gastrintestinais em cães (*Canis familiaris*, Linnaeus, 1758) errantes provenientes da Região Metropolitana do Recife-PE. Biotemas 24, 47–56 [Article in Portuguese].

Otranto, D., Cantacessi, C., Dantas-Torres, F., Brianti, E., Pfeffer, M., Genchi, C., Guberti, V., Capelli, G., Deplazes, P., 2015. The role of wild canids and felids in spreading parasites to dogs and cats in Europe. Part II: Helminths and arthropods. Vet. Parasitol. 213, 24–37.

Otranto, D., Dantas-Torres, F., Mihalca, A.D., Traub, R.J., Lappin, M., Baneth, G., 2017. Zoonotic parasites of sheltered and stray dogs in the era of the global economic and political crisis. Trends Parasitol. 33, 813–825.

Pereira, P.F., Barbosa, A.D.S., Moura, A.P.P., Vasconcellos, M.L., Uchôa, C.M.A., Bastos, O.M.P., Amendoeira, M.R.R., 2017. Gastrointestinal parasites in stray and shelter cats in the municipality of Rio de Janeiro, Brazil. Rev. Bras. Parasitol. Vet. 26, 383–388.

Pivoto, F.L., Lopes, L.F.D., Vogel, F.S.F., Botton, S.A., Sangioni, L.A., 2013. Occurrence of gastrointestinal parasites and parasitism risk factors in domestic cats in Santa Maria, RS, Brazil. Cienc. Rural 43, 1453–1458.

Prates, L., Pacheco, L.S., Kuhl, J.B., Dias, M.L.G.G., Araújo, S.M., Pupulin, A.R.T., 2009. Frequência de parasitos intestinais em cães domiciliados da cidade de Maringá, PR. Arq. Bras. Med. Vet. Zootec. 61, 1468–1470 [Article in Portuguese].

Queiroz, M.L., Simonsen, M., Paschoalotti, M.A., Chieffi, P.P., 2006. Frequency of soil contamination by *Toxocara canis* eggs in the south region of São Paulo municipality (SP, Brazil) in a 18 month period. Rev. Inst. Med. Trop. Sao Paulo 48, 317–319.

Ragozo, A.M.A., Muradian, V., Silva, J.C.R., Caravieri, R., Amajoner, V.R., Magnabosco, C., Gennari, S.M., 2002. Ocorrência de parasitos gastrintestinais em fezes de gatos das cidades de São Paulo e Guarulhos. Braz. J. Vet. Res. Anim. Sci. 39, 244–246 [Article in Portuguese].

Ramos, D.G., Scheremeta, R.G., Oliveira, A.C., Sinkoc, A.L., Pacheco, R.C., 2013. Survey of helminth parasites of cats from the metropolitan area of Cuiabá, Mato Grosso, Brazil. Rev. Bras. Parasitol. Vet. 22, 201–206.

Recuero, J.K., Binda, G., Kiszewski, A.E., 2019. Eosinophilic panniculitis associated with toxocariasis in a child. An. Bras. Dermatol. 94, 250–251.

Regis, S.C., Mendonça, L.R., Silva, N.S., Dattoli, V.C., Alcântara-Neves, N.M., Barrouin-Melo, S.M., 2011. Seroprevalence and risk factors for canine toxocariasis by detection of specific IgG as a marker of infection in dogs from Salvador, Brazil. Acta Trop. 120, 46–51.

Rehbein, S., Knaus, M., Mallouk, Y., Breiltgens, T., Brianti, E., Capári, B., Dantas-Torres, F., Gau, M., Joachim, A., Kaulfuß, K.H., Kirkova, Z., Lechner, J., Mihalca, A.D., Mirabito, R., Petkevičius, S., Rapti, D., Shukullari, E., Sedeilhan, M., Dollhofer, D., Kley, K., Lebon, W., Visser, M., Jeannin, P., 2017. Efficacy against nematode infections and safety of afoxolaner plus milbemycin oxime chewable tablets in domestic dogs under field conditions in Europe. Parasitol. Res. 116, 259–269.

Ribeiro, L.M., Dracz, R.M., Mozzer, L.R., Lima, W.S., 2013. Soil contamination in public squares in Belo Horizonte, Minas Gerais, by canine parasites in different developmental stages. Rev. Inst. Med. Trop. Sao Paulo 55, 229–231.

Rocha, S., Pinto, R.M., Floriano, A.P., Teixeira, L.H., Bassili, B., Martinez, A., Costa, S.O., Caseiro, M.M., 2011. Environmental analyses of the parasitic profile found in the sandy soil from the Santos municipality beaches, SP, Brazil. Rev. Inst. Med. Trop. Sao Paulo 53, 277–281.

Rubinsky-Elefant, G., Hirata, C.E., Yamamoto, J.H., Ferreira, M.U., 2010. Human toxocariasis: diagnosis, worldwide seroprevalences and clinical expression of the systemic and ocular forms. Ann. Trop. Med. Parasitol. 104, 3–23.

Salvador, S., Ribeiro, R., Winckler, M.I., Ohlweiler, L., Riesgo, R., 2010. Pediatric neurotoxocariasis with concomitant cerebral, cerebellar, and peripheral nervous system involvement: case report and review of the literature. J. Pediatr. 86, 531–534.

Santarém, V.A., Sartor, I.F., Bergamo, F.M., 1998. Contaminação, por ovos de *Toxocara* spp, de parques e praças públicas de Botucatu, São Paulo, Brasil. Rev. Soc. Bras. Med. Trop. 31, 529–532 [Article in Portuguese].

Santarém, V.A., Franco Eda, C., Kozuki, F.T., Fini, D., Prestes-Carneiro, L.E., 2008. Environmental contamination by *Toxocara* spp. eggs in a rural settlement in Brazil. Rev. Inst. Med. Trop. Sao Paulo 50, 279–281.

Santarém, V.A., Leli, F.N., Rubinsky-Elefant, G., Giuffrida, R., 2011. Protective and risk factors for toxocariasis in children from two different social classes of Brazil. Rev. Inst. Med. Trop. Sao Paulo 53, 66–72.

Santarém, V.A., Pereira, V.C., Alegre, B.C., 2012. Contamination of public parks in Presidente Prudente (São Paulo, Brazil) by *Toxocara* spp. eggs. Rev. Bras. Parasitol. Vet. 21, 323–325.

Santos, A.O., Costa, V.M., Alfani, R., Carneiro, M.P.M., Oliveira, M.V.S., 2008. Ocorrência de endoparasitas caninos e análise de amostras de solo de parques públicos na cidade de Brasília/DF. Rev. CFMV 44, 70–72 [Article in Portuguese].

Santos, J.L., Magalhães, N.B., Santos, H.A., Ribeiro, R.R., Guimarães, M.P., 2012. Parasites of domestic and wild canids in the region of Serra do Cipó National Park, Brazil. Rev. Bras. Parasitol. Vet. 21, 270–277.

Scaini, C.J., Toledo, R.N., Lovatel, R., Dionello, M.A., Gatti, F.A., Susin, L., Signorini, V.R., 2003. Contaminação ambiental por ovos e larvas de helmintos em fezes de cães na área central do Balneário Cassino, Rio Grande do Sul. Rev. Soc. Bras. Med. Trop. 36, 617–619 [Article in Portuguese].

Serra, C.M., Uchôa, C.M., Coimbra, R.A., 2003. Exame parasitológico de fezes de gatos (*Felis catus domesticus*) domiciliados e errantes da Região Metropolitana do Rio de Janeiro, Brasil. Rev. Soc. Bras. Med. Trop. 36, 331–334 [Article in Portuguese].

Sevá, A.D.P., Pena, H.F.J., Nava, A., Sousa, A.O., Holsback, L., Soares, R.M., 2018. Endoparasites in domestic animals surrounding an Atlantic Forest remnant, in São Paulo state, Brazil. Rev. Bras. Parasitol. Vet. 27, 13–19.

Sianto, L., Souza, M.V., Chame, M., Luz, M.F., Guidon, N., Pessis, A.M., Araújo, A., 2014. Helminths in feline coprolites up to 9000 years in the Brazilian northeast. Parasitol. Int. 63, 851–857.

Silva, H.C., Castagnolli, K.C., Silveira, D.M., Costa, G.H.N., Gomes, R.A., Nascimento, A.A., 2001. Fauna helmíntica de cães e gatos provenientes de alguns municípios do Estado de São Paulo. Semina: Ciênc. Agrár. 22, 67–71 [Article in Portuguese].

Silva, M.B., Amor, A.L., Santos, L.N., Galvão, A.A., Oviedo, V.A.Y., Silva, E.S., Barbosa, C.G., Cooper, P.J., Figueiredo, C.A., Ribeiro, R.C., Alcântara-Neves, N.M., 2016. Data on prevalence and risk factors associated with *Toxocara* spp infection, atopy and asthma development in northeast Brazilian school children. Data Brief 9, 425–428.

Silva, J.C.S., Costa, A.P., Praseres, D.C., Torres, M.A.O., Oliveira-Neta, M.D., Teófilo, T.S., 2017a. Endoparasitas em cães e gatos diagnosticados em São Luís—Maranhão. PUBVET 11, 587–595 [Article in Portuguese].

Silva, M.B., Amor, A.L.M., Santos, L.N., Galvão, A.A., Oviedo Vera, A.V., Silva, E.S., Barbosa, C.G., Gonçalves, M.S., Cooper, P.J., Figueiredo, C.A., Ribeiro, R.C., Alcântara-Neves, N.M., 2017b. Risk factors for *Toxocara* spp. seroprevalence and its association with atopy and asthma phenotypes in school-age children in a small town and semi-rural areas of northeast Brazil. Acta Trop. 174, 158–164.

Souza, R.F., Dattoli, V.C., Mendonça, L.R., Jesus, J.R., Baqueiro, T., Santana, C.C., Santos, N.M., Barrouin-Melo, S.M., Alcantara-Neves, N.M., 2011. Prevalência e fatores de risco da infecção humana por *Toxocara canis* em Salvador, Estado da Bahia. Rev. Soc. Bras. Med. Trop. 44, 516–519 [Article in Portuguese].

Souza, F.B., Nakiri, I.M., Lourenço, N.O., Silva, G.G., Paschoalini, D.R., Guimarães-Okamoto, P.T.C., Melchert, A., 2017. Prevalence of intestinal endoparasites with zoonotic potential in domestic cats from Botucatu, SP, Brazil. Top. Companion Anim. Med. 32, 114–117.

Sprenger, L.K., Green, K.T., Molento, M.B., 2014. Geohelminth contamination of public areas and epidemiological risk factors in Curitiba, Brazil. Rev. Bras. Parasitol. Vet. 23, 69–73.

Stalliviere, F.M., Bellato, V., Souza, A.P., Sartor, A.A., Moura, A.B., Rosa, L.D., 2009. Ectoparasitos e helmintos intestinais em *Felis catus domesticus*, da cidade de Lages, SC, Brasil e aspectos sócioeconômicos e culturais das famílias dos proprietários dos animais. Rev. Bras. Parasitol. Vet. 18, 26–31 [Article in Portuguese].

Strube, C., Heuer, L., Janecek, E., 2013. *Toxocara* spp. infections in paratenic hosts. Vet. Parasitol. 193, 375–389.

Taira, K., Saitoh, Y., Kapel, C.M., 2011. *Toxocara cati* larvae persist and retain high infectivity in muscles of experimentally infected chickens. Vet. Parasitol. 180, 287–291.

Teixeira, C.R., Chieffi, P.P., Lescano, S.A., Silva, E.O.M., Fux, B., Cury, M.C., 2006. Frequency and risk factors for toxocariasis in children from a pediatric outpatient center in southeastern Brazil. Rev. Inst. Med. Trop. Sao Paulo 48, 251–255.

Tesserolli, G.L., Fayzano, L., Agottani, J.V.B., 2005. Ocorrência de parasitas gastrintestinais em fezes de cães e gatos, Curitiba-PR. Rev. Acad. 3, 31–34 [Article in Portuguese].

Tiyo, R., Guedes, T.A., Falavigna, D.L., Falavigna-Guilherme, A.L., 2008. Seasonal contamination of public squares and lawns by parasites with zoonotic potential in southern Brazil. J. Helminthol. 82, 1–6.

Vasconcellos, M.C., Barros, J.S.L., Oliveira, C.S., 2006. Parasitas gastrointestinais em cães institucionalizados no Rio de Janeiro, RJ. Rev. Saúde Pública 40, 321–323 [Article in Portuguese].

Vasconcelos-Santos, D.V., Oréfice, F., Fonseca, C.F., Alencar, L.M., Almeida, P.J., Lenzi, H.L., Pelajo-Machado, M., Volkmer-Ribeiro, C., Batista, T.C., Chieffi, P.P., Lescano, S.Z., Caldeira, R.L., Carvalho, O.S., Pavesio, C.E., 2010. Epidemic of unilateral panuveitis in children from Brazilian Amazonia: clinical and etiological aspects in seven patients. Int. Ophthalmol. 30, 113–125.

Vieira, F.M., Luque, J.L., Muniz-Pereira, L.C., 2008. Checklist of helminth parasites in wild carnivore mammals from Brazil. Zootaxa 1721, 1–23.

Viola, G.R., Giacomin, M.F., França, C.M., Sallum, A.M., Jacob, C.M., Silva, C.A., 2016. Chronic polyarthritis as isolated manifestation of toxocariasis. Rev. Bras. Reumatol. Engl. Ed. 56, 185–187.

Wright, I., Stafford, K., Coles, G., 2016. The prevalence of intestinal nematodes in cats and dogs from Lancashire, north-west England. J. Small Anim. Pract. 57, 393–395.

Zago Filho, H., Barreto, M.P., 1957. Estudo sobre a prevalência e intensidade de infestação por helmintos intestinalis em cães e gatos de Ribeirão Preto, SP. Rev. Bras. Malariol. Doencas Trop. 9, 295–304 [Article in Portuguese].

CHAPTER THIRTY-FOUR

Prevalence of *Toxocara* spp. in dogs and cats in South America (excluding Brazil)

Sara López-Osorio, Felipe Penagos-Tabares, Jenny Jovana Chaparro-Gutiérrez*

CIBAV Research Group, Medicine Veterinary School, Agrarian Sciences Faculty, University of Antioquia, Medellín, Colombia

*Corresponding author: e-mail address: jenny.chaparro@udea.edu.co

Contents

Abstract

Toxocariasis is a worldwide anthropozoonosis caused by *Toxocara* spp. nematodes. High prevalences of the disease has been found in developing countries, particularly in regions with poor sanitary conditions. The definitive hosts of the nematodes are dogs and cats, which play a vital role in the transmission of this parasite as humans are considered a paratenic host. The epidemiology of the disease in South America is not clear as it is usually not diagnosed and is not a notifiable disease. This review summarizes information regarding prevalence reports of *Toxocara* spp. in dog and cats in South America (excluding Brazil). Additionally, and in accordance with the one health approach, reports of contaminated soil in public zones and parks as well as infection/prevalence reports in wildlife species by geographical regions are also included. The findings show the importance of awareness among veterinarians and public health authorities about *Toxocara* spp. as neglected disease.

Advances in Parasitology, Volume 109
ISSN 0065-308X
https://doi.org/10.1016/bs.apar.2020.01.029

1. Introduction

Dogs and cats play an essential role in the transmission of *Toxocara canis* and *Toxocara cati*. Both parasites have a worldwide distribution, being considered endemic in most of the Americas (Bolivar-Mejia et al., 2014; Delgado and Rodriguez-morales, 2009). *Toxocara* spp. infection has been reported in human as well as in definitive hosts such as domestic and/or wild canids/felids in most South American countries (Table 1), suggesting an endemic presence of the parasite in the continent. Typically, the health impact of this parasitosis on definitive hosts is unknown as it tends to be subclinical. Similarly, actual disease occurrence in humans and the role of domestic and wild canid/felid populations in the dissemination of toxocariasis in humans is speculative at best. This review summarizes the currently available data on the epidemiological situation of *Toxocara* spp. infections in dogs, cats and wildlife animals in South America (Fig. 1). Given that this parasite is endemic in several countries of this continent and can be transmitted to humans, it should be considered as a threat to human health. Hereby, we encourage veterinarians to start investigations on these parasites to determine the real importance of the infection and the potential impact on public health.

1.1 Population of dogs and cats in South America

Despite the fact that canine and feline ownership is a controversial but commonly cited risk factor for human toxocariasis, over half of people worldwide have at least one pet living with them, with dogs being the most popular in Latin America (Martin, 2016). Infected cats and dogs pass eggs in faeces, which can contaminate their environment and be a source of infection to humans (Global Health—Division of Parasitic Diseases and Malaria, 2013). In fact, environmental contamination by infected animals is considered the most important risk factor (Lee et al., 2014), which means that even in the absence of a pet in a household, environmental exposure can pose a risk of infection.

In South America, Argentina has the highest population of pet dogs. The number is thought to be above 6.5 million, followed by Colombia with an estimated population of about 5 million (Atitwa, 2018). Nevertheless, data on the number of pet dogs in South America is generally unknown because many dogs are unregistered and there is a lack of national studies on demographics of dog populations. As expected, an increase in the canine

Table 1 Reports of *Toxocara canis* in dogs and wildlife canids in South American countries (excluding Brazil).

Country	Location	Time period	Host	Prevalence	Diagnostic method	References
Argentina	La Plata City	N/A	Dogs	28.9% (1445/5000 anonymous faecal samples)	Coprology—N/A	Martinez et al. (1973)
	La Plata City	N/A	Dogs	10.5% (37/351 pooled faecal samples from streets and parks)	Coprology—N/A	Minvielle et al. (1993)
	Bahía Blanca	1994–1995	Dogs	7% (10/150 faecal samples from the public street)	Coprology—Ritchie's technique	Costamagna et al. (2002)
	Buenos Aires	August 1999	Dogs	9% (5/53) in middle-income neighbourhood (MIN) 19% (10/52) in low-income neighbourhood (LIN) Serological prevalences: 22% (2/9) in MIN 40% (15/37) in LIN	Coprology—modified version of Teleman's concentration–sedimentation formalin/ether method Serology—ELISA	Rubel et al. (2003)
	Mar del Plata	July–September 2001	Dogs	6.67% (1/77 dog faeces samples of public squares from the central zone of the city) 28.2% (11/48 dog faeces samples of public squares from the peripheral zones of the city)	Coprology—Willis Flotation-Sedimentation	Andresiuk et al. (2003)

Continued

Table 1 Reports of *Toxocara canis* in dogs and wildlife canids in South American countries (excluding Brazil).—Cont'd

Country	Location	Time period	Host	Prevalence	Diagnostic method	References
	Corrientes	March 1999–February 2002	Dogs	61.10% (550/900)	Coprology—3 flotation techniques: Willis (with NaCl supersaturated solution), Sheater (with sugar supersaturated solution) and Faust (with zinc sulphate at a density of 1.18–1.20)	Marder et al. (2004)
	Buenos Aires	2003–2004	Dogs	11% (241/2193 anonymous faecal samples)	Coprology—flotation–centrifugation	Fontanarrosa et al. (2006)
	La Plata City	2006	Dogs	General positivity: 42% (105/250) Positivity in ownerless dogs: 51.2% (64/125) Positivity in dogs with owner: 32.8% (41/125)	Coprology—Fülleborn's technique	Radman et al. (2006)
	Neuquén		Dogs (from urban and rural zones)	16.35% (326/1944)	Coprology—flotation and sedimentation conventional methods	Soriano et al. (2010)

	Corrientes	2012	Dogs	86.95% (40/46)	Serology—ELISA	García et al. (2012)
	Corrientes	March–December 2012	Dogs	84.9% (101/119)	Serology—ELISA	García et al. (2014)
	Esperanza	March–December 2012	Dogs	51.2% (42/82)	Serology—ELISA	García et al. (2014)
	Bariloche	2013	Dogs	Neighbourhood Virgen Misionera: 22% (2/9) Neighbourhood Vivero: 33% (3/9) Neighbourhood Los Coihues: 11% (1/9)	Coprology—Telemann's sedimentation and Sheather's flotation techniques	Semenas et al. (2014)
	Santa Fe (La Capital, Castellanos, Garay, Cayastacito, Esperanza), Buenos Aires (Campos del tuyú), Córdoba (PN Quebrada del Condorito)	N/A	Pampas fox (*Lycalopex gymnocercus*)	50%	Coprology—a sedimentation-flotation technique	Moleón et al. (2015)
Bolivia	Santa Cruz de la Sierra	May–October 2004	Dogs	31.44% (104/312)	Coprology—Modified Willis's Flotation Technique	Vega et al. (2006)
	Coroico	2009	Dogs	During dry season: 30.3% (30/98) During wet season: 41.7% (40/98)	Coprology—Willis-Molloy's flotation simple technique with a solution oversaturated of sodium chloride	Llanos et al. (2010)

Continued

Table 1 Reports of *Toxocara canis* in dogs and wildlife canids in South American countries (excluding Brazil).—Cont'd

Country	Location	Time period	Host	Prevalence	Diagnostic method	References
Colombia	Bogotá	July 1987–July 1988	Dogs (Puppies (1–4 months) from a poor neighbourhood)	43.6% (17/39)	Coprology—Ritchie–Frick's concentration technique	Agudelo et al. (1990)
	Medellín	1998	Dogs	12% (30/250)	Coprology	Cañas et al. (1998)
	Popayán		Dogs	4.3% (16/372)	Ritchie–Frick's concentration technique	Vásquez et al. (2005)
	Quindio	2003	Dogs	2.5% (8/324)	Coprology—Ritchie–Frick's concentration technique	Giraldo et al. (2005)
	Bogotá	2013	Dogs (pooled faecal samples from an animal shelter)	7.1% (5/70)	Coprology—direct faecal smears and flotation technique with saturated saline solution	Paredes et al. (2013)
	Bogotá	2000	Dogs	9.6%	Coprology	Cabrera et al. (2003)

	Huila	2003	Dogs	13.6% (83/610)	Coprology	Penagos et al. (2004)
	Envigado	2007	Dogs	7.48% (14/187)	Coprology—Sheather's flotation method	Guzmán et al. (2007)
	Ibague	2014	Dogs	6.72% (8/119)	Coprology—direct faecal smears	Gutiérrez et al. (2014)
	Coyaima	February 2011–March 2013	Dogs	8.6% (15/175)	Coprology—Formaldehyde/ether concentration technique	González and Giraldo (2015)
	Medellín and Eastern Antioquia	April 2014–October 2014	Dogs (from two animal welfare centers)	11.8% (8/68)	Coprology—Sheather's flotation method	Sierra-Cifuentes et al. (2015)
	Bogotá	N/A	Dogs	2% (4/199)	Coprology—Ritchie–Frick concentration technique	Fernandez et al. (2015)
	Caldas, Antioquia	N/A	Dogs	4% (4/97)	Coprology—the saline flotation techniques.	Posada (2014)

Continued

Table 1 Reports of *Toxocara canis* in dogs and wildlife canids in South American countries (excluding Brazil).—Cont'd

Country	Location	Time period	Host	Prevalence	Diagnostic method	References
	Barranquilla	2014–2015	Dogs	12.4% (116/925)	Coprology—flotation technique with saturated saline solution	Sarmiento-Rubiano et al. (2018)
	Medellín	2016	Dogs	0.9% (10/1073)	Coprology—flotation technique with saturated saline solution	Castrillón Salazar et al. (2018)
Chile	Valdivia	March–December 1971	Dogs	13.5% (8/59)	Coprology—modified Telemann's and flotation technique	Torres et al. (1974)
	Santiago City	July–September 1999	Dogs (dog faecal specimens from public places)	13.5% (288/39)	Coprology—modified Telemann's technique	Castillo et al. (2000)
	Santiago	1996–2003	Dogs	11% (101/920 s)	Coprology—Burrows' technique	Lopez et al. (2006)
	Santiago	N/A	Dogs	9.1% (53/582)	Coprology—Zinc flotation method, modified Teleman method and staining of faecal smears with Ziehl–Neelsen	Gorman et al. (2006)

Ecuador	Quito	2015	Dogs (from animal shelters)	24% (30/125)	Coprology—Sheather's flotation method	Suntaxi (2015)
	Ambato City	N/A	Dogs	32.37% (45/139) by spontaneous sedimentation 21.58% (30/139) by Parodi-Alcaraz flotation method	Coprology—Spontaneous sedimentation and Parodi-Alcaraz flotation method	Córdova and Marisol (2015)
	Cuenca City	N/A	Dogs	7.86% (22/280)	Coprology—flotation technique	Sinchi and Dario (2018)
French Guyana (France)		N/A				
Guyana		N/A				
Paraguay				N/A		
Peru	Lima	N/A	Dogs	40% (20/50)	Coprology—N/A	Reyes et al. (1999)
	Chincha Alta	N/A	Dogs	47%	Corpology—N/A	Dávalos et al. (2000)
	Lurigancho	N/A	Dogs	27.7%	Coprology—N/A	García (2001)

Continued

Table 1 Reports of *Toxocara canis* in dogs and wildlife canids in South American countries (excluding Brazil).—Cont'd

Country	Location	Time period	Host	Prevalence	Diagnostic method	References
	Ica	2001	Dogs	19.75% (32/162)	Coprology—Faust Concentration and Spontaneous Sedimentation in Test Tube	Trillo-Altamirano et al. (2003)
	Puno	N/A	Dogs	49.3% (74/150)	Coprology—flotation concentration technique with 33% zinc sulphate solution	de Díaz and Anccasi (2013)
	Lima	2008	Dogs	20.6% (27/131)	Coprology—Spontaneous sedimentation technique in tube	Mocetti et al. (2011)
	Province of Puno		Dogs	49.3% (74/150)	Coprology—simple direct and flotation concentration in zinc sulphate solution at 33.3%	de Díaz and Anccasi (2013)
	Lima	N/A	Dogs (faecal samples taken from surgical patients)	25% (3/12)	Coprology—flotation with saturated saline solution	Villaseca and Socorro (2014)

	Pataz's district, La Libertad region	2016	Dogs	11.6% (19/164)	Coprology—direct and concentration by flotation	Aguilar and Giaminna (2017)
	Province of Puno	December 2011–February 2012	Dogs (Puppies:1–4 months old)	33.1% (51/172)	Coprology—flotation concentration technique with 33% zinc sulphate solution	Añamuro et al. (2019)
Suriname				N/A		
Venezuela	Maracaibo	2001	Dogs	11.4% (70/614)	Coprology—Flotation method	Ramírez-Barrios et al. (2004)
Uruguay	Montevideo and Florida	N/A	Dogs	Total: 26.2% (25/95) In Montevideo (Urban): 30.0% In Florida (Urban): 66.7% In Florida (Rural): 55.4%	Necropsy	Valledor et al. (2006)

N/A, not applicable.

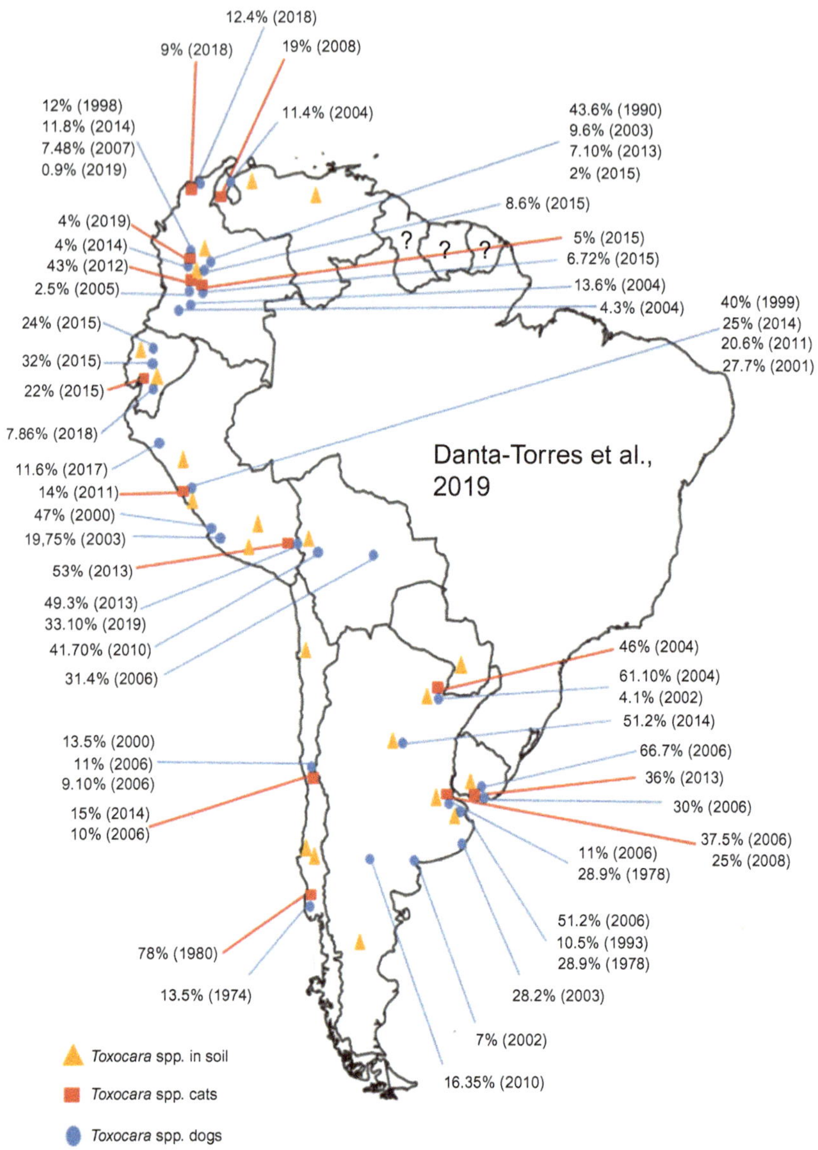

Fig. 1 Distribution of *Toxocara* spp. in dogs, cats and soil from South America. Blue circle: prevalence of *Toxocara canis* dogs. Red square: Prevalence of *Toxocara cati* in cats. Yellow triangle: reports of *Toxocara* spp. in soil.

population would lead to an increase in the interaction between men and dogs, and so increase the risk of disease transmission (Beck, 1975). Furthermore, a change in population dynamics that can also impact public health is the increase of large breed dogs motivated by the fear of urban crime, and the protection that big dogs may provide to their owners (Beck, 1975). The increase in big dog leads to increased stool production. A large breed dog can excrete on average 340 g of faeces per day, and for a city with an estimated population of 500,000 dogs and with no habit of collecting faeces by their owners, there will be approximately 170 tons of excrement per day. Such faecal contamination becomes a public health hazard (Beck, 1975; Salamanca et al., 2011).

On the other hand, cats are less popular pets in Latin and South America. Nevertheless, the trend indicates that cats will be more popular in the future because of the increase in urbanization. Cats are more suited to smaller living spaces than dogs and require less attention, making them less time-consuming (Kurzweil, 2018). Colombia has approximately 1.5 million of cats. Furthermore, in rural areas, cats tend to be allowed to roam freely inside and outside the house. Contact with other cats is common, leading to the risk of pregnancy, fighting and dissemination of diseases.

Apart from the domestic cat, there are at least nine different species of small wild cats and two big wild cats distributed in central and South America (International Society for Endangered Cats (ISEC) Canada). Many of these wild cats are in the IUCN Red List of Threatened Animals as endangered and vulnerable.

Fig. 2 and Table 1 review all the studies on the prevalence of *Toxocara canis* in dogs throughout South American countries with ranges from 0.9% to 61.10% using coprological techniques (Marder et al., 2004, Castrillón Salazar et al., 2018). Similarly, the prevalence of *Toxocara cati* in cat's ranges from 4% to 78% (Fig. 3 and Table 2), (Castrillón Salazar et al., 2018, Bonilla, 1980) while in wild cats the studies reported 16.6–100% of positive faecal samples (Fiorello et al., 2006, Moleón et al., 2015). Next, we summarize the information with regards to the infection in dogs and cats by countries in South America and discuss its impact on public health.

1.2 *Toxocara* spp. in *Argentina*

Argentina has the major number of studies on *Toxocara* spp. in dogs, and its prevalence is quite variable depending on the region and study (Table 1). Approximately 80% of people in Argentina have at least one pet in their home, mostly dogs. This makes Argentina the country with the most pets per capita in the world (Cantó, 2018). The infection by *Toxocara canis* in humans has been studied and described in large cities, where it has been associated with the poor management of the pets' faeces

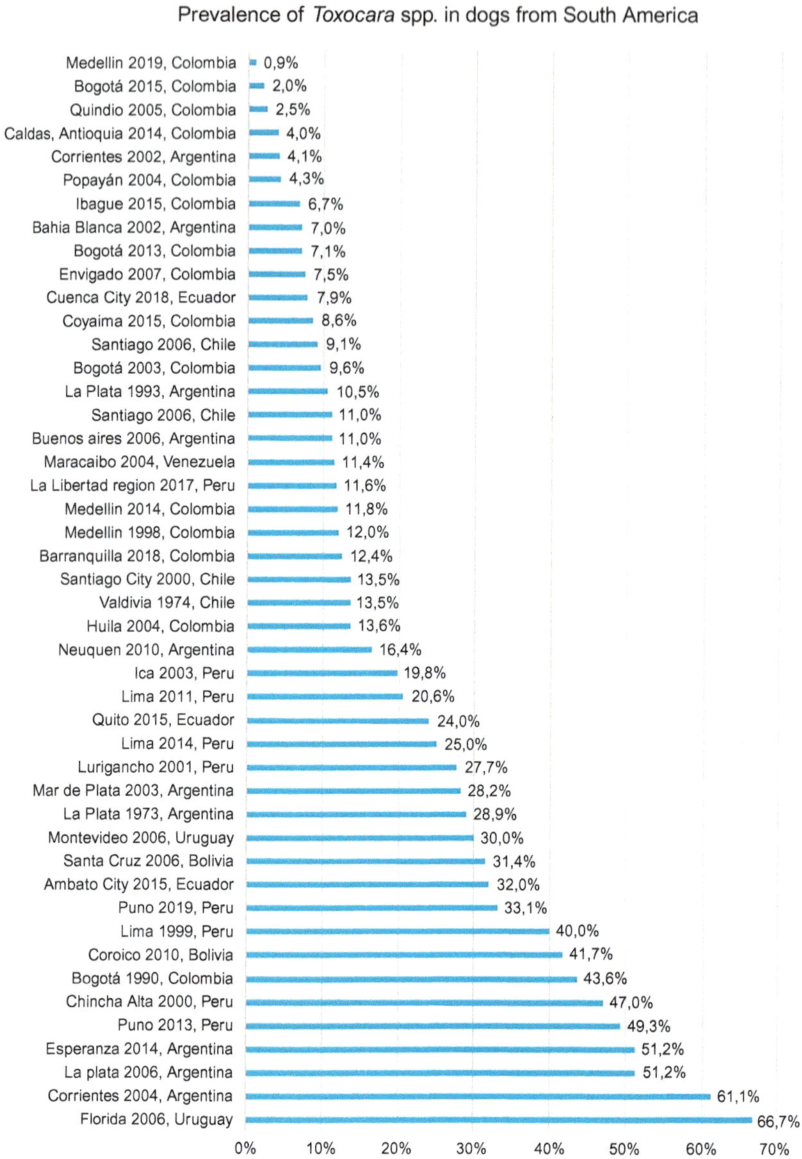

Fig. 2 Prevalence of *T. canis* in domestic dogs in South America. The results are presented from lowest to highest prevalence. Year and country are indicated. All the results are from coprology techniques.

(Kuruc et al., 1995). Reports in different cities across Argentina show the presence of *T. canis* in faeces from dogs to be between 7% and 61.10% (Fig. 2). In 1973, the first large study in La Plata city, revealed a prevalence of 28.9% (1445/5000) of *Toxocara canis*, which in 2006 increased

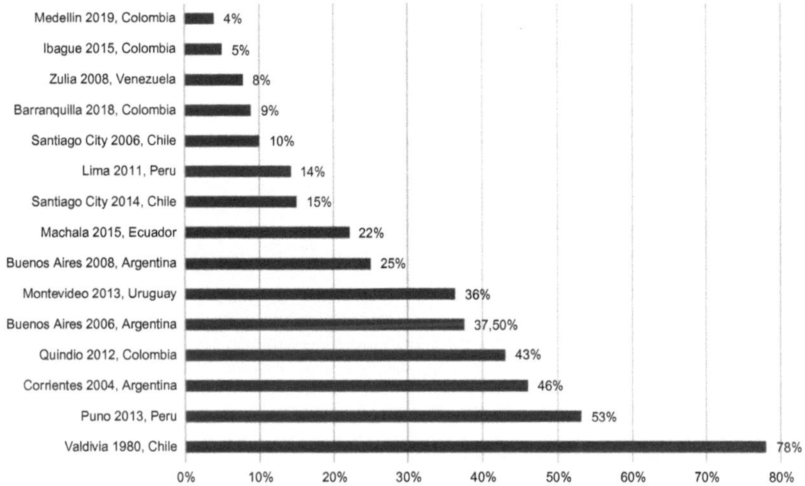

Fig. 3 Prevalence of *Toxocara* spp. in domestic and wild cats from South America. The results are presented from lowest to highest prevalence. Year and country are indicated. All the results are from coprology techniques.

to 42% (105/250) in the same area and using similar methodology (Martinez et al., 1973; Radman et al., 2006). This high prevalence in 2006 was due to the inclusion of animals that were at a greater risk to have the parasite in the sample (no owner, less than 1 year of age). Radman et al. found that stray dogs had a higher prevalence of the infection (51.2%) than dogs with owners (32.8%) in la Plata, Argentina (Radman et al., 2006). On the other hand, Rubel et al. (2003) found a greater prevalence of infection in dogs from low income neighbourhoods (19%), compared with middle income neighbourhood (9%) (Rubel et al., 2003). In addition, another study that evaluated the seroprevalence of *T. canis* in rural dogs in Corrientes, Argentina, showed seroconversion in 80% dogs less than 1 year of age, 94.4% in dogs between 1 and 3 years, and 84.6% in dogs with more than 3 years of age (García et al., 2012), suggesting that coprological techniques may underestimate the real prevalence of the infection (García et al., 2012).

In cats, fewer studies have been published. In 2004, a prevalence of 46% was reported in home cats, and another study in stray cats reported a prevalence of 37.5% in 2006, both using flotation techniques (Marder et al., 2004; Sommerfelt et al., 2006). Cardillo et al. (2008) compared two techniques for *Toxocara* spp. diagnosis in 12 dead cats found on streets. Interestingly, only 3/12 cats were infected by *Toxocara cati* by coprology, whereas 6/12 were positive by artificial digestion of the muscle (Table 2, Fig. 3), revealing that

Table 2 Reports on prevalences of *Toxocara* spp. in felids in South American countries (excluding Brazil).

Country	Region	Period	Prevalence	Diagnostic method	References
Argentina	Corrientes	March 1999–February 2002	Cats 46% (207/450)	Coprology—three flotation techniques: Willis (with NaCl supersaturated solution), Sheater (with sugar supersaturated solution) and Faust (with zinc sulphate at a density of 1.18–1.20)	Marder et al. (2004)
	Monte desert (Lihué Calel National Park, Central Argentina)	N/A	Geoffroy's cat (*Oncifelis geoffroyi*) 85.7% (6/7)	Coprology—a sedimentation-flotation technique.	Beldomenico et al. (2005)
	Buenos Aires	March–June 2005	Cats (faeces from stray cats collected from the open spaces) 37.5% (166/465)	Coprology—flotation technique in saturated sugar solution (ð = 1200–1300) with centrifugation at 1500 rpm during 3 min	Sommerfelt et al. (2006)
	Buenos Aires	N/A	Cats (found dead in the street) 25% (3/12) by coprology 50% (6/12) by necropsy—artificial digestion	Coprology: flotation technique with Benbrook saturated sugar solution Necropsy: macroscopic evaluation and rapid artificial digestion technique (muscle, the lungs, kidneys, liver, mammary gland and brain)	Cardillo et al. (2008)

	La Pampa (PN Lihué Calel, Doblas), Bs.As (Alberti, Berazategui), Entre Ríos (Paraná), Santa Fe (Garay, La Capital)	N/A	Geoffroy's cat (*Lecpardus geoffroyi*) (39%)	Coprology—a sedimentation-flotation technique	Moleón et al. (2015)
	Chubut (PN Los Alerces), Neuquén (PN Lanin)	N/A	kodkod (*Leopardus guigna*) (100%)	Coprology—a sedimentation-flotation technique	Moleón et al. (2015)
	Córdoba (PN Quebrada del Condorito) Santa Cruz (PN Los Glaciares)	N/A	Cougar (*Puma concclor*) (67%)	Coprology—a sedimentation-flotation technique	Moleón et al. (2015)
Bolivia	Tierra Comunitaria de Origen (Bolivian Chaco)	2001–2003	Ocelot (*Leopardus pardalis*) 16.6% (1/6)	Coprology—standard centrifugation concentration flotation techniques with both zinc sulphate and sugar as the flotation media	Fiorello et al. (2006)
Colombia	Department of Quindio	2008	Cats 37.2% (45/121) by Ritchie 43% (52/121) by Kato-Katz	Coprology—modified Ritchie and modified Kato-Katz techniques	Echeverry et al. (2012)
	Ibague, Department of Tolima		Cats 5% (1/20)	Coprology—direct faecal smears	Gutiérrez et al. (2014)

Continued

Table 2 Reports on prevalences of *Toxocara* spp. in felids in South American countries (excluding Brazil).—Cont'd

Country	Region	Period	Prevalence	Diagnostic method	References
	Barranquilla	2014–2015	Cats 8.9% (4/45)	Coprology—flotation technique with saturated saline solution	Sarmiento-Rubiano et al. (2018)
	Medellin, Department of Antioquia	2016	Cats 4.0% (17/428)	Coprology—flotation technique with saturated saline solution (described by Koffoyd and Barber, cited by Restrepo, 1983)	Castrillón Salazar et al. (2018)
Chile	Valdivia	N/A	Cats 78% (39/50)	Coprology—N/A	Bonilla (1980)
	Santiago City	1996–2003	Cats 10% (23/230)	Coprology—Burrows' technique	Lopez et al. (2006)
	Santiago City	April 2009–May 2011	Cats 15% (45/300)	Coprology—modified Telemann's technique	García-Soto (2014)
Ecuador	Machala	November 2014–March 2015	Cats 22.13% (81/366)	Coprology: Faust method	Morales-Rambay (2015)
French Guyana			N/A		

Guyana			N/A		
Paraguay			N/A		
Peru	Lima	2008	Cats 14.3% (7/49)	Coprology—Spontaneous sedimentation technique in tube	Mocetti et al. (2011)
	Puno	N/A	Cats 53.13% (49/96)	Coprology—flotation concentration technique with 33% zinc sulphate solution	de Díaz and Anccasi (2013)
Suriname			N/A		
Venezuela	Zulia	2004	Cats 7.8% (5/64)	Coprology—flotation with saturated saline solution	Ramírez-Barrios et al. (2008)
Uruguay	Montevideo	N/A	Cats 36.36% (8/22)	Necropsy—Coprology	Castro et al. (2013)

coprology underestimates the infection rate when the infection with the parasite is not patent (Deplazes et al., 2016). Nevertheless, specifications of the flotation test for finding *Toxocara* eggs in faeces were calculated as 51% for the specificity and a sensitivity of 100%, using solution with specific gravity of at least 1.18 (M Overgaauw, and Nederland, 1997).

Toxocara spp. has been also found in wild animals from Argentina. Beldomenico et al. (2005) found *Toxocara* spp. in 6/7 (85.7%) Geoffroy's cat (*Oncifelis geoffroyi*) (Beldomenico et al., 2005). *Toxocara cati* was also found in 2015 in Geoffroy's cats (*Leopardus geoffroyi*, 39%), Kodkods (*Leopardus guigna*, 100%), and Cougars (*Puma concolor*, 67%) (Moleón et al., 2015). There are six species of Felidae recognized in Patagonia: *P. concolor*, *L. geoffroyi*, *L. guigna*, *L. colocolo*, *Leopardus jacobita*, and *H. yagouaroundi* (Chebez et al., 2014). The first three are potential hosts for *T. cati*, but for the other species no parasite studies are available. Finally, *Toxocara canis* has been reported in Pampa's foxes (*Lycalopex gymnocercus*, 50%) (Moleón et al., 2015) (Tables 1 and 2).

1.3 *Toxocara* spp. *Bolivia*

To our knowledge, there are few studies about *Toxocara* spp. prevalence in Bolivia. The estimated prevalence of *Toxocara canis* infections in Bolivian dogs varies from 30.3% to 41.7% (Table 1) (Llanos et al., 2010). Llanos et al. found that the prevalence during the wet season (41.7%) was higher than in the dry season (30.3%) in dogs from urban areas from Corpico, La Paz (Llanos et al., 2010). Additionally, in faeces collected from public parks in El Alto, the prevalence of the parasite was 6.22% in Poma et al. (2018), with at least one egg of a *Toxocara* sp. in 80% of the different zones evaluated (Poma et al., 2018). The only report of *Toxocara* sp. in felids, was in 2006, where 16.6% (1/6) of Ocelots (*Leopardus pardalis*) were positive by coprological techniques (Fiorello et al., 2006) (Table 2).

1.4 *Toxocara* spp. in *Colombia*

The prevalence of *T. canis* in different Colombian cities ranges from 0.9% to 43.6% (Agudelo et al., 1990; Castrillón Salazar et al., 2018). The higher prevalence was found in Bogotá, in puppies from a poor neighbourhood (43.6%) (Agudelo et al., 1990). In Medellín, the prevalence in stray dogs from two shelters was 11.68% (Sierra-Cifuentes et al., 2015), while in dogs with owners, it was 0.9% (Castrillón Salazar et al., 2018). In cats, the prevalence in the same study was 4%. Echeverry et al., 2012 compared

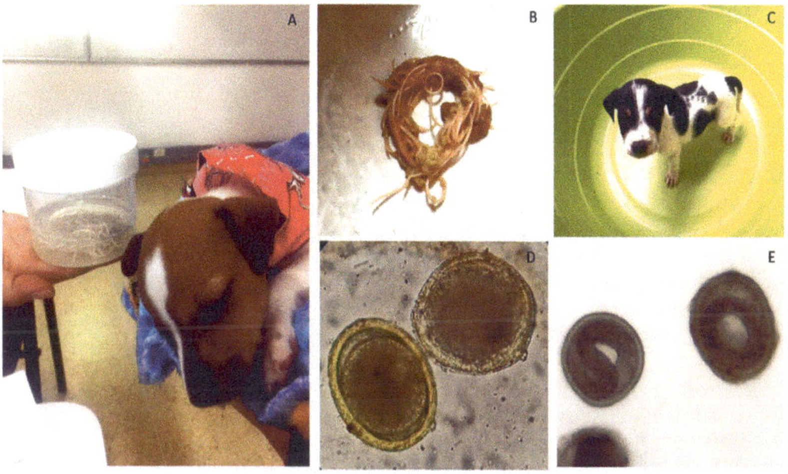

Fig. 4 Excretion of nematodes after first deworming in puppies from rural areas in Colombia. (A) Female puppy and a flask with the specimens of *T. canis* collected after deworming. (B) Faeces with a high burden of adults *T canis* from (C) a 5 weeks old puppy with presence. (D) *Toxocara canis* egg. Magnification 400×. Flotation technique. (E) *Toxocara canis* embryonated egg with larvae 3. Magnification 100×. Flotation technique.

two different coprological techniques in faeces from cats and found 37.2% by Ritchie technique (sedimentation), and 43% with Kato Katz (thick smear) (Echeverry et al., 2012). Most studies in Colombia took place in large cities, so there is little to no epidemiological information from rural areas. Anecdotal cases from veterinarians indicate that puppies from rural areas normally excrete dozens of parasites after the first deworming (Fig. 4). At present, there are no studies about risk factors associated with the presence of the parasite in this country, and in most of the studies the finding of *Toxocara* spp. was incidental.

1.5 *Toxocara* spp. in *Chile*

Toxocara spp. infections has been studied in some of Chilean cities and regions, where the frequency ranges from 15% to 78% in cats (Bonilla, 1980; García-Soto, 2014) and from 9.1% to 13.5% in dogs (Castillo et al., 2000; Gorman et al., 2006) (Fig. 2). In these studies samples from dogs were collected mostly from public parks (Table 1). Nevertheless, as in most of the countries in Latin America, extensive and updated data on real prevalence of *Toxocara* spp. infections in canine and feline populations are lacking.

1.6 *Toxocara* spp. in *Ecuador*

A few studies have been reported in Ecuador during the last decade. In Quito (2015), the prevalence of *T. canis* was 24% by flotation techniques (Suntaxi, 2015). By contrast, Tuasa Córdova (2015) found that with the sedimentation technique the frequency was higher than with flotation techniques (32.37% vs 21.58%) in Ambato City (Tuasa Córdova, 2015) (Table 1, Fig. 2). In cats, the infection was estimated at 22.13% in faeces (Morales-Rambay, 2015) (Table 2).

1.7 *Toxocara* spp. in *Perú*

The epidemiological status of *Toxocara* spp. in dog and cats from Peru is scarce. The prevalence is reported from 11.6% to 47% (Aguilar and Giaminna, 2017; Dávalos et al., 2000), and in puppies (1–4 months) 33.1% (Añamuro et al., 2019) (Table 1). In cats, the frequency of infection detected by coprology was reported in 14.3%, in 2011 (sedimentation) and 53.13% in 2013 (Flotation) (Mocetti et al., 2011, de Díaz and Anccasi, 2013) (Table 2).

1.8 *Toxocara* spp. in *Venezuela*

The current data available in Venezuela is scarce, the two existing reports are from the city of Maracaibo, where the prevalence of *T. canis* in dogs in 2001 was 11.4% (70/614) (Ramírez-Barrios et al., 2004) (Table 1) and the prevalence of *T. cati* in cats in 2004 was 7.8% (5/64) (Ramírez-Barrios et al., 2008) (Table 2).

1.9 *Toxocara* spp. in French Guyana, Guyana, Paraguay and Suriname

To our knowledge, no reports on the prevalence of *Toxocara* spp. in domestic and wild canids and felids populations in these countries were reported. Since the evident endemic status of the parasite in all the South American region, the epidemiological survey on populations of domestic and wild definitive hosts of *Toxocara* spp. is an essential tool to determinate the impact and risk of toxocariasis in their territories.

1.10 Prevalence of *Toxocara* spp. in soil

An epidemiological risk factor that should be considered for the infection in definitive and paratenic host is the contamination of the environment with *Toxocara* eggs. The daily egg production for *T. canis* is approximately 25,000–85,000, and infested puppies can shed >100,000 eggs/g of faeces, causing intense environmental contamination (Deplazes et al., 2016). Furthermore, infected dogs and wild dogs contribute to the spread of the eggs in rural and urban areas, which includes agricultural areas, beaches, playground, public parks and gardens. *Toxocara* eggs are not infectious when shed in the faeces of dogs and cats into the environment. Within a period of between 3 and 6 weeks to several months, depending on soil type and climatic conditions such as temperature and humidity, eggs will develop to an infectious stage that can survive under optimal circumstances for at least 1 year (Overgaauw, 1997). The prevalence of *Toxocara* spp. in soil samples from South America is shown in Table 3. Interestedly, just one study reported 0% presence of *Toxocara* spp. in soil, but it was in an arid zone from Argentina (Bojanich et al., 2015), while more than 25 studies reported the presence of *Toxocara* spp. in up to 90% of the parks or public places evaluated. Alonso et al. (2006) found in Resistencia City, Provincia del Chaco, Argentina, that 61.5% of the eggs in the soil were embryonated. The presence of the eggs in the soil changes according to the zones evaluated and season. Sánchez et al. (2003) found the highest presence of *Toxocara* spp. during the spring (20.9%) versus the winter (12.7%) in faeces of dogs collected from public parks in Argentina. In Uruguay, Hernández et al. (2003) found 52.9% of the parks contaminated (Hernández et al., 2003), similar to what Canese et al. (2003) found in Paraguay (53%) (Canese et al., 2003), but different to what Poma et al. (2018) found in Bolivia (60%) (Poma and Sirpa, 2018). In Bogotá–Colombia, the prevalence of *Toxocara* spp. eggs in soil is reported from 2.67% to 5.4% (Mosquera-Pardo, 2014; Polo-Terán et al., 2007), while in a rural area, Duitama-Boyacá, was reported to be 34.7% (Guarín-Patarroyo et al., 2016). Similar prevalence was found in Quito, Ecuador (33%) (Latorre and Nápoles, 2014). The highest prevalence of *Toxocara* spp. in soil/faeces in public parks was reported in Perú, in Huanuco (90.9%) (Montalvo-Sabino et al., 2014) and Ayacucho (90%) (Cruz et al., 2017; Frisancho Silva, 2016) using flotation techniques.

The presence of *Toxocara* spp. eggs found in the soils of public parks is an environmental indicator of a high presence of infected animals and a source of contamination to human, especially children (Alonso et al., 2006). It is necessary to call the attention of the agencies in charge of the administration of the parks so they take the appropriate control measures on handling the pets and their faeces in recreational spaces. Additionally, decreases in contamination can be achieved by cleaning up faeces from soil by dog owners, preventing access of dogs and cats to public places (especially children's playgrounds) and by use of strategic anthelmintic treatment of dogs and cats (M Overgaauw and Nederland, 1997).

Table 3 Reports of soil contamination of public places and parks with eggs of *Toxocara* spp. in South American countries (excluding Brazil).

Country	Region	Period	Prevalence of contamination	Diagnostic method	References
Argentina	La Plata	N/A	13.2% of soil samples (32/242) 68.2% of squares and parks (15/22)	flotation with sugar solution	Fonrouge et al. (2000)
	Chaco (Salta region)	N/A	17.2% of canine faeces collected in public spaces (19/106)	Direct smear, Willis' flotation method and an enrichment method by centrifugation after filtration by double gauze and homogenized with tap water	Taranto et al. (2000)
	City of Resistencia	April–September 1998	Total contamination of soil in 3.4% of all habitats surveyed (5/146) 20% of public parks (1/5), 5.9% of kindergarten sandpits (1/17) 2.4% of housing estates (3/124)	Flotation-centrifugal method	Alonso et al. (2001)
	Comodoro Rivadavia and Rada Till, Chubut Province, patagonia	July 1999–June 2000	12.7% of canine faeces found in parks during winter (14/110) 20.9% of canine faeces found in parks during spring (27/129) 19.8% of canine faeces found in parks during summer (23/116) 18.3% of canine faeces found in parks during autumn (23/126)	Telemann-modified technique and Willis flotation technique	Sánchez et al. (2003)

	La Plata	March–April 2000	56.5% of public places surveyed (13/23) 22.1% of the collected soil samples (31/140)	Telemann-modified technique	Córdoba et al. (2002)
	Corrientes	2001	0.3% of sand samples (1/300) 1/6 surveyed beaches	Willis flotation technique	Milano and Oscherov (2002)
	Corrientes	May 2002–May 2003	16% of faecal samples found on sidewalks (58/362)	Willis flotation technique	Milano and Oscherov (2005)
	City of Resistencia	August 2003–September 2004	33.3% of big squares (2/6, $n=140/612$) 25% of public parks (1/4, $n=80/612$) 20.6% of small squares (7/34, $n=392/612$)	Flotation-centrifugal method on NaCl solution	Alonso et al. (2006)
	Arid areas. 18 town from 6 provinces central-western region	September 2012	0% of evaluated soil samples (0/76)	Flotation-centrifugal method	Bojanich et al. (2015)
Bolivia	El Alto	October–December 2016	6.22% of canine faeces collected in public parks (300) 60% of public places surveyed (6/10)	Coprology—simple flotation whit saturated glucose solution; modified sedimentation.	Poma and Sirpa (2018)

Continued

Table 3 Reports of soil contamination of public places and parks with eggs of *Toxocara* spp. in South American countries (excluding Brazil).—Cont'd

Country	Region	Period	Prevalence of contamination	Diagnostic method	References
Colombia	Bogotá	July 2005–June 2006	5.4% of soil samples collected (84/1560) in 49 parks	Sheather's flotation technique	Polo-Terán et al. (2007)
	Bogotá	N/A	2.67% canine faeces collected in public parks (4/150)	Willis flotation technique	Mosquera-Pardo (2014)
	Duitama		34.7% of soil samples (25/72)	Sloss technique	Guarín-Patarroyo et al. (2016)
Chile	Santiago	June 1996–January 1998	18.2% of soil samples (29/159) 22.7% of the surveyed places (25/110)	Flotation in saturated zinc solution modified method	Salinas et al. (2001)
	Santiago	July–September 1999	33.3% of squares surveyed (28/84) 66.7% of parks surveyed (8/12)	modified Telemann method	Castillo et al. (2000)
	Temuco	N/A	12.4% of soil samples (24/193) in 87 public parks	Fonrouge's modified method	Armstrong et al. (2011)
	Temuco	April–May 2012	21.5% of the canine faecal samples collected in parks (22/102)	Teuscher's method (modified Faust's method)	Olivares et al. (2014)

	Los Angeles	July 2013	9.2% of canine faecal samples collected in 65 squares and public parks (42/452)	Burrows' technique	Luzio et al. (2015)
	Bío Bío Region	June 2015	29.7% of canine faecal samples collected in squares and public parks (19/64)	Burrows' technique	Luzio et al. (2017)
Ecuador	Cuenca City	N/A	3.66% of canine faecal samples collected in public parks (14/382)	Coprology—spontaneous sedimentation and Parodi-Alcaraz's flotation method	Ramón Lema (2012)
	Quito	N/A	33% of canine faecal samples collected in public parks (165/500)	Coprology—Flotation techniques	Latorre and Nápoles (2014)
French Guyana	N/A				
Guyana	N/A				
Paraguay	Asunción	January–February 2000	53% (27/51 sand from public parks, close to children playgrounds)	Flotation-Centrifugal method on 33% copper sulphate solution	Canese et al. (2003)
Peru	Lima	August 1989–January 1990	80% of public squares surveyed 1989 (8/10) 70% of public squares surveyed in 1990 (7/10)	Flotation method on saturated NaCl solution	Lescano et al. (1998)
	Lima	April–June 1998 January 1999	70.6% of recreational parks surveyed (12/17)	Modified Willis flotation technique	Castillo et al. (2001)

Continued

Table 3 Reports of soil contamination of public places and parks with eggs of *Toxocara* spp. in South American countries (excluding Brazil).—Cont'd

Country	Region	Period	Prevalence of contamination	Diagnostic method	References
	Lima	December 1998–March 1999	29.6% of public parks surveyed (29/98)	Sedimentation and flotation techniques with supersaturated solution of NaCl	Chávez et al. (2000)
	El Callao	December 1998–March 1999	37.2% of public parks surveyed (29/78)	Sedimentation and flotation techniques with supersaturated solution of NaCl	Chávez et al. (2000)
	Lima	November 2007–November 2008	73.8% (62/84) of soil samples and 57.6% (19/33) of the grass samples	Willis-Molloy technique	Iannacone et al. (2012)
	Moquegua and Sameagua	August–September 2010	83.3% of parks surveyed (35/42)	Flotation-Centrifugal method on 33% copper sulphate solution	Torres-Gonzales (2011)
	Huánuco	May–June 2014	90.9% public parks surveyed (10/11)	Flotation with a saturated sugar solution	Montalvo-Sabino et al. (2014)
	Ayacucho	May–June 2015	90% of public parks surveyed (9/10)	Flotation method with oversaturated sodium chloride solution	Frisancho Silva (2016)
	Abancay	June–October 2012	66.7% of public parks surveyed (14/21)	Willis flotation technique	Cáceres Pinto et al. (2017)

	Ayacucho	N/A	90% of the public parks surveyed (9/10)	Flotation method on saturated NaCl solution	Cruz et al. (2017)
	Lima	August 2014–April 2016	0.76% of public parks surveyed (1/131)	Sedimentation and flotation techniques with supersaturated solution of NaCl	Malca Vera (2018)
	Lima	N/A	28.6% of public parks surveyed (8/28)	Willis flotation technique	Carrasco Asín (2015)
Suriname	N/A				
Uruguay	Montevideo	April–December 2000	52.9% of places surveyed (37/70) 12.9% of canine faeces collected in public spaces (99/764)	For soil: Quinn flotation technique For faeces: Willis technique	Hernández et al. (2003)
Venezuela	City of Coro	February–March 2004	63.16% of public parks surveyed (24/38)	Modified Willis-Molloy technique	Perfetti et al., (2007)
	Ciudad Bolívar	N/A	Soil samples from 55% of the public places and parks surveyed (14/25) Canine faeces collected in 16.7% of the public places and parks surveyed (2/12)	Spontaneous sedimentation and flotation in saturated saline	Devera et al. (2008)

2. Conclusions and perspectives

Control of the infection and disease can be done only with the prevention of contamination of the environment, anthelmintic treatment strategies, and education. Dog and cat owners must avoid contamination of the environment with *Toxocara* eggs. Proper information about this zoonosis and the social concept of responsible pet ownership is required. Pet owners should be advised about deworming schemes, and to prevent their animals from defecating on children's playgrounds. More studies should be done on a large scale to determine the real prevalence of the parasite, using the appropriated diagnostic tools, and including risk factor analysis to help to clarify the dynamics of the infections.

Acknowledgements

Thanks to the Strategy for supporting research groups in the process of consolidation et al., 2018–2019, CODI, Universidad de Antioquia.

References

Agudelo, C., et al., 1990. Human and dogs *Toxocara canis* infection in a poor neighborhood in Bogota. Mem. Inst. Oswaldo Cruz 85 (1), 75–78. https://doi.org/10.1590/S0074-02761990000100012.

Aguilar, C., Giaminna, G., 2017. Prevalencia de *Toxocara canis* en caninos domesticos del distrito de pataz, región la libertad, Peru, Enero-Marzo 2016. Available at: http://repositorio.upao.edu.pe/bitstream/upaorep/2925/1/RE_MED.VETE_GIULIANA.CONTRERAS_PREVALENCIA.DE.TOXOCARA_DATOS.PDF%0A.

Alonso, J.M., et al., 2001. Contamination of soils with eggs of *Toxocara* in a subtropical city in Argentina. Journal of Helminthology 75 (2), 165–168. http://www.ncbi.nlm.nih.gov/pubmed/11520441. (Accessed 9 August 2019).

Alonso, J., et al., 2006. Huevos de *Toxocara* en suelos destinados a la recreación en una ciudad argentina. Acta Bioquim. Clin. Latinoam. 40 (2), 219–222. Available at: http://www.redalyc.org/articulo.oa?id=53540209.

Añamuro, C.E., et al., 2019. Prevalencia de enteroparásitos en cachorros comercializados en Puno, Perú. Rev. Investig. Vet. Perú 30 (1), 309–319.

Andresiuk, M.V., et al., 2003. Encuesta coproparasitológico canina realizado en plazas públicas de la ciudad de Mar del Plata, Buenos Aires, Argentina. Parasitol. Latinoam. 58 (1–2), 17–22.

Armstrong, W.A., Oberg, C., Orellana, J.J., 2011. Presencia de huevos de parásitos con potencial zoonótico en parques y plazas públicas de la ciudad de Temuco, Región de La Araucanía, Chile. Arch. Med. Vet. 43 (2), 127–134. Available at: https://scielo.conicyt.cl/scielo.php?script=sci_abstract&pid=S0301-732X2011000200005&lng=pt&nrm=iso.

Atitwa, S.C., 2018. How Many Dogs Are There In The World?—WorldAtlas.com, World Atlas. Available at: https://www.worldatlas.com/articles/how-many-dogs-are-there-in-the-world.html. (Accessed 4 August 2019).

Beck, A.M., 1975. The public health implications of urban dogs. Am. J. Public Health 65, 1315–1318.

Beldomenico, P.M., et al., 2005. Helminths of Geoffroy's cat, *Oncifelis geoffroyi* (Carnivora, Felidae) from the Monte desert, Central Argentina. Acta Parasitol. 50 (3), 263–266.

Bojanich, M.V., et al., 2015. Assessment of the presence of *Toxocara* eggs in soils of an arid area in Central-Western Argentina. Rev. Inst. Med. Trop. Sao Paulo 57 (1), 73–76.

Bolivar-Mejia, A., et al., 2014. Toxocariasis in the Americas: burden and disease control. Curr. Trop. Med. Rep. 1 (1), 62–68, Springer International Publishing. https://doi.org/10.1007/s40475-013-0010-7.

Bonilla, Z., 1980. Study of the helminth fauna of cats from Valdivia, Chile. Arch. Med. Vet. 12 (2), 277.

Cabrera, P., et al., 2003. Determinación de parásitos zoonóticos (helmintos y protozoarios) en caninos del Centro de Zoonosis de Bogotá, D.C. Biomédica 23, 153.

Cáceres Pinto, C.M., Bustinza Cárdenas, R.H., Valderrama Pomé, A.A., 2017. Contaminación con Huevos de *Toxocara* sp y Evaluación Sanitaria de Parques en la Ciudad de Abancay, Perú. Rev. Investig. Vet. Perú 28 (2), 376–386, Universidad Nacional Mayor de San Marcos. https://doi.org/10.15381/rivep.v28.i2.13064.

Cañas, L., et al., 1998. Prevalencia de toxocariosis en caninos del área urbana de Medellín. Infectio 33, 33.

Canese, A., et al., 2003. Huevos infectivos de T*oxocara*, en arenas de plazas y parques de Asunción, Paraguay. Rev. Soc. Bol. Ped. 42 (3), 202–205. Available at: http://www.scielo.org.bo/scielo.php?script=sci_arttext&pid=S1024-06752003000300016. (Accessed 9 August 2019).

Cantó, M., 2018. Argentina, el país con mayor cantidad de mascotas por habitante del mundo—Argentear. In: Novedades del Pais. Available at: https://argentear.com/argentina-mascotas/. (Accessed 4 August 2019).

Cardillo, N., Rosa, A., Sommerfelt, I., 2008. Estudio preliminar sobre los distintos estadios de *Toxocara cati* en gatos. Parasitol. Latinoam. 63, 72–75.

Carrasco Asín, V.G., 2015. Determinación de la presencia de huevos de *Toxocara* sp. y *Ancylostoma* sp. en parques del distrito de Barranco, Lima—Perú 2014. Universidad Científica del Sur. Available at: http://repositorio.cientifica.edu.pe:8080/handle/UCS/418. (Accessed 9 August 2019).

Castillo, D., et al., 2000. Environmental contamination with *Toxocara* sp. eggs in public squares and parks from Santiago, Chile, 1999. Bol. Chil. Parasitol. 55 (3–4), 86–91.

Castillo, Y., et al., 2001. Estudio epidemiológico de *Toxocara canis* en parques recreacionales del distrito de San Juan de Lurigancho, Lima—Perú. Parasitol. Día 25 (3–4), 109–114, Sociedad Chilena de Parasitología. https://doi.org/10.4067/S0716-07202001000300007.

Castrillón Salazar, L.L., et al., 2018. Prevalencia de presentación de algunos agentes zoonóticos transmitidos por caninos y felinos en Medellín, Colombia. Rev. MVZ Cordoba 24 (1), 7119–7126. https://doi.org/10.21897/rmvz.1524.

Castro, O., et al., 2013. Contribution to the knowledge of metazoan parasites of domestic cat in the department of Montevideo, Uruguay. Veterinaria (Montevideo) 49 (190), 28–37.

Chávez, V.A., et al., 2000. Contaminación de parques públicos con huevos de *Toxocara* spp. en los distritos de la provincia constitucional del Callao y del cono sur de Lima metropolitana. Rev. Investig. Vet. Perú 11 (1), 52–57. Available at: https://revistasinvestigacion.unmsm.edu.pe/index.php/veterinaria/article/view/6795/12601.

Chebez, J.C., et al., 2014. Mamíferos terrestres de la Patagonia. CABA, Argentina.

Córdoba, A., et al., 2002. Presencia de parásitos intestinales en paseos públicos urbanos en La Plata Argentina. Parasitol. Latinoam. 57 (1–2), 25–29. https://doi.org/10.4067/S0717-77122002000100007, Sociedad Chilena de Parasitología. Organo Oficial de la Federación Latinoamericana de Parasitólogos.

Córdova, T., Marisol, C., 2015. Prevalencia de helmintos gastrointestinales zoonóticos de caninos en tres parques turísticos de la ciudad de Ambato. (Bachelor's thesis). Available at: http://repositorio.uta.edu.ec/bitstream/123456789/18365/1/Tesis 30 Medicina Veterinaria y Zootecnia -CD 339.pdf.

Costamagna, S.R., et al., 2002. Epidemiología de las parasitosis en Bahía Blanca (Provincia de Buenos Aires) Argentina-1994/1999. Parasitol. Latinoam. 57 (3–4), 103–110.

Cruz, H.M., Blásquez, D.P.G., Monje, M.R., 2017. Contaminación de parques públicos (jesús de nazareno, ayacucho-perú) con huevos de *toxocara*. Biotempo 14 (2), 115–119.

Dávalos, M., Pachas, O., Pérez, V., 2000. Toxocariosis en *Canis familiaris* y suelo en el distrito de Chincha alta. In: Editado en IV Congreso Peruano de Parasitología, Septiembre, Lima, Perú. p. 2.

de Díaz, F.V., Anccasi, M.M., 2013. Enteroparásitos en perros (*canis familiaris*) y gatos (*felis catus*) de la provincia de puno. Rev. Investig. Altoandin. 15 (1), 117–122.

Delgado, O., Rodriguez-morales, A.J., 2009. Aspectos clínico-epidemiológicos de la toxocariasis: una enfermedad desatendida en Venezuela y América Latina. In: Boletín De Malariología Y Salud Ambiental, XLIX(Enero-Julio), pp. 1–33.

Deplazes, P., et al., 2016. Parasitology in Veterinary Medicine. First, Wageningen Academic Publishers, Wageningen, the Netherlands.

Devera, R., et al., 2008. *Toxocara* spp. y otros helmintos en plazas y parques de Ciudad Bolívar, estado Bolívar (Venezuela). In: Enfermedades Infecciosas y Microbiología Clínica. vol. 26. Elsevier Doyma, pp. 23–26. https://doi.org/10.1157/13114391. 1.

Echeverry, D.M., Giraldo, M.I., Castaño, J.C., 2012. Prevalencia de helmintos intestinales en gatos domésticos del departamento del Quindío, Colombia. Biomedica 32 (3), 430–436. https://doi.org/10.7705/biomedica.v32i3.439.

Fernandez, J., Lizarazu, M.C., Forero, J.C., 2015. Parásitos gastrointestinales en caninos domiciliados en la Localidad de Teusaquillo (Bogotá, Colombia). Revista Científica UNINCCA 122, 6150.

Fiorello, C.V., et al., 2006. Parasites of free-ranging small canids and felids in the Bolivian Chaco. J. Zoo Wildl. Med. 37 (2), 130–135.

Fonrouge, R., et al., 2000. Contaminación de suelos con huevos de *Toxocara* sp. en plazas y parques públicos de la ciudad de La Plata. Buenos Aires, Argentina. Bol. Chil. Parasitol. 55 (3–4), 83–85. Available at: https://scielo.conicyt.cl/scielo.php?pid=S0365-94022000000300009&script=sci_arttext.

Fontanarrosa, M.F., et al., 2006. An epidemiological study of gastrointestinal parasites of dogs from southern greater Buenos Aires (Argentina): age, gender, breed, mixed infections, and seasonal and spatial patterns. Vet. Parasitol. 136 (3–4), 283–295.

Frisancho Silva, J.M., 2016. Presencia de huevos de *Toxocara* spp. en parques públicos de los distritos de la provincia de La Mar, Ayacucho—2015. Universidad Nacional de San Cristóbal de Huamanga. Available at: http://repositorio.unsch.edu.pe/handle/UNSCH/2643. (Accessed 9 August 2019).

García, E., 2001. Prevalencia de Helmintos gastrointestinales en *Canis familiaris* en el distrito de Lurigancho, Chosica. Dpto. De Lima. Universidad Nacional Mayor de San Marcos, Lima.

García, L.D., et al., 2012. Detección de IgG anti *Toxocara canis* en perros de la Provincia de Corrientes, Argentina. Rev. Vet. 23 (1), 69–70.

García, L.D., et al., 2014. Seroprevalencia de *Toxocara canis* en perros de las ciudades de Corrientes y Esperanza (Argentina). Rev. Vet. 25 (2), 131–134.

García-Soto, M., 2014. Helmintos y protozoos gastrointestinales de gatos (*Felis catus*) de la ciudad de Santiago, Chile. Available at: http://repositorio.uchile.cl/bitstream/handle/2250/131707/Helmintos-y-protozoos-gastrointestinales-de-gatos-%28Felis-catus%29-de-la-ciudad-de-Santiago%2C-Chile.pdf?sequence=1&isAllowed=y.

Giraldo, M.I., García, N.L., Castaño, J.C., 2005. Prevalencia de helmintos intestinales en caninos del departamento del Quindío. Biomédica 25 (3), 346–352.

Global Health—Division of Parasitic Diseases and Malaria, Toxocariasis (also known as Roundworm Infection), 2013, Centers for Disease Control and Prevention; Atlanta, GA.
González, A.C., Giraldo, J.C., 2015. Prevalencia de parásitos intestinales zoonóticos en caninos (*Canis Lupus Familiaris*) del área urbana del municipio de Coyaima (Tolima). Rev. Med. 23 (2), 24–34.
Gorman, T., Soto, A., Alcaíno, H., 2006. Parasitismo gastrointestinal en perros de comunas de Santiago de diferente nivel socioeconómico. Parasitol. Latinoam. 61 (3–4), 126–132.
Guarín-Patarroyo, C.E., Serrato, M.J., Sánchez-Cuervo, F.R., 2016. *Toxocara canis* eggs determination in Duitama (Boyacá) three public parks soil. Rev. Ciênc. Agron 13 (1), 59–66.
Gutiérrez, V.E.R., et al., 2014. Detección de parásitos intestinales en niños preescolares y animales domésticos del municipio de Ibagué (Tolima). Rev. Colomb. Cienc. Anim. 7 (1), 34–41.
Guzmán, A.C., Jaramillo, A., Loaiza, J., 2007. Prevalencia de parásitos intestinales en caninos atendidos en el Centro deVeterinaria y Zootecnia de la Universidad CES, 2007. CES. Med. Vet. Zoot. 2 (2), 24–31.
Hernández, S., et al., 2003. *Toxocara* spp en muestras de suelo y heces de plazas de la ciudad de Montevideo. J. Trop. Pathol. 32 (1). Available at: https://www.revistas.ufg.br/iptsp/article/download/4355/3813.
Iannacone, J., Flores, L.A., Cárdenas-Callirgos, J., 2012. Contaminación de los suelos con huevos de *Toxocara Canis* en parques públicos de Santiago de Surco, Lima, Perú 2007–2008. Neotrop. Helminthol. 6 (1), 97–108.
Kuruc, J., et al., 1995. Uso de las plazas de la ciudad de Buenos Aires porhumanos y porperros en relación con la transmisión de helmintospor la materia fecal canina. In: 1 Congreso Latinoamericano de Zoonosis (Buenos Aires).
Kurzweil, C., 2018. Cat Ownership Drives Pet Care Growth in Latin America. GlobalPETS, Pets International. Available at: https://globalpets.community/article/cat-ownership-drives-pet-care-growth-in-latin-america. (Accessed 4 August 2019).
Latorre, E., Nápoles, M., 2014. Estudio para determinar la contaminación con Parásitos Zoonóticos Caninos en parquez de la zona urbana del Distrito Metropolitano de Quito. USFQ, Quito. 2014. Available at: http://repositorio.usfq.edu.ec/handle/23000/3119. (Accessed 5 August 2019).
Lee, R.M., et al., 2014. Toxocariasis in North America: a systematic review. PLoS Negl. Trop. Dis. 8 (8), e3116. https://doi.org/10.1371/journal.pntd.0003116, Public Library of Science.
Lescano, S.A.Z., et al., 1998. Soil contamination and human infection by Toxocara sp. in the urban area of Lima, Peru. Mem. Inst. Oswaldo Cruz 93 (6), 733–734. https://doi.org/10.1590/S0074-02761998000600005, Fundação Oswaldo Cruz.
Llanos, M., et al., 2010. Parasitósis entérica en caninos (Canis familiaris) en el área urbana de Coroico, Nor Yungas Departamento de La Paz, Bolivia. J. Selva Andin. Res. Soc. 1 (1), 38–49.
Lopez, J., et al., 2006. Intestinal parasites in dogs and cats with gastrointestinal symptoms in Santiago, Chile. Rev. Med. Chil. 134 (2), 193–200.
Luzio, Á., et al., 2015. Formas parasitarias de importancia zoonótica, encontradas en heces de perros recolectadas desde plazas y parques públicos de la ciudad de Los Ángeles, Región del Bío Bío, Chile. Rev. Chilena Infectol. 32 (4), 403–407.
Luzio, A., et al., 2017. Formas parasitarias gastroentericas de importancia zoonótica, en heces de perros, recolectadas en plazas de armas de las capitales provinciales de la Región del Bío Bío, Chile. Rev. Electrón. Vet. 18 (9), 1–10.
Malca Vera, C.P., 2018. Contaminación con huevos de *Toxocara* ssp. en parques públicos del distrito de La Molina—Lima y su relación con el programa de vigilancia sanitaria de parques y jardines. Universidad Nacional Mayor de San Marcos. Available at: http://cybertesis.unmsm.edu.pe/handle/cybertesis/10091. (Accessed 9 August 2019).

Marder, G., et al., 2004. Infestación parasitaria en suelos y materia fecal de perros y gatos de la ciudad de Corrientes. Rev. Vet. 15 (2), 70–72.
Martin, A., 2016. Pet-Owners Dominate in Latin America, Russia and USA—MarketWatch. Available at: https://www.marketwatch.com/press-release/pet-owners-dominate-in-latin-america-russia-and-usa-2016-05-24-4203228. (Accessed 4 August 2019).
Martinez, A., Led, J., Albariño, M., 1973. Resultados obtenidos sobre 5.000 análisis coproparasitológicos en perros de la ciudad de La Plata y alrededores. Rev. Agron. Vet. 2, 2–10.
Milano, A.M.F., Oscherov, E.B., 2002. Contaminación por parásitos caninos de importancia zoonótica en playas de la ciudad de Corrientes, Argentina. Parasitol. Latinoam. 57 (3–4), 119–123. https://doi.org/10.4067/S0717-77122002000300006, Sociedad Chilena de Parasitología. Organo Oficial de la Federación Latinoamericana de Parasitólogos.
Milano, A.M.F., Oscherov, E.B., 2005. Contaminación de aceras con enteroparásitos caninos en Corrientes, Argentina. Parasitol. Latinoam. 60 (1–2), 82–85. https://doi.org/10.4067/S0717-77122005000100015, Sociedad Chilena de Parasitología. Organo Oficial de la Federación Latinoamericana de Parasitólogos.
Minvielle, M.C., Pezzani, B.C., Basualdo Farjat, J.A., 1993. Frequency of finding helminths eggs in canine stool samples collected in public places in the La Plata City, Argentina. Bol. Chil. Parasitol. 48, 63–65.
Mocetti, N., et al., 2011. Parasitosis zoonóticas en mascotas caninas y felinas de niños de educación primaria del cono norte de Lima, Perú. Rev. Sapuvet Salud Pública 2 (1), 15–24.
Moleón, M.S., et al., 2015. New hosts and localities for helminths of carnivores in Argentina. Zootaxa 4057 (1), 106–114. https://doi.org/10.11646/zootaxa.4057.1.6.
Montalvo-Sabino, E., et al., 2014. Factors associated with contamination of public parks (huánuco, perú) by *Toxocara canis* eggs and other endoparasites of zoonotic importance. Neotrop. Helminthol. 8 (2), 259–268. Available at: http://sisbib.unmsm.edu.pe/bvrevistas/neohel/v8n2/pdf/a07v8n2.pdf. (Accessed 9 August 2019).
Morales-Rambay, A.G., 2015. Prevalencia de nematodos gastrointestinales en felinos de la ciudad de Machala. Universidad Técnica de Machala, Machala. Available at: http://repositorio.utmachala.edu.ec/bitstream/48000/2699/1/CD135_TESIS.pdf.
Mosquera-Pardo, J.J., 2014. Frecuencia de huevos de nematodos gastrointestinales en heces de perros en el parque central simón bolívar de Bogotá. Universidad de la Salle. Available at: https://ciencia.lasalle.edu.co/medicina_veterinaria/230.
Olivares, P., et al., 2014. Descripción de paritos presentes en muestras fecales recolectadas en plazas del sector cítrico de la ciudad de Temuco, Chile. Rev. Investig. Vet. Perú 25 (3), 406–413.
Overgaauw, P.A.M., 1997. Aspects of Toxocara epidemiology: toxocarosis in dogs and cats. Crit. Rev. Microbiol. 23 (3), 233–251. https://doi.org/10.3109/10408419709115138.
M Overgaauw, P.A., Nederland, V., 1997. Aspects of *Toxocara* epidemiology: toxocarosis in dogs and cats. Crit. Rev. Microbiol. 23 (3), 233–258. https://doi.org/10.3109/10408419709115138.
Paredes, L.D.S., Salazar, R.C., Villamarín, A.D.P.P., 2013. Gastrointestinal parasites in street dogs in animal shelter from the Bogota D.C., Colombia. Neotrop. Helminthol. 7 (1), 83–93.
Penagos, J., et al., 2004. Parásitos gastrointestinales en caninos de cinco municipios del Huila y su importancia en salud pública. Infectio 8, 138.
Perfetti, D.J.C., Moreno, P.M., Quintero, M.E.A., 2007. Soil Contamination With *Toxocara* spp. Eggs (Nematoda, Ascaridida) in Public Parks From Coro City, Falcon State, Venezuela. Rev. Cient. 17 (2), 117–122. Universidad Del Zulia. Available at: http://ve.scielo.org/scielo.php?script=sci_arttext&pid=S0798-22592007000200003&lng=es&nrm=iso&tlng=es. (Accessed 9 August 2019).

Polo-Terán, L.J., et al., 2007. Contaminación de los Parques Públicos de la Localidad de Suba, Bogotá con Nemátodos Zoonóticos. Rev. Salud Pública 9 (4), 550–557. https://doi.org/10.1590/S0124-00642007000400007, Instituto de Salud Publica, Facultad de Medicina—Universidad Nacional de Colombia.

Poma, R., Sirpa, N.P., 2018. Presencia de huevos de *Toxocara* spp. en plazas con parques de la ciudad de El Alto, Bolivia. Rev. Estud. Agro-Vet 2 (2), 234–241. Available at: http://ojs.agro.umsa.bo/index.php/AGV/article/download/310/300.

Poma, R., et al., 2018. Presencia de huevos de Toxócara spp. en plazas con parques de la ciudad. Rev. Estud. Agro-Vet 2 (2), 234–241.

Posada, J.O.A., 2014. Descripción de los parásitos intestinales más comunes en caninos llevados a consulta a la Clínica Veterinaria Lasallista Hermano Octavio Martínez López. J. Agric. Anim. Sci. 2 (1), 22–32.

Radman, N.E., et al., 2006. *Toxocara canis* en caninos. Prevalencia en la ciudad de La Plata. Acta Bioquim. Clin. Latinoam. 40 (1), 41–48. Available at: http://www.redalyc.org/articulo.oa?id=53540107.

Ramírez-Barrios, R., Barbosa-Mena, G., Muñoz, J., 2004. Prevalence of intestinal parasites in dogs under veterinary care in Maracaibo, Venezuela. Vet. Parasitol. 121, 11–20.

Ramírez-Barrios, R.A., et al., 2008. Prevalencia de helmintos gastrointestinales en gatos admitidos en la policlínica veterinaria de la Universidad del Zulia. Rev. Cient. 18 (4), 374–380.

Ramón Lema, G.F., 2012. Prevalencia de Helmintos Gastrointestinales (Céstodos y Nematodos) en caninos de la ciudad de Cuenca. Universidad De Cuenca. Available at: http://dspace.ucuenca.edu.ec/bitstream/123456789/383/1/TESIS.pdf. (Accessed 5 August 2019).

Reyes, M., et al., 1999. Relación entre toxocariasis canina domiciliaria y larva migrans en niños del distrito El Agustino. Rev. Estudiantes de Med. UNMSM 1, 5–10.

Rubel, D., et al., 2003. Epidemiology of *Toxocara canis* in the dog population from two areas of different socioeconomic status, greater Buenos Aires, Argentina. Vet. Parasitol. 115 (3), 275–286.

Salamanca, C.A., et al., 2011. Sobrepoblación canina y felina: tendencias y nuevas perspectivas. In: Revista de la Facultad de Medicina Veterinaria y de Zootecnia. Available at: https://revistas.unal.edu.co/index.php/remevez/article/view/21602. (Accessed 4 August 2019).

Salinas, P., Matamala, M., Schenone, H., 2001. Prevalencia de hallazgo de huevos de *Toxocara canis* en plazas de la Región Metropolitana de la ciudad de Santiago, Chile. Bol. Chil. Parasitol. 56 (3–4), 102–105.

Sánchez, P., et al., 2003. Contaminación biológica con heces caninas y parásitos intestinales en espacios públicos urbanos en dos ciudades de la Provincia del Chubut: Patagonia Argentina. Parasitol. Latinoam. 58 (3–4), 131–135. https://doi.org/10.4067/S0717-77122003000300008, Sociedad Chilena de Parasitología. Organo Oficial de la Federación Latinoamericana de Parasitólogos.

Sarmiento-Rubiano, L.A., et al., 2018. Intestinal parasites in dogs and cats with owners of Barranquilla, Colombia. Rev. Investig. Vet. Perú 29 (4), 1403–1410.

Semenas, L., et al., 2014. Helmintos zoonóticos en heces caninas de barrios de Bariloche (Río Negro, Patagonia, Argentina). Rev. Argent. Parasitol. 2 (2), 22–27.

Sierra-Cifuentes, V., et al., 2015. Prevalencia de parásitos intestinales en perros de dos centros de bienestar animal de Medellín y el oriente antioqueño (Colombia), 2014. Rev. Med. Vet. 30, 55–66.

Sinchi, C., Dario, V., 2018. Prevalencia de parásitos intestinales zoonóticos de origen canino en sectores rurales. (Bachelor's thesis). Available at: https://dspace.ups.edu.ec/bitstream/123456789/16266/4/UPS-CT007915.pdf.

Sommerfelt, I.E., et al., 2006. Prevalence of *Toxocara cati* and other parasites in cats' faeces collected from the open spaces of public institutions: Buenos Aires, Argentina. Vet. Parasitol. 140 (3–4), 296–301.
Soriano, S.V., et al., 2010. A wide diversity of zoonotic intestinal parasites infects urban and rural dogs in Neuquén, Patagonia, Argentina. Vet. Parasitol. 167, 81–85.
Suntaxi, I., 2015. Evaluación de la frecuencia de enteroparásitos de caninos en tres refugios del Distrito Metropolitano de Quito. UCE, Quito. Available at: http://www.dspace.uce.edu.ec:8080/bitstream/25000/6786/1/T-UCE-0014-038.pdf.
Taranto, N.J., et al., 2000. Parasitosis zoonóticas transmitidas por perros en el Chaco Salteño. Medicina 60 (2), 217–220.
Torres, P., et al., 1974. Protozoa, helminths and arthropods parasites of domestic dog from Valdivia City, Chile (author's transl). Bol. Chil. Parasitol. 29 (1–2), 18.
Torres-Gonzales, Contaminación de los parques públicos con huevos de parásitos de importancia en salud pública en los distritos de Moquegua y Samegua, 2011, Universidad Nacional Jorge Basadre Grohmann; Tacna, Perú, Available at: http://repositorio.unjbg.edu.pe/handle/UNJBG/612.
Trillo-Altamirano, M., Carrasco, A., Cabrera, R., 2003. Prevalencia de helmintos enteroparásitos zoonóticos y factores asociados en *Canis familiaris* en una zona urbana de la ciudad de Ica, Perú. Parasitol. Latinoam. 58 (3–4), 136–141.
Tuasa Córdova, C. M. (2015) "Prevalencia de helmintos gastrointestinales zoonóticos de caninos en tres parques turísticos de la ciudad de Ambato. Universidad técnica de ambato facultad de ciencias agropecuarias medicina veterinaria y zootécnia. Available at: http://repositorio.uta.edu.ec/bitstream/123456789/18365/1/Tesis 30 Medicina Veterinaria y Zootecnia -CD 339.pdf. (Accessed: 5 August 2019).
Valledor, S., et al., 2006. Relevamiento de helmintos intestinales en perros urbanos de Montevideo y Florida, y perros rurales del departamento de Florida, con el registro de un nuevo género de nemátodo parasitando al canino en nuestro país. 41, Sociedad de Medicina Veterinaria del Uruguay, pp. 43–49, 163–164.
Vásquez, L.R., et al., 2005. Prevalencia de *Toxocara Canis* y Otros Parásitos Intestinales en Caninos en la Ciudad de Popayán, 2004. Rev. FCS. Univ. Cauca. 7 (4), 3–21.
Vega, A.L., Rojas, J.L.G., López, G.M., 2006. Estudio epidemiológico de *Toxocara* sp. y *Ancylostoma* sp. en canes y paseos públicos de los distritos I al V de Santa Cruz de la Sierra. Rev. Electrón. Vet. 7 (9), 1–23.
Villaseca, D., Socorro, Z., 2014. Helmintiasus intestinal y lesiones en *Canis familiaris* atendidos en el laboratorio de técnicas quirúrgicas de la Universidad Nacional Mayor de San Marcos. Universidad Nacional De Piura, Perú. Available at: http://repositorio.unp.edu.pe/bitstream/handle/UNP/432/BIO-DEZ-VIL-14.pdf?sequence=1&isAllowed=y.

CHAPTER THIRTY-FIVE

Prevalence of patent *Toxocara* spp. infections in dogs and cats in Europe from 1994 to 2019

Paul Overgaauw[a,*], Rolf Nijsse[b]

[a]Division of Veterinary Public Health, Faculty of Veterinary Medicine, Institute for Risk Assessment Sciences, Utrecht University, Utrecht, The Netherlands

[b]Department of Infectious Diseases and Immunology, Faculty of Veterinary Medicine, Utrecht University, Utrecht, The Netherlands

*Corresponding author: e-mail address: p.a.m.overgaauw@uu.nl

Contents

Abstract

Objectives: To provide an overview of *Toxocara* prevalences in dogs and cats in Europe from the last 25 years.

Method: Systematic review of the literature.

Results: Over the past 25 years, prevalence studies of *Toxocara* spp. have been published from 26 European countries. The average prevalences were 14.6% for *T. canis* in all dogs and 24.5% for *T. cati* in all cats. Specified for young dogs until 6 months old this was 41.2%, for young cats until 6 months old 25%, adult owned dogs 11.1%, adult owned cats 16.3%, stray dogs 17.6%, and stray cats 33.5%. A recent study in seven European countries showed a prevalence of 3.4% for adult dogs and 4.2% for adult cats. The prevalences seem not to decrease over the years.

Conclusion: The prevalence of patent *Toxocara* infections over the last 25 years did not show a distinct declining trend. Prevalence data provided by recent modern antigen tests showed much lower results than from older studies. Results from studies using less diverse methods and well-defined study-populations could provide more clarity.

Advances in Parasitology, Volume 109
ISSN 0065-308X
https://doi.org/10.1016/bs.apar.2020.01.030

1. Introduction

Toxocara canis and *Toxocara cati* are cosmopolitan roundworms of canids and felids with important public health consequences due to their zoonotic significance. Recent findings suggest that the impact of toxocariasis on human health is increasing in some countries (Ma et al., 2018). Toxocariasis is now considered to be the most common human parasitic infection in the United States, particularly among the impoverished (McManus et al., 2018). The widespread contamination of the environment with *Toxocara* eggs in the faeces of definitive hosts, facilitates infection of both definitive and paratenic hosts (including humans). A good understanding of the epidemiology is required for defining effective strategies for the control of the infection in humans, dogs, and cats. The reported infection rates in the literature vary, however, significantly depending on the country, the life stage of the animals (age groups), the lifestyle of the animals (e.g. feral or household), and the faecal examination method used. Therefore, prevalence rates from different studies cannot directly be compared due to this lack of standardization. To introduce a more standardized approach towards parasite control in companion animals, the European Scientific Counsel Companion Animal Parasites (ESCCAP) published their first Guideline in 2004 (ESCCAP, 2004). This guideline, however, was not about standardization of diagnostics but about a consistent approach for parasitic infection prevention. New guidelines, currently under production, will focus on diagnostic tools.

To provide an overview of *Toxocara* prevalences in dogs and cats in Europe, the results from published studies from the last 25 years will be analysed and discussed in this review.

2. Methods

2.1 Search strategy

A systematic search on the PubMed database was conducted using the following terms and Boolean operators (AND, OR): *Toxocara canis* OR *Toxocara cati,* AND dogs OR cats, AND prevalence; Endoparasites, AND dogs OR cats, AND prevalence; and each search was conducted for the different European countries specified in Section 2.2. The literature search was performed in June and July 2019.

2.2 Inclusion and exclusion criteria

An article was included if it was published in the last 25 years (1994–2019) in a peer reviewed journal and reported on original data on the prevalence of *T. canis* in dogs and/or *T. cati* in cats. Exceptions will be made for any recent dataset that has not been published (Section 2.3.). If the numbers of investigated and/or positive faecal samples were not clearly described, the publication was excluded.

A European country was considered as one of the 44 independent member states on this continent according to the United Nations. This number was expanded to include Kosovo which declared independence in 2008.

The countries Kazakhstan, Azerbaijan, Georgia and Turkey are transcontinental Eurasian countries partially located in both Europe and Asia, while Armenia and Cyprus are often considered European countries politically, although geographically they are located in the West Asia territory. Therefore, these countries were not included in this review.

2.3 Multicentre European studies

To provide directly comparable results between different countries, using the same faecal examination method, two multiple European country studies, performed between 1994 and 2019, were included separately.

3. Results

3.1 European country prevalence studies

Information regarding the prevalence of *Toxocara* spp. in dogs and/or cats was published from 26 countries (Table 1). From the following countries, information could not be found: Andorra, Belarus, Bosnia and Herzegovina, Bulgaria, Croatia, Iceland, Latvia, Liechtenstein, Luxembourg, Malta, Moldova, Montenegro, North Macedonia, Norway, San Marino, Serbia, Slovenia, Ukraine and Vatican City.

Some publications could not be included because information regarding numbers of animals or (positive) samples was not clearly described. This was mostly the case for articles that were published in a local language (mainly Polish and Russian) unknown by the authors and from which, insufficient information was given in the summary. In many cases, only positive *Toxocara* percentages were reported without giving the numbers of investigated animals.

Table 1 Prevalence of *Toxocara* spp. in dogs and cats in Europe.

	Dogs		Cats			
Country	**N**	**%[a]**	**N**	**%[a]**	**Source**	**References**
Albania			18	83	Free-roaming, necropsy	Knaus et al. (2011)
	111	76			Suburban	Xhaxhiu et al. (2011)
			252	48	Semi-domestic feral	Knaus et al. (2014)
	602	8.0			Client-owned	Shukullari et al. (2015)
Austria	1481	1.0			Anonymous faecal samples	Hinney et al. (2017)
Belgium	451	4.4			Household, breeding, GI-problems	Claerebout et al. (2009)
	56	52			Pups pet shops and breeders	Dupont et al. (2013)
Denmark	178	12			Hunting dogs	Al-Sabi et al. (2013)
			99	85	Feral cats	Takeuchi-Storm et al. (2015)
			327	44	Shelter cats	Hansen et al. (2017)
Estonia	454	4.2			Faeces from park lawns	Talvik et al. (2006)
			27	48	Stray	Talvik et al. (2006)
	234	1.7			Faeces from urban areas	Lassen and Jokelainen (2016)
Finland	541	3.1			Household	Pullola et al. (2006)
			411	5.4	Household	Näreaho et al. (2012)

Table 1 Prevalence of *Toxocara* spp. in dogs and cats in Europe.—cont'd

	Dogs		Cats			
Country	**N**	**%[a]**	**N**	**%[a]**	**Source**	**References**
France	420	9.8	98	16	Household dogs and cats	Franc et al. (1997)
	93	5.4	34	2.9	Household dogs and cats	Beugnet et al. (2000)
			133	56	Feral	Fromont et al. (2001)
	18	5.5	93	33	Faeces from kitchen gardens	Poulle et al. (2017)
Germany	8438	22	3167	26	Owned dogs (1999–2002	Barutzki and Schaper (2003)
	1281	2.2	441	3.9	Owned dogs and cats	Epe et al. (2004)
	24,677	6.1	8560	4.7	Owned dogs and cats	Barutzki and Schaper (2011)
	445	4.0	837	27	Stray and fostered	Becker et al. (2012)
	2319	22	1206	11	Young dogs and cats	Barutzki and Schaper (2013)
	2731	2.8	903	3.9	Owned dogs and cats	Raue et al. (2017)
Greece	281	13			Shepherd and hunting dogs	Papazahariadou et al. (2007)
			150	24	Stray and free-roaming	Diakou et al. (2017)
	879	5.9	264	7.6	Shelter, shepherd, household	Kostopoulou et al. (2017)
			1150	24	Household and stray	Symeonidou et al. (2018)
	200	3.5			Owned and sheltered	Diakou et al. (2019)
Hungary	490	27			Urban and rural	Fok et al. (2001)
			235	17	Owned	Capári et al. (2013)

Continued

Table 1 Prevalence of *Toxocara* spp. in dogs and cats in Europe.—cont'd

Country	Dogs N	Dogs %[a]	Cats N	Cats %[a]	Source	References
Ireland	350	83	181	42	Stray	O'Lorcain (1994)
	627	16	289	30	Stray	Garcia-Campos et al. (2018)
Italy	395	34			Rural and urban	Habluetzel et al. (2003)
			139	33	Stray	Spada et al. (2013)
	239	13	81	22	Owned	Riggio et al. (2013)
	318	9.7			Shelter	Simonato et al. (2015)
	502	6.6			Kenneled and privately owned	Paoletti et al. (2015)
	619	12	343	16	Owned dogs and cats	Tamponi et al. (2017)
	1619	5.0			Shelter dogs	Scaramozzino et al. (2018)
	1156	9.3			Household dogs	Scaramozzino et al. (2018)
	639	7.8			Kennel dogs	Sauda et al. (2018)
Kosovo	305	14			Owned dogs	Sherifi et al. (2011)
Lithuania	894	4.0			Village dogs	Vienažindienė et al. (2018)
Netherlands	272	2.9	236	4.7	Owned dogs and cats	Overgaauw (1997)
			337	2.0	Breeding cats and kittens	Overgaauw and Boersema (1998b)
	286	21			Breeding dogs	Overgaauw and Boersema (1998a)
	159	48			Pups of breeders	Overgaauw and Boersema (1998a)
			225	2.0	Breeding cats	Overgaauw and Boersema (1998b)
			112	0	Kittens from catteries	Overgaauw and Boersema (1998b)

Table 1 Prevalence of *Toxocara* spp. in dogs and cats in Europe.—cont'd

	Dogs		Cats			
Country	**N**	**%[a]**	**N**	**%[a]**	**Source**	**References**
	224	8.5			Shelter dogs	Le Nobel et al. (2004)
			305	28	Shelter cats	Robben et al. (2004)
	152	4.4	60	4.6	Household dogs and cats	Overgaauw et al. (2009)
	916	4.6			Household dogs	Nijsse et al. (2015)
	938	4.5			Household dogs	Nijsse et al. (2016a)
			670	7.2	Household cats	Nijsse et al. (2016b)
Poland	249	2.5	91	39	Adult dogs and cats	Luty (2001)
	196	58			Pups up to 3 months old	Luty (2001)
			14	64	Kittens 4–6 months old	Luty (2001)
	110	0.9			Household dogs	Maśnik (2000)
	763	21			Rural and urban Household dogs	Tylkowska et al. (2010)
	108	17			Sled dogs	Bajer et al. (2011)
	95	28	68	17	Stray dogs and cats	Szwabe and Błaszkowska (2017)
Portugal			74	11	Stray cats	Duarte et al. (2010)
	368	6.5			Household dogs	Neves et al. (2014)
			162	38	Stray cats	Waap et al. (2014)
	301	8.0			Rural dogs	Cardoso et al. (2014)
	369	0.5			Faecal samples from parks	Ferreira et al. (2017)
	103	3.9			Faecal samples from parks	Otero et al. (2018)

Continued

Table 1 Prevalence of *Toxocara* spp. in dogs and cats in Europe.—cont'd

	Dogs		Cats			
Country	**N**	**%[a]**	**N**	**%[a]**	**Source**	**References**
Romania			414	20	Household cats	Mircean et al. (2010)
	199	12			Household dogs	Mircean et al. (2017)
	141	11			Kennel dogs	Mircean et al. (2017)
	185	19			Shepherd dogs	Mircean et al. (2017)
	372	21			Shelter dogs	Mircean et al. (2017)
	61	16			Hunting dogs	Mircean et al. (2017)
	356	16			Guard dogs	Mircean et al. (2017)
Russia	35	30			Autopsy dogs North Caucasus	Zhuravlev (2008)
Serbia	65	37			Household dogs	Nikolić et al. (2008)
	11	27			Military working dogs	Nikolić et al. (2008)
	75	25			Stray dogs	Nikolić et al. (2008)
	134	3.0			Shelter dogs	Sommer et al. (2017)
Slovakia	53	32			Stray dogs	Antolová et al. (2004)
	92	7.6			Household dogs	Antolová et al. (2004)
	457	19			Dog faeces from public places	Totková et al. (2006)

Table 1 Prevalence of *Toxocara* spp. in dogs and cats in Europe.—cont'd

	Dogs		Cats			
Country	**N**	**%[a]**	**N**	**%[a]**	**Source**	**References**
Spain			58	55	Stray cats	Calvete et al. (1998)
			231	20	Stray cats	Miró et al. (2004)
			48	25	Farm cats	Miró et al. (2004)
			103	11	Household cats	Miró et al. (2004)
	1161	7.8			Stray dogs	Miró et al. (2007)
	1800	18			Household dogs	Martínez-Moreno et al. (2007)
	125	7.1			Household dogs	Martínez-Carrasco et al. (2007)
	100	13			Shelter dogs	Martínez-Carrasco et al. (2007)
	50	7.0			Stray dogs	Martínez-Carrasco et al. (2007)
			58	35	Stray cats	Millán and Casanova (2009)
	263	8.0			Household dogs	Sanchez-Thevenet et al. (2019)
			278	7.7	Stray cats	Miró et al. (2014)
			76	21	Stray cats	Rodríguez-Ponce et al. (2016)
			263	12	Free-roaming cats	Montoya et al. (2018)
Czech Republic	3780	6.5			Urban dogs	Dubná et al. (2007)
	540	14			Rural area dogs	Dubná et al. (2007)
Sweden			205	21	Outdoor household cats	Grandi et al. (2017)

Continued

Table 1 Prevalence of *Toxocara* spp. in dogs and cats in Europe.—cont'd

	Dogs		Cats			
Country	**N**	**%[a]**	**N**	**%[a]**	**Source**	**References**
Switzerland	217	17			Stray dogs	Deplazes et al. (1995)
	154	14			Shelter dogs	Deplazes et al. (1995)
	505	7.1			Household dogs	Sager et al. (2006)
	402	2.5			Faecal samples from grasslands	Hauser et al. (2015)
	236	1.2			Faecal samples from dog waste bags	Hauser et al. (2015)
			168	55	Stray cats	Zottler et al. (2019)
			197	9.1	Shelter cats	Zottler et al. (2019)
			299	3.0	Household cats	Zottler et al. (2019)
United Kingdom	608	3.3			Hearing dogs	Guest et al. (2007)
	4526	1.4			Owned dogs	Batchelor et al. (2008)
	99	2.0			Privately owned adult	Morgan et al. (2013)
	16	19			3–6 months old	Morgan et al. (2013)
	81	48			0–3 months old	Morgan et al. (2013)
	171	5.3	131	26	Domestic dogs and cats	Wright et al. (2016)
Total	76,722			24,321		
Average	913	14.6	477	24.5		

[a]Prevalences above 10% are rounded to the nearest integer.

3.1.1 Toxocara canis *prevalences*

From the 90 studies found, 66 were investigating in total 76,722 dog faecal samples to establish the presence of *T. canis* eggs. The average prevalence was 14.6% (range: 0.5–83), which has been specified for the different groups in Table 2. The average number of animals per study was 913 and the range of number of animals was 11–24,677.

The average prevalence for pups and young dogs (up to 6 months of age) was calculated as 41.2% (range: 19–58), for owned adult dogs (including household, rural, suburban, breeding, kenneled, domestic, shepherd, sledge or village dogs) as 11.1% (range: 0.5–76), and for stray dogs (including unwanted or shelter dogs) as 17.6% (range: 3–83). In several studies, different animal groups were investigated. A rough impression of the trend of the average prevalence in owned animals can be obtained when comparing the prevalence during the time period from 1994 to 2008 and the prevalence in the years afterwards. This was 11% (range: 0.9–34) from 21,217 dogs in 21 studies and 11.2% (range: 0.5–76) in 45,805 dogs in 40 studies, respectively.

3.1.2 Toxocara cati *prevalences*

In total, 45 studies were investigating in total 24,321 cat faecal samples to establish the presence of *T. cati* eggs. The average prevalence was 24.5% (range: 0–85). The average number of animals per study was 477 and the range of number of animals was 14–8560.

Table 2 *Toxocara canis* and *T. cati* prevalences of dogs and cats in European country studies.

	Number	Average *Toxocara* prevalence %	No. of studies[a]
Dogs			
All	77,895	14.6	60
Pups	2827	41.2	6
Owned dogs	67,022	11.1	61
Stray dogs	6873	17.6	17
Cats			
All	24,321	24.5	45
Kittens	1332	25.0	3
Owned cats	18,539	15.1	23
Stray cats	4702	34.5	25

[a]In several studies, a combination of different animal groups was investigated.

The average prevalence for kittens under 6 months of age was calculated as 25.0% (range: 0–64), for owned cats (including household, domestic and breeding cats) as 15.1% (range: 2–39), and for stray cats (including feral, farm, free-roaming, semi-domestic and shelter cats) as 34.5% (range: 7.6–85). See Table 2. For the owned cats, a trend of the average prevalence can also be calculated. This result is 11.9% (range: 2–39) from 4732 cats in 9 studies before 2008 and 14.8% (range: 3–33) in 13,555 animals in 14 studies after that year.

3.2 Multicentre European prevalence studies

Two multicentre European studies that established the prevalence of *Toxocara* spp. in dogs and cats were included. One study in cats was conducted in seven countries during the period 2012–2013 (Beugnet et al., 2014). In total 1219 cats were included with an average *T. cati* prevalence of 20.0% (Table 3).

The other (unpublished) study has been provided by IDEXX Europe (IDEXX, 2019) that collected the faecal examination results of dogs and cats with the IDEXX Fecal Dx® Antigen Test after the recent introduction in their labs during the period 2017–2019 (Table 4). The samples were sent to these labs by veterinary clinics. The average percentage positive animals combined for all countries and all age groups and life stages, defined as young (up to 1 year for cats and 2 years for dogs), adult (up to 8 years for

Table 3 Prevalence of *Toxocara cati* in cats in a multicentre European study (Beugnet et al., 2014).

Country	Number of cats	Prevalence %[a]
Austria	92	10
Belgium	55	7.3
France	187	9.1
Hungary	300	17
Italy	215	34
Romania	300	27
Spain	70	13
Total	*1219*	*244*
Average		*20.0*

[a]Prevalences above 10% are rounded to the nearest integer.

Table 4 Prevalence of ascarids in dogs and cats in a multicentre European study (IDEXX, 2019).

	Dogs		Cats	
Country	**Number**	**Prevalence %**	**Number**	**Prevalence %**
Austria	1928	4.3	460	4.3
Denmark	1962	4.5	133	6.8
Germany	29,039	2.9	4568	4.2
Italy	927	4.0	95	5.3
Netherlands	1043	2.8	327	4.0
Norway	324	2.2	27	3.7
Sweden	278	1.8	58	8.6
Total	*35,501*		*5668*	
Average		*3.1*		*4.3*

Table 5 Prevalence of *Toxocara* spp. in European dogs and cats per life stage (IDEXX, 2019).

	Dogs			Cats		
Life stage	**Age group**	**Number**	**Prevalence %**	**Age group**	**Number**	**Prevalence %**
Young	0–2 years	2197	3.4	0–1 years	3233	4.8
Adult	3–6 years	7091	3.5	2–8 years	1556	4.6
Senior	7–10 years	4425	1.9	9–13 years	615	2.3
Geriatric	11–15+	2014	1.1	14–15+	264	1.9

cats and 6 years for dogs), senior (up to 13 years for cats and 10 years for dogs), and geriatric (from 14 years for cats and 11 years for dogs), for *T. canis* was 3.1% (range: 1.8–4.5%) in 35,501 dogs and for *T. cati* 4.3% (range: 3.7–8.6%) in 5668 cats (Table 4).

After differentiation for the different life stages of the dogs (Table 5 and Fig. 1), similar prevalences were recorded for young and adult dogs (3.2 and 3.5%, respectively) and cats (4.8 and 4.6%, respectively). In Table 6, the proportion of positive tests in the multicentric studies decreased significantly from adult life stage to senior and geriatric life stages in both dogs ($P < 0.001$, by Fisher's Exact Test) and cats ($P = 0.014$, by Fisher's Exact Test), and remained lower into geriatric life stage.

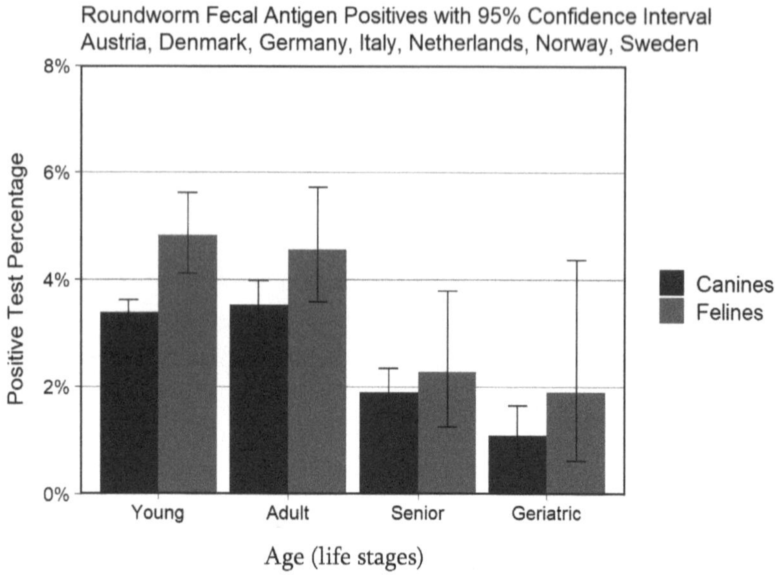

Fig. 1 Prevalence of ascarids in European dogs and cats per life stage.

Table 6 Comparing average roundworm prevalences of *household* dogs and cats in European country and in multicenter studies.[a]

Country	European country cat studies (Table 1)	Multicenter cat study (Beugnet et al., 2014)	Multicenter cat study (IDEXX, 2019)	European country dog studies (Table 1)	Multicenter dog study (IDEXX, 2019)
Austria		10	4.4		4.3
Belgium		7.3			
Denmark			6.8		4.5
France	9.0	9.1			
Germany	9.9		4.2	10	2.9
Hungary	17	17			
Italy	17	34	5.3	11	4.0
Netherlands	4.7		4.0	4.4	2.8
Norway		27	3.7		2.2
Sweden	21	13	8.6		1.8
Romania	20	27			
Spain	11	13			

[a]Prevalences above 10% are rounded to the nearest integer.

4. Discussion

The prevalence studies from the different European countries prove the well-known trend that young and stray animals have the highest infection rates with *Toxocara* spp. (Holland, 2017). When focusing only on owned dogs and cats which are the largest investigated groups, the average prevalence is 11.2% and 15.1%, respectively, in the country studies from the last 25 years. This result was confirmed with the average prevalence rate of 16.8% for cats in the multicentre study in seven European countries (Beugnet et al., 2014). However, this last rate is high mainly due to the high prevalences in Italy and Romania (Table 3). From the 90 studies, 8 investigated only faecal samples from parks and grasslands. This may bias the results because these are not individual animals that were tested. It is possible that several faecal samples originated from the same animals. Finally, the description of the investigated animals is also not standardized. There are many different and overlapping groups mentioned. Kennel dogs may be breeder dogs in one article but shelter or hunting animals in another. Comparison of the different studies is therefore not always consistent.

The latest results of a Roundworm Faecal Antigen Test for dogs and cats in 7 countries show, however, lower prevalences for dogs and cats of 3.2% and 5.4%, respectively. A limitation of this test is that it also detects the other ascarid species *Toxascaris leonina* and *Baylisascaris* spp. These nematodes have, in general, low prevalences in Europe (Beugnet et al., 2014) or are very rare isolated from dogs (Bauer, 2013). On the other hand, there are no false-positive test results as a result of the presence of spurious eggs (Nijsse et al., 2014) because only the parasites will be detected.

Young and adult animals had similar patent infection rates, but senior and geriatric animals showed much lower positive percentages (IDEXX, 2019). It should be considered when interpreting the IDEXX data that, due to the fact that samples were sent in by veterinary clinics, a proportion of the animals tested had clinical problems. These are mostly gastrointestinal and concern younger animals and some may have received an anthelmintic treatment which may partly explain the low prevalence findings. In the other prevalence studies, this bias is not expected.

In some countries, the numbers of cats tested is low (Italy, Norway and Sweden) and such results are less comparable with the other investigated countries.

It is striking that the number of *Toxocara* prevalence studies in dogs are two times higher than in cats. The role of *T. cati* as a zoonotic parasite is still not always clearly recognized. Despite the fact that differentiation between *T. canis* and *T. cati* infections is still not feasible in serological surveys, the majority of reported human cases of toxocariasis have been associated with *T. canis* based on epidemiological considerations (Fisher, 2003). The potential role of *T. cati* in human toxocariasis should not be ignored or underestimated (Overgaauw and Van Knapen, 2013).

In general, the *Toxocara* spp. prevalences in the European studies do not seem to decrease over the years, despite an increase in the amount of education and information given out by vets, governments and organizations such as ESCCAP.

It can be concluded that approximated prevalences for dogs and cats in most European countries are collected. Since the results vary considerably between the classical faecal examination methods and the modern tests, it may be advised to perform a study to compare these two methods in the field. It would also be preferable if the intensity of egg-shedding could also be involved in studies to give more information about the epidemiology and contamination of the environment with eggs by the different groups of animals. A more accurate description of the animals tested is needed in order to make a better assessment for the different risk groups. In the future, higher numbers of animals investigated in different countries using one uniform test method may create more reliable and comparable results leading to better comprehension of the epidemiology of patent *Toxocara* infections.

Acknowledgements

We would like to thank IDEXX, South Portland, Maine, USA for the kind support of faecal antigen test data.

References

Al-Sabi, M.N., Kapel, C.M., Johansson, A., Espersen, M.C., Koch, J., Willesen, J.L., 2013. A coprological investigation of gastrointestinal and cardiopulmonary parasites in hunting dogs in Denmark. Vet. Parasitol. 196, 366–372.

Antolová, D., Reiterová, K., Miterpáková, M., Stanko, M., Dubinský, P., 2004. Circulation of *Toxocara* spp. in suburban and rural ecosystems in the Slovak Republic. Vet. Parasitol. 126, 317–324.

Bajer, A., Bednarska, M., Rodo, A., 2011. Risk factors and control of intestinal parasite infections in sled dogs in Poland. Vet. Parasitol. 175, 343–350.

Barutzki, D., Schaper, R., 2003. Endoparasites in dogs and cats in Germany 1999-2002. Parasitol. Res. 3 (Suppl. 90), S148–S150.

Barutzki, D., Schaper, R., 2011. Results of parasitological examinations of faecal samples from cats and dogs in Germany between 2003 and 2010. Parasitol. Res. 109 (Suppl. 1), S45–S60.

Barutzki, D., Schaper, R., 2013. Age-dependent prevalence of endoparasites in young dogs and cats up to one year of age. Parasitol. Res. 112 (Suppl. 1), 119–131.

Batchelor, D.J., Tzannes, S., Graham, P.A., Wastling, J.M., Pinchbeck, G.L., German, A.J., 2008. Detection of endoparasites with zoonotic potential in dogs with gastrointestinal disease in the UK. Transbound. Emerg. Dis. 55, 99–104.

Bauer, C., 2013. Baylisascariosis-infections of animals and humans with 'unusual' roundworms. Vet. Parasitol. 193, 404–412.

Becker, A.C., Rohen, M., Epe, C., Schnieder, T., 2012. Prevalence of endoparasites in stray and fostered dogs and cats in Northern Germany. Parasitol. Res. 111, 849–857.

Beugnet, F., Guillot, J., Polack, B., Chermette, R., 2000. Enquête sur le parasitisme digestif des chiens et des chats de particuliers de la region Parisienne. Revue Méd. Vét. 151, 443–446.

Beugnet, F., Bourdeau, P., Chalvet-Monfray, K., Cozma, V., Farkas, R., Guillot, J., et al., 2014. Parasites of domestic owned cats in Europe: co-infestations and risk factors. Parasit. Vectors 7, 291.

Calvete, C., Lucientes, J., Castillo, J.A., Estrada, R., Gracia, M.J., Peribáñez, M.A., et al., 1998. Gastrointestinal helminth parasites in stray cats from the mid-Ebro Valley, Spain. Vet. Parasitol. 75, 235–240.

Capári, B., Hamel, D., Visser, M., Winter, R., Pfister, K., Rehbein, S., 2013. Parasitic infections of domestic cats, *Felis catus*, in western Hungary. Vet. Parasitol. 192, 33–42.

Cardoso, A.S., Costa, I.M., Figueiredo, C., Castro, A., Conceição, M.A., 2014. The occurrence of zoonotic parasites in rural dog populations from northern Portugal. J. Helminthol. 88, 203–209.

Claerebout, E., Casaert, S., Dalemans, A.C., De Wilde, N., Levecke, B., Vercruysse, J., et al., 2009. *Giardia* and other intestinal parasites in different dog populations in Northern Belgium. Vet. Parasitol. 161, 41–46.

Deplazes, P., Guscetti, F., Wunderlin, E., Bucklar, H., Skaggs, J., Wolff, K., 1995. Endoparasite infection in stray and abandoned dogs in southern Switzerland. Schweiz. Arch. Tierheilkd. 137, 172–179.

Diakou, A., Di Cesare, A., Accettura, P.M., Barros, L., Lorio, R., Paoletti, B., et al., 2017a. Intestinal parasites and vector-borne pathogens in stray and free-roaming cats living in continental and insular Greece. PLoS Negl. Trop. Dis. 11 (1), e0005335.

Diakou, A., Di Cesare, A., Morelli, S., Colombo, M., Halos, L., Simonato, G., et al., 2019. Endoparasites and vector-borne pathogens in dogs from Greek islands: pathogen distribution and zoonotic implications. PLoS Negl. Trop. Dis. 13 (5) e0007003.

Duarte, A., Castro, I., Pereira da Fonseca, I.M., Almeida, V., Madeira de Carvalho, L.M., Meireles, J., et al., 2010. Survey of infectious and parasitic diseases in stray cats at the Lisbon Metropolitan Area, Portugal. J. Feline Med. Surg. 12, 441–446.

Dubná, S., Langrová, I., Nápravník, J., Jankovská, I., Vadlejch, J., Pekár, S., et al., 2007. The prevalence of intestinal parasites in dogs from Prague, rural areas, and shelters of the Czech Republic. Vet. Parasitol. 145, 120–128.

Dupont, S., Butaye, P., Claerebout, E., Theuns, S., Duchateau, L., Van de Maele, I., et al., 2013. Enteropathogens in pups from pet shops and breeding facilities. J. Small Anim. Pract. 54, 475–480.

Epe, C., Coati, N., Schnieder, T., 2004. Results of parasitological examinations of faecal samples from horses, ruminants, pigs, dogs, cats, hedgehogs and rabbits between 1998 and 2002. Dtsch. Tierarztl. Wochenschr. 111, 243–247.

ESCCAP (European Counsel Companion Animal Parasites), 2004. Guideline 1: Worm Control in dogs and cats, first ed. www.esccap.org.

Ferreira, A., Alho, A.M., Otero, D., Gomes, L., Nijsse, R., Overgaauw, P.A.M., et al., 2017. Urban dog parks as sources of canine parasites: contamination rates and pet owner behaviors in Lisbon, Portugal. J. Environ. Public Health 1, 1–7.
Fisher, M., 2003. *Toxocara cati*: an underestimated zoonotic agent. Trends Parasitol. 19, 167–170.
Fok, E., Szatmári, V., Busák, K., Rozgonyi, F., 2001. Prevalence of intestinal parasites in dogs in some urban and rural areas of Hungary. Vet. Q. 23, 96–98.
Franc, M., Cadiergues, M.C., Marchand, A., Bourdoiseae, G., Bussieras, J., 1997. Le parasitism intestinal des carnivores domestiques: bilan d'une enquête conduit dans les quatre Ecoles Vétérinaires Françaises. Revue Méd. Vét. 148, 247–250.
Fromont, E., Morvilliers, L., Artois, M., Pontier, D., 2001. Parasite richness and abundance in insular and mainland feral cats: insularity or density? Parasitology 123, 143–151.
Garcia-Campos, A., Power, C., O'Shaughnessy, J., Browne, C., Lawlor, A., McCarthy, G., 2018. One-year parasitological screening of stray dogs and cats in County Dublin, Ireland. Parasitology 18, 1–7.
Grandi, G., Comin, A., Ibrahim, O., Schaper, R., Forshell, U., Lind, E.O., 2017. Prevalence of helminth and coccidian parasites in Swedish outdoor cats and the first report of *Aelurostrongylus abstrusus* in Sweden: a coprological investigation. Acta Vet. Scand. 59, 19.
Guest, C.M., Stephen, J.M., Price, C.J., 2007. Prevalence of *Campylobacter* and four endoparasites in dog populations associated with Hearing Dogs. J. Small Anim. Pract. 48, 632–637.
Habluetzel, A., Traldi, G., Ruggieri, S., Attili, A.R., Scuppa, P., Marchetti, R., et al., 2003. An estimation of *Toxocara canis* prevalence in dogs, environmental egg contamination and risk of human infection in the Marche region of Italy. Vet. Parasitol. 113, 243–252.
Hansen, A.P., Skarbye, L.K., Vinther, L.M., Willesen, J.L., Pipper, C.B., Olsen, C.S., et al., 2017. Occurrence and clinical significance of *Aelurostrongylus abstrusus* and other endoparasites in Danish cats. Vet. Parasitol. 234, 31–39.
Hauser, M., Basso, W., Deplazes, P., 2015. Dog and fox faecal contamination of farmland. Schweiz. Arch. Tierheilkd. 157, 449–455.
Hinney, B., Gottwald, M., Moser, J., Reicher, B., Schäfer, B.J., Schaper, R., et al., 2017. Examination of anonymous canine faecal samples provides data on endoparasite prevalence rates in dogs for comparative studies. Vet. Parasitol. 245, 106–115.
Holland, C.V., 2017. Knowledge gaps in the epidemiology of *Toxocara*: the enigma remains. Parasitology 144, 81–94.
IDEXX Europe, 2019. Roundworm Fecal Antigen Test Results 2017-2019 for the countries Austria, Denmark, Germany, Italy, Netherlands, Norway, Sweden. IDEXX Internal Report.
Knaus, M., Kusi, I., Rapti, D., Xhaxhiu, D., Winter, R., Visser, M., Rehbein, S., 2011. Endoparasites of cats from the Tirana area and the first report on *Aelurostrongylus abstrusus* (Railliet, 1898) in Albania. Wien. Klin. Wochenschr. 123, 31–35.
Knaus, M., Rapti, D., Shukullari, E., Kusi, I., Postoli, R., Xhaxhiu, D., et al., 2014. Characterisation of ecto- and endoparasites in domestic cats from Tirana, Albania. Parasitol. Res. 113, 3361–3371.
Kostopoulou, D., Claerebout, E., Arvanitis, D., Ligda, P., Voutzourakis, N., Casaert, S., et al., 2017. Abundance, zoonotic potential and risk factors of intestinal parasitism amongst dog and cat populations: the scenario of Crete, Greece. Parasit. Vectors 10, 43.
Lassen, B., Jokelainen, P., 2016. Survey of the presence of *Toxocara* spp. eggs in dog feces in Tartu, Estonia. Vector Borne Zoonotic Dis. 16, 212–214.

Le Nobel, W.E., Robben, S.R., Döpfer, D., Hendrikx, W.M., Boersema, J.H., Fransen, F., et al., 2004. Infections with endoparasites in dogs in Dutch animal shelters. Tijdschr. Diergeneeskd. 129, 40–44.

Luty, T., 2001. Prevalence of species of *Toxocara* in dogs, cats and red foxes from the Poznan region, Poland. J. Helminthol. 75, 15315–15316.

Ma, G., Holland, C.V., Wang, T., Hofmann, A., Fan, C.K., Maizels, R.M., Hotez, P.J., Gasser, R.B., 2018. Human toxocariasis. Lancet Infect. Dis. 18, e14–e24.

Martínez-Carrasco, C., Berriatua, E., Garijo, M., Martínez, J., Alonso, F.D., de Ybáñez, R.R., 2007. Epidemiological study of non-systemic parasitism in dogs in southeast Mediterranean Spain assessed by coprological and post-mortem examination. Zoonoses Public Health 54, 195–203.

Martínez-Moreno, F.J., Hernández, S., López-Cobos, E., Becerra, C., Acosta, I., Martínez-Moreno, A., 2007. Estimation of canine intestinal parasites in Córdoba (Spain) and their risk to public health. Vet. Parasitol. 143, 7–13.

Maśnik, E., 2000. Relationships between the prevalence of *Toxocara* eggs in dogs' faeces and soil. Wiad. Parazytol. 46, 239–244.

McManus, R., Hamilton, C.M., Holland, C.V., 2018. *Toxocara* spp. In: Rose, J.B., Jiménez-Cisneros, B. (Eds.), Global Water Pathogens Project. www.waterpathogens.org (Robertson, L (eds) Part 4 Helminths) www.waterpathogens.org/book/toxocara Michigan State University, E. Lansing, MI, UNESCO.

Millán, J., Casanova, J.C., 2009. High prevalence of helminth parasites in feral cats in Majorca Island (Spain). Parasitol. Res. 106, 183–188.

Mircean, V., Titilincu, A., Vasile, C., 2010. Prevalence of endoparasites in household cat (*Felis catus*) populations from Transylvania (Romania) and association with risk factors. Vet. Parasitol. 171, 163–166.

Mircean, V., Dumitrache, M.O., Mircean, M., Colosi, H.A., Györke, A., 2017. Prevalence and risk factors associated with endoparasitic infection in dogs from Transylvania (Romania): a retrospective study. Vet. Parasitol. 243, 157–161.

Miró, G., Montoya, A., Jiménez, S., Frisuelos, C., Mateo, M., Fuentes, I., 2004. Prevalence of antibodies to *Toxoplasma gondii* and intestinal parasites in stray, farm and household cats in Spain. Vet. Parasitol. 126, 249–255.

Miró, G., Mateo, M., Montoya, A., Vela, E., Calonge, R., 2007. Survey of intestinal parasites in stray dogs in the Madrid area and comparison of the efficacy of three anthelmintics in naturally infected dogs. Parasitol. Res. 100, 317–320.

Miró, G., Rupérez, C., Checa, R., Gálvez, R., Hernández, L., García, M., et al., 2014. Current status of *L. infantum* infection in stray cats in the Madrid region (Spain): implications for the recent outbreak of human leishmaniosis? Parasit. Vectors 7, 112.

Montoya, A., García, M., Gálvez, R., Checa, R., Marino, V., Sarquis, J., et al., 2018. Implications of zoonotic and vector-borne parasites to free-roaming cats in central Spain. Vet. Parasitol. 251, 125–130.

Morgan, E.R., Azam, D., Pegler, K., 2013. Quantifying sources of environmental contamination with *Toxocara* spp. eggs. Vet. Parasitol. 193, 390–397.

Näreaho, A., Puomio, J., Saarinen, K., Jokelainen, P., Juselius, T., Sukura, A., 2012. Feline intestinal parasites in Finland: prevalence, risk factors and anthelmintic treatment practices. J. Feline Med. Surg. 14, 378–383.

Neves, D., Lobo, L., Simões, P.B., Cardoso, L., 2014. Frequency of intestinal parasites in pet dogs from an urban area (Greater Oporto, northern Portugal). Vet. Parasitol. 200, 295–298.

Nijsse, R., Mughini-Gras, L., Wagenaar, J.A., Ploeger, H.W., 2014. Coprophagy in dogs interferes in faecal examination. Vet. Parasitol. 204, 304–309.

Nijsse, R., Ploeger, H.W., Wagenaar, J.A., Mughini-Gras, L., 2015. *Toxocara canis* in household dogs: prevalence, risk factors and owners' attitude towards deworming. Parasitol. Res. 114, 561–569.

Nijsse, R., Mughini-Gras, L., Wagenaar, J.A., Ploeger, H.W., 2016a. Recurrent patent infections with *Toxocara canis* in household dogs older than six months: a prospective study. Parasit. Vectors 9, 531.

Nijsse, R., Ploeger, H.W., Wagenaar, J.A., Mughini-Gras, L., 2016b. Prevalence and risk factors for patent Toxocara infections in cats and cat owners' attitude towards deworming. Parasitol. Res. 115, 4519–4525.

Nikolić, A., Dimitrijević, S., Katić-Radivojević, S., Klun, I., Bobrć, B., Djurković-Djaković, O., 2008. High prevalence of intestinal zoonotic parasites in dogs from Belgrade, Serbia—short communication. Acta Vet. Hung. 56, 335–340.

O'Lorcain, P., 1994. Epidemiology of *Toxocara* spp. in stray dogs and cats in Dublin, Ireland. J. Helminthol. 68, 331–336.

Otero, D., Alho, A.M., Nijsse, R., Roelfsema, J., Overgaauw, P.A.M., Madeira de Carvalho, L., 2018. Environmental contamination with *Toxocara* spp. eggs in public parks and playground sandpits of Greater Lisbon, Portugal. J. Infect. Public Health 11, 94–98.

Overgaauw, P.A., 1997. Prevalence of intestinal nematodes of dogs and cats in The Netherlands. Vet. Q. 19, 14–17.

Overgaauw, P.A., Boersema, J.H., 1998a. Nematode infections in dog breeding kennels in The Netherlands, with special reference to *Toxocara*. Vet. Q. 20, 12–15.

Overgaauw, P.A., Boersema, J.H., 1998b. A survey of *Toxocara* infections in cat breeding colonies in The Netherlands. Vet. Q. 20, 9–11.

Overgaauw, P.A.M., Van Knapen, F., 2013. Veterinary and public health aspects of *Toxocara* spp. Vet. Parasitol. 193, 398–403.

Overgaauw, P.A., van Zutphen, L., Hoek, D., Yaya, F.O., Roelfsema, J., Pinelli, E., et al., 2009. Zoonotic parasites in fecal samples and fur from dogs and cats in The Netherlands. Vet. Parasitol. 163, 115–122.

Paoletti, B., Traversa, D., Iorio, R., De Berardinis, A., Bartolini, R., Salini, R., et al., 2015. Zoonotic parasites in feces and fur of stray and private dogs from Italy. Parasitol. Res. 114, 2135–2141.

Papazahariadou, M., Founta, A., Papadopoulos, E., Chliounakis, S., Antoniadou-Sotiriadou, K., Theodorides, Y., 2007. Gastrointestinal parasites of shepherd and hunting dogs in the Serres Prefecture, Northern Greece. Vet. Parasitol. 148, 170–173.

Poulle, M.L., Bastien, M., Richard, Y.T., Josse-Dupuis, E., Aubert, D., Villena, I., et al., 2017. Detection of *Echinococcus multilocularis* and other foodborne parasites in fox, cat and dog faeces collected in kitchen gardens in a highly endemic area for alveolar echinococcosis. Parasite 24, 29.

Pullola, T., Vierimaa, J., Saari, S., Virtala, A.M., Nikander, S., Sukura, A., 2006. Canine intestinal helminths in Finland: prevalence, risk factors and endoparasite control practices. Vet. Parasitol. 140, 321–326.

Raue, K., Heuer, L., Böhm, C., Wolken, S., Epe, C., Strube, C., 2017. 10-year parasitological examination results (2003 to 2012) of faecal samples from horses, ruminants, pigs, dogs, cats, rabbits and hedgehogs. Parasitol. Res. 116, 3315–3330.

Riggio, F., Mannella, R., Ariti, G., Perrucci, S., 2013. Intestinal and lung parasites in owned dogs and cats from central Italy. Vet. Parasitol. 193, 78–84.

Robben, S.R., le Nobel, W.E., Döpfer, D., Hendrikx, W.M., Boersema, J.H., Fransen, F., et al., 2004. Infections with helminths and/or protozoa in cats in animal shelters in the Netherlands. Tijdschr. Diergeneeskd. 129, 2–6.

Rodríguez-Ponce, E., González, J.F., Conde de Felipe, M., Hernández, J.N., Raduan Jaber, J., 2016. Epidemiological survey of zoonotic helminths in feral cats in Gran Canaria island (Macaronesian archipelago-Spain). Acta Parasitol. 61, 443–450.

Sager, H., Moret, C.S., Grimm, F., Deplazes, P., Doherr, M.G., Gottstein, B., 2006. Coprological study on intestinal helminths in Swiss dogs: temporal aspects of anthelminthic treatment. Parasitol. Res. 98, 333–338.

Sanchez-Thevenet, P., Carmena, D., Adell-Aledón, M., Dacal, E., Arias, E., Saugar, J.M., et al., 2019. High prevalence and diversity of zoonotic and other intestinal parasites in dogs from eastern Spain. Vector Borne Zoonotic Dis. 19, 915–922.

Sauda, F., Malandrucco, L., Macrì, G., Scarpulla, M., De Liberato, C., Terracciano, G., et al., 2018. Leishmania infantum, Dirofilaria spp. and other endoparasite infections in kennel dogs in central Italy, Parasite 25, 2–8.

Scaramozzino, P., Carvelli, A., Iacoponi, F., De Liberato, C., 2018. Endoparasites in household and shelter dogs from Central Italy. Int. J. Vet. Sci. Med. 6, 45–47.

Sherifi, K., Rexhepi, A., Hamidi, A., Behluli, B., Zessin, K.H., Mathis, A., et al., 2011. Detection of patent infections of *Echinococcus granulosus* ("sheep-strain", G1) in naturally infected dogs in Kosovo. Berl. Munch. Tierarztl. Wochenschr. 124, 518–521.

Shukullari, E., Hamel, D., Rapti, D., Pfister, K., Visser, M., Winter, R., et al., 2015. Parasites and vector-borne diseases in client-owned dogs in Albania. Intestinal and pulmonary endoparasite infections. Parasitol. Res. 114, 4579–4590.

Simonato, G., Frangipane di Regalbono, A., Cassini, R., Traversa, D., Beraldo, P., Tessarin, C., et al., 2015. Copromicroscopic and molecular investigations on intestinal parasites in kenneled dogs. Parasitol. Res. 114, 1963–1970.

Sommer, M.F., Zdravković, N., Vasić, A., Grimm, F., Silaghi, C., 2017. Gastrointestinal parasites in shelter dogs from Belgrade, Serbia. Vet. Parasitol. Reg. Stud. Reports 7, 54–57.

Spada, E., Proverbio, D., Della Pepa, A., Domenichini, G., Bagnagatti De Giorgi, G., Traldi, G., Ferro, E., 2013. Prevalence of faecal-borne parasites in colony stray cats in northern Italy. J. Feline Med. Surg. 15, 672–677.

Symeonidou, I., Gelasakis, A.I., Arsenopoulos, K., Angelou, A., Beugnet, F., Papadopoulos, E., 2018. Feline gastrointestinal parasitism in Greece: emergent zoonotic species and associated risk factors. Parasit. Vectors 11, 227.

Szwabe, K., Błaszkowska, J., 2017. Stray dogs and cats as potential sources of soil contamination with zoonotic parasites. Ann. Agric. Environ. Med. 24, 39–43.

Takeuchi-Storm, N., Mejer, H., Al-Sabi, M.N., Olsen, C.S., Thamsborg, S.M., Enemark, H.L., 2015. Gastrointestinal parasites of cats in Denmark assessed by necropsy and concentration McMaster technique. Vet. Parasitol. 214, 327–332.

Talvik, H., Moks, E., Mägi, E., Järvis, T., Miller, I., 2006. Distribution of *Toxocara* infection in the environment and in definitive and paratenic hosts in Estonia. Acta Vet. Hung. 54, 399–406.

Tamponi, C., Varcasia, A., Pinna, S., Melis, E., Melosu, V., Zidda, A., Sanna, G., Pipia, A.P., et al., 2017. Endoparasites detected in faecal samples from dogs and cats referred for routine clinical visit in Sardinia, Italy. Vet. Parasitol. Reg. Stud. Reports 10, 13–17.

Totková, A., Klobusický, M., Holková, R., Friedová, L., 2006. Current prevalence of toxocariasis and other intestinal parasitoses among dogs in Bratislava. Epidemiol. Mikrobiol. Imunol. 55, 17–22.

Tylkowska, A., Pilarczyk, B., Gregorczyk, A., Templin, E., 2010. Gastrointestinal helminths of dogs in Western Pomerania, Poland. Wiad. Parazytol. 56, 269–276.

Vienažindienė, Ž., Joekel, D.E., Schaper, R., Deplazes, P., Šarkūnas, M., 2018. Longitudinal study for anthelmintic efficacy against intestinal helminths in naturally exposed Lithuanian village dogs: critical analysis of feasibility and limitations. Parasitol. Res. 117, 1581–1590.

Waap, H., Gomes, J., Nunes, T., 2014. Parasite communities in stray cat populations from Lisbon, Portugal. J. Helminthol. 88, 389–395.

Wright, I., Stafford, K., Coles, G., 2016. The prevalence of intestinal nematodes in cats and dogs from Lancashire, north-west England. J. Small Anim. Pract. 57, 393–395.
Xhaxhiu, D., Kusi, I., Rapti, D., Kondi, E., Postoli, R., Rinaldi, L., et al., 2011. Principal intestinal parasites of dogs in Tirana, Albania. Parasitol. Res. 108, 341–353.
Zhuravlev, A.S., 2008. Major Dogs' Helminthosis in North Caucasian Region. 5, Vestn. Krasnojarskogo Gosudarstvennogo Agrarnogo Univ., pp. 257–259.
Zottler, E.M., Bieri, M., Basso, W., Schnyder, M., 2019. Intestinal parasites and lungworms in stray, shelter and privately-owned cats of Switzerland. Parasitol. Int. 69, 75–81.

Further reading

Aubert, D., Villena, I., Knapp, J., 2017. Detection of *Echinococcus multilocularis* and other foodborne parasites in fox, cat and dog feces collected in kitchen gardens in a highly endemic area for alveolar echinococcosis. Parasite 24, 29.

CHAPTER THIRTY-SIX

Toxocara prevalence in dogs, cats and the environment in Russia

Alexander N. Lukashev*, Maria N. Ruzina, Lyudmila V. Akhmadishina
Martsinovsky Institute of Medical Parasitology, Tropical and Vector-Borne Diseases, Sechenov University, Moscow, Russia
*Corresponding author: e-mail address: alexander_lukashev@hotmail.com

Contents

Abstract

The toxocariasis incidence in Russia is relatively low (1.8 cases per 100,000 individuals) and the parasite is not a major healthcare concern. However, the proportion of primary hosts testing positive for the parasite is high and varies between 3% and 100% in dogs (on average 33%), and between 6% and 52% in cats. Higher prevalence was observed in Volga, Urals and Siberia regions. Levels of contamination of soil, children's playgrounds and sandboxes is also high, with up to 100% contamination rates determined in some studies, but more commonly prevalence of contamination around 40% was reported. There is a pronounced seasonality in the prevalence of *Toxocara* in primary hosts and the soil, with peaks in the summer and autumn. Most likely, a lack of permissive conditions for the development of eggs in the winter determines observed seasonal patterns, which are different than those observed in most other countries. *Toxocara* eggs were found in 4–10% of vegetables and greenery samples tested, suggesting that they can contribute to the transmission of *Toxocara*.

Toxocariasis is a globally prevalent parasitic disease. The primary hosts are dogs, cats and a number of carnivores. Men, along with rodents, small mammals and, occasionally, cattle, are paratenic hosts. The life cycle of parasite is complex, and the relative importance of different infection routes (both within the natural cycle and as sources of human infection) is not fully understood (Ma et al., 2018). Dogs and cats are the main infection sources for humans, and the main inoculation route is alimentary by ingestion of eggs that matured in the soil upon excretion by primary hosts. Primary hosts, soil and other environmental objects are commonly contaminated with *Toxocara* eggs (Fakhri et al., 2018), and human infection is ubiquitous.

Advances in Parasitology, Volume 109
ISSN 0065-308X
https://doi.org/10.1016/bs.apar.2020.01.019

However, prevalence of *Toxocara* in the environment and seroprevalence is humans vary across the world (Fakhri et al., 2018; Ma et al., 2018).

About 2500 cases of toxocariasis are reported in Russia each year (1.8 cases per 100,000 individuals), producing only moderate medical concern compared to enterobiosis, ascaridosis and opisthorchiasis. Toxocarosis is a notifiable disease in Russia; therefore, the incidence of overt human infection is documented in statistical reports. Although the awareness and qualifications of medical personnel, as well as the availability of diagnostic tools, are key factors affecting levels of reported incidence, known epidemiological data on overt disease can be viewed as systematic. However, the seroprevalence of toxocarosis in humans in Russia is high (about 20–30%), suggesting that subclinical invasion infections are not reflected in the reported incidence (Akhmadishina et al., 2020). In the meanwhile, the current image of veterinary and environmental toxocariasis is even less clear.

The environmental monitoring is routinely done by the state surveillance system. Alternatively, the prevalence of *Toxocara* in animals and the environment is a common topic of independent research projects. Data from the two types of sources differ significantly, because routine surveillance is more systematic (although it is not carried out in all regions), while scientific studies may provide valuable novel data, but are not systematic and standardized. Prevalence of toxocariasis in final hosts and non-human paratenic hosts is within the scope of veterinary research and does not involve a centralized system of surveillance and reporting similar to incidence surveillance for humans. Nevertheless, the prevalence of animal toxocarosis is commonly studied by regional veterinary institutions, often as graduate or postgraduate projects. There are many more reports on the infection of dogs with *Toxocara canis*, than cats with *T. cati* (still commonly termed *T. mystax* in Russia), likely because obtaining samples from dogs is easier than from cats. Independent environmental and veterinary screening data is only available for some regions of Russia, but, taken together, do provide a fair image of *Toxocara* prevalence.

The method for the microscopic detection of *Toxocara* eggs has been well established. However, approaches for sampling (both collection and processing) differ amongst studies, and may have a decisive effect on the results obtained, especially with respect to studies investigating environmental contamination. Prevalence in a main host can be evaluated by detecting eggs in faeces, live worms in the intestine, or larvae in tissues upon autopsy. While the detection of eggs is more common, the latter approaches have also been used in some studies.

The prevalence of *Toxocara* invasion of dogs in Russia varied between 3% and 100% (Table 1; Fig. 1). A few studies reported a relatively low prevalence

Table 1 Prevalence of *Toxocara* in primary hosts in Russia.

City or region	Group of hosts[a]	Prevalence in dogs (%)	Prevalence in cats (%)	References
Moscow (1)	Pet	3.9	8.0	Budovskoy (2005)
	Shelter	14.3		
Moscow (1)	Pet	2.7	5.9	Kurnosova and Odoevskaya (2017)
Moscow (1)	Stray	25.4	31.6	Panova et al. (2015)
Moscow (1)	n.s.	11.8	13.2	Peshkov (2010)
St. Petersburg (2)	Pet	5.2		Lebedeva (2006)
	Stray	67.4		
Kostroma, Central Russia (3)	n.s.	11.3		Mikhin (2004)
Voronezh, Central Russia (4)	Pets, urban	20		Nikitina (2004)
	Pets, countryside	40		
	Stray	80		
Vologda, North Russia (5)	Urban	16.5		Novikova (2006)
	Rural	14.8		
Ufa, Volga region (6)	Urban	50	38[b]	Suleymanova (2012)
	Rural	15.6		
Cheboksary, Volga region (7)	Urban	40.9		Kosaev and Farhutdinova (2015)
	Rural	53.9		
Saratov, Volga region (8)	n.s.	63.6		Kashkovskaya (2009)
Volgograd, South Russia (9)	Pet	69.5		Akimova (2006)
	Stray	100		
Rostov, South Russia (10)	n.s.	12.7		Shishkanova (2011)
Tyumen, South Urals (11)	n.s.	15.3	11.6	Fadeyeva (2007a)
Tyumen, South Urals (11)	n.s.	30.2	28.2	Fadeyeva (2007b)
Tyumen, South Urals; State surveillance data (11)	n.s.	2.8–6.3		Sabirova et al. (2012)
Omsk, south of West Siberia (12)	Urban and rural	60.7		Berezina et al. (2011)
	Pet, roaming		32.2	
	Pet, strictly home		8.2	

Continued

Table 1 Prevalence of *Toxocara* in primary hosts in Russia.—cont'd

City or region	Group of hosts[a]	Prevalence in dogs (%)	Prevalence in cats (%)	References
Novosibirsk, south of West Siberia (13)	Urban	43.6	38.6	Zubareva (2001)
	Rural	55.1	52.2	
Altay, West Siberia (14)	n.s.	4–33.8		Pautova et al. (2012)
Irkutsk, East Siberia (15)	Pets	19		Kupriyanova (1988)
	Stray	29.5		
Khabarovsk, Far East (16)	n.s.	20		Kozyreva (1999)

[a]As identified in the source.
[b]Group not specified in the source.
n.s., not specified in the source.

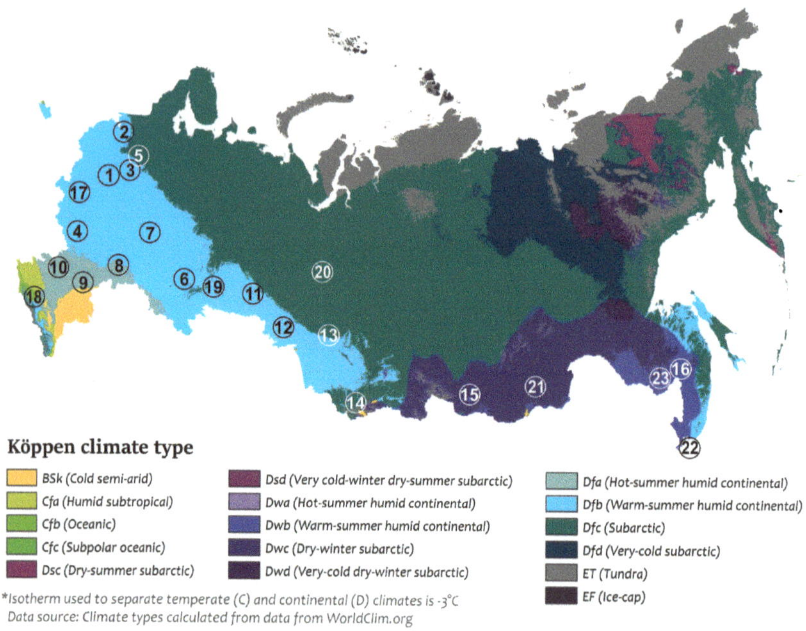

Fig. 1 Sites of published studies on *Toxocara* prevalence in primary hosts (Table 1) and the environment (Table 2). Numbers in circles correspond to Tables 1 and 2. Colour indicates Köppen climate zones according to the legend. *The original image was taken from https://en.wikipedia.org/wiki/Climate_of_Russia.*

of *Toxocara* (3–5%) in pet dogs in Moscow and St. Petersburg. These cities have higher average incomes (180% and 125% of the average in Russia, respectively), higher living standards and relatively good control of the population of stray dogs (or, at least, the spatial overlap between stray and pet dogs is limited). In these areas, dogs are usually kept in apartments and commonly receive prophylactic anthelminthic treatment. *Toxocara* prevalence in stray dogs in Moscow was about five times higher than in pet dogs, but still lower than in most other regions of Russia. Relatively low prevalence in dogs was also reported in Kostroma and Vologda, two cities to the North-East from Moscow. This concurs with results of a 1980s study that reported lower prevalence of *Toxocara* (around 15%) in forest climate zones compared to forest-steppe and steppe zones (Kupriyanova, 1988). *Toxocara* prevalence in other cities was generally higher. Values between 40% and 60% were typical. It is noteworthy that when several studies were done in the same city, the results could concur reasonably well, as, for example, in Moscow, but could also differ several-fold, as in Tyumen (Table 1). The mean of all reported prevalence rates across Russia was 33%; however, due to enormous variance of values reported in different cities, studies and dog groups, this mean value has a limited value.

The *Toxocara* prevalence in dogs in Russia was significantly higher than reported for most other countries. *Toxocara* infection rates for dogs in Germany (Barutzki and Schaper, 2011), the Czech Republic (Dubna et al., 2007) and the USA (Ketzis, 2020; Mohamed et al., 2009) were around or below 5%. In Central and South America, they varied between 7% and 14% (Eguia-Aguilar et al., 2005; Paquet-Durand et al., 2007; Ramirez-Barrios et al., 2004). Interestingly, a relatively high prevalence of egg excretion compared to other North Atlantic countries was observed in Canada, an average of 12.7%, and up to 18.5% in some regions (Villeneuve et al., 2015). This observation could be associated with climatic conditions that are similar to those of Russia. However, prevalence values outside capital cities of Russia and south-east of Moscow (mean 40%, and up to 100% in some areas) were more than twice those observed in Canada and were comparable or exceeded, for example, the 33.8% infection rate reported in Nigeria (Sowemimo, 2009) or the 32.4% prevalence of infection in Malaysia (Ngui et al., 2014). Thus, infection rates of pets in Moscow and St. Petersburg correspond to those of European countries and the USA, but the prevalence of *Toxocara* infestation of dogs from most provincial cities and stray dogs in capital cities is 5–10 times higher than in Europe and the USA, 2–3 times higher than Canada and higher than in most regions of the world (Fakhri et al., 2018). It is likely that both climate and social factors (lack of anthelminthic prophylactics, poor stray dog population control, dog walking habits) contribute to this high level of host infection, and thus, high threat to the human population of Russia.

Recent studies were too diverse in terms of sampling approaches and locations to allow detecting any geographic patterns of *Toxocara* distribution. A comprehensive study done in the 1980s on over 10,000 dogs all across the Soviet Union found that the prevalence of *Toxocara* was the highest (42–44%) in the steppe and desert-steppe climate zones, somewhat lower (31%) in the forest-steppe and even lower in desert and taiga (around 13%). Only the polar zone was devoid of *Toxocara* (Kupriyanova, 1988). The summary of more recent studies (Table 1; Fig. 1) generally corresponds to these historical observations.

Data from studies done in Russia did not support an inverse correlation between *Toxocara* prevalence levels and latitude that was reported recently (Fakhri et al., 2018). That review used just one reference from Russia. It is likely that if all reports of high *Toxocara* prevalence at high latitudes reviewed here were included, the inverse correlation between the latitude and the prevalence might not be supported.

Consistently higher infection rates have been observed in stray dogs, which were 2–12 times more likely to be infected than pets (Starostina and Romanova, 2015). This corresponds to reports from other countries (Moudgil et al., 2016). In Volgograd, 100% of stray dogs were infected throughout the year, and only the infection levels varied across the seasons (Akimova, 2006). This observation suggests that in Russia, stray dogs support the natural lifecycle of the parasite, while the infection of pets is largely a spin-off. For example, in Volgograd, 80% of 1- to 2-month-old stray puppies carried *Toxocara*, while the same age puppies of pets and service dogs were free of infection. These animals became almost totally infected, however, by 6 months of age (Akimova, 2006). Thereafter, the infection prevalence decreases in populations of both stray dogs and pets (Fadeyeva, 2007a). Therefore, it is likely that the vertical transmission is not the key mechanism of infection in pets. The infection prevalence in dogs in rural areas could be higher or lower than in urban ones. It is unclear if this reflects distinct epizootiological patterns in different regions or depends upon study methodology and definition of groups.

The prevalence of infection among cats has been explored to a lesser extent than among dogs. In several published reports prevalence varied between 6% and 52% (Table 1). Similar to the dog infection prevalence, it was lowest in Moscow. Expectedly higher prevalence was observed in freely roaming pet cats and in stray cats.

Longitudinal studies have indicated that there is a high level of seasonal variation in the prevalence of *Toxocara* infection in dogs, with a peak in the summer and autumn and the lowest prevalence in winter and spring (Fig. 2A).

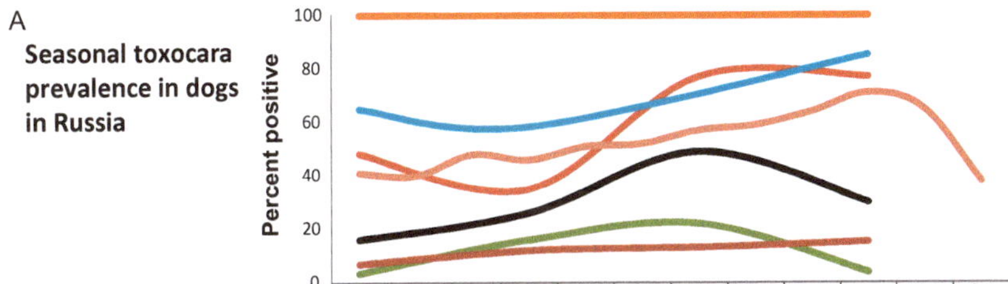

	Jan	Feb	Mar	Apr	May	Jun	Jul	Aug	Sep	Oct	Nov	Dec
Kostroma, North-East Russia (Mikhin, 2004)	3,4			16			22			3,8		
Cheboksary, Central Russia (Kosaev and Farhutdinova, 2015)	48,3			35			77			77		
Volgograd, South Russia, pet (Akimova, 2006)	64,9			58,4						85,2		
Volgograd, South Russia, stray (Akimova, 2006)	100			100			100			100		
Tyumen, South Urals (Fadeyeva, 2007a,b)	16			26			49			30		
Moscow (Peshkov, 2010)	6,9			12			13,1			15,2		
Omsk, South-West Siberia (Efremova, 2011)	41	40	48	46	51	52	57	59	64	71	65	38

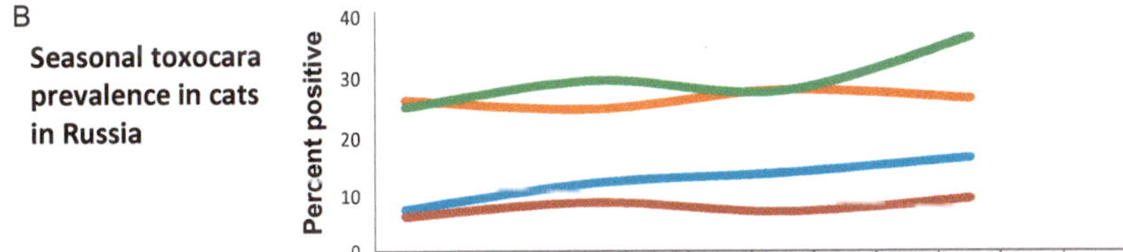

	Jan	Feb	Mar	Apr	May	Jun	Jul	Aug	Sep	Oct	Nov	Dec
Tyumen, South Urals, (Fadeyeva, 2007a,b)	28,3			26,7			30,2			28,55		
Moscow (Peshkov, 2010)	7,8			12,9			14,7			17,5		
Omsk, roaming (Efremova et al., 2011)	27			32			30			40		
Omsk, strictly house (Efremova et al., 2011)	6,5			9,2			7,4			9,9		

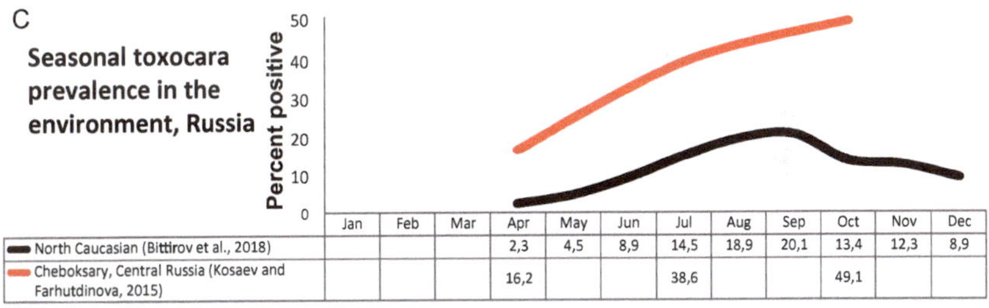

	Jan	Feb	Mar	Apr	May	Jun	Jul	Aug	Sep	Oct	Nov	Dec
North Caucasian (Bittirov et al., 2018)				2,3	4,5	8,9	14,5	18,9	20,1	13,4	12,3	8,9
Cheboksary, Central Russia (Kosaev and Farhutdinova, 2015)				16,2			38,6			49,1		

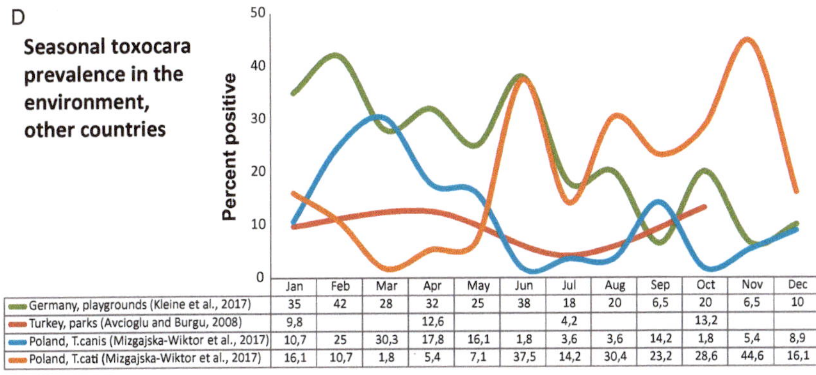

	Jan	Feb	Mar	Apr	May	Jun	Jul	Aug	Sep	Oct	Nov	Dec
Germany, playgrounds (Kleine et al., 2017)	35	42	28	32	25	38	18	20	6,5	20	6,5	10
Turkey, parks (Avcioglu and Burgu, 2008)	9,8			12,6			4,2			13,2		
Poland, T.canis (Mizgajska-Wiktor et al., 2017)	10,7	25	30,3	17,8	16,1	1,8	3,6	3,6	14,2	1,8	5,4	8,9
Poland, T.cati (Mizgajska-Wiktor et al., 2017)	16,1	10,7	1,8	5,4	7,1	37,5	14,2	30,4	23,2	28,6	44,6	16,1

Fig. 2 Seasonal variation in the prevalence of *Toxocara* in dogs (A), cats (B) and the fraction of soil samples contaminated with *Toxocara* eggs in Russia (C) and other countries (D). Results of multi-year studies (Fadeyeva, 2007a) were averaged.

The seasonal variations in the prevalence of *Toxocara* infection observed within a single study have been reported as up to 10-fold. On the contrary, there was almost no seasonal variation observed with respect to the prevalence of infection of cats (Fadeyeva, 2007a). This may be explained by limited access of cats to the infection sources. Indeed, prevalence of infection was four times higher in freely roaming pet cats that in those kept strictly indoors (Berezina et al., 2011), and the summer-autumn prevalence increase was observed only in roaming cats (Fig. 2B). The seasonality patterns of *Toxocara* prevalence in dogs and roaming cats were similar in different regions of Russia, and generally corresponded to seasonal variations in the levels of soil contamination (see below).

In addition to seasonal variation, there are huge year-to-year variations in infection levels, which have been reported to be up to 10-fold and are commonly two- to threefold (Fadeyeva, 2007b; Kosaev and Farhutdinova, 2015). These findings correspond to high year-to-year variation that has been reported with respect to soil contamination levels observed in Poland (Mizgajska-Wiktor et al., 2017) and suggest that reliable longitudinal studies should cover several years or use very extensive sampling.

Environmental surveillance employs a variety of approaches for the collection of samples, including the reporting of the number of eggs per square metre, eggs per cubic metre of sand, or the fraction of contaminated objects. This complicates comparing the results, which should be perceived as general descriptions of contamination levels rather than precise numeric data (Table 2; Fig. 1). A huge variation in the rates of soil samples testing positive for *Toxocara* between districts of Moscow, ranging from 0% to 48.4% within one study (Guzeeva, 2009), highlights limitations of current methodologies (mainly with respect to sampling density, rather than detection efficiency). Interestingly, state surveillance has consistently reported very low soil infestation levels. In all but one report, the fraction of positive soil probes determined by state surveillance sources has been less than 4%. Further, in roughly half of the reports levels have been below 1% (Starostina et al., 2015). Independent studies performed by universities and scientific institutions consistently reported a much higher fraction of contaminated samples, on average 40%, and up to 100% in some studies (Table 2). In some cases, this can be explained by more extensive sampling and the higher sample concentration factors used in research studies, but the motivation of the organizers of different studies may also be questioned. Due to these variations, it is difficult to compare regions and correlate prevalence of *Toxocara* in dogs and in the environment.

Table 2 Prevalence of *Toxocara* eggs in the environment in Russia.

City or region	Sample or soil source	Fraction of contaminated samples	References
Moscow (1)	Community residential	16.2	Vereta and Mamykova (1984)
Moscow (1)	Playgrounds, total	10.1 (0–48.4)	Guzeeva (2009)
	Playgrounds, community	10.8	
	Playgrounds, kindergartens	5.8	
Moscow (1)	Dog keeping sites	15	Aliautdinova et al. (2011)
	Parks	5	
	Community residential	3	
	Kindergartens	2	
Bryansk, Central Russia (17)	Playgrounds	6.7	Avdyukhina (1987)
	Community residential	5	
	Private yards	13.3	
	Mean	8	
Saratov, Volga region (8)	Playgrounds	15.3	Kashkovskaya (2009)
	School yards	4.2	
	Parks	19.8	
	Dog walking sites	49	
	Mean	50.3	
	Soil	54.9	
	Sewage	15–100	
Cheboksary, Volga region (7)	Private yards	24	Kosaev and Farhutdinova (2015)
	Kindergartens	8.1	
Ufa, Volga region (6)	Community yards	30.9	Suleymanova (2012)
	Private yards	44.1	
	School yards	37	
	Kindergartens	26.6	
	Parks	33–38	
	Service dog facility	44.8	

Continued

Table 2 Prevalence of *Toxocara* eggs in the environment in Russia.—cont'd

City or region	Sample or soil source	Fraction of contaminated samples	References
Kabardino-Balkar Republic, North Caucasian (18)	Well-maintained yards	33.0	Bittirov et al. (2018)
	Poorly maintained yards	92	
	Dog keeping sites	100	
	Schools and parks	70–96	
	Private yards	100	
	Animal farms	80–100	
Tyumen, South Urals (11)	Soil	85	Sabirova et al. (2012)
	Playgrounds	61	
Ekaterinburg, South Urals (19)	Stray dog resting sites	23.6	Slobodeniuk et al. (2005)
	Soil	1	
	Sewage	0.7	
	Water in open reservoirs	0.3	
Tyumen, South Urals (11)	Soil	9.3	Fadeyeva (2007a)
Nizhnevartovsk, West Siberia (20)	Parks	21.6	Moskina et al. (2017)
	Playgrounds	0.6	
Novosibirsk, south of West Siberia (13)	Playgrounds	10.3	Zubareva (2001)
	School yards	4.7	
	Parks	12.7	
	Beaches	4.5	
	Dog walking sites	29	
	Mean	15.3	
Chita, Transbaikal region (21)	Community yards	20	Kleusova (2004)
Vladivostok, Far East (22)	Community residential	100	Bozhko et al. (2016)
Khabarovsk, Far East (16)	Community residential	5	Kozyreva (1999)
Jewish autonomous region, Far East (23)	Kindergartens	6.2	Ianovich and Bryunetkina (1999)
	Community yards	5.4	

Similar to prevalence rates in dogs, a clear seasonal pattern for the prevalence of soil contamination has been reported. The peak contamination levels were observed in the autumn season, while the lowest prevalence of *Toxocara* was observed in the spring (Fig. 2C). No data is available describing soil contamination levels in winter months, because there is a permanent layer of snow covering most of the territory of Russia throughout the entire winter season. The seasonality of soil contamination levels in Russia was different from that in Hannover, Germany (Fig. 2D), where peak values were observed in winter and spring (Kleine et al., 2017), or in Turkey, where the lowest rates were observed in the summer (Avcioglu and Burgu, 2008). In Poland, different seasonal profiles were observed for eggs of *T. canis* and *T. cati*. The levels of contamination with *T. canis* eggs peaked in March, similar to overall contamination levels in Hannover, while levels of *T. cati* contamination peaked in the summer and autumn (Mizgajska-Wiktor et al., 2017). Seasonality in Russia is unlikely to be driven by the freezing of eggs in the winter. Although one report demonstrated that *Toxocara* eggs are unable to tolerate freezing below −15 °C (Gillespie, 1988), another study performed in the Altai region of West Siberia (stark continental climate, mean minimum winter temperatures between −20 °C and −24 °C) found that artificially introduced *Toxocara* eggs were able to survive the winter. Experimental incubation of eggs in a freezer at −24 °C also did not kill the eggs (Ponomaryov and Luneva, 2014). A more likely explanation for the pronounced summer-autumn seasonality may be that in winter soil temperatures are not sufficient for maturation of *Toxocara* eggs. Correspondingly, seasonal variation was less pronounced in South Russia (Fig. 2C, black line) than in northern regions. Seasonal variation in the prevalence of *Toxocara* eggs in Germany and Turkey is the inverse of that reported in Russia. This phenomenon could be explained by the effect of insolation or high temperatures on the survival of eggs. Interestingly, no seasonal variation in levels of *Toxocara* contamination has been observed in India (Utaaker et al., 2018). Distinct seasonal patterns reported in different countries suggest that there may be significant differences in epizootiology and epidemiology of toxocariasis around the world, and studies done in one region are not necessarily applicable to another. It is also not clear if a pronounced seasonality of *Toxocara* infection in dogs complements to higher infection levels observed in Russia and in Canada.

Only a few environmental studies have differentiated between *T. canis* and *T. cati* eggs in Russia. Absence of seasonal variation in the levels of cat infection and the correspondence between annual profiles of the excretion of *Toxocara* eggs by dogs and the soil contamination levels suggest that *T. canis* may be a more common contaminant of the soil than *T. cati* in Russia. Seasonal variation in the levels of soil contamination varied 3- to 10-fold between individual studies, which was similar to the variance reported with respect to the level of infestation of dogs. Seasonal profiles can be, in theory, projected for certain territories, but precise predictions are not likely to be accurate. Therefore, cross-sectional studies performed in different regions of Russia might not be directly comparable. August and September could be suggested as optimal months for sampling the environment in Russia, because they provide enough time for contamination levels to peak in all climate zones. Moreover, year-to-year variations in the prevalence of *Toxocara* in dogs (see above) suggests that environmental monitoring should be a systematic, not a one-time activity. It is not clear if the same extent of seasonal and year-to-year variation is typical in other regions, because the number of longitudinal studies performed worldwide is relatively low. From a medical point of view, more than 10-fold seasonal variation in *Toxocara* contamination levels suggest that time of the year could be used as an additional factor that favours or contradicts the diagnosis of human toxocariasis.

Expectedly, the highest levels of soil contamination have been observed at locations with a high prevalence of dogs, especially stray dogs. As discussed above, stray dogs play a key role in maintaining the epizooty in Russia, and areas close to garbage containers, sea ports and beaches are most heavily contaminated. It is noteworthy that the two regions with the highest prevalence of infection and environmental contamination levels, Volgograd and Vladivostok, are coastal cities with extensive industrial zones at the water front. Parks and territories adjacent to communal houses, which are commonly used for walking pets, were also identified as one of the most heavily contaminated types of areas. Interestingly, the contamination of children's sandboxes and kindergarten territories, perhaps the most socially relevant objects, varied between regions, from 0.6% (Moskina et al., 2017) or 3.2% (Aliautdinova et al., 2011) to 44% (Suleymanova, 2012) or 100% (Bozhko et al., 2016), despite comparably high contamination levels in other kinds of areas. The 100% contamination rate was observed in Vladivostok, in the Far Eastern region of Russia, and was accompanied by environmental contamination levels of up to 4500 eggs per kilogram of sand (Bozhko et al., 2016). The high variation of relative contamination levels of playgrounds in different regions indicates that organisational (stray dog control, fencing of kindergarten territories, sand replacement) and cultural factors (dog walking and anthelminthic prophylactic habits) can have a decisive impact on contamination of playgrounds, and thus, on incidence of toxocariasis in children. This was further illustrated by the fact that in Moscow 16% of sandboxes were contaminated in 1984 (Vereta and Mamykova, 1984), a number that dropped to 3.2% in 2011 (Aliautdinova et al., 2011), and the contamination rate of kindergarten playgrounds (which are always fenced in Moscow) was two times lower than that of community playgrounds (Guzeeva, 2009).

Several reports have also addressed the issue of food contamination with *Toxocara* eggs. One such study reported that 4.3% of vegetable samples were contaminated, including 9.5% of greenery specimens (Suleymanova, 2012). Another study reported an average of 13.8 *Toxocara* eggs per kilogram of greenery and cucumbers (Bittirov et al., 2018). In Tyumen, 3.8% (Sabirova et al., 2012) to 7.1% (Fadeyeva, 2007a) of vegetable specimens contained *Toxocara* eggs. Therefore, vegetables and greenery pose a consistent and significant risk as sources of human infection. Screening of paratenic hosts in the North Caucasian region also detected high infection levels: 23–47% in goats (Aliyeva et al., 2016) and 25–67% in cows (Kabardiev et al., 2016). There is no evidence that paratenic hosts are relevant factors in human infection, especially because there are no habits of eating under-cooked meat in these regions, but they can be important sources of infection for farm dogs.

Despite a high number of studies, toxocariasis remains a neglected disease even in high- and medium-income countries. A compete eradication of the parasite is not practically feasible because it is ubiquitously maintained in a natural cycle in feral felids and canid, and up to 34% of soil samples in the steppe regions of Russia are contaminated with eggs (Kupriyanova, 1988). However, published evidence suggests that social factors may have a greater effect on human exposure risk than the zoonotic cycle itself. Contamination levels largely depend upon habits among dog- and cat-owners, such as the administration of prophylactic treatments and walking habits. Another important factor relates to the efficiency of communal services, which includes the control of stray animals and protection of playgrounds, as has also been indicated previously (Blaszkowska et al., 2015).

Results of many studies suggest that significant temporal and spatial variations are typically observed with respect to the prevalence of *Toxocara* in hosts and the environment even within a single municipality. This, together with the lack of standardisation in sampling and screening methods, significantly complicates performing surveillance and comparing between different regions and studies. It is clear that obtaining reliable results requires longitudinal studies (ideally covering at least 3 years) with diversified sampling (thousands of specimens) and varying tested objects, such as natural and paratenic hosts, soil and seroprevalence. Currently, there is a lack of such comprehensive studies, but the high quantity of fragmentary data from smaller and more focused reports provide an image of a ubiquitous and poorly controlled zoonosis with a massive human exposure.

Acknowledgement

This study was supported by the Russian Academic Excellence Project 5-100.

References

Akhmadishina, L.V., Ruzina, M.N., Lukasheva, M.A., Kyuregyan, K.K., Mikhailov, M.I., Lukashev, A.N., 2020. Seroprevalence and incidence of human toxocarosis in Russia. Adv. Parasitol. 109, 419–432.

Akimova, S.A., 2006. Toxocariasis and Toxascaris of Carnivores in the Lower Volga Region: Epidemiology, Pathogenesis and Treatment. PhD in Veterinary Sciences, Volgograd State Agricultural Academy.

Aliautdinova, L.V., Semenova, T.A., Zavoikin, V.D., 2011. Heterogeneity of parasitic contamination of megalopolis soils. Med. Parazitol. (Mosk) 2, 7–10.

Aliyeva, A.A., Bittirov, A.M., Kabardiev, S.S., Aliyeva, Z.R., Bittirova, A.A., Vologirov, A.S., Anahaeva, A.K., Kadyrova, R.K., Ataev, A.M., 2016. Larval toxocarosis of zoned breeds of domestic goats in Kabardino-Balkaria. In: Biodiversity and Natural Resource Management. Proceedings of the IV all-Russian Scientific-Practical Conference With International Participation. Dagestan State Pedagogical University, Makhachkala.

Avcioglu, H., Burgu, A., 2008. Seasonal prevalence of *Toxocara* ova in soil samples from public parks in Ankara, Turkey. Vector Borne Zoonotic Dis. 8, 345–350.

Avdyukhina, T.I., 1987. Comparative Seroepidemiology of Parasitic Zoonoses in Mixed Foci (on Examples of Toxocarosis and Toxoplasmosis). Central Institute of Advanced Medical Education, Moscow, p. 149.

Barutzki, D., Schaper, R., 2011. Results of parasitological examinations of faecal samples from cats and dogs in Germany between 2003 and 2010. Parasitol. Res. 109 (Suppl. 1), S45–S60.

Berezina, E.S., Lobkis, D.V., Starostina, O.Y., 2011. Toxocarosis distribution peculiarities in the populations of small domestic carnivoras and the human being on the territory of Russia. Bull. Krasnoyarsk State Agrarian Univ. 10, 168–177.

Bittirov, A.M., Shakhmurzov, M.M., Kagermazov, T.B., Chilayev, A.S., Bittirova, A.A., 2018. Sanitary state of soil and water of the North Caucasus region in relation to contamination by eggs and larvae of parasitic zoonoses. Agrarian Russ. 12, 36–39.

Blaszkowska, J., Goralska, K., Wojcik, A., Kurnatowski, P., Szwabe, K., 2015. Presence of *Toxocara* spp. eggs in children's recreation areas with varying degrees of access for animals. Ann. Agric. Environ. Med. 22, 23–27.

Bozhko, G.G., Nadelyaev, V.E., Fomin, A.V., 2016. Contamination of sand with *Toxocara* eggs in Vladivostok. Int. J. Exp. Educ. 3–1, 28.

Budovskoy, A.V., 2005. Parasite Diseases of Dogs in Different Types of Keeping and Purpose and Improvement of Anthelmintic Therapy. PhD in Veterinary Sciences, All-Russian Research Institute of Fundamental and Applied Parasitology of Animals and Plants. Named after K.I. Scriabin.

Dubna, S., Langrova, I., Napravnik, J., Jankovska, I., Vadlejch, J., Pekar, S., Fechtner, J., 2007. The prevalence of intestinal parasites in dogs from Prague, rural areas, and shelters of the Czech Republic. Vet. Parasitol. 145, 120–128.

Eguia-Aguilar, P., Cruz-Reyes, A., Martinez-Maya, J.J., 2005. Ecological analysis and description of the intestinal helminths present in dogs in Mexico City. Vet. Parasitol. 127, 139–146.

Fadeyeva, O.V., 2007a. Spread and seasonal dynamics of infesting domestic carnivores with *Toxocara* in Tyumen. Sib. Her. Agric. Sci. 7 (175), 117–119.

Fadeyeva, O.V., 2007b. Toxocariasis of Domestic Carnivores, Tyumen. PhD in Veterinary Sciences, All-Russian Research Institute of Veterinary Entomology and Arachnology.

Fakhri, Y., Gasser, R.B., Rostami, A., Fan, C.K., Ghasemi, S.M., Javanian, M., Bayani, M., Armoon, B., Moradi, B., 2018. *Toxocara* eggs in public places worldwide—a systematic review and meta-analysis. Environ. Pollut. 242, 1467–1475.

Gillespie, S.H., 1988. The epidemiology of *Toxocara canis*. Parasitol. Today 4, 180–182.

Guzeeva, M.V., 2009. The current toxocariasis situation in Moscow. Med. Parazitol. (Mosk) 1, 49–51.

Ianovich, V.A., Bryunetkina, N.M., 1999. Investigation of soil for presence of *Toxocara* eggs in the Jewish Autonomous Region (EAO). Med. Parazitol. (Mosk) 3, 29–30.

Kabardiev, S.S., Alieva, A.A., Bittirov, A.M., Alieva, G.R., Bittirova, A.A., Vologirov, A.S., Anahaeva, A.K., Kadyrova, R.K., Ataev, A.M., 2016. Epizootological features of larval toxocarosis distribution in cattle in Kabardino-Balkaria. Biodiversity and natural resource management. In: Proceedings of the IV all-Russian Scientific-Practical Conference With International Participation, pp. 68–69. Makhachkala.

Kashkovskaya, L.M., 2009. Main Enteric Helminthoses of Dogs in Saratov (Prevalence, Ecological Peculiarities and Combating Measures). PhD in Veterinary Sciences, Saratov State Agrarian University. Named by N.I. Vavilov.

Ketzis, J.K., 2020. *Toxocara canis* and *Toxocara cati* in domestic dogs and cats in the United States, Mexico, Central America and the Caribbean: A review. Adv. Parasitol. 109, 655–714.

Kleine, A., Springer, A., Strube, C., 2017. Seasonal variation in the prevalence of *Toxocara* eggs on children's playgrounds in the city of Hanover, Germany. Parasit. Vectors 10, 248.

Kleusova, N.A., 2004. Spatial Distribution and Surviving of Helminth Eggs at an Urbanized Territory of Eastern Transbaikal Area. PhD in Biological Sciences, Chita State Medical Academy.

Kosaev, N.I., Farhutdinova, A.F., 2015. Distribution of dog's toxocariasis in the Chuvash republic. Agrarian Bull. Urals 8 (138), 33–35.

Kozyreva, T.G., 1999. Ecologo-Epidemiological Basis for Toxocarosis Prophylactics in the Far-Eastern Region of Russia (on an Example of Khabarovsk Region). PhD in Biology, Far-Eastern State Medical University.

Kupriyanova, N.Y., 1988. Areal of Toxocara canis in USSR and Epidemiology of Toxocarosis in East Siberia (on an Example of Irkutsk Region). PhD in Medical Sciences, Central Institute of Advanced Medical Education.

Kurnosova, O.P., Odoevskaya, I.M., 2017. Prevalence of *Toxocara* infestations in domestic dogs and cats in the city of Moscow. Med. Parazitol. (Mosk) 4, 30–34.

Lebedeva, O.V., 2006. Epidemiology of Toxocariasis in St Petersburg. MD, St Petersburg State Medical Academy.

Ma, G., Holland, C.V., Wang, T., Hofmann, A., Fan, C.K., Maizels, R.M., Hotez, P.J., Gasser, R.B., 2018. Human toxocariasis. Lancet Infect. Dis. 18, e14–e24.

Mikhin, A.G., 2004. Toxocarosis of Dogs (Epizootology, Immunodiagnostics, Pathomorphology, Treatment). PhD in Veterinary Sciences, Nizhny Novgorod State Agricultural Academy.

Mizgajska-Wiktor, H., Jarosz, W., Fogt-Wyrwas, R., Drzewiecka, A., 2017. Distribution and dynamics of soil contamination with *Toxocara canis* and *Toxocara cati* eggs in Poland and prevention measures proposed after 20 years of study. Vet. Parasitol. 234, 1–9.

Mohamed, A.S., Moore, G.E., Glickman, L.T., 2009. Prevalence of intestinal nematode parasitism among pet dogs in the United States (2003-2006). J. Am. Vet. Med. Assoc. 234, 631–637.
Moskina, O.V., Malysheva, N.S., Guzeeva, T.M., Samoilovskaya, N.A., 2017. Study of soil, wastewater and sediment contamination by geohelminth eggs (*Toxocara* spp.) in Nizhnevartovsk KhMAO-Yugra. Russ. J. Parasitol. 4, 354–357.
Moudgil, A.D., Mittra, S., Agnihotri, R.K., Sharma, D., Sen, D., 2016. Prevalence of gastrointestinal parasites in dogs of Palampur, Himachal Pradesh. J. Parasit. Dis. 40, 227–229.
Ngui, R., Lee, S.C., Yap, N.J., Tan, T.K., Aidil, R.M., Chua, K.H., Aziz, S., Sulaiman, W.Y., Ahmad, A.F., Mahmud, R., Lian, Y.L., 2014. Gastrointestinal parasites in rural dogs and cats in Selangor and Pahang states in Peninsular Malaysia. Acta Parasitol. 59, 737–744.
Nikitina, E.A., 2004. Toxocarosis of Dogs in Voronezh (Epizootology, Therapy and Prophylactics). PhD in Veterinary Sciences, Voronezh State Agrarian University.
Novikova, T.V., 2006. The Most Important Invasive Diseases of Small Domestic Animals in the Conditions of the North of the European Region of Russia. Doctor of Veterinary Sciences, Saint Petersburg State Academy of Veterinary Medicine.
Panova, O.A., Glamazdin, I.G., Spiridonov, S.E., 2015. Animal toxocariasis in a megalopolis: epidemic aspects. Med. Parazitol. (Mosk) 3, 39–41.
Paquet-Durand, I., Hernandez, J., Dolz, G., Zuniga, J.J., Schnieder, T., Epe, C., 2007. Prevalence of *Toxocara* spp., Toxascaris leonina and ancylostomidae in public parks and beaches in different climate zones of Costa Rica. Acta Trop. 104, 30–37.
Pautova, E.A., Kurepina, N., Dovgalev, A.S., 2012. Toxocariasis in the Republic of Altai. Geoinformation mapping simulation. Med. Parazitol. (Mosk) 4, 11–14.
Peshkov, R.A., 2010. Epizootic Situation on Toxocarosis in Carnivores and Helminthologic Examination of the Environment in the Megalopolis of Moscow. PhD in Veterinary, K.I. Skryabin, All-Russian Scientific Research Institute of Helminthology.
Ponomaryov, N.M., Luneva, N.A., 2014. Survival rate of *Toxocara canis* eggs in the south of West Siberia (case study of the Altai region). Bull. Altai State Agric. Univ. 11, 130–133.
Ramirez-Barrios, R.A., Barboza-Mena, G., Munoz, J., Angulo-Cubillan, F., Hernandez, E., Gonzalez, F., Escalona, F., 2004. Prevalence of intestinal parasites in dogs under veterinary care in Maracaibo, Venezuela. Vet. Parasitol. 121, 11–20.
Sabirova, D.R., Markova, O.P., Belyaeva, M.I., 2012. Incidence of toxocarosis on the territory of Tyumen region. In: 10th VNPOEMP Congress. VNPOEMP, Moscow.
Shishkanova, L.V., 2011. Toxocariasis in the South of Russia (Epidemiological, Sanitary-Parasitological, Serological Characterization). PhD, Rostov Research Institute of Microbiology and Parasitology.
Slobodeniuk, A.V., Kosova, A.A., Rukoleeva, S.I., 2005. Prevalence of toxocariasis in rural and urban areas. Med. Parazitol. (Mosk) 3, 36–38.
Sowemimo, O.A., 2009. The prevalence and intensity of gastrointestinal parasites of dogs in Ile-Ife, Nigeria. J. Helminthol. 83, 27–31.
Starostina, O.Y., Romanova, S.N., 2015. Toxocariasis: current state of the Russian Federation. Message 2: toxocariasis morbidity of the population in various administrative territories of the Russian Federation. Epidemiol. Vaccinal Prev. 3 (82), 54–58.
Starostina, O.Y., Berezina, E.S., Romanova, S.N., 2015. Toxocariasis: current state of the Russian Federation. Message 1: risk of toxocariasis infection of the population on the territory of the Russian Federation. Epidemiol. Vaccinal Prev. 2 (81), 13–18.
Suleymanova, G.F., 2012. Epizootological and epidemiological problems of toxocariasis. Sci. Notes Kazan Bauman State Acad. Vet. Med. 210, 230–234.

Utaaker, K.S., Tysnes, K.R., Krosness, M.M., Robertson, L.J., 2018. Not just a walk in the park: occurrence of intestinal parasites in dogs roaming recreational parks in Chandigarh, Northern India. Vet. Parasitol. Reg. Stud. Rep. 14, 176–180.

Vereta, L.E., Mamykova, O.I., 1984. Soil contamination by *Toxocara* eggs at Moscow pre-school institutions and its sources. Med. Parazitol. (Mosk) 3, 19–22.

Villeneuve, A., Polley, L., Jenkins, E., Schurer, J., Gilleard, J., Kutz, S., Conboy, G., Benoit, D., Seewald, W., Gagne, F., 2015. Parasite prevalence in fecal samples from shelter dogs and cats across the Canadian provinces. Parasit. Vectors 8, 281.

Zubareva, I.M., 2001. Main Helminthoses of Pet Carnivores in Large Cities (on an Example of Novosibirsk). PhD in Veterinary Sciences.

CHAPTER THIRTY-SEVEN

Canine Toxocariosis: Its prevalence, incidence and occurrence in the Indian subcontinent

Manigandan Lejeune[a,*], V. Gnani Charitha[b], C. Mathivathani[c], V.C. Rayulu[b], Dwight D. Bowman[d]

[a]Department of Population Medicine and Diagnostic Sciences, Animal Health Diagnostic Center, College of Veterinary Medicine, Cornell University, Ithaca, NY, United States
[b]Department of Veterinary Parasitology, College of Veterinary Science, Sri Venkateswara Veterinary University, Tirupati, Andhra Pradesh, India
[c]Department of Veterinary Parasitology, Rajiv Gandhi Institute of Veterinary education and Research, Pondicherry University, Puducherry, India
[d]Department of Microbiology and Immunology, College of Veterinary Medicine, Cornell University, Ithaca, NY, United States
*Corresponding author: e-mail address: ml872@cornell.edu

Contents

Abstract

Toxocariosis is an important neglected tropical helminth disease of zoonotic significance for which canids are the definitive hosts. Dogs are also considered the sentinel host for the occurrence of *T. canis* infections in humans. Therefore, understanding its prevalence in canine population is imperative for any effective disease control in humans. A comprehensive review of literature on the prevalence of *T. canis* in canids was lacking from the Indian subcontinent which necessitated our efforts to compile

Advances in Parasitology, Volume 109
ISSN 0065-308X
https://doi.org/10.1016/bs.apar.2020.01.018

available data published on this topic. Data on prevalence, incidence and occurrence of this helminths in canids were presented in this review as tabular format for easy comprehension. Moreover, the data were categorized based on the region where the studies were conducted with an aim to understand the spatial distribution of this parasite in the subcontinent. Factors influencing the regional prevalence/occurrence of *T. canis* such as type of canids (stray or pet), age, sex, breed, season and the choice of analytical methods were also discussed. In addition, data on the prevalence of *T. canis* in environmental samples and in zoo canids were also compiled and presented. We anticipate such an exhaustive review of literature available mostly in the journals published from the subcontinent would become a point source of information necessary for prioritizing future surveillance efforts in this region and for making informed policy decision to control this zoonotic helminth infection.

1. Introduction

Soil-transmitted helminth (STH) infections are estimated to infect 1.45 billion people worldwide (Pullan et al., 2014) which includes the zoonotic *Toxocara canis* for which canids are the definitive host. At present toxocariosis is a highly prevalent neglected helminth disease of the tropics affecting millions of people, pets and stray dogs. Its public health impact remains largely underestimated (Rostami et al., 2019; Zyoud, 2017). Dogs remain a sentinel species for human toxocariosis (Sharma et al., 2015); however, knowledge of the prevalence of *T. canis* in domestic and wild canids, as well as, its associated zoonotic risks have not been well documented for the Indian subcontinent. Recent literature also laments about the lack of prevalence studies of gastrointestinal parasites of dogs in India (Traub et al., 2005). A comprehensive review of literature from the Indian subcontinent is lacking, and therefore, we undertook an earnest attempt to compile data on prevalence and epidemiology of *T. canis* available through print publications in the subcontinent over the last several decades.

The Indian subcontinent encompasses countries namely, India, Pakistan, Bangladesh, Sri Lanka, Nepal, Bhutan, etc. (see Fig. 1).The collective human population in these countries as of 2015 is estimated to be 1.71 billion (Wallace et al., 2017). The dog population is also on the rise in the subcontinent (Chatterjee, 2009; Sharma et al., 2017; Traub et al., 2005). In India, the dog population was quoted in published literatures as 11–30 million (Ahmad et al., 2018; Das et al., 2009b; Sharma et al., 2017; Traub et al., 2005). However, a recent report places the estimate as close to 119 million in India (Wallace et al., 2017). The same report also estimates a collective

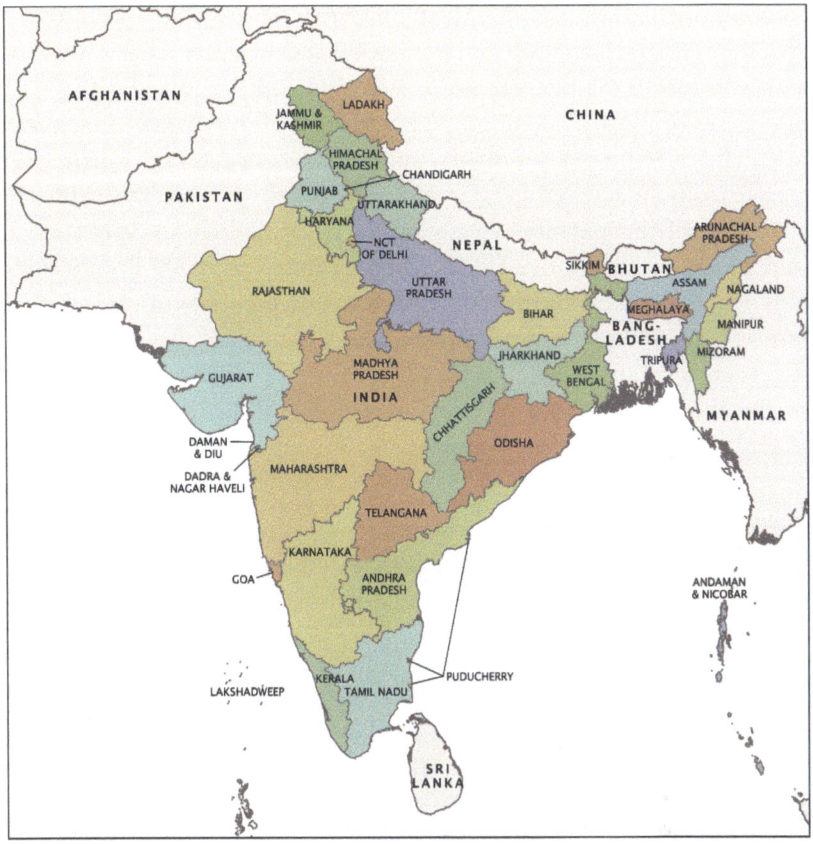

Fig. 1 Map depicting countries in the Indian subcontinent. The states and the union territories of India are demarcated and highlighted. The map was generated using GADM database of Global Administrative Areas version 3.6. *Courtesy: Nicholas A. Hollingshead, Cornell University.*

dog population of 145.6 million in the Indian subcontinent which is approximately 21% of the world's dog population. This amounts to a dog: human ratio of 1:8 which is narrower than noted previously (Das et al., 2009b). There is a possibility that *T. canis* is expanding its range as a consequence of increasing human and canine population coupled with the effect of climatic changes and global warming (Rostami et al., 2019). Despite the uncontrolled increase in stray and pet dog populations, there is a relatively low number of studies pertaining to GI parasites of dogs such as *T. canis*. Understanding the extent to which *T. canis* is prevalent in its definitive hosts across the subcontinent may help mitigate the impact of this zoonotic parasite.

Interestingly, India stood 10th among the most productive countries in toxocariasis research and the University of Peradeniya, Sri Lanka, was listed among the top 10 productive institutes (Zyoud, 2017). However, this ranking pertains to research done on human aspects of this disease. In contrast, the only sizeable number of reports on the animal aspects of the disease that emanate from the subcontinent are mostly about the prevalence/incidence/occurrence of this parasite/disease and its epidemiology in dogs and zoo canids. For this review, we retrieved publications primarily from journals published in the subcontinent. The peer review processes of most of these journals are not clearly known. Nevertheless, compiling these data provide the readers with an overall view of the spread of *T. canis* and might help in gauging the impact of this parasite on definitive hosts, humans and other paratenic hosts, and the environment.

2. Prevalence/incidence/occurrence studies in dog population

2.1 History

To our knowledge, the first report of *T. canis* from the subcontinent was from the parasite collection of the Zoological Survey of India (Baylis and Daubney, 1922). The parasite was reported as *Belascaris marginata,* since this was the binomen known to the scientific community at that time (Hall, 1917). A report of *T. canis* infections in dogs and comments about treatment options appeared in the Indian Veterinary Journal (Velu Pillai, 1924). The worm was mentioned as *Ascaris marginata*, as this was another binomen that was in use at that time (Stewart, 1916). However, it was not clear if Velu Pillai reported his case observation from India or from Malaysia, where he was employed. An unambiguous report on the occurrence of *T. canis* was published in 1933, in 3 stray dogs examined by necropsy at Lucknow, Uttar Pradesh (formerly United Provinces), India (Acharya, 1933). A similar necropsy study identified 82% of 200 dogs at Kolkata (formerly Calcutta) infected with *T. canis* (Maplestone and Bhaduri, 1940). A relative hiatus in reporting occurred until the late 1960s, when there was a surge in publications on toxocariosis in canids (Buscher, 1974; Chhabra and Mahajan, 1978; Misra et al., 1974; Pal et al., 1979; Sahai, 1969). Subsequently, many studies were published providing data on the occurrence/prevalence in pet and stray dogs, wild canids in zoos, and in environmental samples. The three compilations of these reports are presented in the Tables 1–3.

Table 1 Prevalence of *Toxocara canis* in dogs on the Indian subcontinent.

Country	State/Union territory	District/City	Study period	Dog type	Analysis	Number tested	Prevalence %	Remarks	References
India	Andhra Pradesh	YSR Kadapa	2015–2016	Pet	Faecal	236	52.54		Sivajothi and Reddy (2018)
					Hair	236	25.42	36.73% in long haired breed; 17.39% in short haired breed	
		Tirupati				67	58.2		Kumar and Hafeez (1998)
	Assam	Guwahati		Pet	Faecal	905	1.65	Prevalence deduced from the data provided	Dutta et al. (2008)
		Tezpur	2000	Pet + Stray	Faecal	101	11		Traub et al. (2002)
	Bihar	Patna		Pet	Faecal	305	32.13		Sharma et al. (2006)
		Ranchi		Pet	Faecal + Necropsy	126	11.91	Overall prevalence of 21.32% ($n = 197$)	Samantha et al. (1989)
				Stray		71	38.03		
	Chandigarh	Chandigarh	1976–1977	Pet	Faecal	96	8.3	Overall prevalence of 12.2% ($n = 238$)	Chhabra and Mahajan (1978)
				Stray	Faecal	142	14.8		
		Chandigarh	2015	Stray	Faecal	212	2.8		Utaaker et al. (2018)

Continued

Table 1 Prevalence of *Toxocara canis* in dogs on the Indian subcontinent.—Cont'd

Country	State/Union territory	District/City	Study period	Dog type	Analysis	Number tested	Prevalence %	Remarks	References
	Delhi	Delhi		Pet	Faecal	137	9.48		Pal et al. (1979)
		Delhi			Faecal	144	34.7		Dhar et al. (1966)
		Delhi	2008	Stray	Faecal	110	0		Traub et al. (2014)
	Gujarat	Junagadh	2013–2014	Pet	Faecal	223	2.24		Kumar et al. (2015)
		Anand		Pet	Faecal	108	7.4	Prevalence among clinical cases of diarrhoea	Jani et al. (1995)
	Haryana & Delhi	11 Districts in Haryana + Delhi			Faecal	2391	5.06		Kaushik et al. (1978)
	Himachal Pradesh	Kullu, Shimla, Mandi, Kangra, Una	2006		Faecal	236	5.93	0% prevalence Kullu & Shimla; 6.89–9.09% in other districts	Agnihotri et al. (2008)
		Palampur	2010–2011	Pet + Stray	Faecal	246	12.6	Prevalence deduced from the data provided	Moudgil et al. (2016)
	Jammu & Kashmir	Srinagar		Stray	Faecal	150	34	One year study	Wani et al. (2017)
		Jammu		Stray	Necropsy	25	16		Ahmad et al. (2018)
		Hazratbal		Stray	Faecal	652	60.85		Pandit et al. (2008)

	Karnataka	Bangalore	1963–1964	Pet + Stray	Necropsy	61	26.22	Prevalence deduced from the data provided	Malaki (1966)
		Bangalore		Stray	Faecal	140	21.42		Mamatha et al. (2005)
		Bangalore		Pet	Faecal	712	12.13		Hegde and Jagannath (1974)
		Bangalore			Faecal	100	34		D'Souza et al. (2001)
	Ladakh	Ladakh	2008	Stray	Faecal	86	0		Traub et al. (2014)
	Madhya Pradesh			Stray	Necropsy	74	2.7	Study from two towns in MP	Sahasrabudhe et al. (1969)
		Jabalpur		Stray	Faecal	108	16.67		Nath et al. (2011)
		Jabalpur	2008–2009	Pet +Stray	Faecal	325	2.15		Qadir et al. (2012)
		Malwa			Faecal		9.23		Asati et al. (1999)
	Maharashtra	Udgir	2016–2017	Pet + Stray	Faecal	218	26.08		Khillare and Bhangale (2018)
		Nagpur		Pet + Stray		1180	41.94	Prevalence deduced from the data	Khante et al. (2009)
		Miraj		Stray	Faecal	100	55		Joshi et al. (1977)
		Parbhani		Pet	Faecal	56	3.57	Prevalence among clinical cases of gastroenteritis	Masare and Digraskar (2007)

Continued

Table 1 Prevalence of *Toxocara canis* in dogs on the Indian subcontinent.—Cont'd

Country	State/Union territory	District/City	Study period	Dog type	Analysis	Number tested	Prevalence %	Remarks	References
		Parbhani		Stray	Faecal	716	5		Shastri (1991) reported in Kachawha and Tanwar (2007)
		Mumbai	2008–2008	Stray	Faecal	121	0.8		Traub et al. (2014)
	Meghalaya	Shillong	1986–1988		Faecal + Necropsy	135	69	46 faecal + 89 necropsies	Yadav and Tandon (1989)
	Odisha	Bhubaneshwar	2012–2013	Pet	Faecal	154	8.44	Prevalence deduced from the data provided	Panigrahi et al. (2014)
		Bhubaneshwar		Pet	Faecal	32	21.87	Prevalence in dogs with signs of gastritis	Patra and Tripathy (1986)
		Bhubaneshwar		Stray	Necropsy	50	100	Prevalence in puppies	Misra et al. (1974)
	Puducherry	Puducherry	2003–2004	Pet	Faecal	382	4.97	Overall prevalence of 8.44 ($n=545$)	Das et al. (2009b)
				Stray	Faecal	163	16.56		
	Punjab	Ludhiana	1996		Faecal	609	3.6		Chhabra et al. (2001)
	Rajasthan	Bharatpur			Faecal	121	19.83	Prevalence deduced from the data provided	Kumar et al. (2017)
		Jaipur	2007–2008	Pet	Faecal	105	8.6		Godhra et al. (2010)
		Jodhpur	2006	Stray	Faecal	642	4.95		Kachawha and Tanwar (2007)

	Sikkim	Sikkim	2008	Stray	Faecal	94	3.2		Traub et al. (2014)
	Tamil Nadu	Namakkal	1991–1995	Pet	Faecal	812	9.3		Balasubramaniam et al. (2001)
		Chennai		Pet	Faecal	510	5.88	Prevalence deduced from the data provided; only 25 positive by PCR	Suganya et al. (2019)
	Uttar Pradesh	Bareilly		Stray	Necropsy	51	7.84		Sahai (1969)
		Bareilly	2010–2011	Pet		280	17.5	Overall prevalence of 24.3% ($n=558$)	Sahu et al. (2014)
				Stray		278	31.29		
		Bareilly	1994–1996	Pet	Faecal	163	14.72	Overall prevalence of 23.08 ($n=273$)	Samantha and Ghorui (1998)
				Stray	Faecal	110	35.45		
		Lucknow		Stray	Necropsy	50	6		Acharya (1933)
		Mathura	1979–1980	Stray	Necropsy	40	20		Bhatia et al. (1980)
		Mathura	2008–2009	Pet + Stray	Faecal	121	28.93		Kumar et al. (2014)
		Mathura		Stray		108	51.9		Sudan et al. (2015)
	Uttarakhand	Pantnagar	2001–2006	Pet	Faecal	709	2.12		Vatsya et al. (2010)
	West Bengal	Kolkata		Pet + Stray		450	24.4		Biswas et al. (1986)
		Kolkata			Necropsy	200	82		Maplestone and Bhaduri (1940)
		Kolkata					12.66		Beeshmi and Dasgupta (2006)

Continued

Table 1 Prevalence of *Toxocara canis* in dogs on the Indian subcontinent.—Cont'd

Country	State/Union territory	District/City	Study period	Dog type	Analysis	Number tested	Prevalence %	Remarks	References
Pakistan		Faisalabad	1992	Pet	Faecal	240	33.3		Maqbool et al. (1998)
		Karachi		Stray	Necropsy	200	45.4		Maryam and Ahmed (1965)
		Lahore		Pet	Faecal	100	13		Farooqi et al. (2014)
		Lahore	2007–2008	Pet	Faecal	1203	22.44		Shabbir et al. (2010)
		Lahore	1984	Pet + Stray		250	41.2	Prevalence deduced from the data provided	Umar et al. (1986)
		Lahore		Stray		44	45.45	Prevalence deduced from the data provided	Buscher (1974)
		Lahore		Pet + Stray	Faecal	200	39.5	Prevalence deduced from the data provided	Chattha et al. (2009)
		Lahore		Pet	Faecal	200	37		Ahmad et al. (2011)
Bangladesh		Chittagong	2010–2011	Stray	Necropsy	60	23.33		Das et al. (2012)
		Dhaka	2009	Pet		3670	1.93		Tarafder and Samad (2012)

Note: No data were retrieved from literature search from Sri Lanka, Nepal and Bhutan.

Table 2 Prevalence of *Toxocara canis* in environmental samples tested in the Indian subcontinent.

Country	State/union territory	City	Sample type	Number examined	Prevalence %	Comments	References
India	Andhra Pradesh	Tirupati	Soil	179	38.54	12 public parks, 16 school play grounds examined	Kumar and Hafeez (1998)
	Assam	Guwahati	Vegetables	140	45.71	Highest in coriander leaves (90%)	Pathak et al. (2014)
		Tezpur	Soil	130	6.1–12		Singh et al. (2004)
	Chandigarh	Chandigarh	Soil	120	4.16	All positives from one village Kheri. Eggs viable	Grover et al. (2000)
	Karnataka	Bangalore	Soil	208	23		D'Souza et al. (2002)
	Maharashtra	Mumbai	Soil	48	8.33	3 children play grounds, 1 veterinary hospital examined	Kumar et al. (2012)
	Puducherry	Puducherry	Soil	816	12.21		Das et al. (2009a)
	Punjab	Ludhiana	Soil	208	19.71		Harbinder et al. (1997)
	Tamil Nadu	Chennai	Soil	105	4.75	3.75% public places; 8% in kennels	Thomas and Jeyathilakan (2014)
		Chennai	Soil	527	18.41	Highest in parks (46.43%)	Gunaseelan et al. (1985)
		Chennai	Soil	410	6.59	Samples from Madras Vet College	Gunaseelan et al. (1992)
	Uttar Pradesh	Bareilly	Soil	327	12.84	Public parks more contaminated	Sudhakar et al. (2013)
		Bareilly	Vegetables	515	0.77	Contamination in carrots, radish, coriander leaves	Samanta et al. (2011)
	West Bengal	Kolkata	Soil		7.25		Biswas et al. (1986)
Nepal	Central Region	Kathmandu	Soil	122	23		Rai et al. (2000)

Table 3 Prevalence of *Toxocara canis* in zoo animals in India.

Country	State/union territory	City	Animal host	Scientific name	Number examined	Prevalence %	References
India	Assam	Guwahati	Jackal		1	100	Nashiruddullah and Chakraborty (2001)
	Chhattisgarh	Raipur	Jackal	*Canis aureus*	2	100	Thawait et al. (2014)
	Gujarat	Rajkot	Hyaena	*Hyaena striata*	2	0	Parsani et al. (2001)
			Jackal	*Canis aureus*	2	0	
			Indian Fox	*Vulpes bengalensis*	2	0	
	Karnataka	Shimoga	Jackal		6	50	Javaregowda (2016)
	Kerala	Thrissur	Jackal	*Canis aureus*	1	0	Varadharajan et al. (2001)
		Thiruvanathapuram	Hyaena	*Hyaena hyaena*	2	50	Varadharajan and Pythan (1999)
	Maharashtra	Nagpur	Jackal	*Canis aureus*	2	0	Dhoot et al. (2002)
	Odisha	Bhubaneshwar	Jackal			0	Rao and Achariyo (1984)
			Fox			0	
		Bhubaneshwar	Hyaena		11	0	Mahali et al. (2010)

	Punjab	Ludhiana	Jackal	*Canis aureus*	12	0	Singh et al. (2006)
			Hyaena	*Hyaena hyaena*	4	0	
	Tamil Nadu	Coimbatore	Bengal Fox		1	0	Varadharajan and Kandasamy (2000)
			Jackal		10	0	
	Uttar Pradesh	Nainital, Kanpur	Indian Fox, Yellow throated marten	*Vulpes bengalensis*, *Vulpes fulva*	3	0	Gaur et al. (1979)
			Striped hyena	*Hyaena hyaena*	1	0	
		Lucknow	Hyaena	*Hyaena striata*		[a]	Chauhan et al. (1973)
			Wolf	*Canis lupus*		0	
	West Bengal	Darjeeling	Jackal	*Canis aureus*	2	[b]	Pradhan et al. (2011)
			Tibetan wolf	*Canis lupus chanco*	9	0	
		Darjeeling	Himalayan wolf	*Canis lupus chanco*	5[c]	100	Chakraborty and Maity (1995)

[a]Toxocara detected. No prevalence provided.
[b]Two of 19 faecal samples from the 2 jackal tested positive for *Toxocara*.
[c]Necropsy of clinical cases of diarrhoea and death.

2.2 Overview of regional prevalence

In India, of the 37 states/union territories (28 states and 9 union territories), prevalence data are available from 23 (Table 1). Higher prevalence of >25% was reported from Andhra Pradesh (Kumar and Hafeez, 1998; Sivajothi and Reddy, 2018), Bihar (Samantha et al., 1989; Sharma et al., 2006), Jammu & Kashmir (Pandit et al., 2008; Wani et al., 2017), Karnataka (D'Souza et al., 2001; Malaki, 1966), Maharashtra (Khillare and Bhangale, 2018; Joshi et al., 1977; Khante et al., 2009), Meghalaya (Yadav and Tandon, 1989), Odisha (Misra et al., 1974), Uttar Pradesh (Kumar et al., 2014; Sahu et al., 2014; Samantha and Ghorui, 1998; Sudan et al., 2015), and West Bengal (Maplestone and Bhaduri, 1940). Similarly, a prevalence of >15% were never documented from Assam (Dutta et al., 2008; Traub et al., 2002), Chandigarh (Chhabra and Mahajan, 1978; Utaaker et al., 2018), Gujarat (Jani et al., 1995; Kumar et al., 2015), Haryana (Kaushik et al., 1978), Himachal Pradesh (Agnihotri et al., 2008; Moudgil et al., 2016), Punjab (Chhabra et al., 2001), Sikkim (Traub et al., 2014), Tamil Nadu (Balasubramaniam et al., 2001; Suganya et al., 2019) and Uttarkhand (Vatsya et al., 2010). Regional variation among the districts within the state of Himachal Pradesh was reported, wherein, Kullu and Shimla had zero prevalence, whereas, Mandi, Kangra & Una had 2–9% prevalence (Agnihotri et al., 2008). There were only few studies that involved more than one state/union territory. Interestingly, a low prevalences ranging from 0% to 3.2% were recorded in a study that sampled dogs from four different regions in India (Delhi, Ladakh, Mumbai, & Sikkim) (Traub et al., 2014). Negligible prevalence of *T. canis* noted in cities like Delhi and Mumbai was likely due to the low proportion of puppies, pregnant and lactating females sampled.

In Pakistan, higher prevalences were reported in all three cities (Faisalabad, Lahore and Karachi) from where prevalence data was available (Buscher, 1974; Maqbool et al., 1998; Maryam and Ahmed, 1965; Umar et al., 1986). Overall, the prevalence of *T. canis* in both pet and stray dogs ranged from 13% to 45.4% (See Table 1). In Bangladesh, a massive surveillance study involving 3670 pet dogs in Dhaka surprisingly recorded a very low prevalence of 1.93% (Tarafder and Samad, 2012). However, from Chittagong 23.33% prevalence was recorded (Das et al., 2012). No prevalence data for *T. canis* in either pet or stray dogs could be retrieved for Sri Lanka, Nepal and Bhutan. Among metropolitan cities in the subcontinent, recent records show a lower prevalence for cities in India

(Delhi, Mumbai, Kolkata &Chennai), in Pakistan (Lahore) and in Bangladesh (Dhaka) (Beeshmi and Dasgupta, 2006; Farooqi et al., 2014; Suganya et al., 2019; Tarafder and Samad, 2012; Traub et al., 2014). Further studies are required to assess the epidemiological significance of these findings.

2.3 Higher prevalence in stray compared to pet dogs

Prevalence reported in pet dogs ranged from as low as 1.65% (Dutta et al., 2008) to as high as 52.54% (Sivajothi and Reddy, 2018). Similarly, prevalence in stray dogs ranged from 0% (Traub et al., 2014) to 100% (Misra et al., 1974). Seven of 25 studies done in pet dogs report a prevalence of >20%. In contrast, 12 of the 27 studies in stray dogs report a prevalence of >20% (See Table 1). A reporting trend of higher prevalence in stray compared to pet dogs was observed even at studies conducted at the same locality. For example, at Chandigarh, Bareilly and Puducherry, the prevalence between pet and stray dogs were, 8.3 and 14.8, 17.5 and 31.29, 4.97 and 16.56, respectively. Various factors may play role for higher prevalence in stray dogs which include their widespread distribution, scavenging habits, and unrestricted fouling of environment (Samantha and Ghorui, 1998).

2.4 Age as a determinant of *T. canis* infection

The role of age as a factor in *T. canis* infection was noted in various studies. A prevalence of 28.3% in pups compared to 4.7% in older dogs was recorded in a faecal study from dogs at Chandigarh (Chhabra and Mahajan, 1978). A similar study at Haryana & Delhi recorded a prevalence of 10.8% in pups compared to 2.23% in older dogs (Kaushik et al., 1978). In Bangalore, 47.61% of pups and 24.13% of adults were infected with *T. canis* (D'Souza et al., 2001). Similar observations were made from studies conducted at Assam, Uttar Pradesh, Odisha (Dutta et al., 2008; Kumar et al., 2014; Panigrahi et al., 2014; Sahu et al., 2014; Sudan et al., 2015). Transplacental migration, trans-mammary passage coupled with poor immunity could be the main factors for high prevalence in pups (Kumar et al., 2014). As a deviation from the norm, a higher prevalence of 42.10% was recorded from dogs over 6 years of age in comparison to 59.15% prevalence in dogs less than 1 year at YSR Kadapa, Andhra Pradesh (Sivajothi and Reddy, 2018). Interestingly, the same authors also analyzed *T. canis* eggs in the hair coat of dogs and reported no age-specificity in the prevalence of eggs in hair coats in contrast to faecal studies.

2.5 Breed and sex predilection for *T. canis*

In the Indian subcontinent, nondescript and mixed-breed dogs are numerically more than the purebreds. Studies observed no breed predilection for *T. canis* in either nondescript or crossbred dogs (Kumar et al., 2014; Sharma et al., 2006). Among descript breeds, the prevalence rate was 14.74% as compared to 40.68% in local/mixed-breeds; however, large and small descript breeds are equally predisposed (Kumar et al., 2014). Pedigree purebreds were found to be less infected with *T. canis* compared to the mixed-breeds (Sahu et al., 2014). In an interesting study at YSR Kadapa, the authors observed *T. canis* eggs in the hair coats of dogs wherein the incidence was more in long haired compared to short haired dogs (36.73% vs. 17.39%). Sex of either descript or nondescript dogs did not influence the likelihood of *T. canis* infection (Kumar et al., 2014; Samantha et al., 1989). A similar observation was reported for stray and pet pups at Bareilly; however, the prevalence was slightly higher in adult females (Sahu et al., 2014).

2.6 Seasonal variations in *T. canis* prevalence

Seasonal prevalence was noticed for *T. canis* that was in contrast to hookworm infections which occurred throughout the year (Sharma et al., 2006). Incidence of *T. canis* was absent during winter months (Dec–Feb) but peaked during monsoon months (Aug–Sept) (Chhabra et al., 2001). Seasonal variation in the intensity of infection was noticed as *T. canis* egg shedding in monsoon season was more when compared to winter (Utaaker et al., 2018). In contrast, the disease was more prevalent during winters at Mathura, Uttar Pradesh (Kumar et al., 2014). Higher prevalence was also observed in winter (Nov–Feb) at Palampur, Himachal Pradesh (Agnihotri et al., 2008). A study examining 2391 dogs at Haryana and Delhi reported the highest infection rate for *T. canis* in winter (Kaushik et al., 1978).

2.7 Analytical methods as a factor influencing parasite detection

In general, necropsy-based studies were suggested to report a higher prevalence for *T. canis* compared to faecal examination (Chhabra and Mahajan, 1978). Interestingly, prevalence of >20% was reported in 6 of the 10 studies based on necropsy (60%); whereas, only 18 of 52 studies based on faecal examination (~35%) report a prevalence of over 20%. This highlights the variations that could arise based on the surveillance protocol adapted and can be construed as one of the limitations of such studies carried out to ascertain the prevalence of *T. canis*. Moreover, faecal examination may not reveal all positive cases and the real extent of this infection remains greatly underestimated (Chhabra and Mahajan, 1978).

Absence of a standardized parasite surveillance protocols limits meaningful comparison of data from different studies as depicted in Tables 1–3. Importantly, the type of faecal testing methodology is also a factor to consider that could influence the prevalence observed. A wide number of tests were employed by various authors ranging from a simple direct faecal smear to more robust concentration techniques. Some of the faecal testing methods employed are: (1) Direct smear (Chhabra and Mahajan, 1978; Das et al., 2009b; Panigrahi et al., 2014; Vatsya et al., 2010), (2) Formol-ether concentration (Chhabra and Mahajan, 1978), (3) Willi's technique (Das et al., 2009b), (4) Floatation (Moudgil et al., 2016; Panigrahi et al., 2014; Sahu et al., 2014; Samantha and Ghorui, 1998), (5) Sedimentation and floatation (Khillare and Bhangale, 2018; Sudan et al., 2015), (6) Sedimentation and centrifugal floatation (Mamatha et al., 2005; Traub et al., 2002, 2014; Wani et al., 2017), (7) McMaster (Kachawha and Tanwar, 2007; Kumar et al., 2014; Nath et al., 2011; Utaaker et al., 2018), (8) Modified McMaster (Chhabra et al., 2001; Das et al., 2009b; Qadir et al., 2012). The diagnostic performance of many of the abovementioned techniques is not clearly deduced and would have impacted the results from these studies. Nevertheless, molecular surveillance tools are vouched for parasite screening as they provide the level of discrimination that is not often achieved by microscopy (Traub et al., 2005). One study that employed PCR on 30 positive faecal samples by microscopy could confirm *T. canis* in only 25 (Suganya et al., 2019). If this result is to be trusted, it raises the curious question of whether spurious parasitism in dogs was accounted by microscopy in the past studies? Given the fact that dogs are notorious with their feeding habits and high percentage of them are mechanical carriers of other animal parasite stages (Traub et al., 2002, 2005), the prevalence data published from the subcontinent may represent a slight over estimate of the actual.

3. Detection of *T. canis* in environmental sample

Environmental contamination with *T. canis* eggs is inevitable considering that the fact that this helminth is a prolific egg shedder and the parasite stages are viable in the environment normally for 2 years (Kumar et al., 2017;

Parmar et al., 2008; Singla and Juyal, 2005; Thawait et al., 2014). Therefore, analyzing environmental samples may provide information about the risk associated with parasite acquisition from environment for both animals and humans (Thomas and Jeyathilakan, 2014). Interestingly, a sizeable number of studies had looked at the level of environmental contamination with *T. canis* eggs, especially in the soil and in the vegetables grown for human consumption. Table 2 summarize the literatures from the Indian subcontinent in this regard. These studies were mostly from India and one report was from Nepal. Prevalence in soil samples in India varied from 4.16% to 38.54%. Note that the extent of detection of *T. canis* eggs in the soil depends on the sampling and recovery methods, the geographic location, the number and volume of samples examined (Harbinder et al., 1997).

Similar to the limitations with faecal analysis, soil testing is also influenced by the choice of analytical method. Among the 12 studies reported from India, only seven provided reference for the testing method used. They are (1) Zinc Sulphate floatation (Kumar et al., 2012); (2) Dunsmore method (Sudhakar et al., 2013; Thomas and Jeyathilakan, 2014); (3) Dada's method (Gunaseelan et al., 1985, 1992; Harbinder et al., 1997); (4) Habluetzel method (Das et al., 2009a) and (5) O'Lorcain method (D'Souza et al., 2002). The diagnostic performance of most of these methods are not known; however, a recent study compared the three commonly used soil testing methods, namely Kazakos method, O'Lorcain method and Santarem method, and identified O'Lorcain method as more sensitive than the other two (Gnani Charitha et al., 2013). Interestingly, the O'Lorcain method employed to detect *T. canis* from soil samples at Bangalore, India topped the list among the seven above mentioned studies with an egg recovery in 23% of the total 208 soil samples (D'Souza et al., 2002). Soil testing also highlight the state of contamination prevalent in public parks and playgrounds (Gunaseelan et al., 1985; Kumar et al., 2012; Kumar and Hafeez, 1998; Sudhakar et al., 2013). Moreover, a high occurrence of eggs in soil samples from kennels/shelters at Chennai and Bangalore, India supports the notion that heavy infections occur in animal shelters with poor hygienic conditions (D'Souza et al., 2002; Kumar et al., 2014).

4. Prevalence of *T. canis* in zoo canids

Several surveys were conducted to study intestinal parasites of captive wild canids in the subcontinent. However, prevalence of *T. canis* infections were rather low (See Table 3). As there were no appropriate sample size for animals tested, the data mainly indicates the occurrence of this parasite in captive settings. Although the occurrence ranged from 0% to 100%, the low detection of *T. canis* might be due to regular deworming practices employed by zoos (Parsani et al., 2001). Nevertheless, there was one report from Padmaja Naidu Himalayan Zoological Park at Darjeeling which associated *T. canis* with diarrhoea, dehydration and death of 5 Himalayan wolf puppies (Chakraborty and Maity, 1995). Despite the low occurrence for *T. canis*, hookworm infection seems to be more prevalent in zoo canids (Mahali et al., 2010; Rao and Achariyo, 1984; Varadharajan and Kandasamy, 2000; Varadharajan et al., 2001). In general, older canids tend to be infected more with hookworms than pups, which are prone to roundworm infections (Chhabra and Mahajan, 1978; Malaki, 1966). Interestingly, *Toxocara* infection is more common in zoo felids than in canids (Javaregowda, 2016; Mahali et al., 2010; Pradhan et al., 2011; Sutar and Gatne, 2002; Varadharajan et al., 2001).

5. Conclusion

The present review attempts to compile data on the occurrence/incidence/prevalence of *T. canis* infections in canine population and hopefully serves as a guide list on the status of this important canine infection in the Indian subcontinent. Based on the data retrieved, *T. canis* seems to be a widely prevalent helminth parasite of both stray and pet dogs. Despite the lack of uniformity in the methodology used for *T. canis* surveillance, available data points towards the looming threat posed by this zoonotic parasite to burgeoning human population. Accurate parasite detection is a key for monitoring infection in reservoir hosts and for formulating effective control strategies. Therefore, future studies must thoroughly consider the limitations of existing surveillance protocols and design strategies using appropriate classical methodologies complemented with molecular testing tools. Future surveillance must prioritize study regions (Countries/States/Cities) which lack data about this helminth infection. Concerted surveillance efforts in stray, companion and wild canids alongside serological surveillance in human population may benefit the making of informed policy decision to combat this neglected tropical helminth disease.

References

Acharya, S.K., 1933. Incidence of helminth parasites in pariah dogs. Indian Vet. J. 9, 210.

Agnihotri, R.K., Sharma, D., Sharma, Y., 2008. Incidence of gastrointestinal helminths in dogs od Himachal Pradesh. J. Vet. Parasitol. 22, 89–90.

Ahmad, N., Maqbool, A., Saeed, K., Ashraf, K., Qamar, M.F., 2011. Toxocariasis, its zoonotic importance and chemotherapy in dogs. J. Anim. Plant Sci. 21, 142–145.

Ahmad, P.A., Sharma, R., Katoch, R., Yadav, A., Godara, R., Imitiaz, S.R., 2018. Incidence of gastrointestinal helminths of stray dogs: a postmortem study. Haryana Vet. 57, 222–223.

Asati, A.K., Shukla, P.C., Sisodia, R.S., 1999. Faecal prevalence of eggs of gastro-intestinal helminths of dogs in Malwa region of Madhya Pradesh. Indian Vet. Med. J. 23, 237–238.

Balasubramaniam, G.A., Rao, G.V.S., Balachandran, C., George, V.T., Vairamuthu, S., 2001. Incidence of parasitic diseases among domestic animals in Namakkal District of Tamil Nadu. Indian J. Anim. Sci. 71, 340–341.

Baylis, H.A., Daubney, R., 1922. Report on the parasitic nematodes in the collection of the zoological survey of India. Mem. Indian Mus. 7, 264–347.

Beeshmi, P., Dasgupta, C.K., 2006. Studies on occurence of ectoparasites and gastrointestinal parasites of dogs in and around Kolkata. In: XVII National Congress in Veterinary Parasitology, p. 83.

Bhatia, B.B., Chauhan, P.P.S., Agrawal, R., Katara, R.P., 1980. Incidence of parasitic infections amongst stray dogs in Mathura, Uttar Pradesh. Vet. Res. J. 3, 120–123.

Biswas, G., Bhattacharya, A., Sen, G.P., 1986. Dog a source of human visceral larva migrans. Indian J. Public Health 30, 22.

Buscher, H.N., 1974. Intestinal helminths of dog, *Canis familiaris*, in Lahore and their potential as contributors to public health problems. Pak. J. Sci. 26, 12–14.

Chakraborty, T., Maity, B., 1995. Toxocariasis in Himalayan wolf (Canis lupus chanco) pups. Indian J. Vet. Pathol. 19, 136.

Chatterjee, P., 2009. India's ongoing war against rabies. Bull. World Health Organ. 87, 890–891.

Chattha, M.A., Aslam, A., Rehman, Z.U., Khan, J.A., Avais, M., 2009. Prevalence of *Toxocara canis* infection in dogs and its effects on various blood parameters in Lahore (Pakistan). J. Anim. Plant Sci. 19, 71–73.

Chauhan, P.P.S., Bhatia, B.B., Arora, G.S., Agrawal, R.D., Ahluwalia, S.S., 1973. A preliminary survey of parasitic infections among mammals and birds at Lucknow and Delhi zoos. Indian J. Anim. Sci. 43, 163–168.

Chhabra, M.B., Mahajan, R.C., 1978. A note on the prevalence of *Toxocara canis* and other intestinal parasites in Chandigarh. Indian J. Anim. Sci. 48, 929–931.

Chhabra, S., Khabra, S.S., Nauriyal, D.C., 2001. On the prevalence of treatment of helminth parasites of dog. J. Vet. Parasitol. 15, 129–131.

Das, S., Kumar, D., Sreekrishnan, R., Ganesan, R., 2009a. Soil contamination of public places, play grounds and residential areas with ova of *Toxocara*. Indian J. Vet. Res. 17, 13–16.

Das, S., Kumar, D., Sreekrishnan, R., Ganesan, R., 2009b. Gastrointestinal parasitic infection in dogs in Puducherry. J. Vet. Parasitol. 23, 77–79.

Das, S., Alim, M.A., SIkder, S., Das Gupta, A., Masuduzzaman, M., Kelimeler, A., 2012. Prevalence and worm load of enteric helminthiasis in stray dogs of Chittagong metropolitan, Bangladesh. YYU Vet. Fak. Derg. 23, 141–145.

Dhar, D.N., Pattanayak, S., Basu, P.C., 1966. Prevalence of *Toxocara canis* (Werner, 1782) Johnston, 1916 and other intestinal helminth infections in dogs in Delhi and experimental studies on *T. canis* infection in laboratory animals. Bull. Indian Soc. Malar. Other Commun. Dis. 3, 303–311.

Dhoot, V.M., Upadhye, S.V., Kotle, S.W., 2002. Prevalence of parasitism in wild mammals and birds of Maharajbag zoo, Nagpur. Indian Vet. J. 79, 225–227.

D'Souza, P.E., Dhanalakshmi, H., Jagannath, M.S., 2001. Observations on the incidence of worm infestation in dogs and efficacy of different methods in its detection. Blue Cross Book 16, 33–35.

D'Souza, P.E., Dhanalakshmi, H., Jagannath, M.S., 2002. Soil contamination with canine hookworm and roundworm ova in Bangalore. J. Parasit. Dis. 26, 107–108.

Dutta, P.R., Phukan, A., Hazarika, G.G., 2008. Epidemiological study of diarrhoea in dogs. Anim. Sci. Rep. 2, 101–104.

Farooqi, M.T., Maqbool, A., Ashraf, K., Rashid, M.I., Akbar, H., Sheikh, A.A., 2014. Canine zoonosis; its potential and association of soil-borne Helminthes from public parks and its gastro-intestinal helminthes in Lahore, Pakistan. Sci. Int. (Lahore) 26, 771–774.

Gaur, S.N.S., Sethi, M.S., Tewari, H.C., OM, P., 1979. A note on the prevalence of helminth parasites in wild and zoo animals in Uttar Pradesh. Indian J. Anim. Sci. 49, 159–161.

Gnani Charitha, V., Rayulu, V.C., Kondaiah, P.M., Srilatha, C., 2013. Comparative evaluation of flotation techniques for the detection of soil borne parasites. J. Parasit. Dis. 37, 260–263.

Godhra, R., Sharma, R.L., Sharma, C.S., Sharma, D.K., 2010. Parasitic infections in dogs in semi-arid Jaipur (Rajasthan). J. Vet. Parasitol. 24, 83–86.

Grover, R., Bhatti, G., Aggarwal, A., Malla, N., 2000. Isolation of *Toxocara* eggs in and around Chandigarh, India. J. Parasit. Dis. 24, 57–59.

Gunaseelan, L., Ramadass, P., Raghavan, N., 1985. Epidemiological studies on *Toxocara canis* infection in children in Madras city. Cheiron 14, 326–328.

Gunaseelan, L., Ganesan, P.I., Ramadass, P., Basheer, A., Raghavan, N., 1992. Incidence of *Toxocara* ova in the environment. Indian Vet. J. 69, 308–309.

Hall, M.C., 1917. Parasites of dog in Michigan. J. Am. Vet. Med. Assoc. 4, 383–396.

Harbinder, S., Bali, H.S., Arvinderl, K., 1997. Prevalence of Toxocara spp. eggs in the soil of public and private places in Ludhiana and Kellon area of Punjab, India. Epidemiol. Santé Anim. 31, 04.05.1–3.

Hegde, K.S., Jagannath, M.S., 1974. A survey of parasites of digestive tract of dogs in Bangalore. Mysore J. Agric. Sci. 8, 597–601.

Jani, R.G., Jani, B.M., Dave, M.R., 1995. Prevalence of intestinal parasites in dogs at Anand (Gujarat). J. Vet. Parasitol. 9, 51–53.

Javaregowda, A.K., 2016. Studies on prevalence of endo-parasitic infection in wild carnivores maintained under captive state. J. Parasit. Dis. 40, 1155–1158.

Joshi, B.N., Sabne, S.S., Kalkadkar, R.K., 1977. Intestinal helminthic infections in stray dogs—a public health problem. Indian J. Public Health 21, 34–37.

Kachawha, B., Tanwar, R.K., 2007. Prevalence of worm infestations in stray dogs in and around Jodhpur. J. Vet. Parasitol. 21, 171–172.

Kaushik, R.K., Banerjee, D.P., Bali, M.K., 1978. Prevalence of *Toxocara canis* infection among dogs in Haryana and Delhi—a preliminary survey. J. Res. 8, 71–74.

Khante, G.S., Khan, L.A., Bodkhe, A.M., Suryawanshi, P.R., Majed, M.A., Suradkar, U.S., Gaikwad, S.S., 2009. Epidemiological survey of gastro-intestinal parasites of non-descript dogs in Nagpur City. Vet. World 2, 22–23.

Khillare, B., Bhangale, G., 2018. Canine Helminthoses in Udgir: a preliminary prevalence study. TJVR 2, 20–22.

Kumar, B., Hafeez, M., 1998. A study on the prevalence of *Toxocora* spp. eggs at public places in Andhra Pradesh. J. Commun. Dis. 30, 197–198.

Kumar, C., Karabanavar, N., Bhandare, S., Zende, R., Paturkar, A., 2012. Contamination of community soil with ova of *Toxocara* species in Mumbai city. J. Vet. Pub. Hlth. 10, 57–58.

Kumar, M., Sharma, B., Kumar, A., Lal, H.P., Kumar, V., Tripathi, M.K., 2014. Prevalence and Haemato-biochemical studies of *Toxocara canis* infestation in dogs and risk perception of Zooneses by dog owners in Mathura, India. Asian J. Anim. Vet. Adv. 9, 653–663.

Kumar, B., Maharana, B.R., Prashad, A., Hirani, N.D., Joseph, J.P., 2015. Epidemiological survey of gastrointestinal parasites of dogs in South-Western Gujarat (Junagadh), India. J. Vet. Parasitol. 29, 56–60.

Kumar, M., Gaur, N., Sharma, B., Singh, D.P., Kumar, A., 2017. Comparative efficacy of piperazine, ivermectin and levamisole in spontaneous Toxocariasis in Canines based on faecal egg count and haemato-biochemical changes. Intas Polivet 18, 166–173.

Mahali, A.K., Panda, D.N., Panda, M.R., Mohanty, B.N., Sahoo, N., 2010. Incidence and seasonal variation of gastro-intestinal parasitic infections in captive carnivores in Nandankan zoological park Orissa. J. Vet. Parasitol. 24, 111–115.

Malaki, A., 1966. A survey of gastro-intestinal parasites of dogs in Bangalore with notes on some interesting observations. Indian Vet. J. 43, 409–412.

Mamatha, G.S., D'Souza, P.E., Narayana Bhat, M., 2005. Gastrointestinal parasitism in dogs and cats in Bangalore. Intas Polivet 6, 152–153.

Maplestone, P.A., Bhaduri, N.V., 1940. The helminth parasites of dogs in Calcutta and their bearing on human parasitology. Indian J. Med. Res. 28, 595–604.

Maqbool, A., Raza, S.H., Hayat, C.S., Shafiq, M., 1998. Prevalence and chemotherapy of toxocariasis in the dog in Faisalabad (Punjab), Pakistan. Vet. Arhiv 68, 121–125.

Maryam, S., Ahmed, Z., 1965. Intestinal parasites of 200 dogs in Karachi and their potential public health significance. Z. Parasitenkd. 25, 501–505.

Masare, P.S., Digraskar, S.U., 2007. Prevalence of canine parvovirus among haemorrhagic gastroenteritis in dogs. Indian J. Field Vet. 3, 33–34.

Misra, S.C., Sahoo, B., Potel, G.N., 1974. Studies on parasitic problems of puppies. V. Winter populations of helminths and arthropods on puppies at Bhubaneswar. Indian J. Anim. Res. 8, 89–91.

Moudgil, A.D., Mittra, S., Agnihotri, R.K., Sharma, D., Sen, D., 2016. Prevalence of gastrointestinal parasites in dogs of Palampur, Himachal Pradesh. J. Parasit. Dis. 40, 227–229.

Nashiruddullah, N., Chakraborty, A., 2001. Parasites of captive wild carnivores of Assam state zoo. Intas Polivet. 2, 173–181.

Nath, S., Das, G., Roy, B., 2011. Incidence of gastro-intestinal parasitic infection in stray dogs in and around Jabalpur (Madhya Pradesh). Indian J. Field Vet. 7, 49–51.

Pal, M., Nair, R.P.N., Dube, G.D., 1979. Prevalence of helminth parasites in the pet dogs of Delhi metropolitan area. Livestock Adviser 4, 25–28.

Pandit, B.A., Shahardar, R.A., Jeyabal, L., 2008. Prevalence of helminth parasites in stray dogs. J. Canine Dev. Res. 5, 31–34.

Panigrahi, P.N., Gupta, A.R., Behera, S.K., Panda, B.S.K., Patra, R.C., Mohanty, B.N., Sahoo, G.R., 2014. Evaluation of gastrointestinal helminths in canine population of Bhubaneswar, Odisha, India: a public health appraisal. Vet. World. 7, 295–298.

Parmar, B.C., Patel, P.V., Dhami, A.J., Solanki, J.B., 2008. Larva migrans—an overview. Vets Commun. 5, 22–27.

Parsani, H.R., Momin, R.R., Maradia, M.G., Singh, V., 2001. A survey of gastro-intestinal parasites of captive animals at Rajkot municipal corporation zoo, Rajkot, Gujarat. Zoos' Print J. 16, 604–606.

Pathak, P., Bam, J., Parikshit, K., Deka, D.K., 2014. Contamination of vegetables with eggs of certain zoonotic helminths at different market places of Guwahati, Assam. J. Vet. Parasitol. 28, 154–156.

Patra, P.C., Tripathy, S.B., 1986. Gastritis in dogs and its therapy. Indian Vet. J. 63, 940–943.

Pradhan, S., Sharma, D., Subba, B., Chettri, V., 2011. Preliminary investigation on the parasites of mammals at Padmaja Naidu Himalayan Zoological Park, Darjeeling. Zoos' Print 26, 11–13.

Pullan, R.L., Smith, J.L., Jasrasaria, R., Brooker, S.J., 2014. Global numbers of infection and disease burden of soil transmitted helminth infections in 2010. Parasit. Vectors 7, 1–19.

Qadir, S., Dixit, A.K., Dixit, P., 2012. Prevalence and intensity of canine gastrointestinal helminths in Jabalpur, Madhya Pradesh prevalence and intensity of canine gastrointestinal helminths in Jabalpur, Madhya Pradesh. J. Vet. Parasitol. 26, 23–26.

Rai, S.K., Uga, S., Ono, K., Rai, G., Matsumura, T., 2000. Contamination of soil with helminth parasite eggs in Nepal. Southeast Asian J. Trop. Med. Public Health 31, 388–393.

Rao, A.T., Achariyo, L.N., 1984. Diagnosis and classification of common diseases of captive animals at Nandankan zoo in Orrissa (India). Indian J. Anim. Health, 149–152.

Rostami, A., Ma, G., Wang, T., Koehler, A.V., Hofmann, A., Chang, B.C.H., Macpherson, C.N., Gasser, R.B., 2019. Human toxocariasis—a look at a neglected disease through an epidemiological 'prism'. Infect. Genet. Evol. 74, 104002.

Sahai, B.N., 1969. A survey of helminth parasites of stray dogs in and around Bareilly, Uttar Pradesh. Indian Vet. J. 46, 734.

Sahasrabudhe, V.K., Dubey, J.P., Srivastav, H.O.P., 1969. Helminth parasites of dogs in Madhya Pradesh and their public health significance. Indian J. Anim. Health 57, 56–59.

Sahu, S., Samanta, S., Sudhakar, N.R., Raina, O.K., Gupta, S.C., Maurya, P.S., Pawde, A.M., Kumar, A., 2014. Prevalence of canine toxocariasis in Bareilly, Uttar Pradesh, India. J. Parasit. Dis. 38, 111–115.

Samanta, S., Agarwal, R.K., Sahu, S., Sudhakar, N.R., Raina, O.K., Gupta, S.C., Bhilegaonkar, K.N., 2011. Occurrence of parasitic contamination in raw vegetables particularly used in salads. J. Vet. Pub. Hlth. 9, 7–11.

Samantha, S.K., Ghorui, S.K., 1998. Prevalence of *Toxocara canis* in dogs in and around Bareilly. Indian J. Anim. Health 37, 53–54.

Samantha, S., Ansari, M.Z., Sahai, B.N., 1989. Prevalence of *Toxocara canis* in dogs in and around Ranchi, Bihar. J. Res. 1, 201–203.

Shabbir, M.Z., Rabbani, M., Yaqub, T., Ahmad, A., Zia-ur-Rehman, Umair, S., 2010. Comparative clinical epidemiology of toxocariosis in dogs and cats. Pak. J. Zool. 42, 129–133.

Sharma, S.K., Sinha, S.R.P., Sinha, S., Kumar, L., Mahtha, R.K., 2006. Gastrointestinal helminthic parasites and treatment in different breeds of dogs. Indian Vet. J. 83, 834–836.

Sharma, R., Singh, B.B., Gill, J.P.S., 2015. Larva migrans in India: veterinary and public health perspectives. J. Parasit. Dis. 39, 604–612.

Sharma, R., Singh, B.B., Gill, J.P.S., Jenkins, E., Singh, B., 2017. Canine parasitic zoonoses in India: status and issues. Rev. Sci. Tech. 36, 817–830.

Singh, L.A., Das, S.C., Baruah, I., 2004. Observations on the soil contamination with the zoonotic canine gastrointestinal parasites in selected rural areas of Tezpur, Assam, India. J. Parasit. Dis. 28, 1–2.

Singh, P., Gupta, M., Singla, L., Singh, N., Sharma, D., 2006. Prevalence and chemotherapy of gastrointestinal helminthic infections in wild carnivores in Mahendra Choudhury Zoological Park, Punjab. J. Vet. Parasitol. 20, 17–23.

Singla, L.D., Juyal, P.D., 2005. New horizons on clinico-molecular and zoonotic aspects of toxocariosis of dogs and cats. Intas Polivet. 6, 264–273.

Sivajothi, S., Reddy, B.S., 2018. Investigation on *Toxocara* spp. eggs in hair coat of dogs in YSR Kadapa district of Andhra Pradesh, India. J. Parasit. Dis. 42, 550–553.

Stewart, F.H., 1916. Further experiments on Ascaris infection. Br. Med. J. 2, 486–488.

Sudan, V., Jaiswal, A.K., Shanker, D., Kanojiya, D., Sachan, A., 2015. Prevalence of endoparasitic infections of non descript dogs in Mathura, Uttar Pradesh. J. Parasit. Dis. 39, 491–494.

Sudhakar, N.R., Samanta, S., Sahu, S., Raina, O.K., Gupta, S.C., Madhu, D.N., Kumar, A., 2013. Prevalence of *Toxocara* species eggs in soil samples of public health importance in and around Bareilly, Uttar Pradesh, India. Vet. World. 6, 87–90.

Suganya, G., Porteen, K., Sekar, M., Sangaran, A., 2019. Prevalence and molecular characterization of zoonotic helminths in dogs. J. Parasit. Dis. 43, 96–102.

Sutar, A.N., Gatne, M.L., 2002. Incidence of gastrointestinal helminthic parasites of captive wild carnivores in Mumbai and Pune regions. J. Bombay Vet. Coll. 10, 32–34.

Tarafder, M., Samad, M., 2012. Prevalence of clinical diseases of pet dogs and risk perception of zoonotic infection by dog owners in Bangladesh. Bangl. J. Vet. Med. 8, 163–174.
Thawait, V.K., Maiti, S.K., Dixit, A.A., 2014. Prevalence of gastro-intestinal parasites in captive wild animals of Nandan Van zoo, Raipur, Chhattisgarh. Vet. World. 7, 448–451.
Thomas, D., Jeyathilakan, N., 2014. Detection of *Toxocara* eggs in contaminated soil from various public places of Chennai city and detailed correlation with literature. J. Parasit. Dis. 38, 174–180.
Traub, R.J., Robertson, I.A.N.D., Irwin, P., Mencke, N., Thompson, R.C.A., 2002. The role of dogs in transmission of gastrointestinal parasites in a remote tea-growing community in northeastern India. Am. J. Trop. Med. Hyg. 67, 539–545.
Traub, R.J., Robertson, I.D., Irwin, P.J., Mencke, N., Thompson, R.C.A.A., 2005. Canine gastrointestinal parasitic zoonoses in India. Trends Parasitol. 21, 42–48.
Traub, R.J., Pednekar, R.P., Cuttell, L., Porter, R.B., Azaziah, P., Megat, A., Gatne, M.L., 2014. Veterinary parasitology the prevalence and distribution of gastrointestinal parasites of stray and refuge dogs in four locations in India. Vet. Parasitol. 205, 233–238.
Umar, S., Rabbani, A., Mian, M.S., Afzal, M., Saeed, K., 1986. Efficacy of levamisole, mebendazole and pyrantel pamoate against natural infection of *Toxocara canis* in dogs. Pakistan Vet. J. 6, 127–128.
Utaaker, K.S., Tysnes, K.R., Krosness, M.M., Robertson, L.J., 2018. Not just a walk in the park: occurrence of intestinal parasites in dogs roaming recreational parks in Chandigarh, Northern India. Vet. Parasitol. 14, 176–180.
Varadharajan, A., Kandasamy, A., 2000. A survey of gastro-intestinal parasites of wild animals in captivity in the V.O.C. park and mini zoo, Coimbatore. Zoos' Print J. 15, 257–258.
Varadharajan, A., Pythan, C., 1999. Parasites of wildlife—I. A preliminary investigation on the parasites of wild animals at the zoological garden, Thiruvananthapuram, Kerala. Zoos' Print J. 14, 159–164.
Varadharajan, A., Pythal, C., Subramanian, H., 2001. Investigation on the prevalence of helminth parasites of wild mammals in the Thrissur zoo, Kerala. Cheiron 30, 12–15.
Vatsya, S., Garg, R., Kumar, R.R., Yadav, C.L., Banerjee, P.S., 2010. Retrospective study on the incidence of gastrointestinal and blood parasites in dogs at Pantnagar and their public health significance. J. Vet. Pub. Hlth. 8, 29–32.
Velu Pillai, M., 1924. Ascariasis. Indian Vet. J. 3, 124.
Wallace, R.M., Undurraga, E.A., Blanton, J.D., Cleaton, J., Franka, R., 2017. Elimination of dog-mediated human rabies deaths by 2030: needs assessment and alternatives for progress based on dog vaccination. Front Vet. Sci. 4, 1–21.
Wani, Z.A., Allaie, I.M., Shahardar, R.A., Maqbool, I., Gazi, M., 2017. Gastrointestinal parasitism in stray dogs at Srinagar city of Kashmir valley. Indian Vet. J. 94, 18–20.
Yadav, A.K., Tandon, V., 1989. Helminths of public health significance in domestic animals of Meghalaya. Indian J. Anim. Health 28, 169–171.
Zyoud, S.H., 2017. Global toxocariasis research trends from 1932 to 2015: a bibliometric analysis. Health Res. Policy Syst. 15, 1–7.

CHAPTER THIRTY-EIGHT

Epidemiology of *Toxocara* spp. in dogs and cats in mainland China, 2000–2019

Wen-Bin Zheng[a,b], Yang Zou[a], Guo-Hua Liu[b], Xing-Quan Zhu[a,b,*]

[a]State Key Laboratory of Veterinary Etiological Biology, Key Laboratory of Veterinary Parasitology of Gansu Province, Lanzhou Veterinary Research Institute, Chinese Academy of Agricultural Sciences, Lanzhou, China
[b]Hunan Provincial Key Laboratory of Protein Engineering in Animal Vaccines, College of Veterinary Medicine, Hunan Agricultural University, Changsha, China
*Corresponding author: e-mail address: xingquanzhu1@hotmail.com

Contents

Abstract

Toxocariasis is a neglected parasitic zoonosis. Although some studies have reported the *Toxocara* prevalence in dogs and cats in mainland China, there is a lack of comprehensive analysis of these data. Here, we conducted the first systematic review based on relevant literatures published in Web of Science, PubMed and CNKI from January 2000 to July 2019 to assess the prevalence of *Toxocara* infection in dogs and cats in mainland China. A total of 68 eligible papers were retrieved, including 24,490 dogs and 844 cats, with 17.34% (4246/24,490) *Toxocara canis* prevalence in dogs and 22.04% (186/844) *Toxocara cati* prevalence in cats by faecal floatation method. The prevalence and risk factors of *T. canis* and *T. cati* infection in different geographical regions, years, breeds, ages and genders were estimated in this review. This review indicates that there was high prevalence of *Toxocara* infection in dogs and cats in China. This finding calls for measures to reduce the potential risk of *Toxocara* infection and toxocariasis in humans and animals.

Advances in Parasitology, Volume 109
ISSN 0065-308X
https://doi.org/10.1016/bs.apar.2020.01.031

1. Introduction

Toxocariasis, caused by parasites of the genus *Toxocara*, is one of the most neglected zoonoses all over the world, particularly in impoverished communities. *Toxocara canis* and, to a less level, *Toxocara cati* are the main pathogens of toxocariasis in humans (Despommier, 2003). Environment contamination with *Toxocara* eggs is a major threat to humans and animals, and is very common in many countries, especially in urban public parks, with prevalence of soil samples obtained from parks ranging from 14.4% to 20.6% in the USA, 17.4% to 60.3% in Brazil, 6.6% to 63.3% in Asia, 13.0% to 87.1% in Europe and 30.3% to 54.5% in Africa (Chen et al., 2018). The seroprevalence of *Toxocara* infection ranges from 12.25% (351/2866) to 19.3% (281/1458) between 2011 and 2015 in the northeast and east China (Cong et al., 2014; Cong et al., 2015; Yang et al., 2016)

Dogs and cats, the most popular companion animals, have access to playgrounds and other public places. They are also the definitive hosts of *T. canis* and *T. cati*, respectively, serving as the main source of environmental contamination of *Toxocara* eggs, and posing a tremendous risk of human exposure to infective eggs (Glickman and Schantz, 1981). As of August 2017, the number of pet dogs and cats had reached to 87.46 million in China, and the number of pet families had reached to 59.12 million, accounting for 17% of the total number of households in China (Cen, 2018). With the rapid development of economy in China, the number of pet dogs and cats will continue to increase in the future (Cen, 2018). Therefore, it is very necessary to understand the epidemiology of *Toxocara* in dogs and cats in China.

This review summaries and analyses the prevalence of *T. canis* and *T. cati* infection in dogs and cats in mainland China from 2000 to 2019, to provide reference data for the prevention and control of *Toxocara* infection in humans and animals in China.

2. Data sources and data extraction

This review was conducted on the available papers published in English based on the databases of Web of Science and PubMed, as well as papers published in Chinese based on the database of CNKI (http://www.cnki.net) from January 2000 to July 2019. The searches used the key words "*Toxocara*", "prevalence" and "China" in English in Web of Science and PubMed, and "*T. canis*" or "*T. cati*" in Chinese in CNKI.

The abstract and full text of each paper was checked carefully to exclude irrelevant and duplicated studies to assess the prevalence of *T. canis* and *T. cati* infection in dogs and cats. Papers were eligible for this review with the following criteria: (i) they were performed in mainland China; (ii) they used faecal floatation method; (iii) they provided exact total and positive numbers, and (iv) their total sample size was >25. The information of each eligible paper was extracted carefully, including the information of regions, years, breeds, ages, genders as well as the total and positive numbers.

3. Data analysis

All extracted data were implemented to reveal the potential relationship and risk factors of *Toxocara* infection in different regions, years, breeds, ages and genders by chi-square analysis. *P*-value <0.05 was considered as statistically significant. Odds-ratios (OR) with 95% confidence intervals (CI) were analysed in this review. All statistical analyses were performed by SAS 9.1 and GraphPad Prism 5.

4. Results and discussion

A total of 68 eligible papers were retrieved from Web of Science, PubMed and CNKI databases, including 24,490 dogs and 844 cats in mainland China from January 2000 to July 2019 (Table 1). In this review, 17.34% (4246/24,490) of the examined dogs were positive with *T. canis* infection, which was higher than that in some countries, such as the 6.93% (16/231) in dogs in south central West Virginia, USA (Savilla et al., 2011), 7.62% (67/879) in dogs in Crete, Greece (Kostopoulou et al., 2017) and 9.29% (55/592) in dogs in Ponte de Lima, Portugal (Mateus et al., 2014); but lower than the 27.00% (27/100) in domestic dogs in northern Iran (Sarvi et al., 2016) and 29.00% (29/100) in dogs in Egypt (El-Tras et al., 2011). 22.04% (186/844) of the examined cats were positive with *T. cati* infection in this review, which was higher than that in some countries, such as the 7.16% (48/670) in cats in Netherlands (Nijsse et al., 2016), 8.33% (22/264) in cats in Crete, Greece (Kostopoulou et al., 2017), 10.31% (56/543) in stray cats in Peninsular Malaysia (Mohd Zain et al., 2013) and 20.29% (84/414) in household cats in Transylvania, Romania (Mircean et al., 2010); but lower than the 38.27% (62/162) in stray cats in Lisbon, Portugal (Waap et al., 2014).

Table 1 The prevalence of *Toxocara canis* and *Toxocara cati* infection in dogs and cats in mainland China from January 2000 to July 2019

Regions	*T. canis* (%) (a/A)	*T. cati* (%) (a/A)	References
Anhui	7.22 (27/374)	N	Jiang (2003) and Zhou et al. (2014)
Beijing	6.40 (178/2781)	0.53 (1/187)	Yang and Liang (2015), Yu et al. (2006), and Yu et al. (2018)
Chongqing	60.45 (217/359)	N	Kuang et al. (2018), Tang et al. (2003), and Xia and Lai (2001)
Fujian	58.31 (379/650)	N	Lin and Yu (2015) and Lin et al. (2015)
Gansu	8.20 (21/256)	N	Lu et al. (2010)
Guangdong	20.29 (14/69)	N	Zhao et al. (2001)
Guangxi	5.45 (12/220)	5.13 (2/39)	Fang et al. (2015) and Huang et al. (2017)
Guizhou	21.29 (181/850)	N	Wang et al. (2009) and Zhou et al. (2013)
Hebei	9.33 (35/375)	0.00 (0/85)	Huang et al. (2014b), Liu et al. (2011), and Zang et al. (2016)
Henan	18.26 (325/1780)	21.07 (63/299)	Dong et al. (2008), Huo et al. (2013), Qi et al. (2010), Su et al. (2015), Yang and Liang (2015), and Zhang and Dong (2009)
Heilongjiang	30.43 (14/46)	90.63 (29/32)	Jiang and Sun (2001) and Niu et al. (2011)
Hunan	20.26 (660/3257)	N	Dai et al. (2009), Fan (2006), Huang and Chen (2011), Liang (2015), Liu et al. (2009), Sheng (2014), and Tang (2008)
Jiangsu	13.24 (340/2568)	28.30 (15/53)	Huang et al. (2014a); Li and Jia (2017), Li et al. (2011), Pan et al. (2016), Shan and Li (2007), Sun et al. (2018), Wei (2018), and Zhuo et al. (2016)
Liaoning	42.33 (810/1879)	N	Gao et al. (2016), Li (2010), Liu (2012), Liu (2014), Liu et al. (2008), Xiu and Kong (2011), Xu et al. (2010), and Zhou (2014)

Table 1 The prevalence of *Toxocara canis* and *Toxocara cati* infection in dogs and cats in mainland China from January 2000 to July 2019—cont'd

Regions	*T. canis* (%) (a/A)	*T. cati* (%) (a/A)	References
Neimenggu	12.80 (16/125)	N	Liu et al. (2005) and Niu and Wang (2001)
Ningxia	35.71 (20/56)	N	Yang et al. (2012)
Qinghai	29.98 (128/427)	N	Fan et al. (2017), He and Chen (2016), Jing (2017), Li et al. (2014), and Li (2011)
Shandong	8.28 (490/5919)	N	Cui (2009)
Shaanxi	18.59 (111/597)	N	Quan et al. (2016) and Wang (2014)
Shanghai	16.37 (37/226)	N	Dong et al. (2001) and Yang et al. (2010)
Sichuan	10.38 (77/742)	51.01 (76/149)	Feng et al. (2011) and Hu et al. (2011)
Tianjin	15.42 (37/240)	N	Chen and Liu (2017)
Tibet	16.39 (10/61)	N	Gu et al. (2014)
Xinjiang	11.43 (4/35)	N	Su et al. (2013)
Yunan	20.68 (103/498)	N	Jiang et al. (2016)
Zhejiang	0.00 (0/100)	N	Zhou et al. (2014)
Total	17.34 (4246/24,490)	22.04 (186/844)	

N, no information; a, No. positive; A, No. examined

4.1 *T. canis* prevalence in dogs

4246 of 24,490 (17.34%, 95% CI 16.86–17.81) examined dogs were positive with *T. canis* infection, which were distributed in 26 provinces/autonomous regions/municipalities in China with different prevalence, ranging from 0.00% (95% CI 0.00–0.00) in Zhejiang Province to 60.45% (95% CI 55.39–65.50) in Chongqing Municipality (Table 1). However, in some provinces, very low or no *T. canis* infection in dogs were reported, such as Zhejiang Province (0/100), Xinjiang Autonomous region (4/35) and Tibet Autonomous region (10/61).

4.1.1 New understanding of T. canis prevalence in China

In general, *Toxocara* is thought to be mainly popular in tropical and subtropical regions, where the appropriate temperature and humidity can contribute to the development of *Toxocara* eggs (Ma et al., 2018). Fakhri et al. found higher level of *Toxocara* eggs in lower latitudes (0–10° and 11–20°) and lower level of *Toxocara* eggs in higher latitudes (41–50° and 51–60°) (Fakhri et al., 2018). In this review, however, the highest prevalence of *T. canis* infection in dogs was found in northeastern China (118°53′~135°05′E, 38°43′~53°33′N), the coldest area of China, where the prevalence of *T. canis* infection in dogs was as high as 42.81% (824/1925; 95% CI 40.60–45.02). Besides, we found that compared with the northeastern China, the southwestern China and the northwestern China with relatively backward economies, the northern China represented by Beijing Municipality, the southern China represented by Guangdong Province and the eastern China represented by Shanghai Municipality had lower prevalence of *T. canis* infection in dogs, which are the developed areas in China (Table 2 and Fig 1). So, the temperature or humidity did not seem to be the primary reason for increased transmission of *T. canis* in parts of China, but the economic development level was likely the main reason.

4.1.2 Dynamic changes of T. canis prevalence in dogs

In order to explore the dynamic changes of *T. canis* prevalence in dogs in mainland China, the years of 2000–2019 were divided into four statistical time points (Table 2). The fluctuation of *T. canis* prevalence was larger in the four statistical time points in dogs, ranging from 10.94% (95% CI 10.42–11.47) in 2005–2009 to 29.94% (95% CI 28.88–31.00) in 2010–2014. It should be noted that although the prevalence of *T. canis* infection in dogs decreased in 2015–2019 (16.27%, 95% CI 14.95–17.59) compared with 2010–2014 (29.94%, 95% CI 28.88–31.00), it was still at a higher level. Furthermore, compared with 2000–2009 (11.25%, 95% CI 10.73–11.76), the prevalence of *T. canis* infection in dogs increased in 2010–2019 (25.91%, 95% CI 25.06–26.76), which was a decade of rapid development of the pet industry in China (Cen, 2018).

Table 2 Analysis of the variables associated with *Toxocara canis* infection in dogs in mainland China.

Variable	Category	No. examined	No. positive	Prevalence % (95% CI)	*P*-value	OR (95% CI)
Region	Northern China	3521	266	7.55 (6.68–8.43)	Reference	Reference
	Southern China	289	26	9.00 (5.70-12.30)	0.3757	1.21 (0.79–1.84)
	Eastern China	9837	1273	12.94 (12.28–13.60)	<0.0001	1.82 (1.59–2.09)
	Central China	5037	985	19.56 (18.46–20.65)	<0.0001	2.98 (2.59–3.42)
	Northwestern China	1371	284	20.71 (18.57–20.86)	<0.0001	3.20 (2.69–3.81)
	Southwestern China	2510	588	23.43 (21.77–25.08)	<0.0001	3.74 (3.22–4.34)
	Northeastern China	1925	824	42.81 (40.60–45.02)	<0.0001	9.16 (7.96–10.53)
Years	2000–2004	502	98	19.52 (16.06–22.99)	<0.0001	1.97 (1.58–2.47)
	2005–2009	13,815	1512	10.94 (10.42–11.47)	Reference	Reference
	2010–2014	7174	2148	29.94 (28.88–31.00)	<0.0001	3.48 (3.24–3.73)
	2015–2019	2999	488	16.27 (14.95–17.59)	<0.0001	1.58 (1.42–1.77)
	2000–2009	14,317	1610	11.25 (10.73–11.76)	Reference	Reference
	2010–2019	10,173	2636	25.91 (25.06–26.76)	<0.0001	2.76 (2.58–2.95)
Pet dogs	2000–2009	6844	788	11.51 (10.76–12.27)	Reference	Reference
	2010–2019	5435	1105	20.33 (19.26–21.40)	<0.0001	1.96 (1.78–2.16)

Continued

Table 2 Analysis of the variables associated with *Toxocara canis* infection in dogs in mainland China.—cont'd

Variable	Category	No. examined	No. positive	Prevalence % (95% CI)	*P*-value	OR (95% CI)
Breeds	Farm dogs	6931	598	8.63 (7.97–9.29)	Reference	Reference
	Pet dogs	12,279	1893	15.42 (14.78–16.06)	<0.0001	1.93 (1.75–2.12)
	Police dogs	641	118	18.41 (15.41–21.41)	<0.0001	2.39 (1.94–2.95)
	Stray dogs	1042	269	25.82 (23.16–28.47)	<0.0001	3.69 (3.16–4.30)
	N	3597	1405	N		
Age	$0 < yr \leq 1$	4932	790	16.02 (14.99–17.04)	<0.0001	2.60 (2.18–3.09)
	$yr > 1$	2265	155	6.84 (5.80–7.88)	Reference	Reference
	N	17,293	3301	N		
Gender	Male	2912	382	13.12 (11.89–14.34)	Reference	Reference
	Female	2238	342	15.28 (13.79–16.77)	0.0268	1.20 (1.02–1.40)
	N	19,340	3522	N		
Total		24,490	4246	17.34 (16.86–17.81)		

N, no information.

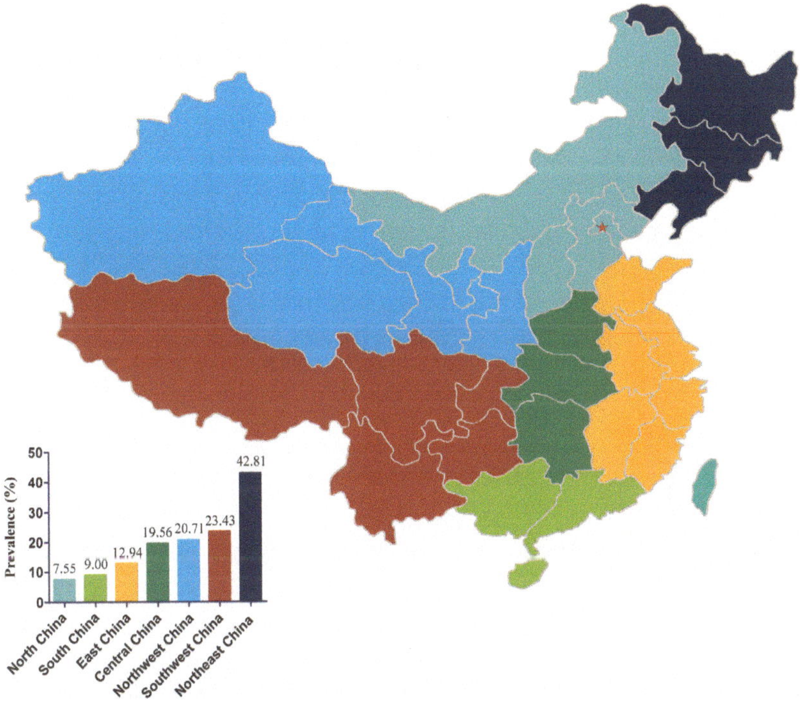

Fig. 1 A map showing the prevalence of *Toxocara canis* infection in seven geographical regions of China. *Northern China:* Beijing Municipality, Tianjin Municipality, Shanxi Province, Hebei Province and Neimenggu Autonomous region; *Southern China:* Guangdong Province, Guangxi Autonomous region and Hainan Province; *Eastern China:* Shanghai Municipality, Jiangsu Province, Zhejiang Province, Anhui Province, Fujian Province, Jiangxi Province and Shandong Province; *Central China:* Henan Province, Hubei Province and Hunan Province; *Northwestern China:* Shaanxi Province, Gansu Province, Qinghai Province, Ningxia Autonomous region and Xinjiang Autonomous region; *Southwestern China:* Sichuan Province, Guizhou Province, Yunnan Province, Chongqing Municipality and Tibet Autonomous region; *Northeastern China:* Heilongjiang Province, Jilin Province and Liaoning Province.

4.1.3 Risk factor analysis of T. canis *prevalence by different breeds of dogs*

In this review, a total of 20,893 (85.31%) dogs were divided into pet dogs, police dogs, farm dogs and stray dogs, according to the information in the eligible papers (Table 2). Stray dogs have the highest *T. canis* prevalence (25.82%, 95% CI 23.16–28.47), which may be the most important resource of *T. canis* transmission in China, following by police dogs (18.41%, 95% CI 15.41–21.41), pet dogs (15.42%, 95% CI 14.78–16.06) and farm dogs (8.63%, 95% CI 7.97–9.29). Compared with farm dogs that were not allowed to roam outside, stray dogs (25.82%) have 3.69 times (OR = 3.69, 95% CI 3.16–4.30) the risk of acquiring *T. canis* infection, police dogs (18.41%) have 2.39 times (OR = 2.39, 95% CI 1.94–2.95) the risk of acquiring *T. canis* infection, and pet dogs (15.42%) have nearly two times (OR = 1.93, 95% CI 1.75–2.12) the risk of acquiring *T. canis* infection, which all have many opportunities to excrete *T. canis* eggs in public places. It was unexpected to find a such high *T. canis* prevalence in police dogs in China.

4.1.4 *Proportion of* T. canis *infection by age and gender in dogs*

The information on ages was only available for 7197 (29.39%) dogs; of which, 4932 were young dogs (under 1 year of age) and 2265 were adult dogs (over 1 year of age) (Table 2). Young dogs (16.02%, 95% CI 14.99–17.04) have 2.60 times (OR = 2.60, 95% CI 2.18–3.09) a risk of acquiring *T. canis* infection, compared with adult dogs (6.84%, 95% CI 5.80–7.88), which is closely related to the life cycle of *T. canis*. Patent infections of *T. canis* often occur in puppies (Dubey, 1978), subsequently, the numbers of eggs excreted gradually decreased with the increase of dog age. That was the reason why *T. canis* eggs are more likely to be detected in young dogs than in adult dogs. Moreover, there was no statistically significant difference in *T. canis* prevalence between male and female dogs ($P > 0.05$, male: 13.12%; female: 15.28%).

4.2 *T. cati* prevalence in cats

The studies on *T. cati* prevalence in cats were less in China than for *T. canis* in dogs. Only 10 papers were eligible with 22.04% (95% CI 19.24–24.83) *T. cati* prevalence in cats, including 844 cats distributed in seven provinces/autonomous regions/municipalities in China (Table 1). Similar to the *T. canis* prevalence in dogs, in this review, the higher prevalence of *T. cati* infection in cats was found in the northeastern China (90.63%, 95% CI 80.53–100.00) and the southwestern China (51.01%, 95% CI 42.98–59.03) that are the areas with relatively backward economies in China. Meanwhile, the lower prevalence was found in the northern China (0.37%, 95% CI 0.00–1.09) and the southern China (5.13%, 95% CI 0.00–12.05) (Table 3 and Fig 2). The prevalence of *T. cati* infection markedly decreased in cats from 26.79% (95% CI 22.40–31.17) in 2000–2009 to 17.92% (95% CI 14.39–21.46) in 2010–2019, which was different from that in dogs. In this review, 346 (41.00%) cats were pet cats, according to the information in the eligible papers, with 30.92% (95% CI 26.06–35.80) *T. cati* prevalence, which was much higher than *T. canis* prevalence in pet dogs (15.42%, 95% CI 14.78–16.06).

Table 3 The prevalence of *Toxocara cati* infection in cats in mainland China.

Variable	Category	No. examined	No. positive	Prevalence % (95% CI)
Region	Northern China	272	1	0.37 (0.00–1.09)
	Southern China	39	2	5.13 (0.00–12.05)
	Central China	299	63	21.07 (16.45–25.69)
	Eastern China	53	15	28.30 (16.17–40.43)
	Southwestern China	149	76	51.01 (42.98–59.03)
	Northeastern China	32	29	90.63 (80.53–100.00)
Years	2000–2009	392	105	26.79 (22.40–31.17)
	2010–2019	452	81	17.92 (14.39–21.46)
Breed	Pet cats	346	107	30.92 (26.06–35.80)
	N	498	79	N
Total		844	186	22.04 (19.24–24.83)

N, no information.

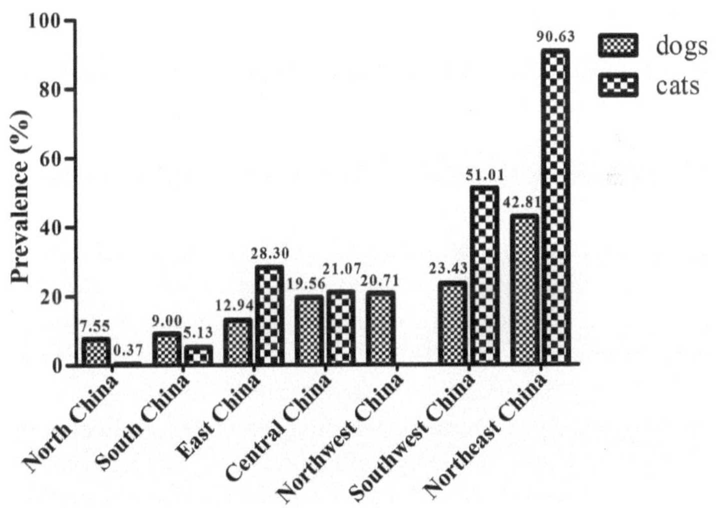

Fig. 2 Comparison of prevalence between *Toxocara canis* in dogs and *Toxocara cati* in cats in seven geographical regions of China.

4.3 *T. cati* infection in felids in zoos

Another three papers were retrieved on *T. cati* infection in felids in zoos in mainland China from 2009 to 2019, including 31 tigers, 13 leopards and 3 lions, which were distributed in 4 zoos (Wang, 2015; Wang et al., 2017;

Table 4 The prevalence of *Toxocara cati* infection in felids in zoos in mainland China.

		Tiger		leopard		Lion		
Years	**Regions**	**No. examined**	**No. positive**	**No. examined**	**No. positive**	**No. examined**	**No. positive**	**References**
2009	Heilongjiang	4	2	13	9	N	N	Zou et al. (2009)
2011–2013	Fujian	7	2	N	N	3	3	Wang (2015)
2015	Heilongjiang	20	5	N	N	N	N	Wang et al. (2017)
Total		31	9	13	9	3	3	

Zou et al., 2009), but there was not a paper about *T. canis* infection in canids in zoos (Table 4). *T. cati* was again detected in tigers in the same zoo in Heilongjiang Province even after 6 years, suggesting that *T. cati* has been a threat to zoo animals (Wang et al., 2017; Zou et al., 2009).

5. Conclusions and future perspectives

In this review, we summarized and analysed the prevalence of *T. canis* infection in dogs and *T. cati* infection in cats in China in the past 20 years, and evaluated the associated risk factors. It was the first systematic review of *Toxocara* prevalence in dogs and cats in mainland China, with 17.34% *T. canis* prevalence in dogs and 22.04% *T. cati* prevalence in cats. We found that the prevalence of *Toxocara* infection in dogs and cats was closely related to different geographical regions, which was related to the economic development levels, suggesting that economic factors seem to be the primary reason for the transmission of *Toxocara* in dogs and cats in China. Because *Toxocara* infections in dogs and cats is asymptomatic or non-pathognomonic for a long time and many veterinarians cannot accurately identify this parasitic disease, thus, misdiagnosis and missed diagnoses often occur. Because human toxocariasis is not a notifiable and not a lethal parasitic disease in China, it is also often neglected by researchers and the general public. Therefore, it is necessary to strengthen the public awareness that prevention of toxocariasis is based on periodic inspection and timely treatment of dogs and cats to stop soil contamination and avoiding direct contact with soil or sand.

The inadequacy of detection methods also restricts the scientific assessment of *Toxocara* prevalence in dogs and cats in China. For example, cats or dogs that carry *Toxocara* larvae without excreting eggs were often determined as negative animals of *Toxocara* infection by faecal examination, causing the prevalence of *Toxocara* infection being underreported or underestimated in animals in China. Therefore, highly sensitive and specific serological diagnostic methods are urgently needed. With the rapidly increasing number of pet dogs and cats, *Toxocara* infection in humans and animals will become more severe in China, if they are continuously neglected.

Acknowledgements

This work was supported by the Planned Programme of Hunan Province Science and Technology Innovation (grant no. 2018RS3085), the Elite Program of Chinese Academy of Agricultural Sciences and the Agricultural Science and Technology Innovation Program (ASTIP) (grant no. CAAS-ASTIP-2016-LVRI-03).

References

Cen, L.H., 2018. Present situation, influencing factors and development trend of pet industry in China. China Anim. Health 20, 4–8. https://doi.org/10.3969/j.issn.1008-4754.2018.08.001. (in Chinese).

Chen, G., Liu, Z.T., 2017. Investigation of intestinal parasites in police dogs in Tianjin municipality. Agric. Jilin 4, 108–109. https://doi.org/10.14025/j.cnki.jlny.2017.04.041. (in Chinese).

Chen, J., Liu, Q., Liu, G.H., Zheng, W.B., Hong, S.J., Sugiyama, H., Zhu, X.Q., Elsheikha, H.M., 2018. Toxocariasis: a silent threat with a progressive public health impact. Infect. Dis. Poverty 7, 59. https://doi.org/10.1186/s40249-018-ica0437-0.

Cong, W., Meng, Q.F., You, H.L., Zhou, N., Dong, X.Y., Dong, W., Wang, X.Y., Qian, A.D., Zhu, X.Q., 2015. Seroprevalence and risk factors of *Toxocara* infection among children in Shandong and Jilin provinces, China. Acta Trop. 152, 215–219. https://doi.org/10.1016/j.actatropica.2015.09.008.

Cong, W., Zhang, X.X., Zhou, N., Yu, C.Z., Chen, J., Wang, X.Y., Li, B., Qian, A.D., Zhu, X.Q., 2014. *Toxocara* seroprevalence among clinically healthy individuals, pregnant women and psychiatric patients and associated risk factors in Shandong Province, Eastern China. PLoS Negl. Trop. Dis. 8, e3082. https://doi.org/10.1371/journal.pntd.0003082.

Cui, Y.J., 2009. Investigation of *Toxocara canis* Infection in Edible Dogs in the Suburbs of Jimo City, China (D). Yanbian University. (in Chinese).

Dai, R.S., Li, Z.Y., Li, F., Liu, D.X., Liu, W., Liu, G.H., He, S.W., Tan, M.Y., Lin, R.Q., Liu, Y., Zhu, X.Q., 2009. Severe infection of adult dogs with helminths in Hunan Province, China poses significant public health concerns. Vet. Parasitol. 160, 348–350. https://doi.org/10.1016/j.vetpar.2008.11.002.

Despommier, D., 2003. Toxocariasis: clinical aspects, epidemiology, medical ecology, and molecular aspects. Clin. Microbiol. Rev. 16, 265–272. https://doi.org/10.1128/CMR.16.2.265-272.2003.

Dong, H.P., Chen, H., Zhang, L.X., Wang, Y.L., Zhu, J.J., Hu, Q.S., 2008. Investigation of the intestinal parasites infection in dogs in Zhengzhou city, China. Chin. J. Vet. Med. 8, 49–50. https://doi.org/10.3969/j.issn.0529-6005.2008.08.024. (in Chinese).

Dong, J., Zhu, L., Chen, Q.B., Jiao, J., Wang, J.J., Zhou, S.J., 2001. Investigation of intestinal nematode infection in dogs in Shanghai, China. Chin. J. Zoonoses 1, 113. https://doi.org/10.3969/j.issn.1002-2694.2001.01.044. (in Chinese).

Dubey, J.P., 1978. Patent *Toxocara canis* infection in ascarid-naive dogs. J. Parasitol. 64, 1021–1023. https://doi.org/10.2307/3279714.
El-Tras, W.F., Holt, H.R., Tayel, A.A., 2011. Risk of *Toxocara canis* eggs in stray and domestic dog hair in Egypt. Vet. Parasitol. 178, 319–323. https://doi.org/10.1016/j.vetpar.2010.12.051.
Fakhri, Y., Gasser, R.B., Rostami, A., Fan, C.K., Ghasemi, S.M., Javanian, M., Bayani, M., Armoon, B., Moradi, B., 2018. *Toxocara* eggs in public places worldwide—a systematic review and meta-analysis. Environ. Pollut. 242, 1467–1475. https://doi.org/10.1016/j.envpol.2018.07.087.
Fan, X.W., 2006. Investigation of parasitic infection in digestive tract of pet dogs. Hum. J. Anim. Sci. Vet. Med. 4, 28–30. https://doi.org/10.3969/j.issn.1006-4907.2006.04.015. (in Chinese).
Fan, P., La, M.C., Gengzang, Z.M., Zhaxi, B.Z., Huang, L., Yang, J.R., Ma, X.Z., Zhang, R.Q., 2017. Investigation of *Toxocara canis* infection in pet dogs in pet market in Xining city, China. Heilongjiang Anim. Hus. Vet. Med. 12, 114–116. https://doi.org/10.13881/j.cnki.hljxmsy.2017.1062. (in Chinese).
Fang, F., Li, J., Huang, T., Guillot, J., Huang, W., 2015. Zoonotic helminths parasites in the digestive tract of feral dogs and cats in Guangxi, China. BMC Vet. Res. 11, 211. https://doi.org/10.1186/s12917-015-0521-7.
Feng, Y., He, Q., Li, J.P., 2011. Investigation of parasites infection in dogs and cats in Tongjiang county, China. Mod. Agric. Sci. Technol. 11, 354–355. https://doi.org/10.3969/j.issn.1007-5739.2011.11.209. (in Chinese).
Gao, D.C., Hao, J.Q., Zhang, P., Han, C.X., 2016. Investigation of parasitic diseases in pet dogs in Shenyang and Tieling cities, Liaoning Province. Heilongjiang Anim. Hus. Vet. Med. 18, 211–212. +300. https://doi.org/10.13881/j.cnki.hljxmsy.2016.1636. (in Chinese).
Glickman, L.T., Schantz, P.M., 1981. Epidemiology and pathogenesis of zoonotic toxocariasis. Epidemiol. Rev. 3, 230–250. https://doi.org/10.1016/0013-9351(81)90172-9.
Gu, Q.Y., Feng, J.W., Cang, M.L., 2014. Investigation of intestinal parasites infection in stray dogs in Lhasa, China. Biotech. World 4, 115. (in Chinese).
He, H.P., Chen, J., 2016. Investigation of parasites infection in Tibetan mastiffs in Tianjun county, Qinghai Province and research of control methods on parasites. Gansu J. Anim. Hus. Vet. Med. 15, 94–95. https://doi.org/10.15979/j.cnki.cn62-1064/s.2016.15.047. (in Chinese).
Hu, L., Qi, M., Peng, G.N., Zhong, Z.J., Dong, H.J., Zhang, L.X., Liu, X.H., 2011. Investigation of intestinal parasites infection in stray dogs in Yaan city. Anim. Hus. Vet. Med. 10, 76–77. (in Chinese).
Huang, J.H., Chen, S.M., 2011. Investigation of parasites infection in digestive tract in dogs in Yongzhou city. Heilongjiang Anim. Hus. Vet. Med. 20, 73–74. https://doi.org/10.13881/j.cnki.hljxmsy.2011.20.024. (in Chinese).
Huang, D.R., Liang, L.Z., Ni, H.Z., 2014a. Investigation of intestinal parasites infection in pet dogs in pet hospital. Anim. Hus. Vet. Med. 2, 121. (in Chinese).
Huang, Z.X., Mi, T.G., Zhang, B.Y., Zhao, X., 2014b. Preliminary investigation on digestive tract worm infection in pet dogs in Handan, China. Heilongjiang Anim. Hus. Vet. Med. 15, 149–151. https://doi.org/10.13881/j.cnki.hljxmsy.2014.0899. (in Chinese).
Huang, J.S., Zhu, X.J., Lu, L.Z., 2017. Investigation and deworming observation of gastrointestinal parasites in dogs. Chin. Livest. Poult. Breed. 6, 16–18. https://doi.org/10.3969/j.issn.1673-4556.2017.06.012. (in Chinese).
Huo, L., Wang, R.D., Tong, Z.X., 2013. Investigation of common intestinal parasites infection in dogs in Zhongmu county, China. Anim. Hus. Vet. Med. 11, 127–128. (in Chinese).
Jiang, H., 2003. Investigation of parasitic infection in dogs in Shi county, Anhui province. Chin. J. Anim. Infect. Dis. 1, 59–60. https://doi.org/10.3969/j.issn.1674-6422.2003.01.023. (in Chinese).

Jiang, C.Y., Sun, S.H., 2001. Parasitic worm in cats from the areas along the Heilong river. Chin. J. Zoonoses 4, 122. https://doi.org/10.3969/j.issn.1002-2694.2001.04.050. (in Chinese).

Jiang, T., Yan, Y.L., Zhang, J.P., Ye, K., Xu, C.X., Wang, G.D., 2016. Investigation of gastrointestinal parasite infection in pet dogs in Qujing in Yunnan Province. Chin. J. Vet. Med. 6, 82–83. (in Chinese).

Jing, F.D., 2017. Investigation of fecal parasite eggs in dogs in Xining city. Chin. Qinghai J. Anim. Vet. Sci. 3, 37–40. https://doi.org/10.3969/j.issn.1003-7950.2017.03.013. (in Chinese).

Kostopoulou, D., Claerebout, E., Arvanitis, D., Ligda, P., Voutzourakis, N., Casaert, S., Sotiraki, S., 2017. Abundance, zoonotic potential and risk factors of intestinal parasitism amongst dog and cat populations: the scenario of Crete, Greece. Parasit. Vectors 10 43 https://doi.org/10.1186/s13071-017-1989-8.

Kuang, C.Y., Jiang, A.G., Li, X.Y., Yang, X.D., Nie, Z.N., Luo, S., Zhou, R.Q., 2018. Survey of epidemiology of alimentary canal parasitosis of dogs in Rongchang district of Chongqing. J. Southwest Univ. (Nat. Sci.) 5, 18–22. https://doi.org/10.13718/j.cnki.xdzk.2018.05.004. (in Chinese).

Li, M., 2010. Epidemiological Investigation on Gastrointestinal Parasites of Dogs in Jinzhou and Treatment Test (D). Jilin University (in Chinese).

Li, C.H., Cai, J.Z., Jia, W.Z., Cairang, Z.X., Lei, M.T., Angba, K.S., Li, J., Tong, Y.J., Renzeng, N.M., Lou, Z.Z., Yan, H.B., Li, C.Y., Xie, Z.Q., Sanmudan, J.C., 2014. Epidemiology investigation of dog parasite in Qinghai pasture. Chin. Qinghai J. Anim. Vet. Sci. 4, 1–4. https://doi.org/10.3969/j.issn.1003-7950.2014.04.001. (in Chinese).

Li, Q.C., Jia, C.L., 2017. Epidemiological investigation and analysis of *Toxoplasma gondii* in Suqian, Jiangsu Province. Graziery Vet. Sci. 10, 9–10. https://doi.org/10.3969/j.issn.2096-3637.2017.10.007. (in Chinese).

Li, X.Z., Yan, R.F., Li, X.R., 2011. Investigation of parasites infection in digestive tract in dogs in Nanjing city. Anim. Hus. Vet. Med. 12, 72–74. (in Chinese).

Liang, X., 2015. Prevalence and Diversity Analysis on ITS and *coxI* of *Toxocara canis* from Dogs in Yiyang (D). Hunan Agricultural University. (in Chinese).

Lin, X.Q., Yu, X.X., 2015. Survey of gastrointestinal parasites in dogs in Fuzhou. Fujian J. Anim. Hus. Vet. Med. 3, 7–10. https://doi.org/10.3969/j.issn.1003-4331.2015.03.004. (in Chinese).

Lin, Z., Zhuang, Y.F., Zhang, W.C., 2015. Investigation of parasites infection in pet dogs. Heilongjiang Anim. Hus. Vet. Med. 12, 135–136. https://doi.org/10.13881/j.cnki.hljxmsy.2015.0907. (in Chinese).

Liu, C., 2012. Investigation of parasites infection and epidemiology in pet dogs. Jilin Anim. Hus. Vet. Med. 6, 27–33. https://doi.org/10.3969/j.issn.1672-2078.2012.06.010. (in Chinese).

Liu, L.K., 2014. Investigation of dominant species of parasites in pet dogs in Pulandian city. Chin. J Anim. Hus. Vet. Med. 12, 20. https://doi.org/10.3969/J.ISSN.1671-6027.2014.12.012. (in Chinese).

Liu, G.W., Cui, Q.Q., Gao, X.T., Meng, B., Guo, L.L., Hao, X.F., Liu, K.Q., Wang, C., Li, J., Tian, X.F., 2011. Investigation of the rate of intestinal parasite infection in dogs and cats in the city of Tangshan. J. Pathogen Biol. 6, 562–563. https://doi.org/10.13350/j.-cjpb.2011.07.004. (in Chinese).

Liu, Q., Wang, Q.G., Yan, S.J., 2009. Investigation of parasites infection in digestive tract in pet dog in Changsha county. Anim. Hus. Feed Sci. 2, 160–162. https://doi.org/10.16003/j.cnki.issn1672-5190.2009.02.047. (in Chinese).

Liu, Z.L., Yang, X.Y., Yang, L.R., Wu, Y.Q.Q.G., Cheng, S.Y., 2005. Investigation of parasites infection in dogs in Hohhot city. Contemp. Anim. Hus. 4, 39–41. (in Chinese).

Liu, X.G., Yu, J.L., Li, B., Xu, P., 2008. Epidemiology of zoonotic parasites in pet dog. Heilongjiang Anim. Hus. Vet. Med. 3, 71–72. https://doi.org/10.13881/j.cnki.hljxmsy.2008.03.034. (in Chinese).

Lu, W.Y., Ha, L., Cao, L.P., 2010. Investigation into intestinal parasites infections in clinic dogs and cats in Lanzhou city. Chin. J. Anim. Infect. Dis. 1, 72–74. https://doi.org/10.3969/j.issn.1674-6422.2010.01.014. (in Chinese).

Ma, G., Holland, C.V., Wang, T., Hofmann, A., Fan, C.K., Maizels, R.M., Hotez, P.J., Gasser, R.B., 2018. Human toxocariasis. Lancet Infect. Dis. 18, e14–e24. https://doi.org/10.1016/S1473-3099(17)30331-6.

Mateus, T.L., Castro, A., Ribeiro, J.N., Vieira-Pinto, M., 2014. Multiple zoonotic parasites identified in dog feces collected in Ponte de Lima, Portugal-a potential threat to human health. Int. J. Environ. Res. Public Health 11, 9050–9067. https://doi.org/10.3390/ijerph110909050.

Mircean, V., Titilincu, A., Vasile, C., 2010. Prevalence of endoparasites in household cat (*Felis catus*) populations from Transylvania (Romania) and association with risk factors. Vet. Parasitol. 171, 163–166. https://doi.org/10.1016/j.vetpar.2010.03.005.

Mohd Zain, S.N., Sahimin, N., Pal, P., Lewis, J.W., 2013. Macroparasite communities in stray cat populations from urban cities in Peninsular Malaysia. Vet. Parasitol. 196, 469–477. https://doi.org/10.1016/j.vetpar.2013.03.030.

Nijsse, R., Ploeger, H.W., Wagenaar, J.A., Mughini-Gras, L., 2016. Prevalence and risk factors for patent *Toxocara* infections in cats and cat owners' attitude towards deworming. Parasitol. Res. 115, 4519–4525. https://doi.org/10.1007/s00436-016-5242-8.

Niu, J.H., Chen, Y.B., Xing, K., Wang, X.T., Wang, H.G., 2011. Investigation of parasites infection in domestic dog in Mudanjiang city. Hubei Anim. Vet. Sci. 5, 31–33. https://doi.org/10.16733/j.cnki.issn1007-273x.2011.05.013. (in Chinese).

Niu, Q.G., Wang, D.J., 2001. Investigation and control of the intestinal parasites infection in dog in Hailar district. Vet Orientation 4, 11–12. (in Chinese).

Pan, W., Jin, L.M., Wu, Q.L., Zhang, Y.H., 2016. Investigation of parasites infection in digestive tract in dogs in Suqian city. Anim. Hus. Vet. Med. 7, 139–140. (in Chinese).

Qi, M., Wang, Q., Sun, Y.R., Dong, H.J., Zhang, J.T., Wang, H.P., Zhang, L.X., Ning, C.S., 2010. Investigation of intestinal parasites in pet dogs and analysis of its public health significance. Anim. Hus. Vet. Med. 4, 81–83. (in Chinese).

Quan, Z.H., Chen, B.J., Zheng, B.F., Ma, X.W., Lv, C.R., Liang, Y.C., 2016. 477 Investigation on the parasite species and infection situation of 477 cases of outpatient dogs. Prog. Vet. Med. 11, 118–122. https://doi.org/10.16437/j.cnki.1007-5038.2016.11.026. (in Chinese).

Sarvi, S., Daryani, A., Sharif, M., Rahimi, M.T., Azami, D., Marhaba, Z., Ahmadpour, E., Mizani, A., 2016. Domestic dog as a human health hazard in north of Iran. J. Parasit. Dis. 40, 930–934. https://doi.org/10.1007/s12639-014-0608-2.

Savilla, T.M., Joy, J.E., May, J.D., Somerville, C.C., 2011. Prevalence of dog intestinal nematode parasites in south central West Virginia, USA. Vet. Parasitol. 178, 115–120. https://doi.org/10.1016/j.vetpar.2010.12.034.

Shan, W.T., Li, B., 2007. The main parasite investigation in the body surface and the intestinal tract of police dog and army dog in the area of Nanjing. China Working Dog 8, 20–21. https://doi.org/10.3969/j.issn.1673-0135.2007.08.010. (in Chinese).

Sheng, X.F., 2014. Epidemiological Investigation of Canine Ascarid and Molecular Biology Identification of Canine (D). Hunan Agricultural University. (in Chinese).

Su, W.Q., Liang, M.M., Wang, X., Yu, S.M., Ou, C.B., Wang, Q.X., 2015. Epidemiological investigation of intestinal parasites in dogs in Xinxiang. J. Henan Inst. Sci. Technol. (Nat. Sci.) 43, 44–47. https://doi.org/10.3969/j.issn.1008-7516.2015.04.009. (in Chinese).

Su, Z.Q., Wang, G.L., Hou, N., Zhang, L., 2013. Application of animal fecal egg diagnostic box in the diagnosis of intestinal parasitic diseases in dogs. Xinjiang Livest Husb. 3, 36–37. https://doi.org/10.16795/j.cnki.xjxmy.2013.03.010. (in Chinese).

Sun, X.H., Liu, D.D., Suding, Z.Y., Cai, W.M., Pan, M.K., Xu, J.J., Tao, J.P., 2018. Investigation on intestinal parasites of stray dogs in Yangzhou city. Anim. Hus. Vet. Med. 2, 131–133. (in Chinese).

Tang, W., 2008. Investigation on domestic dog and cat gastro-intestinal tract parasite etiology of Yongzhou, Hunan Provincev. J. Anhui Agric. Sci. 2008, 9071–9072. https://doi.org/10.13989/j.cnki.0517-6611.2008.21.124. (in Chinese).

Tang, M., Nie, K., Wu, Q.D., Jing, A., Wen, C.L., Sun, T.M., Li, M., Xu, H., Yao, J.P., Huang, W.D., 2003. The survey of parasite faunas on farm animal and poultry in Chongqing city. Chin. J. Anim. Infect. Dis. 2, 35–39. https://doi.org/10.3969/j.issn.1674-6422.2003.02.010. (in Chinese).

Waap, H., Gomes, J., Nunes, T., 2014. Parasite communities in stray cat populations from Lisbon, Portugal. J. Helminthol. 88, 389–395. https://doi.org/10.1017/S0022149X1300031X.

Wang, Y., 2014. Investigation on Species and Infective Status of Enteroparasites of Scattered Dogs in a Town of Huxian (D). Northwest A&F University (in Chinese).

Wang, Y.X., 2015. Investigation of mixed infection of multiple parasites and evaluation of deworming effect in captive carnivores. Chin. J. Tradit Vet. Sci. 10, 21–23. (in Chinese).

Wang, H., Zhu, X., Ji, X.Q., 2009. Preliminary investigation on parasitic infection in digestive tract in outpatients dog. Heilongjiang Anim. Hus. Vet. Med. 22, 73. https://doi.org/10.13881/j.cnki.hljxmsy.2009.22.023. (in Chinese).

Wang, Y., Zou, X.M., Zhang, L.B., Fu, X., Su, X., Gao, Y., Wang, C.R., 2017. Investigation of parasites of the digestine teact infection in ornamental carnivorous animals in four zoos. J. Heilongjiang Bayi Agric. University 1, 42–44. +118. https://doi.org/10.3969/j.issn.1002-2090.2017.01.009. (in Chinese).

Wei, D.X., 2018. Investigation of Intestinal Parasite Infections in Dogs Taizhou and Studies of Efficacy of Drugs against Canine Parasitic Diseases (D). Yangzhou University. (in Chinese).

Xia, D.C., Lai, X., 2001. Investigation of intestinal parasites in dogs in Liangping county. Sichuan Anim. Vet. Sci. 6, 24. https://doi.org/10.3969/j.issn.1001-8964.2001.06.019. (in Chinese).

Xiu, F.X., Kong, Q.B., 2011. Investigation of intestinal parasites infection in police dog base in Shenyang. Anim. Hus. Vet. Med. 3, 81–82. (in Chinese).

Xu, P., Liu, X.G., Li, X., Yu, J.L., Yu, B.L., Li, Y.Z., Chen, Y., 2010. Investigation of parasites infection in pet dogs. Heilongjiang Anim. Hus. Vet. Med. 5, 121–122. https://doi.org/10.13881/j.cnki.hljxmsy.2010.05.036. (in Chinese).

Yang, D.J., Cai, X.N., Chen, Y.J., 2010. Preliminary investigation of the parasites infection in pet dogs in the Shanghai suburb. Shanghai J. Anim. Hus. Vet. Med. 1, 43. https://doi.org/10.3969/j.issn.1000-7725.2010.01.020. (in Chinese).

Yang, Y., Liang, H., 2015. Prevalence and risk factors of intestinal parasites in cats from China. Biomed. Res. Int. 2015 967238 https://doi.org/10.1155/2015/967238.

Yang, D.H., Mian, X.Z., Yan, N., Cheng, Y.N., Wang, N., Gao, N., 2012. Investigation on parasite infection in stray dogs in Guyuan. Ningxia. Sichuan J. Zoology. 2012, 939–941. https://doi.org/10.3969/j.issn.1000-7083.2012.06.021. (in Chinese).

Yang, G.L., Zhang, X.X., Shi, C.W., Yang, W.T., Jiang, Y.L., Wei, Z.T., Wang, C.F., Zhao, Q., 2016. Seroprevalence and associated risk factors of *Toxocara* infection in Korean, Manchu, Mongol, and Han ethnic groups in northern China. Epidemiol. Infect. 144, 3101–3107. https://doi.org/10.1017/S0950268816001631.

Yu, Y.L., Gao, H., Wang, M., 2006. Investigation of gastrointestinal parasites in domestic dogs and cats in Beijing. Chin. J. Vet. Med. 10, 38–39. https://doi.org/10.3969/j.issn.0529-6005.2006.10.020. (in Chinese).

Yu, Z., Ruan, Y., Zhou, M., Chen, S., Zhang, Y., Wang, L., Zhu, G., Yu, Y., 2018. Prevalence of intestinal parasites in companion dogs with diarrhea in Beijing, China, and genetic characteristics of *Giardia* and *Cryptosporidium* species. Parasitol. Res. 117, 35–43. https://doi.org/10.1007/s00436-017-5631-7.

Zang, M., Shen, J.K., Mao, D.Y., Tian, X.F., 2016. Investigation on the intestinal parasite infections in dogs and cats in Tangshan city. J. Trop. Dis. Parasitol. 14, 222–224. https://doi.org/10.3969/j.issn.1672-2302.2016.04.012. (in Chinese).

Zhang, J., Dong, H.P., 2009. Investigation of parasites infection in digestive tract in domestic dogs in Zhengzhou city (C). In: The Fourth Academic Seminar of Association of Small Animal Medicine; the Sixteenth Academic Seminar of Association of Veterinary Surgery. Hohhot, Inner Mongolia, China. (in Chinese).

Zhao, H.Q., Li, C.E., Xie, S.H., Hua, Y.Y., 2001. Investigation of intestinal worm infection in Shapi dogs. Chin. Vet. Sci. 4, 46–47. https://doi.org/10.16656/j.issn.1673-4696.2001.04.037. (in Chinese).

Zhou, J.G., Liu, Z.Z., Cheng, C.Y., 2013. Investigation of parasites infection in dogs in Weining county. Contemp. Anim. Husb. 330, 52–53. (in Chinese).

Zhou, Y., Zhou, L., Chen, C., Chen, T., Han, M.M., Zhang, W., Fan, Z.L., Liu, D.Y., Gu, Y.F., Li, W.C., 2014. Survey on the prevalence of intestinal parasites in pet puppies in Anhui and Zhejiang Province. J. Anhui Sci. Technol. Univ. 1, 15–18. https://doi.org/10.3969/j.issn.1673-8772.2014.01.004. (in Chinese).

Zhuo, G.R., Di, H.S., Liu, J.D., Wang, C.F., 2016. Investigation and treatment of *Toxocara canis* infection in Taizhou. Heilongjiang Anim. Hus. Vet. Med. 2, 134–136. +216. https://doi.org/10.13881/j.cnki.hljxmsy.2016.0143 (in Chinese).

Zou, X.M., Yang, W.H., Zhang, L.B., Wang, C.R., 2009. Investigation of parasitic helminthes in ornamental canrnivorous animals in the northern forfst zoo of Harbin. Chin. J. Anim. Infect. Dis. 3, 73–75. https://doi.org/10.3969/j.issn.1674-6422.2009.03.013. (in Chinese).

Further reading

Li, F.L., 2011. A survey of parasite epidemic zone of Tibetan mastiff in Dariy county, Tibet autonomous region. Chin. Anim. Health Inspection 4, 64. https://doi.org/10.3969/j.issn.1005-944X.2011.04.028 (in Chinese).

Zhou, Z.T., 2014. Investigation of parasites infection in pet dogs in Jinzhou. Chin. Livest. Poult. Breed. 6, 99–100. https://doi.org/10.3969/j.issn.1673-4556.2014.06.075. (in Chinese).

CHAPTER THIRTY-NINE

Prevalence of *Toxocara* in dogs and cats in Africa

Nozyechi Ngulube Chidumayo*
Clinical Studies Department, School of Veterinary Medicine, University of Zambia, Lusaka, Zambia
*Corresponding author: e-mail address: nozyechic@yahoo.com

Contents

Abstract

Dogs and cats have a close association with humans providing companionship; however, pets are reservoirs of zoonotic pathogens such as *Toxocara*. *Toxocara canis* and *Toxocara cati* are small intestinal nematodes found in canids and felids, respectively. Infected pets shed thousands of eggs resulting in environmental contamination. *Toxocara* can infect a wide variety of paratenic hosts including humans, rodents, pigs and chickens. Paratenic hosts become infected by ingestion of the infective eggs containing the third stage larvae or ingestion of dormant larvae in animal tissues. Infected humans may develop visceral larval migrans or ocular toxocariasis. Regular anthelmintic treatment and restricted movement of dogs and cats are recommended to control *Toxocara* environmental contamination. This paper reviews the prevalence and risk factors of *Toxocara* in dogs and cats in Africa; and pet owners' awareness of canine zoonotic helminths.

1. Introduction

Toxocara canis and *T. cati* are cosmopolitan nematodes of canids and felids, respectively (Okulewicz et al., 2012). In Africa, *Toxocara* has been reported in domestic dogs (*Canis familiaris*), wolves (*Canis lupus*), red foxes (*Vulpes vulpes*), wild cats (*Felis silvestris*), Egyptian mongoose (*Herpestes ichneumon*), domestic cats (*Felis catus*), spotted hyenas (*Crocuta crocuta*), African lions (*Panthera leo*) and golden jackals (*Canis aureus*) (Bjork et al., 2000;

Advances in Parasitology, Volume 109
ISSN 0065-308X
https://doi.org/10.1016/bs.apar.2020.01.032

Engh et al., 2003; Lahmar et al., 2014; Lajas et al., 2015; Mukarati et al., 2013; Okoye et al., 2014; Radwan et al., 2009). *Toxocara* is common in Africa and has been reported across different climatic regions including tropical countries such as Nigeria (Okoye et al., 2014; Sowemimo, 2007), Gabon (Davoust et al., 2008) and Ghana (Amissah-Reynolds et al., 2016; Johnson et al., 2015); and arid countries such as Egypt (Ahmed et al., 2014; Awadallah and Salem, 2015; Radwan et al., 2009) and Tunisia (Lahmar et al., 2017).

Toxocara canis and *T. cati* are zoonotic and can infect a wide variety of paratenic hosts such as humans, rodents, pigs, and chickens (Strube et al., 2013). *Toxocara* infections in dogs and cats are usually asymptomatic but some very young animals may develop diarrhoea, vomiting and abdominal distension (Overgaauw and Van Knapen, 2000). Most humans infected with *Toxocara* do not show clinical signs; however, some individuals develop visceral larva migrans and ocular toxocariasis (Despommier, 2003; Overgaauw and Van Knapen, 2000).

Adult *Toxocara* are located in the small intestines of the definitive host and females may produce thousands of eggs per day (Lloyd et al., 1983; Overgaauw and Nederland, 1997), resulting in environmental contamination (Fakhri et al., 2018). Prevalence of *Toxocara* eggs in public places in Africa has been reported at 3.7–75% (Fakhri et al., 2018). Depending on the environmental conditions, the eggs embryonate and become infective over 2–6 weeks or several months (Azam et al., 2012). Definitive and paratenic hosts become infected by ingestion of infective eggs containing the third stage larvae or ingestion of dormant larvae in meat or animal tissues (Okulewicz et al., 2012; Overgaauw and Nederland, 1997). Once ingested the larvae hatch in the small intestines and migrate throughout the body via the blood vessels to localize in the liver, heart, muscles, kidneys and brain (Okulewicz et al., 2012; Overgaauw and Nederland, 1997). Transplacental transmission and rare transmammary transmission also occurs in canines (Burke and Roberson, 1985; Lloyd et al., 1983), and transmammary transmission can occur in cats (Böhm et al., 2015). Regular anthelmintic treatment and restricted movement of dogs and cats are recommended to control *Toxocara* environmental contamination (Overgaauw and Van Knapen, 2000).

2. Prevalence of *Toxocara* in dogs

Dog ownership varies across African communities, ranging from 7.7% to 94% dog-owning households (Chidumayo, 2018b). Reasons for keeping dogs include companionship, hunting, security, and breeding (Johnson et al., 2015; Sowemimo, 2007; Ugbomoiko et al., 2008). Dogs are classified based on ownership and the level of confinement within the owner's property. Based on this classification, dogs belong to one of four categories: owned confined, owned semi-confined, owned free-roaming, and ownerless free-roaming (Amissah-Reynolds et al., 2016; Mekbib et al., 2013; Merga and Sibhat, 2015; Selasie et al., 2013). The majority of dogs in Africa are owned (Chidumayo, 2018b); however, the incidence of owned roaming (semi-confined and free-roaming) dogs varies across communities. Studies investigating the prevalence of canine helminthiasis in Africa have reported the proportion of owned roaming dogs at 61.8% in Ghana (Johnson et al., 2015), and 42.4% in Nigeria (Akeredolu and Sowemimo, 2014). The proportion of owned roaming dogs in Ethiopia has been reported at 75.0% (Selasie et al., 2013) and 71.4% (Mekbib et al., 2013). Despite the low proportion of ownerless dogs, several studies have reported that dogs in Africa do not receive regular anthelmintic treatment. Research by Selasie et al. (2013) in Ethiopia showed that only 2.6% of owners dewormed their dogs. A study investigating the prevalence of canine helminthiasis in Zambia reported that only 5.8% of 292 dogs had been dewormed <3 months before being sampled, while, 3.1% had been dewormed >3–12 months prior to sampling (Bwalya et al., 2011). Another study in Ghana found that 46% of dog owners never dewormed their dogs while 16% and 13% dewormed their dogs once every 3 and 6 months, respectively (Amissah-Reynolds et al., 2016). Ugbomoiko et al. (2008) reported similar trends in Ilorin, Nigeria where 60.6% of dogs had never been dewormed and only 15.7% had a history of deworming 12 months before the study. In addition to the low deworming prevalence, there is generally little awareness of the zoonotic potential of canine helminths. Studies carried out in Ethiopia reported that 0–10% of dog owners were aware of canine zoonotic helminths (Dagmawi et al., 2012; Selasie et al., 2013; Tamerat et al., 2015; Zewdu et al., 2010). A study in Accra, Ghana reported that only 6.3% of dog owners had knowledge of canine parasitic zoonoses (Johnson et al., 2015). Similar results were reported in Nigeria where 38.2% (Akeredolu and Sowemimo, 2014) and 4.0% (Ugbomoiko et al., 2008) of owners were aware of canine zoonotic helminths.

Toxocara canis is the second most common canine helminth in Africa, with *Ancylostoma* species being the most prevalent (Chidumayo, 2018a). The prevalence varies widely with the number of infected dogs reported at 2.2–53.4% in North Africa (Ahmed et al., 2014; Awadallah and Salem, 2015; Lahmar et al., 2017; Radwan et al., 2009), 3.1–40.9% in East Africa (Abere et al., 2013; Awoke et al., 2011; Degefu et al., 2011; Gugsa et al., 2015; Selasie et al., 2013; Zelalem and Mekonnen, 2012), 3.3–95.2% in West Africa (Davoust et al., 2008; Edosomwan and Chinweuba, 2012; Nwoha and Ekwuruike, 2011; Sowemimo and Asaolu, 2008) and 7.5–36.2% in Southern Africa (Alvåsen et al., 2016; Bwalya et al., 2011; Davidson et al., 2017; Minnaar and Krecek, 2001; Mukaratirwa and Singh, 2010). A meta-analysis on canine helminthiasis in sub-Saharan Africa estimated the pooled prevalence and 95% confidence interval (CI) of *Toxocara* at 22% and 16–29%. The pooled regional prevalences for West Africa, East Africa and Southern Africa were estimated at 21% (95% CI: 11–32%), 24% (95% CI: 16–33%) and 12% (95% CI: 3–24%), respectively (Chidumayo, 2018a). The heterogeneity in prevalence has also been observed at country level. For example, the prevalence of *T. canis* in dogs in Ethiopia and Nigeria have been reported at 3.1–40.9% (Abere et al., 2013; Awoke et al., 2011; Degefu et al., 2011; Mekbib et al., 2013; Selasie et al., 2013) and 3.3–95.2% (Edosomwan and Chinweuba, 2012; Ibidapo, 2005; Kutdang et al., 2010; Nwoha and Ekwuruike, 2011), respectively. Table 1 shows the prevalence of *Toxocara* in dogs in Africa.

The majority of studies investigating canine helminthiasis in Africa have found no significant sex-biased *Toxocara* prevalence (Akeredolu and Sowemimo, 2014; Bwalya et al., 2011; Dagmawi et al., 2012; Gugsa et al., 2015; Matthew et al., 2016; Okoye et al., 2011; Udoidung et al., 2018; Zelalem and Mekonnen, 2012). However, a study in Nigeria reported a significant male-biased prevalence with 41% of males and 26.2% of females infected with *T. canis* (Sowemimo, 2007). *Toxocara* is often reported in young animals aged ≤12 months, with this age group having 2.6–11.3 times the odds of infection compared to dogs ≥12 months (Abere et al., 2013; Akeredolu and Sowemimo, 2014; Dagmawi et al., 2012; Degefu et al., 2011; Johnson et al., 2015; Merga and Sibhat, 2015; Sowemimo, 2007; Zelalem and Mekonnen, 2012). The pooled prevalence of *Toxocara* in dogs ≤12 months and >12 months was estimated at 25% (95% CI: 13–39%) and 9% (95% CI: 2–20%), respectively (Chidumayo, 2018a). *Toxocara* infection in young dogs is more common in the ≤6 months age group. Abere et al. (2013) found that in Ethiopia, 54.2% of puppies <6 months, 31.3% of juveniles aged 6–12 months, and 18.5% of adults ≥12 months were infected with *T. canis*. A study in Nigeria by Akeredolu and Sowemimo (2014) found

Table 1 Prevalence of *Toxocara* in dogs in Africa.

Country (study site)	Sample size	Prevalence (%)	Citation
Cameroon (Dschang)	131	34.4	Komtangi et al. (2005)
Egypt (El-Obour city, Fakous city)	130	5.4	Awadallah and Salem (2015)
Egypt (Alexandria)	180	2.2	Ahmed et al. (2014)
Egypt (Giza, Fayoum)	58	53.4	Radwan et al. (2009)
Ethiopia (Bahir Dar)	430	40.9	Abere et al. (2013)
Ethiopia (Gondar)	326	3.1	Awoke et al. (2011)
Ethiopia (Jimma)	334	25.7	Degefu et al. (2011)
Ethiopia (Hawassa)	448	38.8	Selasie et al. (2013)
Ethiopia (Bahir Dar)	384	32.8	Zelalem and Mekonnen (2012)
Ethiopia (Mekelle)	146	23.3	Gugsa et al. (2015)
Ethiopia (Hawassa)	860	23.3	Mekbib et al. (2013)
Ethiopia (Adama)	384	11.7	Merga and Sibhat (2015)
Ethiopia (Hawassa)	455	25.3	Dagmawi et al. (2012)
Ethiopia (Debre Zeit)	120	25.0	Yacob et al. (2007)
Ethiopia (Ambo)	122	17.2	Zewdu et al. (2010)
Gabon (Ogooué-Ivindo)	198	58.6	Davoust et al. (2008)
Ghana (Ashanti)	154	18.8	Amissah-Reynolds et al. (2016)
Ghana (Greater Accra)	380	5.8	Johnson et al. (2015)
Malawi (Lilongwe)	40	7.5	Alvåsen et al. (2016)
Nigeria (Owerri)	554	12.1	Anosike et al. (2004)
Nigeria (Owerri)	284	27.8	Anosike et al. (2006)
Nigeria (Benin)	150	3.3	Edosomwan and Chinweuba (2012)
Nigeria (Lagos)	310	24.5	Ibidapo (2005)
Nigeria (Jos)	1000	38.2	Kutdang et al. (2010)
Nigeria (Zuru)	52	13.5	Magaji et al. (2012)

Continued

Table 1 Prevalence of *Toxocara* in dogs in Africa.—Cont'd

Country (study site)	Sample size	Prevalence (%)	Citation
Nigeria (Sokoto)	40	7.5	Mahmuda et al. (2012)
Nigeria (Makurdi)	400	23.0	Matthew et al. (2016)
Nigeria (Umuahia)	210	95.2	Nwoha and Ekwuruike (2011)
Nigeria (Ibadan)	104	3.8	Odeniran and Ademola (2013)
Nigeria (Obollo-Afor, Ekwulobia)	413	16.5	Okoye et al. (2011)
Nigeria (Sokoto)	272	8.1	Salihu et al. (2013)
Nigeria (Ibadan)	959	9.0	Sowemimo and Asaolu (2008)
Nigeria (Ile-Ife)	269	33.8	Sowemimo (2009)
Nigeria (Ilorin)	396	41.7	Ugbomoiko et al. (2008)
Nigeria (Zaria)	70	5.7	Ugwoke et al. (2011)
Nigeria (Ile-Ife, Ede, Ondo)	474	34.6	Akeredolu and Sowemimo (2014)
Nigeria (Uyo)	250	18.4	Udoidung et al. (2018)
South Africa (Gauteng)	69	36.2	Minnaar and Krecek (2001)
South Africa (Bloemfontein)	63	19.0	Minnaar et al. (2002)
South Africa (Durban)	240	7.9	Mukaratirwa and Singh (2010)
Tanzania (Arusha)	241	13.7	Swai et al. (2010)
Tunisia (Ariana)	271	26.6	Lahmar et al. (2017)
Zambia (Lusaka, Katete)	452	11.3	Bwalya et al. (2011)
Zimbabwe (Harare, Mashonaland East)	246	8.1	Davidson et al. (2017)

that 56.6% of puppies $\leq$6 months, 20.3% of juveniles aged 7–12 months and 15.9% of adults $\geq$13 months were *Toxocara* positive. An age-dependent prevalence was also reported in Ghana, with 25.4% of puppies aged $\leq$6 months, 6.1% of juveniles aged 7–12 months and 0% of adults were

infected (Johnson et al., 2015). However, some studies in Zambia (Bwalya et al., 2011) and Ethiopia (Gugsa et al., 2015; Zewdu et al., 2010) found no significant age-biased prevalence.

Anthelminthic treatment and owner awareness have been reported to have a significant impact on *T. canis* infection. A study in Nigeria found that 28.8% of anthelmintic treated and 39.4% of untreated dogs were infected, while the prevalence in dogs kept by owners with and without knowledge of canine zoonotic parasites was 23.2% and 41.6%, respectively (Akeredolu and Sowemimo, 2014). The study also found that roaming had a significant impact on prevalence with 20.6% of confined and 42.4% of roaming dogs infected. A higher prevalence of *Toxocara* was also found in roaming dogs in Ethiopia (Mekbib et al., 2013; Merga and Sibhat, 2015; Selasie et al., 2013).

3. Prevalence of *Toxocara* in domestic cats

Domestic cats in Africa are kept as pets or to control pests such as rats or snakes (Ogendi et al., 2013). There are limited studies on feline helminthiasis and cat keeping practices; however, there seems to be low deworming prevalence and poor owner awareness of feline zoonotic helminths. A study in Nigeria reported that only 3% of owners dewormed their cats at least once a year and only 17.5% of pet owners were aware of the zoonotic potential of feline helminths (Sowemimo, 2012). *Toxocara cati* is not usually the most prevalent helminth reported in cats in Africa. The helminth was the second most prevalent in cats in Nigeria, Egypt and Kenya (Khalafalla, 2011; Nyambura Njuguna et al., 2017; Sowemimo, 2012). The prevalence of *T. cati* has been reported at 32.5% in Ethiopia (Tamerat et al., 2015), 23.3% in Kenya (Nyambura Njuguna et al., 2017), 48.5% (Sowemimo, 2012) and 47.1% (Okoye et al., 2014) in Nigeria. Research on helminthiasis in ownerless free-roaming cats in Nigeria found 55.9% (Okoye et al., 2014) and 16.7% (Raji et al., 2013) of cats infected, while a study in Egypt reported a prevalence of 9% (Khalafalla, 2011). An age-bias prevalence was reported in Nigeria with cats aged 0–6 months having higher odds of infection; however, no sex-biased prevalence was found (Sowemimo, 2012).

4. Conclusion

Nematodes of the genus *Toxocara* are common zoonotic intestinal helminths of dogs and cats in Africa. These parasites are widely distributed across the continent and have been reported in both domesticated and wild canids and felids. Despite the public significance of these helminths, there is limited public awareness of their zoonotic potential. Regular anthelmintic treatment and restricted movement of dogs and cats are recommended to control *Toxocara* environmental contamination. However, there is poor control of gastrointestinal helminths in pets in Africa which increases the risk of environmental contamination and human exposure.

References

Abere, T., Bogale, B., Melaku, A., 2013. Gastrointestinal helminth parasites of pet and stray dogs as a potential risk for human health in Bahir Dar town, north-western Ethiopia. Vet. World 6, 388–392.

Ahmed, W., Mousa, W., Aboelhadid, S., Tawfik, M., 2014. Prevalence of zoonotic and other gastrointestinal parasites in police and house dogs in Alexandria, Egypt. Vet. world 7, 275–280.

Akeredolu, A., Sowemimo, O., 2014. Prevalence, intensity and associated risk factors for *Toxocara canis* infection in Nigerian dogs. J. Parasitol. Vector Biol. 6, 111–116.

Alvåsen, K., Johansson, S.M., Höglund, J., Ssuna, R., Emanuelson, U., 2016. A field survey on parasites and antibodies against selected pathogens in owned dogs in Lilongwe, Malawi. J. S. Afr. Vet. Assoc. 87, 1–6.

Amissah-Reynolds, P.K., Monney, I., Adowah, L.M., Agyemang, S.O., 2016. Prevalence of helminths in dogs and owners' awareness of zoonotic diseases in Mampong, Ashanti, Ghana. J. Parasitol. Res. 2016, 1715924. https://doi.org/10.1155/2016/1715924.

Anosike, J., Nwoke, B., Ukaga, C., Madu, N., Dozie, I., 2004. Aspects of intestinal helminth parasites of dogs in World Bank-assisted housing estate, New Owerri, Nigeria. Afr. J. Appl. Zool. Environ. Biol. 6, 26–30.

Anosike, J., Ebiziem, N., Ajero, C., Asor, J., Adeiyongo, C., Bolaji, O., Uduji, O., 2006. Prevalence and public health significance of helminth ova in deposited dog feces in Owerri, Nigeria. Anim. Prod. Res. Adv. 2, 34–38.

Awadallah, M.A., Salem, L.M., 2015. Zoonotic enteric parasites transmitted from dogs in Egypt with special concern to *Toxocara canis* infection. Vet. World 8, 946–957.

Awoke, E., Bogale, B., Chanie, M., 2011. Intestinal nematode parasites of dogs: prevalence and associated risk factors. Int. J. Anim. Vet. Adv. 3, 374–378.

Azam, D., Ukpai, O.M., Said, A., Abd-Allah, G.A., Morgan, E.R., 2012. Temperature and the development and survival of infective *Toxocara canis* larvae. Parasitol. Res. 110, 649–656.

Bjork, K.E., Averbeck, G.A., Stromberg, B.E., 2000. Parasites and parasite stages of free-ranging wild lions (Panthera leo) of northern Tanzania. J. Zoo Wildl. Med. 31, 56–61.

Böhm, C., Petry, G., Schaper, R., Wolken, S., Strube, C., 2015. Prevention of lactogenic *Toxocara cati* infections in kittens by application of an emodepside/praziquantel spot-on (Profender®) to the pregnant queen. Parasitol. Res. 114, 175–184.

Burke, T.M., Roberson, E.L., 1985. Prenatal and lactational transmission of *Toxocara canis* and *Ancylostoma caninum*: experimental infection of the bitch before pregnancy. Int. J. Parasitol. 15, 71–75.

Bwalya, E.C., Nalubamba, K.S., Hankanga, C., Namangala, B., 2011. Prevalence of canine gastrointestinal helminths in urban Lusaka and rural Katete Districts of Zambia. Prev. Vet. Med. 100, 252–255.

Chidumayo, N.N., 2018a. Epidemiology of canine gastrointestinal helminths in sub-Saharan Africa. Parasit. Vectors 11, 100. https://doi.org/10.1186/s13071-018-2688-9.

Chidumayo, N.N., 2018b. System dynamics modelling approach to explore the effect of dog demography on rabies vaccination coverage in Africa. PLoS One 13, e0205884. https://doi.org/10.1371/journal.pone.0205884.

Dagmawi, P., Mekonnen, A., Abebe, F., Berhanu, M., 2012. Prevalence of gastrointestinal helminthes among dogs and owners perception about zoonotic dog parasites in Hawassa Town, Ethiopia. Am. J. Public Health Epidemiol. 4, 205–209.

Davidson, A.K., Bhikha, K., Vassilev, G.D., Dhliwayo, S., 2017. Prevalence of intestinal helminth parasites in stray dogs in urban Harare and selected rural areas in Zimbabwe. Zimb. Vet. J. 35, 1–7.

Davoust, B., Normand, T., Bourry, O., Dang, H., Leroy, E., Bourdoiseau, G., 2008. Epidemiological survey on gastro-intestinal and blood-borne helminths of dogs in north-east Gabon. Onderstepoort J. Vet. Res. 75, 359–364.

Degefu, H., Tefera, A., Yohannes, M., 2011. Zoonotic helminth parasites in faecal samples of household dogs in Jimma Town, Ethiopia. Am. J. Public Health Epidemiol. 3, 138–143.

Despommier, D., 2003. Toxocariasis: clinical aspects, epidemiology, medical ecology, and molecular aspects. Clin. Microbiol. Rev. 16, 265–272.

Edosomwan, E., Chinweuba, C., 2012. A survey on helminth parasites of dogs in Benin city, Edo State, Nigeria. J. Vet. Med. Anim. Health 4, 56–60.

Engh, A.L., Nelson, K.G., Peebles, R., Hernandez, A.D., Hubbard, K.K., Holekamp, K.E., 2003. Coprologic survey of parasites of spotted hyenas (Crocuta crocuta) in the Masai Mara National Reserve, Kenya. J. Wildl. Dis. 39, 224–227.

Fakhri, Y., Gasser, R., Rostami, A., Fan, C., Ghasemi, S., Javanian, M., Bayani, M., Armoon, B., Moradi, B., 2018. *Toxocara* eggs in public places worldwide-a systematic review and meta-analysis. Environ. Pollut. 242, 1467–1475.

Gugsa, G., Hailu, T., Kalayou, S., Abebe, N., Hagos, Y., 2015. Study on gastro-intestinal helminth parasites of dogs in Mekelle City Tigray Ethiopia. J. Parasitol. Vector Biol. 7, 29–36.

Ibidapo, C.A., 2005. Prevalence of intestinal helminth parasites of dogs in Lagos, Nigeria. Pak. J. Sci. Ind. Res. 48, 279–283.

Johnson, S.A., Gakuya, D.W., Mbuthia, P.G., Mande, J.D., Maingi, N., 2015. Prevalence of gastrointestinal helminths and management practices for dogs in the Greater Accra region of Ghana. Heliyon 1, e00023. https://doi.org/10.1016/j.heliyon.2015.e00023.

Khalafalla, R.E., 2011. A survey study on gastrointestinal parasites of stray cats in northern region of Nile delta, Egypt. PLoS One 6, e20283. https://doi.org/10.1371/journal.pone.0020283.

Komtangi, M.C., Mpoame, M., Payne, V., Ngufor, M., 2005. Prevalence of gastrointestinal helminths of dogs in Dschang, Cameroon. J. Cameroon Acad. Sci. 5, 11–14.

Kutdang, E., Bukbuk, D., Ajayi, J., 2010. The prevalence of intestinal helminths of dogs (Canis familiaris) in Jos, Plateau State, Nigeria. Researcher 2, 51–56.

Lahmar, S., Boufana, B., Boubaker, S.B., Landolsi, F., 2014. Intestinal helminths of golden jackals and red foxes from Tunisia. Vet. Parasitol. 204, 297–303.

Lahmar, S., Arfa, I., Othmen, S.B., Jguirim, W., Saïd, Y., Dhibi, A., Boufana, B., 2017. Intestinal helminths of stray dogs from Tunisia with special reference to zoonotic infections. Parasitol. Open 3, 1–9.

Lajas, L., Alho, A., Gomes, L., Begg, C., Begg, K., Waiti, E., Otranto, D., Almeida, V., Madeira De Carvalho, L., 2015. Gastrointestinal and respiratory parasites survey in wild African lions (Panthera leo) from Niassa national reserve, Mozambique–preliminary results. In: Proceedings of the International Conference on Diseases of Zoo and Wild Animals, pp. 151–154.

Lloyd, S., Amerasinghe, P., Soulsby, E., 1983. Periparturient immunosuppression in the bitch and its influence on infection with *Toxocara canis*. J. Small Anim. Pract. 24, 237–247.

Magaji, A.A., Mohammed, M.N., Saulawa, M.A., Salihu, M.D., 2012. Survey of zoonotic gastrointestinal parasites of dogs (Canis familiaris) slaughtered at Zuru area, Kebbi state, Nigeria. Sci. J. Vet. Adv. 1, 132–136.

Mahmuda, A., Magaji, A.A., Yakubu, Y., Salihu, M.D., Lawal, M.D., Mahmud, U., Suleiman, N., Danmaigoro, A., 2012. Prevalence of intestinal parasites of dogs slaughtered at Mami market area, Sokoto, Nigeria. Sci. J. Anim. Sci. 1, 126–130.

Matthew, T.T., Seer, I.J., David, O.K., 2016. The prevalence of gastrointestinal helminths (GIH) infection of dogs in Makurdi Metropolis. Imp. J. Interdiscip. Res. 2, 1042–1048.

Mekbib, B., Regassa, A., Sheferaw, D., 2013. Gastrointestinal helminthes of dogs and owners' perception of dogs parasitic zoonoses in Hawassa, Southern Ethiopia. J. Vet. Med. Anim. Health 5, 20–26.

Merga, T., Sibhat, B., 2015. Prevalence of gastrointestinal helminth parasites of dogs and associated risk factors in Adama town, Central Ethiopia. Ethiop. Vet. J. 19, 91–103.

Minnaar, W.N., Krecek, R.C., 2001. Helminths in dogs belonging to people in a resource-limited urban community in Gauteng, South Africa. Onderstepoort J. Vet. Res. 68, 111–117.

Minnaar, W.N., Krecek, R.C., Fourie, L.J., 2002. Helminths in dogs from a peri-urban resource-limited community in Free State Province, South Africa. Vet. Parasitol. 107, 343–349.

Mukarati, N.L., Vassilev, G.D., Tagwireyi, W.M., Tavengwa, M., 2013. Occurrence, prevalence and intensity of internal parasite infections of African lions (Panthera leo) in enclosures at a recreation park in Zimbabwe. J. Zoo Wildl. Med. 44, 686–693.

Mukaratirwa, S., Singh, V.P., 2010. Prevalence of gastrointestinal parasites of stray dogs impounded by the Society for the Prevention of Cruelty to Animals (SPCA), Durban and Coast, South Africa. J. S. Afr. Vet. Assoc. 81, 123–125.

Nwoha, R., Ekwuruike, J., 2011. Prevalence of gastrointestinal parasites in dogs from Umuahia City of Abia State. Glob. J. Med. Sci. 9, 34–42.

Nyambura Njuguna, A., Kagira, J.M., Muturi Karanja, S., Ngotho, M., Mutharia, L., Wangari Maina, N., 2017. Prevalence of *Toxoplasma gondii* and other gastrointestinal parasites in domestic cats from households in Thika region, Kenya. Biomed. Res. Int. 2017, 7615810. https://doi.org/10.1155/2017/7615810.

Odeniran, P.O., Ademola, I.O., 2013. Prevalence of zoonotic gastrointestinal helminth in dogs and knowledge of risk of infection by dog owners in Ibadan, Nigeria. Niger. Vet. J. 34, 851–858.

Ogendi, E., Maina, N., Kagira, J., Ngotho, M., Mbugua, G., Karanja, S., 2013. Questionnaire survey on the occurrence of risk factors for *Toxoplasma gondii* infection amongst farmers in Thika District, Kenya. J. S. Afr. Vet. Assoc. 84, E1–E6. https://doi.org/10.4102/jsava.v84i1.191.

Okoye, I.C., Obiezue, N.R., Okorie, C.E., Ofoezie, I.E., 2011. Epidemiology of intestinal helminth parasites in stray dogs from markets in south-eastern Nigeria. J. Helminthol. 85, 415–420.

Okoye, I.C., Obiezue, N.R., Okoh, F.N., Amadi, E.C., 2014. Descriptive epidemiology and seasonality of intestinal parasites of cats in Southeast Nigeria. Comp. Clin. Pathol. 23, 999–1005.

Okulewicz, A., Perec-Matysiak, A., Buńkowska, K., Hildebrand, J., 2012. *Toxocara canis*, *Toxocara cati* and *Toxascaris leonina* in wild and domestic carnivores. Helminthologia 49, 3–10.

Overgaauw, P.A., Nederland, V., 1997. Aspects of Toxocara epidemiology: toxocarosis in dogs and cats. Crit. Rev. Microbiol. 23, 233–251.

Overgaauw, P.A., Van Knapen, F., 2000. Dogs and nematode zoonoses. In: MacPherson, C.N.L., Meslin, F.X., Wandeler, A.I. (Eds.), Dogs, Zoonoses and Public Health. CABI Publishing, Oxon, NY, pp. 213–256.

Radwan, N.A., Khalil, A.I., Mahi, R.a.E., 2009. Morphology and occurrence of species of Toxocara in wild mammal populations from Egypt. Comp. Parasitol. 76, 273–282.

Raji, A., Magaji, A., Bello, M., Lawal, M., Mamuda, A., Yahaya, M., 2013. Prevalence of gastrointestinal parasites of stray cats: a case study of two hospitals in Sokoto Metropolis, Sokoto, Nigeria. J. Bacteriol. Parasitol. 4, 175. https://doi.org/10.4172/2155-9597.1000175.

Salihu, M.D., Usman, J.A., Alhaji, M.A., Arikpo, H.A., 2013. Zoonotic gastrointestinal helminthes of household dogs in Sokoto, Nigeria. Int. J. Agro Vet. Med. Sci. 7, 50–56.

Selasie, D.G., Mesula, G., Efriem, D., Kassahun, A., Solomon, M., 2013. Gastrointestinal helminthes in dogs and community perception on parasite zoonosis at Hawassa city, Ethiopia. Glob. Vet. 11, 432–440.

Sowemimo, O.A., 2007. Prevalence and intensity of *Toxocara canis* (Werner, 1782) in dogs and its potential public health significance in Ile-Ife, Nigeria. J. Helminthol. 81, 433–438.

Sowemimo, O.A., 2009. The prevalence and intensity of gastrointestinal parasites of dogs in Ile-Ife, Nigeria. J. Helminthol. 83, 27–31.

Sowemimo, O.A., 2012. Prevalence and intensity of gastrointestinal parasites of domestic cats in Ode Irele and Oyo communities, Southwest Nigeria. J. Parasitol. Vector Biol. 4, 7–13.

Sowemimo, O.A., Asaolu, S.O., 2008. Epidemiology of intestinal helminth parasites of dogs in Ibadan, Nigeria. J. Helminthol. 82, 89–93.

Strube, C., Heuer, L., Janecek, E., 2013. *Toxocara* spp. infections in paratenic hosts. Vet. Parasitol. 193, 375–389.

Swai, E.S., Kaaya, E.J., Mshanga, D.A., Mbise, E.W., 2010. A survey on gastro-intestinal parasites of non-descript dogs in and around Arusha municipality, Tanzania. Int. J. Anim. Vet. Adv. 2, 63–67.

Tamerat, N., Abera, D., Teha, R., Terefe, Y., Lemma, F., 2015. Cat and dog gastrointestinal helminth and assessment of community perception on helminthic zoonosis in Haramaya town, eastern Ethiopia. Am. Eurasian J. Sci. Res. 10, 299–306.

Udoidung, N., Adams, E., Ekpo, E., Opara, K., 2018. A survey on intestinal nematodes of dogs in Uyo, Akwa Ibom State, Nigeria. J. Parasitol. Vector Biol. 10, 39–44.

Ugbomoiko, U.S., Ariza, L., Heukelbach, J., 2008. Parasites of importance for human health in Nigerian dogs: high prevalence and limited knowledge of pet owners. BMC Vet. Res. 4, 49. https://doi.org/10.1186/1746-6148-4-49.

Ugwoke, E.V., Audu, P.A., Umoh, J.U., Adakole, J.A., 2011. Prevalence of intestinal helminthes of dogs that have been disposed off at non-descript abattoirs in Zaria, Nigeria. Bayero J. Pure Appl. Sci. 4, 44–47.

Yacob, H.T., Ayele, T., Fikru, R., Basu, A.K., 2007. Gastrointestinal nematodes in dogs from Debre Zeit, Ethiopia. Vet. Parasitol. 148, 144–148.

Zelalem, G., Mekonnen, A., 2012. Prevalence of gastrointestinal helminthes among dogs in Bahir Dar Town, Ethiopia. World Appl. Sci. J. 19, 595–601.

Zewdu, E., Semahegn, Y., Mekibib, B., 2010. Prevalence of helminth parasites of dogs and owners awareness about zoonotic parasites in Ambo town, central Ethiopia. Ethiop. Vet. J. 14, 17–30.

CHAPTER FORTY

Toxocara canis in Australia

David J. Jenkins*
School of Animal and Veterinary Sciences, Charles Sturt University, Wagga Wagga, NSW, Australia
*Corresponding author: e-mail address: djjenkins@csu.edu.au

Contents

Abstract

This review covers reports on prevalence Toxocara in dogs from 2000 to the present and views of the veterinary community as to the importance of it as a zoonosis within Australia. The contamination of soils in public areas with eggs of this parasite seems overall to be minimal for reasons related to required collection of faeces from pets and the use of routine deworming and combination dewormers associated with heart-worm prevention. The potential of other canid hosts being sources of eggs is likely common, especially with the increasing red fox and wild dog populations in more urbanized environs. Human associated disease, e.g., visceral and ocular larva migrans, is reported very rarely in Australia.

Toxocara canis occurs widely in domestic dogs and cats, and also occurs in wildlife (foxes, *Vulpes vulpes*, and dingoes, *Canis lupus dingo*). The locations of recent reports on the occurrence of *T. canis* in Australian dogs and cats are not contiguous, commonly localized in regions around universities housing parasitologists with an interest in canine helminths. To maintain relevance, only data in literature published after 2000 have been reported. For data prior to 2000: re *T. canis* eggs in soil, see Dunsmore et al. (1984) and Bugg et al. (1999); re domestic dogs, see Dunsmore and Shaw (1990) and also Hayward (2004); re wild dogs, see Reichel et al. (1994) and Spratt and Beveridge (2018); re feral cats, see Henderson (2009) and Spratt and Beveridge (2018); re foxes, see Spratt and Beveridge (2018); re Aboriginal community dogs, see Jenkins et al. (1993).

Palmer et al. (2010) also surveyed the opinions of Australian veterinarians regarding the importance of *T. canis* as a veterinary problem in Australian dogs and cats. Most Australian veterinarians did not regard *Toxocara* spp.

Advances in Parasitology, Volume 109
ISSN 0065-308X
https://doi.org/10.1016/bs.apar.2020.01.033

as parasites of particular importance for dogs (89%) or cats (91%). In respect of the zoonotic importance of *T. canis*, only about a quarter (23%) of the veterinarians surveyed were concerned about the zoonotic potential of *T. canis* in pet dogs and fewer (13%) about the zoonotic potential of *T. cati* infection in cats. Awareness of *T. canis* as a zoonosis in Australia has been found to be high amongst dog owners (71.3%) and cat owners (70.7%) (Palmer et al., 2010).

The contamination of public recreation areas with dog faeces containing eggs of *T. canis*, particularly urban parks where dog owners also exercise their pets, is a low potential public health risk. Carden et al. (2003) examined urban recreation areas for the eggs of *T. canis*. One hundred and eighty soil samples were collected from nine suburban locations in Melbourne, Victoria, where domestic dogs are regularly exercised. *Toxocara canis* eggs were recovered from one soil sample only. A faecal flotation study by Gillespie and Bradbury (2017) was conducted on dog faecal samples collected in popular public recreation areas in Central Queensland. Three hundred faecal samples were examined and four (1%) were found infected (Fig. 1).

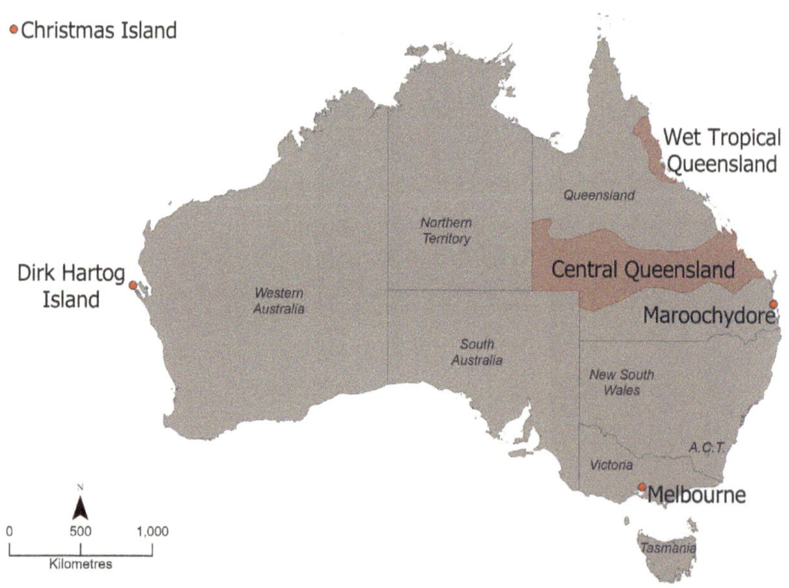

Fig. 1 Map of Australia showing the locations and areas from which *Toxocara canis*, *T. cati* and *Toxascaris leonina*, referred to in the narrative, were found.

The low level of environmental contamination with eggs of *T. canis* reported by Carden et al. (2003) and the low prevalence of faecal samples containing eggs of *T. canis* reported by Gillespie and Bradbury (2017) is a likely reflection of several factors. An increased level of public awareness regarding the importance of *T. canis* (Palmer et al., 2010), the ready availability (in supermarkets) of highly efficient and inexpensive "all-wormers" for dogs and local by-laws in many jurisdictions throughout Australia requiring dog owners to remove faeces deposited by their dogs in public places into the general garbage or containers provided in parks especially for the purpose. In addition, *Dirofilaria immitis* (canine heartworm) is a problem in many parts of Australia and the regular application of heartworm prophylaxis is likely to also influence the presence of intestinal helminths in domestic dogs.

Cases of ocular toxocariasis in humans occur each year in Australia, but they are rare. In Victoria between 1990 and 1997 the incidence of ocular toxocariasis was found to be approximately three cases per year. Based on the population of Victoria in June 2000 (4,765,000 people) the annual incidence of ocular toxocariasis was one case in 1.6 million per head of population per year (Carden et al., 2003).

The most recent study of intestinal helminths in Australian urban domestic dogs (owned pets and refuge dogs) was undertaken by Palmer et al. (2008). In this study 1400 dog and 1063 cat faecal samples were examined. The samples were collected from a wide range of geographical locations around Australia. The prevalence of *T. canis* in refuge dogs was 2.4% (range: 1.2–3.6%); and in owned pets attending veterinary clinics the prevalence was much lower at 0.4% (range: 0–0.8%). The prevalence of *T. canis* in refuge cats was found to be higher than in refuge dogs, at 4.9% (range: 3.0–6.8%) and in owned cats presenting at veterinary clinics the prevalence was lower at 1.7% (range: 0.6–2.8%).

The study of Palmer et al. (2008) also determined the prevalence of *Toxascaris leonina*. In refuge dogs no infections were found, but in owned dogs, presented to veterinary clinics, 0.2% (range: 0–0.5%) were infected. The prevalence of *Toxascaris leonina* in refuge cats was 0.2% (0–0.6%) and in owned cats visiting veterinary clinic cats the prevalence was higher, at 1.75% (range: 0.6–2.8%).

Australian rural dogs (working dogs, hunting dogs, and pet dogs) and cats often receive less veterinary care than their urban counterparts. In a study of intestinal helminths in rural dogs by Jenkins et al. (2014) faecal samples were collected from 1425 rural dogs (farm dogs, hunting dogs, dogs living in small rural centres and dogs from dog refuges in small rural towns) from the eastern side of Australia (1119 from mainland Australia and 306 from Tasmania). Thirty of the dogs were found infected with ascarids. The prevalence of *T. canis* in the rural dogs was 3.1% and slightly lower at 2.8% in the dogs in rural shelters. Of the dogs infected with roundworms, 73.3% (22) were infected with *T. canis* and 26.6% (8) infected with *Toxascaris leonina*.

The top-order predator in Australia is a placental canid, the dingo. In many areas, dingoes have hybridized with domestic dogs (Claridge et al., 2014) and in many local populations, the wild dogs are almost totally dingo/domestic dog hybrids. Also present in Australia are European red foxes (*Vulpes vulpes*) introduced in the late 1700s by European settlers. Parasite-infected wild dogs are currently encroaching into many urban centres in eastern Australia (Jenkins et al., 2008) and foxes have also moved into most urban environments, similarly to the situation seen in Europe. Dingoes, dingo hybrids and foxes are susceptible to infection with *T. canis*. In a study into the prevalence of *Echinococcus granulosus* in urban wild dogs in the Maroochy Shire, eastern Queensland (Jenkins et al., 2008) the presence of other intestinal parasites was also noted. *Toxocara canis* was not recovered from any of 108 wild dog intestines examined but *T. canis* was recovered from 5/7 fox intestines. In a study of intestinal parasites by Smout et al. (2013) the intestines of 26 wild dogs from the wet tropics of north-eastern Queensland were examined. Twelve (46%) of the intestines examined contained *T. canis*. Harriot (2018) examined the intestines of 201 periurban wild dogs collected in south-eastern Queensland and *T. canis* was recovered from 11 (5.4%) of these wild dogs.

Almost all the recent research on the intestinal parasites of feral cats has been undertaken in Western Australia. A study by Adams et al. (2008) investigated intestinal parasites in cats on Christmas Island, their investigation of 28 feral cats found 15 (54%) infected with *T. cati*. A more recent study of feral cats from several locations in south-western Western Australia and on two Islands (Christmas Island and Dirk Hertzog Island) (Dybing, 2017), recovered ascarids from feral cats in all locations. *Toxocara cati* was present in 56% (37 of 56) of feral cats on Christmas Island, 17.4% (4 of 23) on Dirk Hartog Island and 21.3% (23 of 108) in south-western Western Australia. Also present in 4 (3.7%) of the 108 cats from south-western Western Australia was *Toxascaris leonina*.

Domestic dogs residing in and around Aboriginal Communities in the remote parts of Australia often share the environment with wild dingoes. Smout et al. (2018) undertook a study of canine zoonotic intestinal helminths in dogs inhabiting an Aboriginal community in wet tropical north-eastern Queensland and the dingoes living in the surrounding area. *Toxocara canis* infection was detected either at necropsy or by faecal flotation. Fourteen of 39 dingoes (41%) and 25 of 85 dogs (29%) were found to be infected with *T. canis*.

References

Adams, P.J., Elliot, A.D., Algar, D., Brazell, R.I., 2008. Gastrointestinal parasites of feral cats from Christmas Island. Aust. Vet. J. 86, 60–63.

Bugg, R.J., Robertson, I.D., Elliot, A.D., Thompson, R.C.A., 1999. Gastrointestinal parasites of urban dogs in Perth, Western Australia. Vet. J. 157, 295–301.

Carden, S.M., Meusemann, R., Walker, J., Stawell, R.J., MacKinnon, J.R., Smith, D., Stawell, A.M., Hall, A.J.H., 2003. *Toxocara canis*: egg presence in Melbourne parks and disease incidence in Victoria. Clin. Exp. Opthalmol. 31, 143–146.

Claridge, A.W., Spencer, R.J., Wilton, A.N., Jenkins, D.J., Dall, D., Lapidge, S.J., 2014. When is a dingo not a dingo? Hydridisation with domestic dogs. In: Glenn, A.S., Dickman, C.R. (Eds.), Carnivores of Australia. Past Present and Future. CSIRO Publishing.

Dunsmore, J.D., Shaw, S.E., 1990. Clinical Parasitology of Dogs. Veterinary Review No. 31, Published by the University of Sydney Post Graduate Foundation in Veterinary Science.

Dunsmore, J.D., Thompson, R.C.A., Bates, I.A., 1984. Prevalence and survival of *Toxocara canis* eggs in the urban environment of Perth, Australia. Vet. Parasitol. 16, 303–311.

Dybing, N., 2017. Invasive Animals and the Island Syndrome: Parasites of Feral Cats and Black Rats From Western Australia and Its Off-Shore Islands. Thesis for the Degree of Doctor of Philosophy, Murdoch University, Perth, Western Australia.

Gillespie, S., Bradbury, R.S., 2017. A survey of intestinal parasites of domestic dogs in Central Queensland. Trop. Med. Infect. Dis. 2, 60–70.

Harriot, L.C., 2018. Prevalence, Risk Factors and Geographical Distribution of Zoonotic Pathogens Carried by Peri-Urban Wild Dogs. Thesis for the Degree of Doctor of Philosophy, University of Queensland, Australia.

Hayward, M., 2004. Risks of Zoonosis From Dogs on Sporting Fields. Australian Veterinary Association, Centre for Companion Animals in the Community.

Henderson, W.R., 2009. Pathogens in Vertebrate Hosts in Australia. Invasive Animals Cooperative Research Centre, Canberra.

Jenkins, D.J., Allen, L., Goullet, G., 2008. Encroachment of *Echinococcus granulosus* into urban areas in eastern Queensland, Australia. Aust. Vet. J. 86, 204–300.

Jenkins, D.J., Lievaart, J.J., Boufana, B., Lett, W.S., Bradshaw, H., Armua-Fernandez, M.T., 2014. *Echinococcus granulosus* and other intestinal helminths: current status of prevalence and management in rural dogs of eastern Australia. Aust. Vet. J. 92, 292–298.

Jenkins, D.J., Meek, P.D., Ardler, A., Hawksby, R., 1993. Aboriginal community dogs: worms, control and human health. In: Shield, J. (Ed.), Dog Health in Indigenous Communities. Proceedings of a Conference held as part of the Western Pacific Veterinary Conference, Darwin.

Palmer, C.S., Robertson, I.D., Traub, R.B., Rees, R., Thompson, R.C.A., 2010. Intestinal parasites of dogs and cats in Australia: the veterinarian's perspective and pet owner awareness. Vet. J. 183, 358–361.

Palmer, C.S., Thompson, R.C.A., Traub, R.J., Rees, R., Robertson, I.D., 2008. National study of the gastrointestinal parasites of dogs and cats in Australia. Vet. Parasitol. 51, 181–190.

Reichel, M.P., Lyford, R.A., Gasser, R.B., 1994. Hyperendemic focus of echinococcosis in north-eastern Victoria. Med. J. Aust. 60, 499–501.
Smout, F.A., Skerratt, L.F., Johnson, C.N., Butler, J.R.A., Congdon, B.C., 2018. Zoonotic helminths in dogs and dingoes utilising shared resources in an Australian aboriginal community. Trop. Med. Infect. Dis. 3, 110–124.
Smout, F.A., Thompson, R.C.A., Skerratt, L.A., 2013. First report of *Ancylostoma ceylanicum* in wild canids. Int. J. Parasitol. 2, 173–177.
Spratt, D.M., Beveridge, I., 2018. Wildlife parasitology in Australia: past, present and future. Aust. J. Zool. 66, 286–305.

Further reading

Jenkins, D.J., Craig, N.A., 1992. The role of foxes (*Vulpes vulpes*) in the epidemiology of *Echinococcus granulosus* in an urban environment. Med. J. Aust. 157, 754–756.

CHAPTER FORTY-ONE

Toxocariasis: A neglected infection for the Anthropocene epoch

Peter J. Hotez[a,b,c,d,e,*]

[a]Texas Children's Hospital Center for Vaccine Development, Departments of Pediatrics and Molecular Virology & Microbiology, National School of Tropical Medicine, Baylor College of Medicine, Houston, TX, United States
[b]Hagler Institute for Advanced Studies at Texas A&M University, College Station, TX, United States
[c]Department of Biology, Baylor University, Waco, TX, United States
[d]James A Baker III Institute of Public Policy, Rice University, Houston, TX, United States
[e]Scowcroft Institute of International Affairs, Bush School of Government and Public Service, Texas A&M University, College Station, TX, United States
*Corresponding author: e-mail address: hotez@bcm.edu

Contents

Abstract

While ascariasis, trichuriasis, and hookworm infection dominate global efforts to control human soil-transmitted helminth infections, a picture is unfolding to suggest that toxocariasis is now a fourth and perhaps equally important parasitic disease. *Toxocara* eggs are widespread in the environment and practically ubiquitous in the soils of many subtropical and tropical regions of Asia, Africa, and the Americas. Human zoonotic infection is also highly prevalent in these areas, based on serologic studies to detect anti-*Toxocara* antibodies. The relevance of these findings to human and animal disease burden estimates is still largely unknown, but some studies implicate exposure to *Toxocara* eggs and larvae to both pulmonary disease leading to asthma, and neurologic disease resulting in epilepsy and cognitive delays. On that basis, human toxocariasis may emerge as one of the most important neglected parasitic infections of humans. With anticipated global warming and urbanization associated with our modern human-transformed geological epoch, known as the Anthropocene, it is likely that toxocariasis will become a dominant infection and one widely prevalent in our future and projected mega-cities.

Advances in Parasitology, Volume 109
ISSN 0065-308X
https://doi.org/10.1016/bs.apar.2020.03.004

1. Introduction

Soil-transmitted helminth (STH) infections rank among the most prevalent infections of humans and animals. With respect to human STH infections, almost 900 million people are currently infected with *Ascaris* roundworms, *Trichuris* whipworms, or hookworms according to the GBD 2017 Disease and Injury Incidence and Prevalence Collaborators (2018). However, mostly ignored or neglected in any global policymaker discussion regarding STH infections is toxocariasis. We are still missing detailed disease burden estimates for both human and animal toxocariasis, but preliminary evidence based on parasite exposure and positive *Toxocara* antibody levels indicate that this zoonosis may be as common as any STH infection. For example, a systematic review and meta-analysis of studies examining public places, including parks, playgrounds, and beaches, found that up to one-third in East Asia are positive for *Toxocara* eggs, as are one quarter of the public places in Africa and South America (Fakhri et al., 2018).

The fact that *Toxocara* eggs are widespread environmental contaminants is significant. An additional estimate finds that the global seroprevalence of toxocariasis is 19%, but similar to the environmental studies, it is higher in East Asia and Africa (Gasser et al., 2019). Based on these analyses, the prevalence of human toxocariasis is likely to rank closely with the other major human STH infections. There are no published estimates for the global veterinary disease burden of toxocariasis in dogs, cats, or other animal species, although in studies conducted in stray cats and dogs it is common to find the prevalence exceeding 50% (Daryani et al., 2009).

The clinical significance of a positive serologic test for *Toxocara* antibodies in humans is a subject of important debate and discussion. While the full-expression syndromes of toxocariasis—visceral and ocular larva migrans—are relatively rare, there is an increasing evidence to link positive *Toxocara* serologies to human pulmonary and neurologic disease (Hotez and Wilkins, 2009; Ma et al., 2018). Pulmonary findings include asthma and lung dysfunction (Sharghi et al., 2001; Walsh and Haseeb, 2014), while neurologic disease ranges from epilepsy to cognitive delays (Hotez, 2014; Luna et al., 2018; Walsh and Haseeb, 2012). There is an urgent need to understand better the connections between serological diagnosis of human toxocariasis and these clinical findings, but if confirmed toxocariasis could be implicated as one of the most important human parasitic infections.

However, such associations and conclusions might need to wait for further refinements in diagnostic testing and improvements in both assay sensitivity and specificity (Anderson et al., 2015; Zhan et al., 2015).

2. Ideally suited for the Anthropocene

Is the global disease burden of toxocariasis static or it changing? There are reasons to believe that the shifting nature of several social and physical determinants will affect the global epidemiology of toxocariasis. Many characterize our modern Anthropocene geological epoch, referring to the relevance of human activity in effecting global changes, which include climate change, urbanization, and poverty, to name a few (Hotez, 2016b). While human and animal toxocariasis is already widespread and *Toxocara* eggs are practically ubiquitous in some environments, as we advance in the Anthropocene epoch it is likely that the disease prevalence will increase even further (Fig. 1).

For example, climate change predicts a warming planet with rainfall patterns that would be well suited for the survival of *Toxocara* eggs in the soil (Blum and Hotez, 2018). In addition, large populations in tropical and subtropical areas are becoming increasingly urbanized (Hotez, 2017). In cities with substantial areas of urban blight and slums, it is common to find many stray dogs and cats, each releasing thousands of *Toxocara* eggs into the environment. With predictions that the world's population will eventually live

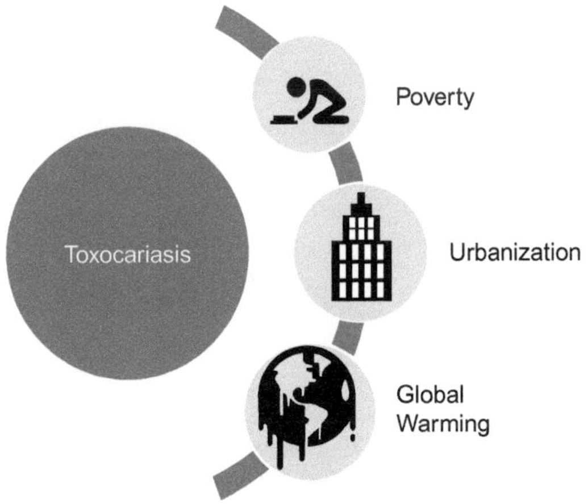

Fig. 1 Three major drivers of human and animal toxocariasis.

mostly in mega-cities affected by warming temperatures, it is reasonable to predict that toxocariasis could become a dominant parasitic and neglected disease by the year 2050 (Hotez, 2018). Still another common factor attributed to high human toxocariasis prevalence is poverty. Today, poverty and poverty-related neglected diseases are surprisingly common in large pockets found in wealthier group of 20 (G20) nations such as Indonesia, India, and Brazil (Hotez, 2016a). However, some projections indicate that by 2050 up to 40% of people living in extreme poverty will live in the sub-Saharan African nations of Nigeria and the Democratic Republic of Congo (Hotez, 2019). Therefore, we might expect a disease like toxocariasis to become widely prevalent in the two mega-cities found in these countries—Lagos and Kinshasa, respectively.

2.1 Moving forward

Despite some ominous projections that toxocariasis will remain widespread or become an even greater public health threat in the coming decades, an wormy future is not inevitable. According to the World Health Organization, approximately 70% of the children at risk for STH infections now receives annual deworming with albendazole or mebendazole (World Health Organization, 2018). Generally, mass deworming is achieved by providing a single dose of these medications on an annual basis. Although, usually several consecutive days of albendazole treatment are required to effectively treat a patient with toxocariasis, we do not know if mass deworming with a single dose might also have some effect in reducing the global prevalence of this infection. We also know that veterinary public health measures, if implemented, could reduce Toxocara egg environmental exposure. They include reproductive control to reduce the numbers of young dogs and cats that typically exhibit the highest *Toxoxcara* worm burdens, in addition to dog and cat deworming programs and enforcement of laws regarding the sanitary disposal of animal faeces (Macpherson, 2013). Therefore, the future global prevalence of toxocariasis will depend significantly on how animal control becomes incorporated into urban planning, especially in Africa, Asia, and the Latin American region.

References

Anderson, J.P., Rascoe, L.N., Levert, K., Chastain, H.M., et al., 2015. Development of a Luminex bead based assay for diagnosis of toxocariasis using recombinant antigens Tc-CTL-1 and Tc-TES-26. PLoS Negl. Trop. Dis. 9, e0004168.

Blum, A.J., Hotez, P.J., 2018. Global "worming": climate change and its projected general impact on human helminth infections. PLoS Negl. Trop. Dis. 12, e0006370.

Daryani, A., Sharif, M., Amouei, A., Gholami, S., 2009. Prevalence of Toxocara canis in stray dogs, northern Iran. Pak. J. Biol. Sci. 12, 1031–1035.
Fakhri, Y., Gasser, R.B., Rostami, A., Fan, C.K., et al., 2018. Toxocara eggs in public places worldwide—a systematic review and meta-analysis. Environ. Pollut. 242, 1467–1475.
Gasser, R.B., Rostami, A., Mohammed, R.S., Holland, C.V., et al., 2019. Seroprevalence estimates for toxocariasis in people worldwide: a systematic review and meta-analysis. PLoS Negl. Trop. Dis. 12, e0007809.
GBD 2017 Disease and Injury Incidence and Prevalence Collaborators, 2018. Global, regional, and national incidence, prevalence, and years lived with disability for 354 diseases and injuries for 195 countries and territories, 1990-2017: a systematic analysis for the Global Burden of Disease Study 2017. Lancet 392, 1789–1858.
Hotez, P.J., 2014. Neglected infections of poverty in the United States and their effects on the brain. JAMA Psychiat. 71, 1099–1100.
Hotez, P.J., 2016a. Blue Marble Health: An Innovative Plan to Fight Diseases of the Poor Amid Wealth. Johns Hopkins University Press, Baltimore MD.
Hotez, P.J., 2016b. Neglected tropical diseases in the Anthropocene: the cases of Zika, Ebola, and other infections. PLoS Negl. Trop. Dis. 10, e0004648.
Hotez, P.J., 2017. Global urbanization and the neglected tropical diseases. PLoS Negl. Trop. Dis. 11, e0005308.
Hotez, P.J., 2018. Human parasitology and parasitic diseases: heading towards 2050. Adv. Parasitol. 100, 29–38.
Hotez, P., 2019. DR Congo and Nigeria: new neglected tropical disease threats and solutions for the bottom 40. PLoS Negl. Trop. Dis. 13, e0007145.
Hotez, P.J., Wilkins, P.P., 2009. Toxocariasis: America's most common neglected infection of poverty and a helminthiasis of global importance? PLoS Negl. Trop. Dis. 3, e400.
Luna, J., Cicero, C.E., Rateau, G., Quattrocchi, G., et al., 2018. Updated evidence of the association between toxocariasis and epilepsy: systematic review and meta-analysis. PLoS Negl. Trop. Dis. 12, e0006665.
Ma, G., Holland, C.V., Wang, T., Hofmann, A., et al., 2018. Human toxocariasis. Lancet Infect. Dis. 18, e14–e24.
Macpherson, C.N., 2013. The epidemiology and public health importance of toxocariasis: a zoonosis of global importance. Int. J. Parasitol. 43, 999–1008.
Sharghi, N., Schantz, P.M., Caramico, L., Ballas, K., et al., 2001. Environmental exposure to Toxocara as a possible risk factor for asthma: a clinic-based case-control study. Clin. Infect. Dis. 32, E111–E116.
Walsh, M.G., Haseeb, M.A., 2012. Reduced cognitive function in children with toxocariasis in a nationally representative sample of the United States. Int. J. Parasitol. 42, 1159–1163.
Walsh, M.G., Haseeb, M.A., 2014. Toxocariasis and lung function: relevance of a neglected infection in an urban landscape. Acta Parasitol. 59, 126–131.
World Health Organization, 2018. Schistosomiasis and soil-transmitted helminthiases: number of people treated in 2017. Wkly. Epidemiol. Rec. 93, 681–682.
Zhan, B., Ajmera, R., Geiger, S.M., Goncalves, M.T., et al., 2015. Identification of immunodominant antigens for the laboratory diagnosis of toxocariasis. Trop. Med. Int. Health 20, 1787–1796.

Kolibri 360 GmbH
Ferdinand-Jühlke-Straße 7
99095 Erfurt, Deutschland
produktsicherheit@kolibri360.de